ST MIDDLESEX UNIVF
MED AL
Twickenham

Withdrawn

Knee Surgery

CONCORDIA DISCORS
Harmony in discord
Horace

Knee Surgery

Current practice

Edited by

Paul M. Aichroth

MS, FRCS

Consultant Orthopaedic Surgeon
Westminster Hospital
Westminster Children's Hospital
Wellington Knee Surgery Unit
Humana Hospital Wellington
London
UK

W. Dilworth Cannon, Jr

MD

Professor of Clinical Orthopaedic Surgery
Director of Sports Medicine
Department of Orthopaedic Surgery
University of California
San Francisco
California
USA

Clinical research by

Dipak V. Patel

MB, MS, MSc Orth, D Orth, FCPS Orth

Assistant Orthopaedic Surgeon
Wellington Knee Surgery Unit
Humana Hospital Wellington
London
UK

Martin Dunitz

© Martin Dunitz Limited 1992

Contribution 4.1 © AAOS 1992
Artwork for contributions 5.5 (1–14), 6.7 (1–11), 8.1 (11a,b,c, 12)
© Peter Cox, reproduced from *Rob & Smith's Operative Surgery:*
Orthopaedics, 4th edn, by permission of the publishers,
Butterworth–Heinemann Ltd

First published in the United Kingdom in 1992 by
Martin Dunitz Ltd, The Livery House, 7–9 Pratt Street, London NW1
OAE

A CIP catalogue record for this book is available from the British
Library.

ISBN 1 85317 090 9

To our wives:

Angela

Helga

Sadhana

Composition by Scribe Design, Gillingham, Kent
Origination, printing and binding by Toppan Printing Company (S)
PTE, Singapore

Contents

vi   **Contents**

List of contributors

Christopher E. Ackroyd

Consultant Orthopaedic Surgeon
Southmead Hospital
Westbury on Trym
Bristol BS10 5NB
UK

Paul M. Aichroth

Consultant Orthopaedic Surgeon
Westminster Hospital

Westminster Children's Hospital

Wellington Knee Surgery Unit
Humana Hospital Wellington
London NW8 9LE
UK

Zaid Al-Duri

Honorary Research Fellow in Orthopaedics
Westminster Hospital
London SW1P 2AP
UK

Paul W. Allen

Consultant Orthopaedic Surgeon
Princess Alexandra Hospital
Hamstel Road
Harlow
Essex CM20 1QX
UK

Brian G. Andrews

Consultant Orthopaedic Surgeon
Queen Mary's University Hospital
Roehampton Lane
London SW15 5PN
UK

Steven P. Arnoczky

Director
Laboratory for Comparative Orthopaedic Research
College of Veterinary Medicine
Michigan State University
East Lansing
Michigan 48827
USA

James A. Arnold

Butterfield Trail Professional Center
1794 Joyce, Suite 3
Fayetteville
Arkansas 72703
USA

Peter R.E. Baird

Consultant Orthopaedic Surgeon
Westminster Hospital
London SW1P 2AP
UK

Richard J. Beaver

Clinical Fellow
Division of Orthopaedic Surgery
Mount Sinai Hospital
Toronto
Ontario M5G 1X5
Canada

Graham J. Belham

Senior Orthopaedic Registrar
Westminster Hospital
London SW1P 2AP
UK

George Bentley

Professor of Orthopaedic Surgery
The Institute of Orthopaedics
University of London

Honorary Consultant Orthopaedic Surgeon
The Royal National Orthopaedic Hospital
Brockley Hill
Stanmore
Middlesex HA7 4LP
UK

Manjit Bhamra

Senior Orthopaedic Registrar
Westminster Hospital
London SW1P 2AP
UK

Nicholas R. Boeree

Orthopaedic Registrar
Bristol Royal Infirmary
Bristol BS2 8HW
UK

Howard R. Brown

Sports Medicine Division
Department of Orthopaedics
University of Florida
JMH Health Center
Gainesville
Florida 32610
USA

Elisabeth Brunet-Guedj

Department of Orthopaedic Surgery and Sports
Medicine
Hôpital Edouard-Herriot
Place d'Arsonval
F-69437 Lyon Cedex 3
France

Timothy D. Bunker

Consultant Orthopaedic Surgeon
Princess Elizabeth Orthopaedic Hospital
Exeter EX2 4UE
UK

P. Adrian Butler-Manuel

Senior Registrar in Orthopaedics
Orthopaedic Academic Unit
Rayne Institute
St Thomas's Hospital
Lambeth Palace Road
London SE1 7EH
UK

W. Dilworth Cannon, Jr

Professor of Clinical Orthopaedic Surgery
Director of Sports Medicine
Department of Orthopaedic Surgery
University of California
San Francisco
California 94143
USA

Brian Casey

Orthopaedic Surgeon
1201 Triple M Tower
500 Oxford Street
Bondi Junction 2022
Sydney
Australia

Guglielmo Cerullo

Orthopaedic Traumatologist
Clinica Valle Giulia
2B via G De Notaris
00197 Rome
Italy

Massimo Cipolla

Orthopaedic Traumatologist
Clinica Valle Giulia
2B via G De Notaris
00197 Rome
Italy

Susan M. Craig

Adjunct Attending Surgeon
Department of Orthopedic and General Surgery
Lenox Hill Hospital
New York
USA

David J. Dandy

Consultant Orthopaedic Surgeon
Addenbrookes Hospital
Cambridge CB2 2QQ
UK

Dale M. Daniel

Associate Clinical Professor of Orthopaedic Surgery
Kaiser Permanente Hospital
San Diego
California 92120
USA

Henri Dejour

Clinique Chirurgicale Orthopédique et
Traumatologique
Centre Hospitalier Lyon-Sud
69310 Pierre-Bénite
Lyon
France

George S.E. Dowd

Consultant Orthopaedic Surgeon
Department of Orthopaedics
St Bartholomew's Hospital
London EC1A 7BE
UK

Scott F. Dye

Assistant Clinical Professor of Orthopaedic Surgery
University of California
San Francisco
California 94143
USA

Stuart C. Evans

Senior Orthopaedic Registrar
Queen Mary's University Hospital
Roehampton Lane
London SW15 5PN
UK

Barry D. Ferris

Consultant Orthopaedic Surgeon
Department of Orthopaedics
Barnet General Hospital
Wellhouse Lane
Barnet EN5 3DJ
UK

Vittorio Franco

Clinica Valle Giulia
2B via G De Notaris
00197 Rome
Italy

Michael A.R. Freeman

Consultant Orthopaedic Surgeon
Bone and Joint Research Unit
The London Hospital Medical College
London E1 2AD
UK

Marc J. Friedman

Southern California Orthopedic Institute
6815 Noble Avenue
Van Nuys
California 91405
USA

Freddie H. Fu

Blue Cross of Western Pennsylvania Professor of
Orthopaedic Surgery
Vice Chairman, Clinical Department of Orthopaedic
Surgery
Chief, Division of Sports Medicine
University of Pittsburgh

Center for Sports Medicine and Rehabilitation
Craig at Baum Boulevard
Pittsburgh
Pennsylvania 15213
USA

Kyosuke Fujikawa

Assistant Professor
Chief of Knee Division
Department of Orthopaedic Surgery
Keio University School of Medicine
35 Shinanomachi
Shinjuku-Ku
Tokyo 160
Japan

John P. Fulkerson

Professor of Orthopaedic Surgery
University of Connecticut School of Medicine
Farmington
Connecticut 06032
USA

John C. Garrett

5671 Peachtree Dunwoody Road NE
Suite 900
Atlanta
Georgia 30342
USA

Edward S. Grood

Noyes-Giannestras Biomechanics Laboratories
University of Cincinnati
Mail Location 48
Cincinnati
Ohio 45221-0048
USA

Allan E. Gross

A.J. Latner Professor and Chairman
Division of Orthopaedic Surgery
University of Toronto
Mount Sinai Hospital
Toronto
Ontario M5G 1X5
Canada

James F. Guhl

Arthroscopic Surgery and Sports Medicine Centers
of Southeastern Wisconsin
St Francis Hospital
Milwaukee
Wisconsin 53215
USA

Rosemary L. Guy

formerly Senior Registrar in Radiology
Orthopaedic Academic Unit
Rayne Institute
St Thomas's Hospital
Lambeth Palace Road
London SE1 7EH
UK

Kevin Hardinge

Consultant Orthopaedic Surgeon
Centre for Hip Surgery
Wrightington Hospital
Appley Bridge
Wigan WN6 9EP
UK

Frederick W. Heatley

Reader and Honorary Consultant in Orthopaedics
Orthopaedic Academic Unit
Rayne Institute and the Department of Nuclear Medicine
St Thomas's Hospital
Lambeth Palace Road
London SE1 7EH
UK

† Charles E. Henning

Mason Hohl

2001 Santa Monica Boulevard
No. 1160
Santa Monica
California 90404
USA

Edward C. Huskisson

Consultant Physician and Senior Lecturer
St Bartholomew's Hospital
London EC1A 7BE
UK

Peter A.N. Hutton

Consultant Orthopaedic Surgeon
Queen Mary's University Hospital
Roehampton Lane
London SW15 5PN
UK

Peter A. Indelicato

Professor of Orthopaedic Surgery
Chief of Sports Medicine
Department of Orthopaedics
University of Florida
JMH Health Center
Gainesville
Florida 32610
USA

Andrew M. Jackson

Consultant Orthopaedic Surgeon
Queen Mary's University Hospital
Roehampton Lane
London SW15 5PN
UK

Roland P. Jakob

Professor of Orthopaedic Surgery
University of Berne
Inselspital
CH-3010 Berne
Switzerland

David Janeway

Department of Orthopaedic Surgery
The Bowman Gray School of Medicine
Wake Forest University
Winston-Salem
North Carolina
USA

Lanny L. Johnson

Department of Surgery
Michigan State University
East Lansing
Michigan 48823
USA

Cledwyn B. Jones

Consultant Orthopaedic Surgeon
Royal United Hospital
Combe Park
Bath BA1 3NG
UK

Ronald P. Karzel

Southern California Orthopaedic Institute
6815 Noble Avenue
Van Nuys
California 91405
USA

Kurt J. Kitziger

Clinical Assistant Professor of Orthopaedics
Tulane University
3322 Canal Street
New Orleans
Louisiana 70119
USA

Carroll A. Laurin

Professor of Surgery
Marthe and Maurice E. Muller Chair of Orthopaedics
McGill University

Surgeon-in-Chief, Division of Orthopaedics
Department of Surgery
Royal Victoria Hospital
687 Pine Avenue West
Montreal
Quebec H3A 1A1
Canada

Jean L. Lerat

Department of Orthopaedic Surgery and Sports
Medicine
Hôpital Edouard-Herriot
Place d'Arsonval
F-69437 Lyon Cedex 3
France

Paul A. Lotke

Professor of Orthopaedic Surgery
Hospital of the University of Pennsylvania
3400 Spruce Street
Philadelphia
Pennsylvania 19104
USA

Malcolm F. Macnicol

Consultant Orthopaedic Surgeon
Princess Margaret Rose Hospital
Fairmilehead
Edinburgh
UK

Mark S. McMahon

Dept of Orthopedic Surgery
Lenox Hill Hospital
New York
USA

David Martin

Department of Orthopaedic Surgery
The Bowman Gray School of Medicine
Wake Forest University
Winston-Salem
North Carolina 27103
USA

Clare L. Marx

Consultant Orthopaedic Surgeon
St Mary's Hospital
Praed Street
London W2 1NY
UK

Richard C. Maurer

Clinical Professor and Vice Chairman
Department of Orthopaedic Surgery
University of California School of Medicine
San Francisco
California 94143
USA

Alan C. Merchant

Clinical Professor of Surgery (Orthopaedic Division)
Stanford University School of Medicine
Stanford

Active Staff Surgeon
Department of Orthopaedic Surgery
El Camino Hospital
2500 Hospital Drive
Building 7
Mountain View
California 94040
USA

Bernard Moyen

Department of Orthopaedic Surgery and Sports
Medicine
Hôpital Edouard-Herriot
Place d'Arsonval
F-69437 Lyon Cedex 3
France

Simon T. Moyes

Senior Orthopaedic Registrar
Westminster Hospital
London SW1P 2AP
UK

John H. Newman

Consultant Orthopaedic Surgeon
Winford Orthopaedic Hospital
Bristol BS18 8AQ
UK

Philippe Neyret

Clinique Chirurgicale Orthopédique et
Traumatologique
Centre Hospitalier Lyon-Sud
69310 Pierre-Bénite
Lyon
France

Jon K. Nisbet

Orthopedic and Sports Medicine Center
3395 N Campbell Avenue
Tucson
Arizona 85719
USA

Thomas O. Nunan

Consultant Physician in Nuclear Medicine
Orthopaedic Academic Unit
Rayne Institute
St Thomas's Hospital
Lambeth Palace Road
London SE1 7EH
UK

Eric J. Olson

Orthopaedic Sports Medicine Fellow
University of Pittsburgh
Pittsburgh
Pennsylvania 15213
USA

Dinesh Patel

Chief of Arthroscopic Surgery Unit
Department of Orthopaedic Surgery
Massachusetts General Hospital
Boston
Massachusetts 02114
USA

Dipak V. Patel

Assistant Orthopaedic Surgeon
Wellington Knee Surgery Unit
Humana Hospital Wellington
London NW8 9LE
UK

Lonnie E. Paulos

The Orthopedic Specialty Hospital
5848 South 300 East
Salt Lake City
Utah 84107
USA

Gary G. Poehling

Professor and Chairman
Department of Orthopaedic Surgery
Bowman Gray School of Medicine
Wake Forest University
Winston-Salem
North Carolina 27103
USA

Giancarlo Puddu

Professor
Department of Orthopaedics and Traumatology
Clinica Valle Giulia
2B via G De Notaris
00197 Rome
Italy

Christoph Rangger

Kaiser Permanente Hospital
San Diego
California 92120
USA

James E. Scott

Consultant Orthopaedic Surgeon
Westminster Hospital
London SW1P 2AP
UK

Richard D. Scott

Associate Clinical Professor of Orthopaedic Surgery
Harvard Medical School
Brigham & Women's Hospital
New England Baptist Hospital
Boston
Massachusetts
USA

W. Norman Scott

Clinical Associate Professor of Orthopaedics
Beth Israel Hospital North
New York
New York 10128
USA

Konsei Shino

Director
Sports Medicine
Rosai Hospital
Nagasone-cho 1179-3
Sakai
Osaka
591 Japan

Neal C. Small

Clinical Assistant Professor
Department of Orthopaedic Surgery
The University of Texas
Southwestern Medical Center
Dallas
Texas
USA

Roger B. Smith

Consultant Orthopaedic Surgeon
Royal Preston Hospital
Sharoe Green Lane North
Fulwood
Preston PR2 4QF
UK

Dennis J. Stoker

Consultant Radiologist
Royal National Orthopaedic Hospital
45–51 Bolsover Street
London W1P 8AQ
UK

David W. Stoller

Assistant Clinical Professor, Skeletal Radiology
University of California
San Francisco

Medical Director
California Advanced Imaging
3440 California Street
San Francisco
California 94118
USA

James W. Stone

Arthroscopic Surgery and Sports Medicine Centers
of Southeastern Wisconsin
St Francis Hospital
Milwaukee
Wisconsin 53215
USA

Mary Lou Stone

Kaiser Permanente Hospital
San Diego
California 92120
USA

Angus E. Strover

President
Droitwich Knee Foundation
Saga House
Sansome Place
Worcester WR1 1UA, UK

Glenn C. Terry

Hughston Orthopaedic Clinic, PC
6262 Hamilton Road
Columbus
Georgia 31995
USA

Joyce M. Vittori

535A Greenwich Street
San Francisco
California
USA

† Jacques Wagner

Gilles Walch

Clinique Chirurgicale Orthopédique et
Traumatologique
Centre Hospitalier Lyon Sud
69310 Pierre-Bénite
Lyon
France

Peter S. Walker

Professor of Biomedical Engineering
Institute of Orthopaedics
Royal National Orthopaedic Hospital
Brockley Hill
Stanmore
Middlesex HA7 4LP
UK

Jonathan S. Wand

Senior Orthopaedic Registrar
Queen Mary's Hospital
Roehampton
London SW15 5PN
UK

Thomas L. Wickiewicz

Assistant Professor of Clinical Surgery
Cornell University Medical College
Hospital for Special Surgery
New York 10021
USA

D. Zukor

Assistant Professor
McGill University
Orthopaedic Surgeon
Royal Victoria Hospital
687 Pine Avenue West
Montreal
Quebec M3A 1A1
Canada

Acknowledgments

We wish to acknowledge with grateful thanks:

Joyce M. Vittori for her dedication and hard work on the American contributions;

Mrs Kerry Isles and Mrs Kate Spratt, our secretaries, for their hard work and devotion; Dina Stanford, who accurately dealt with the computer analysis, for which we are most grateful; the staff of the Medical Photography Department, Westminster Hospital, who have produced, adjusted and configured many of the illustrations;

Mr Reinhard Wentz, assistant librarian at the Westminster Hospital, who has helped with the vast array of references (we are also most grateful to the librarians at the Institute of Orthopaedics in London);

Mrs Lynn Ranscombe, English teacher at Heathfield School, who has corrected some of the English and given us various marks for accuracy (she felt that surgeons 'could do better' at their grammar!);

Robert Peden and his colleagues at Martin Dunitz Ltd for their tremendous dedication to the production of this book and their kind help and encouragement in all stages of its development;

Mr Martin Dunitz himself, who has guided us through difficult times and deadlines – we are most grateful for his knowledge and wisdom during preparation of this book.

Preface

The authors feel that there has been a need to address current problems in knee diagnosis and management. We have brought together 95 contributors, expert in their field. They have recorded their current thoughts, approaches and technique on difficult and sometimes controversial problems in knee surgery. In many instances we have juxtaposed articles that express different approaches to a specific subject. Each chapter includes a review by a contributor or an 'overview' by one of the editors in an effort to find a central channel through the stormy, and at times very contentious, writings of world experts. By this means, it is hoped that the senior resident or registrar will gain practical help in deciding on treatment patterns and trends while the more mature surgeon will be updated on current practice in knee surgery.

The most important current investigation in knee joint pathology is magnetic resonance imaging and there is little doubt that this field will develop greatly in the next few years. The advantages and pitfalls are explored here. The use of the bone scan to detect subtle abnormalities in bone metabolism and vascularity, long before radiographic change, is also discussed.

The most revolutionary change in knee surgery this century has been the development of the arthroscope and the ensuing role of arthroscopic surgery in the treatment of internal disorders of the knee by minimally invasive techniques. This has now led to the development of intricate endoscopic procedures such as meniscal repair, internal fixation of osteochondral defects and a wide range of arthroscopically assisted ligament reconstruction procedures. We have to thank those who pioneered the development of the arthroscope for the stimulus in advancing 'arthroscopic knee surgery' beyond a mere technique into a major discipline within orthopaedic practice.

The transplantation of menisci, ligament tissue and osteochondral surface remains in the developmental phase because of the danger of AIDS and other communicable diseases as well as the inherent immunological effects. Once the treatment of these problems is solved, the use of this technique will become more widespread, but until then one must use caution in recommending allografts.

The emphasis on exact diagnosis has led to the current concepts of knee joint instability and laxity patterns which can now be accurately identified. The development of arthrometer instruments which can measure several parameters of instability has quantified the severity of knee ligament injuries to a degree. A variety of ligament instability reconstruction procedures is recorded in detail here. We make no apology for the length of these chapters, for there is at present wide controversy concerning the merits of different reconstructive operations. We believe that the general trend in these treatment patterns is adequately aired in this volume.

There is much confusion in the diagnosis of extensor apparatus and patellofemoral derangements. Until our investigational tools help delineate these problems in a more precise manner, the question of which treatment technique to adopt will be in dispute. Our various contributors' ideas are included in a very full review and it is hoped that some order will emerge from them.

Knee replacement arthroplasty is not only a successful procedure but is long-lasting, provided that the principles of biomechanical design, operative expertise, limb alignment and rehabilitation are observed. The manner in which these factors have been advanced is fully discussed in this volume. The revision and salvage procedures for complications of arthroplasty remain salutary reminders of the potential for disaster, even in an otherwise straightforward operation; their avoidance must continue to be the main task of the surgeon in this field.

The various knee problems which affect children and adolescents are discussed throughout the various chapters. However, there is a paediatric knee surgery overview, together with specific contributions on problems of congenital abnormalities and growth malalignment.

Knee surgeons must properly document and assess their results. One whole chapter has been devoted to this discipline, which is not merely important but vital in our professional lives, if we are to learn from past experience. Audit is here to stay; consequently every treatment we undertake should be assessed by one of the methods suggested in this chapter.

The speed of change in knee surgery and treatment is such that there will in the future need to be further editions of this book to update the developments and trends discussed here.

Paul Aichroth
W Dilworth Cannon, Jr

1

Investigations

1.1   Investigations in knee disorders

Paul M. Aichroth

In those quiet, idyllic but diagnostically primitive days when knee assessment depended upon hands and simple radiographs, some of our forebears and teachers claimed extravagantly high degrees of accuracy – approaching 100%. When arthrograms and then arthroscopy interrupted this smugness, myself and many others became depressed by our clinical expertise recording accuracy of no more than two-thirds, which sometimes rose to three-quarters with greater concentration and dedication.

There is little doubt that arthroscopy focused the minds specifically on knee disorders and diagnosis. Although arthrography was well established by this stage, the technique of arthroscopy must be considered the 'Renaissance' in producing accurate diagnosis and rational treatment of many knee derangements. In the 1970s arthrography techniques became pre-eminent and accuracy in excess of 90% was achieved.

Dennis Stoker points out in this chapter that magnetic resonance imaging (MRI) is superseding arthrography as the investigation of choice, for it is completely non-invasive and it can show so many more knee structures than those intra-articular features outlined by arthrography. Although MRI is as yet expensive, its cost effectiveness is clearly shown by Nicholas R. Boeree and Christopher Ackroyd in this chapter.

MRI accuracy in the best hands is well in excess of 90%, but there is a learning curve and the technique is definitely operator dependent. In many MRI units there is a high incidence of false positives, and especially so in the posterior segment of the meniscus, when an abnormal signal represents intra-meniscal mucoid degeneration and the anatomical confines of the meniscus are normal. With experience – as in so many knee surgical problems – this inaccuracy decreases but it must keep the clinician on his guard, for patients are turning up in offices and clinics clutching their MRI scans reported as positive posterior segmental meniscal tears and demanding surgical treatment. We all know that knee pain is multifactorial and that the patient must not be pushed into early and unnecessary surgery by the whim of a relatively inexperienced radiologist reporting a signal of dubious significance.

The definitive assessment of MRI technique, together with the most magnificent scans, are presented in this chapter by David Stoller of San Francisco, who is a world expert. The reader is recommended to study this contribution for it clearly shows the present state of the art and indicates future progress. MRI is certainly helpful in such problems as osteonecrosis and osteochondritis dissecans, but the initial pathology is still seen at an earlier stage on isotope scanning, where the three phases of dynamic scintigraphy show focal increased activity.

The enigma of anterior knee pain and the different treatment programmes for reflex sympathetic dystrophy may be helped by isotope scanning, as shown in the contribution by P. Adrian Butler-Manuel et al. in this chapter. Isotopes will also have a great part to play in the future, when our vast numbers of knee replacement arthroplasties require assessment and possibly revision in – we hope – the dim, distant future.

Scott F. Dye from San Francisco points out that radionuclide imaging of the knee has altered our understanding of knee pathology, including abnormal physiology as well as structure. He shows the unexpected scintigraphic activity in anterior knee pain, neurovascular dysfunction, meniscal and ligamentous injury, as well as osseous pathology. He points out that 'the technetium bone scan is the best window into the osseous physiologic status of the knee'.

1.2   Arthrography of the knee

Dennis J. Stoker

Knee arthrography has been practised for over 85 years. Refinement of the technique with fluoroscopic control of a dynamic rather than a static examination has been employed as the standard technique since the work of Butt and McIntyre in 1969.[1] In the last 20 years, therefore, arthrography has established itself as an inexpensive and accurate procedure which rarely gives the patient more than transient discomfort. As late as 1985, Kaye[2] wrote that 'knee arthrography is . . . a simple, safe, very reliable, useful and relatively inexpensive procedure that can be performed by a growing number of interested and capable diagnostic radiologists'; essentially, in the United Kingdom, this is still true today. However, the increasing popularity of arthroscopy has made a major change in diagnostic practice in the United States over the past 10 years. In 1987, Hall[3] canvassed 98 experienced radiologists in the USA and found a significant decrease in knee arthrography over the preceding 5–10 years; in the United Kingdom, at that time, the practice of arthrography had not been affected to such a degree.

At the present time, the introduction of magnetic resonance imaging (MRI) has provided a non-invasive technique which can not only show most of the important features demonstrable by arthrography and arthroscopy, but can also demonstrate lesions of other, hitherto invisible, structures such as the collateral ligaments and the subarticular bone. Each of the three diagnostic methods – arthrography, arthroscopy and magnetic resonance imaging – in expert hands has an accuracy well in excess of 90%, but equally each shows a significant shallow learning curve and has a considerable operator dependency.

There is little doubt that eventually MRI will supplant the other two techniques as a diagnostic procedure, but the widespread use of this imaging technique is limited in most countries by its present cost; it seems that for most of the world's population, to whom even plain radiography is not available, if any investigative procedure at all is to be affordable, arthrography will still offer a cheap accurate diagnostic method.

In current arthrographic practice, most technical success has been achieved by the use of a double-contrast technique using room air or carbon dioxide combined with one of the current water-soluble iodinated contrast media, either ionic, low-osmolar or non-ionic. There is little to be gained by the use of expensive non-ionic media[4] in an examination which essentially causes little pain. Some advantage exists, particularly for the beginner, in the use of a low-osmolar dimer preparation.[5]

The success of the examination depends on the expertise of the arthrographer and the quality of the radiographic image. However, as has been mentioned already, both arthroscopy and MRI also are operator-dependent. Arthrography is an outpatient procedure necessitating local anaesthesia, whereas, even as a day case, arthroscopy requires a hospital bed and theatre time. Whilst this sort of minimal-stay surgery is justified for treatment purposes, it cannot be considered reasonable for diagnosis if other cheaper or less invasive procedures are available.

Technique of arthrography

Synovial puncture requires a strict aseptic technique. Complications of the procedure are few. The one that must be avoided is the production of a joint infection; such an occurrence must suggest an error of technique at the time of puncture, as many thousands of arthrograms have been undertaken without this complication.

The object of a double-contrast arthrogram is to demonstrate the intra-articular structures, by coating them with iodinated contrast medium and allowing controlled stress to separate the articular surfaces after the introduction of gas into the joint. All movements are controlled under fluoroscopic observation; stress is applied by leverage of the leg against a band or post above the knee. Thus it is possible, in turn, to examine the medial compartment and its meniscus and the lateral compartment. Because the lower limb can be rotated easily during the examination through movement of the hip, successive tangential projections of each meniscus are obtained; it is usual to take at least eight views of each meniscus, from the anterior to the posterior horn. These are taken with the meniscus *orthograde*, the tibial

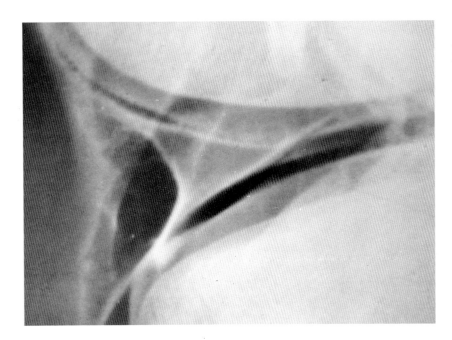

Figure 1

Normal posterior horn of lateral meniscus. The meniscus is shown in triangular cross-section, attached peripherally over the popliteus tendon sheath by a superior and inferior band of synovium. The normal depth of articular cartilage over the femoral and tibial condyles is clearly demonstrated.

plateau in profile, and with minimal overlap of the structures (Figure 1).

Because the techniques and perspectives of arthrography and arthroscopy are different, the examinations are often complementary. Nowadays, many patients are referred for arthrography following an arthroscopic examination with normal findings and when symptoms have persisted. Most of these show normal appearances, or a post-surgical representation which is reasonable, but a sizable minority exhibit meniscal tears. Although some of these tears are in situations where it is expected that the arthroscopist would have difficulty, e.g. far posterior in the medial meniscus (Figure 2) or a tear of the undersurface, in others this is not the case. I believe that these missed tears reflect the problems associated with the small field of view of the arthroscope. Just as when we climb a steep hill the summit is farther on than it appears at first, so the restricted view of the arthroscopist up the slope of the medial meniscus from the free edge may fail to reveal a vertical tear in the peripheral one-third of the meniscus (Figure 2).

Arthroscopy and arthrography share an equal accuracy in the diagnosis of meniscal lesions of about 90–95%. When an error occurs, its nature is often different in the two procedures, so that together an accuracy of 98% may be expected in the difficult case.[6]

Both arthrography and arthroscopy in their different ways share the ability to stress the knee and thereby challenge a suspect meniscus. This is of particular value with a closed tear or a peripherally detached posterior horn of the lateral meniscus (Figure 3). Although cysts of the menisci are essentially intrameniscal and therefore well demonstrated by MRI, when symptomatic they are commonly found to be associated with a tear of the involved meniscus; such lesions are demonstrable at arthro-

graphy (Figure 4), although the glairy contents of the cyst may mean that contrast medium only demonstrates the cyst on a delayed film.

Arthrography is useful in demonstrating the status of a peripheral meniscal tear after arthroscopic repair. It has to be remembered that what the arthrogram shows basically is that the repaired tear has a watertight articular surface; the fibrocartilaginous meniscal tissue could still be unhealed. However, in most cases even MRI cannot differentiate between an unhealed repaired tear and one that has healed but has not produced any reduction of signal as a scar forms. Arthrography following meniscal repair, therefore, can provide evidence that is of clear practical value to the surgeon. In my opinion, the exact detail of the location and orientation of a tear for such purposes also is better demonstrated at arthrography than on magnetic resonance examination.

There is little doubt that arthrography has never been as accurate in the diagnosis of tears of the cruciate ligaments as arthroscopy and now MRI. This is not surprising, because the cruciate ligaments are intra-articular but extrasynovial, so that only the margin of synovial reflection is shown, whilst MRI can indicate the signal within the depth of the ligament or its complete attrition within an intact plica of synovium.

In the demonstration of damage to the articular cartilage, arthrography will enable the grosser evidence of degenerative arthritis to be revealed. This is in contrast to arthroscopy, where the surgeon can demonstrate softening of cartilage or fibrillation of its surface layers; MRI however, when fast gradient-echo sequences are employed, promises to demonstrate changes in the deep subarticular layers of cartilage even when there is no abnormality visible at arthroscopy.

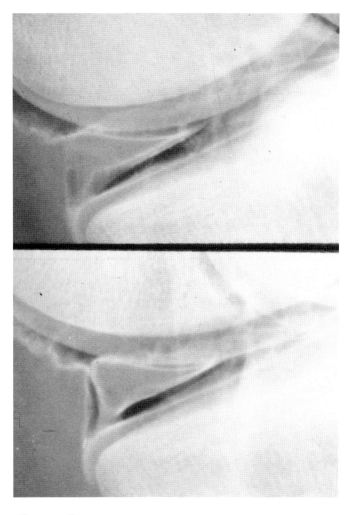

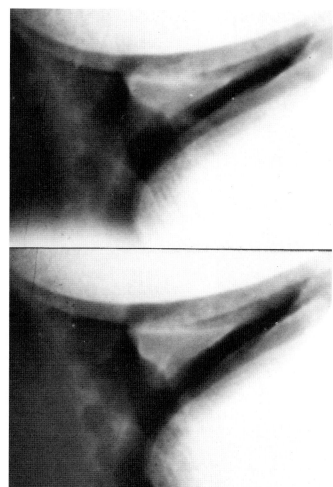

Figure 2

Vertical tear of posterior horn of medial meniscus. Two views of the posterior horn are provided, the lower being farther posterior as indicated by the overlapping of the two femoral condyles. A vertical peripheral tear appears far back in the joint. An injury in such a location is often difficult to demonstrate at arthroscopy.

Figure 3

Peripheral detachment of posterior horn of lateral meniscus. In these views of the posterior horn, the attaching bands shown in Figure 1 have been completely ruptured, so that the posterior horn of the meniscus is hypermobile and unstable. At arthroscopy, testing the mobility of the meniscus with a blunt hook would cause the posterior horn to prolapse abnormally towards the centre of the joint.

Figure 4

Cyst of medial meniscus. A tear of the undersurface of the meniscus has allowed contrast medium to enter the more peripheral cyst. Such tears are not easy to demonstrate at arthroscopy. It is likely that the cyst and associated tear would have been demonstrated by MRI examination.

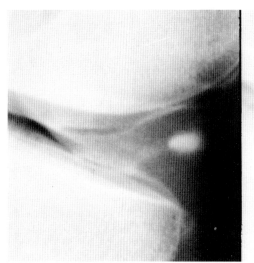
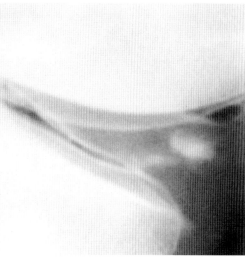

Conclusions

Arthrography of the knee has been a valuable diagnostic aid to the enlightened orthopaedic surgeon. In expert hands, it is still probably as accurate as arthroscopy or MRI in the diagnosis of meniscal tears. Nevertheless, with the advent of a non-invasive diagnostic imaging method (MRI) which is, in addition, capable of the accurate diagnosis of ligamentous damage, arthrography is likely to be superseded. In countries where cost is paramount, and interested radiologists are available, arthrography is likely to persist as an inexpensive, accurate diagnostic method which causes little pain or disturbance to the patient.

References

1. **Butt WP, McIntyre JL**, Double-contrast arthrography of the knee, *Radiology* (1969) **92**: 487–499.
2. **Kaye JJ**, Knee arthrography today, *Radiology* (1985) **157**: 265–266.
3. **Hall FM**, Arthrography: past, present and future, *Am J Roentgenol* (1987) **149**: 561–562.
4. **Belli A, Renton P, Stoker DJ**, Comparative study of iohexol and meglumine iothalamate in double-contrast knee arthrography, *Clin Radiol* (1984) **35**: 375–377.
5. **Ingram C, Stoker DJ**, Contrast media in double-contrast arthrography of the knee: a comparison of ioxaglate and iothalamate preparations, *Br J Radiol* (1986) **59**: 143–146.
6. **Ireland J, Trickey EL, Stoker DJ**, Arthroscopy and arthrography of the knee: a critical review, *J Bone Joint Surg (Br)* (1980) **62**: 3–6.

1.3   Magnetic resonance imaging in the diagnosis and management of knee pathology

Nicholas R. Boeree and Christopher E. Ackroyd

The development of arthroscopy over the past two decades has had a dramatic impact upon the management of soft-tissue injuries of the knee, allowing inspection of the joint without recourse to a far more invasive formal arthrotomy. In skilled hands arthroscopy proved to be accurate,[1-3] and could be combined with therapeutic procedures. None the less, many patients require no operative treatment. As a purely diagnostic tool, arthroscopy exposes such patients to unnecessary discomfort, morbidity and hospitalization. Sherman et al. reported a complication rate of 8.2% in an extensive multicentre study of more than 2500 patients (4.8% representing major complications), and concluded that arthroscopy could no longer be regarded as 'no-problem surgery'.[4]

Arthrography, whilst less invasive, may be painful, and patients often require one or two days off work afterwards. Occasional complications such as infection are reported.[5] Approximately 24 radiographic exposures are required and, for the surgeon, interpretation can be difficult. However, with experience, accurate diagnostic information is obtained in 77–95% of cases.[2,6-10]

In contrast, magnetic resonance imaging (MRI) is entirely non-invasive, causing the patient no discomfort and only the minimum of inconvenience. There do not appear to be any associated risks, and the patient is not exposed to irradiation. Occasionally patients may experience claustrophobia (1–2%), but even this problem could be reduced in the future by the development of 'limb-only' scanners. Whilst experience in interpretation is invaluable, pathology, when demonstrated, is usually easily appreciated.

In June 1987 the Bristol MRI centre was opened. Since that time over 300 patients have been investigated for a variety of knee complaints by means of the Picker 0.5–tesla MRI body scanner. A surface detector coil is used, placed around the slightly flexed and internally rotated knee. The early investigations usually comprised 12 coronal and 16 parasagittal T_1-weighted contiguous sections of 5 mm thickness. Proton density images allow quicker scan times, and this has now become the usual method of investigation.

By comparing the MRI findings with those at arthroscopy, it is possible to assess the reliability of MRI in the diagnosis of soft-tissue injuries of the knee. Over a 2-year period in Bristol 203 patients were investigated for possible meniscal or cruciate injuries. Of these, 133 also underwent arthroscopy, and hence could provide corroborative information about the menisci and cruciate ligaments, allowing an evaluation of the sensitivity, specificity and accuracy of MRI.[11]

Sensitivity may be regarded as the ability of a test to detect pathology. The ability to distinguish normality is defined as *specificity*, while *accuracy* is the ability of a test to determine the true situation.

Meniscal injuries

The normal meniscus, when seen on MRI in cross-section, is a very low-signal (dark) triangular structure (Figure 1). Cross-sectional views of the entire meniscus are obtained by examining both the coronal and parasagittal sections. A common finding is that of internal mucoid degeneration of the meniscus, which is seen as an area of high signal within its substance (Figure 2). This is to be differentiated from a tear, in which an area of high signal clearly communicates with one or both meniscal articular surfaces (Figure 3).[12] Occasionally, in a patient who has not had a prior meniscectomy, a meniscus will be seen which is notably small or absent. Such a finding should be regarded as indirect evidence of a tear.[11]

From Tables 1 and 2 it will be seen that there is very close correlation between the MRI appearances of the menisci and the findings at arthroscopy. In the study undertaken in Bristol, as in other series, there were occasional discrepancies between the appearances of the menisci on MRI and the findings at subsequent arthroscopy. There were three meniscal tears that were not seen on MRI. Two of these were bucket-handle tears that had been displaced into the intercondylar area. Whilst bucket-handle fragments may be visualized, the usual high signal interface between the torn fragment and the remaining meniscus is lost, making diagnosis more difficult. In the remaining case the meniscal tear could not be seen, although it could be inferred on MRI from the presence of an associated meniscal cyst. The opposite

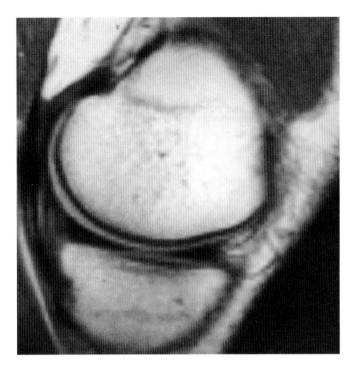

Figure 1

Magnetic resonance image of the knee in parasagittal section showing the appearances of a normal meniscus.

Figure 2

Internal mucoid degeneration of the posterior horn of the medial meniscus, seen as an area of high signal which does not communicate with an articular surface.

situation, with tears being noted on MRI but not confirmed at arthroscopy, occurred in seven cases. Occasionally this may occur because of misinterpretation of normal anatomical structures.[13] More often it is likely to arise from an over-interpretation of the appearances of internal mucoid degeneration, or to result from some tears being missed owing to inadequate arthroscopic technique. In 6 of the 7 cases mentioned above, the arthroscopic examination was

Table 1 The correlation between MRI and arthroscopic findings for the medial meniscus.

MRI	Arthroscopy		
	Normal (%)	Torn (%)	Absent (%)
Normal	47.4	1.5	0.0
Torn	4.5	43.6	0.0
Absent	0.0	2.25	0.75

Table 2 The correlation between MRI and arthroscopic findings for the lateral meniscus.

MRI	Arthroscopy		
	Normal (%)	Torn (%)	Absent (%)
Normal	74.4	0.75	0.0
Torn	1.5	18.8	0.0
Absent	0.0	1.5	3.0

undertaken by a junior member of staff, and the majority of the suspected tears were in the posterior horn. Tears in this region may be missed in approximately 5% of cases.[2]

Other meniscal abnormalities, such as meniscal cysts (Figure 4) or discoid menisci (Figure 5) are also demonstrated clearly by MRI. Meniscal cysts are shown as high signal collections, and, because of their high water content, are particularly bright on STIR (short tau inversion recovery) images.

From Table 3, which shows the sensitivity, specificity and accuracy of MRI in evaluating soft-tissue injuries of the knee, it can be seen that MRI may be relied upon to detect the vast majority of meniscal tears (sensitivity 96.7%), while only occasionally will normal menisci be misinterpreted as torn (specificity 91.3%). Similar results have been reported by other authors.[14,15]

In contrast, clinical assessment of the menisci is entirely unreliable.[2,3,16] This was confirmed in a further comparative study in Bristol.[17] In this report neither the mechanism of injury, as described by the patient, nor any of the traditionally sought symptoms such as locking or giving way, were found to offer any useful guidance as to the likely diagnosis. Clinical examination of the knee was of little further assistance (Table 4). McMurray's test failed to detect approximately 75% of all tears, and, although joint-line tenderness was slightly more sensitive, it lacked

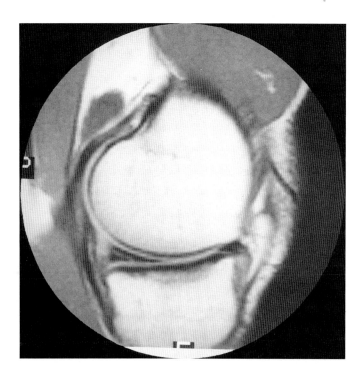

Figure 3

Parasagittal view demonstrating a tear of the posterior horn of the medial meniscus, represented by an area of high signal extending to the inferior articular surface.

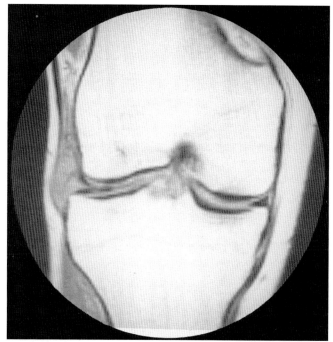

Figure 4

A cyst of the lateral meniscus.

specificity and still failed to detect over one-third of all tears. The finding of a locked knee in outpatients was uncommon, being noted in only 5% of meniscal lesions, and of little diagnostic help since 8% of isolated anterior cruciate ligament injuries were also considered to be locked.

Table 3 The sensitivity, specificity and accuracy of MRI as judged against the findings at arthroscopy.

	Sensitivity (%)	Specificity (%)	Accuracy (%)
Medial meniscus	96.7	91.3	93.8
Lateral meniscus	96.1	98.0	97.6
Anterior cruciate	97.0	89.0	91.0

Table 4 The reliability of clinical signs in the evaluation of the menisci.

	Sensitivity (%)	Specificity (%)	Accuracy (%)
McMurray's test			
Medial meniscus	29.3	87.3	67.4
Lateral meniscus	25.0	89.8	78.3
Joint-line tenderness			
Medial meniscus	63.8	69.4	67.5
Lateral meniscus	27.8	86.8	76.4

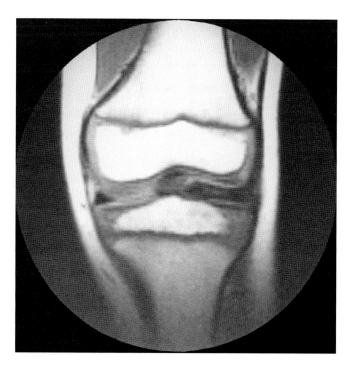

Figure 5

A discoid lateral meniscus in a 9-year-old boy.

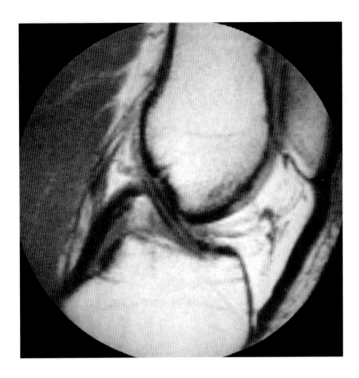

Figure 6

The normal appearance of the posterior and anterior cruciate ligaments.

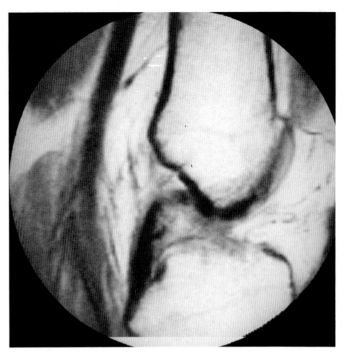

Figure 7

Absence of the anterior cruciate ligament.

Injuries of the cruciate ligaments

The normal anterior and posterior cruciate ligaments may be clearly demonstrated by MRI. The anatomical structure of the anterior cruciate is reflected in its appearances on scanning, characteristically having two or three dark bands which run longitudinally (Figure 6). The posterior cruciate appears as a thicker, low-signal structure (Figure 6).

As a result of its oblique course, the anterior cruciate ligament (and occasionally the posterior) may not be seen in its entirety on one single section, which represents a slice of 5 mm. However, if a cruciate ligament is not visualized at all in its anticipated position (Figure 7), or if it appears only as a diffuse, amorphous area of high signal (Figure 8), it may be presumed to be ruptured.[18]

Using data from the Bristol study, Table 5 demonstrates that there is close agreement between the appearances of the ligament on MRI and the findings at arthroscopy. Once again there were occasional discrepancies. There were 11 patients, thought to have anterior cruciate ruptures on MRI who were found to have an intact ligament at subsequent arthroscopy. However, in these cases MRI may be providing useful information concerning the integrity of the ligament. Although grossly intact, of these 11 ligaments, all of which gave an amorphous high signal on MRI, 7 were found to be evidently lax at arthroscopy and a further 2 had clinical evidence of laxity. Such MRI appearances, in conjunction with evidence of laxity, may thus suggest interstitial rupture of a ligament. Occasionally, because of its oblique course, the anterior cruciate may be inadequately represented on any section, resulting in an erroneous conclusion of rupture. This is a phenomenon known as 'partial voluming', and is more likely with an attenuated or small ligament.

Additional support for suspicion of an anterior cruciate deficiency may be derived from the finding on MRI of a posterior cruciate ligament which appears more curled up than usual (Figure 9).[11] This occurs because the femur, unrestrained by the anterior cruciate ligament, is able to drop posteriorly

Table 5 The correlation between MRI and arthroscopic findings for the anterior cruciate ligament.

	Arthroscopy		
MRI	Normal (%)	Lax (%)	Not seen (%)
Normal	66.9	0.0	0.75
High signal	3.0	1.5	6.0
Not seen	0.0	3.75	18.0

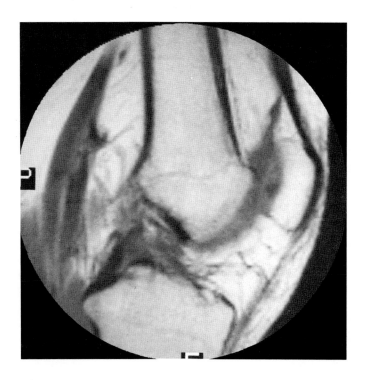

Figure 8

Rupture of the anterior cruciate ligament, which appears as an area of diffuse, amorphous high signal.

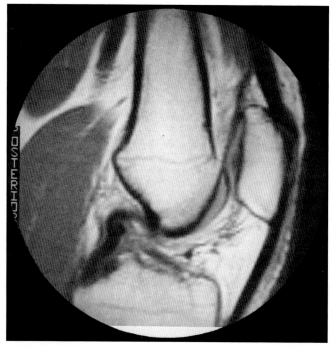

Figure 9

A posterior cruciate ligament appearing more curled up than usual (compare with Figure 6), supporting the diagnosis of rupture of the anterior cruciate ligament where this structure is poorly visualized.

with respect to the tibia when the patient lies with the knee slightly flexed but relaxed on a pillow. This is the position adopted when undertaking a scan.

Magnetic resonance imaging appears to show the posterior cruciate quite clearly. However, this ligament is often not seen at arthroscopy, and is certainly rarely seen in its entirety. In addition, injuries of this ligament are less common than those of the anterior, and surgical repair or reconstruction rarely undertaken. It is therefore difficult to compile sufficient corroborative data to support the accuracy of any form of investigation of the posterior cruciate ligament.

The reliability of MRI in assessing the anterior cruciate ligament is shown in Table 3, and again may be contrasted with clinical evaluation.[17] Anterior cruciate ruptures cannot be predicted from the mechanism of injury, although immediate post-traumatic swelling is strongly suggestive. The symptoms of which the patient may subsequently complain are not helpful in arriving at a diagnosis, and the various tests devised to assess the anterior cruciate are usually quite specific, but very insensitive (Table 6). In other words, a positive test will rarely be elicited in the presence of a normal ligament, but a significant number of ligament ruptures will be missed. Lachman test was the most sensitive, but this will still miss over one-third of all ligament ruptures (sensitivity 62.7%), while more than two-thirds will be missed by the pivot shift test (sensitivity 30.5%).

Articular surface derangements

In addition to demonstrating soft-tissue abnormalities of the knee, MRI can provide valuable information concerning other articular derangements. Joint effusions are clearly seen, and may be demonstrated at a subclinical level. Very early changes associated with osteoarthritis and rheumatoid arthritis may be shown, both in the articular cartilage and in the subchondral bone, the latter perhaps reflecting alterations in the local vascular supply.

Table 6 The reliability of clinical signs in the evaluation of the anterior cruciate ligament.

	Sensitivity (%)	Specificity (%)	Accuracy (%)
Lachman test	62.7	90.3	82.3
Anterior drawer	55.9	91.7	81.3
Pivot shift	30.5	96.5	77.3

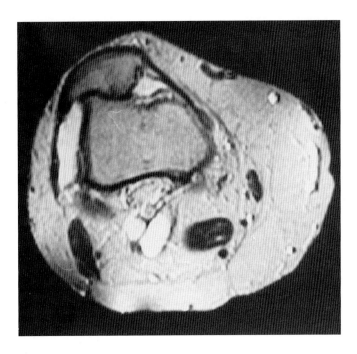

Figure 10

View of the patellofemoral joint showing degenerative changes, with loss of articular cartilage, osteophyte formation, subchondral bone sclerosis and lateral subluxation.

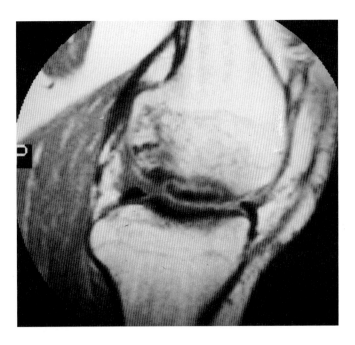

Figure 11

Osteochondritis dissecans of the medial femoral condyle.

In assessing the patellofemoral joint, subluxation may be seen as well as subchondral bone shadowing and loss of articular cartilage (Figure 10). MRI is likely to have an increasing role to play in the evaluation of patients with anterior knee pain, for whom

arthroscopy is very rarely rewarding. In such patients, a scan may exclude significant cartilaginous or subchondral pathology, and may demonstrate the position of the patella with the knee extended.

We are currently exploring the role of MRI in evaluating the changes that occur with osteochondritis dissecans. Such lesions are clearly demonstrated (Figure 11), and information concerning the state of the fragment, the adjacent bone and overlying cartilage, or of the residual defect and any healing that may have occurred, should prove valuable in determining management and in assessing the results of treatment.

Implications for clinical management

If one relies upon clinical evaluation alone, it may be anticipated that at least one-third of all medial meniscal tears and three-quarters of all lateral meniscal tears will be missed, as will over one-third of all anterior cruciate ligament ruptures. Furthermore, because clinical evaluation lacks specificity, particularly in the examination of the menisci, a significant number of patients with normal menisci will erroneously be considered to have a meniscal tear. In Bristol, it was shown that of 203 patients suspected of having meniscal or cruciate injuries, 198 (97.5%) would ultimately have required arthroscopy had the only determinant been clinical diagnosis. Unfortunately, because of errors in diagnosis, 93 patients would have undergone arthroscopy unnecessarily. In a further 33 patients who would not initially have been considered for arthroscopy but who did have meniscal tears, the procedure would have been delayed.

Accurate preoperative diagnosis, available with MRI, can avoid these problems by ensuring that arthroscopy is targeted to those patients likely to obtain therapeutic benefit. Reliance upon clinical diagnosis alone would have resulted in an 89% increase in the number of arthroscopic procedures undertaken had MRI not been available in Bristol.

For the patient, negative arthroscopy entails unnecessary inconvenience, discomfort and hospitalization. Perhaps more importantly, the patient is exposed to an unnecessary risk of morbidity.[4] For the surgeon these unnecessary negative arthroscopies are a waste of limited manpower and operating theatre resources. In Bristol, the average theatre time for arthroscopy was 1 hour and 4 minutes. By confining arthroscopic procedures only to those with proven meniscal tears, it was estimated that MRI allowed more appropriate use of more than 51 hours of theatre time each year.

It may be argued that, whilst desirable, MRI cannot be justified if proper regard is taken of the limited financial resources available to the National Health Service. Closer scrutiny reveals this argument to be flawed.[17] Precise costing of procedures and investigations is difficult, depending upon local practices, costs, and the availability of facilities. However, using the fixed rate of charges applied in the private sector, one may estimate the respective costs of clinical management with or without the benefit of additional investigations. In the study in Bristol of 203 patients, the cost, without additional investigation, of the anticipated 93 unnecessary arthroscopic procedures would have exceeded the cost of investigation by MRI for the entire group. Avoiding further investigation of the knee because of cost therefore represents a false economy.

Conclusion

Through magnetic resonance imaging information about the internal structure of the knee is available which has been shown to agree closely with arthroscopy and which is at least as accurate as the very best results reported with arthrography. Unlike the latter, MRI does not suffer from the drawbacks of an invasive and uncomfortable means of investigation, and offers the surgeon images which are certainly more easily appreciated.

With accurate preoperative information, a significant number of patients need not be exposed to the discomfort and risk of morbidity associated with an arthroscopic procedure that would not prove helpful. As a result the surgeon will achieve a substantial reduction in his arthroscopy workload, liberating theatre time that can be used more productively. Magnetic resonance imaging is already a cost-effective method of achieving these desirable goals, and future developments in both the equipment and in the accompanying software should noticeably improve still further both the efficiency, scope and accuracy of this method of investigation.

Acknowledgments

Many of the data concerning the reliability of MRI and Figures 1 to 9 are reproduced by kind permission of the *Journal of Bone and Joint Surgery*. Data concerning the reliability of clinical assessment are reproduced by kind permission of *Injury*.

References

1. **Dandy DJ, Jackson RW**, The diagnosis of problems after meniscectomy, *J Bone Joint Surg (Br)* (1975) **57**: 349–352.
2. **Ireland J, Trickey EL, Stoker DJ**, Arthroscopy and arthrography of the knee, *J Bone Joint Surg (Br)* (1980) **62**: 3–6.
3. **Jackson RW, Abe I**, The role of arthroscopy in the management of disorders of the knee, *J Bone Joint Surg (Br)* (1972) **54**: 310–322.
4. **Sherman OH, Fox JM, Snyder SJ et al.**, Arthroscopy – "No-problem surgery": an analysis of complications in 2640 cases, *J Bone Joint Surg (Am)* (1986) **68**: 256–265.
5. **Ansell G**, Arthrography, *Complications in diagnostic radiology*, ed Ansell G (Oxford: Blackwell Scientific Publications, 1976) 17: 372–373.
6. **Dumas JM, Eddé DJ**, Meniscal abnormalities: prospective correlation of double-contrast arthrography and arthroscopy, *Radiology* (1986) **160**: 453–456.
7. **Gillies H, Seligson D**, Precision in the diagnosis of meniscal lesions: a comparison of clinical evaluation, arthrography and arthroscopy, *J Bone Joint Surg (Am)* (1979) **61**: 343–346.
8. **Pavlov H, Warren RF, Sherman MF et al.**, The accuracy of double-contrast arthrographic evaluation of the anterior cruciate ligament, *J Bone Joint Surg (Am)* (1983) **65**: 175–183.
9. **Shakespeare DT, Rigby HS**, The bucket-handle tear of the meniscus: a clinical and arthrographic study, *J Bone Joint Surg (Br)* (1983) **65**: 383–387.
10. **Thijn CJP**, Accuracy of double-contrast arthrography and arthroscopy of the knee joint, *Skeletal Radiology* (1982) **8**: 187–192.
11. **Boeree NR, Watkinson AF, Ackroyd CE et al.**, Magnetic resonance imaging of meniscal and cruciate injuries of the knee, *J Bone Joint Surg (Br)* (1991) **73**: 452–457.
12. **Stoller DW, Martin C, Crues III JV et al.**, Meniscal tears: pathologic correlation with MR imaging, *Radiology* (1987) **163**: 731–735.
13. **Watanabe AT, Carter BC, Teitelbaum GP et al.**, Common pitfalls in magnetic resonance imaging of the knee, *J Bone Joint Surg (Am)* (1989) **71**: 857–862.
14. **Mink JH, Levy T, Crues III JV**, Tears of the anterior cruciate ligament and menisci of the knee: MR imaging evaluation, *Radiology* (1988) **167**: 769–774.
15. **Polly DW, Callaghan JJ, Sikes RA et al.**, The accuracy of selective magnetic resonance imaging compared with the findings of arthroscopy of the knee, *J Bone Joint Surg (Am)* (1988) **70**: 192–198.
16. **Simonsen O, Jensen J, Mouritsen P et al.**, The accuracy of clinical examination of injury of the knee joint, *Injury* (1984) **16**: 96–101.
17. **Boeree NR, Ackroyd CE**, Evaluation of the menisci and cruciate ligaments: an audit of clinical practice, *Injury* (1991) **22**: 291–294.
18. **Turner DA, Prodromos CC, Petasnick JP et al.**, Acute injury of the ligaments of the knee: magnetic resonance evaluation, *Radiology* (1985) **154**: 717–722.

1.4   Magnetic resonance imaging of the knee

David W. Stoller

There have been significant advances in magnetic resonance (MR) imaging of the knee since its initial application in the evaluation of the meniscus. Routine examination now encompasses a large spectrum of internal knee derangements and articular disorders. A noninvasive modality, MR has virtually replaced conventional arthrography in the evaluation of the menisci and cruciate ligaments. Arthrography requires an injection of contrast material to evaluate the surface of the meniscus. MR, on the other hand, can evaluate the entire substance and internal structures of the meniscus.[1] The MR techniques involve radial imaging, three-dimensional volume acquisition techniques and kinematic evaluation of the patellofemoral joint.[2,3] Use of intravenous gadolinium contrast (gadolinium DTPA) in inflammatory arthritides can enhance and map areas of pannus tissue.[4]

Imaging protocols for the knee

A circumferential extremity coil provides a uniform signal-to-noise across the knee without the posterior to anterior signal drop-off observed in imaging with flat-surface coils. The protocol for the evaluation of internal derangement uses T_1-weighted images in the axial, sagittal, and coronal planes. Fluid signal intensity is dark on T_1-weighted images and fat signal intensity is bright. T_2 or fast scan T_2-weighted images are performed in the sagittal imaging plane and display fluid signal intensity as bright, and fat marrow as intermediate or dark signal intensity. Images are obtained with a high-resolution acquisition matrix and a small field of view (16 cm or less). The sagittal plane is sensitive for identifying meniscal and cruciate pathology. The coronal plane is best for displaying collateral ligament anatomy.

Place the patient in the supine position with the knee in 15° of external rotation. This realigns the anterior cruciate ligament (ACL) parallel to the sagittal imaging plane. The rotation of the knee does not need to be changed for imaging in either the axial or coronal plane. Sections of 5 mm are routinely obtained in the axial, sagittal, and coronal planes without an interslice gap. Newer 3D volume imaging techniques allow 1 mm imaging that provides greater anatomic coverage of the ACL without having to position the patient in external rotation.

T_2-weighting is helpful in highlighting ligamentous edema in either the coronal (collateral ligaments) or the sagittal (cruciate ligaments) imaging plane. In patients with arthritis, sagittal images provide the most information in early synovial reactions and cartilage erosions. Neoplastic lesions, both benign and malignant, require both T_1- and T_2-weighted images in the axial plane. T_1-weighted sagittal or coronal images demonstrate the proximal and distal extent of a lesion in one section.

Menisci

Imaging protocols for the menisci

T_1-weighted or fast scan T_2-weighted (T_2^*-weighted) protocols are sensitive in detecting meniscal lesions.[5] Gradient echo T_2^* images offer the advantage of effective T_2-weighting without compromising the delineation of meniscal degeneration or tears that may not be as well visualized on conventional T_2-weighted images.[6] Gradient echo techniques are also useful for demonstrating articular cartilage pathology.

Normal MR anatomy of the menisci

The 'C'-shaped fibrocartilaginous menisci attach to the condylar surface of the tibia and provide additional mechanical stability in femoral–tibial rotations. The intact meniscus visualizes with uniform low signal intensity on both T_1, T_2 or T_2^* fast scan techniques (Figure 1). The menisci are triangular in cross-section, with an outer curve and a medially directed apex. They are arbitrarily divided into thirds: the anterior horn, the body, and posterior horn. The lateral meniscus forms a tight 'C' shape and accommodates the popliteus tendon posteriorly. It is separate from the lateral collateral

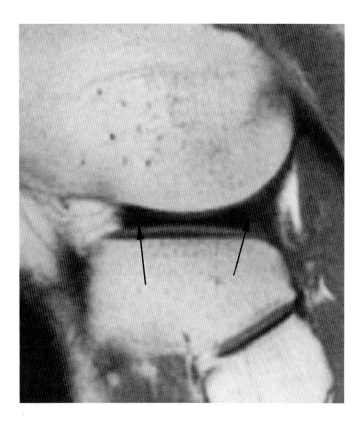

Figure 1

Normal low-signal-intensity lateral meniscal fibrocartilage. Anterior and posterior horns are indicated (arrows).

ligament (LCL). It has posterior horn attachments to the posterior cruciate ligament (PCL) and medial femoral condyle through the ligament of Wrisberg. The medial meniscus is wider, with an open 'C' shape. Besides the intercondylar connections, it attaches to the deep layer of the medial collateral ligament (MCL) through the capsular ligaments, the meniscofemoral, and the meniscotibial ligaments. The posterior horn of the medial meniscus is larger than the anterior horn on sagittal cross-sectional images.

Meniscal pathology

Degenerations and tears – accuracy of MR

The sensitivity of MR in the detection of meniscal tears is reported to be between 75% and 100%.[7,9] In a large series by Mink, Levy and Crues,[10] the accuracy rate of MR in 600 menisci was 92%, with 9 false negatives and 18 false positives. Fast three-dimensional MR of the meniscus produced a 95% concurrence between MR and arthroscopy in detection of meniscal tears and a 100% correlation with meniscal degenerations.[11] The negative predictive value of MR approaches 100% in exclusion of tears in normal MR examinations of the meniscus. The variation in detection rates of meniscal lesions when compared to arthroscopy may be due to multiple factors. These include: (1) a learning curve for the radiologist in interpreting MR signal intensities; (2) the experience of several different arthroscopists participating in correlative studies; (3) false interpretation of areas of fibrillation or fraying as meniscal tears; (4) the inability of arthroscopy to detect degenerative cleavage tears without probing; and (5) the variability in performing examinations with different imagers and surface coils at a variety of field strengths.

MR appearance

An intact meniscus demonstrates homogeneous low signal intensity whatever the pulse sequence. Imbibing synovial fluid causes degenerations and tears of the meniscus to have increased signal intensity.[5] Presignal intensity and synovial fluid gaps have been confirmed in surgically induced tears in animal models.

The development of a grading system that correlates with a pathologic (histologic) model illustrates the significance of increased signal intensity in meniscal abnormalities.[5,8] Increased signal intensity in a spectrum of patterns or grades produces visualization of areas of degeneration. This is due to the signal intensity distribution relative to the articular surface exclusive of the peripheral capsular margin which is nonarticular.

In MR grade 1 there is focal or globular intrasubstance increased signal intensity that is nonarticular. Histologically, grade 1 signal intensity correlates with foci or early mucinous degeneration and chondrocyte-deficient or hypocellular regions. These are pale staining on hematoxylin and eosin (H&E) preparations. The terms mucinous, myxoid, and hyaline degenerations can be used interchangeably to describe the accumulation of mucopolysaccharide ground substance in stressed or strained areas of meniscal fibrocartilage.[12,13] These changes usually occur in response to mechanical loading and degeneration. Grade 1 signal intensity may be observed in asymptomatic athletes and normal volunteers and is not clinically significant.

In MR grade 2 there is horizontal, linear intrasubstance signal intensity that extends from the capsular periphery of the meniscus but does not involve an articular surface. Areas and bands of mucinous degeneration are more extensive in grade 2 than in grade 1. Although no distinct cleavage plane or tear is observed in grade 2 menisci, microscopic clefting and collagen fragmentation have been recorded in hypocellular regions of the fibrocartilaginous matrix. The middle perforating collagen bundle, a structure

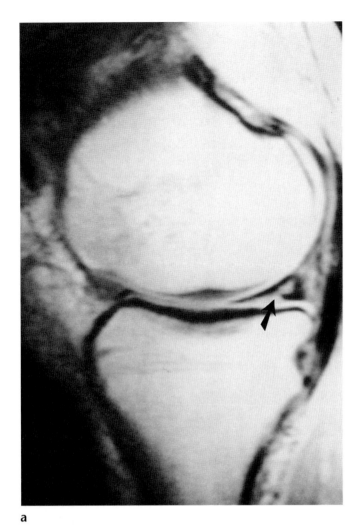

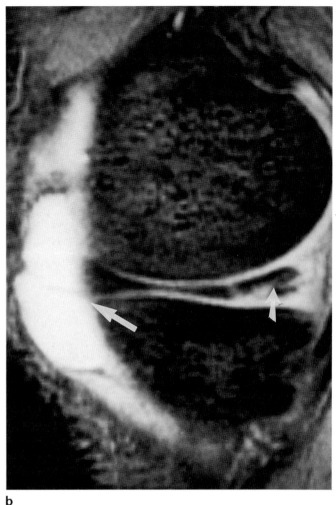

a

b

Figure 2

(a) Grade 3 signal intensity tear in posterior horn of medial meniscus (arrow) on T_1-weighted sagittal images. (b) Separate case with complex grade 3 signal intensity in posterior horn (small arrow) with associated meniscal cyst (large arrow).

not ordinarily seen on MR images, sends out fibers that horizontally divide the meniscus into superior and inferior leaves.[14] A site of preferential accumulation of mucinous ground substance has a grade 2 signal intensity. Patients with grade 2 menisci may or may not present with symptomatic knee pain. These lesions, however, are prone to fibrocartilaginous tears, especially in the posterior horn of the medial menisci. Grade 2 lesions should not be called tears as they represent intrasubstance degenerations.

A meniscus with an MR grade 3 is one in which the area of increased signal intensity communicates or extends to at least one articular surface (Figure 2). Fibrocartilaginous separation or tears are present in all menisci with grade 3 signal intensity. In about 5% of grade 3 menisci these disruptions represent confined intrasubstance cleavage tears.[15] Diagnosis of closed meniscal tears is usually possible by surgical

probing during arthroscopy. These disruptions also may explain in part the 6% false positive interpretations of grade 3 signals when correlated with arthroscopy.[8] Even in the absence of joint locking, the mechanical instability created by confined horizontal cleavage tears may be responsible for acute knee pain.

In a displaced, vertical longitudinal tear of the medial meniscus, the separated central fragment resembles the handle of a bucket[5] (Figures 3 and 4), hence the name bucket-handle tear. This type of tear effectively reduces the width of the meniscus. Peripheral sagittal images fail to demonstrate a normal bow-tie configuration in the body of the medial meniscus. The remaining anterior and posterior horns are often hypoplastic or truncated, with internal signal intensity. A displaced meniscal fragment is frequently found in the intercondylar notch on coronal images.

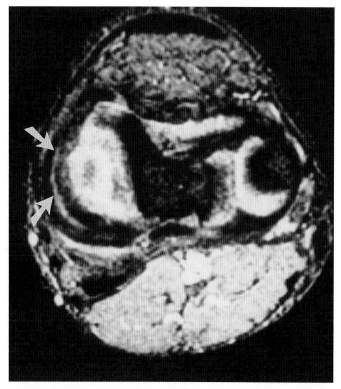

a

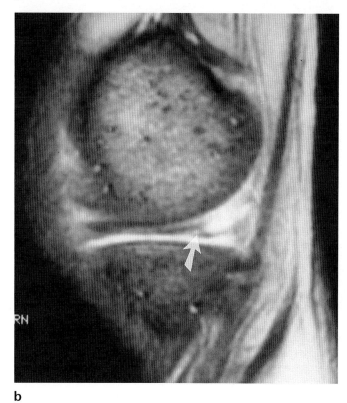

b

Figure 3

Axial image of 0.7 mm demonstrating longitudinal tear (arrows) of the medial meniscus (a) and corresponding T_2*-weighted gradient echo sagittal image (b).

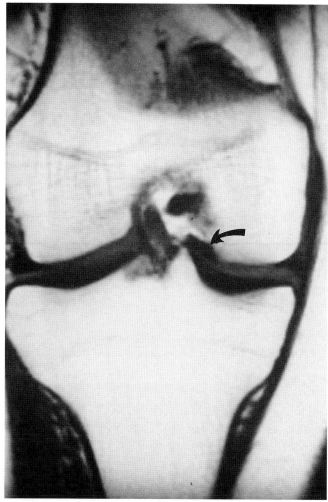

a

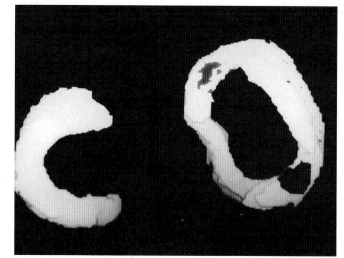

b

Figure 4

(a) T_1-weighted coronal image of a bucket-handle tear with displaced tissue in the intercondylar notch (arrow). (b) Corresponding 3D MR rendering displaying bucket-handle morphology.

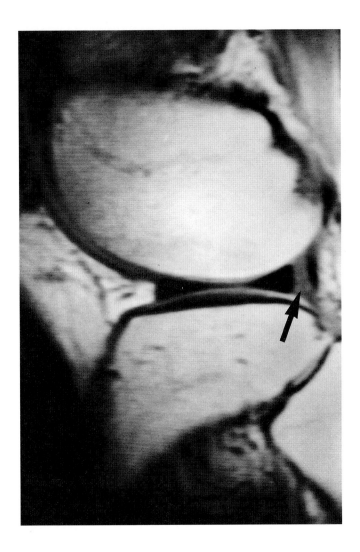

Figure 5

Normal tendon sheath of popliteus tendon on T_1-weighted sagittal image (arrow).

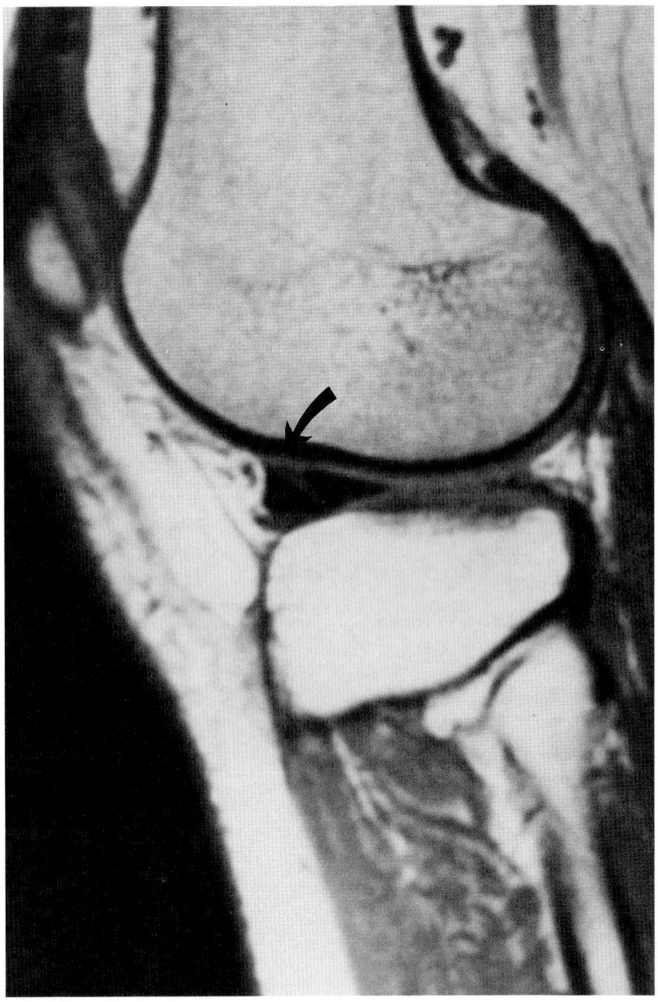

Figure 6

Complex tear of lateral meniscus with posterior horn tissue identified adjacent to anterior horn of lateral meniscus (arrow).

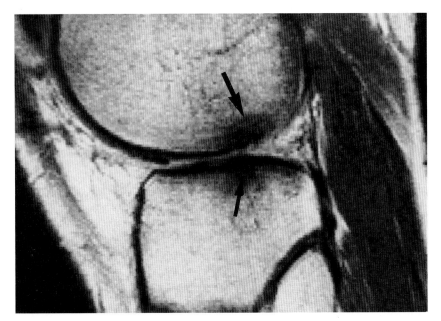

Figure 7

Low-signal-intensity degenerative subchondral sclerosis (arrows) post-lateral meniscectomy. T_1-weighted sagittal image.

Pitfalls in interpretation of meniscal tears

The transverse ligament of the knee connects the anterior horn to the medial and lateral menisci. It can simulate an oblique tear adjacent to the anterior horn of the lateral meniscus.[16] In up to 30% of MR examinations, the fat surrounding the low-signal-intensity ligament mimics grade 3 signal intensity. On serial sagittal images, the round transverse ligament may be traced from the anterior horn to the lateral and medial meniscus in 15% of cases. Isolated tears of the anterior horn of the lateral meniscus are unusual, but can easily be differentiated from the transverse ligament pseudotear.

In the posterior horn of the lateral meniscus, the popliteus tendon sheath may be mistaken for a grade 3 signal intensity and falsely interpreted as a tear (Figure 5). The popliteus tendon sheath is intermediate in signal intensity on T_1- and T_2-weighted images. It courses in an oblique anterosuperior to posteroinferior direction, anterior to the low-signal-intensity popliteus tendon. An absent posterior horn of the lateral meniscus may occur in complex tears (Figure 6).

The meniscofemoral ligaments, consisting of the ligament of Humphrey and ligament of Wrisberg also may simulate meniscal tears.[17] The insertion of the meniscofemoral ligament on the medial femoral condyle may mimic a vertical tear of the posterior horn of the lateral meniscus.

Miscellaneous conditions of the meniscus

Postoperative menisci

MR may be helpful in evaluating patients with pain or mechanical symptoms after partial or total meniscectomy[18,19] (Figure 7). The same criteria can assess meniscal degenerations and tears in native menisci. It may be normal, however, to identify a residual grade 3 signal intensity in a posterior horn remnant after partial meniscectomy. Grade 3 signal intensity after meniscal repair may represent either a retear of the menisci or normal fibrovascular healing.[20] Gadolinium administration may provide a specific diagnosis in the presence of residual grade 3 signal intensity after primary meniscal repair.

Discoid menisci

A discoid meniscus has lost its normal 'C' shape and has a broad disklike form (Figure 8). It has a continuous or bow-tie appearance on three or more successive sagittal MR images.[7,21] Visualization of anterior and posterior horns is limited to one or two sagittal sections near the intercondylar notch. Central taper-

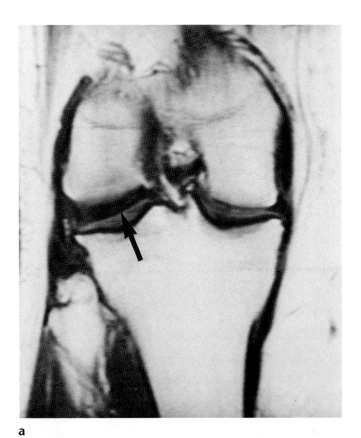

a

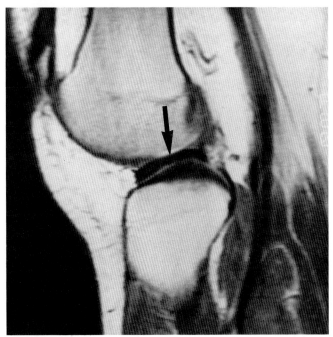

b

Figure 8

Discoid lateral meniscus with loss of normal anterior and posterior horn morphology (arrows) on T_1-weighted coronal (a) and sagittal (b) images.

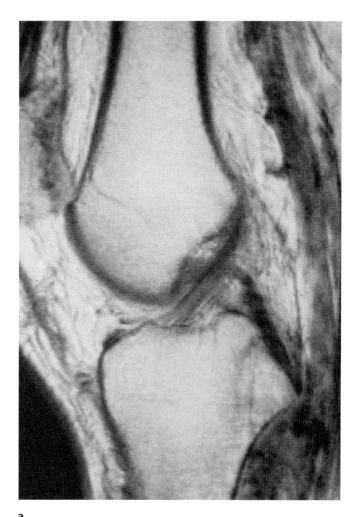

a

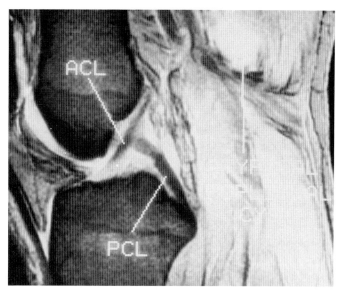

b

Figure 9

Normal cruciate ligament anatomy on T_1 (a) and T_2*
gradient echo (b) sagittal images.

ing, seen in the normal meniscus on sagittal images
is missing in discoid fibrocartilage.

Meniscal cysts

Meniscal cysts are collections of mucinous or
synovial fluid traceable to the joint-line. They have a
uniform low signal intensity on T_1-weighted images
and high signal intensity on T_2-weighted images. A
horizontal tear is usually seen in line with the meniscal cyst, suggesting decompression of synovial fluid.

Meniscocapsular separations

Peripheral meniscocapsular separations or tears usually
involve the less mobile medial meniscus.[22] On sagittal
MR images the tibial plateau cartilage should be
covered by the posterior horn of the medial meniscus
without exposed articular surface. Uncovered tibial
articular cartilage, or fluid interposed between the

peripheral edge of the meniscus and capsule, suggests
peripheral detachment. The meniscofemoral and
meniscotibial attachments of the deep capsular layer
are best seen on either three-dimensional thin section
volume images or radial images of the knee that
display the meniscocapsular junction.

Cruciate ligaments

Anterior cruciate ligament

The ACL is visualized as a band of low signal intensity with separate fiber striations near the tibial
attachment (Figure 9). The ACL may visualize with a
minimally greater signal intensity than the homo-
geneously dark PCL.

In complete tears of the ACL, there is discontinuity in the low-signal-intensity band, with or without
loss of its normally taut parallel margins[23–25] (Figure
10). Partial or complete ligamentous disruptions may

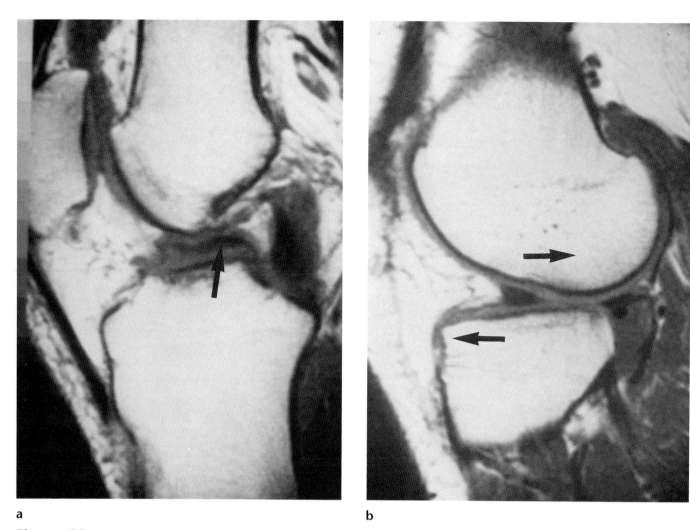

a

b

Figure 10

ACL tear. (a) Complete ACL tear (arrow). (b) Associated anterior translation of the tibia relative to the femur (arrows).

be associated with blurring of the cruciate's fascicles from edema or hemorrhage (Figure 11). Hemorrhagic joint effusions associated with tears of the ACL may incite a synovitic reaction associated with irregularity of the free concave edge of the infrapatellar fat pad.

Accurate assessment of partial ligamentous tears is more difficult than detection of complete disruptions. Posterior bowing of the ACL or buckling of the PCL may be associated with a chronic tear of the ACL. Absence of the ACL on both sagittal and coronal images is diagnostic of ACL disruption. Forward displacement of the tibia on MR is the equivalent of a positive anterior drawer test or Lachman test. Oblique images through the cruciate ligaments may improve visualization of ACL fibers. 3D acquisition techniques with 1 mm sections may be used in place of thin section oblique images through the cruciate ligament. MR also has application in assessing ligamentous reconstructions (Figure 12).

Posterior cruciate ligament

In the sagittal plane, PCL is seen as a uniform dark band usually displayed on a single sagittal image (Figure 13). Cruciate anatomy is also visualized on axial and coronal images (Figures 14–16). An abnormally high arc or buckling in the PCL suggests abnormal laxity or tearing of the ACL.[26] Within this normally low-signal-intensity ligament, any increase in signal intensity, on either T_1- or T_2-weighted images should be interpreted as abnormal (Figure 17). Hemorrhage and edema, seen in acute injuries, are bright on T_2-weighted images and incite less distortion or mass effect than with tears of the ACL. Complete disruption of the PCL has a loss or gap in ligament continuity. Partial tears may be more difficult to assess. Chronic tears with fibrous scarring do not show increased signal intensity on T_2-weighted images.

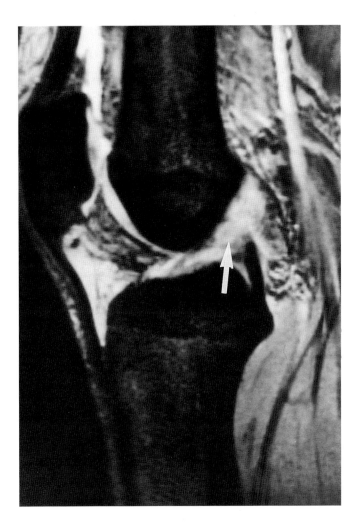

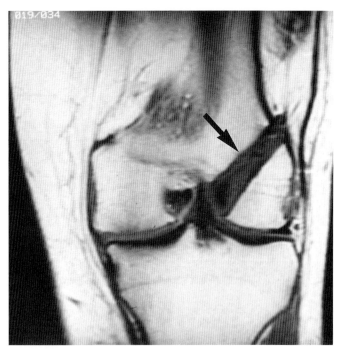

a

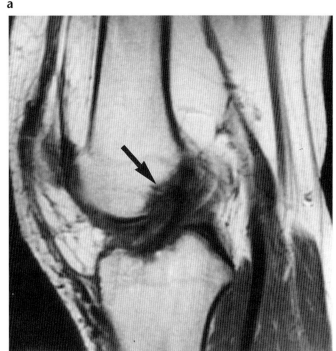

b

Figure 11

High-signal-intensity ACL tear (arrow) on T_2*-weighted gradient echo image.

Figure 12

Synthetic ACL (arrow) reconstruction on T_1-weighted coronal (a) and sagittal (b) images.

Collateral ligaments

Medial collateral ligament

The intact MCL is best demonstrated on T_1- or T_2-weighted coronal images (Figure 18). Partial tears or strains of the MCL are seen with increased distance between the subcutaneous tissue and cortical bone. Mild increases in signal intensity on T_2-weighted images without change in morphology correlate with a grade 1 MCL tear. Increasing ligamentous size and signal intensity with attenuation correlates with a grade 2 MCL tear. Complete disruption of the MCL on MR correlates with a clinical grade 3 disruption (Figures 19–21). T_2 or gradient echo fast scan images demonstrate edema, hemorrhage, or both adjacent to low-signal-intensity fibers. They may also be associated with extensive effusions with extravasation of joint fluid. Focal hemorrhage is common at the femoral intercondylar attachment of the MCL, although tears at its tibial attachment are also identified. MR examination can evaluate associated peripheral tears of the meniscus. Normal menisci in the presence of an MCL tear may obviate the need for arthroscopy.

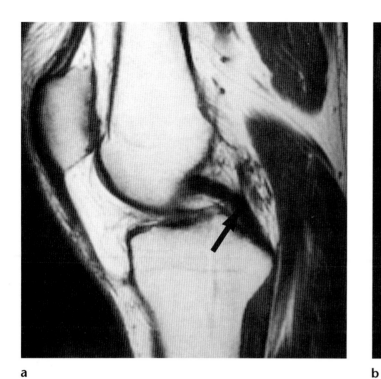

a

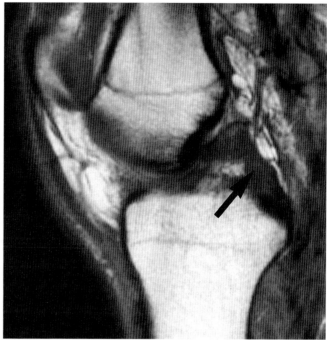

b

Figure 13

PCL tear. (a) Intact low signal intensity PCL (arrow) on T_1-weighted sagittal image. (b) Disrupted PCL (arrow) on T_1-weighted sagittal image.

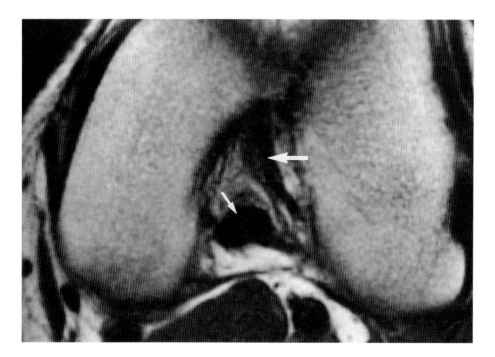

Figure 14

Axial cruciate ligament anatomy. ACL = large arrow; PCL = small arrow.

Lateral collateral ligament

The lateral collateral ligament (LCL) is best visualized on posterior coronal images as a band of low signal intensity. Occasionally, peripheral sagittal images demonstrate LCL anatomy at the level of the fibular head, especially when using less than 3 mm sections (Figure 22). Edema and hemorrhage, although less frequent in this location, are seen as ligamentous thickening with increased signal intensity on T_2-weighted images. In complete disruptions, the LCL may demonstrate a wavy or lax contour with disruption of continuity.

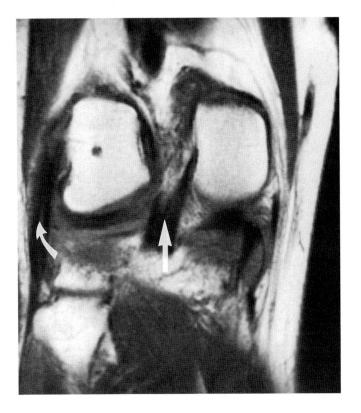

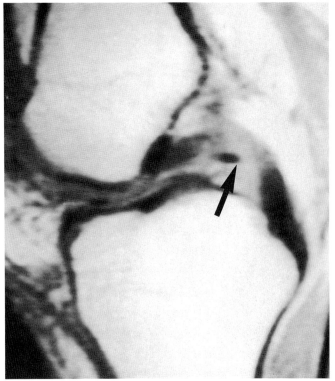

Figure 15

Normal PCL (straight arrow) and LCL (curved arrow) anatomy on posterior coronal T_1-weighted image.

Figure 17

PCL tear with discontinuity of ligament (arrow). T_1-weighted sagittal image.

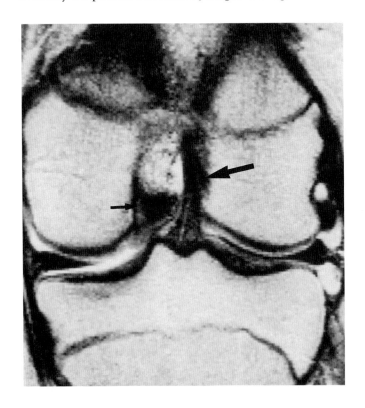

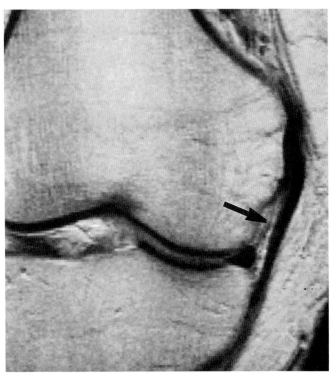

Figure 16

Normal ACL (large arrow) and PCL (small arrow) anatomy on T_2 coronal image.

Figure 18

Intact MCL (arrow) on anterior coronal image.

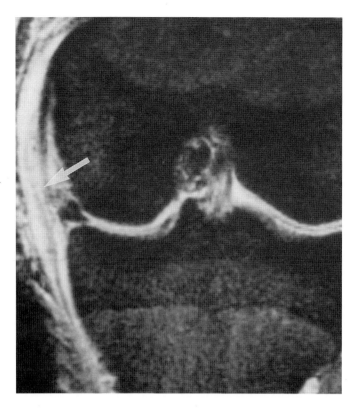

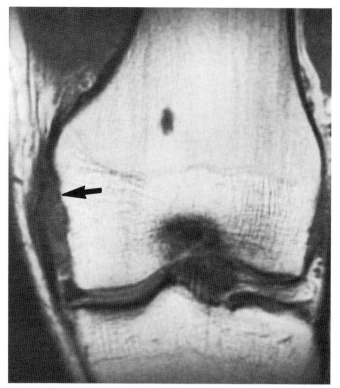

a

Figure 19

Grade 3 MCL with discontinuity of fibers at the level of the joint-line (arrow). No associated meniscal tear is seen.

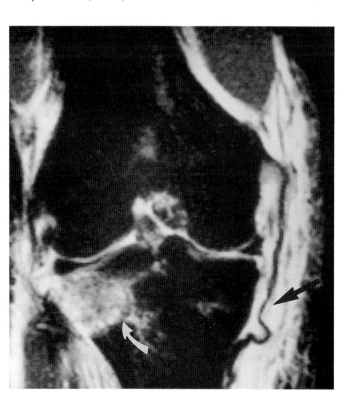

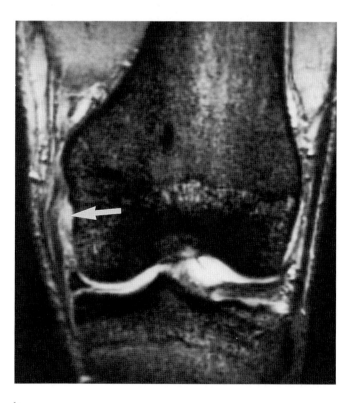

b

Figure 20

Tibial avulsion of medial collateral ligament (straight arrow) associated with severe lateral tibial plateau bone contusion (curved arrow). Fat suppression coronal image.

Figure 21

Thickening of femoral epicondylar attachment in healed grade 3 MCL tear (arrow). (a) T_1-weighted coronal image. (b) T_2*-weighted gradient echo coronal image.

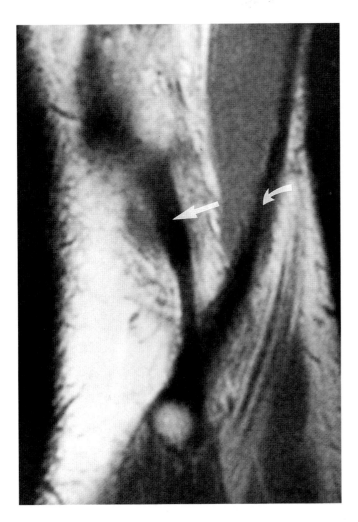

Figure 22

Normal LCL (straight arrow) and biceps femoris tendon (curved arrow) on T_1-weighted sagittal image.

Patellofemoral joint and extensor mechanism

Axial images characterize the patellofemoral articulation accurately. The lateral and medial patellar facets are oblique and cannot be depicted precisely on sagittal or coronal images. Axial sections through the patellofemoral joint can define patellar cartilage and retinacular attachments. Sagittal or axial images can delineate the quadriceps muscles and tendon. Images of the patellar tendon are en face in the coronal plane, in profile in the sagittal plane, and in cross-section on axial planar images.

Chondromalacia patellae

Characteristics of chondromalacia patellae are crepitus and patellofemoral joint pain that is accentuated with knee flexion. On axial MR images, early cartilage attenuation or erosions can be appreciated in either the medial or lateral patellar facets[27] (Figures 23 and 24). Frequently, the opposing femoral cartilage also demonstrates thinning on sagittal images. Sagittal images, which are less sensitive to cartilage erosions, may show a straightening or loss of the normal convex curve seen in patellar hyaline cartilage when viewed in profile. T_2 or gradient echo axial images are useful in demonstrating inhomogeneity of signal intensity from patellar cartilage in areas of focal edema as well as cartilage attenuation and frank erosions. Subchondral low signal intensity, representing sclerosis, may be associated with irregular surface erosions.[28]

Patellar subluxation and dislocation

Patellar subluxation sometimes presents with symptoms of joint locking and may be mistaken for a torn meniscus[29] (Figure 25). The repetitive trauma caused by lateral displacement of the patella accelerates articular surface degeneration. Torn medial retinacular attachments can be identified on axial images following patellar dislocation and traumatic subluxation. Kinematic imaging techniques show the knee in the axial imaging plane from full extension through 40° of flexion. They can evaluate for lateral or medial subluxation secondary to a lateral retinacular release.[30] As faster imaging techniques develop, a true dynamic imaging will be able to evaluate tracking of the patellofemoral joint.

Retinacular attachments

The medial and lateral retinacula are fascicle extensions of the vastus medialis and lateralis muscle groups, respectively.[31] The retinacula reinforce and guide normal patellar tracking. On anterior coronal images, the retinacular attachments display as low-signal-intensity structures converging on the medial and lateral patellar facets.

The medial retinaculum is more frequently torn than the lateral, especially after patellar dislocation (Figure 26). Axial MR images may demonstrate a free-floating retinaculum, without patellar attachment, or they may show a masslike effect of compressed torn retinacular fibers or chondral fragments. Associated edema and hemorrhage produce increased signal intensity on T_2-weighted images.

Patellar tendon abnormalities

Patellar tendon tears, resulting in loss of extension and a high-riding patella, can occur with avulsion injuries of the tibial tubercle or the inferior pole of

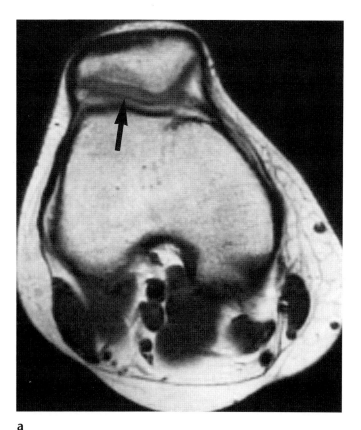

a

Figure 23

Chondromalacia patellae. T_1-weighted axial images. (a) Asymptomatic right knee with preservation of articular cartilage in the lateral patellar facet (arrow). (b) Denuded lateral patellar facet cartilage and subchondral bone in advanced chondromalacia (arrow).

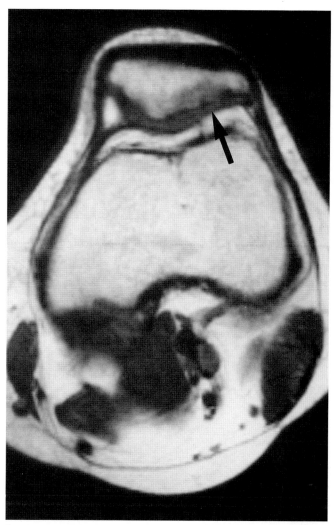

b

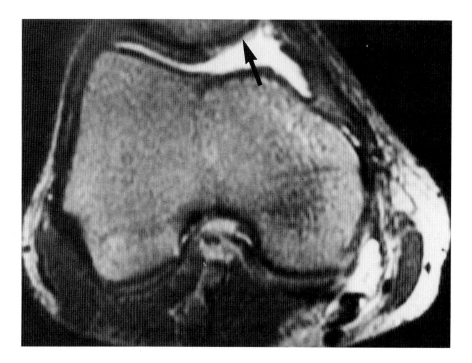

Figure 24

Erosion of medial facet articular cartilage on T_2-weighted axial image (arrow). Joint effusion is of high signal intensity.

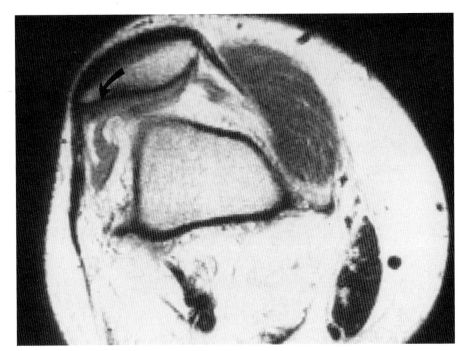

Figure 25

Lateral patellar subluxation demonstrated on T_1-weighted axial image (arrow).

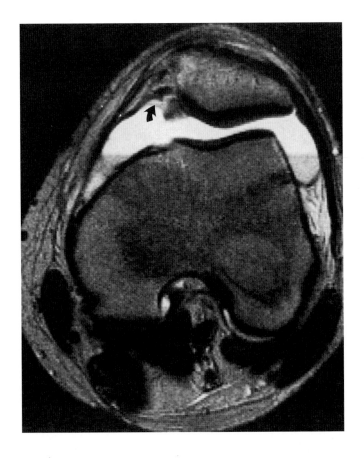

Figure 26

Disruption of medial retinaculum (arrow) subsequent to traumatic patellar dislocation. Associated hemorrhagic joint effusion is identified.

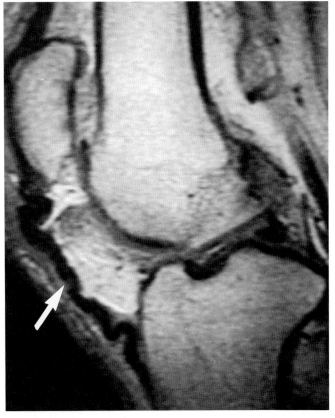

Figure 27

Patellar tendon rupture with lax (arrow) tendon on sagittal image.

the patella.[32] Bony fragments, which visualize with the signal intensity of marrow, may be identified on sagittal MR images. Increased tendon laxity with a wavy or lax contour can present with acute or chronic tears (Figure 27). A thickened patellar tendon may be seen after arthroscopic surgery or trauma. Osgood–Schlatter's disease may be associated with thickening or edema of the adjacent patellar tendon (Figure 28).

Patellar bursa

Prepatellar bursitis appears as a localized soft-tissue mass anterior to the patella. Bursitis has a low signal intensity on T_1-weighted images but signal intensity increases on T_2-weighted images. Infrapatellar bursitis appears posterior to the patellar tendon and inferior to Hoffa's fat pad.[31]

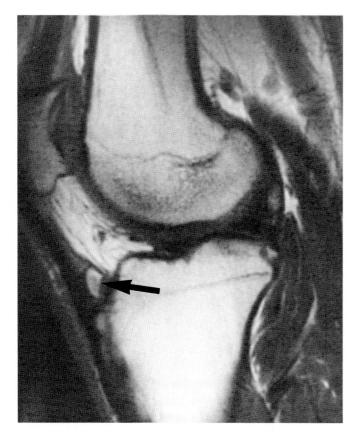

Figure 28

Old Osgood–Schlatter's disease with fragmentation (arrow) of tibial tubercle ossification on T_1-weighted sagittal image.

Pathologic conditions affecting the knee

Arthritis

Assessment of the extent, progression, and therapeutic response in adult arthritic disorders and juvenile chronic arthritis is enhanced by MR of articular cartilage.[33] Even in cases in which conventional radiographs are negative, joint effusions, synovial reactions, popliteal cysts, and osteonecrosis can be demonstrated and evaluated with MR studies.

Cartilage

Cartilage of the patellar, femoral, and tibial articular surfaces is best visualized on T_2-weighted images.[33,35] Because of its hydropic composition, normal hyaline cartilage shows intermediate signal intensity compared with low signal intensity for cortex and fibrocartilaginous menisci. With fast scan gradient echo techniques, articular cartilage has a high signal intensity. The articular cartilage interface is demonstrated with intra-articular administration of gadolinium for precise submillimeter detail.

Synovium and the irregular infrapatellar fat pad sign

Synovial reaction and proliferations appear as changes in the contour of synovial reflections. Irregularity, with loss of the smooth posterior concave free border of the infrapatellar fat pad, can be observed with a variety of synovial reactions. This is called the irregular infrapatellar fat pad sign[33] (Figure 29). Although the synovium cannot be imaged directly in early synovitis, a corrugated surface along Hoffa's fat pad is evident in the initial stages of synovial irritation. This irregular fat pad sign is present in patients with hemophilia, rheumatoid arthritis, pigmented villonodular synovitis, Lyme arthritis, inflammatory osteoarthritis, and in cases of hemorrhagic joint effusion. Synovial hypertrophy and pannus generally has low to intermediate signal intensity on T_1- and T_2-weighted sequences. Fluid associated with synovial masses generates increased signal intensity on T_2-weighted images.

Juvenile chronic arthritis

In juvenile rheumatoid arthritis (JRA), MR studies have characterized early synovitis with an irregular infrapatellar fat pad in the initial stages of clinical presentation.[34] Articular cartilage erosions and synovial hypertrophy can be identified before joint space narrowing is evident on plain film radiography. Popliteal cysts of the gastrocnemius and semimembra-

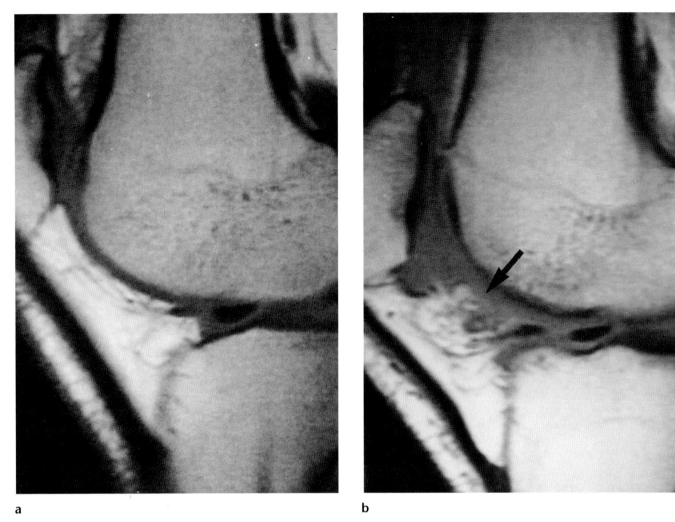

a   b

Figure 29

Infrapatellar fat pad sign. (a) Normal concave contour of infrapatellar fat pad on T_1-weighted sagittal image. (b) Irregular free edge contour of Hoffa's fat pad in a patient with Lyme arthritis and synovitis (arrow). T_1-weighted sagittal image.

nosus bursa are commonly associated with JRA. They appear with low signal intensity on T_1-weighted images and uniform high signal intensity on T_2-weighted images. Thickening of the synovium of the suprapatellar bursa can be visualized with low signal intensity on both T_1- and T_2-weighted images. With MR, subarticular cysts, subchondral sclerosis, and osteonecrosis can be detected on both femoral and tibial surfaces in more advanced disease. These findings are frequently not in evidence on conventional radiographs. Hypoplastic menisci with a small anterior horn, body, and posterior horn have been observed on MR studies in JRA patients. This may be related to an alteration in the composition of synovial fluid, which may impair the development of normal fibrocartilage.

Rheumatoid arthritis

In adult patients with rheumatoid arthritis, bicompartmental and tricompartmental disease displays on MR images through the medial and lateral femorotibial compartments and the patellofemoral joint.[33] Marginal and subchondral erosions with diffuse loss of hyaline articular cartilage are evident on both femoral and tibial surfaces. Large joint effusions and popliteal cysts are commonly seen and demonstrate uniform high signal intensity on T_2-weighted images. Recently, intravenous gadolinium DTPA has been used to selectively enhance the vascularity of pannus tissue in patients evaluated for synovectomy.[36]

Pigmented villonodular synovitis

Pigmented villonodular synovitis (PVNS) is a monoarticular synovial proliferative disorder.[37] It usually presents as a nonpainful soft-tissue mass, and the knee is a frequent site of involvement, especially with the diffuse form of the disease. Hemosiderin-laden macrophages are frequently deposited in hyperplastic synovial masses, and there may be associated sclerotic

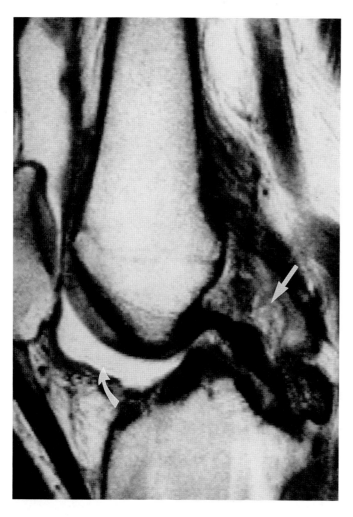

Figure 30

PVNS of the knee characterized by hyperplastic hemosiderin masses (straight arrow) darker than associated joint effusion (curved arrow). T_2-weighted sagittal image.

bone lesions. The hemosiderin-infiltrated synovial masses have a low signal intensity on T_1- and T_2-weighted images because of the paramagnetic effect of iron (Figure 30). Adjacent synovial fluid, however, visualizes with increased signal intensity on T_2-weighted images. MR can prospectively diagnose PVNS.

Hemophilia

In hemophilic arthropathy, hemosiderin and fibrous tissue, formed from repeated episodes of joint hemorrhage, shows with low signal intensity on T_1- and T_2-weighted images.[38,39] Irregular fat pads and markedly thickened hemosiderin-laden synovial reflections are present in these patients.[33] Although conventional radiographs are often normal, articular cartilage irregularities and erosions are detected on MRI scans.

Subchondral and interosseous cysts or hemorrhage can be identified on coronal and sagittal MR images.

Fluid-filled cysts generate high signal intensity on T_2-weighted images. Areas of fibrous tissue remain low in signal intensity on T_1- and T_2-weighted images. Low-signal-intensity synovial effusions can be differentiated from adjacent hemosiderin and fibrosis depositions on T_2-weighted sequences.

Lyme arthritis

Transmission of Lyme disease by the *Ixodes* tick characteristically has a delayed appearance of an oligo- or polyarticular inflammatory arthritis.[40] The knee is commonly affected, with development of inflammatory synovial effusions, synovial hypertrophy, infrapatellar fat pad edema, and, in severe chronic cases, cartilage erosions.

Osteoarthritis

The MR findings in degenerative arthrosis represent a spectrum varying from osteophytic spurring to compartment collapse, denuded articular cartilage, torn and degenerative meniscal fibrocartilage, and diminished marrow signal intensity in areas of subchondral sclerosis.[18,41,42] The ability to assess hyaline cartilage surfaces accurately gives MR an advantage over plain film radiography in preoperative planning for joint arthroplasty procedures. Chondral fragments, of intermediate signal intensity, and loose bodies, with the high signal intensity of marrow fat, may be associated with more advanced degenerative disease.

In synovial chondromatosis, multiple synovium-based chondral fragments appear with low to intermediate signal intensity. In primary chondromatosis, these metaplastic fragments are usually similar to one another in size. In secondary chondromatosis, they have a variety of sizes.

Osteonecrosis and related disorders

Spontaneous osteonecrosis of the knee typically affects an older patient group, predominantly female, and presents with acute medial joint pain.[18,43,44] Commonly, spontaneous osteonecrosis involves the weight-bearing surface of the medial femoral condyle. Cases have been described in which the medial and lateral tibial plateaus and the lateral femoral condyle were involved.[45]

Conventional radiographic evaluation is not sensitive to identification of the osteonecrotic focus prior to development of sclerosis and osseous collapse. Nonetheless, a low-signal-intensity focus can be detected on T_1- and T_2-weighted images in patients with osteonecrosis who have no other demonstrable radiographic findings.

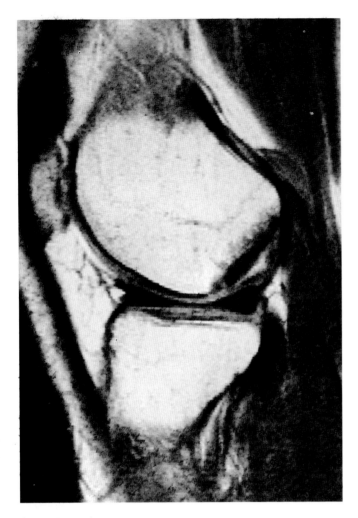

Figure 31

Low-signal-intensity necrotic focus of osteochondritis dissecans on T_2-weighted sagittal image.

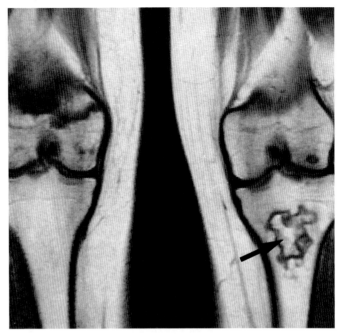

Figure 32

Metaphyseal based bone infarct (arrow) with serpiginous low-signal-intensity sclerotic border and central fat marrow signal intensity. T_1-weighted coronal image.

Osteochondritis dissecans differs from spontaneous osteonecrosis of the knee in that it primarily affects young male patients and involves the non-weight-bearing surface of the medial femoral condyle[46–48] (Figure 31). On MR scans, osteochondritis images with low signal intensity on T_1- and T_2-weighted images prior to detection on conventional radiographs implying loosening of the osteochondral fragment.

Bone infarcts are usually metaphyseal in location but they also image in more epiphyseal and diaphyseal locations[49] (Figure 32). The MR appearance of a bone infarct is characteristic. It has a serpiginous low-signal-intensity border of reactive bone and a central component of high signal intensity equivalent to yellow or fat marrow. Bone infarcts can be differentiated from enchondromas on MR. The latter lack a serpiginous border and have a central region of low signal intensity on T_1-weighted images, which increases with progressive T_2-weighting.

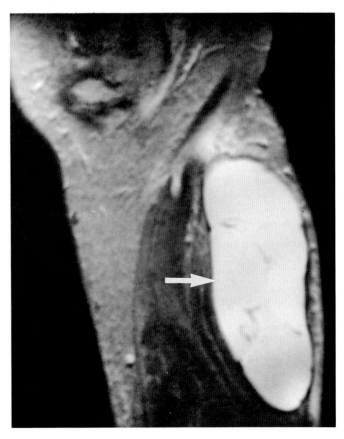

Figure 33

Bright signal intensity popliteal cyst (arrow) dissecting into calf on T_2-weighted sagittal image.

Joint effusions

Joint effusions demonstrate low signal intensity on T_1-weighted images and uniform hyperintense signal intensity on T_2-weighted images. Experience shows that T_1-weighted sequences are adequate for demonstrating small effusions and there is no need for heavy T_2-weighted images. Coronal images are complementary, and the 'saddle bag' distribution of fluid in the medial and lateral gutters of the suprapatellar bursa can be evaluated.

Popliteal cysts

Popliteal or Baker's cysts of the gastrocnemio-semimembranosus bursa arise between the medial head of the gastrocnemius muscle and the semimembranosus[50,51] (Figure 33). These cysts visualize with low signal intensity on T_1-weighted images and are hyperintense on T_2-weighted images. A cyst found in other locations is called an atypical popliteal cyst or ganglion. A cyst at the level of the joint-line is a meniscal cyst. It may communicate with a horizontal meniscal tear or a complex meniscal tear with a horizontal component.

Plicae

Synovial plicae are embryonic remnants of the septal division of the knee joint into three compartments.[52] They are a normal variant in 20–60% of adult knees. Suprapatellar, mediopatellar, and infrapatellar are the common types of plicae. The mediopatellar and infrapatellar plicae are best visualized on axial images. The suprapatellar plicae are seen well on sagittal images traversing the suprapatellar bursa. Plica tissue visualizes with low signal intensity on T_1- and T_2-weighted images.[53] Infrapatellar plicae, the most common, may be confused with the ACL on arthrography.

Fractures

Fractures about the knee can involve the femoral condyle, the tibial plateau surface, or the patella. Fractures can be identified on MR in the face of negative conventional radiographs.[54] Subsequent radiography often shows areas of sclerosis or periosteal reaction at the fracture site initially identified on MR. Type 1, the most frequent MR pattern of fracture, is a diffuse or reticular area of a low signal intensity marrow hemorrhage. Cortical disruption in association with marrow hemorrhage is a type 2 lesion. Localized low signal intensity of a pattern similar to that seen in osteonecrosis or osteochondritis dissecans is a type 3 lesion (Figure 34). Severe bone contusions are often seen in association with a valgus

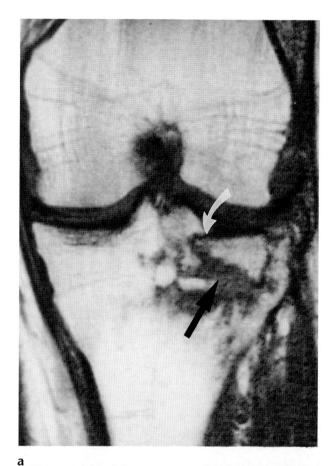

a

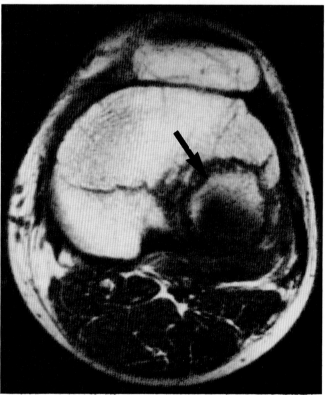

b

Figure 34

Lateral tibial plateau fracture (straight arrow) on T_1-weighted coronal (a) and axial (b) images. Note depression of low-signal-intensity cortex (curved arrow).

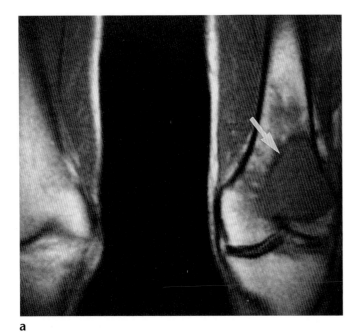
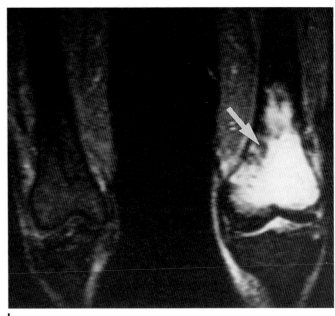

a   b

Figure 35

Distal femoral osteomyelitis (arrow), low signal intensity on T_1-weighted coronal image (a) and high signal intensity on fat suppression image (b).

injury involving rupture of the MCL. Contusions may simulate medial or lateral meniscal pathology. Premature weight-bearing on contusions may lead to development of osteochondral lesions.

MR is also useful in the differentiation of stress fractures, common in the proximal tibia, from neoplastic processes.[55] The linear segment of the stress fracture in the knee is usually accompanied by marrow edema. Lack of a soft-tissue mass, cortical destruction, or characteristic marrow extension effectively excludes a tumor from the differential consideration.

A diffuse or localized pattern of low signal intensity on T_1-weighted images is seen with bone bruises or contusions at sites of impaction or repetitive trauma. In an acute or subacute setting, increased signal intensity is visualized on T_2-weighted images, prior to the appearance of sclerosis on plain films.

Infection

Capsular distension and joint effusion are identified on MR as images of nonspecific joint infection.[56] A septic joint may be further characterized by intra-articular debris and synovitis from hematogenous seeding. In osteomyelitis, a mottled pattern of yellow marrow stores may be identified (Figure 35). Infections or abscesses may be identified on MR in the absence of positive findings on nuclear bone scans.

An infectious tract with fluid may simulate a pathologic or stress fracture. When associated with extensive surrounding edema, it can be confused with tumor.

Neoplastic conditions

MR is used to image benign and primary malignant tumors for staging and limb-salvage procedures and to monitor chemotherapeutic response[57–61] (Figure 36). The longitudinal extent of marrow and cortical involvement is displayed on coronal or sagittal images, facilitating preoperative planning for allograft salvage techniques (Figure 37). T_1- and T_2-weighted axial images define intracompartmental extension and proximity to neurovascular structures. Interval response to preoperative chemotherapy can be assessed. Changes in tumor size; marrow infiltration; cortex, soft tissue, and muscle invasion; hemorrhage, calcification, and necrosis can be recorded. It is important to perform MR studies prior to biopsy because postsurgical inflammation and edema may prolong the T_2 values of uninvolved tissues. Muscle edema is nonspecific and is associated with trauma, infection, and vascular insults. High signal intensity on T_1-weighting in surrounding musculature can be seen in atrophy with fatty infiltration or neuromuscular disorders and should not be mistaken for a tumor.

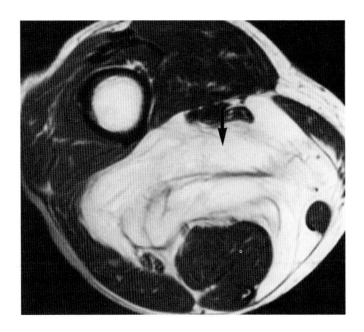

Figure 36

High-signal-intensity infiltrating lipoma (arrow) on T_1-weighted axial image.

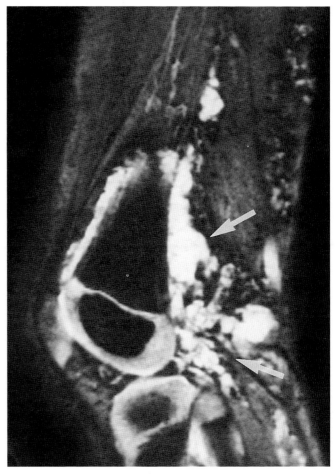

Figure 37

T_2*-weighted gradient echo image displaying neurofibromatosis as bright signal intensity (arrows).

Red to yellow marrow conversion in middle-aged female patients may be seen as low signal intensity in metaphyseal or diaphyseal locations without extension into the epiphysis. These regions become isointense with adjacent marrow on T_2-weighted images. Immature skeletons may exhibit inhomogeneity of metaphyseal red and yellow marrow stores. Marrow infiltrative disorders such as leukemia, lymphoma, and Gaucher's disease extend into the epiphysis or subchondral bone.[62,63] Leukemic infiltrates are detectable on MRI examination of the knee prior to clinical diagnosis and before peripheral blood smears have become abnormal (hairy-cell leukemia). Coarsened nonuniformity of marrow signal intensity is characteristically imaged in Paget's disease.

Artifacts

The presence of orthopedic hardware including plates, screws, pins, and prostheses is not a contraindication for MR examination. Low-signal-intensity artifact is a function of the size, composition, orientation, and design of the device and of the number of devices present within the imaging field.[64–67] MR is successfully used to evaluate tumor recurrence in patients with limb salvage prostheses. A femoral rod or stem does not preclude evaluation of adjacent meniscal or ligamentous structures.

References

1. **Reicher MA, Rauschning W, Gold RH et al.**, High-resolution magnetic resonance imaging of the knee joint: Normal anatomy, *Am J Roentgenol* (1985) **145**: 895–902.
2. **Solomon SL, Totty WG, Lee JKT**, MR imaging of the knee: comparison of three-dimensional FISP and two-dimensional spin-echo pulse sequences, *Radiology* (1989) **173**: 739–742.
3. **Shellock FG, Mink JH, Deutsch AL et al.**, Patellar tracking abnormalities: Clinical experience with kinematic MR imaging in 130 patients, *Radiology* (1989) **172**: 799–804.
4. **Björkengren AG, Geborek P, Rydholm U et al.**, MR imaging of the knee in acute rheumatoid arthritis: synovial uptake of gadolinium-DOTA, *Am J Roentgenol* (1990) **155**: 329–332.
5. **Stoller DW, Martin C, Crues JV III et al.**, Meniscal tears: Pathologic correlation with MR imaging, *Radiology* (1987) **163**: 731–735.
6. **Stoller DW, Helms CA, Genant HK**, Gradient echo MR imaging of the knee, Presented at the Annual Meeting of the Radiologic Society of North America, Chicago, Nov. 29, 1987.
7. **Reicher MA, Hartzman S, Bassett LW et al.**, MR imaging of the knee, Part I: Traumatic disorders, *Radiology* (1987) **162**: 547–551.

8. Crues JV III, Mink J, Levy TL et al., Meniscal tears of the knee: Accuracy of MR imaging, *Radiology* (1987) **164**: 445–448.

9. Mandelbaum BR, Finerman GAM, Reicher MA et al., Magnetic resonance imaging as a tool for evaluation of traumatic knee injuries: Anatomical and pathoanatomical correlations, *Am J Sports Med* (1986) **14**: 361–370.

10. Mink JH, Levy T, Crues JV III, Technical factors, diagnostic accuracy, and further pitfalls, in *Magnetic resonance imaging of the knee*, ed JH Mink, MA Reicher, JV Crues III (New York: Raven Press, 1987).

11. Tyrrell RL, Gluckert K, Pathria M et al., Fast three-dimensional MR imaging of the knee: Comparison with arthroscopy, *Radiology* (1988) **166**: 865–872.

12. Tobler TH, Makroskopische und histologische Befund am kniegelenk Meniscus in verschiedenen Lebensaltern, *Schweiz Med Wochenschr* (1926) **56**: 1359.

13. Ferrer-Roca O, Vilalta C, Lesions of the meniscus. Part I: Macroscopic and histologic findings, *Clin Orthop* (1980) **146**: 289–300.

14. Ferrer-Roca O, Vilalta C, Lesions of the meniscus. Part II: Horizontal cleavages and lateral cysts, *Clin Orthop* (1980) **146**: 301–307.

15. Smillie IS, *Diseases of the knee joint*, 2nd edn (London: Livingstone, 1980) 340–347.

16. Herman LJ, Beltran J, Pitfalls in MR imaging of the knee, *Radiology* (1988) **167**: 775–781.

17. Vahey TN, Bennett HT, Arrington LE et al., MR imaging of the knee: pseudotear of the lateral meniscus caused by the meniscofemoral ligament, *Am J Roentgenol* (1990) **154**: 1237–1239.

18. Burk DL, Kanal E, Brunberg JA et al., 1.5-T Surface-coil MRI of the knee, *Am J Roentgenol* (1986) **147**: 293–300.

19. Smith DK, Totty WG, The knee after partial meniscectomy: MR imaging features, *Radiology* (1990) **176**: 141–144.

20. Deutsch AL, Mink JH, Fox JM et al., Peripheral meniscal tears: MR findings after conservative treatment or arthroscopic repair, *Radiology* (1990) **176**: 485–488.

21. Silverman JM, Mink JH, Deutsch AL, Discoid menisci of the knee: MR imaging appearance, *Radiology* (1989) **173**: 351–354.

22. Mink JH, Pitfalls in interpretation, In: *Magnetic resonance imaging of the knee*, ed JH Mink, MA Reicher, JV Crues III (New York: Raven Press, 1987).

23. Li DK, Adams ME, McConkey JP, Magnetic resonance imaging of the ligaments and menisci of the knee, *Radiol Clin North Am* (1986) **24**: 209–227.

24. Turner DA, Prodromos CC, Pitasnick JP et al., Acute injury of the ligaments of the knee: Magnetic resonance evaluation, *Radiology* (1985) **154**: 717–722.

25. Moeser P, Bechtold RE, Clark T et al., MR imaging of anterior cruciate ligament repair, *J Comput Assist Tomogr* (1989) **13**: 105–109.

26. Grover JS, Bassett LW, Gross ML et al., Posterior cruciate ligament: MR imaging, *Radiology* (1990) **174**: 527–530.

27. Stoller DW, MRI of the patella and patellofemoral joint, Presented to American Roentgen Ray Society, San Francisco: May 8–13, 1988.

28. Hayes CW, Sawyer RW, Conway WF, Patellar cartilage lesions: in vitro detection and staging with MR imaging and pathologic correlation, *Radiology* (1990) **176**: 479–483.

29. Resnick D, Niwayama G, *Diagnosis of bone and joint disorders*, 2nd edn, vol 5. (Philadelphia: WB Saunders, 1988) 2896–2897.

30. Shellock FG, Mink JH, Fox JM, Patellofemoral joint: Kinematic MR imaging to assess tracking abnormalities, *Radiology* (1988) **168**: 551–553.

31. Mink JH, Reicher MA, Crues JV III, *Magnetic resonance imaging of the knee* (New York: Raven Press, 1987).

32. Rockwood CA, Green CP, *Fractures* (Philadelphia: JB Lippincott, 1975).

33. Stoller DW, Genant HK, MR imaging of knee arthritides, *Radiology* (RSNA 1987 scientific program) abstr 165, p. 233.

34. Stoller DW, MRI in juvenile rheumatoid (chronic) arthritis, Presented to Association of University Radiologists. Charleston, SC, March 22–27, 1987.

35. Mink JH, Deutsch AL, Occult cartilage and bone injuries of the knee: detection, classification and assessment with MR imaging, *Radiology* (1989) **170**: 823–829.

36. König H, Sieper J, Wolf K-J, Rheumatoid arthritis: Evaluation of hypervascular and fibrous pannus with dynamic MR imaging enhanced with Gd-DTPA, *Radiology* (1990) **176**: 473–477.

37. Steinbach LS, Neumann CH, Stoller DW et al., MRI of the knee in diffuse pigmented villonodular synovitis, *Clin Imag* (1989) **13**: 305–316.

38. Kulkarni MV, Drolshagen LF, Kaye JJ et al., MR imaging of hemophilic arthropathy, *J Comput Assist Tomogr* (1986) **10**: 445–449.

39. Yulish BS, Lieberman JM, Strandjord SE et al., Hemophilic arthropathy: Assessment with MR imaging, *Radiology* (1987) **164**: 759–762.

40. Johnston YE, Duray PH, Steere AC et al., Lyme arthritis· Spirochetes found in synovial microangiopathic lesions, *Am J Pathol* (1985) **118**: 26–34.

41. Hartzman S, Reicher MA, Bassett LW et al., MR imaging of the knee, Part II: Chronic disorders, *Radiology* (1987) **162**: 553–557.

42. Beltran J, Noto AM, Mosure JC et al., The knee: Surface-coil MR imaging at 1.5 T, *Radiology* (1986) **159**: 747–751.

43. Ahlbäck S, Bauer GCH, Bohne WH, Spontaneous osteonecrosis of the knee, *Arthritis Rheum* (1968) **11**: 705–733.

44. Williams JL, Cliff MM, Bonakdarpour A, Spontaneous osteonecrosis of the knee, *Radiology* (1973) **107**: 15–19.

45. Lotke PA, Ecker ML, Osteonecrosis-like syndrome of the medial tibial plateau, *Clin Orthop* (1983) **176**: 148–153.

46. Lindén B, The incidence of osteochondritis dissecans in the condyles of the femur, *Acta Orthop Scand* (1976) **47**: 664–667.

47. Mesgarzadeh M, Sapega AA, Bonakdarpour A, Osteochondritis dissecans: Analysis of mechanical stability with radiography, scintigraphy, and MR imaging, *Radiology* (1987) **165**: 775–780.

48. De Smet AA, Fisher DR, Graf BK et al., Osteochondritis dissecans of the knee: Value of MR imaging in determining lesion stability and the presence of articular cartilage defects, *Am J Roentgenol* (1990) **155**: 549–553.

49. Ehman RL, Berquist TH, McLeod RA, MR imaging of the musculoskeletal system: A 5-year appraisal, *Radiology* (1988) **166**: 313–320.

50. Guerra J, Newell JD, Resnick D et al., Gastrocnemio-semimembranosus bursal region of the knee, *Am J Roentgenol* (1981) **136**: 593–596.

51. Lindgren PG, Willen R, Gastrocnemius-semimembranosus bursa and its relation to the knee joint: I. Anatomy and histology, *Acta Radiol [Diag] (Stockh)* (1977) **18**: 497–512.

52. Apple JS, Martinez S, Hardaker WT et al., Synovial plicae of the knee, *Skeletal Radiol* (1982) **7**: 251–254.

53. Passariello R et al., CT and MR imaging of the knee joint in the "plica syndrome," *Radiology* (RSNA 1986 scientific program) abstr 161, p. 240.

54. Crues JV III, MR imaging of bone injuries of the knee, *Radiology* (1990) **176**: 296.

55. Stafford SA, Rosenthal DI, Gebhardt MC et al., MRI in stress fracture, *Am J Roentgenol* (1986) **147**: 553–556.

56. Resnick D, Niwayama G, *Diagnosis of bone and joint disorders*, 2nd edn, vol 1. (Philadelphia: WB Saunders, 1988) Chap 18.

57. Stoller DW, Waxman A, Rosen J, Comparison of T1-201, GA-67, Tc-99m MDP, and MR imaging of musculoskeletal sarcoma, *Radiology* (RSNA 1987 scientific program) abstr 165, p. 223.

58. Bloem JL, Bluemm RG, Taminiau AH et al., Magnetic resonance imaging of primary malignant bone tumors, *Radiographics* (1987) **7**: 425–445.

59. Wetzel LH, Levine E, Murphey MD, A comparison of MR imaging and CT in the evaluation of musculoskeletal masses,

Radiographics (1987) **7**: 851–874.

60. **Petasnick JP, Turner DA, Charters JR et al.**, Soft-tissue masses of the locomotor system: Comparison of MR imaging with CT, *Radiology* (1986) **160**: 125–133.

61. **Totty WG, Murphy WA, Lee JKT, Soft-tissue tumors: MR imaging,** *Radiology* (1986) **160**: 135–141.

62. **Lanir A, Hadar H, Cohen I et al.**, Gaucher disease: Assessment with MR imaging, *Radiology* (1986) **161**: 239–244.

63. **Olson DO, Shields AF, Scheurich CJ et al.**, Magnetic resonance imaging of the bone marrow in patients with leukemia, aplastic anemia, and lymphoma, *Invest Radiol* (1986) **21**: 540–546.

64. **Porter BA, Hastrup W, Richardson ML et al.**, Classification and investigation of artifacts in magnetic resonance imaging, *Radiographics* (1987) **7**: 271–287.

65. **Pusey E, Lufkin RB, Brown RK et al.**, Magnetic resonance imaging artifacts: Mechanism and clinical significance, *Radiographics* (1986) **6**: 891–911.

66. **Augustiny N, von Schulthess GK, Meier D et al.**, MR imaging of large nonferromagnetic metallic implants at 1.5 T, *J Comput Assist Tomogr* (1987) **11**: 678–683.

67. **James R, Bartlett CR, Renicker J et al.**, Unusual MR metallic artifact due to steel threads, *J Comput Assist Tomogr* (1987) **11**: 722–723.

1.5   Radionuclide imaging of the knee

Scott F. Dye

The knee is one of the most complex systems in all of biology. This assemblage of billions of cells with its genetically controlled mechanisms of homeostasis acts, in concert, as a type of biologic transmission or torque converter. It is the largest vertebrate joint and must accept and redirect very high loads in multiples of body weight during activities of daily living. Thus, injuries to the knee are common, and as orthopedists we have the challenge of diagnosing and treating a variety of injuries of this system.

The available diagnostic modalities determine to a great extent the way in which the knee and its pathologic conditions are understood. Most current diagnostic imaging methods, including radiography, computed tomography, magnetic resonance imaging, and even arthroscopy, provide primarily structural information regarding the musculoskeletal system. Consequently, our concepts of musculoskeletal injury are often described in terms of structural disruption of tissue (e.g., meniscal tears, rupture of the anterior cruciate ligament, osteochondral fracture, chondromalacia, etc.) rather than in physiologic terms.

Our research group has over 10 years of experience with the use of technetium-99 methylene diphosphonate scintigraphic imaging of the knee in a clinical setting. The use of the bone scan has altered our understanding of knee pathology to include physiologic as well as structural characteristics. It is the only current imaging method that can provide a dynamic geographic manifestation of osseous metabolic activity. Thermography is more an indication of surface blood flow, and positron emission tomography (PET scanning) is only in a nascent research phase.

Historical perspective

The current use of scintigraphic information about the knee is relatively limited. Besides the occasional patient with either tumor, infection, or reflex sympathetic dystrophy, its utility is most accepted in delineating sites of increased osseous stress and/or degenerative changes in the older patient evaluated for arthroplasty. To the present, little mention has been made in the literature regarding the evaluation

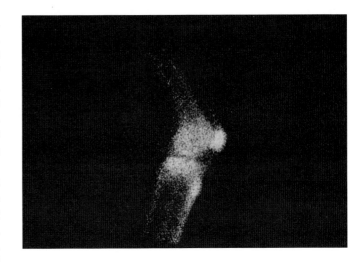

Figure 1

Example of a technetium bone scan of a patient with anterior knee pain, showing increased patellar activity.

of common knee symptoms of young and middle-aged adults with scintigraphic techniques. The clinical conundrum of patients with anterior knee pain, where there is often a lack of objective findings using standard diagnostic methods, was the first area in which scintigraphic data revealed a previously unappreciated alteration of osseous metabolic characteristics. Nearly one-half of a group of 113 adults with anterior knee pain demonstrated abnormally increased osseous metabolic activity of the patella as compared to controls – often in the presence of normal radiographs and grossly normal articular cartilage (Figure 1).[1]

Scintigraphic examination of controls

At the time of our initial research work into this area, no published reports describing normal scintigraphic activity about the knee were available. To delineate

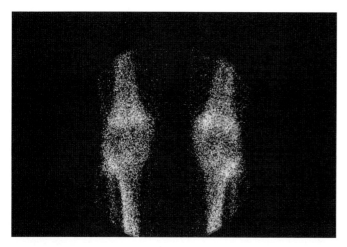

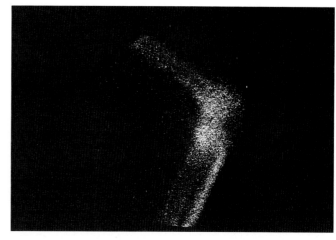

a

b

Figure 2

(a) Control technetium A–P knee scan with indistinct joint margins and slight increase in the physeal region of the femur and lateral proximal tibia. (b) Control lateral knee scan with patellar activity roughly equal to the distal femoral diaphysis and indistinct joint margins.

the pattern of normal scintigraphic activity about the knee, a series of bone scans were obtained in 39 patients between the ages of 18 and 49 years who had had technetium imaging for reasons other than lower extremity symptoms. Physical examinations and radiographic evaluations of their knees were within normal limits. Anterior, posterior, and lateral static imaging of both knees were obtained 3 hours after injection of 20 mCi of technetium-99 methylene diphosphonate. Review of these scans revealed that 94% of this asymptomatic control group had shared characteristics of osseous homeostasis.

Normal scintigraphic examination of the knee

A classically normal bone scan of the knee is represented in Figure 2a and 2b. The anterior–posterior view shows diffuse activity of the femur and tibia, with the femoral activity fading imperceptibly into the tibial activity. One may see mild increased uptake at the distal femoral physis in young adults as well as the lateral border of the tibia, including the inferior lateral plateau and proximal tibiofibular joint. On the lateral view the patella is poorly visualized with indistinct separation from the anterior femur. This activity should be roughly equal to that of the distal femoral diaphysis. The contour of the femoral condyle is barely discernible, with fading of the femoral activity imperceptibly into the tibial activity.

Abnormal patellar activity in patients with anterior knee symptoms

Abnormally increased scintigraphic activity of the patella in anterior knee pain patients correlated well with symptoms, and sequential data indicated that if the increased osseous metabolic activity was present it was often difficult to resolve. The average time for resolution of symptoms and bone scan activity was 10 months, with some individuals not improving until 26 months, most without surgery.[2] Patterns of uptake associated with a more benign course were those with normal patellar activity, increased focal activity (Figure 3) (except for the inferior pole), and diffusely increased patellar activity (Figure 4). Those scintigraphic patterns that correlated with a worse prognosis were focal inferior pole uptake and increased trochlear and patellar activity (Figures 5 and 6).

Osseous pathology

A variety of clinical conditions manifest increased scintigraphic activity of bone, including tumors[3] and infection.[4,5] To establish the microscopic nature of the osseous process detected by the bone scan in anterior knee pain patients, a series of sagittally oriented bone biopsies 3 mm in diameter were obtained from 17 patients with positive patellar scans and persistent

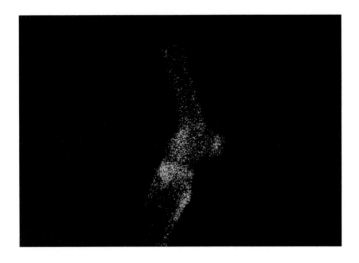

Figure 3

Bone scan of the knee, showing increased focal retropatellar activity.

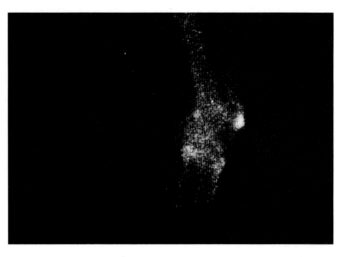

Figure 5

Bone scan of the knee, showing increased focal activity of the inferior pole.

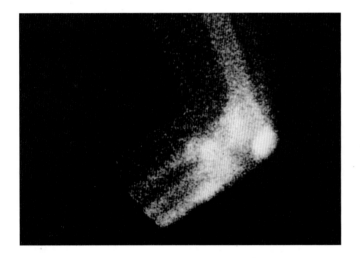

Figure 4

Bone scan of the knee, showing diffuse increased patellar activity.

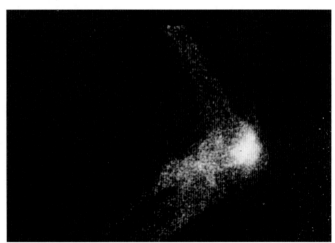

Figure 6

Bone scan of the knee, showing increased activity of the femoral trochlea and patella.

symptoms. Six age-matched cadaver patellae obtained from a tissue transplant bank served as controls.[6]

A typical microscopic appearance of a control patella manifests articular cartilage, calcified cartilage, and a thin subchondral bone layer with projecting spicules of patellar trabeculae from the subchondral region (Figure 7). Under polarized light this section reveals even lamellations of the trabeculae, which we feel to be a histologic indicator of osseous homeo-

stasis. The whorled lamellar pattern in the area deep to the calcified cartilage zone represents a normal region of slightly increased metabolic activity. Biopsy of a symptomatic patella with a positive bone scan shows thickened trabeculae with a whorled burled-walnut appearance of the lamellar pattern on polarized light, which we feel indicates recent remodeling activity (Figure 8). On occasion we have seen evidence of classic cutting cone activity and

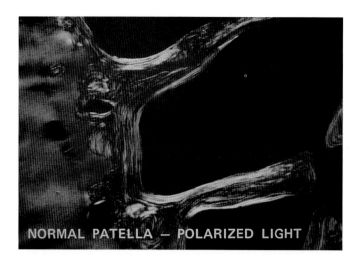

Figure 7

Microscopic section of control patella with polarized light, revealing articular cartilage, calcified cartilage, subchondral bone and thin trabeculae with even lamellations indicative of osseous homeostasis.

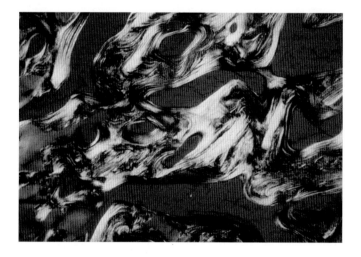

Figure 8

Microscopic section of a biopsy of a symptomatic patella with a positive bone scan, showing thickened trabeculae, vascular invasion into articular cartilage and whorled lamellar patterns indicative of increased osseous remodeling activity.

Howship's lacunae with multinucleated osteoclastic giant cells as well as metabolically active woven bone.

In none of the 17 biopsies did we find any evidence of tumor, infection, bone cysts, or necrosis. In no instance was the sedimentation rate or white blood cell count elevated. We believe that the osseous process detected by the bone scans in these patients is one of increased bone turnover and remodeling, not associated with tumor or infection.

Etiology of increased osseous metabolic activity

What then are the likely etiologic factors to account for the alterations of osseous homeostasis detected in these patients? There are three clinical areas associated with increased osseous scintigraphic activity that as archetypes may provide some insight into the nature of this process. *Osseous trauma* – mechanical bone overload – either through a single event (an overt fracture) or repetitive submaximal loading (an incipient stress fracture) can initiate the increased metabolic activity of bone detectable by scintigraphic methods.[7-9] *Neurovascular dysfunction* as exemplified by the clinical syndrome of reflex sympathetic dystrophy (RSD) is an etiologic factor well known to cause intense osseous remodeling activity detectable by scintigraphic techniques in bones that may have been initially uninvolved in the original injury that initiated the process.[10] It is our impression that many individuals with only a mild to moderate retinacular strain who subsequently demonstrated intense patellar activity on bone scan represent a 'mini-RSD process' with alteration of the normal neurovascular osseous supply resulting, by some unknown mechanism, in an increased osseous turnover.

A third clinical area associated with increased metabolic activity of bone detectable by scintigraphy is *hormonal dysfunction*. The osteoclastic activity induced by increased circulating levels of parathyroid hormone[11] from primary or secondary parathyroid disorders, for example, is associated with increased scintigraphic activity. As indicated by MacKinnon and Holder,[12] experimental evidence has shown that prostaglandins act as a potent stimulator of bone resorption. Speculation exists that the powerful action of prostaglandins on bone metabolism may be a process common to both traumatic and neurovascular etiologies of increased bone remodeling, with prostaglandins released from sites of osteocyte injury or soft-tissue inflammation providing a physiologic stimulus to induce increased bone turnover.

A schematic representation of a theoretical model that appears to account for the clinical findings in the patellofemoral group is shown in Figure 9. Several etiologic factors may act through a common trigger to initiate the remodeling detectable by the bone scan. Following appropriate therapy, although the majority will eventually become asymptomatic, some patients' scans will remain positive, indicating a continuous osseous remodeling process that may with time return to normal. A minority of patients, despite the best therapeutic attempts, may remain symptomatic and continue to have positive scintigraphic findings. Undefined factors acting as repetitive triggers are felt to continue the abnormal remodeling process. It is my opinion that the high biomechanical loading activities of daily living, such

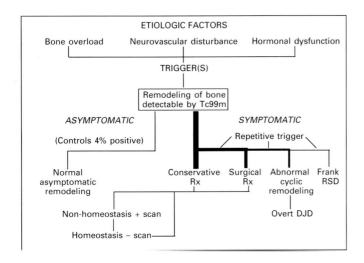

Figure 9

Schematic of a theoretical model of osseous homeostasis in knee patients.

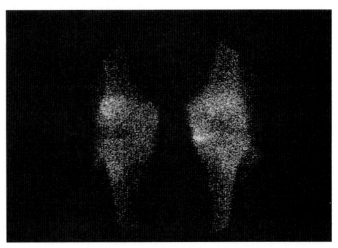

a

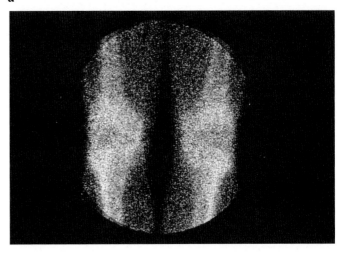

b

Figure 10

(a) Bone scan of a knee with a flap tear of the medial meniscus, showing increased subchondral activity of the medial tibial plateau. (b) Bone scan of the same knee 18 months following careful partial medial meniscectomy, revealing normal activity indicative of osseous homeostasis.

as climbing stairs, squatting, etc., can act as repetitive triggers to subvert the underlying attempts of stressed bone to come to homeostasis in many individuals. The closest familiar clinical analogy is the osseous process that occurs in an incipient stress fracture.

Scintigraphic activity in patients with meniscal tears

We now have gained experience with common scintigraphic patterns associated with other established diagnoses of the knee, including tears of menisci, chronic anterior cruciate ligament insufficiency, and osteochondral fractures. Over 80% of a group of 31 patients with documented tears of the menisci had an associated increased scintigraphic pattern of subchondral bone activity in the involved compartment, often with normal radiographs and normal-appearing articular cartilage.[13] We have also demonstrated that following appropriate careful surgical and postsurgical management, most patients can achieve normal or nearly normal bone scan activity within 18 months (Figures 10a and 10b). Of interest is that subset of patients whose bone scan remains abnormal or worsens. This group has been identified as a subset 'at risk' for early degenerative changes with the continuing abnormal scintigraphic activity predictive of eventual Fairbank changes in greater than 40% within 3 years.

Scintigraphic activity in patients with ACL insufficiency

Over 80% of patients with symptomatic chronic anterior cruciate ligament insufficiency demonstrated abnormal scintigraphic activity about the knee involving at least one of the compartments.[14] The medial compartment is most often involved, followed by the lateral and patellofemoral compartments. The restoration of normal osseous metabolic activity is also possible in such patients following careful guidance and therapy, sometimes without surgical

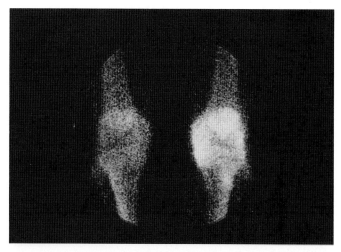

a

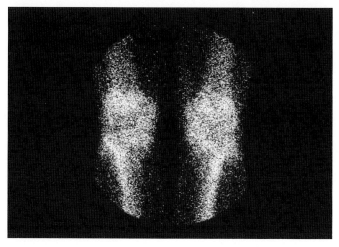

b

Figure 11

(a) Bone scan of an anterior cruciate ligament-deficient knee shows generalized increased activity. (b) Bone scan of the same knee 25 months following reconstructive surgery, showing normal activity indicative of osseous homeostasis.

Significance of scintigraphic data

The technetium bone scan is the *best window* into the osseous physiologic status of the knee. It is clear from our experience that many common diagnoses thought to be mere structural disruption of tissues, e.g., meniscal tears, have an associated widespread osseous physiologic stress resulting in at least temporary loss of osseous homeostasis. The same osseous events that later manifest themselves as irreversible structural changes of degenerative joint disease, e.g., Fairbank changes, can be detected early by scintigraphic methods. We have evidence that restoration of anatomy and kinematics in such patients can lead to restoration of osseous homeostasis as manifested by a normal bone scan post-therapy. We feel, therefore, that the earliest phases of the natural history of post-traumatic arthritis can be reversible in many patients. The main goal of therapy for patients with any knee problem should be not only resolution of symptoms but also *restoration of homeostasis* of the joint.

After extensive experience with blood flow and blood pool scans in patients and controls, we do not routinely obtain these studies as they usually add little information. We also do not feel that single photon emission computed tomography (SPECT) is needed in the evaluation of most knee patients, since a good-quality standard 3-hour delayed static image provides sufficient data.

Scintigraphic evaluation of the knee offers an excellent objective method for assessing the results of various therapeutic approaches following traumatic injury. For example, the current standard of successful anterior cruciate ligament surgery is laxity equal to the normal, uninjured knee. Perhaps an adjunctive standard should be a normal technetium scan at 1–2 years following treatment, indicating osseous homeostasis with implied restoration of normal functional mechanics and subsequent decreased probability of degenerative changes barring new injury.

intervention (Figures 11a and 11b). We feel it is crucial for those patients to realize they have 'linkage failure' of their biologic transmission and that gaining functional control of the knee and remaining in their envelope of load acceptance are the most important factors in resolution of homeostasis as evidenced by a normal scintigraphic examination.

Osteochondral fractures are easily identified by the technetium bone scan with characteristic intense focal activity of the involved region of the knee. Surprisingly, even patients with a significant injury can achieve eventual osseous homeostasis.

Conclusions

The use of the bone scan with other clinical and experimental data has provided a new and previously unappreciated perspective of a dynamic osseous process occurring about the knee of symptomatic adults. Delineating sites of increased osseous metabolic activity geographically and sequentially can define a significant aspect of the early natural history of post-traumatic osteoarthritis of the knee. Further studies may aid in identifying those therapeutic approaches to the knee that are most helpful and least physiologically damaging.

References

1. **Dye SF, Boll DA**, Radionuclide imaging of the patellofemoral joint in young adults with anterior knee pain, *Orthop Clin N Am* (1986) **17**: 249–262.
2. **Dye SF, Peartree PK**, Sequential radionuclide imaging of the patellofemoral joint in symptomatic young adults, *Am J Sports Med* (1989) **17**: 727.
3. **McNeil, B**, The value of bone scanning in neoplastic disease, *Semin Nucl Med* (1984) **14**: 277–286.
4. **Duszynski DO, Kuhn JP, Afshani E et al.**, Early radionuclide diagnosis of acute osteomyelitis, *Radiology* (1975) **117**: 337–340.
5. **Hirsch H, Leonards R**, The bone scan in inflammatory osseous disease, *Semin Nucl Med* (1976) **6**: 95–105.
6. **Dye SF, Daniel JA, Fry PJ et al.**, The correlation of increased scintigraphic activity and patellar osseous pathology in young patients with patellofemoral pain, *Orthop Trans* (1986) **10**: 480.
7. **Matin P**, Bone scintigraphy in the diagnosis and management of traumatic injury, *Semin Nucl Med* (1983) **13**: 104–121.
8. **Matin P**, Bone scanning of trauma and benign conditions, *Nuclear Medicine Annual*, 5th edn, ed L. Freeman, H. Weissman (New York: Raven Press, 1982) 81–118.
9. **Rosenthall L, Hill RO, Chuang S**, Observation on the use of 99m Tc-phosphate imaging in peripheral bone trauma, *Radiology* (1976) **119**: 637–641.
10. **Kozin F, Ryan LM, Carerra GF et al.**, The reflex sympathetic dystrophy syndrome (RSDS) – III. Scintigraphic studies, further evidence for the therapeutic efficacy of systemic corticosteroids, and proposed diagnostic criteria, *Am J Med* (1981) **70**: 23–30.
11. **Sy W**, Bone scan in primary hypoparathyroid, *J Nucl Med* (1974) **15**: 1089–1091.
12. **MacKinnon S, Holder L**, The use of three-phase radionuclide bone scanning in the diagnosis of RSD, *J Hand Surg* (1984) **9A**: 556–563.
13. **Dye SF, McBride JT, Chew M et al.**, Unrecognized abnormal osseous metabolic activity in patients with documented meniscal pathology, *Am J Sports Med* (1989) **17**: 723–724.
14. **Dye SF, Andersen CT, Stowell MT**, Unrecognized abnormal osseous metabolic activity about the knee of patients with symptomatic anterior cruciate ligament deficiency, *Orthop Trans.* (1987) **11**: 492.

1.6 Bone scanning in the assessment of the painful knee

P. Adrian Butler-Manuel, Rosemary L. Guy, Frederick W. Heatley and Thomas O. Nunan

When presented with a knee problem, the clinician usually needs to know more than just the diagnosis. For instance, it is not enough to decide that a patient has a torn meniscus, since this immediately poses the questions (a) Which meniscus is torn? and (b) Are the symptoms sufficient to warrant surgery? The triad of diagnosis, site and severity are all required for a proper assessment. Thus, in the knee even comparatively simple problems such as osteoarthritis can easily deceive the unwary clinician owing to the complex anatomy of the joint. What assistance, if any, can be expected from an investigation such as a bone scan, which by its very nature is non-specific? Has bone scintigraphy anything additional to offer over standard radiographs, arthrograms, computed tomography (CT), magnetic resonance imaging (MRI) and arthroscopy? What does it tell us and how should we use it? Before attempting to answer these questions, let us briefly first consider how the image is actually derived, since it is necessary to have this basic scientific knowledge before we can interpret what we see.

Technetium diphosphonate bone scanning

The radiopharmaceuticals used in bone scanning are technetium-99m (^{99m}Tc) diphosphonates. There are several different diphosphonates in use, the commonest being methyl diphosphonate (MDP). However, we prefer to use hydroxymethyl diphosphonate (HMDP) because we feel it gives a better-quality image.

Diphosphonates are taken up by the metabolically active bone. Two main factors determine the degree of uptake – the blood flow to the region under study and the metabolic activity of that region. Since increased metabolic activity is usually associated with increased blood flow, the uptake in a lesion is a function of both factors.

It is possible using a three-phase (dynamic) bone scan to image the blood flow. For this the patient is positioned under the gamma camera prior to the injection. Sequential images are acquired every 5 seconds immediately after the injection, thus enabling the blood flow in the region of interest to be compared with that in the opposite side. The images are usually of rather poor quality because of the low count rate. A second blood pool image is taken at 5 minutes. This is a better-quality image and, if there is a significant increase in blood flow and blood pool, this image is easier to interpret. The third part of the study is the delayed 3-hour image. There has been some debate in nuclear medicine circles recently regarding the use of three-phase scans. The consensus is that they do not give very much added information over the standard static images. Although we initially did some three-phase scans, we did not find them of any additional use and so we routinely only perform static scans.

In order for bone scanning to be of value, it is necessary to produce high-quality images that the clinician can interpret and thus have confidence in. In this respect attention to detail is crucial. In all nuclear medicine investigations there is a conflict between resolution (ability to distinguish between two separate points) and sensitivity (the ability to detect counts). For knee scanning a high-resolution collimator (focusing device) is used which enables regions of increased diphosphonate uptake to be localized accurately. The trade-off is a low count rate which will itself degrade the image. To overcome this problem the image is acquired for a relatively long time, typically 400 seconds (compared to approximately 200 seconds for a conventional whole-body scan). It is important that the patient keeps absolutely still during this time and therefore the patient must be kept comfortable. Foam wedges and sandbags may be used to support the knees for this purpose.

It is possible with most modern gamma cameras to perform tomography (SPECT, single photon emission computed tomography). The patient lies on a couch and the camera rotates stepwise around the patient, acquiring a series of images. This typically takes 20–30 minutes and again the patient must keep still throughout this period. Standard computed tomography reconstruction techniques are used to reconstruct the image. These images can then be viewed in axial, sagittal and coronal planes. We have not found that these images provide any additional information over good-quality planar images of the knees.

Interpreting a scan

Although quantitative methods for measuring uptake have been described,[1] in practice the scans are usually assessed qualitatively. In the normal adult the appearances are symmetrical, with greater activity around the knee in the femoral condyles and in the proximal tibia and the patella (Figure 1). In the immature skeleton there is also markedly increased epiphyseal uptake (Figure 2). There are two main pathological patterns of uptake: there can either be a diffuse increase throughout the affected knee (Figure 3), or focal uptake which may affect the patellofemoral (Figure 1), the medial or lateral tibiofemoral compartments (Figure 4) or less commonly the metaphysis.

As long ago as 1968 Bauer, in his review of radionuclides in orthopaedic practice, showed that increased scintigraphic uptake was associated with fractures, osteonecrosis, osteoarthritis, rheumatoid arthritis, osteomyelitis, primary and secondary bone tumours and Paget's disease.[2] Subsequently other workers have shown scintigraphy to be specifically of value in the diagnosis of osteoid osteoma,[3] osteochondritis dissecans and other rarities. Bone scintigraphy is widely available and inexpensive[4] and the radiation doses are low and well within the accepted ranges for diagnostic investigations.[5] Its value has hitherto been underestimated in the investigation of common knee problems.

Scintigraphy in specific conditions

Osteoarthritis

Osteoarthritis of the knee can be a very deceptive condition. Varus and valgus deformities can be missed or underestimated in patients with fat legs and even in slim patients clinical examination can often be misleading and fail to localize the affected compartments of the knee. The 'agony test', in which a compressive force is applied to the medial and then to the lateral compartment as the knee is flexed and extended, is perhaps the most reliable clinical test for localizing osteoarthritis.[6]

Unfortunately, in the majority of the hospitals in the UK, it is still standard practice to take routine radiographs with the patient supine. These 'lying' radiographs do indeed lie, frequently showing a joint space when in reality there is eburnated bone. Even routine standing anteroposterior (AP) radiographs taken in extension may not tell the whole truth, as

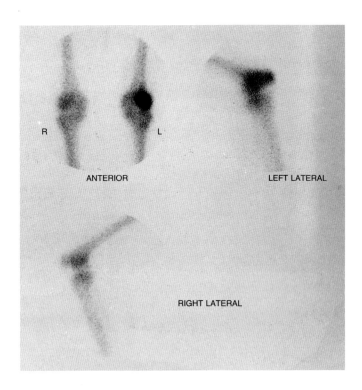

Figure 1

Normal appearance of the right knee. Focal uptake in the left patellofemoral joint following a recent patellar dislocation.

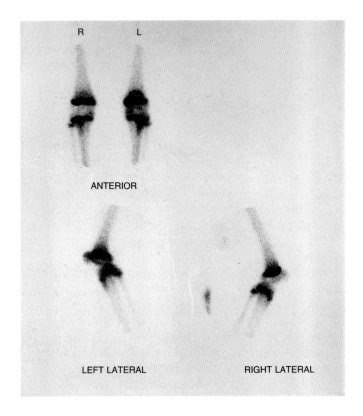

Figure 2

Normal epiphyseal uptake in the knees of a 14-year-old girl. There is also abnormal focal uptake in the left patella due to chondromalacia patellae.

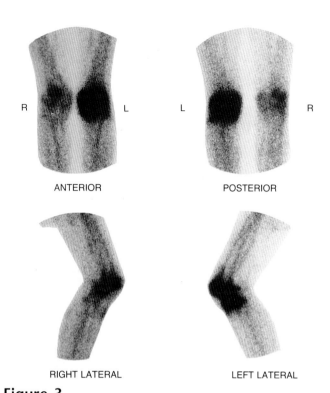

ANTERIOR   POSTERIOR

RIGHT LATERAL   LEFT LATERAL

Figure 3

Diffusely increased uptake in the left knee of a patient with rheumatoid arthritis.

osteoarthritic change is often most marked in the mid or posterior part of a compartment and consequently the surviving anteriorly placed articular cartilage will still show a joint space. The loss of joint space in these circumstances is best shown on an AP standing radiograph taken in 30° of flexion.[7]

Another source of error arises because clinicians do not always appreciate that osteophytosis is a generalized response. Thus, osteophytes may be present in all three compartments, but this does not mean that there is a loss of articular cartilage throughout the knee. True tricompartment osteoarthritis is in fact uncommon. Similarly, osteoarthritis of the medial or lateral compartments rarely occurs in the absence of the appropriate varus or valgus deformity, which is best shown by a long leg standing film.[8]

What then is the reason for doing a bone scan? The answer is that scintigraphy is not deceived as easily as many clinicians are. In a series of 30 knees with osteoarthritis the authors found that all 30 had abnormal scans. In 26 the scans showed focal uptake which clearly localized the affected compartments of the knees (Figure 4). The remaining four patients had generalized increased uptake throughout the knee due to widespread osteoarthritis affecting all three compartments.

Bone scintigraphy has been shown to have a greater sensitivity than radiography[9] in detecting early degenerative changes and Thomas et al.[10] have

also demonstrated its ability to delineate the distribution of the degenerative changes throughout the three compartments of the knee joint.

This ability to localize the compartments affected by osteoarthritis is important in determining surgical treatment. For example, a corrective angular osteotomy or a unicompartmental knee replacement would be the procedure of choice if only one of the tibiofemoral compartments were involved, whereas a total knee replacement would be more appropriate if both of the tibiofemoral compartments were affected. Similarly, the scans can be helpful in identifying patients with pure patellofemoral osteoarthritis who would be suitable for treatment aimed solely at the patellofemoral joint, for example a tibial tubercle advancement osteotomy. Bone scintigraphy is therefore an alternative to arthroscopy in the assessment of patients being considered for major knee surgery. In comparison to arthroscopy it is cheap, readily available and does not use up scarce surgical expertise. It also provides a simple, easily filed permanent record.

Rheumatoid arthritis

Rheumatoid arthritis can be distinguished from osteoarthritis by the differing pattern of scintigraphic uptake. Patients with rheumatoid arthritis have generalized increased uptake in the affected knee (Figure 3) in contrast to the predominantly focal pattern in osteoarthritis.[2] This would be expected because the rheumatoid process is a synovitis affecting the whole joint rather than specific joint compartments.

Anterior knee pain

Anterior knee pain is the commonest condition affecting the knee in adolescents and young adults, and is particularly common in females. The aetiology is diverse and includes chondromalacia patellae, patellofemoral maltracking, patellar tendinitis, the plica syndrome, the post-patellectomy syndrome and reflex sympathetic dystrophy (RSD). However, quite frequently no definitive diagnosis can be made even after arthroscopic examination.

Reflex sympathetic dystrophy

Most reports of the use of bone scintigraphy in anterior knee pain have been concerned with reflex sympathetic dystrophy (RSD). Several studies have shown that the majority of knees with RSD have increased scintigraphic uptake, although the timing of the scan with respect to the onset of symptoms has not always been indicated.[11-13] In a series reported

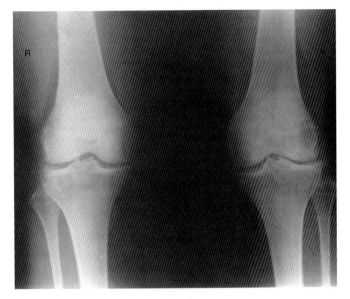

a

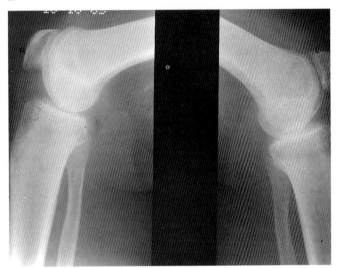

b

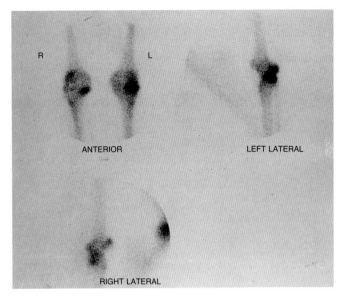

c

Figure 4

This 79-year-old female was seen as a second opinion complaining of severe lateral pain in the left knee, mild medial pain in the right knee and a declining walking distance. The standing anteroposterior radiograph (a) showed an apparently well-preserved joint space and her complaints had been largely dismissed by the surgeon who had seen her initially.

The left knee was in valgus and had a positive agony test. The bone scan shows marked increased uptake in the lateral compartment. On close inspection, the lateral radiograph (b) shows some posterolateral loss of joint space.

Although there are small osteophytes along the margin of the medial compartment of the right knee, the standing radiograph (a) shows an apparently well-preserved joint space and the lateral radiograph (b) shows only minor changes in the patellofemoral joint. However, the bone scan (c) shows a definite increase in uptake in the medial compartment, in keeping with the patient's symptoms.

by Ogilvie-Harris and Roscoe, all 6 knees investigated within 6 months of the onset of symptoms had positive scans, whereas 6 out of 8 knees scanned after 6 months had positive scans.[14] We have found that scans of knees that initially show diffusely increased radionuclide uptake may also subsequently return to normal, although this is not necessarily associated with resolution of symptoms. Hence a normal scan does not preclude the diagnosis of sympathetically mediated pain, particularly if the scan has been done late in the course of the disease.

Scintigraphic uptake is usually of the diffuse pattern in RSD[13,15] and in patients with anterior knee pain diffusely increased uptake can be taken to indicate RSD, provided other diagnoses such as synovitis, as in infection or rheumatoid arthritis, or widespread arthrosis can be excluded. Although focal patellar uptake may also occur in RSD it is not diagnostic of this condition as it is also seen in mechanical conditions of the patella such as chondromalacia, dislocations and fractures.

Dynamic scintigraphy is of limited additional value in the syndrome of sympathetically mediated pain. Although the characteristic scintigraphic appearance in RSD is increased uptake in the involved knee on the immediate, blood pool and the static images,[14] the immediate and blood pool images do not enable any additional patients with RSD to be diagnosed.

The vasomotor disturbance in RSD of the knee is usually less florid than in RSD of the upper limb[12] and we have found that some patients with anterior knee pain syndrome, but without the classical clinical features of RSD, have increased scintigraphic uptake. The knee pain in these patients shows a good response to lumbar sympathetic blockade, indicating that they do have a sympathetic component to their pain. Patients with anterior knee pain who have a normal bone scan do not respond to lumbar sympathetic blockade. Hence bone scintigraphy can be used to identify those patients most likely to benefit from sympathetic blockade, which can be used as a definitive treatment for their pain.

These findings may explain why orthopaedic surgeons have found anterior knee pain syndrome such an unpredictable and unrewarding condition to treat by purely surgical techniques. The majority of patients with anterior knee pain syndrome have mechanical problems which may be amenable to surgical correction. However, if they also have a sympathetically mediated component to their pain, it is unlikely that they will be cured by any operation. Our experience has been that when a sympathetically mediated component to the pain has been identified, this should be treated prior to considering any surgical treatment. In some cases, particularly in those with only minor mechanical problems such as mild chondromalacia patellae, sympathetic blockade has proved successful when used as the only form of treatment. In other cases where there has been a more serious mechanical problem, good results have been obtained when surgery was performed after sympathetic blockade.

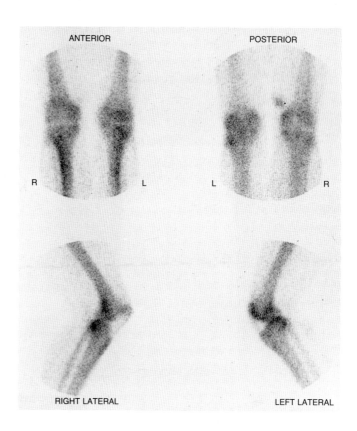

Figure 5

The typical appearance in the post-patellectomy syndrome with increased uptake in the left femoral groove.

Chondromalacia patellae

The relationship between bone scan appearance and chondromalacia patellae reported in the literature is confusing. This may be due to differences in the populations studied, but equally important is the fact that some authors have studied the incidence of chondromalacia in 'hot' bone scans[16] whilst others have studied the incidence of 'hot' bone scans in chondromalacia patellae.[1,17,18] Only in the latter group can the value of scintigraphy in chondromalacia be truly assessed.

There is a wide variation in reports of how many patients with chondromalacia have positive bone scans. Kohn et al. found that in a population of sportsmen and sportswomen diagnosed as having chondromalacia patellae on clinical grounds, 97 out of 100 had positive bone scans.[16] Hejgaard and Diemer studied 64 knees with chondromalacia patellae and found that 39 had positive bone scans.[18] However, Kaufman and Langlotz found that only 2 out of 9 arthroscopically proven cases of chondromalacia patellae had abnormal findings on scintigraphy.[17] In our own series, only 7 out of 18 cases of chondromalacia had positive bone scans.

If the bone scan is abnormal in chondromalacia, it typically shows focal uptake localized to the patella (Figure 2). However, there may be diffuse uptake if there is an associated sympathetic component to the pain. Kohn et al. reported a correlation between the severity of the chondromalacia on arthroscopy and the intensity of the patellar uptake.[16] However, Hejgaard and Diemer showed no correlation between the intensity of abnormal uptake and the severity of the chondromalacia, but found that the proportion of positive scans increased with the severity of the chondromalacia.[18] In contrast, we were not able to demonstrate a correlation between the severity of the chondromalacia patellae and the scan appearance.

In conclusion, the value of scintigraphy in chondromalacia is unclear. The important point is that a normal bone scan does not exclude this condition.

Post-patellectomy knees

We have noted increased uptake in the femoral groove (Figure 5) in patients with anterior knee pain following patellectomy.[15] This is unlikely to have been due to the patellectomy itself, as this had been performed at least 3 years prior to the bone scan in all cases. Although the scintigraphic appearance following patellectomy in an asymptomatic patient (a good post-patellectomy result) is not known, it is likely that this increased uptake was due to increased stress from continued maltracking or subluxation of the patellar tendon, or from chondromalacia of the femoral groove itself. Indeed, chondromalacia of the femoral groove was confirmed in 2 out of 6 patients who were arthroscoped.

Traumatic causes of anterior knee pain

Patients with traumatic soft-tissue injuries around the knee, such as jumper's knee (patellar tendinitis) and quadriceps tendinitis, may have normal scans,[15] although focal uptake in the lower pole of the patella has been reported in three cases of jumper's knee.[19] As elsewhere in the skeleton, bone scintigraphy is especially useful in the detection of stress fractures and unsuspected fractures or dislocations occurring around the knee joint (Figure 1). In the case of the patella, it may not be at all obvious that a stress fracture is the diagnosis. In the past many army recruits presenting with acute onset of severe knee pain with the joint held rigid a few degrees off full extension have, not surprisingly, been wrongly diagnosed as a meniscal tear! These patellae have markedly increased uptake.

The negative scan

In knees in which no organic diagnosis was made despite thorough investigation including arthroscopy, we have found that the scan appearances were normal.[15] Although a normal scan by itself cannot rule out chondromalacia patellae, sympathetic mediated pain or other conditions such as jumper's knee, it would appear that when combined with a normal clinical examination and a normal arthroscopy, the chances of making an organic diagnosis are small. As a corollary, although it is not specific to any one condition, a positive scan is one indication for a repeat arthroscopy where no diagnosis has previously been made, as it may indicate that a mechanical disorder has been missed.

Osteonecrosis

Idiopathic osteonecrosis usually affects the medial femoral condyle or medial tibial plateau and the differential diagnosis includes medial compartment osteoarthritis, medial meniscal pathology and osteoid osteoma. Plain radiography may be normal, particu-

larly early in the course of this condition.[20] In the acute stage all three phases of the dynamic scintigram show focal increased activity, but later only the delayed images remain abnormal. Dynamic scintigraphy is useful in differentiating osteonecrosis from osteoarthritis, which shows increased uptake only on the delayed images and also involves both the femoral and tibial sides of the affected joint compartment.

In steroid-induced osteonecrosis there is initially decreased uptake at the site of the necrosis, progressing to the more usual scan appearance of intense focal uptake occurring during the stage of repair.[21]

In osteochondritis dissecans there is also a focus of increased activity associated with repair on the static scans. The devitalized osteochondral fragment is too small to be identifiable as having decreased uptake. In a study of 11 patients with symptomatic osteochondritis dissecans, McCullough et al. demonstrated a diagnostic rate of only 29% with static bone scans, improving to 57% when dynamic scans were also used.[22] However, in our opinion a radiographic appearance of osteochondritis dissecans in the presence of a normal scan usually means that the radiographic lesion is a coincidental finding and is not the cause of the pain.

Osteonecrosis is a rare but important diagnosis to make because the patient should immediately cease weight bearing. There is also some evidence that early arthroscopic drilling relieves the symptoms and lessens the need for subsequent major surgery. In renal transplant patients with steroid-induced osteonecrosis, the prognosis is much better in the knee than in the hip.

Infection

The role of bone scintigraphy in the diagnosis of septic arthritis of the knee is limited because infection is easily and readily diagnosed by aspiration of the joint. Gilday et al. showed that bone scintigraphy is more sensitive than plain radiography in the detection of septic arthritis.[23] In a series of 9 patients with septic arthritis, 8 had diffusely increased uptake around the joint and blood pool images showed increased blood flow to the affected joint. In clinical practice scintigraphy is of greater value in osteomyelitis, especially in infants, as it will accurately localize the site of infection.

Assessment of the painful arthroplasty

The numerous reports on the evaluation of the painful arthroplasty have mostly referred to the hip, although the findings can be extrapolated to the knee. Following arthroplasty, there is normally decreased uptake overlying the prosthesis and increased activity surrounding it. This increased activity has usually returned to normal around the femoral component by 6–9 months with a cemented prosthesis, but abnormal uptake may remain indefinitely around an uncemented prosthesis.

The two important conditions to be differentiated are loosening of the prosthesis and infection, both of which cause a similar diffuse pattern of uptake on ^{99m}Tc MDP scintigraphy.[24] Gallium-67 citrate and indium-111 leukocyte scanning have been used to try to differentiate these two conditions. From a review of the literature, Mido et al. have concluded that a normal bone or gallium scan makes infection in a prosthetic joint very unlikely.[25] A diffuse pattern on a bone scan, with more abnormality on the gallium scan, is highly suggestive of infection, and a positive white cell scan makes the diagnosis reasonably certain, although uptake in residual bone marrow can be a source of confusion.

Tumours and tumour-like conditions

Plain radiography, CT and MRI, with bone biopsy, are the most useful means of diagnosing primary bone tumours and demonstrating their extent. Although bone scintigraphy may have a characteristic appearance in some tumours, its main role is where the appearances on plain radiography are equivocal or in certain lesions such as osteoid osteoma which can be notoriously difficult to identify on plain radiographs.

About half of all osteoid osteomas occur in the femur or tibia. The sensitivity of bone scanning is greater than that of plain radiography and a normal bone scan virtually excludes the diagnosis of osteoid osteoma. On scintigraphy there is marked uptake of tracer at the site of the tumour on the early and delayed phases of the dynamic scintigram.[3] Bone scintigraphy may also be used in the intraoperative localization of osteoid osteoma.[26]

Metastases generally affect the axial skeleton and the limbs are not usually included in a routine bone scan for metastatic disease. However, if there is pain around the knee this may be included in the examination. Metastases will usually show the typical pattern of focal increased scintigraphic uptake, often before a radiographic abnormality is apparent, although they may occasionally appear as 'cold' areas on high-resolution scans. It is important to remember that multiple myeloma does not normally give increased uptake.

Other conditions affecting the knee

Metabolic conditions such as Paget's disease and the brown tumours of hyperparathyroidism when they occur around the knee result in increased activity. Fibrous dysplasia is also a cause of increased uptake.

The injection of very small traces of radionuclide into the knee joint has been used for arthrography. Synovial tears, bursitis and ruptured Baker's cysts may be evaluated in this way, although its use is limited.

In conclusion we, like other authors, have found bone scintigraphy to be useful in the diagnosis of unusual conditions, but we have also found it very helpful in the assessment of the two common conditions, osteoarthritis and anterior knee pain. This investigation is safe, straightforward, reliable and cost-effective. It merits wider use in everyday clinical practice.

References

1. **Dye SF, Boll DA**, Radionuclide imaging of the patello-femoral joint in young adults with anterior knee pain, *Orthop Clin North Am* (1986) **17:** 249–262.
2. **Bauer GCH**, The use of radionuclides in orthopaedics. Part IV. Radionuclide scintimetry of the skeleton, *J Bone Joint Surg (Am)* (1968) **50:** 1681–1709.
3. **Smith FW, Gilday DL**, Scintigraphic appearances of osteoid osteoma, *Radiology* (1980) **137:** 191–195.
4. **Harding LK**, The cost of x-rays and nuclear medicine investigations, *Br J Radiol* (1985) **58:** 101–102.
5. **Holder LE**, Current concepts review: Radionuclide bone-imaging in the evaluation of bone pain, *J Bone Joint Surg (Am)* (1982) **64:** 1391–1396.
6. **Heatley FW, Butler-Manuel A**, Osteoarthritis of the knee: (i) Assessment, *Curr Orthop* (1990) **4:** 79–87.
7. **White SH, Ludkowski P, Goodfellow JW**, Observations on the pathological anatomy of primary osteoarthritis of the knee, *J Bone Joint Surg (Br)* (1989) **71:** 885.
8. **Maquet PGJ**, Biomechanics of the knee: with application to the pathogenesis and the surgical treatment of osteoarthritis (Berlin: Springer-Verlag, 1976).
9. **Egund N, Frost S, Brismar J et al.**, Radiography and scintigraphy in the assessment of early gonarthrosis, *Acta Radiol (Diagn)* (1988) **29:** 451–455.
10. **Thomas RH, Resnick D, Alazraki NP et al.**, Compartmental evaluation of osteoarthritis of the knee, *Radiology* (1975) **116:** 585–594.
11. **Tietjen R**, Reflex sympathetic dystrophy of the knee, *Clin Orthop* (1986) **209:** 234–243.
12. **Coughlan RJ, Hazleman BL, Page Thomas DP et al.**, Algodystrophy: a common unrecognised cause of chronic knee pain, *Br J Rheumatol* (1987) **26:** 270–274.
13. **Katz MM, Hungerford DS**, Reflex sympathetic dystrophy affecting the knee, *J Bone Joint Surg (Br)* (1987) **69:** 797–803.
14. **Ogilvie-Harris DJ, Roscoe M**, Reflex sympathetic dystrophy of the knee, *J Bone Joint Surg (Br)* (1987) **69:** 804–806.
15. **Butler-Manuel PA, Guy RL, Heatley FW et al.**, Scintigraphy in the assessment of anterior knee pain, *Acta Orthop Scand* (1990) **61:** 438–442.
16. **Kohn HS, Guten GN, Collier BD et al.**, Chondromalacia of the patella: Bone imaging correlated with arthroscopic findings, *Clin Nucl Med* (1988) **13:** 96–98.
17. **Kaufman J, Langlotz M**, Is it possible to diagnose idiopathic chondromalacia patellae using radiologic methods? *ROFO* (1984) **141:** 422–426.
18. **Hejgaard N, Diemer H**, Bone scan in the patellofemoral pain syndrome, *Int Orthop* (1987) **11:** 29–33.
19. **Kahn D, Wilson MA**, Bone scintigraphic findings in patellar tendinitis, *J Nucl Med* (1987) **28:** 1768–1770.

20. **Lotke PA, Ecker ML,** Osteonecrosis of the knee: Symposium on idiopathic osteonecrosis, *Orthop Clin North Am* (1985) **16:** 797–808.

21. **Burt RW, Matthews TJ,** Aseptic necrosis of the knee: Bone scintigraphy, *Am J Roentgenol* (1982) **138:** 571–573.

22. **McCullough RW, Gandsman EJ, Litchman HE et al.,** Dynamic bone scintigraphy in osteochondritis dissecans, *Int Orthop* (1988) **12:** 317–322.

23. **Gilday DL, Paul DJ, Paterson J,** Diagnosis of osteomyelitis in children by combined blood pool and bone imaging, *Radiology* (1975) **117:** 331–335.

24. **Williamson BRJ, McLaughlin RE, Wang GJ et al.,** Radionuclide bone imaging as a means of differentiating loosening and infection in patients with a painful total hip prosthesis, *Radiology* (1979) **133:** 723–726

25. **Mido K, Navarro DA, Segall GM et al.,** The role of bone scanning, gallium and indium imaging in infection. *Bone scanning in clinical practice,* ed Fogelman I (New York: Springer-Verlag, 1987), 9: 105–120.

26. **O'Brien TM, Murray TE, Malone LA et al.,** Osteoid osteoma: excision with scintimetric guidance, *Radiology* (1984) **153:** 543–544.

2

Arthroscopy and meniscal surgery

2.1 Basic arthroscopy

W. Dilworth Cannon, Jr and Joyce M. Vittori

Masaki Watanabe in 1957 developed the Number 21 arthroscope in Japan. Visualization was accomplished by a light bulb placed at the end of the arthroscope. Also in 1957, Watanabe, Takeda, and Ikeuchi published an *Atlas of Arthroscopy* based on their early observations of knee arthroscopy.[1] In 1962, Watanabe performed the first partial meniscectomy. In 1964, Robert W. Jackson spent a year in Tokyo, and brought back this technique to North America.[2] In 1969, Ikeuchi performed the first arthroscopic meniscal repair[3] and the first excision of a discoid lateral meniscus. Thereafter, arthroscopy spread rapidly around the world and is now the commonest operation performed in the United States and Canada. Few techniques are left for open surgery. Caspari has even developed a technique for arthroscopic unicompartmental hemiarthroplasty.[4]

Critics of the technique previously said that arthroscopy was 'akin to looking into a room through the keyhole rather than opening the door.' Now there is little question that arthroscopy allows 90–95% of the knee joint to be inspected. Magnification up to tenfold or more allows for precise surgery to be performed. Partial meniscectomy is more accurately performed than through open surgical techniques. Morbidity is markedly lower because arthroscopy is a minimally invasive procedure. Patients rarely need to be admitted to the hospital as most arthroscopic procedures take place in an ambulatory surgery center on a come-and-go basis. Patients are able to return to desk-type work within days, and often may begin to run after 14 days. Athletes commonly return to sports after 3–4 weeks. There is an economic advantage not only with reduced hospitalization costs, but also in the reduced sick leave during recovery. Arthroscopically assisted anterior cruciate ligament (ACL) reconstruction is being done in some centers as outpatient surgery. Complications are far fewer than with open techniques. Infection is extremely rare. Knee arthroscopic techniques will continue to improve in the 1990s, and many of these techniques will spill over into arthroscopy of other joints.

Basic set-up

Place the patient supine on the operating table with the knee joint beyond the last break of the table. Although the senior author (W.D.C.) prefers to keep both legs supine on the table, other surgeons prefer to break the end of the table. To access the posteromedial corner of the knee, the knee must extend an ample distance beyond the break in the table. Although it is not routinely used, a tourniquet is placed on the high thigh. With the extremity in a thigh holder and abducted, there is ample room to stand between the table and the leg and exert valgus

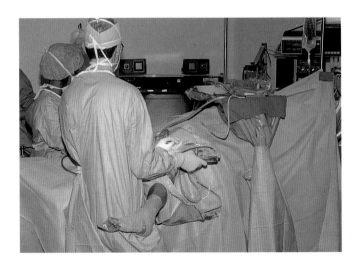

Figure 1

With the table completely flat, and the leg abducted in the leg holder, there is ample room for the surgeon to stand between the table and the leg to exert a valgus force for medial compartment surgery.

stress for medial compartment surgery (Figure 1). If ACL reconstructive surgery, meniscal repair or both are to be done, flex the thigh 45°. A well-padded leg holder is placed distal to the tourniquet. If the leg holder is placed too proximal, there will be excessive leverage on the thigh, and a transient sciatic nerve palsy may result. In the 45° position, excellent access to the posterior corners of the knee can be accomplished. Paint the entire leg with 1% or 2% tincture of iodine. Take care not to let any iodine run down under the tourniquet or leg holder.

Almost all surgeons today use a small television camera coupled to the arthroscope. Both the arthroscope and the camera can be soaked in Cidex but early wear and tear changes may occur. To avoid this, the TV camera can be sterilely bagged (Figure 2). It is preferable to sterilize arthroscopes in ethylene oxide.

As a general principle, the TV monitor should be placed directly in front of the arthroscope. Hand–eye coordination deteriorates if the surgeon must look over his shoulder to the monitor, or if the arthroscope is introduced through a proximal portal and is pointing away from the monitor. Coordination is also improved if the TV image is oriented to the true position of the knee, and not necessarily oriented to the horizontal. To avoid having to turn to obtain an instrument, it is recommended that the Mayo stand be placed over the patient's abdomen. In this way, the surgeon also can keep his eyes on the monitor.

Surgeons should document their cases. At a minimum, documentation should cover the pathology and a final look at the joint at the end of the procedure. This can be done using a video printer, but it does not give as true an accounting as videotape or a 35-mm camera. For good color resolution and color balance ¾ inch video works best. Super VHS and Hi-8 formats also are vying for attention. Video also provides documentation for teaching and the surgeon can review it before performing 'second-look' surgery.

An arthroscopic pump with both pressure and flow regulation is recommended for routine use. The pump is especially important when performing surgery in a tight lateral compartment with the knee flexed 70–90°, or in a knee with florid synovitis, where fluid circulation through the joint can be markedly impaired. The primary advantage of a pump is its ability to clear blood from the joint compartment quickly by increasing the pressure and flow rate. It also offers an advantage in its ability to flush debris at the end of a case with a high flow rate. To facilitate this, a second cannula is inserted into another portal for the effluent. It is important that the pump has the safety feature of a shut-off valve to protect against overpressurization of the joint.

To avoid excessive fluid collection on the floor, a mat with suction can be placed on the floor. An alternative would be to use a collection pouch placed about the knee.

Portal placement

The conventional portal is anterolateral. This portal should be one thumb-breadth above the joint-line, measured with the knee flexed, and adjacent to the lateral border of the patellar tendon (Figure 3). Either a transverse or vertical incision is acceptable. However, a transverse incision heals better. I prefer to make the incision approximately ⁵⁄₁₆ to ⅜ inch long to allow less tethering on the arthroscopy. This also allows some fluid to exit adjacent to the arthroscope if there is excessive pressure in the joint. Fluid collection in the subcutaneous tissue with subsequent imploding of the synovium into the joint can be minimized.

Place the anteromedial portal one thumb-breadth above the medial joint-line, adjacent to the medial border of the patellar tendon (Figure 3). This portal,

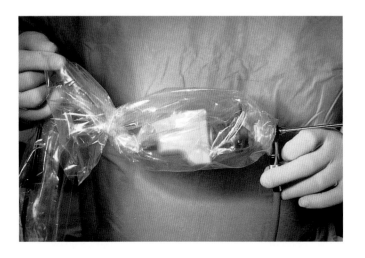

Figure 2

If Cidex soaking is not done, the arthroscope–TV camera connection can be sterilely draped as shown. This draping technique not only provides greater sterility, but also eliminates fogging of the camera, and will result in prolonged camera life.

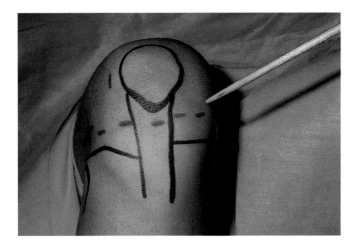

Figure 3

The standard arthroscopic portals are marked on this right knee. The anterolateral portal is one thumb-breadth above the joint-line immediately adjacent to the patellar tendon. The anteromedial portal is comparably placed on the medial side of the patellar tendon. The central portal is placed 1 cm below the inferior pole of the patella and midway between the medial and lateral femoral condyles. The mid-patellar lateral portal provides excellent visualization of the anterior aspect of the joint. The accessory anterolateral and anteromedial portals are also shown. The pointer is indicating the accessory anteromedial portal.

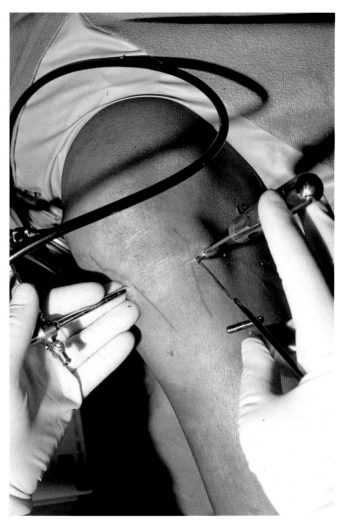

Figure 4

By introducing two instruments through one portal, a third anterior portal can be avoided. This technique is especially useful for pulling the lateral meniscus anteriorly and making surgery on the lateral meniscus easier.

when viewed from in front of the knee, should be slightly more proximal than the anterolateral portal. It is the commonest portal for probing and instrument introduction. It is also an alternative arthroscopic portal.

The central portal, which the senior author rarely uses, is transpatellar tendon, approximately 1 cm below the inferior pole of the patella, and midway between the medial and lateral femoral condyles (not the midpoint of the patellar tendon) (Figure 3). This portal was popularized by Oretorp and Gillquist.[5] The arthroscope should be introduced in a slightly upward direction to avoid skewering the fat pad and dragging it around for the rest of the case. It is a good portal for viewing through the intercondylar notch posteromedially and posterolaterally. For meniscal surgery one can use grasping and cutting instruments through the other two inferior portals. However, if necessary one can use three instruments through the standard two inferior portals without making a central portal (Figure 4). A disadvantage of the central portal is the injury that it causes to the patellar tendon. It might weaken the patellar tendon if it were to be used later for an ACL reconstruction.

The mid-patellar lateral portal was popularized by Patel[6] (Figure 3). He used it as his primary portal,

giving him excellent visualization of the anterior aspect of the knee joint, and allowing him also to introduce the arthroscope into the popliteus hiatus. Although the author does not use this portal, it is a reasonable alternative.

Superolateral and superomedial portals. Use of the superolateral portal for placement of the pressure-sensing cannula for the pump is more easily accomplished than the superomedial portal. Go 1–2 cm above the superior pole of the patella, and place it well laterally to get under the patella and not damage the quadriceps tendon. If the superomedial portal is used, the vastus medialis obliquus has to be penetrated and the suprapatellar plica may interfere. Arthroscopic introduction through either one of these superior portals allows excellent assessment of

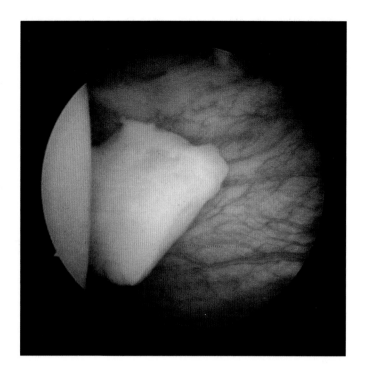

Figure 5

This osteochondritis dissecans fragment was lying in the posteromedial portion of the joint and was only detected by passing the arthroscope from the anterolateral portal through the intercondylar notch medial to the posterior cruciate ligament.

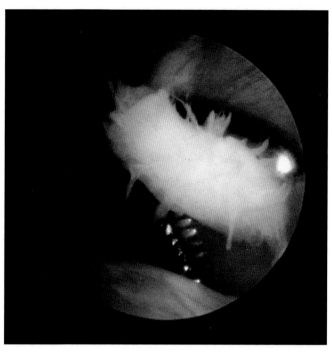

Figure 6

A small grasping clamp has been introduced through the posteromedial compartment and the loose body secured.

the congruency of the patellofemoral joint during extension to flexion motion.

The primary use of posteromedial and posterolateral portals is for instrument introduction to remove loose bodies or meniscal fragments (Figures 5 and 6). The effective use of the portals requires planning. The patient's knee should extend well beyond the footbreak of the table, and the leg should be abducted to access the posterior portals with instruments. Establish this portal by visualizing the posteromedial corner of the knee with the arthroscope medial to the posterior cruciate ligament through the intercondylar notch from the anterolateral portal. Digital palpation of the posteromedial corner should identify on the TV screen the best location for this portal. A spinal needle will confirm the selection, and then a sharp and blunt trochar can produce the opening. Following this, whatever instrument may be indicated can be passed into the posteromedial compartment through this portal. If visualization of the posteromedial compartment with the 30° arthroscope from the anterolateral portal is inadequate, then a 70° arthroscope should be inserted. In some instances, one can introduce the arthroscope through the posteromedial compartment for direct visualization of this part of the knee (Figures 7 and 8). An adjacent

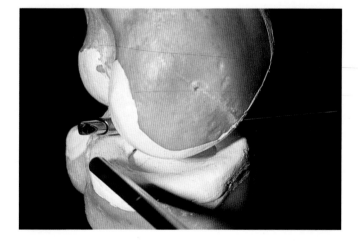

Figure 7

This knee model shows two methods for visualizing the posteromedial compartment. The 30° arthroscope in the foreground may be introduced posterior to the medial collateral ligament for direct visualization of this part of the joint. A 70° arthroscope is shown passing through the intercondylar notch medial to the posterior cruciate ligament from an anterolateral portal.

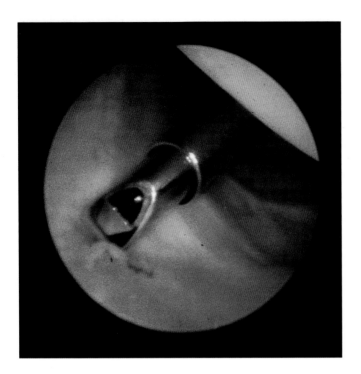

Figure 8

The intra-articular view of the posteromedial compartment from a 30° arthroscope introduced posteromedially. A 70° arthroscope is shown lying medial to the posterior cruciate ligament and was introduced through an anterolateral portal.

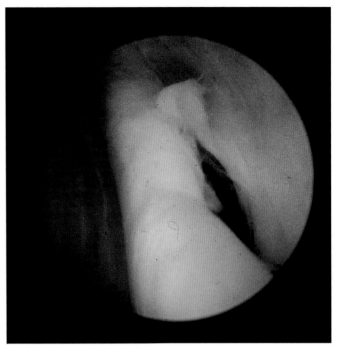

Figure 9

The orifice of a popliteal cyst is seen on the posteromedial capsular wall of this right knee. The arthroscope was easily directed through this orifice to look for loose bodies within the cyst.

second portal can be used for instruments. On several occasions, the senior author has passed the arthroscope through the posteromedial portal and into the orifice of a popliteal cyst (Figure 9). Through a second instrument portal, loose bodies have been removed from the cyst.

The sweep of the knee

After inserting the pressure-sensing and outflow cannula for the pump through the superolateral portal, introduce the arthroscope through the anterolateral portal with the knee in a 90° flexed position. The sharp trochar should be used to bring the sheath to but not through the synovium. Use a blunt obturator to penetrate the synovium and, with the knee in extension, deliver the arthroscope into the suprapatellar pouch. After establishing orientation and focus on the TV camera, move the arthroscope into the lateral recess and sweep the lateral gutter down to the popliteus hiatus. Visualization in the hiatus permits one to visualize the superior and inferior fasciculi of the lateral meniscus. With the knee still in extension, view the meniscosynovial junction of the middle third of the lateral meniscus up to the

anterolateral corner of the knee. With the knee flexed approximately 25° and a varus force applied, the arthroscope can literally be 'walked' along the anterior horn of the lateral meniscus, and the ACL can be seen in the intercondylar notch. One can obtain better visualization of the anterior horn by using this method than when the arthroscope is looking laterally from the anterolateral portal with the knee in the 'figure of 4' position. In this 'peripheral lateral view,' focal degenerative changes of the lateral femoral condyle can be better appreciated.

Pass the arthroscope over to the medial recess, and continue the sweep proximally into the suprapatellar pouch. A normal suprapatellar plica should be present in approximately 80–89% of people.[7,8] Occasionally, it can cross the suprapatellar pouch to the lateral sidewall. Rarely, it may compartmentalize the suprapatellar pouch. It is an uncommon cause of symptomatology.

With the knee in extension, and the arthroscope positioned between the patella and the medial femoral condyle, look for a medial parapatellar plica (Figure 10). Approximately 50% of normal people have one,[9] and Patel[7] stated that 19% have a large one. Occasionally, it can overlap the medial femoral condyle and appear to impinge underneath the medial facet of the patella. Look for a groove on the

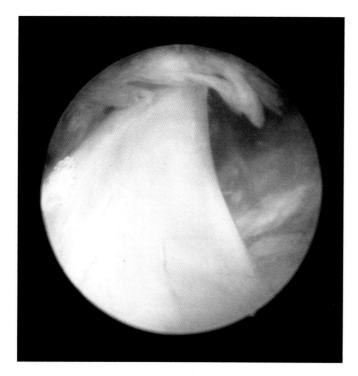

Figure 10

A large fibrotic medial parapatellar plica in a left knee. Large plicas like this one are found in only approximately 19% of people.

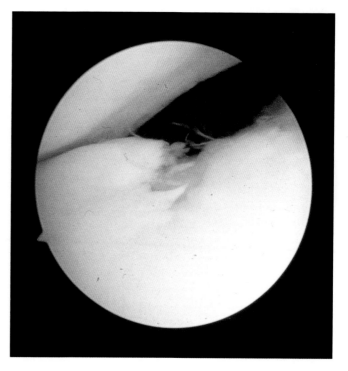

Figure 11

At 30° of flexion, this right patella has not yet seated in the trochlear groove. The medial facet should articulate by 45–55° of flexion. Moderately severe fissuring is shown in the trochlear groove of this patient.

medial femoral condyle underneath the plica where it articulates during flexion. The adjacent articular cartilage may be degenerative, and this can be an indication that the plica is symptomatic and may have to be excised. Excision is best accomplished by passing a basket rongeur across the joint from a superolateral portal.

Inspect the patellofemoral joint by directing the orientation of the arthroscope upward. Place a hand on the patella and move it medially while inspecting the lateral facet, and laterally while inspecting the medial facet. This facilitates 100% visualization of the articular surface of the patella. Now look down onto the trochlear surface, and sweep from lateral to medial, inspecting the integrity of the articular cartilage. Positioning the arthroscope just distal to the midpoint of the trochlear groove, begin to flex the knee. Articulation between the medial side of the groove and the medial facet of the patella normally should occur between 45° and 55° of flexion (Figure 11). Beyond 55°, lateral subluxation exists.

Move the arthroscope over to the medial femoral condyle and sweep down into the medial compartment, looking in a posterior direction. Enter the medial compartment with the orientation of the arthroscopic line of sight tangential to the tibial plateau. The knee should be flexed only approxi-

mately 15–20°, and a valgus load applied by the surgeon will further open the medial compartment. The surgeon has better control of this visualization in a standing position than in a sitting position. Starting at the posterior horn origin of the medial meniscus, move around to the anterior horn. To appreciate better the anterior horn, orient the arthroscope so that its line of sight is looking downward. An appreciation of the integrity of the articular cartilage of the medial femoral condyle, and the medial tibial plateau, is accomplished by gradually flexing the knee through an arc of 70°.

Move the arthroscope to the medial edge of the intercondylar notch. Trace the junction of the notch and articular cartilage upward in an inverted 'U' over the ligamentum mucosum, which attaches at the top of the intercondylar notch. Continue down on the lateral side of the notch. At this point, the arthroscope can be moved into the notch to inspect the ACL.

Next, in the 'figure of 4' position, inspect the lateral compartment. In contrast to the 'peripheral lateral view' vantage point, position the arthroscope close to the intercondylar notch with a 30° view directed posterolaterally and tangential to the plateau. At this point, a probe is introduced through the anteromedial portal and directed to the posterior horn of the lateral meniscus. Starting at the posterior horn origin, probe the entire meniscus both superiorly and inferiorly. By hooking the probe onto the inner edge of the anterior horn and pulling it anteriorly, circumferential hoop stresses can be generated to display any radial split tears of the middle third of the lateral meniscus that may have previously been hidden.

To probe the ACL, beginners might place the probe on the posterior horn of the lateral meniscus in the 'figure of 4' position. Flex the knee to 90°, and the probe will fall right onto the anterior cruciate making probing of the ligament easy.

Remove the probe from the joint and place the knee again in approximately 15–20° of flexion and apply a valgus load. Introduce the probe into the medial compartment through a new synovial puncture to prevent tethering. Occasionally, the posterior horn may be difficult to visualize. Further extension of the knee may help, and the surgeon may increase the valgus stress to the knee. It is better for the surgeon to do this rather than an assistant. The surgeon has better control of the total forces applied to prevent a medial collateral ligament tear.

After probing the medial meniscus, place the probe underneath the posterior horn origin. Pass the arthroscope through the intercondylar notch to the posteromedial compartment, medial to the posterior cruciate ligament. If this cannot be accomplished under direct vision with a valgus force applied to the knee in 60° of flexion, then a blunt obturator should be placed in the sheath to direct it through the notch. Only in approximately one in ten knees is this maneuver unsuccessful, usually owing to a stenotic notch in an arthritic knee. Figure 12 shows the angle of view with a 30° arthroscope introduced anterolaterally versus centrally. Notice that the field of view is good enough through the anterolateral portal that the use of a 70° arthroscope usually is not necessary. Digital palpation at the posteromedial corner of the

knee while viewing posteromedially can dislodge any loose bodies that would otherwise not be apparent. The probe, previously tucked under the posterior horn origin, can easily be brought out and over the top of the meniscus to palpate the posterior horn (Figures 13 and 14).

To complete the sweep, introduce the arthroscopic sheath through the anteromedial portal in the 'figure of 4' position. Direct it to the posterolateral compartment lateral to the posterior cruciate ligament. This entry is usually easier than the entry into the posteromedial compartment. The probe can be introduced anterolaterally and the posterior horn of the lateral meniscus further palpated.

Loose bodies

Removal of loose bodies is one of the easiest arthroscopic procedures to perform (Figure 15). It also can be frustrating if a loose body cannot be found in a patient with characteristic symptoms. Never promise a patient that a loose body will definitely be found and removed. There are some nooks and crannies in the knee joint that are difficult to visualize. The senior author has had at least two cases where loose bodies have been residing anterior to the anterolateral tibial plateau underneath the anterior horn of the lateral meniscus. It is mandatory that if a loose body is not seen after an initial sweep, that both posteromedial and posterolateral compartments be inspected. This is a favorite place for loose bodies to come to rest, and it usually requires a posteromedial or posterolateral portal to remove them. Make sure that the incision is almost as big as the loose body, otherwise further frustration will ensue when they slip away during the attempt to remove them.

If a loose body is found near the intercondylar notch, instead of making a larger anteromedial or

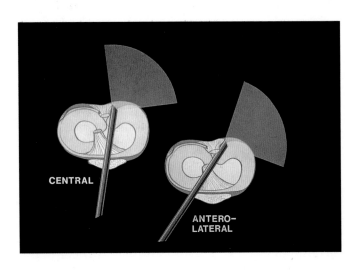

Figure 12

The angle of view with a 30° arthroscope as introduced anterolaterally is contrasted with a centrally placed arthroscope. Notice that the field of view through the anterolateral portal is good enough to make the routine use of a 70° arthroscope unnecessary. (Drawing courtesy of Jeanne Koelling.)

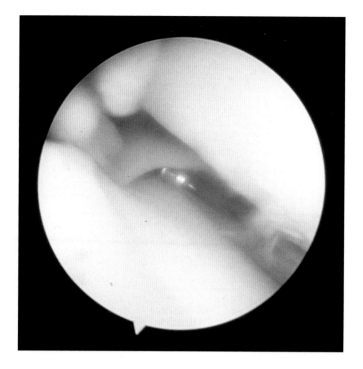

Figure 13

The view of the posterior horn of the medial meniscus in this right knee is seen from the anterior aspect of the intercondylar notch. Note the improved visualization in Figure 14.

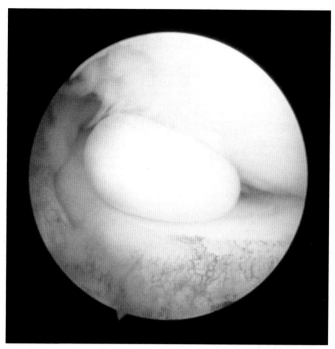

Figure 15

A symptomatic loose body rests on the anterior horn of the medial meniscus in this right knee.

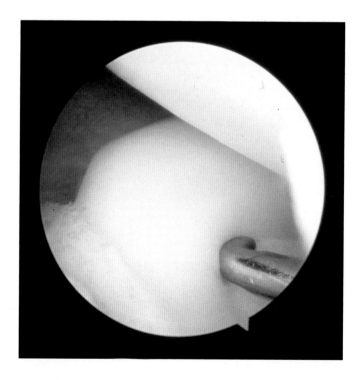

Figure 14

In the same case shown in Figure 13, the arthroscope has been advanced from an anterolateral portal through the intercondylar notch for direct visualization and probing of the posterior horn of the medial meniscus in this right knee.

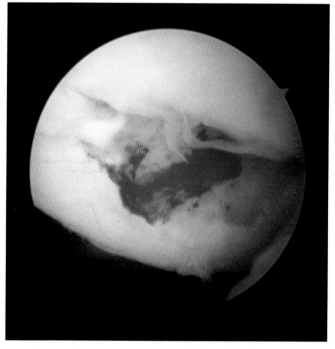

Figure 16

A fresh crater in a patient with osteochondritis dissecans involving the lateral femoral condyle is shown. The loose fragment was found in the posteromedial compartment (see Figure 5).

anterolateral portal it is sometimes easier to direct the loose body into the suprapatellar pouch with the knee in extension and remove it through a superolateral incision.

The senior author has seen a loose body encapsulated in a pseudopod of the fat pad that caused intermittent locking as it flopped in and out of the medial compartment. The loose body was released and removed from the joint after incision of the fat pad.

The source of a loose body should be looked for. Many of them come from an osteochondritis dissecans lesion (Figure 16). This subject is covered in another contribution (9.2).

Meniscal problems

Meniscal tears can be classified into flap tears, vertical longitudinal tears including displaced bucket-handle tears, broken bucket-handle tears, double and triple vertical longitudinal bucket-handle-type tears, horizontal cleavage tears, radial split tears, and complex degenerative tears.

Flap tear

The flap tear is the commonest meniscal tear encountered. It is especially common in patients in their fourth decade and older. It usually involves the inner edge of the avascular portion of the meniscus and is irreparable. It consists of a complex oblique tear, usually involving the inferior surface of the posteromedial corner of the medial meniscus, and is typically anteriorly based. It behooves the surgeon to inspect the posterior horn origin to make sure there is not an additional flap tear in this location, which might be overlooked if inspection is carried out only from the anterior aspect of the joint. The steps in the removal of a flap tear at the posterior horn origin consist of inspection of the tear with the arthroscope through the anterolateral portal through the notch, and positioned next to the PCL, and probing the tear with a nerve hook introduced anteromedially (Figure 17). A 1-mm basket rongeur can be introduced and the tear, if lying in a vertical direction, can be transsected through 90% of its base (Figure 18). Avulse the remainder with a grasping clamp. If the flap is in a horizontal plane, then it can be morsalized.

The flap tear (Figure 19) at the posteromedial corner of the meniscus is best approached by initially switching portals. With the arthroscope anteromedially, and looking down on the tear site, a 1-mm basket rongeur can be brought in through the anterolateral portal. By starting the cut in the mid to anterior region of the meniscus, it can be blended into the remaining central portion of the meniscus

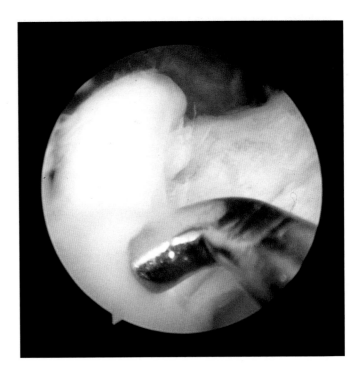

Figure 17

Unless specifically looked for, a posterior horn flap from the origin of the medial meniscus may be missed unless the arthroscope is passed through the intercondylar notch as shown in Figure 14 (From ref. 13.)

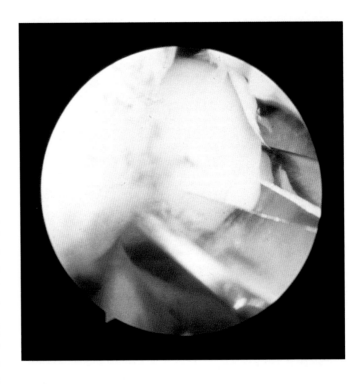

Figure 18

The flap tear shown in Figure 17 is cut across its base until only 10% of its attachment remains. It may then be easily avulsed. (From ref. 13.)

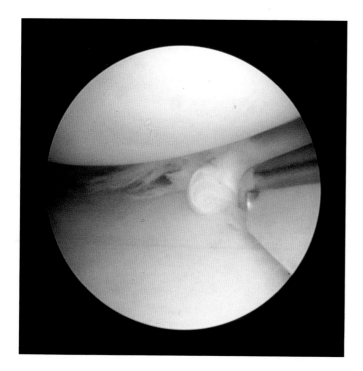

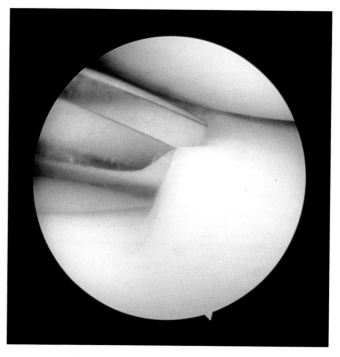

Figure 19

This flap tear of the medial meniscus in this right knee is being probed. It is the commonest meniscal tear encountered. (From ref. 13.)

Figure 20

The initial step in resection of the flap tear shown in Figure 19 is accomplished by switching the arthroscope to the anteromedial portal and bringing a small basket rongeur in from the anterolateral portal. This technique provides an excellent means of starting the cut in the mid-central portion of the medial meniscus, leaving a balanced and contoured rim behind. (From ref. 13.)

without creating an unstable step cut in the meniscus (Figure 20). Aim the cut to the base of the flap, having ascertained the depth of the cut previously during probing. The flap of meniscal tissue can either be released completely from this approach, or with the rongeur back in the anteromedial portal the cut can be further directed posteriorly around the unstable meniscal fragment. A grasper can be used to avulse the fragment and remove it through the anterolateral portal. If some irregularity of the inner edge of the meniscus remains, it can be trimmed with a rongeur or shaver (Figures 21 and 22). If the remaining inner rim of the meniscus has a vertical orientation, it may be beveled on the superior surface to create a triangular appearance. If the remaining superior leaf of the posterior horn of the meniscus is irregular and needs to be partially resected, an up-angled rongeur may be able to access it. If the medial compartment is tight, completing this resection may be difficult. Digital palpation from the popliteal fossa can occasionally translate the meniscus further anteriorly into the joint. Alternatively, introduction of a 18-gauge spinal needle followed by a nerve hook through an accessory anteromedial portal approximately 2 cm medial to the usual anteromedial portal

may be necessary to pull the meniscal fragment anteriorly into the joint to complete the meniscal resection (Figure 23). Flap tears of the lateral meniscus (Figure 24) can be resected by introducing the appropriate rongeur from the anteromedial portal (Figure 25). It is more difficult to obtain the proper angle of resection for anterior flaps. Typically, the tear extends to the posterolateral corner of the meniscus and further trimming may be necessary (Figures 26 and 27). A right-angle basket rongeur is frequently useful for contouring the anterior horn of the lateral meniscus.

There are alternative methods for accomplishing flap resection. Some surgeons prefer to use a motorized shaver. However, hand-held instruments are usually faster. Electrocautery has been advocated by some, but may risk damage to underlying articular cartilage. O'Brien[10] has shown retardation of meniscal healing after electrocautery in the animal model.

There is an increasing interest among orthopedic surgeons in laser surgery. It is still in its developmental phase and is too expensive for most surgeons to place in their operating room. Advocates of laser surgery argue that difficult-to-reach posterior horn pathology can be handled easily with the laser probe.

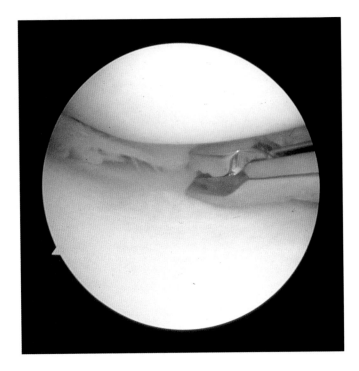

Figure 21

In the same case as shown in Figures 19 and 20, the irregularly torn posterior horn is further resected back using a broad rongeur. (From ref. 13.)

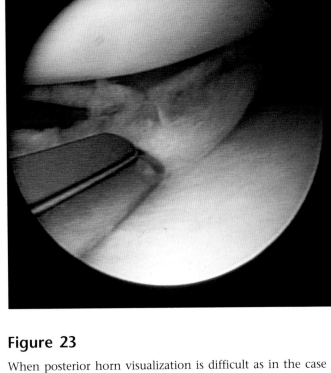

Figure 23

When posterior horn visualization is difficult as in the case of this torn left medial meniscus, a nerve hook can be introduced through an accessory medial portal in order to pull the posterior horn fragment anteriorly for better visualization. Note the nerve hook in the photograph located to the left just above the rongeur. (From ref. 13.)

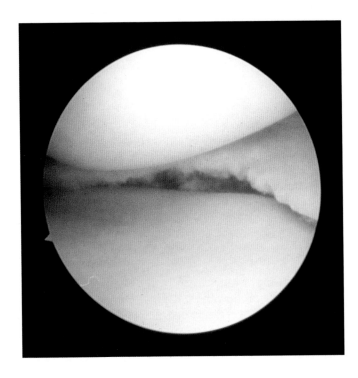

Figure 22

The final appearance of the medial meniscus after partial meniscectomy in the case shown in the preceding three figures. (From ref. 13.)

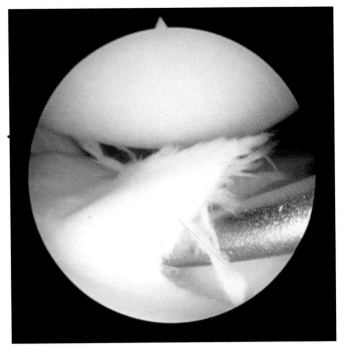

Figure 24

A complex flap tear in the central portion of the lateral meniscus in this right knee is shown.

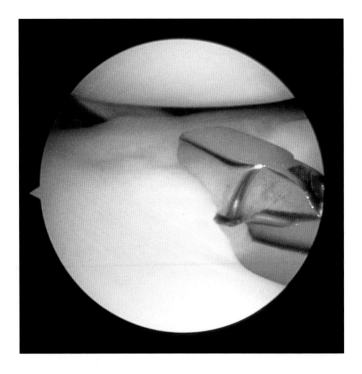

Figure 25

Resection of the tear begins by bringing a small straight basket rongeur, as shown in this case, or a right-angle rotatory rongeur in from the anteromedial portal to resect the anterior portion of the flap tear.

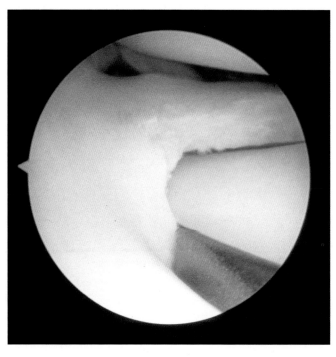

Figure 27

The final appearance of the lateral meniscus after partial meniscectomy in the case shown in Figures 24–26.

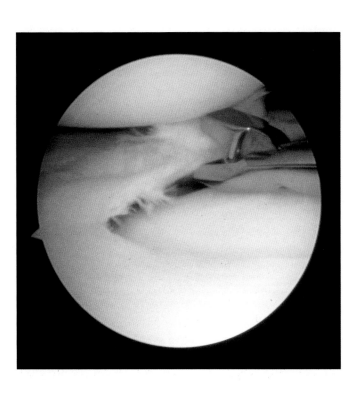

Figure 26

After the anterior flap has been resected (see Figures 24 and 25), further torn meniscal tissue is resected from the lateral meniscus immediately in front of the popliteus hiatus.

However, it is rare that resection of the posterior horn of the medial meniscus cannot be accomplished by conventional techniques as described above. Further investigations will be necessary before a general recommendation of laser surgery can be made.

Displaced bucket-handle tears

The diagnosis of a displaced bucket-handle tear of the medial meniscus can be made preoperatively in most instances. This will allow the alternatives of treatment, including the possibility of meniscal repair, to be discussed with the patient. In patients under age 50 years, serious consideration should be given to meniscal repair unless the anatomic aspects of the tear would dictate excision. Therefore, excision might include: (1) a significant radial split tear in the substance of the displaced bucket-handle fragment; (2) a rim size of 5 mm or greater, which would place the tear well within the avascular zone of the meniscus; or (3) a grossly deformed chronic tear twisted on itself, where the meniscus cannot be pushed back to its normal position.

Excision of a bucket-handle fragment of a medial meniscus (Figure 28) can be divided into a series of steps. The displaced bucket-handle fragment should be pushed back to its normal orthotopic position

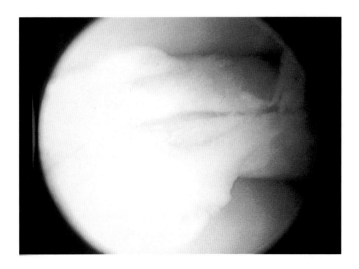

Figure 28

Anterior visualization of a displaced bucket-handle tear of the medial meniscus in the right knee (From ref. 13.)

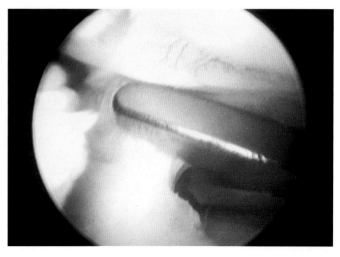

Figure 30

Resection of the bucket-handle tear should start at the posterior horn origin after reduction of the fragment. The arthroscope is situated adjacent to the posterior cruciate ligament and provides excellent visualization of the posterior horn origin. Resection of the posterior horn attachment is accomplished with a small rongeur introduced through the anteromedial portal. (From ref. 13.)

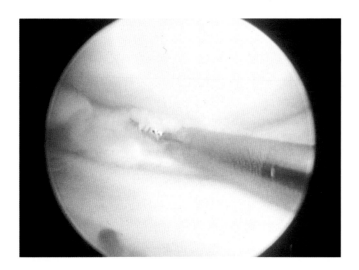

Figure 29

Reduction of the displaced bucket-handle tear is accomplished with a nerve hook, and with the knee in approximately 10–15° of flexion. (From ref. 13.)

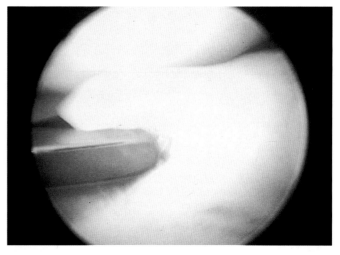

Figure 31

After the posterior horn attachment of the fragment has been resected, the anterior horn attachment is cut with a rongeur introduced through the anterolateral portal. (From ref. 13.)

using a nerve hook through the anteromedial portal (Figure 29). Rarely is this difficult to accomplish if the knee is extended to 15° or less of flexion. Difficulty in accomplishing reduction is usually the result of too much knee flexion. Pass the arthroscope through the intercondylar notch to the posteromedial compartment to visualize the origin of the posterior horn of

the medial meniscus. Probing should determine the exact origin of the vertical longitudinal tear. Introduce a 1-mm basket rongeur. Make an incision from the posterior horn origin to line up and coincide with the origin of the tear (Figure 30). Once the fragment is free posteriorly, switch the arthroscope to the antero-medial portal and palpate the anterior origin of the

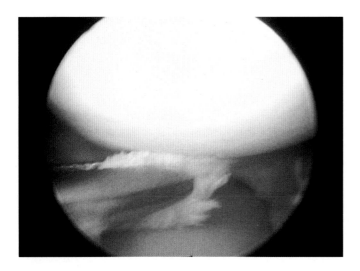

Figure 32

The bucket-handle fragment is now free in the joint, and a rongeur is shown grasping its cut anterior end. (From ref. 13.)

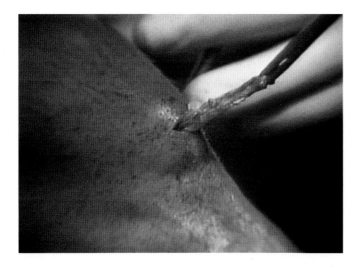

Figure 33

The bucket-handle fragment shown in Figure 32 is being removed through the anterolateral portal. (From ref. 13.)

handle fragment. Bring a 1-mm straight basket rongeur, or a 15° up-biter across from the anterolateral portal. A cut is made at the anterior horn and aimed at the origin of the tear (Figure 31). The fragment should now be completely mobile, and can be removed through the anterolateral portal by grasping the end of the fragment (Figures 32 and 33).

Usually a nubbin of meniscal tissue is left at the anterior horn origin of the tear and this can be trimmed back with the use of a straight basket rongeur or a right-angle basket rongeur.

In the less common displaced bucket-handle tear of the lateral meniscus, the same approach may be used. Start by reducing the displaced fragment. Usually the posterior horn resection is more easily accomplished while viewing from the anterior aspect of the joint. The anterior horn attachment is more difficult owing to the smaller radius of curvature of the lateral meniscus. Use a right-angle biting rongeur to release the anterior horn attachment. One may use an accessory anterolateral portal a centimeter or two lateral to the conventional anterolateral portal. This may allow a better angle of attack on the anterior horn attachment.

Single vertical longitudinal tears

Most vertical longitudinal tears, unless macerated or with a large rim size, may be arthroscopically repaired. Again, proper discussion with the patient before surgery is necessary so that the different postoperative regimens of the two techniques are familiar to the patient. If excision is elected, the same technique described for the displaced bucket-handle tear should be used.

Double and triple bucket-handle tears

For the double bucket-handle tear (Figure 34) and the more rare triple bucket-handle tear, we recommend using the same approach as with the single vertical longitudinal tear. Remove each handle fragment in an anterior to posterior order. Do not exclude the possibility of meniscal repair in the double bucket-handle tear. The senior author has had several successful outcomes in this category documented by 'second-look' arthroscopy.

Horizontal cleavage tears

Horizontal cleavage tears can be present both in the medial meniscus and the lateral meniscus. They are frequent residual tears in the rim segment in instances of displaced bucket-handle tears of the medial meniscus. Shear patterns in the meniscus may predispose to horizontal cleavages. A central zone of mucoid degeneration may also be a factor. The horizontal cleavage tear should be probed to determine the more substantial and stable leaf. The unstable or torn segment can then be resected back with basket rongeurs. The resection does not usually have to be carried back to the periphery of the meniscus. If the remaining segment is stable, it should remain

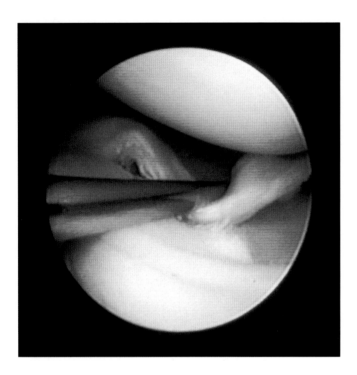

Figure 34

There is a displaced double bucket-handle tear of the medial meniscus in this left knee. The probe is on the posterior section of the two fragments. It was deemed irreparable and excision of both fragments was carried out. (From ref. 13.)

asymptomatic. Leaving a tear of up to 3 mm depth is usually quite acceptable provided the rim is stable (Figure 35).

Radial split tears

Many radial split tears involving the medial or lateral meniscus may be asymptomatic and may be discovered as an incidental finding. Figure 36 shows an example of a radial split tear in a young adult 4 years after a previous arthroscopy at which this tear was observed and left alone, and the patient remained asymptomatic. His arthroscopies were for another problem.

If a radial split tear is symptomatic, then simple trimming back of the anterior and posterior leaves immediately adjacent to the tear site should suffice. Radial split tears near the posterior horn origin of the lateral meniscus are frequently associated with ACL tears. Every attempt should be made to repair rather than excise them. There is a rich blood supply to the posterior horn of the lateral meniscus, and repair is frequently successful and can result in the maintenance of meniscal function. Some radial split tears may be part of a complex tear where the peripheral component of the tear is part of a vertical longitudinal tear. In the contribution on 'Meniscal Repair' (2.2), the details of the technique for repair are shown.

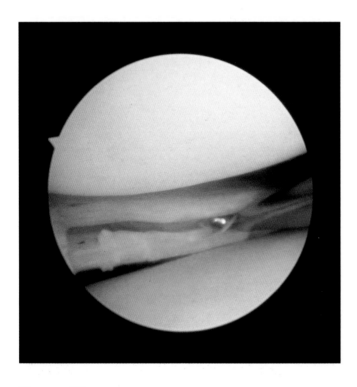

Figure 35

A probe is shown in a residual horizontal cleavage tear in the posterior horn of the lateral meniscus in this right knee. It is usually acceptable to leave a residual tear of up to 3 mm depth provided the rim is stable.

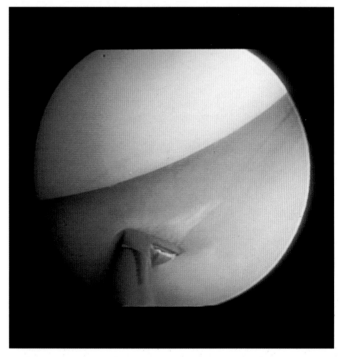

Figure 36

A 'second-look' 4 years after noting a radial split in the middle third of this right lateral meniscus revealed no change in its appearance, and was asymptomatic. (From ref. 13.)

Degenerative tears

Degenerative tears typically occur in the arthritic knee with associated joint space narrowing documented on a P–A bent-knee weight-bearing radiograph.[11] Patients may present with loading type pain or mechanical symptoms such as catching.[12] Be conservative when approaching this type of tear pattern, keeping in mind the preservation of as much meniscal tissue as possible (Figures 37 and 38). Patients with significant joint space narrowing should be warned beforehand that partial meniscectomy does not offer as high a degree of success as in the younger patient with an intact joint space. If it is indicated, an extensive synovectomy and removal of any impinging osteophytes should be part of the procedure.[12]

Soft-tissue impingement

Occasionally, patients may present with pain during terminal extension localized to the anterior portion of the joint. Not uncommonly, they have had a previous unsuccessful arthroscopy. Sometimes, there can be clicking during terminal extension (Figure 39). The diagnosis is more one of exclusion, since neither

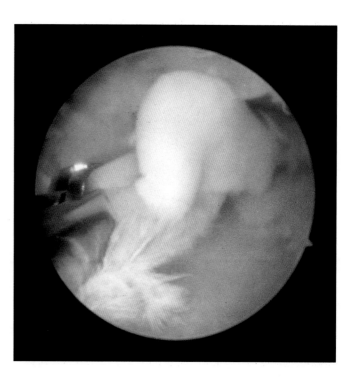

Figure 38

The dominant flap tear in Figure 37 is shown being resected.

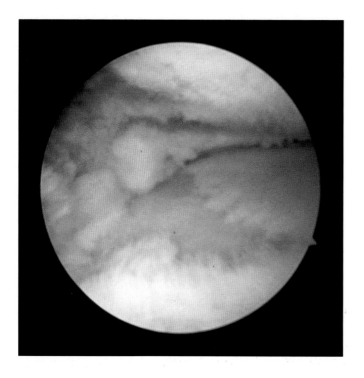

Figure 37

In this degenerative left medial compartment, a complex tear of the medial meniscus is shown.

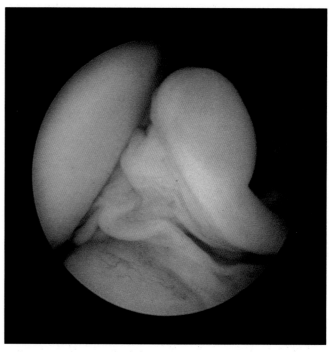

Figure 39

The scar tissue in the intercondylar notch of the right knee after ACL reconstruction was causing clicking and pain during terminal extension. Resection was easily accomplished and the patient was markedly improved.

magnetic resonance imaging nor arthrography will show it. This syndrome of soft-tissue impingement should not be confused with patellofemoral pathology, since the pain pattern is near the joint-line, not in the subpatellar or parapatellar region. Arthroscopy should be carried out on patients presenting with unrelenting pain that has not responded to rest and nonsteroidal anti-inflammatory medication. The findings at arthroscopy may be subtle. Now and then, all that one may find is a tag of synovial tissue overlapping the anterior horn of the medial meniscus and projecting into the medial compartment joint space. If it has been impinging, the tip of the synovium may be white and avascular. Simple debridement with a motorized shaving unit usually suffices.

Impinging soft tissue also may occur in the parapatellar region. In contrast to the previous location, these symptoms are definitely associated with patellofemoral pain. Parapatellar debridement with a motorized shaver, including projecting tissue from the fat pad area under the inferior pole of the patella, may provide symptomatic relief.

Patellar disorders, meniscal repair, chondral lesions, osteochondritis dissecans, synovial disorders

These subjects are covered in other contributions.

References

1. **Watanabe M, Takeda S, Ikeuchi H**, *Atlas of arthroscopy* (Tokyo Igaku Shoin Ltd., 1957).
2. **Jackson RW**, History of arthroscopy, *Operative arthroscopy*, ed McGinty JB (New York: Raven Press, 1991) 1–4.
3. **Ikeuchi H**, Surgery under arthroscopic control, *Proceedings of the Societé Internationale d'Arthroscopie 1975, Rheumatology* (1976) (special issue) 57–62.
4. **Caspari RB**, An arthroscopic modular prosthetic knee replacement, *Operative Arthroscopy*, UCLA Extension, Kauai, Hawaii 25 Oct., 1990.
5. **Gillquist J, Hagberg G**, A new modification of the technique of arthroscopy of the knee joint, *Acta Chir Scand* (1976) **142**: 123–130.
6. **Patel D**, Proximal approaches to arthroscopic surgery of the knee, *Am J Sports Med* (1981) **9**: 296–303.
7. **Patel D**, Arthroscopy of the plicae: synovial folds and their significance, *Am J Sports Med* (1978) **6**: 217–225.
8. **Joyce JJ III, Harty M**, Surgery of the synovial fold, *Arthroscopy: diagnosis and surgical practice*, ed Casscells SW (Philadelphia: Lea and Febiger, 1984).
9. **Iino S**, Normal arthroscopic findings in the knee joint in adult cadavers, *J Jpn Orthop Assoc* (1939) **14**: 467–523.
10. **Miller DV, O'Brien SJ, Arnoczky S et al.**, Use of the contact Nd:YAG laser in arthroscopic surgery: Effects on articular cartilage and meniscal tissue, *Arthroscopy* (1989) **5**: 245–253.
11. **Rosenberg TD, Paulos LE, Parker RD et al.**, The forty-five-degree posteroanterior flexion weight-bearing radiograph of the knee, *J Bone Joint Surg (Am)* (1988) **70**: 1479–1483.
12. **Baumgaertner MR, Cannon WD, Vittori JM et al.**, Arthroscopic debridement of the arthritic knee, *Clin Orthop* (1990) **253**: 197–202.
13. **Cannon WD**, Meniscal problems and treatment, *The knee: Form, function, pathology and treatment*, ed Larson RL, Grana WA (Philadelphia: WB Saunders, 1992).

2.2 Meniscal repair

W. Dilworth Cannon, Jr and Joyce M. Vittori

The history of meniscal repair

Great achievements are often not recognized at the time they occur. Frequently, they are ridiculed. The evolution of meniscal repair has had its share of geniuses and scoffers. In 1883, Thomas Annandale performed the first meniscus repair, on a mine worker.[1] Ten weeks later, the man was able to return to work with a fully functioning knee. In 1897 Sutton, a contemporary of Annandale, dismissed menisci as the 'functionless remains of leg muscle origins.'[2] This thinking would dominate orthopedic medicine for another 53 years. Annandale did not live to see his achievement acknowledged.

In 1936, Don King did his experiments on canine menisci and published his results. In 'The function of semilunar cartilages,' King was the first to associate degenerative arthritis with meniscectomy.[3] In another publication, 'The healing of semilunar cartilages,' he showed that intrasubstance meniscal tears would not heal.[4] Nevertheless, tears did heal in the avascular portion of the menisci if they extended to the vascularized synovial membrane. Decades went by before surgeons began to understand the importance of King's work. Eventually, surgeons began to develop techniques to salvage the torn meniscus.

DeHaven and others began doing open meniscal repair in the late 1970s.[5] Price and Allen reported on 36 repairs of peripheral medial meniscal tears associated with medial collateral ligament disruption in 1978.[6] Thirty-three of their repairs were successful.

In Tokyo in 1969, Ikeuchi did the first arthroscopic meniscal repair. He reported on four repairs done from 1969 to 1974.[7] Since that time, arthroscopic meniscal repair has evolved to the sophisticated and exacting technique it is today. The first American to do an arthroscopic meniscal repair was Henning in 1980. Henning's arthroscopic meniscal repair technique is difficult and its widespread acceptance has been slow.[8]

---

* This contribution is dedicated to Chuck Henning. All too often genius is too late acknowledged.

Open meniscal repair

Open meniscal repair is used today as an established alternative to arthroscopic meniscal repair of vertical longitudinal peripheral tears with rim sizes of less than 2.5 mm. DeHaven is perhaps the most prominent surgeon in the field of open meniscus repair. His repair technique is well established and his results are based on long-term follow-up examinations.[9]

DeHaven's technique for open meniscal repair

Medial meniscus repair

To repair a peripheral medial meniscus tear begin by making a 5-cm (2-inch) vertical posteromedial skin incision. Starting just posterior to the trailing edge of the medial collateral ligament, make an oblique capsular incision. With a curette, debride the edges of the meniscus. This technique calls for double-armed 4–0 vicryl sutures threaded with a small needle on one end and a larger needle on the other (Figure 1). Pass the small needle inferiorly through the meniscal rim. Advance the larger needle below the meniscus and through the capsular bed. Tie the suture. DeHaven recommends using a King stitch in the most vulnerable portion of the tear site. This box-like horizontal mattress suture calls for 2–0 vicryl.

Lateral meniscus repair

The repair of the posterior horn of the lateral meniscus varies little in technique to the medial side (Figure 2a–d). Split the iliotibial band in line with its fibers and open the capsule vertically along the posterior border of the popliteus tendon. Again, using double-armed 4–0 vicryl sutures, pass the first suture through the superior surface of the meniscus. When it emerges inferiorly, pass the suture through the fibers that connect the popliteus tendon to the lateral meniscus and continue on through the synovial bed.

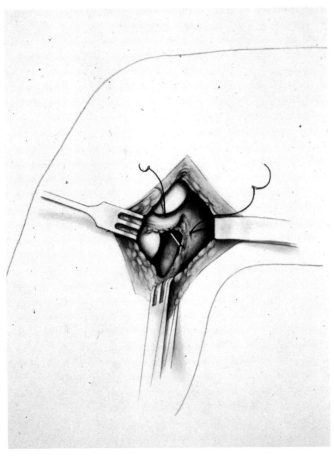

a

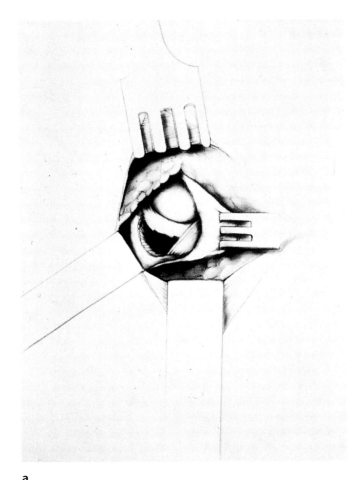

a

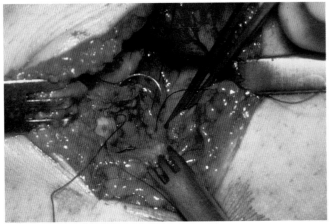

b

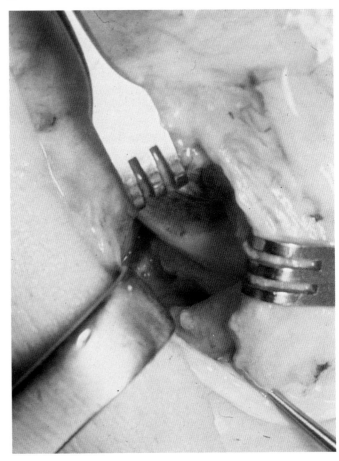

b

Figure 1

DeHaven's technique of open medial meniscal repair. The meniscal rim is sutured to its attached synovial bed using vertically placed absorbable 4–0 mattress sutures. Using double-armed sutures, a small needle is passed from the inferior to the superior surface of the meniscus, and a larger needle is passed from below up through the capsular bed. (From ref. 9.)

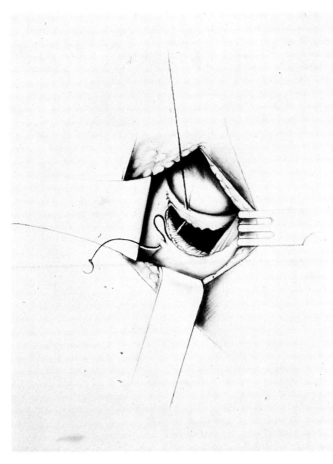

c

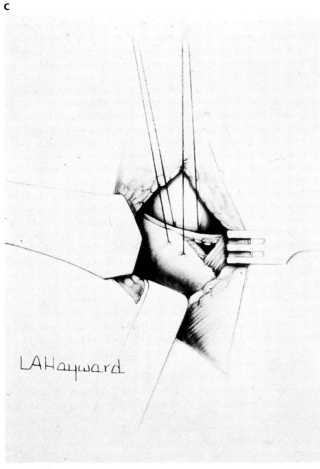

LAHayward

d

Figure 2

(a,b) DeHaven's technique for a repair of a peripheral tear of the posterior horn of the lateral meniscus which extends to the popliteus hiatus. (c,d) The suture is passed from the superior to the inferior surface of the meniscus through the popliteal fibers to the lateral meniscus, and then through the synovial bed. (From ref. 23.)

Postoperative rehabilitation

Patients begin touch-down weight bearing immediately and continue it until 6 weeks following surgery. Limited active motion from 30° to 70° is initiated at 2 weeks after surgery. Free motion is allowed at 4 weeks. Patients may jog and swim at 3–4 months and all sports are resumed 6 months postoperatively.

Results

DeHaven has an 11-year follow-up of results of 33 open meniscus repairs.[10] He divided these repairs into three groups. Knees were classified as stable if there was less than a 3 mm, involved minus uninvolved, anterior displacement difference. Knees were considered nearly stable if the involved minus uninvolved difference was greater than 3 mm and less than 4.5 mm. Knees with a greater than 4.5 mm involved minus uninvolved anterior displacement difference were defined as unstable.

Of 9 menisci in stable knees, there was 1 retear (11%). In contrast, among the 12 menisci in the unstable group, there were 5 retears (42%). Repair of 21 acute tears resulted in 3 retears (14%). Of 12 chronic meniscal tears, there were 4 retears (33%). Overall, there was a 79% meniscal survival rate. The average time from surgery to retear was 4 years.

Follow-up radiographic results revealed that none of the patients had moderate or severe degenerative changes. All 33 patients had either no radiographic changes or mild changes (less than 2 mm joint space narrowing or sclerosis).

Arthroscopic meniscal repair

Arthroscopic meniscal repair is believed by many surgeons to be easier to perform than open meniscal repair. In truth, arthroscopic meniscal repair, if done correctly, and if fibrin clot is used, is technically more difficult. For other types of tears, arthroscopic repair is preferable and for rim sizes that are larger than 2.5 mm there is no alternative (Figure 3).

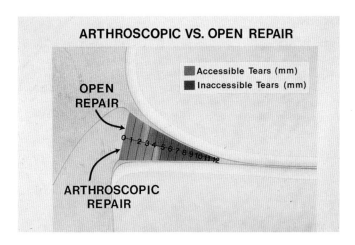

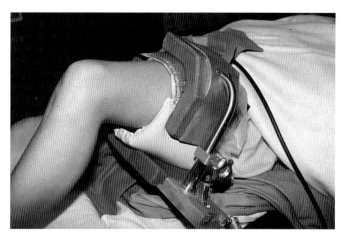

Figure 3

Arthroscopic vs. open repair. The upper half of the meniscus shows the accessibility of the meniscus to open repair, the green area demonstrating that the surgeon cannot gain access to tears that have rim widths greater than 2.5–3.0 mm. In contrast, arthroscopic techniques can repair meniscal tears with rim widths greater than 4.0 mm. (From ref. 24.)

Figure 4

A thigh holder placed distal to the tourniquet and well padded posteriorly maintains thigh flexion at 45°, providing excellent access to the posteromedial and posterolateral corners of the knee. (From ref. 24.)

The three generic repair techniques for arthroscopic meniscal repair are the inside–outside,[11] the outside–outside,[12] and the inside–inside.[13] To handle any eventuality, the surgeon should be proficient with more than one repair technique. The occasion may arise when a particular meniscal tear pattern can be repaired more efficiently by a technique other than the surgeon's usual one. The surgeon should also have the instrumentation for each technique at his disposal.

Modified Henning arthroscopic meniscal repair technique

Medial meniscus repair

Place the tourniquet high on the patient's thigh, just proximal to a well-padded leg holder. Although, the tourniquet is rarely used during meniscal repair, it is usually used for the ACL reconstruction part of the case. Meniscal repairs are frequently done concurrently with ACL reconstruction because most meniscal repairs are associated with ACL deficiency. In the senior author's series, 80% were associated with an ACL reconstruction. To lessen the possibility of well-leg nerve palsies or thromboemboli, it is preferable to keep the patient supine and not break the end of the table. To allow for good access to the posteromedial and posterolateral corners of the knee and to distribute pressure evenly, flex the hip 30–45° and

place a gel-filled pad posteriorly to alleviate pressure on the sciatic nerve (Figure 4).

View the meniscus arthroscopically and probe it completely, including the posterior horn, to ascertain the need and feasibility of repair. Make a 5–6-cm longitudinal incision posteromedially centered at the joint-line. It is critical that the incision avoids the saphenous vein and the sartorial branch of the saphenous nerve. The dissection should be anterior to the sartorius. It continues between the posteromedial capsule and the direct head of the semimembranosus and across the medial head of the gastrocnemius. Place a popliteal retractor in an extra-articular position, behind the posterior horn of the medial meniscus. The direct head of the semimembranosus may push the retractor in a proximal direction, complicating needle retrieval. Therefore, it may be necessary to cut part of the attachment of the direct head of the semimembranosus. When repairing an extensive bucket-handle tear, anteriorly placed sutures may be especially difficult to retrieve. Then, it may be necessary to make a second small incision midway between the posteromedial incision and the anteromedial portal to retrieve these needles (Figure 5).

While viewing the posteromedial corner of the knee, introduce a 3-mm or smaller rasp through the synovium (Figure 6). Abrade the meniscosynovial junction over the superior surface of the meniscus and rasp both sides of the tear. It is important to freshen all surfaces of the tear to remove any superfluous material that can interfere with meniscal healing. The neovascular response that rasping produces provides

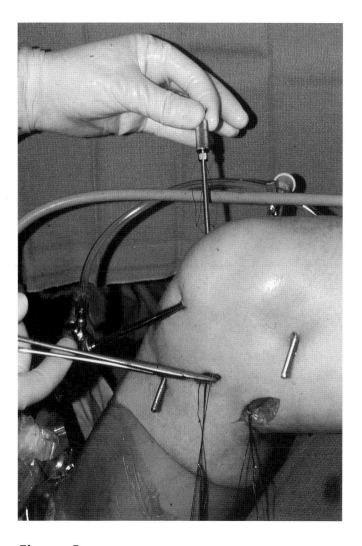

Figure 5

When suturing the middle third of the medial meniscus, occasionally a second incision may be made anterior to the posteromedial incision and sutures brought directly through this wound. These sutures have a more radial orientation than if they had been brought through the posteromedial incision. The knee distractor has been temporarily removed. (From ref. 24.)

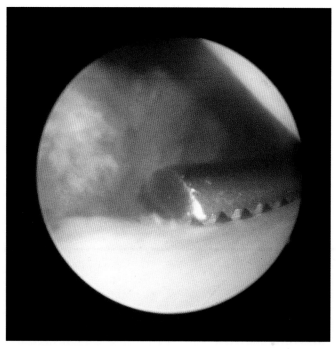

Figure 6

A 2-mm burr-type rasp has been introduced through the posteromedial incision while viewing through the intercondylar notch in this left knee. Parameniscal synovial abrasion is carried out over the superior surface of the meniscus and in the tear site.

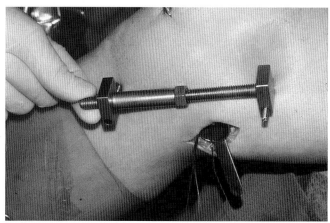

Figure 7

A knee distractor is used for medial meniscal repairs. This enables better visualization of the posterior horn. The popliteal retractor can be seen in the posteromedial incision. (From ref. 24.)

an adjunct to the meniscal healing process. To abrade the inferior surface of the meniscus, pass a burr through a small nick made in the synovium at the posteromedial corner and under the meniscus. Another approach is to introduce a small angled burr (Bowen & Co., Inc., Rockville, MD, USA) from the anteromedial portal and under the posterior horn of the meniscus.

When placing more than two sutures through the posterior horn of the medial meniscus, use an external joint distractor (Figure 7). This will usually ensure adequate visualization of the posterior horn. If visualization is inadequate following joint distraction, wait a few minutes and distract the joint further.

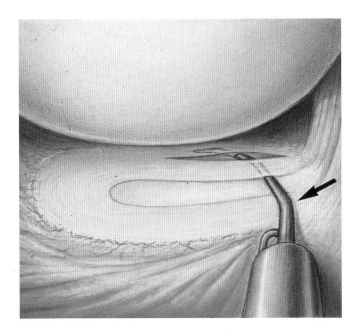

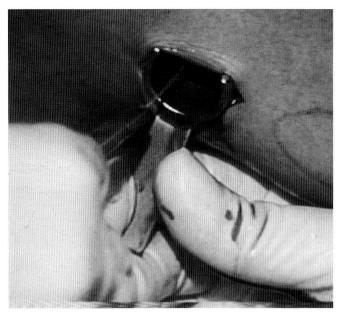

Figure 8

The first suture is placed close to the posterior horn origin of either medial or lateral meniscus and may be difficult to retrieve posteriorly. Hence, a third bend in the needle is made by levering the cannula and needle holder into the intercondylar notch. The additional bend in the needle will allow the surgeon to guide the needle into the popliteal retractor with greater ease. (From ref. 24.)

Figure 9

When the tip of the needle has penetrated through the posterior horn and capsule, it is deflected off of the popliteal retractor and retrieved with a needle holder.

All meniscal suturing is done with non-absorbable 2-0 Ethibond (Ethicon, Inc., Somerville, NJ, USA; Special order D-6702) with double-armed taper-ended Keith needles. Most surgeons believe that nonabsorbable suture material should be used for meniscal repair. Meniscal healing goes on for many months, so it is important for the suture material to remain intact during the healing process.

To ensure that the needle is angled into the meniscus and directed to the posteromedial corner of the knee, the needle is bent. Bend the needle approximately 10–15° 4 mm from the tip. A second bend is made 10–15° 1 cm away from the first bend. Press-fit the needle into a needle holder designed for the Henning technique (Stryker Corporation, San Jose, CA, USA). Insert the cannula into the anteromedial portal just above the superior surface of the anterior horn of the meniscus. Make certain that the knee is maintained in approximately 10–15° of extension. Carefully pass the needle through the cannula and aim it into the intercondylar notch. When the needle is seen to exit the cannula, direct it to the posterior horn of the medial meniscus. The first suture should go from the inferior surface and be directed superiorly to lie near the posterior horn origin. To keep the needle from getting lost in the midline structures behind the joint, a third bend in the needle is needed

(Figure 8). Introduce the needle into the meniscus up to its second bend. Create the third bend by levering the cannula along with the needle holder into the intercondylar notch. Advance the needle from close to the inner border of the intercondylar notch. The needle should deflect off the popliteal retractor and exit posteromedially. Grasp the needle point and release the needle holder. Retrieve the needle and tag the suture (Figure 9).

Pass the second needle of the first suture into the joint. Vertical mattress sutures (Figure 10) are more biomechanically sound and are therefore preferable to horizontal mattress sutures (Figure 11) in meniscal repair. The second throw goes under the meniscus and out through the meniscosynovial junction. The needle is retrieved in the way previously described. Stagger the sutures superiorly and inferiorly every 3–4 mm (Figure 12).

In repairing a vertical longitudinal tear that extends anterior to the posteromedial corner, move the arthroscope to the anteromedial portal. Suturing should be done from the anterolateral portal through a long cannula (Figure 13).

Displaced bucket-handle tears are also amenable to repair. After reducing the handle fragment and rasping both sides of the tear, suturing is begun at the posterior horn origin and carried anteriorly (Figures 14, 15).

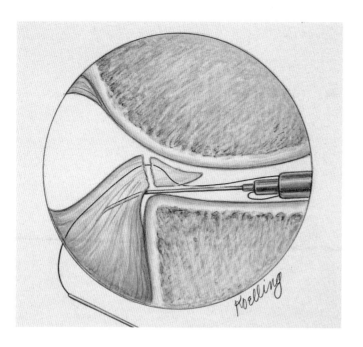

Figure 10

This diagram demonstrating the Henning technique shows the placement of divergent vertically oriented mattress sutures. (From ref. 24.)

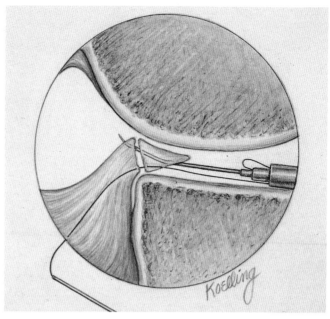

Figure 11

This diagram shows the placement of a horizontal mattress suture through the posterior horn with divergent passes of the two needles. (From ref. 24.)

Lateral meniscus repair

Lateral meniscus repair, although similar in technique to medial meniscal repair, is easier to do. Execution of the posterolateral dissection is not as complex as the posteromedial incision. Begin by flexing the patient's knee 90° and splitting the biceps from the posterior border of the iliotibial band. Locate the lateral head of the gastrocnemius and dissect deep to the lateral head. The peroneal nerve will lie posterior to the biceps and will be out of harm's way. Dissect the lateral head of the gastrocnemius off the posterior capsule. Initiate this dissection at or below the joint-line and advance it proximally. Place the popliteal retractor behind the posterior horn of the lateral meniscus. Insert the arthroscope into the anteromedial portal through the intercondylar notch. This will allow optimum visualization during parameniscal rasping of the tear site. Although Henning's technique traditionally calls for a joint distractor on the lateral side, it is not necessary. With the arthroscope in the anterolateral portal, lateral meniscal suturing is done from the anteromedial portal. Take care to avoid the popliteal artery when placing sutures at the posterior horn origin (Figure 16). Although it is sometimes unavoidable, one should try not to pass sutures through the popliteus tendon.

Do not hesitate to repair tears of the posterior horn of the lateral meniscus. The profuse vascularity of this area makes it particularly amenable to successful repair of complex tears, including radial split tears.

Fibrin clot

Canine studies by Arnoczky, reported in 1986, demonstrated that fibrin clot, with its growth factors, can stimulate fibrochondrocytes when injected into a torn meniscus. Since that time, fibrin clot has become an important adjunct to some meniscal repairs.[14]

Under strict sterile conditions, have the anesthesiologist remove approximately 50–75 ml of venous blood from the patient. On the operative field, place the blood in a plastic or glass container and stir it with two glass barrels from syringes (Figure 17). Fibrin clot will adhere to the sintered glass barrels after continuous stirring for approximately 5 minutes. Remove and blot the clot with moistened pads. Elongate the clot until it forms a tubelike structure. Sew a 2–0 Ethibond meniscal repair suture into each end (Figure 18). Pass the needles inferior to the meniscus at the extreme anterior and posterior poles of the tear. Pull the clot through a 5–6-mm cannula into the joint. Evacuate the joint of fluid. Loosen the

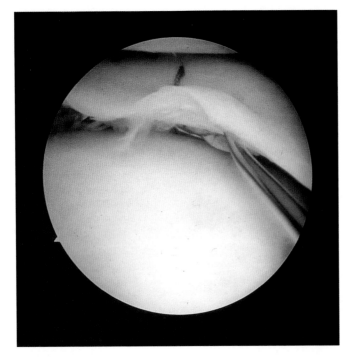

a

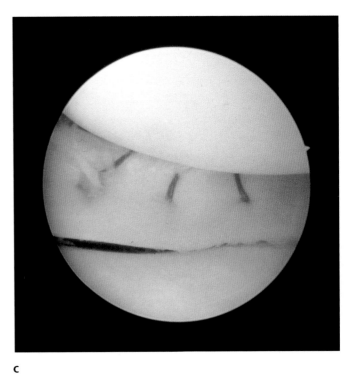

c

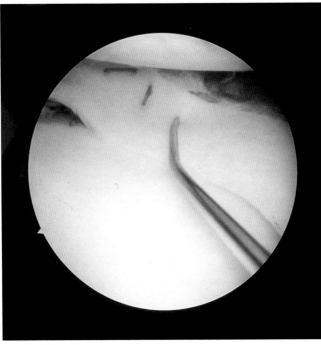

b

Figure 12

Vertically oriented mattress sutures are shown being placed through both inferior and superior aspects of the posterior horn of the medial meniscus in this right knee. Sutures are placed every 3 mm. (From ref. 24.)

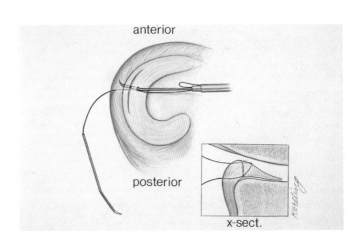

Figure 13

This diagram shows the technique for repairing the middle third of the medial meniscus. The scope has been moved to the anteromedial portal and suturing is carried out through the anterolateral portal. Note again the divergent needle placement, creating excellent coaptation of the meniscus. (From ref. 24.)

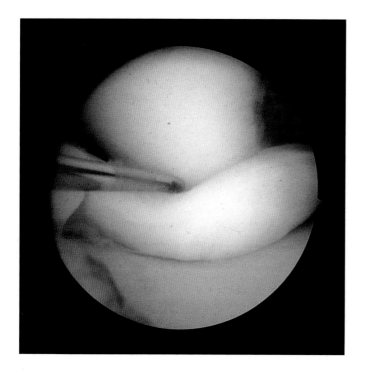

Figure 14

Most displaced bucket-handle tears such as this one can be successfully repaired. (From ref. 24.)

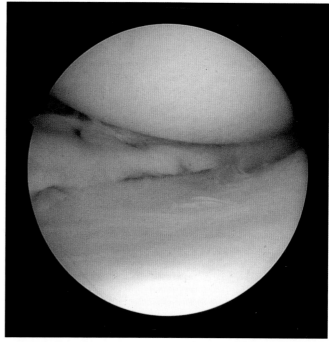

Figure 15

The displaced bucket-handle tear shown in Figure 14 was repaired with eight sutures. (From ref. 24.)

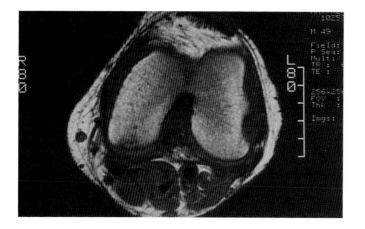

Figure 16

This magnetic resonance image demonstrates the intimate association of the popliteal artery to the posterior horn of the lateral meniscus. Without the insertion of a popliteal retractor in back of the posterior horn of the lateral meniscus, the artery can be easily injured. The black arrow indicates popliteal artery. (From ref. 24.)

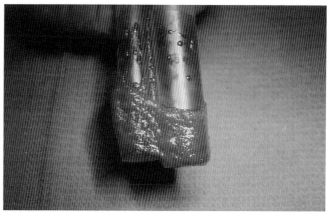

Figure 17

The appearance of the fibrin clot adhering to two glass syringe barrels after stirring 75 ml of venous blood for 5 min. (From ref. 24.)

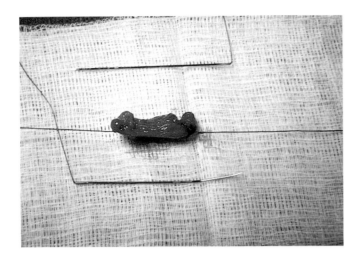

Figure 18

A 2–0 Ethibond suture has been placed through either end of the fibrin clot facilitating its stable placement under the inferior surface of the meniscus at the tear site.

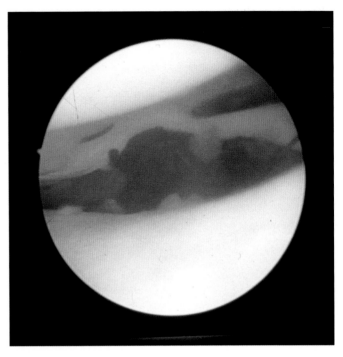

Figure 19

The fibrin clot has been placed under the meniscus throughout the tear length, and the sutures then pulled tight. Notice the right-hand suture actually holding the clot under the meniscus. (From ref. 24.)

previously placed meniscal sutures. Place the clot throughout the length of the inferior surface of the meniscus and into the opened tear cleft. Pull the sutures tight to trap the clot in the tear site (Figure 19).

Fibrin clot should be inserted into the tear clefts of isolated meniscal repairs. The satisfactory healing rate for isolated meniscal repairs without the use of fibrin clot is disappointing. In contrast to isolated repairs, meniscal repairs associated with ACL reconstruction have a high rate of satisfactory healing. Therefore, in ACL-associated meniscal tears, the senior author uses fibrin clot only when repairing complex tears or tears with a rim size of 4 mm or more. Clot is always used to repair isolated meniscal tears.

Complex tears

Radial split tears of the medial and lateral meniscus can be repaired by placing a horizontal mattress suture through the anterior and posterior leaves of the tear (Figures 20–22). Place these sutures close to the inner edge to approximate the tear. Radial split tears of the avascular middle third of the meniscus have a poor incidence of healing. Therefore, fibrin clot should be used in these repairs. If the tear is asymptomatic, often it can be left alone.

Fibrin clot should be used as an adjunct for repair of flap tears and broken bucket-handle tears. Henning developed a difficult and exacting technique for repair of these complex tears. It consists of sewing a piece of fascial sheath over the tear and attaching it superiorly and inferiorly before injecting it with fibrin clot.[15]

Other arthroscopic meniscal repair techniques

There are other meniscal repair systems available that are not as difficult to master as the Henning technique. Rosenberg's design introduces single needles through zone-specific curved cannulas.[16] This system allows for divergent suture placement for better meniscal coaptation. Needles are retrieved through a posterior incision.

Perhaps the most popular technique available is Clancy and Graf's double-barrel curved-cannula system.[17] It uses a pair of long needles linked by 2–0 PDS suture. This technique is faster than Henning's, but the surgeon has less control over suture placement. It is difficult to create divergent sutures that are so important to a well done repair.

Warren was the developer of the outside–inside technique.[12] Spinal-gauge needles are advanced through the skin and into the meniscal tear. PDS suture passes through the needle, is retrieved anteriorly, and is tied in a double knot before being pulled back into the joint to snug up against the meniscus. Pairs of sutures are tied subcutaneously.

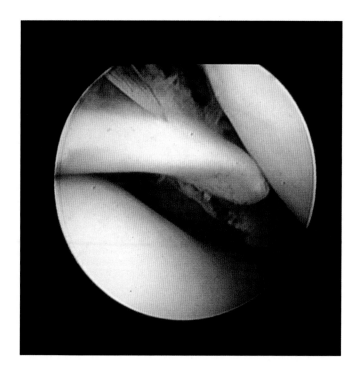

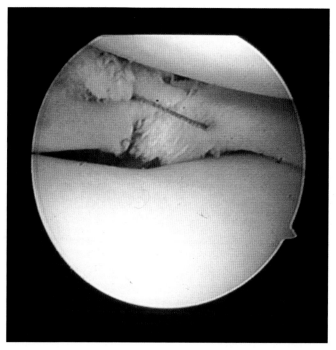

Figure 20

There is a radial oblique flap tear at the posterior horn origin of this left lateral meniscus associated with a vertical longitudinal tear extending in front of the popliteus hiatus in this 21-year-old basketball player's left knee. He also had a medial meniscal tear in addition to a torn ACL. (From ref. 24.)

Figure 21

Five sutures were used to repair the tear shown in Figure 20. Note the technique of repair of the radial split tear; one throw of the suture is placed through the posterior leaf and the second through the anterior leaf and the tear is approximated. (From ref. 24.)

Morgan's inside–inside technique is a new approach to meniscus repair.[13] Curved suture needles are used and suturing is similar to that of open technique. Knot tying is done with a special tier and passed down a posterior cannula.

There are other good meniscal repair techniques that are variations of those described above.

Postoperative rehabilitation

Whether the meniscal repair is isolated or one associated with ACL reconstruction, the postoperative regimens are identical. The patient is allowed to move his knee immediately. Crutches are used for the first 6–8 weeks with the patient not weight bearing for the first 4 weeks. Weight bearing progresses from 23 kg (50 lb) at 4 weeks to almost full weight bearing at the sixth week. Once full weight bearing is achieved, patients usually remain on crutches for another 2 weeks. At 6 weeks, closed kinetic chain quadriceps and unlimited hamstring exercises are begun. The patient may start to run at 5 months. No contact sports are allowed before 9 months but some sports are permitted at 6 months postoperatively.

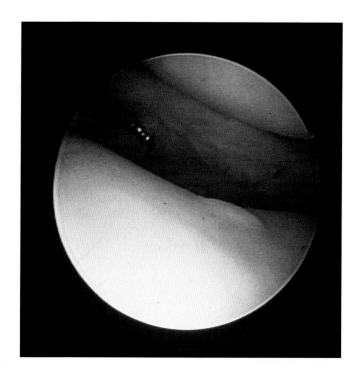

Figure 22

Seven months after meniscal repair (shown in Figure 21), the posterior horn of the lateral meniscus appears healed. (From ref. 24.)

Results

Henning did not assess the results of his meniscal repairs by clinical examination alone. He recognized that an anatomical assessment would more truthfully reveal the incidence of healing. Therefore, Henning recommended that at 6 months postoperatively a 'second-look' arthroscopy be done for all lateral meniscal repairs, and an arthrogram be performed for medial meniscal repairs. He established strict criteria for evaluating healing incidence. A meniscus is considered healed if there is a 10% or less residual cleft at the tear site. A partially healed meniscus is one in which the cleft is less than 50% of the thickness of the meniscus. A repair is considered a failure if at any point along the tear site the cleft is greater than 50% of the thickness of the meniscus (Figure 23). Sometimes anatomical failures are clinically asymptomatic. Approximately half of our anatomical failures and two-thirds of Henning's were clinically asymptomatic. This is an important finding, as many surgeons are reporting results based on clinical assessments alone. They are biasing their studies and probably underestimating the incidence of meniscal repair failure.

The senior author has done 145 arthroscopic meniscal repairs since 1982. There were 64 medial meniscal repairs, 51 lateral meniscal repairs, and 15 bilateral repairs. There were 42 acute and 73 chronically torn menisci repaired at an average time from injury of 19 months. Most of the repairs were associated with ACL deficiency (80%). The average patient age was 27 years.

Follow-up anatomical assessment was done on 115 patients. Eighty-four patients had a 'second-look' arthroscopy and 31 had an arthrogram. If both medial and lateral meniscal repairs were done, they were assessed arthroscopically. Patients requiring arthroscopic debridement after ACL reconstruction had meniscal repair evaluation done at this time. Magnetic resonance imaging (MRI) studies are not done to evaluate the incidence of meniscal healing. The accuracy of MRI in assessing meniscal healing is still under investigation. Early studies show the presence of type III signals in anatomically healed menisci.[18] This may indicate that meniscal repairs do not heal perfectly, or MRI may be misreading healed or partially healed menisci as failures.

Our data concur with Henning's in finding that partially healed menisci do as well as the completely healed menisci. Therefore, we define the healed and the partially healed groups as satisfactorily healed. In our series, overall there was a 76% incidence of satisfactory healing. Assessment of these patients clinically resulted in a 92% incidence of healing. The incidence of satisfactory meniscal repair healing (84%) when associated with an ACL reconstruction stands in sharp contrast to a 52% healing rate in isolated meniscal repairs. The use of fibrin clot may

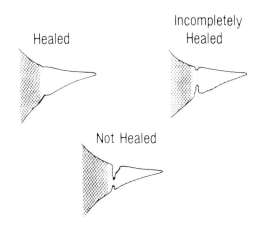

Figure 23

Six months after repair, the degree of healing can be determined by arthrogram for the medial side and arthroscopy for the lateral side. A meniscus is classified as 'healed' (upper left figure) if it is healed over the full length of the tear with a residual cleft less than 10% of the thickness of the meniscus. A tear that is healed over its full length with a residual cleft that is less than 50% of its vertical height is classified as 'incompletely healed' (upper right figure). A residual cleft of greater than 50% of the thickness of the meniscus at any point over the length of the tear is classified as 'failed' (lower figure). (From ref. 24.)

improve the incidence of healing in isolated meniscal repairs. Since clot has only been used since late 1987, this will not be evaluated until the data base is large enough for statistical analysis. Henning, however, reported that with the use of fibrin clot his incidence of successful healing of isolated repairs rose from 59% to 92%.[19]

The size of the tear rim width has a direct effect on repair results. Menisci with rim widths of 3.9 mm or less had an 80% incidence of satisfactory healing. Rim widths of 4 mm or greater had only a 50% healing success.

Increasing tear lengths also have an adverse effect on meniscal healing. Tears with lengths of 2 cm or less have an excellent healing incidence (91%). Tears greater than 2 cm and less than 4 cm have a 77% incidence of satisfactory healing, but this drops to 41% when tear lengths are 4 cm or more.

Patient age is an important factor. Oddly enough, the older the patient, the better the incidence of healing in our series. Patients 18 years of age or younger had a 65% incidence of successful healing compared with 78% of patients who were 19 years or older. Patients who were 36 years or older did particularly well, with an 86% incidence of successful healing.

Acute tears are defined for this study as 8 weeks or less from the date of injury. Meniscal repairs done while in the acute stage had an 83% incidence of successful healing. Repair of chronic meniscal tears (any tear greater than 8 weeks from injury) had a 71% satisfactory healing rate.

There were no vascular complications, infections, or wound healing problems in our series. One patient had a partial peroneal nerve palsy. A suture had passed through 25% of the nerve, but it was released within a week of surgery and the patient had a full recovery. One case of transient phlebitis occurred 4 weeks after surgery. There was no loss of motion that was attributable to meniscal repair.

Discussion

Meniscal repairs associated with concomitant ACL reconstruction do significantly better than isolated meniscal repair. One theory as to why this occurs is that a patient who has an ACL disruption experiences a major anterior subluxation of the tibia. The femoral condyle crunches down on the posterior horn of one or both of the menisci and creates a tear. Successful ACL reconstruction stabilizes the knee, prevents the subluxation from recurring, and protects the meniscal repair site. Conversely, the biomechanical forces that created the isolated meniscal tear are still present after repair and could cause the meniscus to re-tear. A second theory is that the trauma of an ACL reconstruction produces additional fibrin clot in the joint which can further stimulate meniscal healing. Tiling (personal communication) in a study of acute meniscal tears (less than 12 days old), found that histologic and electron-microscopic analysis of biopsies taken from the tears revealed degenerative changes consistently in the isolated tear group, in contrast to no degenerative changes in the torn ACL group. This is consistent with our results in that the two tear groups seem to be different entities. We once thought that meniscal tears resulting from ACL disruption were more peripheral and in a more vascularized area of the meniscus than isolated tears. Data analysis did not bear this out. In our series, ACL-associated meniscal tears have an average rim width of 2.4 mm and isolated tears of 2.3 mm.

A surprise finding in our series was that older patients had more successfully healed meniscal repairs than those under 18 years of age. This may be attributed to poor patient compliance among youngsters. Nevertheless, most reparable meniscal tears occur in the second and third decades of life. Older patients tend to have more complex and oblique flap tears and a higher frequency of mucoid degeneration within the meniscus. Yet, the incidence of healing among patients 36 years and older was 86%. Perhaps, when deciding whether or not to repair the meniscus

of an older individual, the need for ACL reconstruction should be the pivoting factor. A patient up to 50 years of age with an ACL-deficient knee who wants ACL reconstruction should also have meniscal repair.

Both arthroscopic or open meniscal repair techniques provide an invaluable service in reducing the incidence of degenerative arthritis that is the frequent result of meniscectomy. Henning's studies showed a fourfold reduction in arthritic changes in ACL-reconstructed patients who had meniscal repair as compared with partial or total meniscectomy.[20]

Rosenberg radiographed his meniscal repair patients 2 years after surgery using a 45° bent knee view.[21] He reported that 96% of his patients had less than 1 mm of joint space narrowing.[22]

The advantages of arthroscopic over open meniscal repair are apparent. Complex tear patterns inaccessible to open techniques can be repaired arthroscopically. Tears with a rim width of more than 2.5 mm cannot be repaired with open meniscal repair but are routinely arthroscopically repaired. Knowing what we do of the predisposition to arthritis following meniscectomy, it is reasonable to try to salvage torn menisci, even those occurring in the avascular zone.

References

1. **Annandale T**, An operation for displaced semilunar cartilage, *Br Med J* (1885) 779.
2. **Sutton JB**, *Ligaments, their nature and morphology*, 2nd edn (London: HK Lewis & Co, 1897).
3. **King D**, The function of semilunar cartilages, *J Bone Joint Surg (Am)* (1936) 18: 1069–1076.
4. **King D**, The healing of semilunar cartilages, *J Bone Joint Surg (Am)* (1936) 18: 333–342.
5. **DeHaven KE, Hales W**, Peripheral meniscus repair: An alternative to meniscectomy, *Orthop Trans* (1981) 5: 399–400.
6. **Price CT, Allen WC**, Ligament repair in the knee with preservation of the meniscus, *J Bone Joint Surg (Am)* (1978) 60: 61–65.
7. **Ikeuchi H**, Surgery under arthroscopic control, *Proceedings of the Societé Internationale d'Arthroscopie 1975, Rheumatology* (1976) (special issue) 57–62.
8. **Henning CE**, Arthroscopic repair of meniscus tears, *Orthopedics* (1983) 6: 1130–1132.
9. **DeHaven KE**, Open meniscus repair, *Operative arthroscopy*, ed McGinty JB (New York: Raven Press, 1991) 253–260.
10. **DeHaven KE, Lohrer WA, Lovelock JE**, Long-term results of meniscus repair, Presented at International Arthroscopy Association, Toronto, Canada, 14 May 1991.
11. **Scott GA, Jolly BL, Henning CE**, Combined posterior incision and arthroscopic intra-articular repair of the meniscus, *J Bone Joint Surg (Am)* (1986) 68: 847–861.
12. **Warren RF**, Arthroscopic meniscus repair, *Arthroscopy* (1985) 1: 170–172.
13. **Morgan CD**, The "all-inside" meniscus repair, *Arthroscopy* (1991) 7: 120–125.
14. **Arnoczky SP, Warren RF, Spivak JM**, Meniscal repair using an exogenous fibrin clot – an experimental study in dogs, *J Bone Joint Surg (Am)* (1988) 70: 1209–1220.
15. **Henning CE, Yearout KM, Vequist SW et al.**, Use of the fascia sheath coverage and exogenous fibrin clot in the treatment of complex meniscal tears, *Am J Sports Med* (1991) 19: 626–631.

16. **Rosenberg TD, Scott S, Paulos LE**, Arthroscopic surgery: Repair of peripheral detachment of the meniscus, *Contemp Orthop* (1985) **10:** 43–50.

17. **Clancy WG, Graf BK**, Arthroscopic meniscal repair, *Orthopedics* (1983) **6:** 1125–1128.

18. **Deutsch AL, Mink JH, Fox JM et al.**, Peripheral meniscal tears: MR findings after conservative treatment or arthroscopic repair, *Radiology* (1990) **176:** 485–488.

19. **Henning CE, Lynch MA, Yearout KM et al.**, Arthroscopic meniscal repair using an exogenous fibrin clot, *Clin Orthop* (1990) **252:** 64–72.

20. **Lynch MA, Henning CE, Glick KR**, Knee joint surface changes: Long-term follow-up meniscus tear treatment in stable anterior cruciate ligament reconstructions, *Clin Orthop* (1983) **172:** 148–153.

21. **Rosenberg TD, Paulos LE, Parker RD et al.**, The forty-five-degree posteroanterior flexion weight-bearing radiograph of the knee, *J Bone Joint Surg (Am)* (1988) **70:** 1479–1483.

22. **Rosenberg TD, Paulos LE**, Clinical results of arthroscopic meniscal repair after a minimum of 2 years follow-up, Presented at American Orthopaedic Society for Sports Medicine Las Vegas, 12 Feb., 1989.

23. **DeHaven KE, Black JP, Griffiths HJ**, Open meniscus repair: technique and two to nine-year results, *Am J Sports Med* (1989) **6:** 788.

24. **Cannon WD**, Arthroscopic meniscal repair, *Operative arthroscopy*, ed McGinty JB (New York: Raven Press, 1991) 237–251.

2.3 The use of local anesthesia in knee arthroscopy

Gary G. Poehling, David Martin and David Janeway

The transformation of routine knee procedures from the inpatient setting to the outpatient setting has fostered the development of effective local anesthetic techniques. The control of bleeding had been an issue because a tourniquet cannot be used effectively with local anesthesia. Now, the accurate control of pressure from within the knee using pumps allows control of bleeding without the need for a tourniquet, and the pressure generated by the pump is easily tolerated with local anesthetic.

In the early 1970s, initial attempts to utilize local anesthesia for diagnostic arthroscopy were made with lidocaine for both the extra-articular portion and the intra-articular portion of the block. Although one could accomplish a short procedure, the patient was not comfortable, and the technique was abandoned.

With the availability of bupivacaine, a dramatic change in patient tolerance was seen. In order to understand the greater effectiveness of bupivacaine as well as the benefits and risks of both anesthetics, a closer look at their actions and toxicity is necessary.

Lidocaine is an amide that stabilizes the normal membrane and prevents initiation of the action potential. The onset of action is rapid, but because lidocaine does not fix to tissues well it is washed out of the joint if used intra-articularly, and its greatest usefulness is to block the extra-articular skin, the subcutaneous tissue, the capsule, and the fat pad. The commercial preparation of lidocaine is acidic and it tends to burn when injected. The pH can be adjusted by using 1 ml of standard sodium bicarbonate solution (8.4%) in each 10 ml of lidocaine. The duration of action can be prolonged by using 1:100 000 concentration of epinephrine, which will also diminish subcutaneous bleeding.

Bupivacaine is an amide derivative of lidocaine, and it increases the threshold of excitation, thereby slowing the propagation of action potentials. The onset of bupivacaine action is slow, but it fixes to tissues well and is not susceptible to being washed out. It is used to block intra-articularly during or after knee arthroscopy,[1,2] and is combined with a 1:100000 concentration of epinephrine to prolong its effect and to decrease its absorption in order to improve its safety.

As for toxicity, that of lidocaine is first noticed in the central nervous system, manifested as excitation or depression. Ultimately, there is cardiovascular collapse, but the safety margin between the initial onset of symptoms and cardiovascular collapse is nearly twice the dosage. The toxicity of bupivacaine is also in the central nervous system, with excitation or depression developing, followed by cardiovascular collapse. However, in contrast to that of lidocaine, the safety margin of bupivacaine is extremely narrow. That is, once excitation or depression develops, cardiovascular collapse is imminent. The toxicity level of bupivacaine generally is accepted to be 1000 ng/ml, although blood levels of bupivacaine as high as 3000 ng/ml have been reported following blocks in the knee, without evidence of toxicity.[3]

In one of our studies, 9 patients had bupivacaine blocks only: 0.25% with epinephrine used in a volume of 40 ml. Bupivacaine levels averaged 33.3 ng/ml and ranged from 6.8 to 125 ng/ml. Seven patients having 0.25% bupivacaine blocks without epinephrine had levels that reached 515 ng/ml, with a range of 46–875 ng/ml. Peak levels occurred at the 30–40-min interval with no toxic symptoms. The maximal suggested bupivacaine dose for injection is 2 mg/kg, and for standard arthroscopy a total of 150 mg of bupivacaine is considered the upper limit.[4] This corresponds to 30 ml of 0.5% or 60 ml of 0.25% bupivacaine. We have noted no difference in the quality of anesthesia with the 0.5% and 0.25% concentrations, and therefore recommend the lower dosage.

Our present procedure is to use lidocaine for surface anesthesia and for infiltration of the portals and the anterior infrapatellar fat pad. The dose used is 1% lidocaine with epinephrine buffered with 1 ml of standard sodium bicarbonate solution in each 10 ml of lidocaine. This is followed by an intra-articular infiltration of 40 ml of 0.25% bupivacaine with 0.4 ml of epinephrine. Most patients are given short-acting sedation just before the block, and anxious patients (about 25%) can be given mild doses of intravenous sedation during the procedure.

Current contraindications to the use of a local anesthetic for knee arthroscopy are obesity, arthrofibrosis, reflex sympathetic dystrophy, personal preference for spinal or general anesthesia, or an inexperienced surgical team. Local anesthesia is being used successfully in 95% of our routine arthroscopic knee cases. We have found that its use allows our patients to better understand their problem and the approach used to correct that problem. The overall experience is much more pleasant because the nausea, headache, and immobility necessitated by other techniques are avoided. Local anesthesia for knee arthroscopy is well suited to the outpatient surgical center.

References

1. Kaeding CC, Hill JA, Katz J et al., Bupivacaine use after knee arthroscopy: Pharmacokinetics and pain control study, *Arthroscopy* (1990) 6: 33–39.
2. Chirwa SS, MacLeod BA, Day B, Intra-articular bupivacaine (Marcaine) after arthroscopic meniscectomy: A randomized double-blind controlled study, *Arthroscopy* (1989) 5: 33–35.
3. Wasudev G, Smith BE, Limbird TJ, Blood levels of bupivacaine after arthroscopy of the knee joint, *Arthroscopy* (1990) 6: 40–42.
4. Meinig RP, Holtgrewe JL, Wiedel JD et al., Plasma bupivacaine levels following single dose intra-articular instillation for arthroscopy, *Am J Sports Med* (1988) 16: 295–300.

2.4   Complications in arthroscopic surgery

Neal C. Small

Arthroscopic surgery has evolved from a curiously innovative surgical technique in the early 1970s to the definitive technique for much knee and shoulder surgery in the 1990s. As the technical equipment and surgical skills continue to improve, more avenues for utilizing arthroscopic surgical techniques are being implemented. It seems evident that these arthroscopic techniques will replace open surgical techniques now still being performed on various joints. Additional innovations, including the use of lasers in arthroscopy, will add even further to the usefulness and effectiveness of the surgical technique.

When surgical techniques evolve, complications resulting directly from these techniques can occur. Arthroscopic surgery is certainly no exception. Complications can and will happen and may be catastrophic.

Tabulation of complications in arthroscopic surgery is still relatively new.[1-7] Mulhollan was the first to report the incidence of complications in arthroscopy. In 1983, a retrospective survey was sponsored by the Arthroscopy Association of North America (AANA) and was completed.[8] The types of procedures reported in this survey were the early procedures that arthroscopists could perform at that time. These included partial meniscectomies, partial synovectomies, excision of plicae, lateral retinacular releases and procedures of a similar limited nature. The complication rate was found to be 0.6%. A second retrospective survey was completed in 1986.[9] For the first time, procedures on joints other than the knee were surveyed. More difficult procedures were being performed at that time, including meniscal repair, anterior cruciate ligament procedures, subacromial space procedures and stabilization procedures for shoulder instability. Procedures were also reported for the first time on joints such as the elbow, wrist and ankle. Once again, the overall complication rate was 0.6%. When the newer procedures were isolated in this overall survey, however, it was apparent that most of the more technically demanding procedures had a higher complication rate than the overall rate of 0.6%. There were a number of deficiencies in these retrospective studies. Despite these deficiencies, however, a starting point for further scrutiny of complications in arthroscopy was established.

It was felt that the bias of the retrospective study, including the tendency to overestimate the numbers of procedures being performed and to underestimate the numbers of complications, would be eliminated with a prospective multicenter study. This multicenter prospective study was begun in 1986. Twenty-one arthroscopic surgeons in various centers in North America participated in this study. Monthly reporting included the number of procedures performed, the types of procedures performed and any complications that occurred. Each complication was studied in significant detail. The study was begun in 1986 and completed in 1988.[10] In all, 10 262 procedures were reported. There were 173 complications. The overall complication rate was 1.7%. This confirmed the suspicions that the retrospective studies had provided an artificially low complication rate. The types of procedures recorded in this prospective study were similar to those in the 1986 retrospective survey. A large number of meniscal repair procedures, anterior cruciate ligament procedures and shoulder procedures were reported. Arthroscopic surgery of the hip was added to that of the other joints where complications from arthroscopic surgery had been reported.

The participants in the multicenter prospective study were all experienced arthroscopic surgeons (Table 1). The average participant had performed

Table 1 Experience level of participating surgeons.

	Average number of years diagnostic arthroscopy	Average number of years surgical arthroscopy
Knee	14.5	11.0
Shoulder[a]	7.2	6.1
Elbow[a]	7.2	6.6
Ankle[a]	7.1	6.6
Wrist[a]	9.6	9.3
Hip[a]	7.8	7.8

[a] Not all respondents performed arthroscopy on these joints.

diagnostic arthroscopy for 13 years and surgical arthroscopy for 10 years at the time the multicenter prospective study was initiated.

Types of complications (Table 2)

Hemarthrosis

The most frequent complication noted in both retrospective studies and in the prospective multicenter study is hemarthrosis. In the multicenter study, 1% of arthroscopic procedures resulted in a significant hemarthrosis. A significant hemarthrosis, for the purposes of the complications study, was defined as intra-articular bleeding that required either aspiration or surgical evacuation. The vast majority of hemarthroses occurred in the knee joint.

Infection

Infection is more common in arthroscopic surgery than the previous retrospective surveys suggested. The infection rate was previously estimated to be 0.07%. This would indicate one in 1500 procedures based on data obtained in the 1983 and 1986 retrospective surveys. In fact, however, the complication rate reported in the prospective study among this experienced group of arthroscopic surgeons was 1 in 500 procedures. The organism identified most frequently in infections was *Staphylococcus aureus* coagulase-positive.

Thromboembolic disease

Thromboembolic disease was found to be a significant problem in both retrospective surveys in the early and mid 1980s.[11] Thromboembolic disease continues to be a frequently reported complication in arthroscopy. Thromboembolic episodes have been studied, searching for a possible correlation with tourniquet usage. In addition, tourniquet time and inflation pressure of the tourniquet have been studied. No correlation has been found thus far. In the multicenter prospective study, four pulmonary emboli were reported but none was fatal.

Miscellaneous complications

In the earlier studies, instrument failure was reported quite frequently. The incidence has been dropping in recent years. The incidence was 0.05% in the recent multicenter prospective study. Reasons for a lower instrument failure rate may include new manufacturing techniques and quality-control improvements

Table 2 Types of complications (173 complications).

Complications	Incidence (%)	Number of complications
Hemarthrosis/hematoma	60.1	104
Infection	12.1	21
Thromboembolic disease	6.9	12
Anesthetic	6.4	11
Instrument failure	2.9	5
Reflex sympathetic dystrophy	2.3	4
Ligament injury	1.2	2
Fracture	0.6	1
Neurologic injury	0.6	1
Miscellaneous	6.9	12
Vascular injury	0	0
Total	100	173

among the various arthroscopic instrument manufacturers. In addition to instrument failure, other complications included medial collateral ligament ruptures. These are rather uncommon. Two were reported in the multicenter study. Both occurred during medial meniscal procedures. Eight anesthesia complications were reported. Two reflex sympathetic dystrophies were reported. One followed a knee procedure and the other followed a shoulder procedure.

Neurologic injuries

In both the 1983 and the 1986 retrospective surveys, neurologic injuries were reported with a frequency that was cause for significant concern. In the 1988 multicenter prospective study only one neurologic injury was reported. This particular occurrence was a saphenous nerve injury that occurred during a medial meniscus repair. The significantly lower incidence of neurologic complications among the experienced group of arthroscopic surgeons participating in the multicenter study is a reflection of improved knowledge of the anatomical positions and technical innovations. The location of the peroneal and saphenous nerves with various degrees of knee flexion has allowed meniscal repair techniques to develop that expose these neurologic structures to very little risk of injury from the needle or suture material. The use of accessory posteromedial and posterolateral incisions for meniscal repair, with retraction of the peroneal and saphenous nerves when necessary, has also contributed to a lower injury rate.

Vascular injuries

There was a small but significant incidence of vascular complications reported in the early retrospective surveys. The catastrophic nature of this complication is well known to all arthroscopic surgeons. No vascular complications were reported in the series of 10 262 procedures reported in the prospective study. Once again, improvements in meniscal repair techniques and techniques of anterior cruciate ligament reconstruction have led to this lowered incidence. Knee positioning during various procedures, along with the use of accessory posteromedial and posterolateral portals, has been a major factor. Techniques emphasizing suturing through contralateral portals while viewing through ipsilateral portals have also lessened the likelihood of injury to the popliteal artery.

Table 3 Incidence of complications for specific procedures (in decreasing order of frequency).

Complication	Incidence (%)
Lateral retinacular release	7.17
ACL synthetic reconstruction	3.7
ACL allograft reconstruction	3.3
Shoulder staple capsulorrhaphy	3.3
Arthroscopic synovectomy	3.12
Abrasion arthroplasty	1.89
Outside-in meniscal repairs	1.89
Medial meniscectomy	1.78
Plica excision	1.71
ACL autogenous reconstruction	1.71
Shaving chondroplasty	1.6
Medial meniscal repair	1.52
Lateral meniscectomy	1.48
Anterior acromioplasty	1.1
Debridement of glenoid labrum tear	0.5
Lateral meniscal repair	0

Complications in individual types of procedures (Table 3)

The single procedure with the highest complication rate is the lateral retinacular release. The complication rate for this procedure is 7.2%.[12,13] Almost all of these complications have been hemarthroses. A study of the complication rate in lateral retinacular release procedures was performed using the data obtained in the multicenter prospective study from 1986 to 1988.[13] Factors which correlated with an increased risk of complication during and following a lateral retinacular release procedure included the use of a tourniquet, a subcutaneous release under arthroscopic control, and use of a suction drain for more than 24 hours. The use of electrocautery did not correlate with a lesser incidence of hemarthrosis. The complication rate for meniscectomy was found to be slightly higher than that for meniscal repair in the multicenter prospective study. This reflected the experienced nature of the participants in this study and the improvements in meniscal repair techniques.

Among anterior cruciate ligament procedures, the complication rate overall was found to be 2%. The highest complication rate was in the synthetic ACL reconstructions. The complication rate for these procedures was 3.7%. For allograft reconstructions the complication rate was 3.3%. For autogenous ACL reconstructions the complication rate was 1.7%.

The anterior staple capsulorrhaphy of the shoulder had the highest complication rate among shoulder procedures. The majority of these complications were noted to be impingement or loosening of the staple. This often resulted in abrasion of the humeral head.

Because the number of procedures performed in joints other than the knee and shoulder were few, no significant conclusions could be drawn regarding the incidence of complications in these joints.

Conclusions

The complication rate in arthroscopic surgery is approximately 1.7% as determined in a multicenter prospective study concluded in 1988. The most frequent complication in arthroscopy is hemarthrosis. This occurs in approximately 1% of procedures. The infection rate in arthroscopic surgery is approximately 1 in 500 cases. The highest complication rate among individual procedures was found in the lateral retinacular release procedure (7.2%). The complication rate for meniscal repair has diminished compared to previous studies. This is related to improvements in meniscal repair techniques, including the use of posteromedial and posterolateral accessory incisions. The complication rate for meniscectomy has been found to be slightly higher than that for meniscal repair among this experienced group of arthroscopic surgeons. The highest complication rate found in procedures on joints other than the knee was the anterior staple capsulorrhaphy of the shoulder.

References

1. **DeLee J**, Complications of arthroscopy and arthroscopic surgery: results of a national survey, *Arthroscopy* (1985) **1**: 214–220.

2. **Fiddian NJ, Poirier H**, The morbidity of arthroscopy of the knee, *J Bone Joint Surg (Br)* (1981) **63**: 630.

3. **Gillquist J, Oretorp N**, Arthroscopic partial meniscectomy: technique and long-term results, *Clin Orthop* (1982) **167**: 29–33.

4. **Hershman E, Nisonson B**, Arthroscopic meniscectomy: a follow-up report, *Am J Sports Med* (1983) **11**: 253–257.

5. **Jackson RW**, Current concepts review: arthroscopic surgery, *J Bone Joint Surg (Am)* (1983) **65**: 416–420.

6. **Lindenbaum BL**, Complications of knee joint arthroscopy, *Clin Orthop* (1981) **160**: 158.

7. **Rorabeck CH, Kennedy JC**, Tourniquet-induced nerve ischaemia complicating knee ligament surgery, *Am J Sports Med* (1980) **8**: 98–102.

8. **Mulhollan JS**, Symposium: Arthroscopic knee surgery, *Can Orthop* (1982) **5**: 79–112.

9. **Small NC**, Complications in arthroscopy: the knee and other joints, *Arthroscopy* (1986) **2**: 253–258.

10. **Small NC**, Complications in arthroscopy, Presented at the AANA Annual Meeting, Washington DC, 25–27 March, 1988.

11. **Walker RH, Dillingham M**, Thrombophlebitis following arthroscopic surgery of the knee, *Contemp Orthop* (1983) **6**: 29–33.

12. **Small NC**, Complications in arthroscopic surgery performed by experienced arthroscopists, *Arthroscopy* (1988) **(4)3**: 215–221.

13. **Small NC**, An analysis of complications in lateral retinacular release procedures, *Arthroscopy* (1989) **(5)4**: 282–286.

2.5   Knee joint infection following arthroscopic surgery

Richard C. Maurer

Open orthopedic procedures have an overall postoperative infection rate of 1–2%. The infection rate following arthroscopy of the knee is lower. It is reported to be approximately 1 in 500 procedures, or 0.2%.[1] This low rate of postoperative infection does not warrant the prophylactic use of antibiotics. On the other hand, knowing that the risk is small may serve to assuage suspicion that postoperative pain is due to infection.

Certain arthroscopic procedures are associated with a higher risk of postoperative infections. This is true of arthroscopic lateral retinacular release procedures where postoperative infection rates range from 0.6% to 0.7%.[2] Extensive arthroscopic procedures, such as anterior cruciate ligament reconstruction and synovectomy, carry infection rates lower than those of lateral retinacular releases but greater than 0.2%.

Expectations are high with arthroscopic procedures. Patients and surgeons expect a minor procedure and good results. Unfortunately, postoperative pyarthrosis can quickly eliminate the advantages of minimal disability and rapid recovery normally associated with arthroscopy. As most arthroscopic procedures are done on an outpatient basis, it is sometimes difficult for the surgeon to be kept apprised of a patient's postoperative course. Patients should be instructed to contact their surgeons in the event of severe pain, increased swelling, or fever beginning the night of surgery and for 5 days postoperatively. The destruction of articular cartilage and the development of intra-articular adhesions progress from the onset of infection until the initiation of treatment. Therefore, in the event of an adverse outcome, the time of diagnosis and the beginning of active therapy may become a legal question.

The pathophysiology of postoperative knee joint infection includes a latent period of 24–72 hours. During this time the small inoculum of bacteria multiplies before becoming an invasive infection. Infections caused by most pyogenic organisms require 24–48 hours to become clinically symptomatic. The use of prophylactic antibiotics may delay the onset of overt symptoms. Some infections with organisms such as streptococci may become symptomatic within the first 24-hour period. The symptoms include increased pain with motion and swelling.

Since these symptoms also might be explained by postoperative hemarthrosis, it is not uncommon to confuse the two conditions within the first 24 hours.

Once a postoperative pyarthrosis is established, the organisms, the degradation of white blood cells, and the release of lysosomes further evoke a synovial inflammatory response. This will eventually degrade the articular cartilage ground substance. The damaged cartilage is susceptible to abrasive wear. This results in the joint space narrowing and the postinfection arthritis seen in the radiographs of advanced cases. In extreme cases of untreated pyarthrosis, total loss of articular cartilage, spontaneous bony ankylosis, and adjacent osteomyelitis may occur. The goal of therapy is to prevent this sequence of events by draining the inflammatory and enzymatic products from the joint and to provide appropriate antibiotic therapy to the joint space in bactericidal levels.

Aspirate the joint at the first suspicion of infection and send a specimen for a Gram's stain and cell count. If the Gram's stain is negative but the cell count is greater than 1000 white cells per high power field, start a broad-spectrum antibiotic such as a cephalosporin. This will cover Gram-positive cocci while the culture results are awaited. Staphylococcus is the most commonly infecting agent. In an otherwise healthy patient, an aminoglycoside might be added until the culture report rules out a Gram-negative organism. If the Gram's stain reveals Gram-positive cocci, then cephalosporin is sufficient. When the culture results and sensitivities are known, the antibiotic regimen can be adjusted.

The initiation of joint drainage is critical and should be started when the diagnosis of pyarthrosis is established. There are various methods of knee joint drainage, varying from repeated daily needle aspiration to the insertion of a drain tube for continuous or intermittent suction drainage, and finally an open drainage procedure. I have found that insertion of a 16-French sterile nasogastric tube through an arthroscopic sheath allows for the inspection of the joint and the irrigation removal of any hemarthrosis clot. The large size of the drainage tube maintains patency. The tube attaches to a closed intermittent suction system. Use of this closed suction drainage system avoids contamination with adjacent skin bacteria, which may result in a secondary infection, a risk in an open drainage procedure.

Intravenous antibiotic administration will usually achieve sufficient intra-articular concentrations. Antibiotics generally reach the intra-articular space in approximately the same concentrations as found in the blood. It has been my experience that the use of intermittent instillation of antibiotics within the knee joint, via a closed suction drainage system, is beneficial in increasing the efficiency of the tube drainage system.[3] It keeps the tubes open and increases the concentration of locally active antibiotics that would not be achievable by a systemic route. I have used gentamicin 0.1% and polymyxin 0.1% as a local antibiotic combination that covers both cocci and Gram-negative rods. Up until recently, 1% kanamycin was used rather than gentamicin, but kanamycin is no longer available. Instillation is done via the suction drainage tube at the maximum of 10 ml twice a day. The suction drainage is turned off for a 3–6-hour period to allow the antibiotics to bathe the synovial and articular surfaces. Suction is re-instituted for 6–9 hours between antibiotic instillations. This local antibiotic protocol is generally well-tolerated in patients with normal renal function. Antibiotic balance studies have shown that 50% of the antibiotic is removed by the suction drainage system and 50% is absorbed. In previous studies, there was no traceable level of kanamycin on testing blood levels at the dosage used. Approximately 25%

of the antibiotic is excreted in the urine. The remaining 25% is either metabolized or excreted in stool. The tube method of suction drainage and intermittent antibiotic instillation allows for drawback cultures of joint fluid for monitoring of the bactericidal effect of therapy. Cultures are usually negative by 7 days of therapy and tube instillation and drainage may be discontinued by 10–14 days after three negative cultures.

Protect the joint from both weight bearing and a vigorous range of motion until the patient has clinically responded to the treatment. A gentle range of motion should be encouraged during therapy to avoid restraining adhesions. After responding to therapy, if the knee has a limited range of motion, consider a manipulation under anesthesia or an arthroscopic debridement with lysis of adhesions. Non-weight-bearing range of motion exercises and the use of a continuous passive motion device may facilitate rehabilitation and recovery of motion.

References

1. **Small NC**, Complications in arthroscopic surgery performed by experienced arthroscopists, *Arthroscopy* (1988) **4:** 215–221.
2. **Small NC**, An analysis of complications in lateral retinacular release procedures, *Arthroscopy* (1989) **5:** 282–286.
3. **Jergesen F, Jawetz E**, Pyogenic infections in orthopaedic surgery, *Am J Surg* (1963) **106:** 152–163.

3

Meniscus disorders and transplants

3.1   Meniscal transplantation — Where do we stand?

Steven P. Arnoczky

The importance of the menisci to the well-being of the knee joint has been well documented and has provided the impetus for preserving these structures whenever possible. Although meniscal repair has become an accepted mode of treatment for selected injuries, it is not applicable in every instance, and partial and even total meniscectomy may still be necessary. Because of the deleterious effects of total meniscectomy on the knee joint, the orthopaedic surgeon has looked toward the possibility of replacing the severely damaged or absent meniscus with an allograft.

Basic science investigation into the preservation, healing, and function of meniscal allografts has demonstrated that meniscal transplantation is feasible and provides an attractive alternative to total meniscectomy. However, many considerations, including the need for a viable cell population, the development of appropriate preservation techniques, the use of immunologic assays to examine the antigenicity of the allografts, and the long-term biomechanical and biochemical analyses of the transplanted tissues, must be explored in detail before the potential of using allografts to replace the meniscus can be fully understood. In addition, more practical questions such as donor criteria, sizing, and surgical technique must be addressed.

As can be seen in Dr Garrett's contribution (3.2), the use of meniscal allografts to replace absent or severely injured menisci has been taken from the experimental laboratory to the clinical patient. Although long-term results will tell us whether this transition has occurred too quickly, the initial results appear promising. Hopefully, meniscal transplantation will continue to evolve through the careful and controlled application of basic science data and clinical experience.

3.2   Meniscal transplantation

John C. Garrett

A new appreciation of the function of the meniscus has altered the philosophy regarding surgery. Three decades ago total extirpation was advised to obviate the possibility that residual pathology might linger within the depths of the knee. Total meniscectomy was accepted and considered the norm. However, although the short-term effect of complete meniscectomy was relatively innocuous, the long-term effect could not be ignored.[1-11]

Laboratory studies have revealed the importance in load bearing and the effect of meniscectomy in increasing point contact stress and wear in articular cartilage.[12-23] These findings prompted partial rather than total meniscectomy.[24] Short-term morbidity measured in terms of pain, stiffness and swelling is less, as are long-term degenerative changes. If partial is to be preferred over complete meniscectomy, then repair is still better.[25,26] The majority of repairs withstand the long-term rigors of physical activity, especially in a stable knee. Although studies have not demonstrated a protective effect of meniscal repair against degenerative changes, it is assumed that a repaired and competent meniscus will work similarly to a previously undamaged one.[27,28]

A second important meniscal function is that of enhancing stability. In an anterior cruciate deficient knee, loss of a major portion of the medial meniscus, even simply of the posterior horn, increases antero-posterior instability.[29,30] The same is not true of the lateral meniscus.[31] Thus it seems logical that when reconstructing for anterior cruciate ligament deficiency there are occasions when the medial meniscus should be replaced as well.

If retention of competent meniscal tissue is considered desirable, then philosophically it is a short leap from meniscal suture to meniscal transplantation. Certainly there is little difference between suture of a long, fresh, peripheral bucket-handle meniscal tear and suture of a meniscal transplant. The number of sutures is nearly the same. The difference lies between suturing an avascular portion of the patient's own meniscus – which might be construed as an autograft – and suturing that of a distant donor – an allograft. This logic was what led orthopedic surgeons in Australia and Germany and more recently in the United States to initiate the transplant process.[32,33]

A short history of meniscal transplantation

Meniscal transplantation began in a limited sense when surgeons began to transplant large segments of the bony skeleton in order to replace defects left after resection for benign and low-grade malignant tumors or trauma.[34] When the entire proximal tibia was replaced the menisci were transplanted as well. Such extensive procedures are beset with a multitude of problems: sizing, balancing of collateral ligaments, and cruciate ligament reconstruction. Postoperatively, fracture and collapse are common. Meniscal grafts are subject to stresses that even in the best of knees would be detrimental to function. Nevertheless, cryopreserved menisci often retain shape and substance. Similar observations have been made of fresh menisci transplanted with fresh osteochondral allografts for treatment of malunion after tibial plateau fracture. Subsequent arthroscopy has revealed that 75% of these exhibited reasonable morphology.[35]

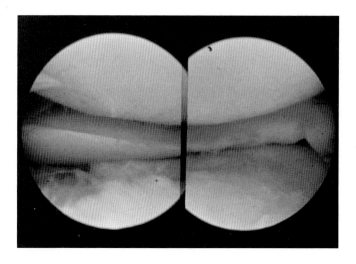

Figure 1

Follow-up arthroscopy at 6 months. Courtesy of Gregory Keene, Adelaide.

Legitimate free meniscal transplantation began May 24, 1984, when Milachowski transplanted deep-frozen and lyophilized menisci into the medial compartment of knees in 20 patients.[32] Subsequent arthroscopy in 14 revealed healing to the meniscal rim in all but one. However, shrinkage was sometimes noted and, subsequently some meniscal grafts have vanished entirely. In August 1985, Keene implanted a fresh, lateral meniscus in the knee of a soccer player with the hope of reversing problems of pain and degenerative disease noted after complete meniscectomy. Six months following implantation, arthroscopy revealed the meniscus had healed and retained its usual shape[33] (Figure 1). Thus, meniscal transplantation began with some success and optimism as well as noticeable failures that led clinicians to wonder whether technical details, tissue rejection, or lack of cryopreservation was at fault.

Laboratory experience of meniscal transplantation

Laboratory verification of the success of meniscal transplantation has been performed in dogs and sheep.[33,36,37] Arnoczky transplanted deep-frozen, cryopreserved menisci into the medial compartment of dogs with standard arthrotomy, the menisci being secured with multiple interrupted sutures[36] (Figure 2). When sacrificed at 3 months, 24 of the 25 menisci were noted to be healed. Cytologic studies reveal a diminished cell viability, but those that survived exhibited metabolic hyperactivity with ^{32}S uptake studies returning towards normal at 12 weeks. Instron testing of meniscal segments revealed normal tensile strength. Articular cartilage changes were minimal, whereas meniscectomized controls exhibited gross fraying and fissuring of articular cartilage of the medial femoral condyles. (The precise extent to which these menisci functioned in load bearing and preserved stability was not evaluated.) Thus, with relatively simple experiments, healing of meniscal tissue and reasonable preservation of cell viability and strength were demonstrated.

Immunology

Menisci, like heart valves and corneas, are felt to be 'immunologically privileged.'[36] This, however, is more assumption than fact. It is extrapolated from studies on articular cartilage where humoral and cell-directed antibodies can be detected but the rejection process is weak, presumably because antibodies are filtered by the cartilaginous ground substance and fail to reach their target, the chondrocyte. Although skin transplants exhibit necrosis and kidneys a diminution

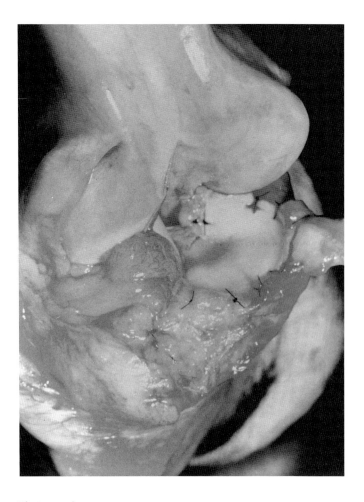

Figure 2

Medial meniscal transplantation in a dog. Courtesy of Steven P. Arnoczky, Hospital for Special Surgery, New York.

in glomerular filtration rate, it is uncertain how menisci might exhibit rejection. No specific reaction such as synovitis, pannus formation or necrosis has been observed with free fresh meniscal transplantation either in humans or in the laboratory. Whether more subtle manifestation may be present is a matter of conjecture. If, indeed, menisci are 'immunologically privileged,' then tissue typing is irrelevant and immunologic suppression is unnecessary.

Biologic glue

Although menisci are sutured in place, they ultimately bond by virtue of the normal healing process. This necessitates a vascularized bed. The vascular pattern of the normal meniscus appears to be largely dependent upon the geniculate system,[38] which may be damaged significantly by meniscectomy whether open or arthroscopic, leaving the remaining rim with hypovascular or avascular segments. The recipient rim probably 'sees' the collagen network of the transplant as it would that of its own meniscus. Healing occurs via a complex process, including a number of intermediary substances such as fibronectin and thrombospondin. Whether this process is altered by use of an allograft rather than autograft is unknown. The extent to which it might be enhanced by the use of autogenous clot or more specific 'activators' has not been studied.

Microscopic anatomy of transplantation

In transplantation there is a desire to transfer 'normal' meniscus into a deficient department. Microscopically, the anatomy includes a collagen framework, the intervening ground substance and the chondrocytes themselves, all of which are extremely important for function[39] (Figure 3). Longitudinal collagen fibers are thought to participate in the transfer of hoop stresses. Transverse fibers act to preserve the integrity of the meniscus by binding longitudinal fibers one to another and preventing cleavage. The ground substance probably participates in absorption of compressive loads as well as filtration of metabolites and antibodies. The chondrocytes sustain

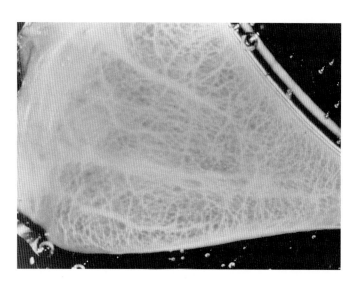

Figure 3

Cross-section of the mid-portion of the medial meniscus illustrating the intricate pattern of longitudinal and transverse collagen fiber bundles. Courtesy of Van C. Mow, Columbia College of Physicians and Surgeons, New York.

both of these structural elements. In meniscal transplantation it is desirable to have all three function optimally. If one is to have a robust, resilient meniscus then a young collagen framework is preferable to an old one. Similarly, it is desirable to have a meniscus that, because of viable chondrocytes, can replenish ground substance. It is a matter of conjecture whether viable chondrocytes must be transplanted with the meniscus or can be stimulated to migrate into a 'dead' meniscus.

Macroscopic anatomy of transplantation

If a meniscus is to continue to function, then it must be inserted into the normal load-bearing mechanism of the knee. The manner in which the meniscus interacts mechanically with the other parts of the knee is not completely understood. Meniscotibial attachments at the anterior and posterior horns probably act as firm anchors that aid in the creation of hoop stresses. The remaining rim, except where firmly attached to ligaments, may simply serve as a 'skirt' guiding anteroposterior motion, which may be enhanced in the case of the more mobile lateral meniscus by the popliteal muscle tendon unit. Theoretically it is desirable to restore as many of these mechanical linkages as possible. Suture of the meniscus to a reasonable recipient rim that is attached to the adjoining ligaments and tendons, and insertion of the anterior and posterior meniscal horn attachments, appears to achieve these goals.

Candidates for meniscal transplantation

Who is a reasonable candidate for meniscal transplantation? The matter is undecided. Undoubtedly the strongest argument can be made for the young individual who has undergone complete meniscectomy and predictably will develop significant degenerative changes in middle age. This is especially true of individuals who undergo removal of the lateral meniscus, which, when compared to the medial, seems more sorely missed and sooner to result in degenerative changes, especially in large, active persons. A second category for transplantation includes those who have an anterior cruciate deficient knee and lack a major portion of the medial meniscus. To fully stabilize these knees, anterior cruciate ligament reconstruction can be supplemented with meniscal transplantation. Some individuals also have significant chondral lesions that may prompt three-part reconstruction: meniscus, anterior cruciate ligament, and osteochondral graft of a femoral condyle, each transplant helping to preserve the function and integrity of the others. A reasonable argument can be made for transplanting menisci into a middle-aged individual in which no more than partial-thickness articular lesions are present. In these cases transplantation is used to decelerate degenerative changes and forestall the need for osteotomy or joint replacement. Similarly, transplantation may be of some value to the middle-aged individual with full-thickness articular lesions. Although significant meniscal abrasion by the rough articular surface is anticipated, the transplant is used to improve the load-bearing characteristics of the compartment and enhance the effect of osteotomy.

Matching

Donors are matched with recipients according to age. If transplantation is to achieve long-term success, it seems prudent to use young, robust menisci from donors in their second or third decade of life rather than risk the use of potentially frayed or fragile menisci from those in the fifth or sixth decade, when 20% exhibit degenerative tears. Similarly, menisci are matched according to size. A small meniscus is of little value when transplanted into a large individual: it simply will not fully fill the void and properly transmit loads. The reverse, transplantation of a large meniscus into a small individual, has somewhat greater value because trimming of the outer margin of the meniscus can be performed in order to 'down-size' the meniscus. However, to avoid undue damage to the intricate structure of the meniscus, sizing to within 5% is preferable.

Numerous techniques are currently available for sizing. Measurement of the diameter of the proximal tibia with a standard anteroposterior radiograph is a rough but pragmatic means of matching donor and recipient, especially when live material is used. In these cases, the potential donor is typically located in an intensive-care unit. Although standard radiographs can be taken, the transportation of the critically ill donor to a computed tomography (CT) or magnetic resonance imaging (MRI) scanner is medically undesirable and exorbitantly expensive. With cryopreserved tissue, direct measurements of the specimen can be matched with MRI or CT imaging for sizing of the menisci in the recipient's contralateral limb.

The desire to reproduce optimum joint mechanics argues for the isotopic (i.e. transplantation of right medial meniscus for right medial meniscal deficiency) rather than heterotopic transplantation, which requires that the meniscus from the contralateral limb be flipped upside-down to be used. Similarly, the difference in the shape between medial and lateral menisci suggests that they not be interchanged.

Screening of donors

Donors are screened by a multifactorial process according to the guidelines of the American Council of Tissue Banks. Screening begins with a careful social history to rule out high-risk groups, including intravenous drug users, prostitutes, runaways, homosexuals, and high-risk national groups. It continues with a medical history to rule out the possibility of systemic disease, including infection, neoplasia, and degenerative disease. Blood is screened for syphilis, types B and C hepatitis, and HIV disease, including antigen antibody testing. Donor tissues are cultured for bacterial and fungal infection. Finally, autopsy with lymph node evaluation is performed. As of 1989, the risk of transmission of HIV disease was calculated as 1 in 1 500 000.[40]

Harvesting

Harvesting is performed under sterile operating-room conditions immediately after the kidneys, heart, and lungs have been removed and life-support systems have been terminated. Knees are often excised en bloc from mid-femur to mid-tibia, ligaments and capsule included. Alternatively, they may be divided immediately to accommodate multiple transplantations: of femoral condyles, menisci, tibial plateaus, and ligaments.

Specimens are preserved in sterile tissue culture solution at 4°C (39°F) until transplantation occurs. No specific studies have been performed to determine how long menisci remain viable, but extrapolation from data on articular cartilage suggests that a major loss of viability of chondrocytes occurs after 7 days.[41]

Currently, a number of groups are working with cryopreservation. Using techniques similar to those used with heart valves, menisci treated with dimethyl sulfoxide are frozen at –196°C (–321°F) for unlimited periods. Studies by CryoLife, Inc., indicate a cell viability of 35%, the greatest number of viable cells residing on the surface of the transplants as opposed to the core.[42]

Transplant registry

As with soft organ transplantation, a number of individuals typically await transplantation at any given center. Requirements differ according to age and size, and the specific requirements of the transplant process. For instance, when a meniscus is transplanted with an anterior cruciate ligament, cryopreserved tissue may suffice. If it is combined with an osteochondral graft, then fresh rather than cryopreserved transplants must be utilized. Once the donor tissue has been identified and matched, recipients are gathered to the transplant site, which with modern air travel can be achieved within a day or two. Surgery can be performed during normal operating hours when the complement of transplantation team, anesthetists, and operating room personnel is available.

Transplantation procedure

Menisci have been transplanted by arthrotomy and arthroscopy. Arthrotomy has been utilized in order to firmly secure menisci and establish the feasibility of the transplantation procedure. It is necessary when menisci are transplanted with osteochondral allografts that cannot be implanted with arthroscopic technique. When menisci are transplanted alone or in conjunction with anterior cruciate ligament reconstruction, then arthroscopic technique offers the distinct advantage of lesser morbidity.

Technique: arthrotomy

For medial meniscal replacement, standard medial arthrotomy is carried out with lateral dislocation of the patella. With lateral meniscus replacement, exposure is facilitated with lateral arthrotomy combined with osteotomy of the tibial tubercle and medial dislocation of the patella. In either case reflection of the ipsilateral collateral ligament from its femoral origin facilitates exposure by permitting a greater distraction of the femoral and tibial articular surfaces. If the collateral ligament is detached with a flake of bone, it can easily be reattached with a 6.5-mm AO cancellous screw. With an anterior cruciate deficient knee, detachment of the collateral ligament and the ipsilateral arcuate complex permits gross forward subluxation of the tibial plateau, delivering the entire rim for transplantation and making the procedure quite straightforward. Once exposure is achieved, the meniscal rim is prepared. Assuming that the individual has previously undergone complete or near complete meniscectomy, a varying amount of rim remains. If 3–4 mm is left, it is trimmed until punctate bleeding, evidence of vascularity, is noted. Often the meniscus has been resected beyond the rim and only the fibrous meniscotibial attachment remains. This is trimmed without excessive resection so as to assure both vascularity and adequate residual tissue to secure the transplant.

When possible, it is desirable to insert the meniscal tibial horn attachments. These can be implanted in a conjoined manner with a bridge of bone and articular cartilage that is inserted into the tibial plateau, or separately with bone plugs secured with sutures (Figure 4). Occasionally the donor situation

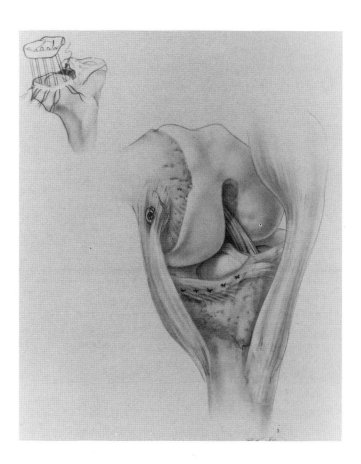

Figure 4

Free medial meniscal transplantation – arthrotomy technique. The medial collateral ligament is detached for exposure. The transplanted meniscus in this case is inserted with a bone bridge connecting the anterior and posterior meniscal horns. The remaining portion of the meniscus is then sutured to the residual rim with multiple permanent sutures of 00 Mersilene.

may dictate that no bony tissue is left for the meniscal tibial attachments, as is the case when anterior and posterior cruciate ligaments are harvested.

The meniscus is sutured in a standard fashion. Exposure dictates the type of suture utilized. Because of superior extraction strength, interrupted, vertically oriented sutures are utilized when possible. They can be used with anterior cruciate ligament deficiency when the collateral ligament is taken down and exposure is maximal. When intact then multiple, preplaced, interrupted vertical sutures may be placed through the posterior horn of the meniscus and rim. The meniscus is inserted, and the sutures are tied with a knot 'pusher' over the substance of the meniscus. Typically 2-0 or 0 meniscal sutures are used. Debate persists as to whether absorbable or nonabsorbable types are appropriate. In the author's experience, permanent sutures have been effective in securing the menisci without obvious detrimental

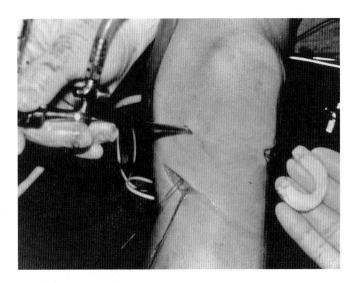

Figure 5

Arthroscopic insertion of a lateral meniscus.

suggests that reasonable healing occurs early, although the strength of this bond has not been tested in the laboratory. Continuous passive motion is desirable to facilitate nutrition of the transplanted meniscus. Motion is doubly useful when osteochondral grafts are also used and nourishment of the articular segment is also necessary. Whether weight bearing can be permitted immediately is a matter of debate. When the meniscus has been transplanted alone or in conjunction with an anterior cruciate ligament, weight-bearing has been initiated as comfort allows, typically within the first few days or weeks. When osteochondral allografts are implanted, it is delayed for 6 weeks.

Experience with free fresh meniscal transplantation

Over the past 5 years, the author has performed meniscal transplantation using fresh specimens. The desire has been to side-step problems of shrinkage as witnessed with frozen menisci. Menisci have been matched according to age and size, harvested under sterile operating-room conditions, maintained at 4°C (39°F) in tissue culture solution, and transplanted within 5 to 7 days. Because meniscal loss is often associated with a torn anterior cruciate ligament or chondral damage, almost all transplantations have been multiple, with one or both menisci transplanted in conjunction with anterior cruciate ligament reconstruction and osteochondral allografts of one or both femoral condyles.

effect to the joint. Timing of meniscal insertion depends upon the number of other transplantations to be performed. The best sequence seems to be meniscus, anterior cruciate, osteochondral allograft.

Arthroscopic insertion

With arthroscopic insertion, only a small, limber meniscus can be inserted. Therefore, it is impossible to insert the meniscotibial bony attachments as a conjoined unit with an intervening bony bridge. Instead, the meniscotibial ligaments may be inserted with bone plugs into drillholes and anchored with sutures led out anteriorly through the tibial metaphysis (Figure 5). Meniscal suture can be achieved by standard means. Some surgeons prefer a small posterior arthrotomy for suture of the posterior horn attachment. Interrupted vertical sutures tied over the meniscus with a knot passer from the anterior direction achieve the same end. Typically a dozen sutures suffice to secure the meniscus and permit early motion. To date, clot has not been utilized to enhance healing.

Postoperative care

Securing the menisci with a myriad of sutures seems to allow for early passive and active motion, although long-term studies are needed to determine the wisdom of this approach. Arthroscopy performed as early as 6–8 weeks following meniscal transplantation

Verification of success and transplant viability has been achieved. Although theoretically of value, arthrograms have not been utilized. MRI scans have been compromised because of the proximity of hardware in the ipsilateral femoral condyle at the site of reattachment of the collateral ligament. Arthroscopy has been performed after transplantation in 13 cases and it has demonstrated healing of all cases. Healing is complete from the superior to inferior surface of the graft. No statement can be made about the strength of the bond, but there is no indication that there would be any less than that achieved with standard meniscal suture. In contrast to the experience with frozen menisci, no shrinkage has been noticed. The crispness of the free meniscal edge is maintained and the substance of the meniscus appears to be normal (Figure 6).

In 8 of the 17 cases, meniscal transplantation has been combined with anterior cruciate ligament reconstruction utilizing a patellar tendon allograft. KT-1000 measurements at 15 lbs force revealed an average 1.8 mm side-to-side difference. This compared most closely to a group of 20 consecutive cases of anterior cruciate ligament reconstruction with an intact medial

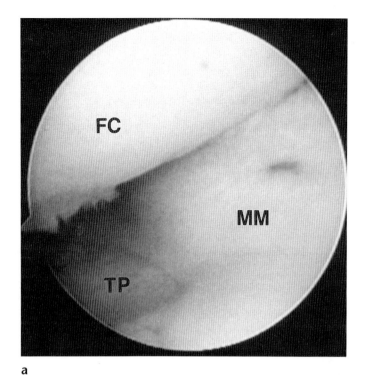

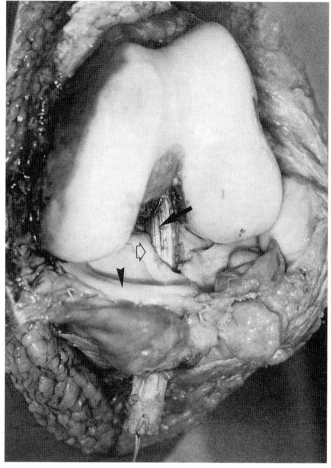

b

Figure 6

(a) Follow-up arthroscopy at 1 year. Note the sharp meniscal rim and absence of shrinkage. FC, femoral condyle; TP, tibial plateau; MM, medial meniscus. (b) Medial meniscal transplantation and anterior cruciate ligament reconstruction in a 42-year-old male.

meniscus, which had a 1.5 mm difference, and was a marked contrast to a second group of 20 patients with anterior cruciate ligament reconstruction who had undergone complete medial meniscectomy and in which the difference averaged 4.8 mm. These data suggest that medial meniscal implantation indeed enhances stability after anterior cruciate ligament reconstruction when performed in the face of deficiency of the major portion of the medial meniscus. Whether even better values might have been maintained with reconstruction utilizing an anterior cruciate rather than patellar tendon allograft is a matter of conjecture.

A more difficult question is whether medial meniscal transplantation restores normal load bearing and articular wear, thus reversing the trend toward degenerative arthritis typical of meniscal deficiency. Of the cases subjected to arthroscopy, one exhibited partial dissolution of an osteochondral allograft inserted in the ipsilateral femoral condyle, but otherwise none has exhibited any advancing articular damage. However, arthroscopy is usually performed some weeks to a year following meniscal transplantation;

only once has it been performed 2 years following meniscal transplantation, an interval too brief to permit any significant statement about articular wear.

The future of meniscal transplantation

Even at this early date several important trends are obvious. Having menisci of appropriate sizes banked and available when a recipient appears is preferable to waiting months or years for a donor. Thus cryopreservation has great appeal. As arthroscopic techniques advance, more menisci will be implanted with less morbidity. This will increase the appeal of and therefore probably the indications for the procedure. Conceivably, a given individual may undergo multiple transplants over the course of a lifetime. Allografts will always be in short supply even with the best of transplant programs. This, coupled with the fear of hepatitis and HIV infection, will create a demand for a meniscal prosthesis. A number of types have been utilized in small numbers.[43] Initial animal research with a collagen ingrowth type of prosthesis is currently being undertaken,[44] but as yet no satisfactory prosthesis is available for use in humans.

Conclusion

In general, meniscectomy results in degenerative arthritis. Medial meniscectomy increases instability in the anterior cruciate-deficient knee. Meniscal transplantation has been instituted for these two reasons. Menisci are transplanted fresh in order to maintain chondrocyte viability and minimize matrix degeneration and subsequent fraying and shrinkage. Rejection is felt to be trivial negating the need for tissue typing and immunosuppression. Follow-up studies reveal that menisci heal to the recipient ring, maintain normal morphology and increase stability. Laboratory studies suggest that metabolic and structural integrity is maintained and that the tendency to develop arthritis is aborted.

References

1. Medlar RC, Mandiberg JJ, Lyne ED, Meniscectomies in children: Report of long-term results (mean, 8.3 years) of 26 children, *Am J Sports Med* (1980) 8: 87–92.
2. Lynch MA, Henning CE, Glick KR, Jr, Knee joint surface changes: Long-term follow-up meniscus tear treatment in stable anterior cruciate ligament reconstructions, *Clin Orthop* (1983) 172: 148–153.
3. Tapper EM, Hoover NW, Late results after meniscectomy, *J Bone Joint Surg (Am)* (1969) 51: 517–526.
4. Johnson RJ, Kettelkamp DB, Clark W et al., Factors affecting late results after meniscectomy, *J Bone Joint Surg (Am)* (1974) 56: 719–729.
5. Allen PR, Denham RA, Swan AV, Late degenerative changes after meniscectomy: factors affecting the knee after operation, *J Bone Joint Surg (Br)* (1984) 66: 666–671.
6. Jørgensen U, Sonne-Holm S, Lauridsen F et al., Long-term follow-up of meniscectomy in athletes: A prospective longitudinal study, *J Bone Joint Surg (Br)* (1987) 69: 80–83.
7. Krause WR, Pope MH, Johnson RJ et al., Mechanical changes in the knee after meniscectomy, *J Bone Joint Surg (Am)* (1976) 58: 599–604.
8. Allen PR, Denham RA, Swan AV, Late degenerative changes after meniscectomy: Factors affecting the knee after operation, *J Bone Joint Surg (Br)* (1984) 66: 666–671.
9. Jackson JP, Degenerative changes in the knee after meniscectomy, *Br Med J* (1968) 2: 525–527.
10. Appel H, Late results after meniscectomy in the knee joint: A clinical and roentgenologic follow-up investigation, *Acta Orthop Scand* (1970) Suppl. 133: 1–111.
11. Huckell JR, Is meniscectomy a benign procedure? A long-term follow-up study, *Can J Surg* (1965) 8: 254–260.
12. Baratz ME, Fu FH, Mengato R, Meniscal tears: The effect of meniscectomy and of repair on intra-articular contact areas and stress in the human knee: A preliminary report, *Am J Sports Med* (1986) 14: 270–275.
13. Kurosawa H, Fukubayashi T, Nakajima H, Load-bearing mode of the knee joint: Physical behaviour of the knee joint with or without menisci, *Clin Orthop* (1980) 149: 283–290.
14. Radin EL, De Lamotte F, Maquet P, Role of the menisci in the distribution of stress in the knee, *Clin Orthop* (1984) 185: 290–294.
15. Bourne RB, Finlay JB, Papadopoulos P et al., The effect of medial meniscectomy on strain distribution in the proximal part of the tibia, *J Bone Joint Surg (Am)* (1984) 66: 1431–1437.
16. Maquet PG, Van De Berg AJ, Simonet JC, Femorotibial weight-bearing areas: experimental determination, *J Bone Joint Surg (Am)* (1975) 57: 766–771.
17. Walker PS, Erkman MJ, The role of the menisci in force transmission across the knee, *Clin Orthop* (1975) 109: 184–192.
18. Ahmed AM, Burke DL, In vitro measurements of static pressure distribution in synovial joints. Part I: Tibial surface of the knee, *J Biomech Eng* (1983) 105: 216–225.
19. Brown TD, Shaw DT, In vitro contact stress distributions on the femoral condyles, *J Orthop Res* (1984) 2: 190–199.
20. Fukubayashi T, Kurosawa H, The contact area and pressure distribution pattern of the knee: A study of normal and osteoarthritic knee joints, *Acta Orthop Scand* (1980) 51: 871–879.
21. King D, The function of semilunar cartilages, *J Bone Joint Surg* (1936) 18: 1069–1076.
22. Seedhom BB, Dowson D, Wright V, Functions of the menisci: A preliminary study, *J Bone Joint Surg (Br)* (1974) 56: 381–382.
23. Shrive N, The weight-bearing role of the menisci of the knee, *J Bone Joint Surg (Br)* (1974) 56: 381.
24. McGinty JB, Geuss LF, Marvin RA, Partial or total meniscectomy: A comparative analysis, *J Bone Joint Surg (Am)* (1977) 59: 763–766.
25. DeHaven KE, Peripheral meniscus repair: An alternative to meniscectomy, *Orthop Trans* (1981) 5: 399–400.
26. Scott GA, Jolly BL, Henning CE, Combined posterior incision and arthroscopic intra-articular repair of the meniscus: An examination of factors affecting healing, *J Bone Joint Surg (Am)* (1986) 68: 847–861.
27. Baratz ME, Rehak DC, Fu FH et al., Peripheral tears of the meniscus: The effect of open versus arthroscopic repair on intra-articular contact stresses in the human knee, *Am J Sports Med* (1988) 16: 1–6.
28. Cabaud HE, Rodkey WG, Fitzwater JE, Medial meniscus repairs: An experimental and morphologic study, *Am J Sports Med* (1981) 9: 129–134.
29. Levy IM, Torzilli PA, Warren RF, The effect of medial meniscectomy on anterior–posterior motion of the knee, *J Bone Joint Surg (Am)* (1982) 64: 883–888.
30. Shoemaker SC, Markolf KL, The role of the meniscus in the anterior–posterior stability of the loaded anterior cruciate-deficient knee: Effects of partial versus total excision, *J Bone Joint Surg (Am)* (1986) 68: 71–79.
31. Levy IM, Torzilli PA, Gould JD et al., The effect of lateral meniscectomy on motion of the knee, *J Bone Joint Surg (Am)* (1989) 71: 401–406.
32. Milachowski KA, Weismeier K, Wirth CJ et al., Meniscus transplantation – experimental study and first clinical report, *Am J Sports Med* (1987) 15: 626.
33. Keene GCR, Paterson RS, Teague DC, Advances in arthroscopic surgery, *Clin Orthop* (1987) 224: 64–70.
34. Locht RC, Gross AE, Langer F, Late osteochondral allograft resurfacing for tibial plateau fractures, *J Bone Joint Surg (Am)* (1984) 66: 328–335.
35. Zukor DJ, Brooks PJ, Gross AE et al., Meniscal allografts— experimental and clinical study, *Orthop Rev* (1988) 17: 522.
36. Arnoczky SP, McDevitt CA, Cuzzell JZ et al., Meniscal replacement using a cryopreserved allograft: An experimental study in the dog, *Orthop Trans* (1984) 8: 293.
37. Canham W, Stanish W, A study of the biological behaviour

of the meniscus as a transplant in the medial compartment of a dog's knee, *Am J Sports Med* (1986) **14:** 376–379.

38. **Arnoczky SP, Warren RF,** Microvasculature of the human meniscus, *Am J Sports Med* (1982) **10:** 90–95.

39. **Beaupré A, Choukroun R, Guidouin R et al.,** Knee menisci: Correlation between microstructure and biomechanics, *Clin Orthop* (1986) **208:** 72–75.

40. **Buck BE, Malinin TI, Brown MD,** Bone transplantation and human immunodeficiency virus: An estimate of risk of acquired immunodeficiency syndrome (AIDS), *Clin Orthop* (1989) **240:** 129–136.

41. **Tomford WW, Henry WB, Trahan CA et al.,** The fate of allograft articular cartilage: fresh and frozen, *Transactions of the 30th Annual Meeting of the Orthopaedic Research Society,* February 6–9 (1984) 217.

42. **Brockbank KGM, McCaa C, Dawson PE et al.,** Warm ischemia limits: Protein synthesis/viability of cryopreserved menisci, *J Transplant Coordination* (1991) **1:** 121–123.

43. **Toyonaga T, Uezaki N, Chikama H,** Substitute meniscus of teflon-net for the knee joint of dogs, *Clin Orthop* (1983) **179:** 291–297.

44. **Stone KR, Rodkey WG, Webber RJ et al.,** Future directions: Collagen-based prostheses for meniscal regeneration, *Clin Orthop* (1990) **252:** 129–135.

3.3 Observations on the meniscus

Frederick W. Heatley

One of the remarkable features of a synovial joint is that it is capable of withstanding large stresses over many years but its articular surfaces have minimal capacity for repair. It is well known that if a knife cut is made in error in the top of the tibial plateau while doing an open meniscectomy, or a defect is put in the femoral surface with an arthroscopic scissor, both remain as permanent marks of the surgeon's lack of expertise. A respect for hyaline articular cartilage is one of the first things taught in surgical training. That same respect is unfortunately not always given to meniscal fibrocartilage although the response to trauma in the meniscus is similar, if not identical, to that of hyaline cartilage. Macroscopically, the meniscus appears tough and strong, but this is very misleading since at microscopic level it can readily be demonstrated that cartilage cells are very vulnerable. The standard response to trauma is for a zone of cell death to be surrounded by a zone of chondrocyte activity. Figure 1 shows the response to the simple experiment of merely putting a skin hook in the anterior horn of a rabbit's meniscus and applying a little gentle forward traction. The disruptive pathway of the skin hook is obvious, as is the zone of cell death and the chondrocyte activity, shown here with periodic acid–Schiff (PAS) staining. This chondrocyte response may produce large chondrocyte clusters (Figure 2). It is, however, very important to understand that this chondrocyte activity and division has very limited capacity, if any, for a functional repair. The cluster illustrated in Figure 2 lies adjacent to an experimental cut placed in the substance of the meniscus, but there has been no attempt at any repair of the cut itself. Although chondrocytes react and produce mucopolysaccharides, there seems to be no evidence that they are able to reconstruct the fibrous architecture of the meniscus or even to promote healing by fibrosis. The chondrocytes respond but they do not repair.

Is there any other biological capability, in or around the meniscus, that surgeons could possibly utilize to promote repair? Although a number of papers have been published over the last decade, the most important paper remains of King,[1] which was written over 50 years ago. In a series of simple experiments performed on dogs, he established the scien-

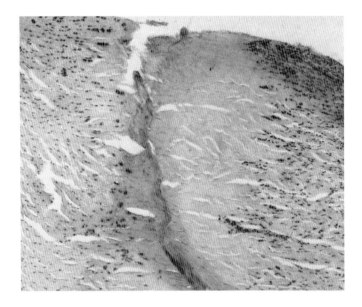

Figure 1

Response to a skin hook placed in the anterior horn of a rabbit's meniscus. Note the track of the hook, the zone of acellularity and the reaction of the chondrocytes surrounding the acellular zone. Stained PAS technique, ×40.

tific basis for treating meniscal injuries. He demonstrated the following three facts:

1. A cut in the body of the meniscus does not heal.
2. A cut through the periphery of the meniscus at or near its synovial attachments will heal.
3. A cut in the substance of the meniscus which extends peripherally into the synovium may sometimes heal.

The first of King's observations confirmed what orthopaedic surgeons had found in clinical practice. Although the first operation performed on the meniscus by Annandale in 1885[2] had been an apparently successful suturing of a torn meniscus, this operation had fallen into disrepute by the turn of the century and was condemned by Sir Robert Jones.[3] The clinical importance of King's second observation was not appreciated until 20 years after he published his

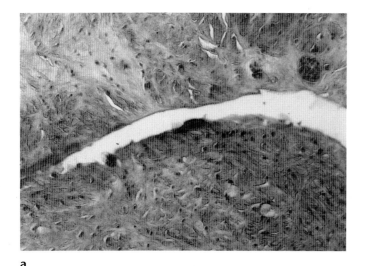

a

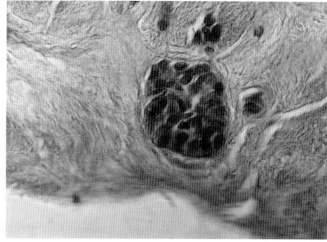

b

Figure 2

A large chondrocyte cluster lies adjacent to an experimental cut placed in a rabbit's meniscus. Although the chondrocytes have divided, there is no evidence of any attempt at repair. (a) ×51; (b) ×340.

findings. Hughston and Barrett[4] eventually proved not only that it was unnecessary to excise a peripherally detached meniscus when carrying out an acute repair for complete rupture of the medial ligament, but that the long-term results were superior when the meniscus was retained. It is only in the last decade that surgeons have shown an interest in King's third observation, namely that there was a possibility of healing if a cut in the substance of the meniscus extended to the peripheral synovial margin. In the rabbit, Heatley[5] achieved healing of an experimental bucket-handle tear by excising the peripheral rim of the meniscus. He believed that there were two basic requirements for successful repair:

1. A cellular ingrowth which was derived from the peripheral synovial and subsynovial cells.
2. Stability of the retained bucket-handle, which he achieved by suturing it to the synovium to close the peripheral gap.

He also demonstrated that when this technique of peripheral excision was applied to incomplete bucket-handle tears (in his experiments a vertical incision had been placed through the substance of the anterior horn and the meniscus between the incision and the peripheral margin excised) not only could the resulting defect heal with fibrous tissue but this tissue resumed the shape of the original meniscus (Figure 3). Arnoczky and Warren,[6] in a series of elegant experiments in the dog, achieved healing by creating a vascular 'channel' through partial excision of the peripheral part of the meniscus lying between

the experimental cut and the synovium. Ghadially et al.[7] experimented with a synovial flap which they rotated down into the experimental incision.

Whilst none of these techniques was entirely reliable, they did demonstrate that there were biological possibilities which surgeons might be able to manipulate. In essence both Heatley, and Arnoczky and Warren were exploiting the same biological response as leads to the regeneration of a peripheral fibrous rim following a total meniscectomy. This response had been experimentally investigated in the 1930s by Bruce and Walmsley,[8,9] who demonstrated in a series of studies on rabbits and dogs that meniscal regeneration only occurred if a total meniscectomy was carried out. It was of course this observation which was used for many years to support the operation of total meniscectomy in man. Unfortunately, the clinical evidence in man is that meniscal regeneration occurs only to a very limited extent. The regrown structure rarely equals the size of the normal meniscus and very rarely, if ever, matches the thickness.

However, whilst man may be less good than the dog at regenerating a meniscus-like structure, there is clinical evidence that man may respond rather better and more reliably than experimental animals to surgical repair. Certainly on an experimental basis one would expect a very high incidence of failure from simple suturing. Clinically, meniscal repair was pioneered by DeHaven,[10] who carried out his first repair in 1976 and reported a series of 55 operations with a 5-year follow-up in 1985. He had an 11% re-

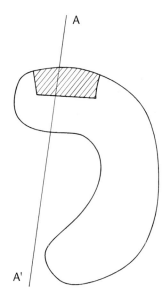

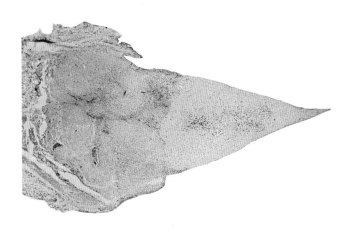

a   b

Figure 3

(a) A diagram to illustrate the area excised from the anterior horn of a rabbit's meniscus. Line A–A' illustrates the plane of the section of Figure 3(b). The shape of the anterior horn has been reformed but the tissue is much more cellular. It is fibrous tissue rather than fibrocartilage. ×19.5.

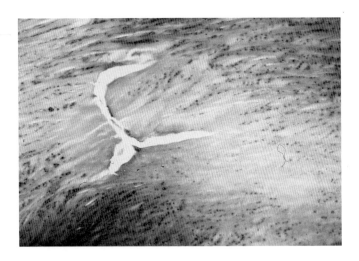

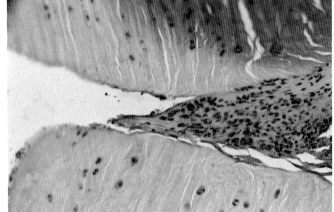

Figure 4

A gauge-22 hypodermic needle has been passed through the meniscus in a vertical direction. Six weeks later a zone of cell death surrounds the needle track. There is no attempt at repair. ×80.

Figure 5

The needle has been passed transversely into the meniscus via the capsule, that is through the meniscosynovial junction. Note the proliferation of cells penetrating into the needle track from the subsynovial region. ×120.

tear rate and all his failures occurred in cases in which he had carried out late repair. One of the most informative papers is that of Hamberg et al;[11] they used DeHaven's technique, but their follow-up protocol included a repeat arthroscopy. Whilst 8 of their 50 patients required further meniscal surgery, only 4 were failures of the surgical technique since the other 4 had a new tear in another part of the meniscus. Most of the patients in this series had anterior cruciate deficient knees and this probably remains the best indication for considering meniscal repair.

A number of surgeons have reported similar good results from arthroscopic repair. A recent paper by Hanks et al.[12] found no statistical difference between open repair, done in 26 cases, and arthroscopic repair, done in 45 cases. The overall failure rate was 9.8% (11% in the open repair group and 8.8% in the arthroscopic repair group). Interestingly, this study contained a subset of 23 patients with anterior cruciate ligament (ACL) deficient knees who elected not to have a ligament repair but to have a meniscal repair only. The re-tear rate in this group was 13% in comparison to 8% for ACL stable knees. However, because of the small number of patients this result did not produce any statistical difference between the two groups.

Most surgical repair techniques, whether open or arthroscopic, involve the passage of sutures out through the meniscosynovial junction and into the capsule of the joint. What actually happens at cellular level to the suture track is not only interesting but may have considerable importance.[13] As with other forms of trauma, merely passing a needle vertically through the substance of the meniscus will create a standard response, namely the persistence of the needle track, a surrounding zone of cell death and more peripherally a zone of cell reaction (Figure 4). However, when a needle is passed from the periphery into the meniscus, that is through the subsynovial layer, then this needle track will form a microscopic channel down which the peripheral cells can penetrate and invade into the body of the meniscus (Figure 5). Absorbable sutures may well increase this capacity and assist in cellular migration since it is the incitement of a cellular response that leads to suture absorption. It may well be this mechanism which explains the fact that the results of suture in man are rather better than one would expect on the basis of experimental findings in animals.

It is also of note that, following the work of Arnoczky and Warren,[14] nearly all the articles published about meniscal repair have laid great stress on the meniscus being vascular in its outer third and assumed that because it is vascular it will therefore repair. However, the distance that blood vessels penetrate into the meniscus is variable and there are

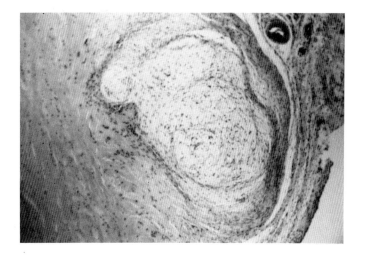

Figure 6

An example of a cyst arising at the meniscosynovial junction in a rabbit's knee at the site where a needle had been passed transversely through the capsule into the meniscus. ×120.

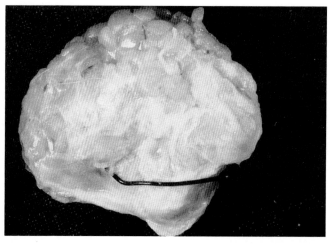

Figure 7

A meniscal cyst plus nylon suture. This clinical specimen was obtained by kind permission of Mr Adrian Henry, to whom the patient had been referred for a second opinion. He had previously undergone a simple suturing of a bucket-handle tear. Not only had the suture failed but the trauma to the synovial tissues at the periphery had resulted in the formation of this meniscal cyst. From *Current Orthop* (1987) **1**: 163, by kind permission of Churchill Livingstone.

zones, such as the posterolateral corner of the lateral meniscus adjacent to the popliteus tendon, which are avascular. One would expect a high failure rate from simple suturing in any avascular zone and the reported clinical success rate is perhaps circumstantial evidence that the penetration of cells and blood vessels along suture tracks is an important repair mechanism. Biologically, therefore, there are advantages and disadvantages in passing a suture through the meniscus.

Current advances in arthroscopic technique appear to be enabling surgeons to suture vertical posterior horn tears that lie further from the synovial margin. Using the 'all-inside' technique, Morgan[15] has repaired tears up to 4 mm from the periphery, with the suture being placed first through the peripheral meniscal rim and secondly through the mobile meniscal fragment. Morgan stresses the importance of adequate debridement of the peripheral rim and excoriation of the local synovium. If other surgeons merely follow his actual suture technique and ignore the debridement, they may well provide only temporary stability and not permanent healing. However, having advocated 'damaging' the meniscosynovial junction it is important to realize that there is also a biological price to be paid for inflicting this insult. Both experimentally and clinically it has been shown that damage to this junction can result in the development of a meniscal cyst (Figures 6, 7). Fortunately, this only seems to be a rare complication. Pathologically, meniscal cysts are similar if not identical to other ganglia and in the author's opinion there has been a great tendency to overtreat them. Unless there are intra-articular symptoms, it seems unnecessarily destructive to carry out any form of meniscectomy. As the first line of treatment, rupture of the cyst with a large needle under local anaesthetic as an outpatient procedure, seems preferable and usually more in keeping with the extent of the patient's symptoms than an anaesthetic and arthroscopy!

Over the last decade, surgeons have demonstrated a very innovative ability to manipulate biology, but it is all too easy for us to be beguiled by our own technical brilliance. Whilst the argument in favour of repairing a peripheral vertical meniscal tear in a knee with instability would seem to be valid, the long-term benefit of repairing a meniscus in a knee with normal alignment and no instability most certainly remains to be proved. The argument always put forward for meniscal repair is that it will lower the incidence of osteoarthritis later in life. Unfortunately, we do not yet know this figure in a stable, well-aligned knee.

The previous generation of knee surgeons were, with some notable exceptions, very poor at diagnosing anterior cruciate instability, and furthermore there is only one retrospective study which makes any attempt to relate the incidence of a post-meniscectomy osteoarthritic change to leg alignment radiographs.[16] From the world literature one can cull a figure of approximately 20% for post-meniscectomy radiological change with half that number, only 10% of the total, having significant clinical symptoms some 20 years after their meniscal surgery. However, it is most important to realize that this figure is derived from patients having meniscectomies for a variety of reasons. Straightforward arthroscopic excision of a bucket-handle tear of a meniscus in a patient with normal leg alignment and no ligamentous instability probably has a very low chance, much less than 10%, of developing clinically significant osteoarthritis. One must, therefore, pause and question whether the technically more demanding procedure of meniscal repair, which has a longer recuperative period and in inexperienced hands a significant complication rate, is in fact valid in the stable, well-aligned knee even though it is biologically and technically feasible.

In their excellent post-mortem study on the incidence of degenerative change in the meniscus, Noble and Hamblen[17] used the following histological criteria for the basis of the diagnosis: mucoid degeneration, chondrocyte proliferation with the production of clusters, chondrocyte degeneration and areas of acellularity. With the exception of mucoid degeneration, all these features can be noted in a meniscus a few weeks after it has been subjected to experimental trauma. One cannot help wondering whether our present advances of both diagnostic arthroscopy combined with the use of a probe and meniscal repair will actually lead to an increase in the incidence of horizontal cleavage tears and even osteoarthritic change later in life. Certainly, the hypothesis that repair will lead to a lower incidence of degenerative change than partial or even total excision remains to be proved.

Acknowledgments

My grateful thanks are due to my colleague William Revell for his skilled assistance with the experimental studies and to Miss Kate Hampton for preparing the manuscript.

References

1. **King D**, The healing of semilunar cartilages, *J Bone Joint Surg* (1936) **18**: 333–342.
2. **Annandale T**, An operation for displaced semilunar cartilage, *Br Med J* (1885) **1**: 779.
3. **Jones Sir Robert**, Notes on derangements of the knee, *Ann Surg* (1909) **50**: 969–1001.
4. **Hughston JC, Barrett GR**, Acute anteromedial rotatory instability: Long-term results of surgical repair, *J Bone Joint Surg (Am)* (1983) **65**: 145–153.
5. **Heatley FW**, The meniscus – can it be repaired? An experimental investigation in rabbits, *J Bone Joint Surg (Br)* (1980) **62**: 397–402.

6. **Arnoczky SP, Warren RF,** The microvasculature of the meniscus and its response to injury: an experimental study in the dog, *Am J Sports Med* (1983) **11:** 131–141.

7. **Ghadially FN, Wedge JH, Lalonde J-MA,** Experimental methods of repairing injured menisci, *J Bone Joint Surg (Br)* (1986) **68:** 106–110.

8. **Bruce J, Walmsley R,** Replacement of the semilunar cartilages of the knee after operative excision, *Br J Surg* (1937) **25:** 17–28.

9. **Walmsley R, Bruce J,** Early stages of replacement of semilunar cartilages of knee joint in rabbits after operative excision, *J Anat* (1938) **72:** 260–263.

10. **DeHaven KE,** Meniscus repair in the athlete, *Clin Orthop* (1985) **198:** 31–35.

11. **Hamberg P, Gillquist J, Lysholm J,** Suture of new and old peripheral meniscus tears, *J Bone Joint Surg (Am)* (1983) **65:** 193–197.

12. **Hanks GA, Gause TM, Sebastianelli WJ et al.,** Repair of peripheral meniscal tears: Open versus arthroscopic technique, *Arthroscopy* (1991) **7:** 72–77.

13. **Heatley FW,** Mini Symposium. Soft tissue injuries of the knee – treatment – menisci, *Current Orthop* (1987) **1:** 160–164.

14. **Arnoczky SP, Warren RF,** The microvasculature of the human meniscus, *Am J Sports Med* (1982) **10:** 90–95.

15. **Morgan CD,** The "all-inside" meniscus repair, *Arthroscopy* (1991) **7:** 120–125.

16. **Allen PR, Denham RA, Swan AV,** Late degenerative changes after meniscectomy: factors affecting the knee after operation, *J Bone Joint Surg (Br)* (1984) **66:** 666–671.

17. **Noble J, Hamblen DL,** The pathology of the degenerate meniscus lesion, *J Bone Joint Surg (Br)* (1975) **57:** 180–186.

3.4   Cysts of the meniscus

Giancarlo Puddu, Guglielmo Cerullo, Massimo Cipolla and Vittorio Franco

Cysts can occur commonly at the lateral meniscus and very unusually at the medial meniscus, probably owing to the thickness of the peripheral portion of the lateral meniscus in relation to the medial, and to the fact that the central part is less vascular (Figure 1).

Injuries that produce tangential or compression forces on the lateral meniscus may start avascular necrosis in the central part of the lateral border, resulting in subsequent mucoid degeneration and development of a cyst. If the mucoid degeneration propagates only peripherally, it may leave the meniscus intact but with an external cyst. This is very unusual in the case of lateral meniscus but very frequent with the medial meniscus.

Generally (in 90% of cases) the lateral meniscus with cyst has a parrot-beak type flap tear or a horizontal lesion. Sometimes, tears occur centrally and spread peripherally; for example, the radial tears could cause cystic degeneration when they reach the periphery of the meniscus.

A cyst of the lateral meniscus normally spreads out in front of the collateral ligament or between the collateral ligament and the popliteus tendon, because at this level the capsule of the knee is thinner; a medial meniscal cyst can be located beneath the medial collateral ligament or in the posteromedial corner beneath the posterior obliquus ligament. More rarely, the cyst can be situated anterior to the medial collateral ligament.

Usually the medial menisci with cysts are intact, probably because the medial meniscus is more stable than the lateral and so less susceptible to horizontal tears. In such cases, when cystic degeneration begins in the periphery, it develops eccentrically and not towards the central border of the meniscus.

Symptoms

The symptoms of a lateral meniscal cyst are quite different from those of a medial meniscal cyst. Patients with a lateral meniscal cyst complain of lateral pain, especially during sporting activities; they often feel clicking, have occasional swelling and, very rarely, locking. Objectively, they present a lateral intumescence with tenderness on the joint-line. In contrast, patients with a medial meniscal cyst do not complain of any problems if the presence of the intumescence is excluded. Sometimes, especially in athletes, the cyst becomes painful owing to subsequent tendinitis of the semimembranosus that passes over it.

Surgical management

Medial meniscal cyst

Arthroscopic evaluation is performed under general anaesthesia with accurate probing of the posterior horn of the meniscus. Of the 12 patients of our series, 11 had an intact medial meniscus and only one had a complex degenerative tear that required arthroscopic subtotal meniscectomy.

Once the arthroscopic examination is over, we proceed to an *open cystectomy*. With the patient lying supine, the knee is flexed at 90° and the hip abducted and externally rotated ('figure of four' position), a longitudinal skin incision is made over the cyst. The posterior fibres of the medial collateral ligament and the anterior fibres of the posterior obliquus ligament are gently divided longitudinally, and the cyst that lies under this ligament is isolated. Often, it is possible to find a vascular pedicle originating from the periphery of the posterior horn of the meniscus. In this case, it is important to cut the pedicle after having tied it; otherwise, if the cyst has a large area of contact with the meniscal wall, it should be divided from the meniscus and if a horizontal tear is present, it should be freshened and closed with absorbable sutures (Figure 2).

Between 1982 and 1988, we treated 12 patients with this technique. There were 10 males and 2 females; their average age at operation was 35 years. At a follow-up of 4 years (range 2–8 years), there was no recurrence and the results were 100% good or excellent according to Tapper and Hoover's criteria.[1]

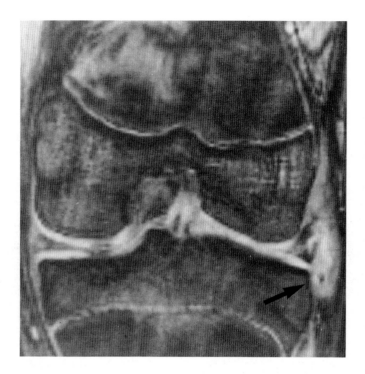

Figure 1

Magnetic resonance image showing a lateral meniscus cyst (arrow).

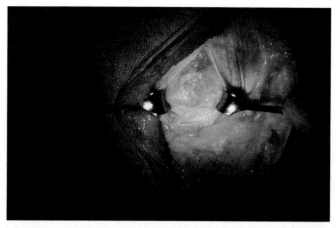

a

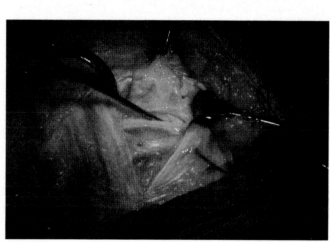

b

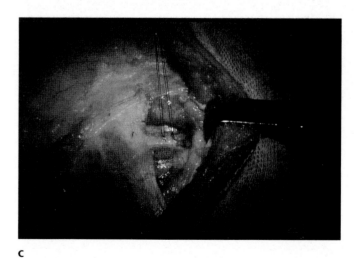

c

Lateral meniscal cyst

Arthroscopic evaluation is performed under general anaesthesia with a standard anterolateral portal and vastus medialis obliquus inflow. Of the 29 patients of our series, operated on between 1982 and 1989, 27 had a torn meniscus that required partial or subtotal arthroscopic meniscectomy. Two menisci were apparently intact. The lesions were horizontal tears (70%), parrot-beak type flap tears (20%) and radial tears (10%).

Whenever possible, we tried to leave an intact rim of the meniscus overlying the popliteus tendon, thereby providing more stability to the naturally unstable posterior horn of the lateral meniscus. This is in contrast to the technique suggested by Seger and Woods.[2] In very few cases, when an asymmetrical horizontal tear was found in which one of the two strips was thicker than the other, we removed only the thinner strip, hoping to retain as much as possible of the function of the meniscus.

Figure 2

Medial meniscal cyst. (a) The cyst. (b) The horizontal tear. (c) The tear is freshened and closed with absorbable sutures.

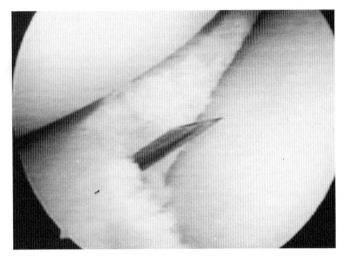

a

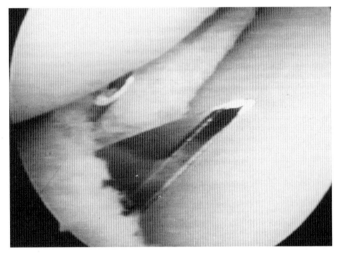

b

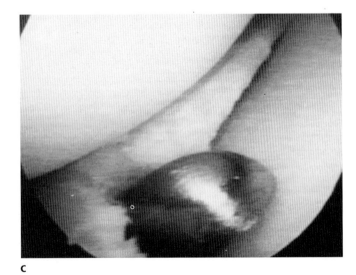

c

Figure 3

Arthroscopic treatment of the lateral meniscal tear and cyst.

Multiple percutaneous needle punctures were performed under arthroscopic control in all the cases and in many cases percutaneous curettage of the cyst and of the meniscus was undertaken. We prefer to freshen the meniscus by introducing a No. 11 scalpel blade right into the centre of the cyst, passing through the meniscus with the blade parallel to the joint-line ('out to in' technique) (Figure 3). If at this point the cyst can be easily decompressed, no further intervention is necessary. This was possible in 10 of the 27 torn menisci. In other cases, and especially when the meniscus was apparently intact, we proceeded to an open cystectomy.

Open cystectomy is performed through a small Bruser incision.[3] The iliotibial tract is divided along the line of its fibres with the knee flexed at 90°. The capsule is incised perpendicular to the joint-line, exposing the cyst, which usually has a narrow neck communicating with the meniscal tear. Following the cyst excision, the meniscal wall is freshened and, if necessary, repaired with a couple of absorbable sutures. Recently, Reagan et al. have published a paper showing almost the same technique.[4]

Postoperatively, the patient is kept non-weight-bearing for 1 week and then the routine management for arthroscopic meniscectomy is carried out.

Between 1982 and May 1988 we treated 29 patients (18 males and 11 females) with this technique; their average age at operation was 26.3 years (range 15–54 years). The mean postoperative follow-up was 4.2 years (range 2–8 years). We had 24 (82.7%) good or excellent results according to Tapper and Hoover's criteria.[1] Of the five poor results, four had a recurrence of the cyst 6–12 months after surgery, requiring open meniscectomy. The fifth case had persistence of pain and occasional swelling that required a second arthroscopic meniscectomy.

Before 1982 we treated the lateral meniscal cyst with open total meniscectomy technique, with no recurrences in 14 knees. At follow-up of less than 5 years we had nearly 95% good or excellent results. At follow-up of more than 10 years, five patients (35.7%) presented with radiological evidence of arthrosis in the lateral compartment with ingrowing functional disturbances.

The *open lateral meniscectomy*, when necessary, was made through the same approach (Bruser) as used for cystectomy[3] (Figure 4). Once the capsule is opened, the anterior one-third of the meniscus is resected with a scalpel and grasped with a Kocher. The freed part is then pulled and the middle one-third of the meniscus is released from the capsule with a Smillie knife. Great care must be exercised where the popliteus tendon separates the meniscus from the capsule. The excision of the meniscus is completed up to the posterior peripheral attachment, keeping the knee in a 'figure of four' position for better visualization of the lateral compartment.

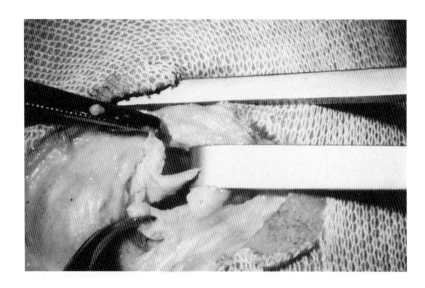

Figure 4

Open lateral meniscectomy.

References

1. Tapper EM, Hoover NW, Late results after meniscectomy, *J Bone Joint Surg (Am)* (1969) **51:** 517–526.
2. Seger BM, Woods GW, Arthroscopic management of lateral meniscal cysts, *Am J Sports Med* (1986) **14**(2): 105–108.
3. Bruser DM, A direct lateral approach to the lateral compart-

ment of the knee joint, *J Bone Joint Surg (Br)* (1960) **42:** 348–351.
4. Reagan WD, McConkey JP, Loomer RL et al., Cysts of the lateral meniscus: arthroscopy versus arthroscopy plus open cystectomy, *Arthroscopy* (1989) **5**(4): 274–281.

4

Biomechanics of ligamentous disorders of the knee

4.1   Placement of knee ligament grafts

Edward S. Grood

The knee is a complex mechanism in which the ligaments, capsular structures, menisci, joint cartilage, and bones all interact to provide normal motion and function. Following knee ligament injuries, it is impossible to precisely restore the normal anatomy and mechanical properties of the injured structures or the joint as a whole. Thus, some deficit in the properties and function of the knee always remains after surgery. As a result, controversy exists regarding the optimum surgical technique to stabilize the knee following ligament injuries.

The outcome of knee ligament reconstruction is influenced by numerous factors. Not all of the factors are well understood and some of them are not readily controllable. One factor that is under direct control of the surgeon is placement of the ligament graft. A variety of ligament replacements are currently available. They include various autograft and allograft tissues, grafts combined with synthetic augmentation devices, and total synthetic ligaments. The reader should understand that the reference to 'grafts' in the text is meant to be generic and that the information presented is applicable to many types of ligament replacements.

In this contribution, the term 'placement' is used to mean all the geometrical considerations pertaining to where the graft is implanted within the knee. This includes the route employed in passing the graft from tibia to femur (for example, 'over-the-top' versus through bone tunnels), the location of the intra-articular entrance of any bone tunnels or troughs (also called the attachment location), the orientation of the tunnels within the bones, any twists placed in the graft, and the site of its fixation to bone. Related factors that cannot be considered independent of placement are the amount of pretension applied prior to fixation and the position of the knee at the time of pretensioning.

Improper placement and tensioning are known to result in a number of post-surgical complications.

This contribution reproduced with permission from *Biology and Biomechanics of the Synovial Joint*, ed G Finerman, to be published in November 1992 by the American Academy of Orthopaedic Surgeons, Park Ridge, Ill.

These include a reduced range of motion immediately postoperatively, failure of the graft's attachment to bone, and incomplete removal of pathological laxity.[1] ('Laxity', as used here, is meant to connote joint displacements induced by the application of a force or moment without reference to the specific degree of freedom or direction of the displacement.) Other complications, such as the return of pathological joint laxity over time, might also result in part from improper placement.

Placement goals

A major goal of recent surgical placement techniques has been to locate attachments that yield an isometric graft.[2–10] The concept of isometry is a misnomer, since not all graft fibers are expected to remain isometric as the knee is flexed. The primary objective of isometric placement is to prevent excessive elongation or slackening of the graft as the knee is flexed or extended from the angle where the graft is pretensioned and fixed to bone. Excessive elongation produces graft forces that can limit the full range of motion, fail attachments to bone, and cause permanent stretching over time. Excessive slackening results in pathological laxity.

The achievement of intraoperative isometry is not the only goal sought in the selection of appropriate placement of a graft. Other goals include the avoidance of deleterious bone impingement, the restoration of normal relationship between physiological laxity and flexion angle, and the restoration of normal load-sharing among the ligaments.

It has not yet been established that locating isometric attachments is the proper or most important goal of placement. There are two possibilities that need to be considered in this regard. The first possibility is that intraoperative determination of isometric attachments might yield locations that are not isometric in the intact knee. Indeed, a number of factors have been identified which affect the intraoperative determination of isometric attachments. The second possibility is that since the majority of fibers in normal ligaments are not isometric, an isometric graft might not restore normal knee mechanics. A recent study by Galloway et al.,[11,12] in fact, suggests that a non-isometric intraoperative posterior cruciate graft is better in this regard than an isometric one.

In addition to attachment location, both the amount of pretension applied and the flexion angle where the graft is fixed (tensioning angle) are important variables,[13,14] since they establish the initial mechanical state of the graft and of the knee.

Lewis and co-workers[15–17] have also demonstrated abnormal load-sharing among the ligaments following reconstruction and have developed improved methods for tensioning that might allow the surgeon to more completely restore normal knee mechanics. Clearly, the goals of placement should not be limited to just obtaining isometric placement at the time of surgery.

Organization of this contribution

The remainder of the contribution is divided into three major sections. The first section, 'Basic concepts,' presents and discusses some of the properties of ligaments and ligament length patterns which underlie the concept of isometric placement.

The second section, 'Extra-articular reconstructions,' reviews studies on the isometry of both medial and lateral capsular and collateral ligament reconstructions. This section also includes a discussion of Burmester curves, which have been used to explain the attachments of the collateral ligaments and capsular structures as well as to predict appropriate bone attachments for extra-articular reconstructions.

The third section, 'Intra-articular reconstructions,' considers the cruciate ligaments. Emphasis is placed on the anterior cruciate ligament (ACL) because it is more frequently injured and reconstructed than the posterior cruciate ligament (PCL). As a result, the majority of published studies also focus on the ACL. The section begins with a summary of studies on the primary fibrous bands within the cruciate ligaments, since these studies provide the scientific foundation for their surgical restoration. The remainder of the section reviews studies on graft placement. This includes consideration of bone impingement, isometry and the effect of both placement and tensioning on the ability of the graft to restore normal joint motions (kinematics) and ligament forces. An important part of this section is a review of what is known about the factors that affect the intraoperative determination of isometric placement.

Basic concepts

As early as 1911, Fick[18] recognized that ligaments do not act as a single uniform structure. Rather, ligaments are comprised of fibers, often described as being grouped into two or three bands, that are not all tense at the same time. Fick noted that knee flexion angle was an important variable that determined which bands are tense and which are slack.

In the period since Fick's work it has been demonstrated that the location where ligament fibers attach to bone plays an important role in how knee flexion affects fiber tension. Fiber tension is important because it is an indicator that the fiber has been recruited to resist joint motions. The relationship between fiber tension, flexion angle, and attachment location is mediated by three separate relationships. The first is how the tension in a fiber depends on its length. The second is how the length of a fiber varies with knee flexion angle. The third is how the relationship between length and flexion angle depends on the fibers' attachment location.

Length–tension relation

The elastic properties of ligaments allow them to stretch and develop the tension needed to resist further tibiofemoral displacements or become slack and nonfunctional. An important concept to recognize is that ligament fibers develop tension only within a small range of lengths. This is illustrated in Figure 1, which shows a length–tension curve reconstructed from tensile failure test data on young human ACL fiber bundles.[19] When the distance between bone attachments is less than L_0, the fiber bundle is slack and nonfunctional. If the distance between attachments is more than $1.12–1.16L_0$, the fiber bundle fails and becomes nonfunctional. Thus, the fiber bundle can only function when its length is within a small range of lengths beginning at L_0 and ending with failure at lengths 12–16% greater than L_0. Since failure initiates in the upper region of this range, it is likely that normal function utilizes only the lower region of the range. This is shown by the shaded region in Figure 1. The size of this region has been estimated to include strains of 5% and less.[20] This estimate is supported by recent in-vivo measurements of strain in the ACL's anteromedial band. A strain of $4.0\% \pm 0.8\%$ was measured when a 150-N anterior shear force was applied to the knee at 30° flexion.[21] It is not yet known what strains and tensions are developed by locomotor and other activities of daily living.

Length–flexion angle relation

An important consequence of the fact that ligament fibers are only functional within a small range of lengths is that most fibers only function over a limited range of flexion angles. This results from the fact that the fiber's length varies with flexion angle. A curve that shows how the fiber's length depends on flexion angle is called a length pattern.

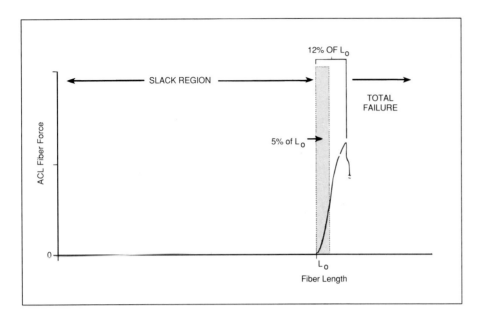

Figure 1

Force–length curve for human ACL fibers. Fiber force is shown as a function of the distance between attachments (length). The fiber is slack if the distance is less than L_0. Complete failure occurs when the distance between attachments is larger than about $1.16L_0$. In-vivo functional activities are thought to occur within the shaded region, which corresponds to fiber strain of only 5%.

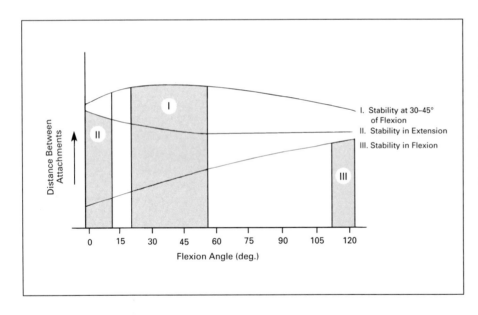

Figure 2

Three types of length patterns. Type I is appropriate for combating instability between 30° and 45° of flexion as this is the region in which the ligament, so positioned, would be tightest. Curve II would be appropriate for a situation where stability was sought in full extension, and curve III would be appropriate for achieving stability in flexion. Other patterns are also possible. (Revised from ref. 22.)

Length patterns of ligament fiber bundles and bands have been studied by numerous investigators. Because the actual length of a fiber bundle is hard to measure directly, investigators have often used the distance between attachments (DBA) in place of length. The distance between attachments and fiber length is only the same when the fiber follows a straight-line path between its attachments.

Figure 2 shows three different fiber length patterns described by Krackow and Brooks[22] based on studies of extra-articular reconstructions. Other length patterns are also possible. The shaded regions show the range of flexion angles within which the fiber is expected to develop a tension and be functional. The size of the region estimated by assuming the longest length on a curve corresponds to a fiber strain of 5%. When the length falls to a strain of zero, the fiber becomes slack and nonfunctional. Note that some fibers will function in extension (Type II), others primarily in flexion (Type III), or within an intermediate range of angles (Type I).

Dependence of length pattern on femoral attachment location

While a fiber's length pattern is affected by many factors, it is particularly sensitive to the location of the fiber's femoral attachment location and much less sensitive to the fiber's tibial attachment location.

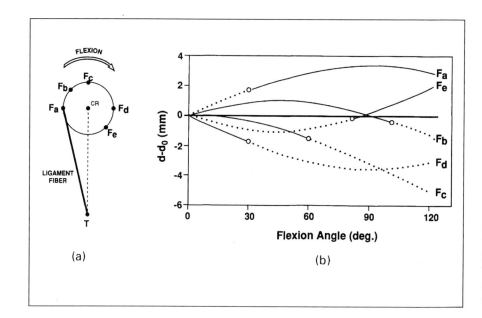

Figure 3

Length patterns are determined by the femoral attachment location. (a) A ligament fiber is shown with tibial attachment, T, and femoral attachment F_a. Other femoral attachments are represented by points F_b through F_e. The femur is assumed to flex about a fixed center of rotation, CR. (b) The graph shows how the distance between attachments (d) referenced to the distance between attachments at 0° (d_0) varies with flexion to 120°. The curves are solid in the region over which the ligament fiber is tense and dotted in the region they are slack. The functional region is obtained by assuming that the fiber is strained 5% at its maximum length.

Bartel et al.,[23] studying medial reconstructions, was probably the first to note this. Similar results have also been reported for the cruciate ligaments[24] and lateral extra-articular reconstructions.[22]

A simple model that explains these experimental findings and also shows how the length pattern is altered by a change in femoral attachment location was described by Grood et al.[3] The model is illustrated in Figure 3.

The tibia and tibial attachment (T) of a fiber are stationary in the model. It is assumed, for the sake of simplicity, that flexion of the femur occurs about a fixed center of rotation (CR). This fixed center is considered to be located at the average center of rotation for real knee flexion. With this simplification, all femoral attachments will follow circular paths about the center of rotation. The size of the circle (radius) is determined by the distance from the femoral attachment to the center of rotation. The circular path followed by the femoral attachments makes it easier to visualize how the length of any fiber changes with knee flexion.

Consider the fiber shown that attaches anterior to the CR at location F_a. This fiber will lengthen during the first 90° of flexion as its femoral attachment rises up the circle until it is directly above the center of rotation. Further flexion causes the fiber to shorten as its femoral attachment follows the descending portion of the circle. The length pattern for this fiber is shown in the graph. The curve is drawn as a solid line when the fiber length is within 5% of its maximum length (and assumed to be tense) and as a fine dotted line when it is shorter (and assumed to be slack).

In a similar fashion, length patterns were drawn for the four other femoral attachments (F_b–F_e). A wide diversity of patterns results with only small changes of the femoral attachment location. A fiber attached at site F_b lengthens during the first 45° of flexion and shortens during the last 90°. The opposite occurs with a fiber attached at site F_d.

The model shows that the overall shape of a fiber's length pattern depends upon where around the circle the fiber attaches. Further, it is easy to verify that the shape of the length pattern is not affected by the circle's radius. However, the magnitude of the change in length will be in direct proportion to the distance between the femoral attachment and the center of rotation.

The effect of changing the tibial attachment can also be studied with the model. Moving the attachment directly towards or away from the center of rotation (CR) will not change the basic shape of the length pattern, nor will it change the flexion angle where the fiber is longest and shortest. Moving the tibial attachment perpendicular to the line connecting it to the CR will also have only a small effect.

This small effect is primarily caused by how the change in tibial attachment location alters the relative position of the femoral attachment around the circle. The relative position is measured from the bottom of the circle, defined by the intersection of the circle with the line connecting the CR to the tibial attachment. If the tibial attachment of the fiber shown in Figure 3 is moved to the left, the bottom of the circle also shifts to the left, causing the femoral attachment site F_a to be located at a lower point on the rising side of the circle. This causes a small change in the flexion angles where the fiber is longest and shortest without changing the basic shape of the length pattern.

The model presented above is only approximate because the knee does not have a fixed center of rotation. Still, the basic features described can be seen in length patterns measured on human knees in vitro.

Contour plots

The finite size of a ligament's femoral attachment makes it impossible for all fibers within a ligament to have the same length pattern. To map out the behavior of the fibers requires a large number of length pattern curves. An even greater number of curves are required if one is interested in studying potential graft attachments that lie outside the anatomic insertion of the injured ligament. Sidles et al.[10] and others[3,4] have avoided this problem by using contour plots to illustrate the effect of femoral attachment location. A typical contour plot (Figure 4) is comprised of a series of contour lines. A single contour line contains all attachments that produce the same maximum fiber strain. The region bounded by the contour line with the smallest maximum strain contains the most isometric attachments. Thus, contour plots show both the shape and size of the region of most isometric attachments. The contour plots also show the directions along which a change in attachment location has the smallest and largest effect on maximum strain. These directions correspond to the direction along and perpendicular to the contour lines, respectively. Further the spacing between lines provides a visual clue as to how rapidly the changes occur. A disadvantage of contour plots is that they do not show the shape of the underlying length pattern curve. Thus, the flexion angles at which fibers are tense or slack are not presented. Further, each contour plot assumes a single tibial attachment.

Extra-articular reconstructions

Medial reconstructions

The earliest studies of placement[22,23,25,26] focused on extra-articular repairs and reconstructions. Bartel et al.[23] was probably the first investigator to recognize that length patterns were more sensitive to the femoral attachment site than to the tibial attachment site. They found that advancing the medial collateral ligament's (MCL's) femoral origin produced large ligament strains, while advancing the tibial attachment did not produce such strains. Since tibial advancements are more difficult to perform, some surgeons now choose to recess the MCL's femoral attachment into the medial condyle, thereby removing the slack in the ligament without changing its attachment location.

While most studies on placement have been based on the measurement or computation of length patterns, Menschik[25,26] has developed an alternate approach for determining acceptable attachments. This approach is based on both the four-bar mechanism model of the knee first proposed by

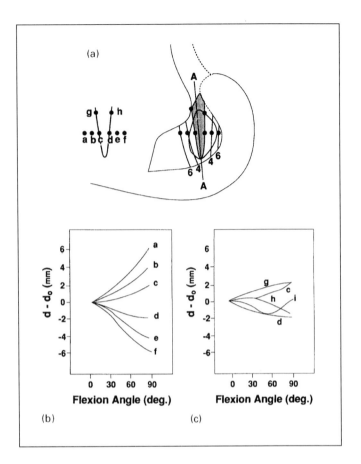

Figure 4

Typical contour plot for the anterior cruciate ligament in the lateral condyle. This figure was determined for knee flexion from 0° to 90° while an anterior force of 100 N was applied to the tibia. The tibial attachment site used in the analysis was located in the geometric center of the ACL's tibial insertion. (Reproduced with permission from ref. 4.)

Strasser,[27] (Figure 5), and on a mathematical theory for analyzing mechanism motion developed by Burmester.[28] In simple terms, Burmester's theory allows the determination of all pairs of femoral and tibial attachments that remain the same distance apart (i.e., the attachments are isometric) as the mechanism is moved through small (infinitesimal) motions. Collectively, the pairs of attachment points comprise two curves. These curves are called cubics because of their mathematical form. One cubic contains all possible femoral attachments, the other all possible tibial attachments (Figure 6). A single pair of attachments is obtained by drawing a straight line through the instant center for knee flexion. (In the four-bar mechanism model of the knee, the instant center for flexion is located at the point where the cruciate links cross each other.) The tibial and femoral attachments are the points where this line crosses the tibial and femoral cubics. All other pairs

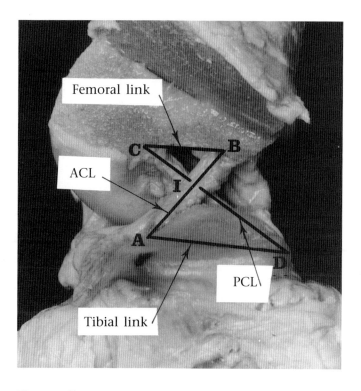

Figure 5

A human knee with the lateral femoral condyle removed, exposing the cruciate ligaments. Superimposed is a diagram of a four-bar linkage comprising the anterior cruciate ligament AB, the posterior cruciate ligament CD, the femoral link CB joining the ligament attachment points on the femur, and the tibial link AD joining their attachment points on the tibia. (Reproduced with permission from ref. 47.)

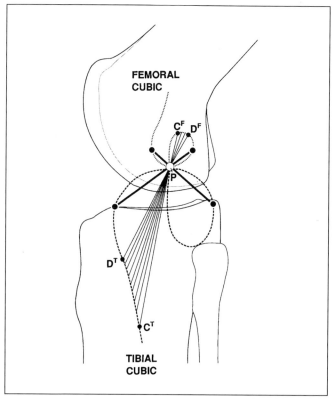

Figure 6

Burmester's curves for the four-bar mechanism. There are two separate curves, a femoral cubic and a tibial cubic. Pairs of nearly isometric attachments can be obtained by passing a line through instant center, P, and extending the line until it crosses both cubics. The points C^F and C^T where the line crosses the cubics are nearly isometric. Other pairs of nearly isometric attachments can be found by rotating the line about the instant center. The lines shown here represent theoretical fibers of the medial collateral ligament. (Redrawn with permission from ref. 29.)

can be obtained by rotating the line about the center of rotation.

Müller[29] has used Burmester's curves to explain the attachment locations of the collateral ligaments and capsular structures. This use of Burmester's curves appears to be supported by the good agreement between attachment locations found in Müller's dissections and the shape of Burmester's curves. There are several reasons, however, for believing Burmester's curves cannot be used to explain ligament attachments.

Müller[29] recognized that Burmester's theory is based on small motions of the four-bar mechanism. This led him to question whether the distance between pairs of Burmester's attachments remains isometric over a full range of knee flexion. J.A. Sidles (personal communication) found that while Burmester's attachments were not isometric, the change in length was indeed small. However, he also found tibial attach-

ments off Burmester's curve that were more isometric when the full range of knee motion was studied. While the region which contained these attachments was only a few millimeters wide in the proximal–distal direction, it covered nearly the entire width of the tibia in the anterior–posterior direction. Thus, the tibial Burmester's attachments are not more isometric than other attachments when a large range of knee motion is considered.

There is a second, and perhaps more significant, problem in the clinical application of Burmester's curves. Their shape is not unique and it depends strongly on the flexion angle assumed when they are computed. Menschik only published the curve for 43° flexion. Figure 7 shows curves computed for three flexion angles. The one for 43° agrees well with Menschik's curves. The others demonstrate the widely varying shapes that are possible with only small changes in flexion angle. None of the others

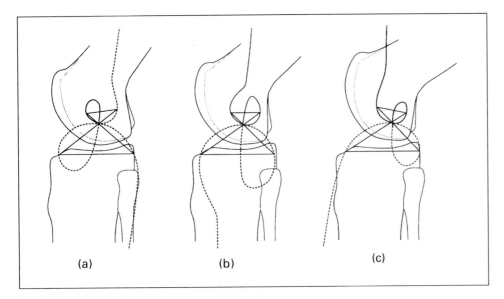

(a)   (b)   (c)

Figure 7

Burmester's curves computed for flexion angles of 33° (a), 43° (b), and 53° (c). The curve for 43° flexion is nearly identical to the curves published by Menschik[25,26] and Müller.[29] Note that most of the tibial cubics for 33° and 53° flexion are not even on the tibia, so that they are not possible ligament attachments.

shows any similarity to the attachments of the normal collateral ligaments. Further, there is no criteria for why the curve for 43° flexion should be used over the other curves.

Lateral reconstructions

Krackow and Brooks[22] measured the length patterns of a large number of tibial and femoral attachments for lateral extra-articular reconstructions and found that no pair of attachments was isometric. In order to eliminate a positive pivot shift sign, they recommended a pair of attachments whose length pattern was longest near 20–30° flexion. This ensures that the reconstruction will be under tension and able to resist tibial subluxation near these angles. The recommended femoral attachment was located at the junction of the lateral femoral condyle and the femoral shaft at site F_9 (Figure 8). The tibial attachment was located at Gerdy's tubercle, T_3 site. A length pattern for this pair of attachments is shown in Figure 9 along with several other femoral attachments paired with the same tibial attachment. The closest other femoral attachment studied, F_4, demonstrated a length pattern that was longest near 60° flexion.

Krackow's results are consistent with contour plots of maximum absolute strain (MAS) for lateral extra-articular reconstructions determined by Sidles.[10] These contour plots were determined from measurements of three-dimensional motion and bone anatomy of human cadaveric specimens. The resulting contour plots are shown in Figure 10 rotated and scaled to the same size as the adjacent figure from Krackow and Brooks. As noted above, the most isometric region is the one with the smallest MAS. This region is close to Krackow and Brooks' site F_4 and

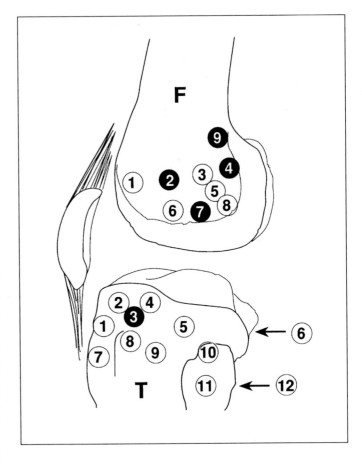

Figure 8

Extra-articular attachments studied by Krackow and Brooks. F = femur, T = tibia. Point F-5 is the origin of lateral collateral ligament at lateral epicondyle, T-10 is the insertion of lateral collateral ligament and T-3 is Gerdy's tubercle. (Reproduced with permission from ref. 22.)

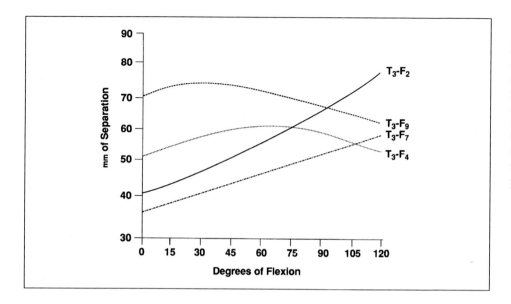

Figure 9

Each curve shown has been averaged over the five specimens after normalizing to a common mean. The widely differing contours of these four curves show the influence of changing the femoral attachment while the tibial connection, T-3, remains the same. (Reproduced with permission from ref. 22.)

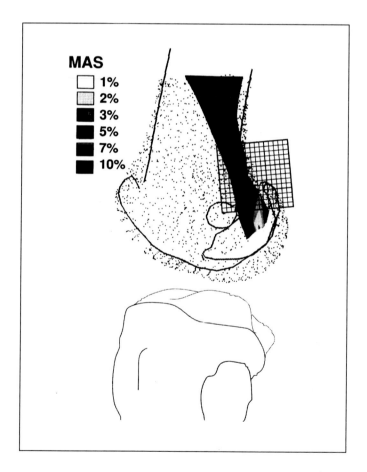

Figure 10

Extra-articular isometry map of Sidles for 0° to 110° of flexion. Tibial load is anterior during flexion. Articular surface and lateral aspect of knee are shown as scattered points. Lateral articular margin, lateral collateral ligament attachment, notch roof, lateral notch margin, and posterior femoral midline are continuous lines. The squares in the grid are 2 mm on a side. (Reproduced with permission from ref. 10. Additionally, the tibia has been added.)

is directly posterior to the femoral attachment of the lateral collateral ligament, and about 6 mm from the cartilage margin (Figure 10). However, the position of the region of smallest MAS varied greatly between knees. Sidles speculated that this variation was due to an observed sensitivity of extra-articular length patterns to axial tibial rotation.

Engebretsen et al.[30] studied the effect of an iliotibial band tenodesis, fixed at Krackow's F_9 site, on knee mechanics. The tenodesis was performed before and after an intra-articular reconstruction with a patellar tendon graft. The tenodesis held the tibia in an abnormal externally rotated position whether performed before or after the intra-articular reconstruction. In contrast, the intra-articular reconstruction did not alter tibial rotation. The tenodesis also unloaded the patellar tendon graft. The ability to unload the patellar tendon graft was greater when the tenodesis was performed after the intra-articular reconstruction.

Intra-articular reconstructions

Normal anatomy and length patterns

Knowledge of fiber function in a normal cruciate ligament is a prerequisite to the development of ligament substitutes or reconstructive procedures that mimic their function. Even after numerous studies,[6,18,31–38] there is no consensus on the anatomy of either cruciate ligament. In the ACL, some investigators identify two[18,31,33] or three[34,38] primary bands, while others maintain that the ACL is comprised of a continuum of fibers.[6,35–37] It is not surprising, therefore, that there is also disagreement on the flexion angles where fibers are tense and functional.

A point of general agreement is that the most isometric ACL fibers originate anteroproximally on the femur and insert anteromedially on the tibia.[4,10,36,38] However, disagreement still exists over the remainder of the ligament's anatomy and function. Fuss[36] has proposed that the ACL's fibers are progressively recruited, with only the most antero-medial fibers being tight in full flexion. With exten-sion, the remainder of the fibers become pro-gressively tense, starting with the most anterior fibers and moving toward the most posterior fibers, which are only tense in full extension. Amis,[38] however, reports that some posterior fibers are also tense in full flexion. Kurosawa et al.[39] describe the anteromedial band as being longest between 60° and 70° flexion, becoming shorter as the knee is brought to full flexion or full extension. A recent study by Blankevoort et al.[40] shows the anterior portion of the ACL to have a variable length pattern. In three knees it was slack in extension and in one knee it was tense only in extension.

Some of the disagreement in the literature was explained by Hefzy and Grood[24] who noted that ligament length patterns depend strongly on the location of the femoral attachment. They used this finding to show how differences among prior studies[41–45] could be caused by small differences in the femoral attachment locations used.

Regions of fiber lengthening and shortening

A number of investigators have more thoroughly studied how femoral attachment location affects length patterns of both the ACL[4,10,46,47] and the PCL.[3,10] These investigators found, for each cruciate ligament, that the femoral surface could be divided into two regions. Within one region the primary fiber response was lengthening, so that fibers were longer in flexion than extension. The reverse occurred for the other region. Fibers that attach at the boundary where the two regions meet have the same length in extension as in flexion. Bradley et al.[46] further subdi-vided each region on the basis of whether the initial length change with flexion was shortening or length-ening.

The line dividing the primary shortening and lengthening regions has a different orientation for the two cruciate ligaments (Figure 11). The line for the ACL is oriented primarily in the proximal–distal direction, so that anterior fibers are longer in flexion while posterior fibers are shorter.[4,10,24] The line for the PCL is oriented primarily in the anterior–posterior direction. Fibers proximal to the line are shorter in flexion, while those distal to the line are longer in flexion.

The amount of fiber lengthening and shortening was found to depend strongly on the distance between the fiber's origin and the line that separated the shortening and lengthening regions. This can be appreciated from the contour plots in Figure 4. The further the attachment is from this line, the greater the length change. In contrast, fibers attached along the line separating the regions had the smallest changes in length.

These findings have important implications for surgical reconstruction. They show that the effect of an error in placement depends on the direction of the error. Errors in placement perpendicular to the line will produce a much larger effect than the same error made in the direction of the line. For ACL grafts, placement errors in the anterior–posterior direction have the largest effect. Similarly, placement errors for PCL grafts are largest if the error is in the proxi-mal–distal direction.

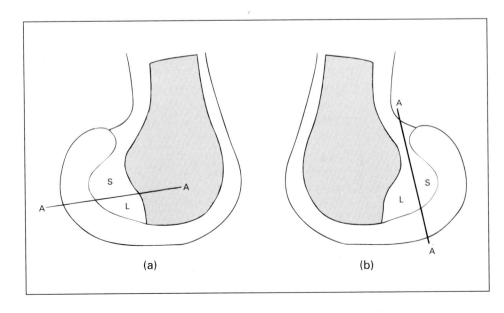

(a)　　　　(b)

Figure 11

The division of the femoral surface into shortening and lengthening regions. The line A–A dividing the regions has a different orientation for the two cruciate ligaments. Small errors in placement along the direction of the line have only small effects on length patterns. In contrast, placement errors perpendicular to the line cause large changes in length patterns. The text explains how the orientation of this line can be determined for other ligaments. (a) Shows the medial condyle; (b) the lateral condyle.

Similar rules for other ligaments of the knee, and the ligaments of other joints, can easily be obtained. All that is needed is to determine the orientation of the line that separates regions of fiber lengthening from regions of shortening. This is obtained from the orientation of the line connecting the average center of rotation and the center of the ligament's tibial attachment when the knee is midway in its range of flexion.

Studies on intra-articular graft placement

The preceding two sections considered studies conducted on intact knees. This section deals with placement studies where the anterior cruciate ligament was removed and reconstructed. Surprisingly, there are relatively few such studies. In analyzing the literature, the effect of femoral attachment location is considered first, followed by the effect of tibial attachment location.

Femoral attachment location

There are two basic approaches to the femoral attachment of grafts. The graft can either be fixed within a femoral tunnel or it can be pulled 'over-the-top' (OTT) of the lateral femoral condyle and fixed to the femur extra-articularly. Several investigators and clinical experience have shown that OTT reconstructions become slack with flexion, causing excessive anterior translation.[1,6,13] As a result, many clinicians place a trough in the femoral condyle so that the graft passes closer to the ACL's anatomical insertion. This technique has been shown to be more isometric than OTT alone and also to eliminate the excessive anterior translation with flexion. At the same time, the technique eliminates two advantages of the OTT alone approach. The first is the lack of rough bone edges that can cause abrasion. The second is the lower sensitivity of the result to surgical technique.[13] Instead of the reproducible and consistent graft shortening with flexion, the length pattern will depend on the variable depth of the trough. As a result, there is probably little difference between using the OTT technique with a trough and a properly placed femoral tunnel. The studies that support these statements and provide further information on femoral placement are described below.

Melhorn and Henning,[1] in a retrospective clinical review, showed that the pattern of A–P translation correlated with the graft's femoral attachment location. Twelve previously reconstructed knees were divided into three groups, based on femoral attachment location as determined from X-rays: anterior tunnel, OTT, and OTT with a deep bone trough. Anterior laxity of each group was measured in exten-

sion (20°) and flexion (90°). The authors found that (1) the anterior placement group was loose in extension but tight in flexion, (2) the OTT group showed the opposite pattern, being tight in extension and lax in flexion, and (3) only the deep bone trough group was tight at both flexion angles.

Penner et al.[7] showed that changes in the distance between graft attachments were associated with changes in graft tension. The greater the distance between attachments, the greater the tension. Tension was measured during knee flexion in four groups differing in femoral placement: anterior tunnel, posterior tunnel, OTT, and OTT plus trough. For each route they determined how much of the graft had to be withdrawn (or inserted) into the tibial tunnel in order to maintain a constant graft tension. Large tension changes were associated with the anterior tunnel and OTT groups. In the OTT group the graft had to be withdrawn from the tunnel as the knee was flexed to maintain a constant tension. The anterior tunnel group exhibited the opposite behavior. The extra-articular part of the graft had to be inserted into the tibial tunnel as the knee was flexed to maintain a constant tension. The smallest changes occurred for the OTT plus trough and the posterior tunnel groups. Unfortunately, the precise location of the femoral tunnels was not clearly described.

The results of these studies are, for the most part, consistent with each other and with the results of Bylski-Austrow et al.,[13] who measured length patterns in the intact knee and knee laxity and graft tension in the reconstructed knee. Three tunnel locations, anterior, distal, and posterior, were studied along with an OTT routing combined with four extra-articular attachment locations. Once the graft was passed 'over-the-top,' the results did not depend on where it was fixed to bone. Further, the variation in results for all OTT groups combined was much less than for any of the femoral tunnel locations. This suggests that the outcome of OTT reconstructions may be more consistent and reproducible than those of femoral tunnel reconstructions.

Overall, Bylski-Austrow et al., found that the knee had the least anterior laxity and the graft the largest tensions under conditions where the distance between attachments was longest. The only significant difference from the results of Penner were for the posterior tunnel. Where Penner et al.[7] found little change in tension with knee flexion, Bylski-Austrow et al. found both decreased tension and increased anterior translation with flexion. This disagreement might be due to differences in the location of the posterior tunnel used or to Bylski-Austrow's use of a fine cable substitute and Penner's use of the Kennedy LAD as a substitute.

Schutzer et al.[9] measured the length patterns in knees reconstructed with a 6-mm diameter synthetic replacement. They investigated the intact knee and reconstructions at three femoral attachments: anatomic, OTT, and anterior. The length pattern that was most similar to the intact knee was the anatomical tibial attachment combined with the anatomical femoral attachment. OTT femoral attachment produced significant shortening with flexion, while the anterior tunnel produced significant lengthening.

Tibial attachment location

Schutzer et al.[9] also reported on three tibial attachments: anterior, anatomic, and posterior. While none of the effects was statistically significant, there were a few possible trends. With an anteriorly placed femoral graft, a smaller length change could be obtained by moving the tibial attachment posterior. With an OTT placement, moving the tibial attachment posterior had the opposite effect and increased the length change. The effect of a posterior tibial attachment combined with an OTT placement was also noted by Penner et al.[7] Their observations, however, were based on only a few specimens and the statistical significance of the results was not tested.

Graf[2] also reported an effect of tibial attachment based on measurement made in cadaveric knees with a clinical isometer. A nearly isometric femoral attachment was used. A tunnel at the anterior edge of the ACL's tibial attachment resulted in about 2 mm of shortening with flexion. In contrast, a central tibial tunnel produced 4 mm of shortening, and the posterior tunnel just over 8 mm of shortening.

Overall, the data on the effect of tibial attachment are sparse and the effects produced are much smaller than those produced by similar changes in the femoral attachment location. On the basis of the available data, it does not appear that an error in femoral placement can be successfully compensated by changing the tibial attachment.

Intraoperative determination of isometric attachments

A number of commercial devices are now available to assist the surgeon in determining the location of isometric femoral and tibial tunnels.[2,48] Typically, these devices allow the surgeon to measure how the intra-articular distance between potential attachment points changes with knee flexion. Any pair of points for which the distance between attachments changes less than 2 mm over a full range of motion is considered clinically acceptable. Clancy[49] has noted that bone tunnels should be drilled eccentric to these points because grafts, once implanted, lie along one edge of the tunnel.

Existing commercial devices use one of three methods to determine isometric attachments intra-operatively. The first method is to pass a suture through small-diameter trial holes in each bone. The proximal end of the suture is attached to the femur. The distal end is attached to an isometer that measures relative motion between the suture and the tibia as the knee is flexed and extended. The isometer applies a small force to the suture to ensure that all slack is removed. The surgeon applies an external force to the tibia to ensure that it is fully reduced. If the relative motion between suture and tibia is too large, the location of the pilot hole is changed and the measurements are repeated.

The second method is to use a six-degree-of-freedom instrumented spatial linkage that measures both the intra-articular distance between selected attachments and knee flexion angle. This approach is considerably more expensive than the use of isometers as it requires, in addition to the instrumented linkage, a dedicated computer to collect and display the measurements.

The third approach is to use the drill-guide developed by Odensten and Gillquist.[50] The design of this guide is based on the authors' observations that isometric attachments have an intra-articular distance of 32 mm.[6] When compared to visualization and hand drilling, this drill guide reduced the variability of locating isometric attachments.[51]

Recent evidence shows that the use of isometers does not guarantee restoration of normal knee motion. Galloway et al.[11,12] found that PCL reconstruction whose placement was determined by using an intraoperative isometer resulted in poor control of posterior translation at 90° flexion. In contrast, a nonisometric placement restored normal posterior translation in both extension and flexion.

There are several possible explanations for these findings. A likely one is that intraoperative use of isometers might yield bad estimates of the isometric region.

Factors affecting isometric attachments

Blankevoort[52] noted that the isometric point may change postoperatively because the reconstruction itself alters knee motions. Many other factors affect knee motion, so it is reasonable to expect that these factors also affect length patterns and the location of the isometric region. Hefzy and Grood[24] stated that ACL length patterns should be determined in the intact knee while applying an anterior force to the tibia to ensure that the ligament is always under tension. Unfortunately, this is not possible at the time of reconstruction because the ligament has been ruptured.

Both Sidles et al.[10] and Hefzy et al.[4] found that the location of the most isometric region depended on whether an anterior or posterior shear force was applied to the tibia. Posterior forces, like those used to reduce the joint at surgery, caused the proximal portion of the isometric region to move anteriorly.

Sapega et al.[8] measured length patterns under operative conditions when both gravity and the surgeon applied a posterior shear force to the tibia. Three ACL bands were studied: anteromedial, central, and posterior. Corresponding femoral insertions were aligned from proximal (anterior band) to distal (posterior band). They concluded that the most isometric femoral attachment was located just superior to where the anteromedial fibers originate. However, they stated that these fibers will not appear isometric intraoperatively because the posterior shear force causes the fibers of the ACL to slacken during early knee flexion. Finally, Schutzer et al.[9] found that length patterns are affected by other injuries that are present. This effect was minimized when the other injuries were repaired prior to testing for isometry.

Pretensioning

Once placement is selected, proper pretensioning is required to ensure elimination of abnormal joint laxity. Since some joint laxity returns postoperatively, there is a tendency to obtain maximal reduction and tensioning at the time of surgery. However, excessive pretensioning might overconstrain the knee, producing high graft tensions that can stretch the graft and thereby contribute to the return of knee laxity.

Bylski-Austrow et al.[13] found that ACL graft tensions depended on the femoral attachment site, the tensioning angle, and the amount of pretension applied. No single level of pretension was found appropriate for restoring normal limits to anterior translation. Further, these authors found that the tensioning angle was as important as the amount of pretension in obtaining full reduction of the knee. Both the tensioning angle and the amount of pretension also affected graft tension when an anterior force was applied to the tibia. The highest graft tensions occurred when the knee was overconstrained and laxity was less than normal. An overconstrained condition was easiest to create (lowest pretension) at 30° flexion. This is where the intact knee has its greatest physiological A–P translation. Bylski-Austrow et al.[13] hypothesized that both tensioning angle and pretension magnitude exerted their influence by changing the ligament graft's initial intra-articular length.

Burks and Leland[53] found that the tissue used as a graft also affected the amount of pretension needed to obtain a normal 20-lb (90 N) KT-1000 test. The stiffest tissue used, patellar tendon, required the least pretension (3.6 lb; 16 N). The least-stiff tissue used, iliotibial band, required the largest pretension (13.6 lb; 60 N). Lewis et al.[14] found that joint position and graft force were highly variable, even when one surgeon performed all reconstructions and a constant 67 N (15 lb) pretension was used.

Ligament load sharing

Lewis and coworkers[15-17,54] have suggested that the primary goal of placement and pretensioning is not only to restore laxity to normal, but also to restore the forces in all joint tissues to normal. In support of this goal they noted that large changes in ACL graft force are associated with only small changes in knee laxity.[14] Thus, even if the joint laxity returns to normal, ligament forces may be abnormal. To obtain surgical control of graft force, Hunter et al.[17] developed a new tensioning device that enabled the adjustment of graft pretension while an anterior force of 90 N was applied to the tibia. In comparison to pretensioning with no anterior force applied to the tibia, they found that pretensioning with an anterior force returned all ligament forces closer to normal, and also reduced the size of the knee-to-knee variability.

Bone impingement

A major goal of proper placement is to avoid deleterious impingement of the ligament substitute with bone. Impingement becomes deleterious when it excessively stretches the graft, causes abrasion, or induces a fibrocartilaginous remodeling due to large compressive stresses. There are two primary locations of impingement. The first is against the roof and walls of the intercondylar fossa. The second is at the intra-articular exits of bone tunnels.

Impingement with the intercondylar roof

A normal anterior cruciate ligament lies along the roof of the intercondylar fossa when the knee is fully extended. Further, the distal portion of the ACL fans out and the most anterior fibers appear to curve around the junction of the fossa and trochlear groove prior to insertion into the tibia (D.L. Butler, personal communication, 1991). The fiber curvature just prior to the tibial insertion does not exist in grafts or synthetic replacements. Thus, a graft placed at the anterior edge of the ACL's tibial attachment can impinge on the roof of the intercondylar fossa at full extension. Impingement can also occur with the wall of the intercondylar fossa. The extent of this impingement is affected by the shape of the fossa, the presence of osteophytes, and the size of the ligament graft.

Impingement at tunnel exits

A second location of impingement occurs at the intra-articular exits of bone tunnels. Impingement at this location is probably not completely avoidable.

This is an area of potential severe abrasion because knee flexion causes the graft to bend and rub at the tunnel exit. Clinically, this impingement problem is reduced by putting a generous radius at the tunnel exit. Drill-guides have also been developed[50] that allow the surgeon to drill both tunnels at once so that they align with each other. Odensten and Gillquist[50] recommended drilling the tunnels with the knee at 90° flexion. Doing so would avoid impingement at the posterior exit of the tibial tunnel because the graft will pull away from this edge as the knee extends. The interaction between grafts and the tunnel edges has virtually been ignored by basic scientists. The only work to date on this subject appears to be that of Sidles,[55,56] who has measured large pressures within the graft at the tunnel exits. This pressure is induced by curvature of fibers as they wrap around the bone edge at the tunnel exit.

Biological effects of impingement

In addition to large internal pressures, a lateral compressive stress applied to tendons has been shown to induce a fibrocartilaginous response.[57,58] This response includes increased proteoglycan (aggrecan) content, and the cells become more rounded and appear to live in lacunalike chondrocytes.[57,58] Recently Howell[59] has reported radiographic changes in ACL grafts that impinge on the roof of the intercondylar notch. The significance of these changes to the long-term viability of the graft remains to be determined.

Acknowledgment

I would like to thank Kimberly Hamilton for her assistance. This manuscript was also prepared for an AAOS/NIH/AOSSM workshop entitled 'Biology And Biomechanics Of The Synovial Joint: The Knee As A Model.' Partial support was provided by NIH Grants AR 39703-03 and AR 21172-13 from the National Institute of Arthritis, Musculoskeletal, and Skin Diseases, and from the Cincinnati Sportsmedicine Research and Education Foundation.

References

1. **Melhorn JM, Henning CE,** The relationship of the femoral attachment site to the isometric tracking of the anterior cruciate ligament graft, *Am J Sports Med* (1987) **15**: 539–542.

2. **Graf B,** Isometric placement of substitutes for the anterior cruciate ligament, Jackson DW, Drez D Jr (eds): *The anterior cruciate deficient knee – new concepts in ligament repair* (St Louis: CV Mosby, 1987) 102–113.

3. **Grood ES, Hefzy MS, Lindenfield TN,** Factors affecting the region of most isometric femoral attachments. Part I: The posterior cruciate ligament, *Am J Sports Med* (1989) **17**: 197–207.

4. **Hefzy MS, Grood ES, Noyes FR,** Factors affecting the region of most isometric femoral attachments. Part II: The anterior cruciate ligament, *Am J Sports Med* (1989) **17**: 208–216.

5. **Hoogland T, Hillen B,** Intra-articular reconstruction of the anterior cruciate ligament: An experimental study of length changes in different ligament reconstructions, *Clin Orthop* (1984) **185**: 197–202.

6. **Odensten M, Gillquist J,** Functional anatomy of the anterior cruciate ligament and a rationale for reconstruction, *J Bone Joint Surg (Am)* (1985) **67**: 257–262.

7. **Penner DA, Daniel DM, Wood P et al.,** An in vitro study of anterior cruciate ligament graft placement and isometry, *Am J Sports Med* (1988) **16**: 238–243.

8. **Sapega AA, Moyer RA, Schneck C et al.,** Testing for isometry during reconstruction of the anterior cruciate ligament: Anatomical and biomechanical considerations, *J Bone Joint Surg (Am)* (1990) **72**: 259–267.

9. **Schutzer SF, Christen S, Jakob RP,** Further observations on the isometricity of the anterior cruciate ligament: An anatomical study using a 6-mm diameter replacement, *Clin Orthop* (1989) **242**: 247–255.

10. **Sidles JA, Larson RV, Garbini JL et al.,** Ligament length relationships in the moving knee, *J Orthop Res* (1988) **6**: 593–610.

11. **Galloway MT, Mehalik JN, Grood ES et al.,** Posterior tibial translation following PCL reconstruction, *Trans 1st Combined Meeting of the US, Canadian, and Japanese Orthopaedic Research Societies, Banff, Canada* (1991) 263.

12. **Grood ES, Mehalik JN, Galloway MT et al.,** Posterior cruciate ligament reconstruction: Effect of femoral attachment site location on posterior tibial translation, *Trans 1st Eur Orthop Res Soc* (1991).

13. **Bylski-Austrow DI, Grood ES, Hefzy MS et al.,** Anterior cruciate ligament replacements: A mechanical study of femoral attachment location, flexion angle at tensioning, and initial tension, *J Orthop Res* (1990) **8**: 522–531.

14. **Lewis JL, Lew WD, Engebretsen L et al.,** Factors affecting graft force in surgical reconstruction of the anterior cruciate ligament, *J Orthop Res* (1990) **8**: 514–521.

15. **Lewis JL, Lew WD, Hill JA et al.,** Knee joint motion and ligament forces before and after ACL reconstruction, *J Biomech Eng* (1989) **111**: 97–106.

16. **Lew WD, Engebretsen L, Lewis JL et al.,** Method for setting total graft force and load sharing in augmented ACL grafts, *J Orthop Res* (1990) **8**: 702–711.

17. **Hunter RE, Lew WD, Lewis JL et al.,** Graft force-setting technique in reconstruction of the anterior cruciate ligament, *Am J Sports Med* (1990) **18**: 12–19.

18. **Fick R,** Anatomie und Mechanik der Gelenke unter Berücksichtigung der Bewegenden Muskelen, *Handbuch der Anatomie des Menschen* (Karl von Bardeleben, 1911) Band II, Teil III.

19. **Butler DL, Kay MD, Stouffer DC,** Comparison of material properties in fascicle-bone units from human patellar tendon and knee ligaments, *J Biomech* (1986) **19**: 425–432.

20. **Crowninshield R, Pope MH, Johnson RJ,** An analytical model of the knee, *J Biomech* (1976) **9**: 397–405.

21. **Howe JG, Wertheimer C, Johnson RJ et al.,** Arthroscopic strain gauge measurement of the normal anterior cruciate ligament, *Arthroscopy* (1990) **6**: 198–204.

22. **Krackow KA, Brooks RL,** Optimization of knee ligament position for lateral extra-articular reconstruction, *Am J Sports Med* (1983) **11**: 293–302.

23. **Bartel DL, Marshall JL, Schieck RA et al.,** Surgical repositioning of the medial collateral ligament: An anatomical and mechanical analysis, *J Bone Joint Surg (Am)* (1977) **59**: 107–116.

24. **Hefzy MS, Grood ES,** Sensitivity of insertion locations on length patterns of anterior cruciate ligament fibers, *J Biomech Eng* (1986) **108**: 73–82.

25. **Menschik A**, Mechanik des kniegelenks, Tiel 3, *Z Orthop* (1974) 3–24.

26. **Menschik A**, The basic kinematic principles of the collateral ligaments, demonstrated on the knee joint, *Injuries of the ligaments and their repair*, ed Chapchal G (Stuttgart: Thieme, 1977).

27. **Strasser H**, *Lehrbuch der Muskel- und Gelenkmechanik* (Berlin, Springer, 1913).

28. **Burmester L**, *Lehrbuch der Kinematik* (Leipzig: A Felix Verlag, 1888).

29. **Müller W**, *The knee: Form, function, and ligament reconstruction* (Berlin: Springer-Verlag, 1983).

30. **Engebretsen L, Lew WD, Lewis JL et al.**, The effect of an iliotibial tenodesis on intra-articular graft forces and knee joint motion, *Am J Sports Med* (1990) **18**: 169–176.

31. **Girgis FG, Marshall JL, Al Monajem ARS**, The cruciate ligaments of the knee joint: anatomical and experimental analysis, *Clin Orthop* (1975) **106**: 216–231.

32. **Kennedy JC, Weinberg HW, Wilson AS**, The anatomy and function of the anterior cruciate ligament, *J Bone Joint Surg (Am)* (1974) **56**: 223–235.

33. **Furman W, Marshall JL, Girgis FG**, The anterior cruciate ligament: A functional analysis based on postmortem studies, *J Bone Joint Surg (Am)* (1976) **58**: 179–185.

34. **Norwood LA, Cross MJ**, Anterior cruciate ligament: functional anatomy of its bundles in rotatory instabilities, *Am J Sports Med* (1979) **7**: 23–26.

35. **Arnoczky SP**, Anatomy of the anterior cruciate ligament, *Clin Orthop* (1983) **172**: 19–25.

36. **Fuss FK**, Anatomy of the cruciate ligaments and their function in extension and flexion of the human knee joint, *Am J Anat* (1989) **184**: 165–176.

37. **Clark JM, Sidles JA**, The interrelation of fiber bundles in the anterior cruciate ligament, *J Orthop Res* (1990) **8**: 180–188.

38. **Amis AA, Dawkins GPC**, Functional anatomy of the anterior cruciate ligament: Fibre bundle actions related to ligament replacements and injuries, *J Bone Joint Surg (Br)* (1991) **73**: 260–267.

39. **Kurosawa H, Yamakoshi KI, Yasuda K et al.**, Simultaneous measurements of changes in length of the cruciate ligaments during knee motion, *Clin Orthop* (1991) **265**: 233–240.

40. **Blankevoort L, Huiskes R, de Lange A**, Recruitment of knee joint ligaments, *J Biomech Eng* (1991) **113**: 94–103.

41. **Edwards RG, Lafferty JF, Lange KO**, Ligament strain in the human knee joint, *Trans Am Soc Mech Eng* (1970) **92**: 133–136.

42. **Wang CJ, Walker PS**, The effects of flexion and rotation on the length patterns of the ligaments of the knee, *J Biomech* (1973) **6**: 587–596.

43. **Kennedy JC, Hawkins RJ, Willis RB**, Strain gauge analysis of knee ligaments, *Clin Orthop* (1977) **129**: 225–229.

44. **Dorlot JM, Christel P, Meunier A et al.**, The displacements of the bony insertion sites of the anterior cruciate ligament during flexion of the knee, In: *Biomechanics: principles and applications*, ed R Huiskes (The Hague: Martinus Nijhoff, 1982).

45. **Van Dijk R**, The behaviour of the cruciate ligaments in the human knee, Ph.D. Dissertation (Amsterdam: Rodopi, 1983).

46. **Bradley J, FitzPatrick D, Daniel D et al.**, Orientation of the cruciate ligament in the sagittal plane: A method of predicting its length-change with flexion, *J Bone Joint Surg* (1988) **70B**: 94–99.

47. **O'Connor J, Shercliff T, FitzPatrick D et al.**, Geometry of the knee. In: *Knee ligaments – structure, function, injury, and repair*, ed Daniel D, Akeson W, O'Connor J (New York: Raven Press, 1990) 163–199.

48. **Raunest J**, Application of a new positioning device for isometric replacement in anterior cruciate ligament repair and reconstruction, *J Trauma* (1991) **31**: 223–229.

49. **Clancy WG Jr, Nelson DA, Reider B et al.**, Anterior cruciate ligament reconstruction using one-third of the patellar ligament, augmented by extra-articular tendon transfers, *J Bone Joint Surg (Am)* (1982) **64**: 352–359.

50. **Odensten M, Gillquist J**, A modified technique for anterior cruciate ligament (ACL) surgery using a new drill guide for isometric positioning of the ACL, *Clin Orthop* (1986) **213**: 154–158.

51. **Good L, Odensten M, Gillquist J**, Precision in reconstruction of the anterior cruciate ligament: A new positioning device compared with hand drilling, *Acta Orthop Scand* (1987) **58**: 658–661.

52. **Blankevoort L**, ACL reconstruction: Simply a matter of isometry? In: Passive motion characteristics of the human knee: Experiments and computer simulation, Ph.D. Dissertation (The Catholic University of Nijmegen, 1991).

53. **Burks RT, Leland R**, Determination of graft tension before fixation in anterior cruciate ligament reconstruction, *Arthroscopy* (1988) **4**: 260–266.

54. **Hanley P, Lew WD, Lewis JL et al.**, Load sharing and graft forces in anterior cruciate ligament reconstructions with the ligament augmentation device, *Am J Sports Med* (1989) **17**: 414–422.

55. **Sidles JA, Clark JM, Huber JD**, Large internal pressures occur in ligament grafts at bone tunnels (abstract), *Transactions of the 36th Annual Orthopaedic Research Society Meeting, New Orleans, Louisiana, February 5–8* (1990).

56. **Sidles JA, Clark JM, Garbini JL**, A geometric theory of equilibrium mechanics of fibers in ligaments and tendons, *J Biomech* (1991) **24**: 943–950.

57. **Gillard GC**, The influence of mechanical forces on the glycosaminoglycan content of the rabbit flexor digitorum profundus tendon, *Connect Tiss Res* (1979) **7**: 37–46.

58. **Vogel K**, Proteoglycans accumulate in a region of human tibialis posterior tendon subjected to compressive force in vivo and in ligaments, *Trans 1st Combined Meeting of the US, Canadian, and Japanese Orthopaedic Research Societies, Banff, Canada* (1991) 58.

59. **Howell SM, Berns GS, Farley TE**, Unimpinged and impinged anterior cruciate ligament grafts: MR signal intensity measurements, *Radiology* (1991) **179**: 639–643.

5

Acute anterior cruciate ligament injury

5.1 Acute anterior cruciate ligament reconstruction: A review

Paul M. Aichroth

Reconstruction of the anterior cruciate ligament is required in the acutely injured knee when the diagnosis is confirmed, when the associated meniscal problem has been dealt with, and if the patient's activities, sports pursuits and general philosophy suggest that this is the right way to proceed. Full counselling is most desirable, for many patients with limited sports output will opt for muscle and knee joint rehabilitation and subsequent bracing of their knee joint for games and sports. The arguments and details of conservative management are outlined in contribution 6.2 by Malcolm Macnicol of Edinburgh.

It is now well accepted that direct repair of the anterior cruciate ligament in mid-substance is a total waste of time and that stability of the knee cannot be restored by this procedure. The replacement of a bony ossicle at the ligament's distal end (rarely proximal) will restore the cruciate length and anatomy adequately if the accuracy and stability of the bone reposition can be assured by internal fixation.

The two main procedures used for the acute anterior cruciate reconstruction are (1) patellar tendon transfer and (2) transfer of the medial hamstring tendons.

Patellar tendon graft

Bone–patellar tendon–bone grafting with accurate isometric position is successful. The procedure may be undertaken open and an 'over-the-top' technique is usually used. The arthroscopically assisted closed procedure is now the operation of choice for most knee surgeons. The procedure gives a very strong reconstruction and excellent stability as long as the anchorage at the proximal and distal ends is perfect. The bone segments of the graft are impacted into bone tunnels into the femur and the tibia and the addition of an interference screw secures the structure. Ronald Karzel and Mark Friedman's contribution on reconstruction using the central one-third of the patellar tendon is important. It is comprehensive, with exact details of technique and results which are carefully reported and analysed. Dilworth Cannon's comments are apt and should be read in association with this contribution.

One disadvantage is the size of the graft, for a large percentage of the intercondylar notch is taken up by the patellar tendon segment graft and adhesions in the notch may be substantial, preventing full extension in spite of all efforts to prevent it. A notchplasty will allow adequate room for the graft, but again adhesions may form at this site with local fibrosis. The revascularization of the large patellar tendon segment is very prolonged and may be incomplete. Nevertheless, this procedure appears to be the most popular throughout the world's knee surgery fraternity at the present time.

Medial hamstring transplant

An excellent alternative is the transplantation of the medial hamstring tendons: semitendinosus and gracilis. The technique is described in this chapter, both open and closed. Giancarlo Puddu and his co-workers from Rome report on the open and arthroscopic techniques and they found no significant difference between the two results.

The advantage of this technique is that the inferior fixation of the transplant is the natural tendon/bone insertion at the pes anserinus. The proximal anchorage may be with a double-staple buckle-type fixation and this again is as strong as the combined tendons. The combined tendon transplant produces an excellent reconstruction of the anterior cruciate ligament, approximately the same size, thickness and elasticity as the original. In most hands, it produces less arthrofibrosis. The main disadvantages are that it is a little less strong than the patellar tendon transplant and there is some variability in the size of the transplanted tendon.

It is not thought that with present knowledge prosthetic primary reconstruction is correct, although this operation is gaining ground in Europe. Bernard Moyen, Jean Lerat and Elisabeth Brunet-Guedj review the Lyon protocol in contribution 5.7. Their radiographic assessment of anterior cruciate laxity is important.

Practical points in the management of a patient with an acute anterior cruciate ligament tear

If a lesion of the anterior cruciate ligament is suspected from the history, the examination will usually confirm a haemarthrosis. This may be enormous and very painful, but in a partial tear the effusion is usually minor. The pain and irritability will modify the examination, for a routine Lachman and drawer test will be too painful to be undertaken and the production of a pivot shift or jerk may be impossible. However, with great gentleness of manual examination, an impression of laxity will frequently be present and sometimes the above signs are elucidated with clarity.

Counsel the patient!

If an anterior cruciate ligament rupture is definite or suspected, the patient must be fully counselled at this stage. The possible definitive options must be discussed – conservative treatment or final operative reconstruction. The patient's age, occupation, sports and sports ambitions must be considered and discussed. It is also necessary to point out that the anterior cruciate ligament ruptures frequently have associated meniscal damage and examination under anaesthetic and arthroscopy is necessary to finalize the diagnosis, the pattern and extent of instability and to deal with the meniscal derangement.

This examination under anaesthetic, together with arthroscopy, is indicated at a fairly early stage, and this usually means the next convenient operating list. The physical knee examination will now be possible, and especially so after aspiration of the haemarthrosis. Arthroscopy confirms the diagnosis and will allow the definite treatment of the associated meniscal lesion by arthroscopic technique. It may, however, be very difficult because of this haemarthrosis. With patience and good irrigation, the surgeon will be rewarded with adequate visualization of all areas of the knee. An arthroscopic irrigation pump and a large-bore outlet cannula will certainly help the blood clearance, but caution must be observed, for a full capsular and synovial tear may allow fluid to be extravasated at pressure and a compartment syndrome may result. Luckily this is very rare but must always be considered.

Dilworth Cannon points out in contribution 2.2 the indications and technique for peripheral meniscal repair and re-suture. This procedure is usually best undertaken at the same time as the arthroscopic anterior cruciate reconstruction, but if the latter is to be undertaken by open operation at a later stage, the meniscal re-suture may be performed at this time of initial arthroscopy. If meniscal re-suture is carried out, then the anterior cruciate ligament reconstruc-

tion becomes mandatory and the patient must be firmly told this fact.

The patient must be counselled again!

After the examination under anaesthetic and arthroscopy, the diagnosis is confirmed and the patient must be clearly put in the picture as to the significance of the injury. His activities and sporting ambitions must again be assessed, and his thoughts concerning the future of his injured knee considered. There is no doubt that in sportsmen, the anterior cruciate ligament complete tear is 'the beginning of the end' for this knee's function and stability, for in the long run the secondary restraints will loosen and the sports function will progressively and then grossly deteriorate. We all know of sportsmen who maintain good function with superb musculature and anterior cruciate ligament deficiency. The author has one patient who scored a goal in the last Soccer World Cup with a complete ACL tear. Nevertheless, with time, the knee loosens and deteriorates progressively with eventual degenerative change.

Bracing of the knee is an alternative and many patients with anterior cruciate ligament deficiency rely on this external support to maintain good sports function. The more mature patient who plays a little tennis and goes skiing once a year will often opt for a brace and, as long as repeated rotary incidents are avoided, no significant degenerative change supervenes.

Most sportsmen with continued ambition in this respect, and most active younger patients, now opt for operative reconstruction—especially as they see and hear of good results now universally accepted.

When should the reconstruction be performed?

Most knee surgeons will wait until the effusion and irritability have settled and the mobility of the knee joint is restored. Initial crutch support may be necessary and the assistance of a physiotherapist is strongly advised to help with this management and also to advise the surgeon on the progress. I do not proceed until these criteria are fulfilled, and although this usually means a wait of 2–3 weeks, it is time well spent. There is no doubt that the smoothness of rehabilitation, the maintenance of muscle power and bulk and the rapid return to full motion depend upon this knee 'quiescence'. The complete absence of arthrofibrosis postoperatively is essential, and this is most easily achieved if the preoperative state is ideal.

The preoperative preparation may take longer in some timid patients and anti-inflammatory medication may be helpful. It is wise to wait, and the absence of intra-articular oedema will reward the operator with an easier task and a better result with a smooth and easy rehabilitation course. It is realized that waiting for a few weeks transfers the patient's category from acute to subacute, but this does not matter as long as their activities during this period are adjusted to prevent rotary strains and to maintain the integrity of the secondary restraints.

There has been a great debate over the past decade as to the best management of the patient with an acute tear of the anterior cruciate ligament. ESKA (European Society of Knee Surgery and Arthroscopy) arranged an eminent International group to attempt a consensus on current definitions, aims and trends in the surgery and treatment of this enigmatic ligament. The final statement from ESKA is printed here.

Treatment of acute knee injuries with anterior cruciate lesions (ACL-injuries) (Report from the Consensus Conference during the Fourth ESKA Congress, Stockholm, Sweden)

The following statement is directed to all physicians and surgeons involved in the diagnosis and treatment of knee injuries.

A. Definition of an acute ACL injury

An ACL injury is defined as the disruption of ACL fibres, which usually results in an increase in anterior displacement of the tibia. *Acute* is defined as the period within 2 weeks of injury, and *subacute* 2–8 weeks after injury. The term acute also implies that there has been no previous history suggestive of an ACL injury.

B. Diagnosis

The diagnosis and treatment of the acute ACL rupture is based on the following:

1. *Careful evaluation of the patient's history:*
   (a) Injury history: ACL injury is suspected if there is a history of twisting, bending, contact or deceleration injury; a sensation of pain, a sudden 'pop', the knee 'giving way', and an acute painful swelling of the knee within a few hours (up to 24 hours).
   (b) The patient's preinjury and desired postinjury activity (functional level, intensity and exposure – *see IKDC format*).
2. The clinical knee examination includes (*see IKDC format*):

   (a) Estimate the effusion. *Arthrocentesis (puncture) of the knee joint* may be performed to relieve pain and facilitate examination
   (b) The active and passive range of motion (ROM)
   (c) The Lachman test (anterior displacement at 25° of flexion
   (d) The anterior–posterior drawer test (at 90° flexion)
   (e) The Pivot shift or rotary-drawer test (when allowed by pain)
   (f) The abduction/valgus, medial joint-line opening (MJLO) test at 25° of flexion and full extension
   (g) Adduction/varus, lateral joint-line opening (LJLO) test at 25° of flexion and full extension
   (h) Patellofemoral joint investigation
3. *A plain, standard radiograph* (AP, lateral and patellar view) should be taken.

In most cases a diagnosis of an ACL injury should be based on the history and the demonstration of an abnormal anterior tibial displacement by clinical examination, alone, or in combination with *instrumented measurement* or *stress radiographs*. MRI may be used to determine associated lesions. The cost–benefit value of MRI has to be determined, but the increasing use of MRI in diagnosis is expected to occur in the future.

Once the preliminary diagnosis is made, the alternative treatments should be discussed with the patient.

Arthroscopy is not essential to diagnose an ACL rupture; however, if this procedure is recommended it may be used for surgery on the ACL and also to diagnose and treat concomitant intra-articular injuries. *If* arthroscopy is planned, it should be performed by an experienced knee ligament surgeon.

The initial step in any surgical procedure is to *examine the knee under anaesthesia.*

C. Treatment

The treatment of an acute ACL injury should be individualized – not all patients require surgery. Factors that affect the decision include:

(a) the patient's age;
(b) work and sports activities (present and future – *see the included IKDC format*), and the patient's willingness to participate in a rehabilitation programme, etc.;
(c) *knee-related and medical factors* – associated injuries, degree of pathological motion, general joint laxity, and disadvantageous biomechanical or health factors.

Factors that also influence the type of treatment offered to the patient include sex and open growth plates. Acute ACL injuries in children deserve special attention since injury to epiphysis may occur during repair or reconstruction.

The surgeon's goal is to identify the patient at risk for future injuries and try to guide the patient into safe activities. The patient should be informed about the benefits versus the risks of treatment: complications, future re-injuries and joint arthrosis. Together, the surgeon and the patient develop a treatment plan.

(I) *Non-operative treatment of acute ACL injuries* should also be individualized. It should include early mobilization and active, guided rehabilitation of joint movement, muscular strength, endurance and coordination. The patient should be monitored and counselled on occupation and activity level and intensity to prevent episodes of giving-way and recurrent effusions.

(II) *Surgery for acute ACL injuries* is a relatively low risk type of operation when performed by an experienced knee ligament surgeon. The operation can be expected to decrease the risk for future injuries and complications and prolong activity. Surgical treatment is not an emergency operation and its timing should consider the patient's needs and emotions.

The optimal procedure cannot be identified at present, but it should:

- follow anatomical principles;
- allow early, full range of motion;
- utilize a technique and fixation method appropriate for the tissues and structures used or repaired;
- consider the issues affecting excessive elongation of repaired or reconstructed structures.

Currently used surgical procedures include the following:

1 *Simple suture repair* should be reserved for avulsion fractures and detachments and should be performed during the acute period (<2 weeks).
2 *Intra-articular augmented repair.* In most cases an ACL repair should be augmented with autologous tissue since the ruptured ends of an ACL ligament do not heal satisfactorily.
3 *Primary reconstruction* is preferred by some surgeons instead of augmented repair.
4 *Allograft reconstruction* is a clinical investigational procedure.
5 *Ligamentous augmenting devices and prosthetic devices* are clinical investigational devices.

The place of *functional braces* to protect the ACL injured knee against further secondary knee injury has yet to be established. At the moment, no studies support the absolute necessity for bracing in the non-operative or postoperative treatment of acute ACL injuries. In some situations physicians and surgeons may determine that the use of braces is indicated.

The use of *prophylactic braces* (single or double-hinged) to prevent ACL injuries has not been proved to date. In some situations physicians and surgeons may determine that brace-use is indicated.

D. Rehabilitation

(I) The rehabilitation of non-operated ACL injuries should aim to safely guide the patients back to their chosen level of activity while avoiding giving-way and recurrent effusions. The rehabilitation should avoid immobilization and restriction of ROM. The goal is to restore full ROM, regain full strength (at least 80–90% before returning to high-risk activity). The training progression should be individualized. The patient should be continuously reassessed, preferably using an objective evaluation method.

(II) The rehabilitation of surgically treated ACL injuries should follow the same principles and have the same goal as (I), cf above. However, you have to consider the healing properties of the tissue graft used in the surgical procedure. Protection of the graft is recommended for at least 6 months; the patient should not be advised to return to high-risk activities during this period of time. The role of bracing during the postoperative rehabilitation needs further study but individualized programmes may require bracing.

E. Prophylaxis

At the present time there are no documented studies on the prevention of acute ACL ruptures, but research into this important area is necessary. However, there are many non-medical factors: strength and co-ordination conditioning, coaching, and the rules in different sports may be important in the prophylaxis of injuries and provides the stimulus for additional studies in the prevention of knee injuries.

F. Need of future knowledge

Many areas in the treatment of acute ACL injuries remain to be clarified. Important areas for future research and validation include:

- the randomized, prospective, comparative evaluations of long-term results of various surgical techniques;
- the use of extra-articular procedures alone or as reinforcement;
- the value of different rehabilitation methods and regimens;
- the role of bracing and protective equipment;
- the healing and remodelling of tissues;
- the ability to re-establish normal kinematics.

Conclusion

The general management of the patient with an acute anterior cruciate ligament tear is difficult. The variety of surgical reconstructions is such that none as yet is considered perfect, although improvement continues apace. It is hoped that with this review and the individual contributions in this chapter the reader will gain some help in the management of his patients with this severe knee injury.

5.2 Overview of treatment of acute tears of the anterior cruciate ligament using middle-third patellar tendon

W. Dilworth Cannon, Jr

Incredible advances in anterior cruciate ligament (ACL) surgery have transpired over the past twenty years. In the early 1970s, surgery of the ACL was considered an exercise in futility. Not only did we lack the surgical techniques to reconstruct the ACL, but there was little regard for its function or for the role of the meniscus. Untreated ACL tears resulted in a higher incidence of meniscal tears and meniscectomies. An appreciation of the biomechanics of the ACL, as well as enhanced surgical techniques, have led to markedly improved surgical results.

John Feagin initially recommended primary repair of acute ACL tears, but found that by 5 years 94% had recurrent episodes of giving-way and 76% were impaired in athletic activity. Eriksson modified the Jones and Brostrom technique and began to report satisfactory surgical results. Eriksson was also one of the first surgeons to appreciate the importance of early functional rehabilitation after surgery. Instead of 6–8 weeks of casting after surgery, patients were fitted with light-weight braces. Currently, limited range-of-motion exercises are replaced by an immediate full range-of-motion program.

The 1980s also had some modifications in the grafts used for ACL reconstruction. Butler, Grood, and Noyes reported on the relative strengths of tissues used for augmentation or substitution of the ACL. Cho and Mott popularized the use of the semitendinosus. Iliotibial band and gracilis grafts were also used. A debate ensued over the merits of an extra-articular reconstruction with or without an accompanying intra-articular reconstruction in the treatment of acute ACL lesions. Clancy devised a vascularized pedicle bone–patellar tendon–bone graft, but a few years later animal studies showed that free tendon grafts did just as well. Significant complications continued, which added support to the surgeon's espousal of conservative treatment consisting of a hamstring exercise program and functional bracing.

Shino pioneered the use of allografts. Initially, he performed the surgery through an arthrotomy backed up with an extra-articular reconstruction and followed with 2 months of casting. Nevertheless, his results were very good. Further improvement came with the elimination of the extra-articular procedure, the development of arthroscopically assisted ACL reconstruction, and the institution of a more aggressive rehabilitation program.

In the early to mid-1980s, synthetic ACL prostheses were developed. Initial excitement was dampened when the frequency of graft breakage increased with follow-up. Particulate debris, usually resulting from graft impingement and inadequate notchplasty, caused annoying synovitis leading to graft removal. Presently, most knee surgeons feel that synthetics should be used only as a salvage procedure.

Today, knee surgeons can expect better than 90% good and excellent results after ACL reconstruction in the acute patient. The most commonly performed procedure in the world for this condition is the middle-third patellar tendon replacement of the ACL. Karzel and Friedman have described their technique in the following contribution (5.3).

5.3   Anterior cruciate ligament reconstruction using central one-third of the patellar tendon

Ronald P. Karzel and Marc J. Friedman

The most popular procedure for reconstruction of the anterior cruciate ligament (ACL) uses a graft harvested from the central one-third of the patellar tendon. Jones first described this procedure in 1963, and he subsequently reported favorable long-term results.[1] In his technique, the patellar tendon was left attached distally, and a 13-mm strip of patellar tendon with a patellar bone plug was used.[1,2] Later, the technique was modified to include bone plugs from both the tibial tubercle and the patella. Initial attempts were made to maintain the vascularity to the patellar tendon graft through the retinaculum.[3–5] Recently, the central one-third of the patellar tendon has been used as a free graft. Originally performed as an open technique, it can now be done as an arthroscopically assisted technique.[6–8] New technology allows placement of the patellar tendon graft through a single tibial drill tunnel. This method has been called 'endoscopic reconstruction' of the ACL.[9] Use of the patellar tendon has become so widespread that many authors consider it the 'gold standard' for ACL reconstruction.

Use of the patellar tendon for ACL reconstruction has several distinct advantages. Biomechanical studies performed by Noyes and coworkers showed that a 14-mm patellar tendon graft was 158% as strong as the normal ACL, and significantly stronger than other available autogenous sources for ACL reconstruction.[10] Another advantage is that the bone plugs within bone tunnels allow for very stable fixation using interference screws,[11] and this allows for faster rehabilitation. In addition, bone-to-bone healing is thought to be more reliable than bone-to-soft-tissue healing. Bone plug fixation within a bony tunnel is also an adaptable method for endoscopic reconstruction. Finally, the removal of the central third of the patellar tendon allows easy access through the fat pad at the time of arthroscopy. This will facilitate the positioning of instruments and guide-wires for endoscopic ACL reconstruction.

Use of the central third of the patellar tendon also has some disadvantages. Most of these disadvantages concern possible damage to the extensor mechanism of the knee. Reported complications have included patellar fracture[12] and rupture of the patellar tendon.[13] A less dramatic but significantly more common problem is the development of quadriceps weakness and patellofemoral pain after ACL reconstruction. One study found that patients with patellar tendon reconstruction were significantly more likely to have persistent quadriceps deficits 1 year after surgery than those undergoing semitendinosus and gracilis reconstruction.[14] Irritation and scarring in the patellar tendon following removal of the central third may also lead to persistent patellar tendinitis. Also, the immediate postoperative morbidity is usually greater in patients with patellar tendon reconstruction than in those with hamstring tendon reconstruction. The former procedure may require a larger incision and patients may have pain at the sites of bone harvesting.

Nevertheless, the advantages of graft strength and improved fixation makes patellar tendon reconstruction of the ACL the procedure of choice for most young active patients. These patients often have no history of patellofemoral pain or subluxation, and they will place high demands on their knees in the future. Semitendinosus and gracilis tendon reconstruction of the ACL is generally used in older patients, those with degenerative arthritis and less instability, and in those with fewer functional demands. In addition, many younger patients with a history of significant patellofemoral pain or subluxation are treated with hamstring tendon reconstruction. An alternative is the use of patellar tendon allografts. These allow the advantages of patellar tendon reconstruction without the increased morbidity or patellofemoral joint problems. Initial results have been encouraging.[15] Nevertheless, the use of allografts also carries the risk of disease transmission, subclinical rejection of the graft tissue, and the possibility that the donor allograft tissue may not revascularize. Use of allograft therefore remains experimental at this time.

Technique of ACL reconstruction

Do a careful clinical evaluation of both lower extremities to determine any associated pathology prior to surgery, such as posterolateral instability. Administer perioperative antibiotics for 24 hours. Perform a

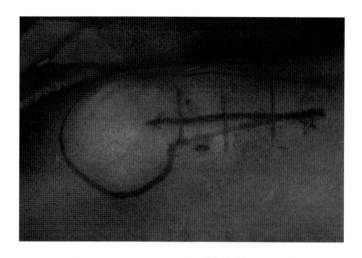

Figure 1

An incision is made 1 cm above the inferior pole of the patella and slightly medial to the tibial tubercle.

thorough arthroscopic evaluation of the involved knee with the tourniquet not inflated. Arthroscopic meniscectomy, meniscal repair, shaving, or loose-body removal are done without a tourniquet. If a meniscal repair is done, sutures are clamped but they are not tied until after the ACL reconstruction is completed.

Harvesting of the patellar tendon

Under most circumstances the tourniquet is not inflated at this time. Make an incision 1 cm above the inferior pole of the patella and carry it down slightly medial to the tibial tubercle (Figure 1). Keep the patellar tendon retinaculum intact for later repair (Figure 2).

Cut the central third portion of the patellar tendon and place a hemostat beneath it (Figure 3). With a bovie, outline the proximal patellar bone and distal tibial bone blocks. Use a 25-mm saw marked at 7 mm (Figure 4) to cut a 60° angle around the patellar bone block. Tap the bone minimally with a ½-inch osteotome to release it. It is important to avoid excessive use of an osteotome in harvesting the patellar graft. It is also possible to harvest this graft in a cylindrical fashion either with a Stryker 10-mm plug cutter or with an oscillating gouge made by Instrument Makar (Figure 5).

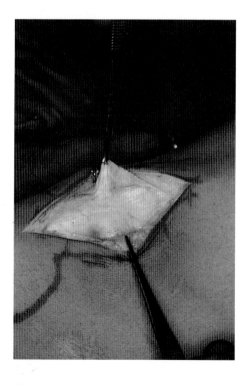

Figure 2

Flaps are developed and patellar tendon retinaculum is kept intact for later repair.

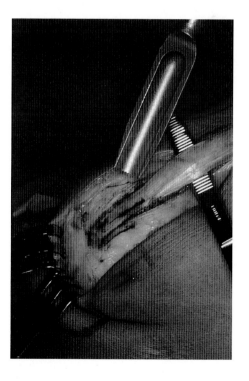

Figure 3

The central-third portion of the patellar tendon is cut sharply and a hemostat is placed beneath it.

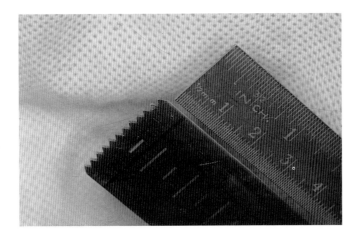

Figure 4

A 25-mm saw is marked at 7 mm to give that depth of cut.

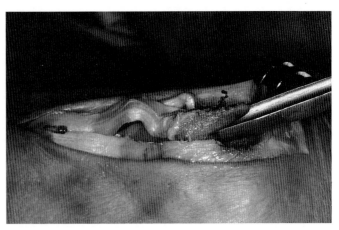

Figure 5

An oscillating 10-mm gouge by Instrument Makar.

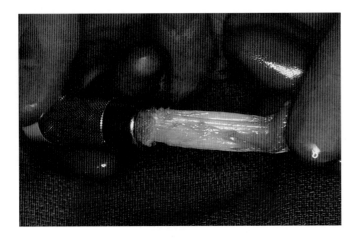

Figure 6

The bone plug is passed through a cylindrical tunnel for sizing.

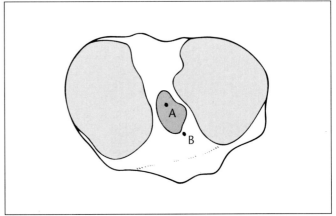

Figure 7

Point B is anteromedial to the actual anterior cruciate stump. Our preferred location is Point A in the central medial aspect of the old anterior cruciate ligament stump.

Harvest the tibial bone graft with a 3-cm straight osteotome. Pack cancellous bone from the tibial harvesting site into the patellar bone defect. Close the prepatellar bursal tissue, but leave the tendon defect open. If there is a decrease in patellar glide, an abnormal patellar tilt angle, or both, do an arthroscopic lateral release.

Place 2-mm-diameter drill holes in each bone block. Pass no.5 Ticron sutures through the drill holes in each bone block. Contour the graft with rongeurs so that it fits snugly in the 10-mm tunnel (Figure 6).

Debride the notch, removing the remnants of ACL tissue from the femur to afford a better view of the 'over-the-top' position. To start the notchplasty, use a ¼-inch curved gauge followed by a 4.5-mm-diameter abrader and shaver. Place a nerve hook through the anteromedial portal posterior to the 'over-the-top' position by palpating the femoral condyle.

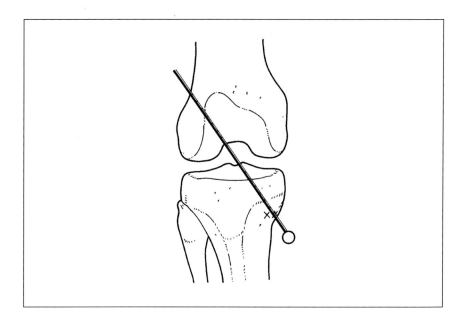

Figure 8

Isotak in place on the femur.

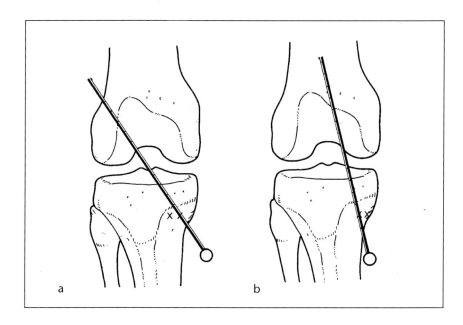

Figure 9

In order to exit the femur in a 'lateral' fashion and avoid proximal migration of the K-wire, one should start the tibial tunnel slightly 'medial.' The correct placement is shown in (a), the incorrect in (b).

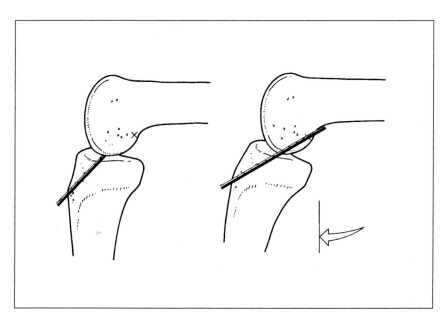

Figure 10

If a normal 45° angle 'vertical' tibial tunnel is drilled, one must often *extend* the knee to hit the isometric point on the femur. With extension, this K-wire will then exit *posteriorly*.

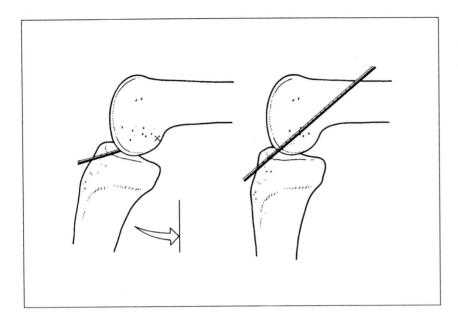

Figure 11

With a more *horizontal* tibial tunnel, one can easily go directly from the tibia to the posterior isometric point of the femur and simply flex the knee, and have the guide-wire exit on the anterolateral aspect of the femur.

Tibial tunnel

Historically, the location of the guide-wire would be at the anterior medial portion of the ACL. It will lessen impingement in extension, however, if the guide-wire goes directly in the center of the old ACL stump. This will also eliminate the need for an aggressive notchplasty (Figure 7).

A 10-mm cannulated reamer is placed over the guide-wire with a curette limiting wire migration. Using the Acufex isotak system, pick an isometric point on the femur 5 mm anterior to the 'over-the-top' position. For a right knee, the point of isometricity is located at the 1 o'clock position and for a left knee, at the 11 o'clock position (Figure 8).

There are two techniques for drilling a guide-wire for the femoral tunnel.

Technique no.1

Drill a guide-wire with an eyelet for sutures across the tibial tunnel to the isometric point of the femur and then through the femoral condyle. To accomplish this, two factors must be modified: (1) the tibial starting point (Figure 9) and (2) the superior/inferior direction of the tibial tunnel. Normally, the ACL tunnel begins at the level of the tibial tubercle, 4–5 cm below the joint-line. The guide-wire will be in a vertical alignment. Therefore, to get posterior on the femoral condyle to the isometric point, extend the knee as shown in the figure. Unfortunately, this drives the K-wire posteriorly into an unacceptable position (Figure 10). Acufex has designed an endoscopic system to produce a tibial tunnel which originates at 2.5 cm

below the joint-line. This will give the tunnel a more horizontal orientation. It will now be easier to go from the tibia to the posterior isometric point of the femur. Simply flex the knee and the guide-wire will exit on the anterior lateral aspect of the femur (Figure 11). Use a no. 11 blade to make a 5-mm hole through the skin. Leaving the guide-wire in place, use an endoscopic reamer to drill across the joint. Take care to walk the reamer across the area of the posterior cruciate ligament to avoid damaging it. It is helpful to introduce an arthroscopic shaver through the standard anteromedial border to shave any debris that blocks visualization of the numbers on the reamer. Usually a 30-mm tunnel is adequate.

At this point, place no. 5 sutures in the tibial bone graft and through the eyelet of the guide-wire. Gently rotate the sutures across the joint with a pair of pliers. Apply tension with a hemostat. Under direct vision, guide the graft across the joint, pulling it up snugly into the femoral socket. Place the cortex posteriorly so that the functional part of the tendon is as posterior as possible, to avoid any potential damage from the screw.

Technique no. 2

Using the Instrument Makar endoscopic fixation set, one does not have to drive the K-wire out the femur. Instead, with a series of socket sizers, starting with 7 mm to 12 mm, compact the cancellous bone and tunnel. Drive a lollipop K-wire with threads on one end parallel to the tibial bone plug (Figures 12 and 13), up the tibial tunnel into the femoral tunnel.

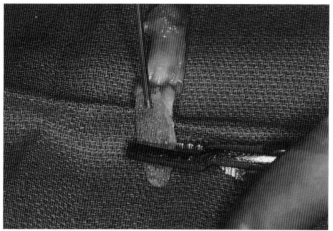

Figure 12

A threaded K-wire made by Instrument Makar is used to drill down the central portion of the femoral graft.

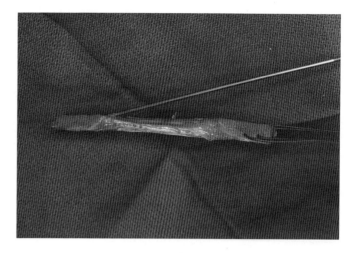

Figure 13

Sutures are placed around the tibial end and the threaded K-wire is then used to 'pass' the graft through the tibia into the femoral tunnel.

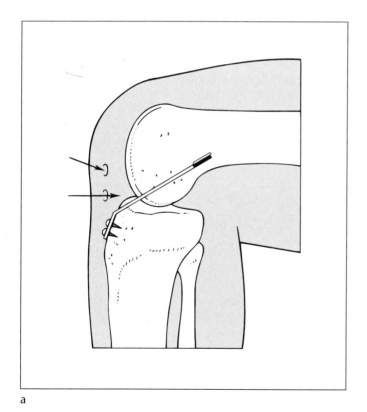

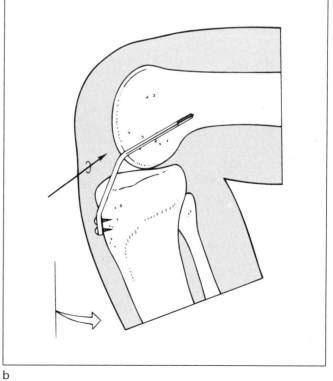

a   b

Figure 14

(a) An *accessory* anteromedial portal is used so that the screw 'parallels' the bone graft and posterior cortex of the femur. (b) The knee is further flexed.

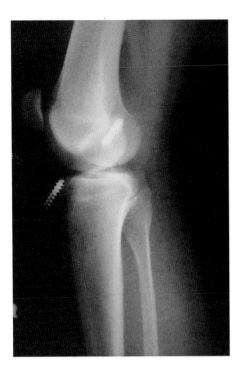

Figure 15

Radiographs show incorrect positioning of the screw.

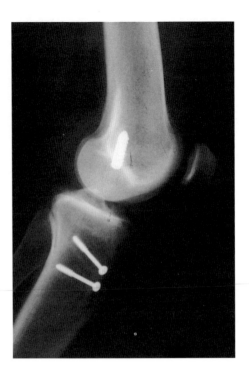

Figure 16

Correct positioning of the screw paralleling the posterior femoral cortex.

Endoscopic screw fixation

It is important to use an accessory anterior medial portal through the autogenous patellar tendon defect. That way the angle of the screw parallels the bone graft and the posterior cortex of the femur (Figure 14). Radiographs illustrate incorrect (Figure 15) and correct (Figure 16) positioning of the screw.

Use either cannulated cancellous screws or Instrument Makar threaded screws. Flex the knee 110–120° to place the screw parallel to the bone graft. Instrument Makar screws have threads that allow for screw insertion and removal with relative ease and safety should fixation be less than ideal. Should the screw come off during insertion, it can be retrieved through the fat-pad incision and reinserted. After fixation, take a lateral radiograph while still in the operating room, to ascertain the screw's direction, length, and depth.

Femoral fixation

After securing femoral fixation, bring the knee through a full range of motion. With the knee in extension, apply approximately 3–5 lb (13–22 N) of tension to the tibial bone graft. Apply a posterior drawer and fix the bone graft with interference screws or sutures around a 6.5-mm screw post. If the bone graft protrudes too far out of the tunnel, use a curved gauge to deepen the trough. Insert two 4-mm cancellous screws level with the cortex into the 2-mm holes placed anterior to posterior into the graft (Figure 17).

Acufex has an arthroscopic drill-guide that enables one to measure the length of the tibial tunnel to make it long enough to accept an interference screw. When the tibial tunnel is too vertical, transfemoral positioning of the guide-wire is difficult. One can get around this difficulty by utilizing the Acufex guide with the Instrument Makar lollipop. Since one does not have to come out the femur with the Instrument Makar system, a larger and more vertical tunnel can be made that still allows interference screw fixation. If, however, the posterior cortex of the femoral tunnel is violated, all efforts at endoscopic fixation must stop, and sutures are taken 'over-the-top' and tied around a screw post (Figure 18).

Release the tourniquet, close the wounds, and apply dressings and TED stockings. Place the knee in an immobilizer in complete extension.

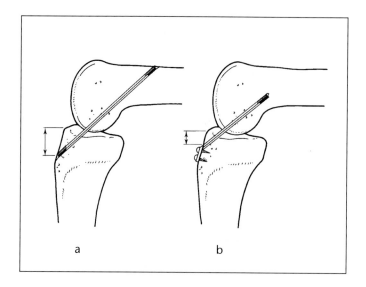

Figure 17

Two 4.0 cancellous screws fix the bone plug to the anterior tibia. In (a) the tibial tunnel is standard, in (b) it is horizontal.

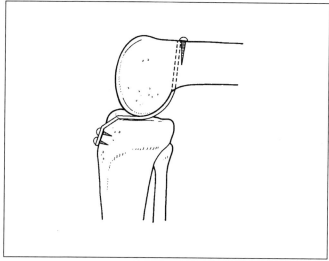

Figure 18

If the posterior cortex of the femoral tunnel is violated, all efforts at endoscopic fixation must stop. Sutures are taken 'over-the-top' and tied around a screw.

Postoperative rehabilitation

The use of a patellar tendon graft with its strong initial fixation and graft strength allows for rapid rehabilitation postoperatively. Recent rehabilitation protocols have challenged many previously held beliefs about ACL postoperative rehabilitation. These beliefs were based on animal studies on revascularization and tensile strength of ligament replacements. Arnoczky and coworkers reported that in dogs a patellar tendon graft underwent initial avascular necrosis, although some viable cells remained in the periphery of the graft.[16] By 8–10 weeks, intrinsic vascularization was noted within the patellar tendon graft, but a central area of necrosis remained. Complete revascularization of the graft required 20 weeks. The graft was found to weaken significantly prior to complete maturation.[17] Laboratory research also suggests that full active knee extension places excessive stress on the newly reconstructed ACL. These findings led researchers to recommend initial immobilization of the knee without weight bearing, and prolonged protection from terminal active quadriceps extension.[18-20] Recently, however, the development of stronger graft fixation, the use of arthroscopy to minimize postoperative morbidity, the improved knowledge of isometric graft placement, and the increased confidence in graft strength have led to a significant acceleration of the postoperative rehabilitation program. Accelerated rehabilitation leads to faster return of full knee motion, strength, and overall function.

Shelbourne has been a proponent of an aggressive rehabilitation program after patellar tendon reconstruction.[21] Rehabilitation is divided into three phases. The goals of Phase 1 (the initial 2 weeks after surgery) are wound healing, full extension of the operative leg equal to that of nonoperated leg, minimization of swelling, and regain of active leg control and quadriceps function. The patients are placed in a passive range of motion machine from 0 to 30°, and maintained at bed rest for 3 days to minimize swelling. Cryotherapy is applied to the leg to diminish swelling. Patients are instructed in early straight leg raising for quadriceps control. They are allowed to ambulate with weight bearing as tolerated while wearing a knee immobilizer. Patients perform passive range of motion exercises to achieve terminal extension and 90° of flexion. They are encouraged to extend the knee fully with a pillow behind the ankle and with the knee unsupported at least 10 minutes per hour during this period. At the end of 2 weeks, patients should be able to extend their knees completely and to perform straight leg raises with a minimal lag. Swelling should be minimal.

Phase 2 begins approximately 2 weeks postoperatively. The emphasis is on regaining a full range of motion. Patients begin closed-chain kinetic activities such as unilateral knee bends, leg presses, Stairmaster, bicycling, and swimming. Patients are encouraged to walk with a normal gait without a brace. A full range of motion should be achieved by approximately 6 weeks. At the end of Phase 2, patients should be comfortable with activities of daily living.

Cybex testing for quadriceps muscle strength is performed. If at least 70% of the nonoperated leg strength has been attained in the operated leg at this time, Phase 3 begins. If strength is less than 70% of the noninjured leg, an additional 4 weeks of strengthening exercises is initiated.

Retesting is done prior to advancing to Phase 3, the final stage. Here, patients gradually return to athletic activities. Jumping rope, lateral shuffles, and cariocas commence along with sports-specific activities. Most athletes are allowed to return to sports at approximately 6–9 weeks after beginning Phase 3, provided their quadriceps strength is satisfactory. A brace is recommended for use during sports activities. Shelbourne states that they have had no failures of graft fixation or loss of graft strength following this rehabilitation protocol.

Our own protocol is more conservative. We agree with the importance of regaining full passive knee extension immediately. Patients are placed in a knee immobilizer for ambulation with weight bearing as tolerated. They are encouraged to perform straight leg raises and to achieve full passive extension immediately. Active flexion as tolerated is also encouraged. If ambulation is comfortable without the brace, the brace is discarded. We generally defer resisted quadriceps activities until 6 weeks to allow the bone plugs to incorporate securely into the bone tunnels. Patients begin closed-chain kinetic exercises, and activities such as Stairmaster and bicycling, at 3–6 weeks. Running is allowed at approximately 3 months. If swelling increases, the rehabilitation is slowed. Patients return to athletic competition at 6 months if they have quadriceps strength equal to at least 85% of the strength in the nonoperated leg. There should be a full range of motion, with no significant pain or swelling. Patients are fitted with a derotation brace prior to resuming sports activities. This brace is worn for sports activities during the first 2 years after surgery. We have found that this rehabilitation protocol allows patients to return rapidly to their activities of daily living. There is a reduction of quadriceps atrophy, the incidence of flexion contracture, and the loss of range of motion after ACL surgery. There is also a reduction in the incidence of patellofemoral problems.

Prevention of complications

Complications may occur after patellar tendon reconstruction of the ACL. Many of these complications may be averted through attention to technical details. To avoid patellar fracture, limit the depth of the patellar bone plug to approximately 5–6 mm. The donor site on the patella is filled with bone graft obtained from contouring the bone plugs and from the tibial graft site prior to wound closure. This appears to speed the healing of the bony defect, as noted on postoperative skyline views.

To avoid patellar tendon rupture, measure the width of the patellar tendon prior to graft harvesting. Do not use more than one-third of the width of the tendon, and limit the graft taken to 10 mm. Carefully cut the graft from the tibial tubercle to avoid inadvertently detaching the insertion of the remaining medial or lateral band of the patellar ligament. Preserve the paratenon during exposure of the patellar tendon and close it over the defect to provide a new vascularized bed for healing to occur.

Circumventing patellofemoral problems is important after patellar tendon reconstruction. Arthroscopic surgery significantly reduces the overall insult to the extensor mechanism and decreases the frequency of patellofemoral problems. Also, the avoidance of prolonged immobilization helps to prevent quadriceps shortening and flexion contracture, both of which contribute to postoperative patellofemoral symptoms. Do not close the defect in the patellar tendon, to avoid shortening and a possible subsequent increase in patellofemoral joint pressure.

Arthrofibrosis is common after ACL reconstruction with patellar tendon. The incidence is higher with patellar tendon grafts than with semitendinosus and gracilis grafts. Arthrofibrosis is also prevalent if surgery is performed within 7–10 days after injury, especially if primary ACL repair is done. Since the results of primary ACL repair are not as good as of those using middle-third patellar tendon, there is no urgency to the surgery. The best results after ACL reconstruction occur in patients in which at least 2–3 weeks have elapsed since injury. In an acutely injured knee in which locking is not present, defer surgery until swelling has decreased, a full range of motion has been regained, and there is active quadriceps control. By waiting several weeks before performing ACL reconstruction, and by using an early rehabilitation program, the incidence of arthrofibrosis in our practice has dramatically diminished. When arthrofibrosis does occur, we take an aggressive approach to treatment. If the patient has not regained at least 60° of motion by 6 weeks after surgery, he is returned to surgery for manipulation of the knee and arthroscopy. The graft is evaluated and the adhesions are lysed. The patient is hospitalized overnight in a continuous passive motion machine. He is sent home with the machine for 1–2 weeks until motion is regained.

A slight flexion contracture following surgery is a common problem. An early flexion contracture of 10° will respond to further passive stretching. A gradual improvement in the flexion contracture is noted up to 1 year after surgery. In patients with a significant flexion contracture greater than 10° at 3 months after surgery, manipulation of the knee and repeat arthroscopy are performed. If the notchplasty is inadequate it can be expanded. If scar tissue is impinging on the graft and preventing full extension it can be debrided. Loss of motion after patellar tendon reconstruction is less likely if an adequate notchplasty is performed initially. Isometric placement of the graft will prevent entrapment of the knee. Early full passive extension will prevent posterior capsular contraction or scar tissue from forming within the intercondylar notch.

Results of patellar tendon reconstruction

Several recent reports have documented good results following patellar tendon reconstruction of the ACL. Clancy and coworkers reported their results in a group of patients with acute ACL tears treated with open repair of the torn ligament augmented with patellar tendon graft.[22] Of 70 patients, 42 had an excellent result, 26 had a good result, and only 2 patients had a fair result. There were no failures. Results were significantly better than in a group of 22 patients treated nonoperatively, only half of whom were satisfied with their results.

In another study, the results of acute ACL reconstruction using a patellar tendon graft through an arthrotomy was reported.[23] These patients had an average difference of 1.3 mm between the injured and noninjured knees at 20 lb (89 N) of force on KT-1000 arthrometer testing at final follow-up. Mean quadriceps strength was 90% of the noninjured knee. All patients had a full range of motion, and 60 of 69 university athletes returned to their preinjury competition level the following season. Out of 140 patients, 131 did not have any sensation of knee instability following the reconstruction. The average knee score was 92.7 out of a maximum of 100 points.

In another recent study, 45 patients underwent arthroscopically assisted reconstruction of the ACL using bone–patellar tendon–bone autograft.[24] Forty-five patients had at least 2 years of follow-up examinations. One ligament graft failed during later sports activity. The average KT-1000 difference between the operative and nonoperative knee was 1.2 mm. Thirty-six of the patients had less than or equal to 3 mm difference in the injured and noninjured knees. Forty-two patients returned to their same level of athletic and occupational activities without restriction. The patients had an average Cincinnati knee score of 94 and an average Lysholm score of 95. Overall, 97.7% had a good or excellent result.

The studies reported above are preliminary, with short follow-up examinations. Further studies will be needed to determine more accurately the efficacy of bone–patellar tendon–bone grafting for ACL deficiency. The results are expected to improve as the understanding of the technical factors involved increases, and faster rehabilitation is emphasized. When used in properly selected patients with careful attention to operative techniques and postoperative rehabilitation, central-third patellar tendon grafts are an excellent method for restoring stability and function to patients with an ACL deficient knee.

References

1. **Jones KG**, Reconstruction of the anterior cruciate ligament using the central one-third of the patellar ligament: A follow-up report, *J Bone Joint Surg (Am)* (1970) **52**: 1302–1308.
2. **Jones KG**, Reconstruction of the anterior cruciate ligament: A technique using the central one-third of the patellar ligament, *J Bone Joint Surg (Am)* (1963) **45**: 925–932.
3. **Clancy WG Jr, Nelson DA, Reider B et al.**, Anterior cruciate ligament reconstruction using one-third of the patellar ligament augmented by extra-articular tendon transfers, *J Bone Joint Surg (Am)* (1982) **64**: 352–359
4. **Noyes FR, Butler DL, Paulos LE et al.**, Intra-articular cruciate reconstruction. Part I: Perspectives on graft strength, vascularization and immediate motion after replacement, *Clin Orthop* (1983) **172**: 71–77.
5. **Paulos LE, Butler DL, Noyes FR et al.**, Intraarticular cruciate reconstruction: Replacement with vascularized patellar tendon, *Clin Orthop* (1983) **172**: 78–84.
6. **Bach BR**, Arthroscopically assisted patellar tendon substitution for anterior cruciate ligament insufficiency: surgical technique, *Am J Knee Surg* (1989) **2**: 3–20.
7. **Jackson DW, Jennings LD**, Arthroscopically assisted reconstruction of the anterior cruciate ligament using a patellar tendon bone autograft, *Clin Sports Med* (1988) **7**: 785–800.
8. **Karzel RP Jr, Friedman MJ**, *Arthroscopic diagnosis and treatment of cruciate and collateral ligament injuries*, ed Scott WN (Philadelphia: WB Saunders, 1990) 131–154.
9. **Rosenberg T**, *Technique for Endoscopic Method of ACL Reconstruction* (Norwood, Mass.: Acufex Microsurgical, 1989).
10. **Noyes FR, Butler DL, Grood ES et al.**, Biomechanical analysis of human ligament grafts used in knee ligament repairs and reconstructions, *J Bone Joint Surg (Am)* (1984) **66**: 344–352.
11. **Kurosaka M, Yoshiya S, Andrish JT**, A biomechanical comparison of different surgical techniques of graft fixation in anterior cruciate ligament reconstruction, *Am J Sports Med* (1987) **15**: 225–229.
12. **McCarroll JR**, Fracture of the patella during a golf swing following reconstruction of the anterior cruciate ligament: A case report, *Am J Sports Med* (1983) **11**: 26–27.
13. **Bonamo JJ, Krinick RM, Sporn AA**, Rupture of the patellar ligament after use of its central third for anterior cruciate reconstruction: A report of two cases, *J Bone Joint Surg (Am)* (1984) **66**: 1294–1297.
14. **Sachs RA, Daniel DM, Stone ML et al.**, Patellofemoral problems after anterior cruciate ligament reconstruction, *Am J Sports Med* (1989) **17**: 760–765.
15. **Noyes FR, Barber SD, Mangine RE**, Bone–patellar ligament–bone and fascia lata allografts for reconstruction of the anterior cruciate ligament, *J Bone Joint Surg (Am)* (1990) **72**: 1125–1136.
16. **Arnoczky SP, Tarvin GB, Marshall JL**, Anterior cruciate ligament replacement using patellar tendon: An evaluation of graft revascularization in the dog, *J Bone Joint Surg (Am)* (1982) **64**: 217–224.
17. **Clancy WG, Narechania RG, Rosenberg TD et al.**, Anterior and posterior cruciate ligament reconstruction in rhesus monkeys, *J Bone Joint Surg (Am)* (1981) **63**: 1270–1287.
18. **Arms SW, Pope MH, Johnson RJ et al.**, The biomechanics of anterior cruciate ligament reconstruction and rehabilitation, *Am J Sports Med* (1984) **12**: 8–18.

19. **Paulos L, Noyes FR, Grood ES et al.**, Knee rehabilitation after anterior cruciate ligament reconstruction and repair, *Am J Sports Med* (1981) **9**: 140–149.

20. **Grood ES, Suntay WJ, Noyes FR et al.**, Biomechanics of the knee-extension exercise, *J Bone Joint Surg (Am)* (1984) **66**: 725–734.

21. **Shelbourne KD, Nitz P**, Accelerated rehabilitation after anterior cruciate ligament reconstruction, *Am J Sports Med* (1990) **18**: 292–299.

22. **Clancy WG, Ray JM, Zoltan DJ**, Acute tears of the anterior cruciate ligament: Surgical versus conservative treatment, *J Bone Joint Surg (Am)* (1988) **70**: 1483–1488.

23. **Shelbourne KD, Whitaker HJ, McCarroll JR et al.**, Anterior cruciate ligament injury: Evaluation of intraarticular reconstruction of acute tears without repair: Two to seven year followup of 155 athletes, *Am J Sports Med* (1990) **18**: 484–489.

24. **Andrews JR, Moran DJ**, Arthroscopically assisted reconstruction of the anterior cruciate ligament using bone–patellar tendon–bone autograft: Results after two years, Presented at the 58th Annual Meeting of the American Academy of Orthopedic Surgeons, Anaheim, Calif., March 7–12, 1991.

5.4 Acute anterior cruciate ligament reconstruction with semitendinosus and gracilis transfer

Giancarlo Puddu, Guglielmo Cerullo, Massimo Cipolla and Vittorio Franco

There is still considerable difference of opinion as to the technique of reconstructing the anterior cruciate ligament (ACL) in acute instabilities.

We present a simple method of ACL reconstruction using the semitendinosus and gracilis tendons. This technique has been used since 1979 using only the semitendinosus tendon, and since 1981 using both the semitendinosus and gracilis tendons.[1] In patients with anteromedial rotatory instabilities, the ACL reconstruction was combined with repair of the medial compartment tears in selective cases.

In cases of anterolateral rotatory instability, we have combined the ACL reconstruction with repair of the middle one-third of the lateral capsular ligament and tenodesis of the iliotibial tract to the linea aspera, as advocated by Hughston. Since 1981, we have augmented the semitendinosus and gracilis tendons with a 7.5-mm wide Vicryl band (Ethicon) and, since 1983, with a 7.5-mm wide PDS band (Ethicon) in order to protect the graft for at least 30 days after surgery.

Reconstruction of the ACL with pes anserinus tendons is not a new idea. In fact, Lindemann,[2] Ramadier and Benoit,[3] Ficat,[4] Cho[5] and more recently Bousquet[6] and Rosenberg[7] have used the semitendinosus tendon to reconstruct the ACL. Lindemann and Ficat detach the semitendinosus from its tibial insertion and pass it through the posteromedial aspect of the capsular ligament in order to recreate the course of the ACL. Bousquet lets the semitendinosus pass both ways in the knee joint.

On the other hand, the techniques of Merle d'Aubigné and Cho section the semitendinosus at its musculotendinous junction, leaving it inserted on the tibia, and use it to retrace the normal course of the anterior cruciate, first with a transtibial and then with a transfemoral drillhole. More recently, Rosenberg has been using the semitendinosus tendon as a free graft. In all cases where this technique is used, the semitendinosus loses its function of internal rotation and flexion.

With our technique, the semitendinosus and gracilis keep their physiological function, whereas the more distal part of the tendons substitutes for the ACL (Figure 1).

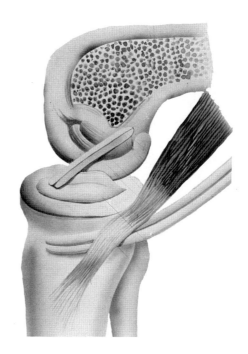

Figure 1

The technique.

Surgical technique

Between 1979 and 1987, we performed ACL reconstruction for acute tears by open surgery, while using the arthroscope to evaluate the intra-articular lesions. From 1987 until now, we have been doing arthroscopically assisted ACL reconstructions.

When the tear of the medial or lateral compartment is large and lets the irrigation solution overflow into the subcutaneous tissue, the intra-articular vision and the subsequent open surgery become difficult owing to the oedema of the tissues. In such circumstances, we use arthroscopy only to evaluate and treat

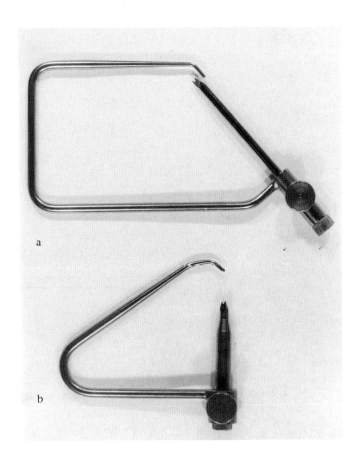

Figure 2

(a) The femoral guide. (b) The tibial guide.

the lesions of the menisci, and to drill and prepare the femoral and tibial tunnels. Thereafter, we proceed with open surgery.

If there is no or minimal extravasation of fluid, we continue the ACL reconstruction with the aid of arthroscopy.

Arthroscopically aided ACL reconstruction using semitendinosus and gracilis tendons

The guides

Since 1979 we have been using two simple guides to make the femoral and tibial tunnels in the so-called 'isometric position'. During these 11 years, our femoral guide has undergone some modifications to arrive at the latest model, which we use endoscopically and is

now available (Figure 2a). The characteristic of our guide is the offset between its point and the emergence of the Kirschner wire from the lateral femoral condyle.

The point of the guide must be positioned behind the lateral femoral condyle. The Kirschner wire can emerge 4–6 mm from the posterior cortex, depending upon which sleeve is used, to obtain a 10–12-mm or 9–10-mm or 7–8-mm hole. The femoral insertion of the 'new' ACL is posterior and it is placed in the so-called 'anatomical position'. The remnant of the ACL from the intercondylar notch is excised and a notchplasty is performed. The femoral guide is then inserted in the joint through the anteromedial portal and is positioned behind the lateral femoral condyle. With our guide, since 1979 we have performed at least 800 open ACL reconstructions and 200 arthroscopically assisted ACL reconstructions. In the majority of cases, we have succeeded in obtaining an isometric reconstruction.

The tibial guide has a characteristic triangular shape that makes it easy to manoeuvre (Figure 2b).

Technique

The patient is placed in a supine position under general anaesthesia. Three standard portals are used for arthroscope, instruments and inflow (anterolateral, anteromedial and superomedial, respectively) in order to evaluate and treat the meniscal pathology, to clean the intercondylar notch and the tibial insertion from the ACL remnant. In acute cases, the notchplasty is usually not necessary. We perform notchplasty only in knees with congenital narrowing of the intercondylar notch.

The semitendinosus and gracilis tendons are identified and dissected through a small vertical incision, 3–4 cm long, just medial to the tibial tuberosity. At this level, the two tendons run parallel and almost perpendicular to the medial aspect of the tibia. With the knee flexed at 90°, it is easy to palpate the two tendons under the fascia. This fascia should be divided in the interval between the two tendons with a parallel incision.

The tendons are detached from the tibial insertion with a small flake of bone and secured by passing two non-absorbable sutures through the free ends (Figure 3a). Then the tendons are pulled and the proximal dissection is completed by dividing three thick adhesions between the semitendinosus and the deep fascia. Only after the cutting of these insertions will the tendons be sufficiently long to achieve the length of the ACL and to enter at least a couple of centimetres into the femoral tunnel.

We usually augment the graft with a 7.5-mm wide PDS band (Ethicon) that is sutured between the tendons like a sandwich, with eight stitches of No. 0 non-absorbable material (Figure 3b).

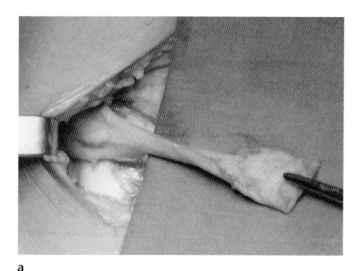
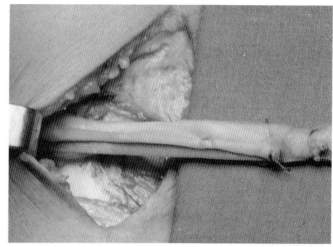

a

b

Figure 3

(a) The semitendinosus and gracilis tendons are detached from the tibial insertion with a small flake of bone. (b) The tendons are augmented with a 7.5-mm PDS band.

Once the graft is prepared, it is passed deep to the sartorius to exit 2 cm distal to the joint-line. A small incision (5 cm) is made on the lateral aspect of the thigh and the iliotibial tract is divided along the direction of its fibres. The vastus lateralis muscle is retracted and the lateral femoral metaphysis is exposed. A Kirschner wire is inserted through the lateral femoral condyle with the aid of a femoral guide and its isometric position in the intercondylar notch is confirmed via the arthroscope. A bone tunnel is prepared with a 7-mm cannulated drill.

Once the femoral tunnel is made and its emergence into the joint is chamfered, a Kirschner wire is passed through the upper tibia using the tibial guide. The entrance of the Kirschner wire into the tibia is positioned 2–3 cm below the joint-line and 1 cm anterior to the medial collateral ligament.

The position of the Kirschner wire is checked in flexion and particularly in extension (the point of the wire has to be totally covered by the notch in full extension). Then the tibial tunnel is drilled using the same 7-mm drill point.

In some cases where a good remnant of the ACL is present, we conserve it in order to reattach it to the femur. Much care is required in drilling the tibial

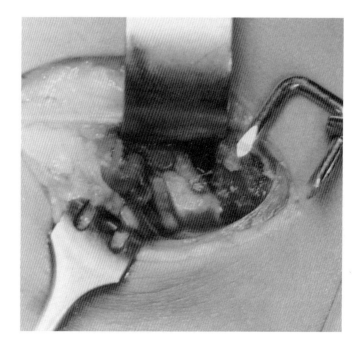

Figure 4

The graft is fixed, tying the PDS band over a staple inserted on the emergence of the femoral tunnel.

hole without damaging the remaining fibres of the ruptured ACL and the tunnel is drilled just posterior to the remnant.

It is very important not to overchamfer the emergence of the tunnels into the joint; this might make the femoral hole too anterior and the tibial hole too posterior, loosening the so-called 'isometricity' of the ACL.

The loss of fluid from the bone tunnels can be minimized by use of suitable plugs.

A loop of wire is now used to thread the graft, which is passed into the tunnels, pulling it from the femoral exit with the knee flexed at 90°. If there is resistance in this passage, it is advisable to check that the graft is free from adhesions in its extra-articular portion near the tibial hole and to look arthroscopically to ensure that the bone flake freely enters the femoral tunnel.

The semitendinosus and gracilis tendons are now re-inserted into the tibia by two absorbable transperiosteal sutures just posterior to the tibial hole. On the femoral side the graft is fixed, tying the PDS band on a staple previously inserted over the emergence of the femoral hole (Figure 4).

With *open surgery*, the technique is the same, the only difference being a medial parapatellar skin incision and naturally a miniarthrotomy, leaving intact as far as possible the vastus medialis obliquus insertion over the patella.

Postoperative management

The knee is protected in a Don Joy ROM splint after surgery. On the first day, postoperative continuous passive motion (CPM) is begun with a range of movement between 40° and 80°, and this is progressively augmented.

The gracilis and semitendinosus muscles are initially very tight but in 3 days they relax completely. Partial weight bearing is permitted on the 25th postoperative day and full weight bearing on the 40th day. Swimming and cycling are encouraged after 7–8 weeks. The patient begins running at the 5th month. Light sports activity and training are allowed after 6 months, while competitive non-contact sports can be played after 8 months and contact sports after 10 months.

In conclusion, we have found no significant difference in our results between the arthroscopically assisted ACL reconstruction and the open technique.

References

1. **Puddu G**, Method for reconstruction of the anterior cruciate ligament using the semitendinosus tendon, *Am J Sports Med* (1980) 8(6): 402–404.
2. **Lindemann K**, Über den plastischen Ersatz der Kreuzbänder durch gestielte Sehnenverpflanzung, *Z Orthop* (1950) **79**: 316–334.
3. **Ramadier JO, Benoit J**, Laxités post-traumatiques du genou: Reconstruction des ligaments lateraux et croisés, Syndesmoplasties du genou, *Rev Chir Orthop* (1972) **58**: 78–84.
4. **Ficat P, Cuzachq JP, Ricci A**, Chirurgie reparatrice des laxités chroniques des ligaments croisés du genou, *Rev Chir Orthop* (1975) **61**(2): 89–100.
5. **Cho KO**, Reconstruction of the anterior cruciate ligament by semitendinosus tenodesis, *J Bone Joint Surg (Am)* (1975) **57**: 608–612.
6. **Bousquet G**, *Chirurgia del ginocchio* (Rome: Verduci Editore, 1979) 191–194.
7. **Rosenberg TD**, Endoscopic technique of ACL reconstruction, *Abstracts of the 16th Meeting of American Orthopedic Society for Sports Medicine* (1990) 79–82.

5.5 Anterior cruciate ligament reconstruction using tendon transfers — medial hamstrings: Open technique

Paul M. Aichroth

Incision

A medial parapatellar incision with inferior extension is made to allow access to the pes anserinus. A routine medial parapatellar arthrotomy is undertaken through the upper end of this incision. In the second part of the operation, a lateral incision is made to allow access to the lateral supracondylar region. (See Figure 1.)

Dissection of the pes anserinus

The semitendinosus and gracilis tendons are identified by careful dissection. These two tendons are felt and seen beneath the superficial fascial sheet which makes up the whole pes structure. The isolated tendons are traced back into the posteromedial thigh and using a tenotome the maximal length of the tendon is stripped and divided as high as possible. If

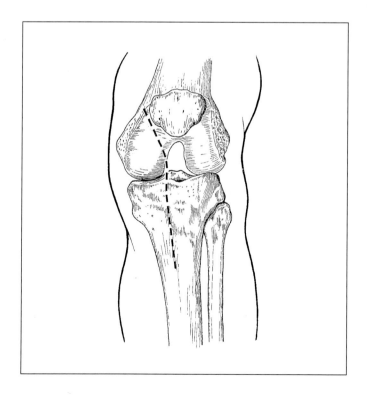

Figure 1

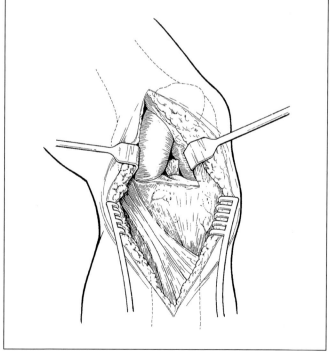

Figure 2

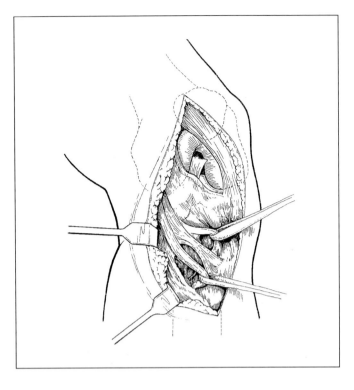

Figure 3

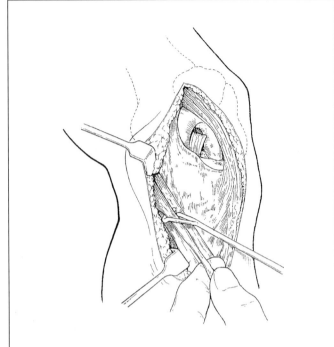

Figure 4

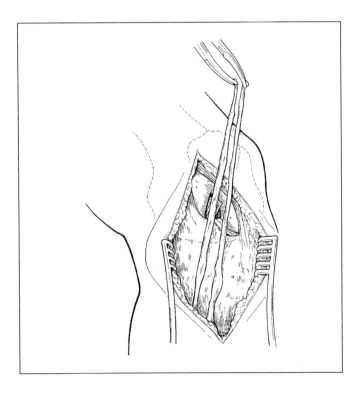

Figure 5

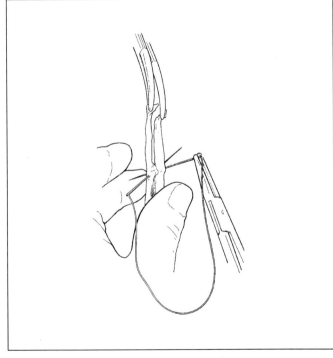

Figure 6

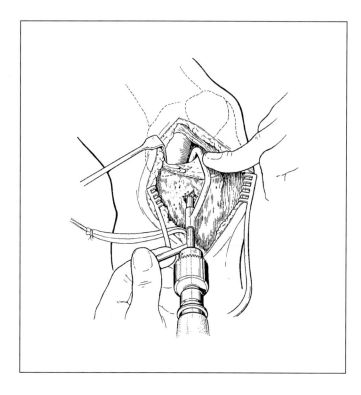

Figure 7

a tenotome is not available a small incision is made in the posteromedial thigh, the tendons are dissected free, and isolated, and they are separated from the surrounding muscle and divided as high as possible. (See Figures 2, 3, 4.)

Suture

The gracilis and semitendinosus tendons are sutured together. A 'tendon leader' is positioned over their free ends, or alternatively a Bunnell type suture is inserted. (See Figures 5, 6.)

Drilling the tunnel

A jig is used to drill the tibial tunnel. The drill enters the tibia just above the insertion of the two tendons and emerges at the tibial plateau at the normal inferior attachment of the anterior cruciate ligament – just at, and slightly behind, the bifid anterior tibial spine. This exact point is often better felt than observed. (See Figure 7.)

Transferring the tendons

The tendons are then brought through the tibial tunnel using the stiff tendon leader or alternatively a malleable probe is passed down the tibial tunnel and the Bunnell suture is pulled through with the tendons following. (See Figure 8.)

The lateral dissection

Incision

The incision follows the supracondylar line. The iliotibial tract is exposed and split vertically. The vastus lateralis is retracted forwards. (See Figure 9.)

Dissection

The dissection then proceeds beneath the lateral gastrocnemius, separating it from the lateral capsule. A curved director is passed through the capsule in the intercondylar region and over the top of the lateral femoral condyle. A long curved artery forceps may then be passed into the main knee joint to pick up the tendon leader. Alternatively, a tape may be taken down with the curved director into the knee joint cavity and the Bunnell suture is attached. The conjoint tendon is brought through and over the top of the lateral femoral condyle. (See Figure 10.)

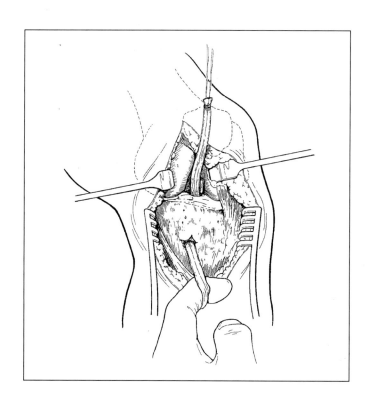

Figure 8

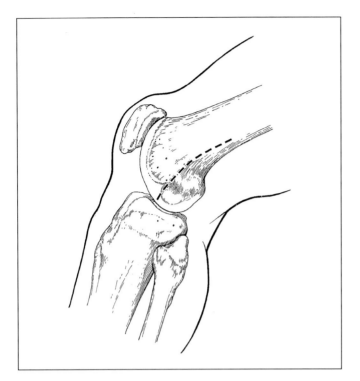

Figure 9

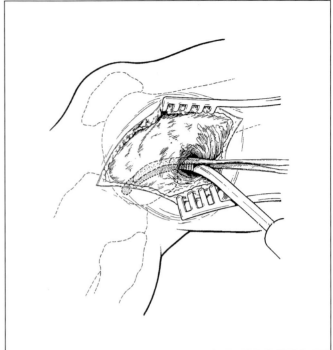

Figure 10

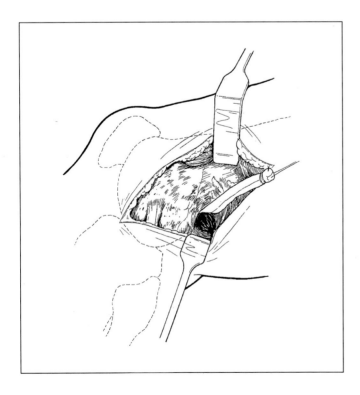

Figure 11

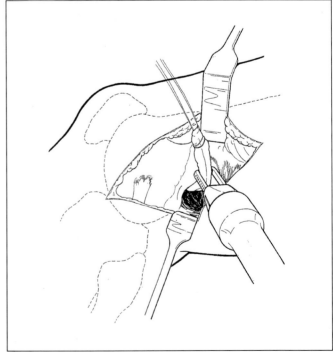

Figure 12

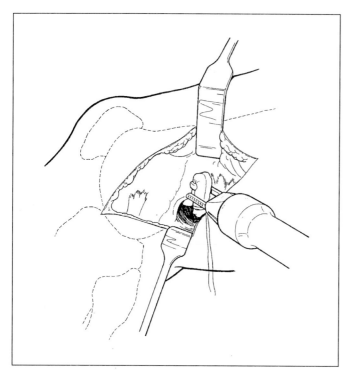

Figure 13

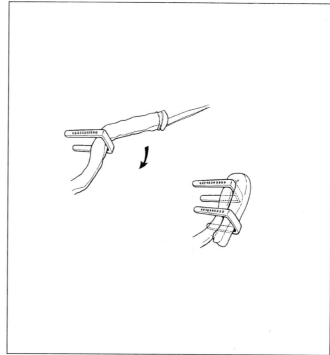

Figure 14

Figure 15

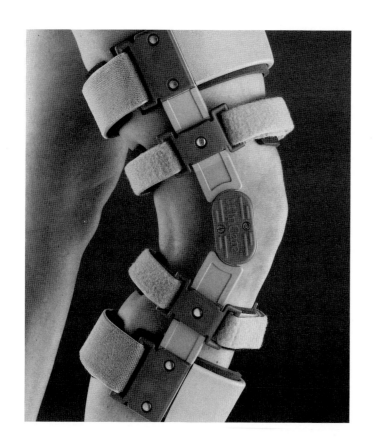

Attachment

The next stage is attachment of the tendons to the lateral supracondylar femur. The tendons are strongly attached to the exposed supracondylar bone using a double-barbed staple technique. This produces a buckle effect and the attachment is extremely firm. (See Figures 11, 12, 13, 14.)

Postoperative management

The wounds are closed in layers with appropriate drains. The limb is placed on the constant passive motion machine and in the first few hours movement from 0° to 40° is obtained. There is progressive increase in the flexion range, which should reach 90° over the next 4–5 days with the physiotherapist's help.

A brace is then applied to allow movement from 0° to 90° (Figure 15) and the patient must remain not or minimally weight bearing on crutches until the sixth week postoperatively.

It is thought that earlier weight bearing may be allowed in some cooperative patients if the reconstruction is of good strength.

Further rehabilitation

The brace is removed and weight bearing commences at the sixth week. From 6 to 12 weeks postoperatively a specific physiotherapy rehabilitation programme is undertaken with progressive knee movement and strengthening. Increasing walking will lead to cycling, swimming and other smooth activities. At 3 months postoperatively jogging commences. At the 6th month gentle recreational sports such as tennis may re-start. At 9 months competitive game training commences and all competitive sports are resumed at 1 year.

5.6 Semitendinosus and gracilis tendon reconstruction for acute anterior cruciate ligament injuries

Dipak V. Patel, Paul M. Aichroth and Graham J. Belham

The management of acute anterior cruciate ligament (ACL) injuries is controversial. The natural history of untreated ACL injury has been reported by various authors.[1-6] Anterior cruciate insufficiency usually results in progressive, symptomatic instability, and there is increasing risk of injury to the menisci and the articular cartilage with subsequent onset of early osteoarthrosis of the knee. Early surgical intervention has been suggested for acute ACL injuries in selected patients.[7-9]

The treatment of acute mid-substance tear of the ACL by direct repair is unsatisfactory and, therefore, augmentation is necessary. The most commonly used autogenous tissues for augmentation are the patellar tendon,[10-13] the iliotibial tract,[14,15] and semitendinosus tendon.[16-20] The semitendinosus tendon can be used with or without the addition of the gracilis tendon. The purpose of this study was to evaluate the clinical results of semitendinosus and gracilis tendon reconstruction for acute ACL injuries in young, athletically active individuals with high sporting demand on the knee.

Table 1 The mode of injury in 40 patients.

Mode	Number of knees	Percentage
Skiing	32	80
Football and rugby	6	
Tennis	1	20
Horse riding	1	

Table 2 The associated procedures.

Procedure	No. of knees
Medial collateral ligament repair	3
Arthroscopic partial medial meniscectomy	3
Arthroscopic partial lateral meniscectomy	4
Arthroscopic medial meniscal repair	1
Arthroscopic lateral meniscal repair	2
Osteochondral fracture of the medial femoral condyle	1
Chondral fracture of the lateral tibial plateau	1

Material and methods

Between January 1986 and April 1989, 40 patients underwent semitendinosus and gracilis tendon reconstruction for acute ACL injury to the knee. All operations were either performed or supervised by the senior author (P.M.A.). There were 17 males and 23 females. The right knee was involved in 12 cases and the left in 28. The mean age of the patients at the time of operation was 28.8 years (range 16–57 years). The average follow-up was 36.4 months (range 24–64 months). The mean interval between the injury and the operation was 6 days (range 2–42 days). However, with the advent of arthroscopically assisted technique, this interval has increased. We now prefer to do the arthroscopically assisted ACL reconstruction using the medial hamstrings tendons, at 2–8 weeks following the injury, when the effusion has settled and the knee is mobile.

The majority of the patients participated in some form of sport prior to the injury. The majority of the female patients were involved in recreational sports and most of the male patients were participating in competitive sports. Each patient's sporting activities were documented with attention to the level of intensity of participation. The details of the mode of injury are given in Table 1. Skiing accounted for 80% of the injuries.

The incidence of the associated surgical procedures in patients with an ACL tear is shown in Table 2. Three patients required medial collateral ligament repair for grade III tears. Seven patients had arthroscopic partial meniscectomy (3 medial and 4 lateral) and three had arthroscopic repair of the meniscus for peripheral detachment (1 medial and 2 lateral).

The preoperative Lysholm-II knee score, the Tegner activity level, the clinical signs of instability and the KT-1000 assessment were carefully recorded. The Lysholm-II knee score (Table 3) is a slight modification of the Lysholm knee score originally described

Table 3 The Lysholm-II score.

	Points
Limp	
None	5
Slight or periodic	3
Severe and constant	0
Support	
None	5
Stick or crutch needed	2
Weight bearing impossible	0
Locking	
None	15
Catching sensation, but no locking	10
Locking occasionally	6
Locking frequently	2
Locked joint at examination	0
Instability	
Never	25
Rarely during athletic activities	20
Frequently during athletic activities	15
Occasionally during daily activities	10
Often during daily activities	5
Every step	0
Pain	
None	25
Inconstant and slight during strenuous activities	20
Marked during or after walking >2 km	10
Marked during or after walking <2 km	5
Constant	0
Swelling	
None	10
After strenuous activities	6
After ordinary activities	3
Constant	0
Stairs	
No problem	10
Slight problem	6
One step at a time	3
Impossible	0
Squatting	
No problem	5
Slight problem	4
Not beyond 90° of flexion of the knee	2
Impossible	0

by Lysholm and Gillquist.[21] Patients with a score between 91 and 100 were considered excellent; between 77 and 90 as good; between 68 and 76 as fair; and less than 68 as poor.[22]

The pre-injury, the preoperative and the postoperative Tegner activity levels[23] were also documented. The mean preoperative Lysholm score was 36 points (range 13–53 points). The average pre-injury Tegner activity level was 7 (range 5–10) and the average preoperative Tegner activity level was 1.8 (range 0–4).

The Lachman test,[24] the anterior drawer sign and the pivot shift sign[30] were graded from 0 to III (0 being normal) by comparison with the opposite uninjured knee. Preoperatively, 32 knees (80%) had grade III Lachman test and 8 knees (20%) had grade II Lachman test (Figure 1). Thirty-three knees (82.5%) had grade II pivot shift and 7 knees (17.5%) had grade III pivot shift sign (Figure 2).

The instrumented measurement of the anterior tibial displacement was performed using the KT-1000 arthrometer (MEDmetric Corp., San Diego, Calif., USA) with application of an 89-N load (20 lb) at 20° of knee flexion.[25] The mean side-to-side difference in the anterior tibial translation was recorded both preoperatively and postoperatively.

All patients were independently reviewed by one of the authors (D.V.P.). The postoperative assessment included the Lysholm-II score, the Tegner activity level, the clinical signs of instability and the KT-1000 assessment as recorded preoperatively. Routine radiographs (AP weight-bearing, lateral, 'tunnel' and skyline views) were obtained to assess possible degenerative changes in the patellofemoral and tibiofemoral joints.

The data were analysed using the chi-squared test and Student's *t*-test.

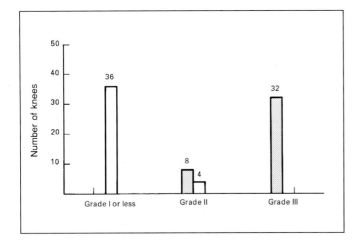

Figure 1

The preoperative (solid) and postoperative (open) details of the Lachman test.

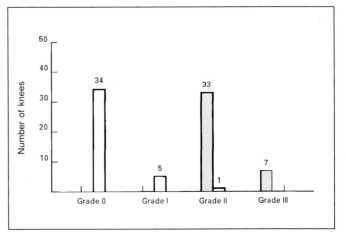

Figure 2

The preoperative (solid) and postoperative (open) details of the pivot shift sign.

Indication for surgery

It is difficult to define the indications for surgery in the acute situation. In our series, all patients were carefully counselled preoperatively. The reconstruction was advised in young, well-motivated, athletically active patients who wished to return to competitive or recreational sports. In addition, those patients who were reluctant to wear a knee brace or those who were totally unwilling to modify their sporting lifestyle were also considered.

Operative technique

All patients had an examination under anaesthetic and arthroscopic assessment prior to or at the time of surgery. An open technique of ACL reconstruction using the semitendinosus and gracilis tendons was performed. The tendons were detached proximally, keeping the distal insertion intact. The tendons were routed 'over-the-top' of the lateral femoral condyle and secured with two staples. The surgical procedure is described in detail by Paul Aichroth in contribution 5.5. Currently, the same operation is being performed using the arthroscopically assisted technique. The preliminary results of the ACL reconstruction using the arthroscopically assisted technique seem to be encouraging and the postoperative rehabilitation is faster and easier.

Postoperative management

Immediate continuous passive mobilization (CPM) was commenced while the patient was in the recovery room. Initially, the CPM machine was set with range of movement blocked between 0 and 40° depending upon the tolerance of the patient. Gradually the degree of flexion was increased and by about 7–10 days, 90° of knee flexion was achieved. After 5–7 days, a knee brace was applied. On the 2nd or 3rd postoperative day, non-weight-bearing mobilization was started using elbow crutches.

The brace was discontinued at 6 weeks from the date of operation and partial weight bearing was allowed, followed by full weight bearing. All patients underwent a well-supervised quadriceps and hamstrings rehabilitation programme for the first 6–8 weeks. Between 3 and 6 months, swimming, cycling and fast walking were permitted. Between 6 and 9 months, gentle recreational sports were encouraged. Athletic training began at 9 months, and contact sports and skiing were allowed after 12 months. A Don–Joy knee brace was used for the first season of skiing. A few anxious patients felt more secure with the Don–Joy brace while participating in recreational or competitive sports.

Results

Eighteen patients (45%) had an excellent result, 19 (47.5%) had a good result and 3 (7.5%) had a fair result. None of the patients had a poor result. At the time of latest review, the Lachman test was grade I or less in 36 patients (90%) (details in Figure 1) and the pivot shift sign was eliminated in 34 patients (85%) (details in Figure 2). Five patients (12.5%) had a grade I pivot shift (minimal glide but no jerk) and one patient had grade II pivot shift.

The mean postoperative Lysholm-II knee score was 91 (range 68–100) and the average Tegner activity level was 5.5 (range 4–10). Thirty patients (75%) returned to their previous sports with a pre-injury level of performance (including four international football players) and 5 (13%) were participating in pre-injury sports at a reduced intensity level. Three patients were playing different sports and two had changed their lifestyle.

Seven patients complained of occasional swelling on strenuous exertion. However, on clinical examination, a minimal effusion was noted in only two knees. Residual quadriceps wasting of <1 cm was seen in eight knees; four knees had 1–2 cm of quadriceps wasting and two knees had >2 cm of quadriceps atrophy. Thirty-six patients had a full range of knee movement (0–140°), three had 10° limitation of terminal flexion and one had 15° restriction of flexion.

The KT-1000 assessment (measured at 20° of knee flexion at 89-N load) showed that 37 patients (92.5%) had side-to-side difference values of 3 mm or less (details are shown in Table 4). The clinical findings of knee stability correlated well with the instrumented measurements ($P<0.05$).

Table 4 KT-1000 arthrometer findings.

Side-to-side difference[a] (mm)	Number of knees	Percentage
≤1 mm	22	55
1.1–2.0 mm	8	20
2.1–3.0 mm	7	17.5
>3 mm	3	7.5

[a]At 89 N (20 lb) load, with the knee in 20° of flexion.

On radiological assessment, no significant degenerative changes were seen in any of the knees. On critical analysis of the radiographs, mild subchondral sclerosis was seen in six knees and inferior patellar pole spurring was noted in five.

Patient satisfaction

Thirty-eight patients (95%) were pleased or satisfied with the functional result of their knees and two patients expressed reservation about the outcome.

Complications

One patient had a superficial stitch infection which settled with a course of broad-spectrum antibiotics. There were no cases of deep sepsis in this series. Manipulation under anaesthetic was performed in three patients at an average of 3 weeks postoperatively. Two of these patients had 130° of knee flexion and one had 125° of flexion when last reviewed.

One patient subsequently underwent arthroscopic partial lateral meniscectomy 26 months following the primary reconstruction. At 'second-look' arthroscopy, the 'neoligament' was found to be stable on probing, with good superficial vascularity.

Discussion

The central one-third of the ligamentum patellae is the most commonly used autogenous tissue for the management of the anterior cruciate deficient knee. However, there are numerous problems associated with its use, such as persistent patellofemoral pain, rupture of the ligamentum patellae, patellar fracture, or rarely medial subluxation of the patella.[26-28] Therefore, alternative autologous tissues such as semitendinosus and gracilis tendons were advocated for the reconstruction of the ACL. These tendons are accessible and their use involves less dissection in the acutely injured knee.

In our series, we used the semitendinosus and the gracilis tendons for ACL reconstruction. Lipscomb et al.[29] reported that after harvesting the semitendinosus and gracilis tendons, the hamstrings strength averaged 99% compared to the normal knees using Cybex isokinetic dynamometer testing at an average follow-up of 26.2 months. When the semitendinosus tendon alone was used, there was no difference (102%) from the normal knee. This study confirms that there is no significant loss of hamstring strength when the semitendinosus and gracilis tendons are used for reconstruction of the ACL.

In the present series, the ACL reconstruction was undertaken using an open technique. Eighteen patients (45%) had an excellent result and 19 (47.5%) had a good result at an average follow-up of 36.4 months (range 24–64 months). However, in the past 3 years, our operative technique has changed and we now perform the ACL reconstruction using the arthroscopically assisted technique. The postoperative pain

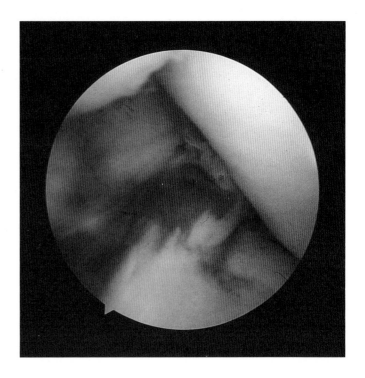

Figure 3

Arthroscopic appearance of an acute ACL tear in a 24-year-old patient.

and morbidity is much less following the arthroscopically assisted ACL reconstruction and the rehabilitation much quicker. To date, the preliminary results of this technique appear to be most encouraging.

We believe that arthroscopic examination of the acutely injured knee is vital in order to confirm the clinical diagnosis of the ACL tear (Figure 3), to identify any associated meniscal injury (tear or peripheral detachment) and to assess the extent of damage, if any, to the articulating surfaces of the knee. In our study, 3 patients had an associated grade III injury of the medial collateral ligament which required surgical repair; 7 patients had meniscal tears (3 medial and 4 lateral) requiring arthroscopic partial meniscectomies, and 3 patients underwent arthroscopic repair for peripheral detachment of the meniscus (1 medial and 2 lateral). There was no statistically significant difference in the subjective or objective outcome in patients with associated meniscal or collateral ligament injuries as compared to those without such injuries.

At the time of latest follow-up, the Lachman test was grade I or less in 90% of the patients and the pivot shift was eliminated in 85%. These findings were supported by the objective KT-1000 assessment, in which 92.5% of the knees had side-to-side difference values of 3 mm or less of anterior tibial translation, as compared to the opposite uninjured knee.

We believe that early reconstruction of the ACL in young, athletically active patients with high sporting demand on the knee is necessary to minimize the risk of further meniscal or articular cartilage damage. Careful preoperative counselling is vital before surgery is undertaken.

Summary

A prospective study of 40 patients with acute anterior cruciate ligament injury who underwent reconstruction using the semitendinosus and gracilis tendons is reported. The average age of the patients at operation was 28.8 years (range 16–57 years) and the average follow-up was 36.4 months (range 24–64 months). Skiing accounted for 80% of the injuries.

All patients had an examination under anaesthetic and arthroscopic assessment prior to or at the time of surgery. The mean preoperative Lysholm score was 36 (range 13–53). The average pre-injury Tegner activity level was 7 (range 5–10).

Eighteen patients (45%) had an excellent result, 19 (47.5%) had good result, and 3 (7.5%) had a fair result. None of the patients had a poor result. The mean postoperative Lysholm score was 91 (range 66–100) and the average postoperative Tegner activity level was 5.5 (range 4–10). Thirty patients (75%) returned to their previous sports with a pre-injury level of performance and 5 (13%) were participating in pre-injury sports at a reduced activity level. Thirty-eight patients (95%) were pleased or satisfied with the result of surgery.

We recommend semitendinosus and gracilis tendon reconstruction for acute anterior cruciate ligament injuries in young, athletically active individuals who wish to return to competitive or recreational sports. The results on a short-term basis are encouraging. A long-term follow-up study is necessary.

References

1. Arnold JA, Coker TP, Heaton LM et al., Natural history of anterior cruciate tears, *Am J Sports Med* (1979) **7**: 305–313.
2. Fetto JF, Marshall JL, The natural history and diagnosis of anterior cruciate ligament insufficiency, *Clin Orthop* (1980) **147**: 29–38.
3. Jacobsen K, Osteoarthrosis following insufficiency of the cruciate ligaments in man, *Acta Orthop Scand* (1977) **48**: 520–526.
4. McDaniel WJ Jr, Dameron TB Jr, Untreated ruptures of the anterior cruciate ligament: a follow-up study, *J Bone Joint Surg (Am)* (1980) **62**: 696–705.
5. Noyes FR, Mooar PA, Matthews DS et al., The symptomatic anterior cruciate-deficient knee: Part 1. The long-term functional disability in athletically active individuals, *J Bone Joint Surg (Am)* (1983) **65**: 154–162.
6. Satku K, Kumar VP, Ngoi SS, Anterior cruciate ligament injuries: to counsel or to operate? *J Bone Joint Surg (Br)* (1986) **68**: 458–461.
7. DeHaven KE, Decision-making in acute anterior cruciate ligament injury, *Instructional Course Lectures* (1987) **36**: 201–203.
8. Jackson DW, The future of anterior cruciate ligament surgery, *The anterior cruciate deficient knee: new concepts in ligament repair*, ed Jackson DW, Drez D Jr. (St Louis: C.V. Mosby, 1987) 315–318.
9. Noyes FR, McGinniss GH, Controversy about treatment of the knee with anterior cruciate laxity, *Clin Orthop* (1985) **198**: 61–76.
10. Clancy WG, Nelson DA, Reider B et al., Anterior cruciate ligament reconstruction using one third of the patellar ligament, augmented by extra-articular tendon transfers, *J Bone Joint Surg (Am)* (1982) **64**: 352–359.
11. Eriksson E, Reconstruction of the anterior cruciate ligament, *Orthop Clin North Am* (1976) **7**: 167–179.
12. Johnson RJ, Eriksson E, Haggmark T et al., Five- to ten-year follow-up evaluation after reconstruction of the anterior cruciate ligament, *Clin Orthop* (1984) **183**: 122–140.
13. Paulos LE, Butler DL, Noyes FR et al., Intra-articular cruciate reconstruction: II. Replacement with vascularised patellar tendon, *Clin Orthop* (1983) **172**: 78–84.
14. Bertoia JT, Urovitz EP, Richards RR et al., Anterior cruciate reconstruction using the McIntosh lateral-substitution over-the-top repair, *J Bone Joint Surg (Am)* (1985) **67**: 1183–1188.
15. O'Donoghue DH, A method for replacement of the anterior cruciate ligament of the knee, *J Bone Joint Surg (Am)* (1963) **45**: 905–924.
16. Cho KO, Reconstruction of the anterior cruciate ligament by semitendinosus tenodesis, *J Bone Joint Surg (Am)* (1975) **57**: 608–612.
17. Ferretti A, Conteduca F, De Carli A et al., Results of reconstruction of the anterior cruciate ligament with the tendons of semitendinosus and gracilis in acute capsulo-ligamentous lesions of the knee. *Ital J Orthop Traumatol* (1990) **16**: 451–458.
18. Lipscomb AB, Johnston RK, Snyder RB, The technique of cruciate ligament reconstruction, *Am J Sports Med* (1981) **9**: 77–81.
19. Mott HW, Semitendinosus anatomic reconstruction for cruciate ligament insufficiency, *Clin Orthop* (1983) **172**: 90–92.
20. Zaricznyj B, Reconstruction of the anterior cruciate ligament using free tendon graft, *Am J Sports Med* (1983) **11**: 164–176.
21. Lysholm J, Gillquist J, Evaluation of knee ligament surgery results with special emphasis on use of a scoring scale, *Am J Sports Med* (1982) **10**: 150–154.
22. Odensten M, Lysholm J, Gillquist J, Long-term follow-up study of a distal iliotibial band transfer (DIT) for anterolateral knee instability, *Clin Orthop* (1983) **176**: 129–135.
23. Tegner Y, Lysholm J, Rating systems in the evaluation of knee injuries, *Clin Orthop* (1985) **198**: 43–49.
24. Torg JS, Conrad W, Kalen V, Clinical diagnosis of anterior cruciate ligament instability in the athlete, *Am J Sports Med* (1976) **4**: 84–93.
25. Daniel DM, Malcolm LL, Losse G et al., Instrumented measurement of anterior laxity of the knee, *J Bone Joint Surg (Am)* (1985) **67**: 720–726.
26. Bonamo JJ, Krinick RM, Sporn AA, Rupture of the patellar ligament after use of its central third for anterior cruciate reconstruction: a report of two cases, *J Bone Joint Surg (Am)* (1984) **66**: 1294–1297.
27. Hughston JC, Complications of anterior cruciate ligament surgery, *Orthop Clin North Am* (1985) **16**: 237–240.
28. Langan P, Fontanetta AP, Rupture of the patellar tendon after use of its central third, *Orthop Rev* (1987) **16**: 317–321.
29. Lipscomb AB, Johnston RK, Snyder RB et al., Evaluation of hamstring strength following use of semitendinosus and gracilis tendons to reconstruct the anterior cruciate ligament, *Am J Sports Med* (1982) **10**: 340–342.
30. Galway RD, Beaupré A, MacIntosh DL, Pivot shift: a clinical sign of symptomatic anterior cruciate ligament insufficiency, *J Bone Joint Surg (Br)* (1972) **54**: 763–764.

5.7 Acute anterior cruciate ligament rupture and reconstruction: The Lyon concept

Bernard Moyen, Jean L. Lerat and Elisabeth Brunet-Guedj

Acute anterior cruciate ligament rupture is a common injury. Our experience is mainly related to two major sports injury: soccer and skiing.

Diagnosis

In our experience, the accurate diagnosis of the isolated rupture of the anterior cruciate ligament (ACL) is based on the following steps.

Careful assessment of the patient's injury

The way the knee is bent, twisted or flexed during the injury, the magnitude of contact deceleration and quadriceps contraction are good indicators of what ligamentous structures are eventually stretched or torn.

The injury history should be noted. For the ACL, according to our data:
   a sudden 'pop' is noticed in 93% of cases
   a giving way in 83%
   the sport is not resumed immediately in 85%
   haemarthrosis is significantly noticed in 83% of cases.

Careful knee examination

The tests which are *always possible* are:
   Lachman test (using the Feagin technique)
   Valgus test (medial joint-line opening) at 25° and in full extension
   Varus test (lateral joint-line opening) at 25° and in full extension.
The tests which are often more difficult are:
   Pivot-shift test
   Anterior drawer test at 90° of flexion.

Radiographs

AP, lateral and patellar views should be taken and examined at seven levels:
   Tibial spines (2)
   Femoral, tibial and fibular collateral ligament insertions
   Anterolateral Segond fracture.
Arthrometer KT 1000
Passive stress radiographs according to our protocol.

Patient selection for surgery

Not all patients require surgery and the treatment must be well accepted by the patient. Specifically, the patient has to be informed of the risks of surgery and the need for a rehabilitation programme.

Patients who require surgery are those young (skeletally mature) patients involved in high-level sporting activities with hard cutting, jumping, etc.

Patients who do not require surgery are skeletally immature patients; those with a history of knee infection; patients who are unable to follow the postoperative rehabilitation programme for personal or professional reasons; older patients; those with disadvantageous general health factors.

Examination of the knee under general or epidural anaesthesia with arthroscopy is the first recommended step before surgery. Arthroscopy must be extremely carefully performed when associated peripheral lesions are present because of the risk of compartment syndrome.

Surgery

Two questions must be answered: when and how to operate? For us, this depends mainly on whether the

ACL is torn in a so-called isolated fashion or not.

From our previous surgical experience, we will prospectively consider as significant a differential peripheral laxity that is one plus (5 mm) on the lateral side, two plus on the medial side, unless the patient has a morphotype in valgus (one plus in this situation).

When to operate?

Isolated ACL rupture

We will delay the operation until the knee has minimal or no effusion, using appropriate anti-inflammatory drugs and physiotherapy. The operation will take place at 3–4 weeks.

ACL rupture with associated peripheral capsuloligamentous structures

The operation is done in the first 2 weeks. We recommend that it should not be done immediately after the injury when there is a large subcutaneous haematoma. In this case, the risk of skin necrosis is increased.

What kind of surgery?

For isolated ACL rupture

We use an intra-articular bone–patellar tendon–bone autologous graft as a primary reconstruction. In few cases, ACL is repaired (avulsion fractures, femoral detachments) and augmented with a smaller graft. We consider an additional lateral extra-articular procedure when our passive stress radiographs indicate a large amount (more than 15 mm) of differential advancement of the lateral knee compartment.

For ACL rupture with associated peripheral capsuloligamentous structures

ACL is reconstructed as previously described. Medial and lateral capsulo-menisco-ligamentous structures are repaired and augmented using semitendinosus for the medial side and a strip of either biceps or fascia lata for the lateral side.

Rehabilitation

Non-operated ACL rupture

After a short period of knee splinting, with weight bearing, patients regain their normal range of movement, increasing their muscular strength and knee muscular control (co-contraction hamstrings, quadriceps). Patients are encouraged to do at least 3 months of rehabilitation prior to resuming any sports training. They are also strongly recommended to change the sport level in terms of intensity exposure and functional level, in order to avoid giving-way episodes, effusions and damage to menisci or articular cartilage.

Operated ACL rupture

Immediate protected weight bearing is allowed with a non-rigid knee immobilizer and two crutches for 3–4 weeks. Range of movement from zero to full flexion is initiated with continuous passive motion for the first 10 days. Flexion of 130° should be obtained by 6 weeks. Slow running is resumed at 3 months, and full sports participation at 5–6 months.

In case of peripheral repair, there is no change in the rehabilitation programme except for medial repair on a valgus knee. In these cases, a rigid knee immobilizer is used for walking for 4–6 weeks.

5.8 Preoperative evaluation of anterior knee laxity by dynamic radiographs

Jean L. Lerat and Bernard Moyen

The anterior cruciate ligament (ACL) is the main restraint of the anterior tibial translation. Butler's experiments[1] have shown that it absorbs nearly 90% of the constraints due to this motion, whatever the angle of knee flexion.

Experimentally, Fukubayashi et al.[2] showed that the ACL section induces an increase in this translation, without a modification in the amplitude of the posterior translation. This increase is for Markolf et al.[3] more distinct at a flexion angle of 20° than on complete extension or at 90° of flexion. Numerous clinical tests have confirmed that the Lachman test, or anterior drawer at 20° of flexion, is the most reliable diagnostic sign for an ACL lesion. But an evaluation of the importance of the laxity is impossible by simple clinical tests, which are subjective, imprecise and scarcely reproducible.[4-7]

Several instrumental techniques have been developed to fill this deficiency[8-10] but have no regular clinical application because of their complexity. Except for the Daniel[11] and Sherman[12] apparatus, radiographic techniques are currently the simplest and most reliable, especially when effected at a flexion of 20°.[13-16]

This study describes a protocol for the measurement of radiological laxity by passive dynamic lateral views in anterior and posterior drawer at a flexion angle of 20° and with a load of 9 kg, allowing the proposal of a classification of the pathological anterior laxity with objective foundations.

Material and methods

One hundred consecutive patients operated on for an ACL insufficiency have benefited from an identical protocol evaluation of the importance of the laxity. This protocol consisted of passive dynamic radiographs in anterior and posterior drawer with a 9-kg load, bilateral and comparative, according to the technique described by one of our research team.[17,18]

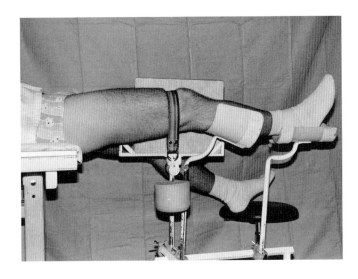

Figure 1

Anterior drawer: positioning of the patient.

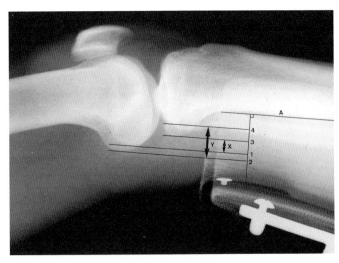

Figure 2

Radiological analysis.

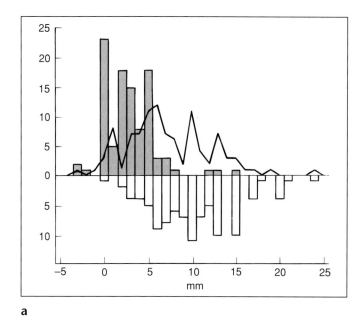

a

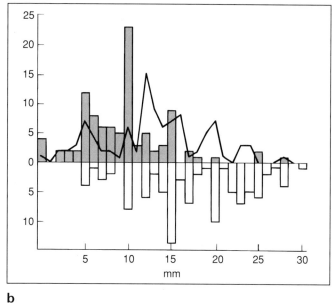

b

Figure 3

(a) Anterior translation of medial compartment values for uninjured knees (solid), injured knees (open), and pathological laxity (line). (b) Anterior translation of lateral compartment values for uninjured knees (solid), injured knees (open), and pathological laxity (line).

Radiological technique

Anterior drawer

The patient is supine on the radiological table, hips on the edge of the table (Figure 1). The examined limb is placed on a special support: the thigh is free, and the leg is placed in a rigid splint fixed to the floor, the edge of which is placed just underneath the knee joint. The foot rests on a second support, which is height-regulated and the ankle is fixed by a strap. The opposite limb rests on a stool in the inferior plane. The tested knee is flexed at 20° by the fixed inclination of the splint. The 9-kg load is applied to the thigh using a strap placed above the patella. This load therefore pushes down the distal femur, while the proximal tibia is maintained in place by the splint, causing an anterior tibial displacement. The radiography cassette is fixed to a support and placed against the medial face of the knee. The X-ray source is set up at 1 m from the cassette, following the exact profile incidence of the knee. (See Figure 1.)

Posterior drawer

The installation of the patient on the radiological table and of the opposing limb is identical. The proximal end of the support is turned by 180°; the thigh then rests on the splint, the edge of which is placed just above the knee joint. The leg is free, the ankle and the foot are in the same position as above. The tested knee is flexed at 20° by the fixed inclination of the splint. The 9-kg load is applied to the leg by a strap placed on the tibial tubercle. This load therefore pushes down the proximal tibia, while the distal femur is held in place by the splint, causing a posterior tibial displacement. The radiological technique is identical.

Radiological analysis

Bone contours

The medial femoral condyle has a rather insignificant notch at its junction with the trochlea, which is relatively anterior; it is rounded at its posterior end; the adductor tubercle can be visible above its posterior edge if the radiograph is not a perfect profile. The condylotrochlear notch of the lateral condyle is larger, deeper and more posterior; its posterior edge is more angled.

The posterior edge of the medial tibial plateau is vertical, and its junction with its superior edge makes a right angle. The posterior edge of the lateral tibial plateau is rounded, and follows a gentle slope towards the posterior tibial spine. (See Figure 2.)

Displacement measurement

The reference line is the posterior tibial cortex. The respective positions of the femur and tibia are determined for each medial and lateral compartment by two parallels to the reference line, passing by the most posterior point of the condyle and the corresponding tibial plateau. The position which corresponds to the superposition of the two homologous lines in each compartment can be defined as neutral, or 'radiologically zero'. The anterior or posterior displacements are measured by the distance in millimetres between the two lines in each compartment on the respective pictures in anterior or posterior drawer, it being possible to measure negative values.

Four measurements are obtained for each knee: anterior translation of medial compartment (ATMC) or lateral compartment (ATLC), and posterior translation of medial compartment (PTMC) or lateral compartment (PTLC). It is then possible to calculate the differential values between the injured and the uninjured knee of the same patient, that is the pathological laxity (abbreviated respectively PATMC, PATLC, PPTMC and PPTLC).

Results

Anterior translation

The average ATMC value for uninjured knees is 2.9 ± 2.9 mm with a range from –3 to +15 mm. The average value for injured knees changes to 10.2 ± 4.8 mm, with a range from 0 to 24 mm (P <0.001). The average pathological laxity PATMC is then 7.3 ± 4.8 mm with a range from –3 to +24 mm. (See Figure 3a.)

The average ATLC value for uninjured knees is 9.4 ± 5.2 mm, with a range from 0 to 28 mm. The average value for injured knees changes to 17.3 ± 6.2 mm, with a range from 5 to 30 mm (P <0.001). The average pathological laxity PATLC is then 7.9 ± 5.8 mm with a range from –5 to +23 mm. (See Figure 3b.)

A statistical correlation exists between the paired values of the anterior pathological laxities of both compartments of the same patients, which do not follow the same variation curve (Figure 4): the pathological laxity of the lateral compartment is greater than that of the medial compartment for lower values, and this relationship becomes inverted for higher values (correlation coefficient r = 0.32, P <0.001).

Posterior translation

The average PTMC value for uninjured knees is 2.7 ± 2.5 mm, with a range from –2 to +10 mm. The average value for injured knees is 2.8 ± 2.9 mm, with

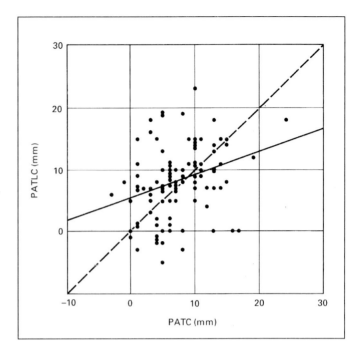

Figure 4

Statistical correlation between pathological laxity of anterior translation of lateral compartment (PATLC) and pathological laxity of anterior translation of medial compartment (PATMC). Ideal correlation, dotted line; calculated correlation, solid line.

a range from –2 to +14 mm (no statistical difference). The average pathological laxity PPTMC is then practically zero: 0.1 ± 3.2 mm, with a range from –9 to +7 mm. (See Figure 5a.)

The average PTLC value for uninjured knees is 1.7 ± 4.1 mm, with a range from –10 to +13 mm. The average value for injured knees is 1.3 ± 3.7 mm, with range from –10 to +10 mm. The average pathological laxity PPTLC is also practically zero: –0.4 ± 5.1 mm with a range from –15 to +14 mm. (See Figure 5b.)

No correlation exists between the paired values of the pathological posterior translations of both compartments in the same patient.

Discussion

The evaluation of the preoperative knee laxity must provide three items of information: the conclusive diagnosis of the ACL rupture, a reference value of the efficiency of surgical treatment, and a detailed study of the pathological displacements, leading to a better comprehension of laxity physiopathology, and perhaps to an adapted treatment.

Radiographic methods have been most described because they are easy to use, and involve no sophisticated apparatus. As the tibial displacement is at its

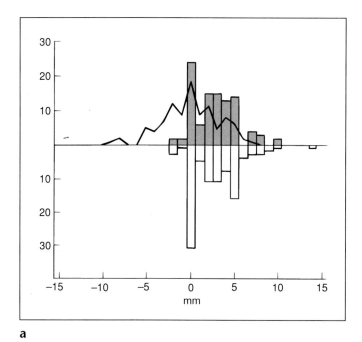

a

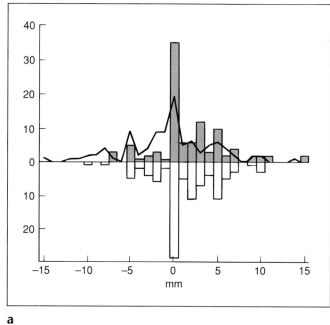

a

Figure 5

(a) Posterior translation of medial compartment values for uninjured knees (solid), injured knees (open), and pathological laxity (line). (b) Posterior translation of lateral compartment values for uninjured knees (solid), injured knees (open), and pathological laxity (line).

maximum at 20° of flexion, it is preferable to perform the radiological examination in this position.

The intensity of the applied load causes a variation in the measured values of not negligible proportions: the displacements are moderate, and sometimes even negative for the uninjured knee, in the study by Hooper[13] with a load of 3 kg. But a load of 20 kg, recommended by Stäubli et al.[15] hardly modifies the results in relation to those of the present research, for the uninjured knees as well as the injured ones. The choice of a load of 9 kg therefore seems a satisfactory compromise between the sensitivity of the test and the patient's comfort. Nevertheless, it is necessary, because of its variability, to carry out the examination using a fixed, known load, and this seems to us a contraindication for the utilization of active radiographs as recommended by Dejour et al.[19]

In these conditions, the normal radiological values of anterior translation are compatible to those obtained by more sophisticated apparatus, which vary between 3 and 10 mm.[11,12,20] Values for the pathological knees are difficult to compare from one study to another because the recruitment may not be homogeneous.

In agreement with Hooper[13] and Stäubli et al.,[15] this series shows the presence of a clear increase in the anterior displacement of the two compartments of the knee in the absence of the ACL (P <0.001).

The ATMC measurement is the most reliable for the diagnosis of the ACL lesion, the statistical limit being situated at 5 mm: 90% of uninjured knees do not exceed this value (specificity), whereas 84% of injured knees exceed it (sensitivity). The predictive positive value (probability that a value over 5 mm corresponds to an ACL lesion) is 89%, whereas the predictive negative value (probability that a value under 5 mm corresponds to an intact ACL) is 85%.

As a result of the variability of constitutional laxity in patients, the study of the differential, or pathological, values in relation to the uninjured knee, which Shino et al.[10] showed to be near to zero in normal patients, allows a more accurate diagnosis. On choosing arbitrarily a normality limit of 2 mm, as proposed by Markolf et al.[9] the sensibility of PATMC for the diagnosis of an ACL lesion is 87%. The other figures (specificity and predictive values) cannot be calculated in the absence of a comparative series of normal subjects, but it is probable that they are also better than those of the isolated ATMC. The comparative dynamic radiographs are therefore an appreciable diagnostic test.

However, their principal interest lies in the possibility of visualizing not only a global displacement of the tibia, but of differentiating the displacements of the medial and lateral compartments. Therefore, it is possible to carry out a more precise study of the pathological anterior laxity. The curve of the paired values (PATLC as a function of PATMC – Figure 4) can be statistically reduced to a line of slope $p = 0.66$, with a correlation coefficient $r = 0.32$ ($P < 0.001$). It appears, in comparison with the neutral line of slope 1, that the pathological displacement of the lateral compartment is superior to that of the medial one for low values, whereas this relationship inverts for higher values, the transition occurring for values of about 10 mm for the two measurements. In other words, an increase in the internal rotation of the injured knee can be observed when the anterior translation is low; in contrast, a reduction of the internal rotation can be observed when the anterior translation becomes higher. The measurement of the pathological translation of the lateral compartment is therefore always high, even for a low distension of the medial compartment: it is the classical consequence of an isolated rupture of the ACL, and it is the basis for all the dynamic tests in internal rotation. But a more marked distension of the medial compartment, probably resulting from a lesion of the posteromedial corner, is not accompanied by an analogous increase in the lateral distension, and can become preponderant.

Two types of anterior laxity can therefore be distinguished (Figure 6):

– The anterolateral laxity, with a moderate pathological anterior translation predominating in the lateral compartment, and which corresponds to an isolated ACL lesion.

– The global anterior laxity, with a large pathological anterior translation predominating in the medial compartment, and which corresponds to the association of the ACL lesion with damage to the posteromedial corner.

The posterior drawer radiographs were aimed at detecting an associated posterior laxity, in particular posterolateral, by lesion of the corresponding corner. No significant statistical difference has been discovered in this series between the values of the posterior translation depending on the condition of the ACL. No posterior or posterolateral laxity can therefore be discovered at 20° of flexion with dynamic radiographs.

Conclusion

If the diagnostic contribution of dynamic radiographs can be useful in the case of an ACL lesion, especially in cases where the clinical examination is difficult to interpret, their principal interest is to allow, by visualization of the displacement of each compartment, a detailed study of their anterior pathological drawers. This can lead to a distinction between two types of laxity, depending on their respective relationships. The anatomical difference between

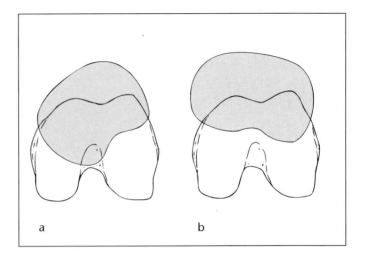

Figure 6

(a) Anterolateral laxity; (b) global anterior laxity.

anterolateral and global anterior laxity probably results, in the second case, from damage to the posteromedial corner. This study, confined to a single preoperative examination, cannot confirm whether there is a progressive deterioration with time for a given patient, from one category to another. However, the posterior drawer radiographs at 20° of flexion cannot identify damage to the posterolateral corner.

It would now be desirable to define for each type of laxity a surgical treatment adapted to the lesions of peripheral formations, a judicious surgical repair of which could be a basis for the better treatment of ACL insufficiency.

References

1. **Butler DL, Noyes FR, Grood ES**, Ligamentous restraints to anterior–posterior drawer in the human knee: a biomechanical study, *J Bone Joint Surg (Am)* (1980) **62**: 259–270.
2. **Fukubayashi T, Torzilli PA, Sherman MF et al.**, An in vitro biomechanical evaluation of antero-posterior motion of the knee: tibial displacement, rotation and torque, *J Bone Joint Surg (Am)* (1982) **64**: 258–264.
3. **Markolf KL, Mensch JS, Amstutz HC**, Stiffness and laxity of the knee – The contributions of the supporting structures: a quantitative in vitro study, *J Bone Joint Surg (Am)* (1976) **58**: 583–594.
4. **Galway HR, MacIntosh DL**, The lateral pivot shift: a symptom and sign of anterior cruciate ligament insufficiency, *Clin Orthop* (1980) **147**: 45–50.
5. **Hughston JC, Andrews JR, Cross MJ et al.**, Classification of knee ligament instabilities, *J Bone Joint Surg (Am)* (1976) **58**: 159–179.

6. Slocum DB, James SL, Larson RL et al., Clinical test for anterolateral rotatory instability of the knee, *Clin Orthop* (1976) **118**: 63–69.

7. Torg JS, Conrad W, Kalen V, Clinical diagnosis of anterior cruciate ligament instability in the athlete, *Am J Sports Med* (1976) **4**: 84–93.

8. Kennedy JC, Fowler PJ, Medial and anterior instability of the knee: An anatomical and clinical study using stress machines, *J Bone Joint Surg (Am)* (1971) **53**: 1257–1270.

9. Markolf KL, Graff-Radford A, Amstutz HC, In vivo knee stability: A quantitative assessment using an instrumented clinical testing apparatus, *J Bone Joint Surg (Am)* (1978) **60**: 664–674.

10. Shino K, Inoue M, Horibe S et al., Measurement of anterior instability of the knee: a new apparatus for clinical testing, *J Bone Joint Surg (Br)* (1987) **69**: 608–613.

11. Daniel DM, Malcom LL, Losse G et al., Instrumented measurement of anterior laxity of the knee, *J Bone Joint Surg (Am)* (1985) **67**: 720–726.

12. Sherman OH, Markolf KL, Ferkel RD, Measurements of anterior laxity in normal and anterior cruciate absent knees with two instrumented test devices, *Clin Orthop* (1987) **215**: 156–161.

13. Hooper GJ, Radiological assessment of anterior cruciate ligament deficiency: a new technique, *J Bone Joint Surg (Br)* (1986) **68**: 292–296.

14. Iversen BF, Sturup J, Jakobsen K, Stress radiographic comparison of drawer symptoms measured in 90 degrees versus 15 degrees of knee flexion, *Surgery and arthroscopy of the knee*, ed Müller W, Hackenbruch W (Berlin: Springer, 1988) 91–92.

15. Stäubli HU, Jakob RP, Noesberger B, Anterior–posterior knee instability and stress radiography: A prospective biomechanical analysis with the knee in extension, *Biomechanics: current interdisciplinary research* (The Hague: Nijhoff, 1984) 397–402.

16. Torzilli PA, Greenberg RL, Hood RW et al., Measurement of anterior–posterior motion of the knee in injured patients using a biomechanical stress technique, *J Bone Joint Surg (Am)* (1984) **66**: 1438–1442.

17. Lerat JL, Moyen B, Dupre La Tour L et al., Measurement of the anterior laxity of the knee with dynamic X-rays and with the KT1000 arthrometer, *Rev Chir Orthop* (1988) **74** (suppl. II): 194–197.

18. Lerat JL, Moyen B, Dupre La Tour L et al., Measurement of laxities by stress radiography and by KT1000 arthrometer, *Surgery and arthroscopy of the knee*, ed Müller W, Hackenbruch W (Berlin: Springer, 1988) 85–90.

19. Dejour H, Walch G, Neyret P et al., Résultats des laxités chroniques antérieures opérées. A propos de 251 cas revus avec un recul minimum de 3 ans, *Rev Chir Orthop* (1988) **74**: 622–636.

20. Markolf KL, Kochan A, Amstutz HC, Measurement of knee stiffness and laxity in patients with documented absence of the anterior cruciate ligament, *J Bone Joint Surg (Am)* (1984) **66**: 242–253.

5.9 Anterior cruciate ligament injuries in childhood and adolescence

Zaid Al-Duri, Dipak V. Patel and Paul M. Aichroth

Injuries to the anterior cruciate ligament in the growing child and adolescents require careful consideration. Such injuries are extremely unusual in children under the age of 14 years.[1-4] The increased participation in sports by the younger age groups and the increased interest in the cruciate ligaments demand an awareness on the part of the surgeon and an improvement in the means of diagnosing such injuries. Adolescence is a unique phase of physical and emotional change. It is the time for testing the individual's capabilities and tuning the athletic skills and as such moderation or curtailing of activity secondary to injury is not realistic.

The purpose of this chapter is to present an overview to the current perception and understanding of the injured anterior cruciate ligament in the skeletally immature individual.

Types of anterior cruciate ligament insufficiency

It is essential that the broad spectrum of anterior cruciate ligament insufficiency is clarified at the outset of the discussion. The assumption that anterior cruciate ligament insufficiency per se would cause a notable laxity in the knee joint is not strictly true but will help here to group the lesions satisfactorily.

A modification of the DeLee and Curtis scheme[5] is presented here.

Non-traumatic anterior cruciate ligament insufficiency

This group includes children who have no history of trauma and yet whose anterior cruciate ligament is lax. They fall into two groups.

Generalized non-pathological joint laxity

The necessity of an overall assessment of a patient cannot be overemphasized, with the knees being a part of the whole. Here bilaterality of the involvement and absence of symptoms are important. It has also been reported that no correlation could be found between ligamentous laxity and the occurrence or the type of injury in secondary-school athletes.[6] However, individuals who are unaccustomed to regular training develop rheumatic symptoms, particularly in hypermobile joints, after performing aerobics in keep-fit classes. Excessive straining of the knees by exercising may lead to a significant increase in joint laxity.[7]

Congenital absence of the anterior cruciate ligament

There is now increasing awareness of this rare condition. Some of these children may have wildly unstable knees on the examination couch while, surprisingly, their performance is little impaired.[5,8] The anterior cruciate ligament is rarely absent in an otherwise normal knee.[9] The condition may occur in association with tibial or femoral dysplasia or congenital dislocation of the patella, habitual anterior subluxation of the tibia as the knee extends, congenital dislocation of the knee, and in patients with a valgus knee and leg-length discrepancy.[8,10] The long-term future of these knees is unknown.

Post-traumatic anterior cruciate ligament insufficiency

In children the knee ligaments are known to be stronger than the adjacent physeal plate.[5,11-13] Trauma that might rupture the anterior cruciate ligament in an adult will usually cause an avulsion fracture because the incompletely ossified tibial eminence fails before the ligament.[11,28] The pattern of injuries that emerges is as follows:

1. Avulsion of the intercondylar eminence of the tibia[14]
2. Avulsion of the femoral attachment of the anterior cruciate ligament[2]

3. Avulsion of both femoral and tibial attachments of the anterior cruciate ligament[3]
4. Mid-substance tears of the anterior cruciate ligament[5,12,13,16-18]

Classification of avulsion fractures of the anterior tibial eminences

Meyers and McKeever[19,20] developed the time-honoured classification into three types based on the amount of displacement of the avulsed fragment on the lateral radiographic view.

Type I. The avulsed fragment of bone is minimally displaced, with only slight elevation of its anterior margin.
Type II. There is greater displacement, with the anterior third to half of the avulsed fragment being elevated from its bone bed. This produces a beak-like deformity on the lateral radiograph.
Type III. The avulsed fragment is completely elevated from its bed on the tibia. There is total lack of bony apposition. In some instances, the avulsed fragment is rotated.

Zaricznyj[4] modified the classification as follows:

Type 1. There is minimal anterior elevation of the fragment.
Type 2. There is up to 50% anterior elevation of the fragment.
Type 3A. The fragment is completely displaced from its bony bed in the intercondylar eminence.
Type 3B. The fragment is completely displaced and rotated.
Type 4. The fragment is comminuted, possibly extending into the medial and lateral tibial plateaux.

Incidence

Knee injuries account for 12–22% of sports injuries in school children.[21-23] Anterior cruciate ligament insufficiency is distinctly unusual in children under the age of 14 years with open physes. Clanton et al.[1] reviewed 1749 cases of knee ligament injuries and found only 9 cases of anterior cruciate ligament injuries in children under the age of 14 years.

Avulsion of the anterior intercondylar eminence of the tibia

Fracture of the intercondylar eminence of the tibia was not seen under the age of 7 years. It occurred most frequently in children between the ages of 8 and 13 years.[19]

In an analysis of 91 consecutive metaphyseal fractures, physeal injuries and ligament ruptures in children aged 14 years, there were 18 fractures of the anterior tibial spine with an annual incidence of 2.7 per 100 000,[15] The incidence of the types was as follows: Type I 28%, Type II 50%, Type III 22%. It is worth mentioning here that avulsion fracture of the posterior intercondylar eminence is a rare injury in children. The ratio of fracture of the anterior eminence to that of the posterior one is 10:1.[3] For all reported cases of tibial spine avulsions in patients with open physes, the incidence of associated ligament injury is 2.6%.

Mid-substance tears of the anterior cruciate ligament

Mid-substance tears of the anterior cruciate ligament alone or in association with other knee ligament injuries in children are distinctly unusual.[5] DeLee and Curtis reported on three mid-substance anterior cruciate ligament tears in 338 knee ligament injury cases, making the incidence of this group 0.9% of the total.[5]

Engebretsen et al.[16] found only 6 cases of childhood rupture of the substance of the anterior cruciate ligament in the literature. They reported on another 8 cases. Lipscomb et al.[17] reviewed 710 patients with anterior cruciate ligament tears. Twenty-four of them were between the ages of 12 and 15 years, making the incidence of adolescent involvement with such tears 3.4% of the total. McCarroll et al.[12] reported on 57 patients under the age of 14 years with anterior cruciate ligament tears out of a total of 1722 anterior cruciate ligament injuries, making the incidence of adolescent involvement 3.3%.

Structural and functional aspects of the cruciates

It is well known that the structures of the knee develop in an orderly succession, beginning with the chondrification of the femur and tibia and development of the patella. The cruciate ligaments develop at a later stage.[24] On the basis of a mechanical model, followed later by a mathematical one, Kapandji[25] believes that the outlines of the femoral trochlea and condyles are geometrical entities determined on the one hand by the interaction between the cruciate ligaments and their femoral and tibial attachments and, on the other, by the relationships among the ligamentum patellae, the patella and patellar retinaculum. Biologically few points of interest have emerged on this issue. Johansson and Aparisi[10] reported on a patient with congenital absence of the anterior cruciate ligament. With treatment for leg-length inequality, it was eventually clear that there was a congenital absence of the cruciate ligaments in his right knee. At the age of 7 years, a decreased height of the intercondylar fossa and a flattening of the intercondylar eminence of his right knee were seen on radiographs. At arthroscopy, there were no cruciate ligaments, the intercondylar notch was hypoplastic and the intercondylar eminence was rounded to fit the shallow notch and prevent the scope from passing through.

It is believed that atrophy of the anterior cruciate ligament follows detachment such as in an avulsion fracture, because tension is important in stimulating ligament growth[9,19,20,26] as well as the intercondylar eminence growth.[9] On the basis of clinical observations by Giorgi,[9] the hyperplasia or hypoplasia of the intercondylar eminences do not cause alterations in the mechanics of the knee joint productive of symptoms. Complete aplasia, however, which is probably associated with a morphological and functional alteration of the cruciate ligaments, is the cause of an abnormal mechanical relationship which can lead to joint symptoms.

The natural history

It is only fair to say here that long-term studies are not yet available to give the answers to several important questions. These questions include the following: Does the child and/or the adolescent have a better power of healing of the ligaments in general and the cruciates in particular compared to adults? Could the child compensate an anterior cruciate ligament deficiency better than an adult? Do various surgical procedures affect the growth plate and therefore lead to growth arrest? Are lesions of the ligaments and menisci in association with an anterior cruciate ligament rupture in the child a bigger burden on the knee joint that would eventually augment the bad influence of an anterior cruciate ligament tear or avulsion?

When an injury to the anterior cruciate ligament does occur in a child, the ligament usually fails at its insertion into the tibia,[5] rarely at its femoral attachment,[2] or within its substance.[11] There is no evidence to suggest that knee ligaments in children have the potential to heal any better than those in adults.[1,5]

Avulsion fracture of the intercondylar eminence

It is essential that the proper anterior cruciate ligament tension is restored in these cases by anatomical reduction of the displaced fragment. Therefore, only displaced fracture separations need surgical fixation.[3,19,27-29] Although displaced fractures not treated by anatomical reduction will heal, there will be effective lengthening of the anterior cruciate

ligament and, therefore, excessive anteroposterior instability.[4] If the displacement is allowed to persist, then atrophy, shortening, and laxity of the ligament will result.[4,29] No evidence of arthrosis was found on radiographs in the cases that were anatomically reduced whether treated by closed or open methods on follow-up.[3,19] All these patients have normal knee function in 2–3 months, the operative group taking slightly longer to recover.

Instability of the knee following avulsion of the anterior intercondylar eminence is due to an associated undiscovered tear of the medial collateral ligament or secondary to meniscectomy for an associated meniscal tear.[1,3,5,28,29] Repair and reattachment of menisci may contribute to stability of the knee, thus improving the results of the surgical treatment in cases of ligamentous injuries.[1] The possible complications of joint infection, arthrofibrosis and quadriceps atrophy are more likely to follow operative treatment of this injury.[3]

Mid-substance tears of the anterior cruciate ligament and associated ligamentous and meniscal lesions

The outcome of the conservative treatment of ligament injuries in adolescents has been disappointing. Kannus and Järvinen[13] reviewed 32 adolescents with an age range of 10–18 years with knee ligament injuries, of whom there were 7 cases of isolated anterior cruciate ligament ruptures and 5 cases of combined anterior cruciate ligament and medial collateral ligament injuries. All the patients were treated conservatively by plaster immobilization and followed up for an average of 8 years. The outcome of Grade II injuries was acceptable, even though static knee stability failed to improve when compared to that found at the time of the initial examination and in some even increased during follow-up, owing to stretching of the secondary restraints. However, the patients with Grade II injury tolerated mild or moderate residual instability quite well.

The long-term outcome of unrepaired Grade III injuries of the knee ligaments was poor and not acceptable. It seems that, in adolescents, the severity of the damage to ligaments is the most important factor in long-term prognosis and that which individual ligaments are involved is of only secondary importance.

In conclusion, substantial Grade II injuries of the knee ligaments in adolescents can be treated satisfactorily without operation, but this cannot be recommended for Grade III injuries. Primary repair alone is not recommended, and it may be that either primary repair with augmentation or primary reconstruction will become established as the best methods of treatment.

Waldrop et al.[28] treated a disruption of the mid-substance of the anterior cruciate ligament in a 3-year-old girl by POP immobilization in 45° flexion. They could not repair the anterior cruciate ligament and acknowledge the fact that primary repair of the mid-substance tear of the anterior cruciate ligament led to poor healing in any case. Reconstruction was viewed cautiously for fear of growth arrest in such a young patient; however, they agree that reconstruction might well produce good results in older children.[1,5]

Primary repair of the mid-substance tear of the anterior cruciate ligament has not produced satisfactory results. Mid-substance anterior cruciate ligament tear in an 11-year-old that was reported by Bradley et al.[30] resulted in only a fair result at a 13-year follow-up.

Engebretsen et al.[16] performed primary repair of the anterior cruciate ligament in 8 patients with an age range of 13–16 years. There were 3 associated medial collateral ligament ruptures that were also repaired within the first week. Meniscal injuries also occurred and were treated by medial meniscectomy in three cases and meniscal reattachment in a case of a peripheral tear of the lateral meniscus. They were all followed up for an average period of 5 years (range 3–8 years). The activity level of the group as a whole dropped from strenuous to moderate, and only three knees were stable. Five knees had anterolateral rotatory instability that was severe (in one patient), moderate (in three patients), and trace positive (in one patient). All of them had a moderately positive Lachman test. There were no complications in the immediate postoperative period. At the time of the follow-up, there were no cases of arthrosis or disturbance of growth. However, five knees had osteophytes or slight subchondral sclerosis. Therefore, they concluded that primary repair should not be used in children.

Lipscomb et al.[17] reported on the reconstruction of the mid-substance anterior cruciate ligament tear in 24 adolescent athletes with ages ranging from 12 to 15 years using the semitendinosus and gracilis tendons plus extra-articular augmentation using the Ellison procedure (in 3 patients) and the Losee procedure (in 18 patients). There were other associated procedures such as medial meniscectomy (in 12 patients) and lateral meniscectomy (in 7 patients). Two medial and two lateral menisci were repaired. The follow-up period ranged from 24 to 66 months with an average of 35 months. All patients were skeletally mature at the time of follow-up. Sixteen patients stated that the involved knee was normal; the remaining 8 stated that it was improved.

Regarding the post-operative level of activity:

- 15 patients returned to participation in all sports that they had engaged in preoperatively, with an equal level of performance.
- 3 patients returned to participation in all sports but their performance was not as good postoperatively as it had been before the injury.

- 1 patient complained of being less aggressive.
- 1 patient had some stiffness.
- 1 patient noted loss of speed.
- 5 patients returned to sports other than football (owing to their parents' advice) but their level of performance was equal to that before injury.

The overall evaluation showed that there were 16 excellent, 7 good, and 1 fair-plus result. Only one patient showed a significant growth abnormality.

The semitendinosus and gracilis were used because they were stronger than most other substitutes, with the exception of one-third of the patellar tendon (120% compared with 160% of the normal tensile strength of the anterior cruciate ligament) and in terms of their stiffness characteristics they match the anterior cruciate ligament better than the patellar tendon does, which is 3–4 times stiffer. Also the use of the semitendinosus and gracilis tendons to reconstruct the anterior cruciate ligament did not significantly affect the strength of internal rotation of the tibia or knee flexion evaluated with the Cybex-II dynamometer.

It is also believed that a static extra-articular reconstruction procedure (such as the Losee procedure) for anterolateral rotatory instability controls stability better than other dynamic stabilization procedures (such as the transfer of the long head of the biceps) advocated by Clancy et al. in 1979.

Reconstruction of the anterior cruciate ligament in children and adolescents by drilling across the open tibial physis and through the femoral epiphysis has not been reported previously. The obvious concern here is that the operative trauma might result in a disturbance of growth of the knee. A limb-length inequality of 1.3 cm or less was considered physiologically normal on the basis that 77% of the normal population had an average limb-length discrepancy of 7 mm and that 7–8% of adults have a limb-length discrepancy of 1.25 cm or more.

There was no important difference in the amount of inhibition of growth in the 12-year-old patients compared with those who were 14 or 15 years old at the time of the anterior cruciate ligament reconstruction. They have not followed to maturity any patient who was younger than 12 years of age at the time of operation and, therefore, they cannot advise whether this procedure should be done in younger patients. Restoration of the end-point compliance of the knee seems important in preventing symptomatic giving-way. There was a 68% prevalence of the changes after meniscectomy described by Fairbank in his patients. Those changes adversely affected the results. Consequently, meniscal repair should be performed whenever possible, in preference to meniscectomy.

McCarroll et al.[12] reported the result of their experience with 40 patients under the age of 14 years with mid-substance tears of the anterior cruciate ligament:

16 were treated conservatively with rehabilitation, bracing and counselling on activity modification; the remaining 24 patients underwent arthroscopic examination and either an extra-articular or intra-articular reconstruction based on growth potential. The average follow-up was 27 months for the conservative group and 26 months for the surgical group. In the conservative group, only 7 patients returned to sports, all experiencing recurrent episodes of giving-way, effusion and pain. Six patients underwent arthroscopy for meniscal tears, four medial and two lateral. In the surgical group, there were 10 extra-articular reconstructions and 14 intra-articular reconstructions. All returned to sports activity, and 22 of the 24 are still competing. The two remaining patients both suffered reinjury 3 years after the surgery.

DeLee and Curtis[5] reported on three mid-substance tears of the anterior cruciate ligament in 9, 11, and 12-year-old patients. All three patients underwent primary repair of the anterior cruciate ligament by a method modified from the technique of Marshall et al. 1979. They concluded that primary repair of these injuries has permitted the patients to return to preinjury activities, but the resultant clinical laxity strongly suggests that anterior cruciate ligament repair fares little better in children than in adults. However, since the long-term results of unrepaired anterior cruciate ligament injuries in children are unknown, surgical repair is still considered the treatment of choice.

Mode of injury in anterior cruciate ligament avulsions and ruptures

Avulsion fractures of the tibial or femoral attachment of the anterior cruciate ligament

Such injuries occur mainly in children as a result of a fall from a bicycle or a motorbike.[15,19,31] Meyers and McKeever[19] believed that this fracture occurred so frequently in bicycle accidents that they felt it reasonable to state that a child between the ages of 8 and 13 years who has a painful swollen knee after falling from a bicycle must be assumed to have a fracture of the intercondylar eminence of the tibia until it is proved otherwise. The injury can also occur following a fall while participating in sports such as running or playing baseball or football.[19]

Mid-substance tears of the anterior cruciate ligament

Most mid-substance tears of the anterior cruciate ligament occur as a result of sporting activities mainly in adolescents. Contact sports such as football and basketball seem to cause the brunt of these injuries.[12,16,17] In a series of 24 patients between the ages of 12 and 15 years reviewed by Lipscomb et al.,[17] football and basketball accounted for 90% of the injuries. Similarly McCarroll et al.[12] reported on 40 patients under the age of 14 years with mid-substance tears of the anterior cruciate ligament in which football and basketball accounted for 60% of the cases. Motorcycle accidents and a fall from a height can also cause the injury.[5,17]

Severe knee ligament disruption injuries tend to be associated with motor vehicular accidents.[1]

Mechanism of injury

In general, children are not engaged in the same traumatic activities that produce such ligament injuries in adolescents. Anterior, posterior, and rotatory stresses in children result in avulsion of the tibial eminence, while in the adult they result in cruciate ligament stretching or disruption.[5]

Isolated osteochondral avulsion fractures of the tibial intercondylar eminence in children are thought to be caused by abduction and internal rotation.[15,19]

Diagnosis

Symptoms

The history is not always clear in the cases of children, but some idea can be formed from the nature of the accident, whether a motor vehicular accident, a fall, or contact sports. The bicycle accident in a child with haemarthrosis is strongly suggestive.[19,20] Therefore, a high index of suspicion should alert the surgeon to such a possibility.

Signs

In an acute injury, a rapidly developing effusion of the knee occurs. In an avulsion injury to the tibial eminence, the knee joint is held in a position of flexion and there may be lack of full extension partly because of the haemarthrosis and partly owing to the muscular spasm. Meyers and McKeever[19] insist that it is the muscular spasm and not the avulsed fragment impinging upon the articular surfaces of the tibia or femur that leads to the knee being held in flexion. In children a thorough knee evaluation may not be possible in the emergency room.[1]

Meyers and McKeever[19] insist that anteroposterior instability is rarely present in the case of the avulsed intercondylar eminence fracture and if present it is minor. It is generally believed that a positive anterior drawer test sign in a patient with tibial spine avulsion indicates an associated collateral ligament injury.[1,27,32] Peripheral meniscal detachments have been reported to have a high incidence of association with avulsion fractures of the tibial spines.[1,27]

Aspiration of the involved knee joint and instillation of a local anaesthetic agent need not necessarily be done in the operating room. It allows for an easier examination of the knee joint.[1]

Many surgeons recommend *examination under anaesthesia* as a routine procedure for those cases in whom the diagnosis is unclear on the completion of the standard history, physical examination and radiography.[1,2,12] It not only helps in confirming the diagnosis in the frightened child and apprehensive adolescent but also allows a proper evaluation of associated injuries.

Arthroscopy has been recommended by many as an aid in the diagnosis of anterior cruciate ligament injuries in children and adolescents.[11,12,33,35] They do not consider the young age of the patient or the slight build of children a hindrance to the use of standard arthroscopic techniques. The value of arthroscopy is not simply diagnostic but therapeutic as well.

Investigations

Plain radiography in the form of anteroposterior and lateral views is a must in all cases of suspected ACL injury in the skeletally immature. An avulsion fracture of the intercondylar eminence is characteristically seen on the lateral radiographic view and is the basis of the classification of Meyers and McKeever.[19] Intercondylar plain views (also called the notch view) were recommended by Robinson et al.[3] to help visualize the detached femoral osteochondral attached anterior cruciate ligament fragment, and suggested that such an injury might have been missed in the past owing to the lack of awareness of the importance of this view. Oblique views may come to the rescue at times.[29]

Stress radiology has been advocated by many and some perform it routinely while examining the patient under anaesthesia. Opening at the joint-line on stress radiograph 8 mm or greater than that in the stressed normal knee has been their criterion for operative treatment in cases of combined anterior cruciate ligament and medial collateral ligament injury.[1]

Magnetic resonance imaging is helpful in the depiction of both the avulsed fragment of the intercondylar eminence and the mid-substance tear.[29]

Treatment of the childhood and adolescent anterior cruciate ligament avulsions and ruptures

It is important here to discuss a few points of relevance to the treatment philosophy. It is the aim of the surgeon in whatever method of treatment he uses to try to restore the anatomical and functional integrity of the anterior cruciate ligament and repair an associated meniscal lesion whenever that is feasible.

Avulsion fracture of the tibial spine

Treatment of this particular injury is based on the type of avulsion fracture of the tibial spine. Meyers and McKeever[19] believe that treatment of types I and II consists of aspirating the haemarthrosis followed by immobilization of the knee in a well-fitting toe-to-groin cast. This cast should be applied with the knee in a comfortable, flexed position. Tachdjian[33] advises a 20–30° of knee flexion position. Others believe that the injured knee can be immobilized in a position of extension but not hyperextension.[3] Some believe immobilization needs to be for 12 weeks.[19] Others advise immobilization for 6–8 weeks in a child that may be prolonged to 12 weeks in the older adolescent.[28] It is best that immobilization is continued until there is radiographic evidence of healing of the fragment to its bed. Since the anterior cruciate ligament is taut in hyperextension, manipulating the knee into hyperextension is not advised and may actually displace the avulsed fragment.[19,28] After removal of the cast, active exercises and gradual weight bearing are allowed. Two to three months is the required period, as a rule, to restore normal motion to the knee and normal activity to the child.[3,19,28]

Lisser and Weiner[29] recommended the following scheme of conservative treatment for types I and II avulsion fractures of the tibial spine. A long-leg hinged brace is used for 6 weeks. Hinges are set at 30–60° for 3 weeks. At this point the brace is exchanged for a short knee brace for 6 weeks, limiting to 15° of extension. Throughout this period the patient performs quadriceps and hamstring exercises in the motion allowed by the brace. Arthroscopy is indicated when persistent locking or concomitant meniscal injury is the case.

Surgical treatment of avulsion fractures of the tibial spine

Indications
1. Type II fractures with residual displacement after attempting closed reduction.[4,29]
2. Associated collateral ligament injuries or meniscal detachment.[1,29]

3. Type III Meyers and McKeever [Types 3 and 4 Zaricznyj].[3,4,19,28,29]
4. Malunited fracture[3] and old non-united fractures of the intercondylar eminence.[19,34]

Open reduction and internal fixation can be performed either through an arthrotomy[3,19,20,28] or via arthroscopy.[28,29] Should arthroscopic reduction prove difficult, then arthrotomy should be done through the anterolateral approach as the pathology is lateral.[3,28,29]

Failure of closed reduction is usually due to interposition of the anterior horn of the lateral meniscus.[22,29,33] Meyers and McKeever[19] described a case in which the avulsed area was partially under the medial meniscus. It can be gently extracted with forceps or a small hook. Once the interposing soft tissue is cleared, it should be easy to reduce the avulsed fragment either by pushing down on the superior aspect of the fragment or by extending the knee under direct vision.[3]

Internal fixation can be done using a variety of methods. Whatever method is used, crossing the proximal growth plate of the tibia should be avoided.[3,19,28,29] A wire loop may be passed over the top of the fragment behind the anterior cruciate ligament and through drillholes in the proximal tibial epiphysis, exiting anteriorly.[3,28] Small threaded pins or screws can be used to transfix the fragment into the epiphysis.[3,28,29] Meyers and McKeever[19] insist that metallic fixation and drilling holes through the upper end of the tibia are not necessary. A simple absorbable suture passed through the thin edge of the avulsed fragment and through the meniscus near its sharp margin with a cutting needle will give adequate fixation.

Some feel that not all reductions whether through arthrotomy or arthroscopy, need to be followed by internal fixation.[19,28] If the fragment is reduced operatively, then the knee can be tested for stability by attempting to extend the knee. If it is found to be stable, then no internal fixation is necessary. With the knee in extension, the apposed distal femur maintains the reduction.[3,28]

Roberts[22] advises that every attempt should be made to treat a fracture of the intercondylar eminence of the tibia by closed methods, whether the fragment is displaced or not. Reduction of even a markedly displaced fragment is possible by lifting the foot and allowing gravity to extend the knee. Roberts' criterion for successful reduction is a degree of knee extension symmetrical with the opposite knee. The fragment may appear to be slightly tilted upwards, but that is accepted if there is full knee motion.

Malunited avulsion fractures and non-united avulsion fractures

The choice in this type of fracture is between excision of the fragment or freshening of the fragment and its bed in the intercondylar eminence area.[27] It goes without saying that an attempt at the latter is the option of choice. However, the outcome of the decision depends on a few factors. First, an avulsed fragment of the intercondylar eminence may enlarge by maturation of the epiphyseal cartilage contained in it; therefore, the size of the fragment on radiography may not be the real size.[20] Second, atrophy of the anterior cruciate ligament follows detachment, because tension is important in stimulating ligament growth[9,19,20,26] as well as the intercondylar eminence growth.[9]

Late open reduction was reported by Meyers and McKeever[19] in a child treated 5 months after the injury by freshening of the fragment. Sullivan et al.[23] reported on a 29-year-old adult who had the injury untreated for 2 years from the date of the accident. The bony fragment was freshened and the intercondylar eminence bed was curetted. Sutures were then passed in drillholes both in the fragment and proximal tibia. Both patients returned to normality within the year.

Mid-substance tears of the anterior cruciate ligament

The majority of such injuries tend to occur in adolescents.[5,11] The desire of this age group to continue their sporting activities is understandable and their increasing participation on a competitive level and at times a professional level is increasingly evident. Such injuries may occur combined with other knee ligaments.[5,13,16,17,30]

Surgical indications for adolescents

In the acute anterior cruciate ligament rupture:

1. The patient is unwilling to modify his physical activity.[12,17]
2. A positive Lachman and pivot-shift tests and/or a repairable meniscal lesion.[12]
3. Associated collateral ligament injuries.

In the chronic anterior cruciate ligament rupture: positive physical findings plus a history of repeated episodes of giving-way, pain and effusion.

In order to avoid iatrogenic growth arrest, McCarroll et al.[12] tried to determine the growth potential in the following way:

1. Bone age was compared to chronological age with an anteroposterior radiographic view of the left hand.
2. A thorough history was taken of the family's growth characteristics.
3. Tanner's classification of maturation was used to determine puberty.

Surgical procedures employed in the treatment of the adolescent anterior cruciate ligament rupture

1. Primary repair.[16]
2. Combined intra-articular reconstruction using the semitendinosus and gracilis tendons with extra-articular augmentation performed routinely.[17]
3. Combined intra-articular reconstruction using the patellar tendon with extra-articular augmentation used in selected cases.[12]
4. Extra-articular procedures such as the A–O tenodesis of the iliotibial band or the modified Andrews' iliotibial band tenodesis performed as the main procedure.[12]

The procedures were performed using standard bony tunnels that cross either the femoral epiphysis or the tibial epiphysis or both.[1,12,17,30] The 'over-the-top' method has been used as well.[29]

Primary repair of the mid-substance tear of the anterior cruciate ligament

Engebretsen et al.[16] performed primary repair of the mid-substance tear of the anterior cruciate ligament in 8 adolescents with an age range of 13–16 years. The patients were operated on within the first week. Non-absorbable suture material was used as four U-sutures were passed in the ligament stump and pulled out through two drill channels in the femur, taking care not to cross the physeal plate. Three cases with associated medial collateral ligament ruptures were repaired as well. In one of the cases, there was a peripheral lateral meniscal tear that was reattached. Postoperative immobilization in a long-leg cast for 6 weeks in 30–40° of flexion was employed. The patient was allowed no weight bearing while in the cast.

Combined intra-articular reconstruction using the semitendinosus–gracilis unit with extra-articular augmentation

Lipscomb et al.[17] reported on 24 adolescent athletes of ages ranging from 12 to 15 years with interstitial anterior cruciate ligament tears. Eleven of them had completely open physes while 13 had partially open physes. These lesions were acute in 10 patients (seen within 2 weeks after injury), subacute in 8 patients (seen within 2 weeks to 3 months after injury), chronic ruptures in 6 patients. In each patient, the anterior cruciate ligament was reconstructed using the semitendinosus–gracilis tendons. Extra-articular augmentation procedures were routinely combined with the anterior cruciate ligament reconstruction after the first three patients were operated on. Such

procedures included the Ellison procedure in 3 patients, replaced by the Losee procedure in the last 18 patients.

At least one other associated procedure was performed. Such procedures included removal of the torn medial meniscus in 12 patients, removal of the torn lateral meniscus in 7 patients, repair of 4 peripheral tears of the medial and lateral menisci.

Selective combined intra-articular reconstruction using the patellar tendon and extra-articular augmentation versus extra-articular augmentation performed as the sole procedure

McCarroll et al.[12] reviewed 24 out of 40 mid-substance tears in patients under the age of 14 years who were treated surgically. Growth potential was determined (vide supra). Accordingly, extra-articular augmentation alone was chosen, to avoid the possibility of growth arrest if any one of the following existed:

1. The patient was 13 years of age or younger.
2. The bone age was 6 months or greater below the chronological age.
3. A family history of growth potential was present.
4. Maturation level was not complete.

Ten extra-articular procedures were performed on 8 acute and 2 chronic injuries; 3 were A–O tenodesis of the iliotibial band, and 7 were modified Andrews' iliotibial band tenodesis. The remaining 14 patients had intra-articular patellar tendon reconstruction, combined with dynamic transfer of the biceps tendon in 6 patients and iliotibial band tenodesis in the remaining 8 patients for reinforcement. The 10 extra-articular reconstructions were allowed to return to full activity at 6 months following surgery if they had 90% strength return on Cybex testing. The 14 intra-articular reconstructions (7 acute and 7 chronic) were allowed to return to full activity after 12 months of rehabilitation if they met the same criteria.

From the above account, one can conclude that avulsion injuries of the anterior intercondylar eminence can be successfully treated by conservative measures in most patients. Only if there is soft-tissue interposition, or block to extension, does the surgeon need to attempt an arthroscopic or open reduction. Reduction of the fragment can be maintained by simple suturing of the fragment to the anterior horn of a near meniscus.

Regarding mid-substance tears, it seems that immobilization in a cast or primary repair are inadequate treatment modes. While work is still being carried out on assessing reconstruction with or without augmentation, it appears to be the preferred method of treatment.

References

1. **Clanton TO, DeLee JC, Sanders B et al.**, Knee ligament injuries in children, *J Bone Joint Surg (Am)* (1979) **61**: 1195–1201.
2. **Eady JL, Cardenas CD, Sopa D**, Avulsion of the femoral attachment of the anterior cruciate ligament in a seven-year-old child, *J Bone Joint Surg (Am)* (1982) **64**: 1376–1378.
3. **Robinson SC, Driscoll SE**, Simultaneous osteochondral avulsion of the femoral and tibial insertions of the anterior cruciate ligament, *J Bone Joint Surg (Am)* (1981) **63**: 1342–1343.
4. **Zaricznyj B**, Avulsion fracture of the tibial eminence: treatment by open reduction and pinning, *J Bone Joint Surg (Am)* (1977) **59**: 1111–1114.
5. **DeLee JC, Curtis R**, Anterior cruciate ligament insufficiency in children, *Clin Orthop* (1983) **172**: 112–118.
6. **Grana WA, Moretz JA**, Ligamentous laxity in secondary school athletes, *J Am Med Assoc* (1978) **240**: 1975–1976.
7. **Beighton P, Grahame R, Bird H**, *Hypermobility of joints*, 2nd edn (London: Springer-Verlag, 1989) 143–144.
8. **Jackson AM**, The knee and leg, *Orthopaedics in infancy and childhood*, 2nd edn, ed Lloyd-Roberts GC and Fixen J (London: Butterworth-Heinemann, 1990) 180–181.
9. **Giorgi B**, Morphologic variations of the intercondylar eminence of the knee, *Clin Orthop* (1956) **8**: 209–217.
10. **Johansson E, Aparisi T**, Congenital absence of the cruciate ligaments, *Clin Orthop* (1982) **162**: 108–111.
11. **Wiley JJ, Baxter MP**, Tibial spine fractures in children, *Clin Orthop* (1990) **255**: 54–60.
12. **McCarroll JR, Rettig AC, Shelbourne KD**, Anterior cruciate ligament injuries in the young athlete with open physes, *Am J Sports Med* (1988) **16**: 44–47.
13. **Kannus P, Järvinen M**, Knee ligament injuries in adolescents: Eight year follow-up of conservative management, *J Bone Joint Surg (Br)* (1988) **5**: 772–776.
14. **DeLee JC**, Anterior cruciate ligament insufficiency in children, *The crucial ligaments*, ed Feagin JA (New York: Churchill Livingstone, 1988) 439–447.
15. **Skak SV, Jensen TT, Poulsen TD et al.**, Epidemiology of knee injuries in children, *Acta Orthop Scand* (1987) **58**: 78–81.
16. **Engebretsen L, Svenningsen S, Benum P**, Poor results of anterior cruciate ligament repair in adolescence, *Acta Orthop Scand* (1988) **59**(6): 684–686.
17. **Lipscomb AB, Anderson AF**, Tears of the anterior cruciate ligament in adolescents, *J Bone Joint Surg (Am)* (1986) **68**: 19–28.
18. **Suman RK, Stother IG, Illingworth G**, Diagnostic arthroscopy of the knee in children, *J Bone Joint Surg (Br)* (1984) **66**: 535–537.
19. **Meyers MH, McKeever FM**, Fracture of the intercondylar eminence of the tibia, *J Bone Joint Surg (Am)* (1959) **41**: 209–222.
20. **Meyers MH, McKeever FM**, Fracture of the intercondylar eminence of the tibia, *J Bone Joint Surg (Am)* (1970) **52**: 1677–1684.
21. **Backx FJG, Erich WBM, Kemper ABA and Verbeek ALM**, Sports injuries in school-aged children: An epidemiologic study, *Am J Sports Med* (1989) **17**: 234–240.
22. **Roberts JM**, Fractures and dislocations of the knee, *Fractures in children*, ed Rockwood CA Jr, Wilkins KE, King RE (Philadelphia: JB Lippincott, 1984) 940–941.
23. **Sullivan DJ, Dines DM, Hershon SJ et al.**, Natural history of a Type III fracture of the intercondylar eminence of the tibia in an adult: A case report, *Am J Sports Med* (1989) **17**: 132–133.
24. **Hosea TM, Tria AJ Jr, Bechler JR**, Embryology of the knee, *Ligament and extensor mechanism injuries of the knee: diagnosis and treatment*, ed Scott WN (St Louis: Mosby-Year Book, 1991) 9.
25. **Kapandji IA**, *The physiology of the joints*, 5th edn, vol. 2 (Edinburgh: Churchill Livingstone, 1987) 82.
26. **Girgis FG, Marshall JL, Al Monajem ARS**, The cruciate ligaments of the knee joint: Anatomical, functional, and experimental analysis, *Clin Orthop* (1975) **106**: 216–231.
27. **Garcia A, Neer CS**, Isolated fractures of the intercondylar eminence of the tibia, *Am J Surg* (1958) **95**: 593–598.
28. **Waldrop JI, Broussard TS**, Disruption of the anterior cruciate ligament in a three-year-old child, *J Bone Joint Surg (Am)* (1984) **66**: 1113–1114.
29. **Lisser S, Weiner LS**, Ligament injuries in children, *Ligament and extensor mechanism injuries of the knee; diagnosis and treatment*, ed Scott WN (St Louis: Mosby, 1991) 195–200.
30. **Bradley GW, Shives TC, Samuelson KM**, Ligament injuries in the knees of children, *J Bone Joint Surg (Am)* (1979) **61**: 588–591.
31. **Nichols JN, Tehranzadeh J**, A review of tibial spine fractures in bicycle injury, *Am J Sports Med* (1987) **15**: 172–174.
32. **Hayes JM, Masear VR**, Avulsion fracture of the tibial eminence associated with severe medial ligamentous injury in an adolescent, *Am J Sports Med* (1984) **12**: 330–333.
33. **Tachdjian MO**, Fractures of the intercondylar eminence of the tibia, *Pediatric orthopedics*, 2nd edn, vol. 4, ed Tachdjian MO (Philadelphia: W.B. Saunders, 1990) 3286–3290.
34. **Sullivan JA**, Ligamentous injuries of the knee in children, *Clin Orthop* (1990) **255**: 44–50.
35. **Hayes AG, Nageswar M**, The adolescent painful knee: The value of arthroscopy in diagnosis, *J Bone Joint Surg (Br)* (1977) **59**: 499–500.

5.10 A review of anterior cruciate reconstruction with open epiphyses

W. Dilworth Cannon, Jr

The child or young adult with open epiphyses and an ACL tear always presents a quandary to the orthopaedic surgeon. One can usually find someone who recommends drilling through the epiphyseal plate and has personally vouched never to have had a growth deformity problem. With the medicolegal climate being what it is, one should approach this problem with considerable forethought before embarking on a surgical procedure with potentially serious complications.

Dr Henning's analysis of this issue is superb and reflects his usual careful approach to a problem. Dr Henning has always considered the status and preservation of the meniscus as paramount in his decision-making process. Knowing that the meniscus is at risk in this age group of patients, and that meniscus repair alone does not assure a good result, he has devised an intriguing surgical plan. By staying above the epiphyseal growth plate on the tibia and making his tunnel exit anteriorly, not only has he provided a better mechanical advantage to the graft, but also improved isometry when committed to an 'over-the-top' position on the femur. Of course a generous superior notchplasty must be done. By not using the patellar tendon as a graft, he has saved it for later use in case of failure. Since the results of extra-articular reconstruction are not as successful as a well-performed intra-articular reconstruction, he has not advocated performing it. His results in a small series of patients were excellent.

On a personal note, Charles Henning has had immeasurable influence in directing my interests in meniscal repair and ACL reconstruction. His approach to these challenging problems has been innovative. The scientific reporting of his results has attested to his incredible surgical skills and advanced thinking. Some surgeons could not understand how Dr Henning could spend more than six hours meticulously repairing a meniscus. Many patients, however, are thankful for the time he spent working on their knees, providing them with a better chance of being free of arthritis, tibial osteotomies, and total knee replacements.

Dr Henning died in a glider crash on June 13, 1991, shortly after completing his dictation of the following contribution, his final testimony to the advancement of knee surgery. He will be sorely missed.

5.11 Anterior cruciate ligament reconstruction with open epiphyses

Charles E. Henning

Tears of the anterior cruciate ligament (ACL) in children with open epiphyses and significant long-bone growth potential are uncommon. Only 11 of 998 ACL reconstructions performed in our unit between 1983 and 1989 were in growing children. These young anterior cruciate deficient patients are typically more loose-jointed than the older adolescent but experience a similar incidence of giving-way. Also, meniscus tears occurred in 5 of the 11 adolescents, an incidence similar to that in an adult population. Therefore, it is desirable to reconstruct the ACL in the patient with open epiphyses to decrease the incidence of meniscal tears and development of late arthritis.

Factors affecting success of ACL reconstruction include graft selection, tibial attachment position, femoral attachment position, adequate anterior notch clearance, conditioning, preloading, and provision for revascularization. In addition, in the patient with open epiphyses, epiphyseal closure must be avoided. The graft must be of sufficient size and strength to withstand the rigors of adult athletic participation. This is an important consideration, in that the structure used for replacement is proportionately smaller in these young patients. Finally, the condyles will get bigger and the attachment sites will become farther apart, so the graft must adapt gradually to this increase in length.

Because of the potential for partial closure of an epiphysis, it is essential to follow the patients closely during the first year: clinically, note any changes in leg length and alignment; obtain bilateral knee radiographs at 6 months and 1 year; adhere to the usual motion and stability follow-up protocol.

Patient selection

The surgeon must determine the potential growth both clinically and radiographically. In males, the patient's height may be compared to the parents' and older siblings'. Use dominant hand films to estimate bone age.

The average increase in patients' height from surgery to maturity in this series was 4.6 inches (117 mm). The maximum increase was 5 inches (127 mm) and the minimum was 4 inches (102 mm). Significant growth potential correlated with open phalangeal epiphyses and small thumb sesamoids. Other attributes of immaturity are the absence of secondary sexual characteristics and menstruation in the female.

Technique

Graft selection

Grafts used in this series are limited to the central one-half of the iliotibial band and semitendinosus and gracilis tendons. Use of the bone–tendon–bone patellar tendon would have the potential risk of closure at the donor site. Also, the bone block could traverse an epiphyseal line.[1,2]

When using the iliotibial tract, take special care when harvesting it from Gerdy's tubercle. To ease graft handling, take a small 3-mm length fragment of cartilage from the lateral proximal surface of the proximal tibial epiphysis. Peel off the iliotibial band like a piece of tape across the epiphyseal line for another centimeter. This will give more area for attachment of the anchoring sutures. The exposed epiphyseal plate may not be touched or traumatized with instruments.

A length of 25 cm is necessary when using either the iliotibial band graft or the semitendinosus and gracilis tendons. Anchor the iliotibial band graft distally, passing it through the knee. Turn the remaining proximal portion of the fascia down over the lateral aspect of the joint. Use the semitendinosus as a double loop. It is critical that the graft be of sufficient length to anchor the ends proximally. The gracilis becomes so small proximally that it is suitable only for a single length through the joint.

Tibial attachment

Two methods are used for creating the tibial attachment. In the first portion of the series, the iliotibial band graft was taken through a vertically made tibial hole, crossing the tibial epiphyseal plate just deep to the surface at the epiphyseal line.[3] The present method is to make the holes in the tibial epiphysis alone. Via a suture superficial to the epiphysis anchor the graft to a staple more distal in the metaphysis.

The older transepiphyseal drillhole method requires that the hole begin distally in the metaphysis. A 5/16-inch drill passes deep to the epiphyseal line as the drill enters the proximal tibial epiphysis. Pass the iliotibial band through the hole in the conventional manner. This method avoids crossing the epiphyseal line and reduces the risk of partial epiphyseal arrest.[1] There are several disadvantages to this method. There is a risk that a drillhole may cross the epiphyseal line, and it is difficult to get the hole forward enough on the tibia. Also, the turn angle of the graft increases as it exits the tibial hole to its intra-articular pass.

The preferred method is to make two holes in the tibial epiphysis, entering it proximal to the epiphyseal line (if using the double-looped semitendinosus), or to connect these holes creating a transverse slot if the iliotibial band graft is used. A good method is to use the A-O cannulated drill for the 4.5-mm cannulated screw. This allows careful placement of the small guide-wire and control of the small drill when creating these holes. The periphery of the proximal tibial epiphysis is largely cartilage. Take care to avoid having the guide-wire migrate during drilling.

The first hole must be immediately adjacent to the articular surface of the medial tibial condyle and a second hole must converge. This places the tibial attachment very far forward and medial. It is just under cover of the medial meniscus and its transverse ligament. This places the graft central axis in the axis of the anterior portion of the anteromedial fibers, resulting in maximum mechanical advantage. This attachment site has been studied in vitro by O'Brien and Henning.[4] They found that after an applied Lachman's load, the anteriorly placed graft was subjected to a 30% lower load than a graft placed more posteriorly toward the central area. Maximizing the mechanical advantage for this smaller graft is better accomplished with this anterior tibial attachment.

Anterior notchplasty

Anterior notchplasty is mandatory with an anteriorly placed tibial graft. With the drill in the anteromedial tibial epiphyseal hole, hold the knee at 20° flexion. Advance the drill through the intercondylar notch to the palpating finger behind the posterior capsule posterolaterally. Memorize this line. The drill is then carefully backed up to be just flush with the articular surface of the tibial epiphysis. With the knee fully extended, the drill advances in this line, marking the position for the anterior femoral notchplasty.

Do the notchplasty by passing a guide-wire through an anteromedial capsular portal *proximal* to the anterior horn of the medial meniscus. Advance the guide-wire a few millimeters into this marking hole. Advance the 5/16-inch drill 1 cm to create the most anterior and proximal element of the anterior femoral notchplasty. A small isthmus of bone will remain in the area of the original anterior shelf. Remove this with a 1/4-inch osteotome. Pass the 5/16-inch drill again through this anteromedial capsule portal and with the knee flexed 20° pass it through the notch to the palpating finger. (Again memorize this line.) Back the drill up so that the tip extends about 10 mm into the joint. Extend the knee until the drill just fits in the anterior notchplasty. Continue the notchplasty posteriorly 60% of the distance to the posterior outlet.

Notch impingement occurs from the anterior contact of the intercondylar notch, not the lateral femoral condyle. It is not necessary to remove significant bone from the lateral femoral condyle. It is essential that the notchplasty is not continued posteriorly to intersect the distal femoral epiphyseal line. No significant impingement occurs from the more posterior aspect of the intercondylar notch and the only requirement is a smooth transition. The notchplasty can be progressively widened appropriately to the condyle size of the patient. Minimum width is 3/8 inch and maximum width is 7/16 inch.

The middle and anterior bundles of the posterior cruciate ligament insert all the way to the roof of the intercondylar notch. It is important not to disturb the fibers of the posterior cruciate. If done properly, the continuity of the lateral femoral condyle–lateral wall of the notchplasty will be a smooth, continuous line. It is important to palpate the posterior cruciate fibers and the lateral margin of the notchplasty to make certain that the alignment is correct. When widening the notch anteriorly, each successively larger drill is taken not quite as high as the one before. This is to preserve the 'A-frame' contour to the new notchplasty. Bevel the patellofemoral margin of the notchplasty slightly with a rasp.

The notchplasty must be sufficiently large to accommodate both the graft and its later fat-pad coverage. Failure to make the notchplasty large enough anteriorly results in lack of full extension, and trauma to the fat-pad coverage or even to the graft. Making the notchplasty larger than necessary will provoke patellofemoral crepitus. Place a probe in the tibial epiphyseal hole along the path of the anterior cruciate and extend the knee to observe the graft clearance.

The femoral attachment is an 'over-the-top' route with *no* trough. It is simply a perforation of the posterior capsule in the superolateral posterior outlet of the inner condylar notch. The distal femoral epiphyseal line converges at the roof of the posterior outlet and it would be risky to make any bony attachment.

If the semitendinosus is used, pass the ends of the tendons through the posterior capsule. Weave the ends into the lateral origin of the gastrocnemius, superficial to the epiphysis.

Unfortunately, good isometry is difficult to achieve with this technique. In-vitro work by Graf[5] demonstrates that a very far anterior tibial position and an 'over-the-top' femoral position gives satisfactory tracking characteristics. Long-term follow-up of the patients done with this technique confirms that it works satisfactorily.

Fat-pad coverage

Revascularization of the graft may be important to aid change in the cross-sectional area with increasing age and demands. It may also help to increase graft length with increasing patient stature. Make a tunnel through the fat pad using the ligamentum mucosum lobe or an infrapatellar lobe. Pull the graft through from the tibial epiphysis, proximal through the fat pad, and out via the small lateral arthrotomy. Suture the graft and fat pad together. Inject 1–2 ml of autogenous blood clot into the seam between the graft and fat-pad cover to stimulate the vascular fibrosis and revascularization. Typically, all but the most proximal 10 mm of the graft can be covered with the fat pad. Follow-up arthroscopy has demonstrated that vascular fibrosis and vascular adhesions will adequately cover this remaining proximal 10 mm.

Pull the three Bunnell sutures in each end of the semitendinosus (and a single strand of gracilis) through the 'over-the-top' route. About 2 cm of each end of the tendon extends beyond the posterior capsule. Weave these into the lateral gastrocnemius origin. Tension the sutures proximally to an A-O malleolar screw in femoral metaphysis. The screw will be 3–4 cm proximal to the distal femoral epiphysis. Distally, a single No. 5 Ethibond suture is placed at the mid-point of the semitendinosus.

Graft conditioning

A load of 8–10 lb (36–45 N) is applied on the proximal graft. Check the fat pad again for clearance with the knee in full extension. If there is still a tight web in the fat pad, it should be released at this time.

Ten to twenty flexion–extension cycles are sufficient to condition the graft. Tie the proximal sutures to the malleolar screw in the femoral metaphysis.

Further stabilize the tibial attachment by tying the single No. 5 Ethibond suture to a staple in the proximal tibial metaphysis. This suture serves only to restrain the small transverse length of the mid-point of the semitendinosus graft. It will prevent it from breaking out the thin superior cartilage walls of the drill holes. Tie this suture to a staple in the proximal tibial metaphysis. This staple must be placed both distal to the tibial epiphysis and medial to the tuber-

cle tongue. The final preload of approximately 5 lb (23 N) can be established with this suture.

Postoperative management

Postoperatively, the patients are treated just like adult patients. Begin continuous passive mobilization (CPM) on the second postoperative day, going from 0 to 90°. Monitoring range of motion at frequent intervals is essential. If full extension is not regained right away, clot will sit in the notchplasty. Scar tissue will form and the notchplasty will fill in. If this occurs, it is necessary to do an arthroscopic clearing-out of the notchplasty. A cast can be used for a few days to regain any extension lost within the first 10 days. Any extension lost during the first month should be recognized and treated promptly. Any attempt at forced extension after the notchplasty has filled will result in the rupture of the reconstructed ACL.

Rehabilitation

None of the 11 patients in this series had a meniscectomy. Meniscus repairs were done in 5 of the 11 patients. There is no difference in the rehabilitation program with or without meniscus repair.

Crutch walking to touch weight bearing is allowed during the first month and weight bearing is progressively increased to full weight at the end of 3 months. Begin cycling as soon as flexion reaches 120°. Patients begin cycling in 5-minute intervals, increasing as tolerated. At 2 months postoperatively, cycling progresses to 30 minutes. Hamstring progressive resistance exercise begins immediately postoperatively and continues indefinitely. Begin with closed-chain kinetic quadriceps exercises and bent-knee leg lifts. Progress to cycling, and then to leg presses and squats. Never prescribe open-chain quadriceps exercises. Quadriceps strength testing is done statically at 60°, with the patient doing a series of maximum effort isometric contractions. Patients can begin running at 6 months; lateral movement skills begin at 9 months; and sports are permitted after 1 year.

Results

This is a small series but it differs from Lipscomb's[3] in that all of the torn menisci were repaired. Follow-up examinations range from 1 year to 9 years. Leg length, standing leg alignment, arthrometry (including the Lachman's and incremental measurements from 0 to 90°) and standing weight-bearing radiographs were done. Leg lengths were symmetrical for one patient who had overgrowth of 3 mm. The leg length changes noted by Lipscomb[3] were not seen in this series. This may be due to avoiding drilling across the epiphyseal lines, especially in the femur.

Leg alignment was symmetrical in all patients. Arthrometry, using the Knee Laxity Tester and applying a manual maximum load, indicated a side-to-side difference of −2.5 mm to 2 mm. No patient had greater than 2 mm increased laxity of the operated knee. Incremental arthrometry indicated symmetrical stability of the knee at 0, 10°, 20°, and 90°, suggesting satisfactory graft tracking at follow-up.

Standing radiographs showed no epiphyseal closure or tilting defects. Joint spaces were symmetrical and the only radiographic finding was minimal ridging of a femoral condyle that did not correlate with meniscal repair. In this series, the incidence of degenerative changes was less than in Lipscomb's[3] series, where 50% of the patients had a meniscectomy.

Return to activity was satisfactory in all patients. One patient with an incompletely healed lateral meniscus was advised not to wrestle or play football. He did, however, take sixth rank in the state track competition in discus in his senior year.

All patients are instructed in proper habits of rounded turns, three-step stops, and bent knee landings at our monthly injury prevention meeting at the gymnasium.[6] No patient incurred reinjury of the reconstructed ligament.

References

1. **Peterson HA**, Partial growth plate arrest and its treatment, *J Pediatr Orthop* (1984) **4**: 246–258.
2. **Siffert RS**, Injuries to the growth plate and the epiphysis, *AAOS Instructional Course Lectures* (1980) **29**: 62–77.
3. **Lipscomb AB, Anderson AF**, Tears of the anterior cruciate ligament in adolescents, *J Bone Joint Surg (Am)* (1986) **68**: 19–28.
4. **O'Brien WR, Henning CE**, Anterior cruciate ligament substitute load versus tibial positioning: an in-vitro study, Presented at the interim meeting of the American Orthopedic Society for Sports Medicine, San Francisco, California (21 January, 1987).
5. **Graf B, Simon T, Jackson DW**, Isometric placement of cruciate ligament substitutes: a new technique, Presented at the Annual Meeting of the International Society of the Knee, Salzburg, Austria (May 1985).
6. **Griffis ND, Vequist SW, Yearout KM et al.**, Injury prevention of the anterior cruciate ligament, Presented at the 15th Annual Meeting of the American Orthopedic Society for Sports Medicine, Traverse City, Michigan (20 June, 1989).

6

Chronic anterior cruciate ligament deficiency

6.1 Chronic anterior cruciate insufficiency of the knee: A review

Paul M. Aichroth

The chronic anterior cruciate-deficient knee problem with instability is increasing rapidly, and especially so in the United Kingdom and some parts of Europe where acute injuries of the knee are often not treated comprehensively, nor aggressively. The assessment of chronic ligament injuries is fully described in the contributions by Dale Daniel and Dilworth Cannon. It is quite obvious that in the right hands and with appropriate training, instrumented evaluation of cruciate laxity is relatively accurate and certainly reproducible, with the side-to-side difference being the most important measurement.

The patient may not require operative reconstruction and especially so if the secondary restraints are not too lax, if the musculature is good and if the games and sports ambitions are low. Malcolm Macnicol's contribution is important here, and the bracing review by Dilworth Cannon is practical.

If activities of everyday living are interfered with by knee instability or if the young athletes' sports output is high, then operative reconstruction will usually be demanded. What technique is the surgeon to advise?

Extra-articular reconstructions have been readily undertaken over the past 20 years and the Toronto School remains fairly happy with this tenodesis in isolation. However, many reconstructions of this type stretch and the knee becomes lax again. The development of the extra-articular tenodesis together with various modifications is reported by James Arnold and the concept of a combined intra-articular reconstruction plus extra-articular tenodesis is raised.

Hey-Groves in London in 1917 first reconstructed the anterior cruciate ligament with the iliotibial tract and recognized in his patients the concept of rotary instability. Although one may argue that there is nothing new in surgical concept, the plethora of intra-articular reconstructions over the past 15 years has blossomed—some would even say 'exploded'—and especially so if the initial results of prosthetic ligaments are observed. The early carbon-fibre ligament reconstructions literally exploded, with a mass of liberated carbon fibres staining the whole of the synovium. Quite rightly, this gave carbon fibre a bad name. Nevertheless, Angus Strover defends strongly the concept of prosthetic ligaments and outlines the pros and cons of various materials. A scaffold-type ligament replacement is of importance, but it may be most appropriate to use these materials as an augmentation rather than as the primary intra-articular prosthesis in isolation. My own technique—reported in this chapter—was previously to use a composite of a woven Dacron tube with a central core of carbon fibre to augment a combined intra-articular reconstruction with a tubulated iliotibial tract, plus an extra-articular tenodesis. This technique, started 10 years ago, gave consistent results in the grossly unstable knees we see so frequently in England. The central core of carbon fibre was withdrawn in the second series, using polyester alone as the augmentation material. The operative technique and the results are included (contributions 6.7 and 6.8).

The Leeds–Keio prosthesis is a combined UK/ Japanese concept. The ligament consists of an open-weave Dacron and the results and problems are outlined by Roger Smith. Some series are reporting a greater incidence of rupture, but the originators, and especially Dr Fujikawa from Tokyo, are still very happy with this technique and especially so if an extra-articular strut is added.

The most important intra-articular prosthesis alone is the Gore-Tex ligament developed over the past 10 years and more than 18 000 cases have been so treated worldwide. The technique, development, results and complications are comprehensively recorded by Peter Indelicato and Howard Brown from Florida. There is an increasing failure rate with time and the authors do not strongly recommend the technique.

The caution with which synthetic ligaments should be used is fully revealed by Freddie Fu and Eric Olson of Pittsburgh. They point out that we have insufficient knowledge concerning the synovial and the para-articular reaction in vivo with intra-articular synthetic ligaments. For the moment we are surely unwise to use prosthetic materials purely as a primary ligament prosthesis in isolation. The most dramatic development over the past few years is the anterior cruciate ligament allograft, now experimentally under way in many units throughout the world. Konsei Shino from Osaka has a large experience of this technique and his results, biological assessment and cautions are well stated. The risk of transmission of communicable diseases such as AIDS and hepatitis is a great worry. So problematic is the AIDS fear that this technique must be restricted to experimental units at the present time.

Again, what is the surgeon to recommend? The various contributions in this chapter will certainly enlighten the reader on the advantages and disadvantages of various techniques. The trainee, resident or registrar will no doubt be totally confused. The whole concept of stabilization of the chronic anterior cruciate ligament deficiency is an on-going development and the present status will look naive in ten years time—probably even in five.

The ACL Study Group meets every two years and reviews the development of all techniques and the trends in great depth. There is a noticeable trend in this organization towards suggesting that a combined intra-articular and extra-articular reconstruction together is perhaps the ideal for an anterior cruciate ligament-deficient knee with great instability. Primary synthetic prostheses alone are too problematic at the present time. Perhaps a combined intra-articular reconstruction together with extra-articular tenodesis, combined with some kind of synthetic augmentation, will take the prize over the next few years. We shall see!

6.2   Instrumented measurement of anterior–posterior knee motion

Dale M. Daniel, Mary Lou Stone and Christoph Rangger

Ligaments limit joint motion. In-vitro ligament sectioning studies have documented that disruption of a specific ligament results in a characteristic change in motion.[1] One indicator of a successful ligament repair or reconstruction is the reestablishment of the normal motion limits. Instrumented measurement of joint motion (1) assists the clinician in diagnosing ligament disruptions by detecting pathologic motion, (2) documents the amount of pathologic motion, and (3) measures the success of ligament surgery in establishing the normal motion limits. Motion measurements consist of:

1. Positioning the limb in a specified manner
2. Applying a displacing force
3. Measuring the resultant joint motion

The testing devices may perform one, two, or all of the above tasks. The early reports of instrumented testing consisted of positioning the limb, applying a standard displacement force, and documenting change in joint position by comparing photographs[2] or radiographs[3-7] of the unstressed and stressed knee. Although stress radiography techniques are widely known to the clinician, they have not been widely used. This may be due to a concern about the resultant radiation exposure, the expense of multiple radiography, and the attention to detail needed when positioning the patient and when measuring the films.

Instrumented measurement systems that document anterior–posterior tibial displacement by tracking the tibial tubercle in relation to the patella have become popular in the orthopedic community relatively recently. Markolf (USA),[8] Shino (Japan),[9] and Edixhoven (Netherlands)[10] developed stationary testing systems. Portable testing systems commercially available were developed by Cannon and Lamoreux (Knee Laxity Tester, Stryker Ligament Tester) and by Malcom and Daniel (KT-1000 MEDmetric, San Diego, Calif., USA).[11,12] More recently, commercial devices have been introduced that simultaneously measure motion in several directions (Genucom, Faro Medical Technologies, Champlain, New York, USA, and KSS Acufex, Norwood, Mass., USA).

Motion measurements depend on:

1. Joint position at the initiation of the test[8,13-16]
2. Motion constraints imposed by the testing system[17]
3. Displacing force[8,10,17]
4. Measurement system[17]
5. Muscle activity[8-10,18]
6. Passive motion constraints

The role of the testing device is to minimize the variability between factors 1 through 5 so that the difference in measurements between two knees or one knee tested at time intervals indicates a true change in the passive motion constraints.

KT-1000 Testing technique

We have used the KT-1000 arthrometer in our clinic to measure anterior–posterior displacement since 1982. Measurements are routinely performed on patients with acute injuries and chronic instabilities. Patients who have knee ligament surgery are measured in the clinic at the time of their preoperative examination, under anesthesia prior to surgery and under anesthesia after wound closure. An adhesive drape is placed over the leg during testing to maintain wound sterility. Postoperative displacement measurements are performed at 6 weeks, 3 months, 6 months, 1 year, and 2 years. We have used instrumented measurements to diagnose a cruciate ligament disruption, to document the amount of pathologic laxity, and to evaluate the success of cruciate ligament reconstruction surgery. Testing technique is as follows.

The arthrometer is placed on the anterior aspect of the leg and held with two circumferential Velcro straps (Figure 1). There are two sensor pads: one in contact with the patella and the other in contact with the tibial tubercle. These move freely in the anterior–posterior plane in relation to the arthrometer case. The instrument detects the relative motion in millimeters between the two sensor pads and, therefore, motion of the arthrometer case (as the calf

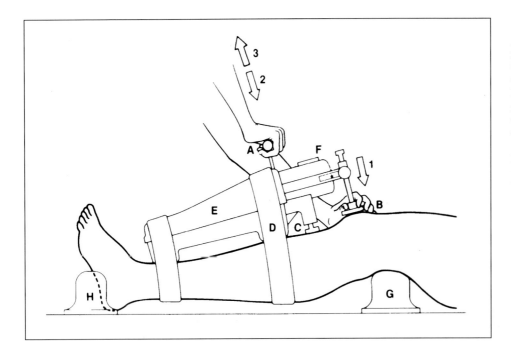

Figure 1

KT-1000 Arthrometer. A: Force handle (posterior force [2] or anterior force [3] is applied). B: Patellar sensor pad (a constant force [1] is applied to stabilize the patellar sensor pad). C: Tibial sensor pad. D: Velcro straps. E: Arthrometer body. F: Displacement dial. G: Thigh support. H: Foot support.

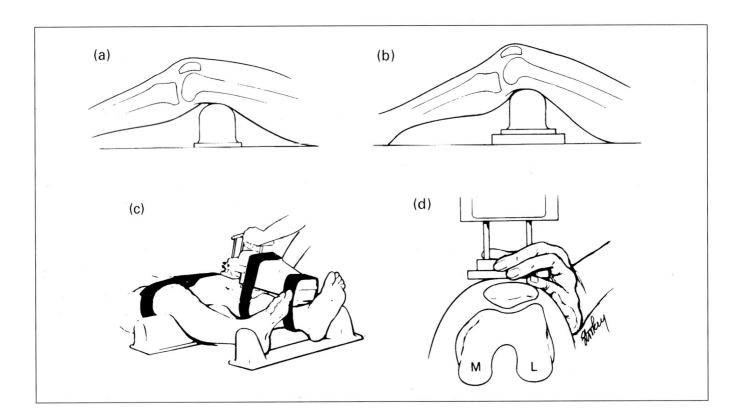

Figure 2

The knee is supported in a flexed position to engage the patella in the femoral trochlea (a). In some patients the thigh support must be raised an additional 3–6 cm to provide sufficient knee flexion to engage the patella in the femoral trochlea. This may be done by placing a board under the thigh support (b). The thigh should be supported so the patella is facing up. Occasionally, a thigh strap is used to accomplish this task (c). The foot support is not used to internally rotate the limb, but simply to support the feet. The examiner stabilizes the patellar sensor with manual pressure. Prior to establishing the testing reference position, sufficient pressure should be applied to the patella to press it firmly into the femoral trochlea (2–6 lb; 9–27 N), so the increase in pressure on the patellar pad that will inevitably occur while stabilizing the instrument and limb during testing will not change the position of the patella and patellar sensor. The hand stabilizing the patellar sensor should rest against the lateral thigh to help stabilize the testing instrument and prevent instrument rotation during testing (d).

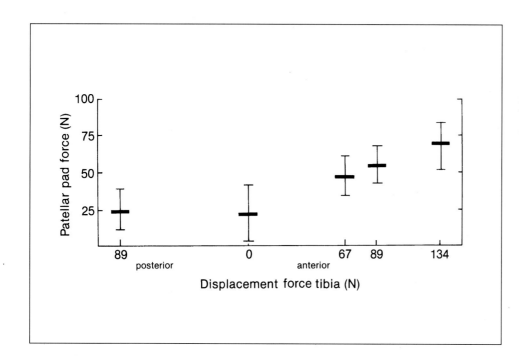

Figure 3

Patellar pad force versus force applied through the force handle. The mean and range at four force handle levels recorded by seven examiners testing the same patient.

compresses under the Velcro straps) does not affect the instrument's output. Displacement loads are applied through a force-sensing handle that is located 10 cm distal to the joint-line.

The precision of A–P displacement measurements is dependent on a standardized method of placing the measuring device on the leg and securely stabilizing the patella in the femoral trochlea. With adequate patellar stabilization, tibial tubercle motion relative to the patella accurately reflects the motion of the tibia relative to the femur. It is necessary to flex the knee 20–30° in order to engage the patella in the femoral trochlea. In patients with patella alta or lateral tracking patella, the knee may need to be flexed to 40° or more by placing a board under the standard thigh support (Figure 2) or using the MEDmetric adjustable thigh support. The patella is stabilized in the femoral trochlea by direct pressure, which should be oriented to seat the patella. A recent evaluation of seven examiners using a KT-1000 instrument, modified to include a patellar pad pressure sensor, revealed that all examiners increased the patellar pad pressure as they increased the force through the force handle (Figure 3). The examiners did not know that patellar pad pressure was being measured during the test. Patellar pad pressure changes from 5 N to 75 N in most patients. If the patellofemoral geometry and condition of the subject's two knees are symmetrical and the same examiner tests both knees with a similar technique, patellar depression during the test with increasing patellar pressure will have a negligible effect on the right/left displacement differences. However, if the patella is not well seated in the femoral trochlea as shown in Figure 4, varying the patellar pad pressure may have a significant effect on the patellar sensor position (Patient 1, Figure 5).

Rotation of the instrument during the test will alter the position of the displacement sensors and alter the direction of the displacement force. Rotation of the instrument during the test should be avoided. To evaluate instrument rotation during testing, a KT-1000 instrument was modified to include a pendulum inside the instrument, which recorded rotation around the longitudinal axis. Ten experienced examiners tested the same patients. The examiners did not know that instrument rotation was being measured. Instrument rotation during a complete anterior–posterior cycle varied from 0 to 7°; the mean was 2°. One examiner tested 45 patients. Instrument rotation varied from 0 to 10° and the mean was 1.7°.

To stabilize the instrument on the limb, the hand stabilizing the patella in the femoral trochlea should rest on the thigh and prevent the instrument from rotating during the test (Figure 2). During the test the patient should be comfortable and relaxed. Gentle manual A–P oscillation may assist in obtaining muscle relaxation (Figure 6). The arthrometer is applied to the leg and oriented in a position so that pressure on the patellar sensor pad will stabilize the patella within the femoral trochlea (Figure 2). This usually places the force handle parallel to the foot axis. While watching the dial, patellar pressure should be applied until the dial motion stops. If the patella cannot be securely stabilized, the knee should be flexed in order to bring the patella farther down into the femoral trochlea. A 20-lb (89-N) anterior–posterior cycle is performed to condition the joint. The measurement reference position is then obtained by repeatedly applying and releasing a 20-lb posterior load until a reproducible unloaded knee position is obtained. The instrument dial is then set at 0. After each anterior load cycle is performed, a 20-lb

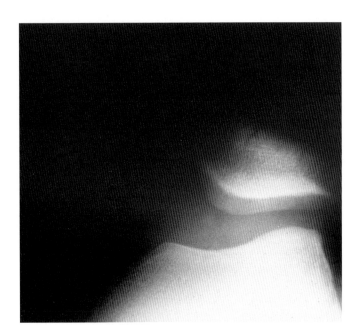

Figure 4

Radiograph with the knees in 45° of flexion.

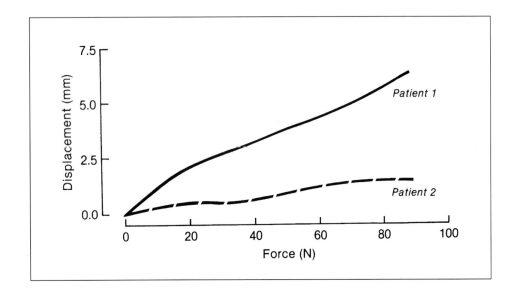

Figure 5

Patellar pad posterior displacement versus patellar pad force. Patient 1, patient with lateral patellar subluxation (Figure 4). Patient 2, patient with normal patellar position.

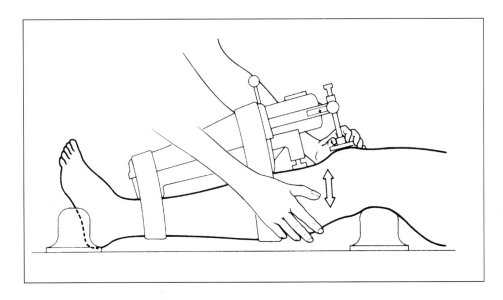

Figure 6

Gentle manual oscillation of the leg may assist in obtaining muscle relaxation.

posterior force is applied and released. Return of the dial to 0 ± 0.5 mm confirms that the instrument's orientation on the leg has not been altered and the quadriceps is relaxed. Confirmation of a stable reference position should be performed after each test. The mean of three tests rounded to 0.5 mm is recorded as the measurement.

Posterior cruciate screen

Prior to performing 30° displacement measurements, the 90° active quadriceps test is performed to determine whether there is posterior tibial subluxation. The examination is performed with the patient supine. The examiner sits lightly on the patient's foot to stabilize the limb with the knee flexed 90° as when performing a 90° drawer test. The arthrometer is placed on the leg. With the hand stabilizing the arthrometer patellar sensor pad, the examiner also supports the patient's knee so that the patient may completely relax the leg musculature (Figure 7a). When examining larger patients we frequently have an assistant sit by the side of the table and support the limb (Figure 7b). It is critical that the muscles crossing the knee are completely relaxed. The testing reference position is established: this is the resting position after a 20-lb posterior force is applied and then released. The patient then performs an isolated quadriceps contraction. We have found that the most helpful command is to tell the patient "Gently try to slide your foot down the examining table." The examiner palpates the hamstring tendons to confirm that there is no hamstring contraction. The test is repeated until the patient performs an isolated quadriceps contraction without concomitant knee extension. The arthrometer documents the anterior or posterior tibial displacement. Anterior tibial

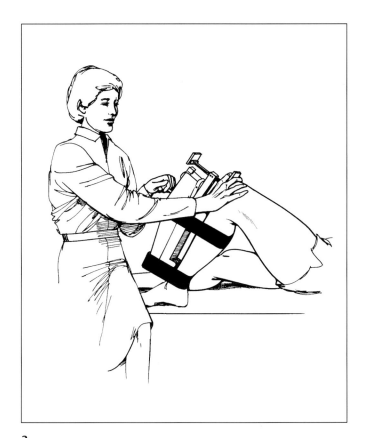

a

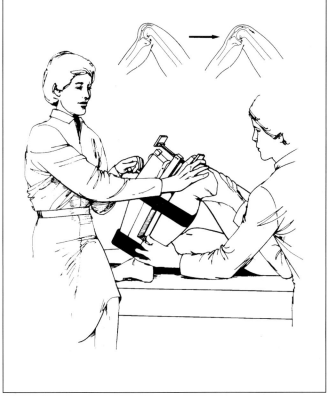

b

Figure 7

Measurement of anterior and posterior displacement using a knee ligament arthrometer and a 20-lb (89-N) displacing force. (a) The examiner supports the subject's limb by sitting lightly on the foot and stabilizing the knee laterally. Alternatively, an assistant may support the limb, as is shown in (b). The support must be comfortable to ensure complete relaxation. The quadriceps neutral angle in the normal knee is located and measured. Anterior and posterior displacements are measured at this angle using the displacing force. The injured knee is then supported at the angle that has been identified as the quadriceps neutral angle in the normal knee. A posterior displacing force is applied and released to establish a reproducible reference position. Anterior and posterior displacements from the reproducible reference position are measured using the displacement force. The quadriceps active test is used to measure posterior subluxation of the tibia at the reproducible reference position.

motion greater than 1 mm is abnormal and probably indicates a PCL injury. If the anterior tibial motion is greater than 1 mm, then the quadriceps neutral angle test should be performed. This is described later. If there is no anterior tibial motion, the tibial position is normal and the examination should proceed to the 30° tests.

Passive 30° tests

An anterior cruciate ligament disruption is best revealed by testing the patient with the knee in slight flexion.[8,15,16] An 11-cm thigh support and a foot rest position both limbs in an equal position of flexion (30 ± 5°) and limb rotation (10–30° of external rotation). If insufficient flexion is obtained by the thigh support to stabilize the patella in the femoral trochlea, further knee flexion is obtained by placing a board under the standard thigh support or raising the MEDmetric adjustable thigh support. The lateral aspect of the foot rests against the foot support. If the limb lies in an externally rotated position with the patella facing laterally, the thigh should be internally rotated and supported with a restraining strap to face the patella anteriorly (Figure 2). Positioning the limb to place the patella anteriorly and engaged in the femoral trochlea optimizes stabilization of the patella in the femoral trochlea. Pressure is placed on the patellar sensor to stabilize the patella. A 20-lb anterior–posterior cycle is performed to condition the joint. The measurement reference position is then obtained by repeatedly applying and releasing a 20-lb posterior load until a reproducible unloaded knee position is obtained. The instrument dial is then set at 0. A 30-lb anterior force followed by a 20-lb posterior force is applied and the displacements are read directly off the dial as the tone is heard.

After each anterior load cycle is performed, a 20-lb posterior force is applied and released. The dial should return to 0 ± 0.5 mm to confirm that the instrument orientation on the leg has not been altered and the quadriceps is relaxed. Confirmation of a stable reference position should be performed after the manual maximum test, the quadriceps active test, and those tests where the anterior load is applied through the force handle. The mean of three tests rounded to 0.5 mm is recorded as the measurement.

Five passive displacement measurements are recorded for each limb at 30°:

1. *20-lb (89-N) posterior displacement.* The posterior excursion from the measurement reference position with a 20-lb push.
2. *15-lb (67-N) anterior displacement.* The anterior excursion from the measurement reference position with a 15-lb pull.
3. *20-lb (89-N) anterior displacement.* The anterior excursion from the measurement reference position with a 20-lb pull.
4. *30-lb (134-N) anterior displacement.* The anterior excursion from the measurement reference position with a 30-lb pull.
5. *The manual maximum anterior displacement.* The anterior displacement with a high anterior force applied directly to the proximal calf just distal to the knee joint-line (Figure 8). The manual maximum test produces greater displacement due to a higher applied load and a more proximally applied load. In our clinic, manual loads applied are estimated to be 30–40 lb (134–178 N).

Anterior joint compliance may be measured by calculating the anterior displacement between any two load levels recorded in the same cycle; for example, the displacement difference between the 15-lb and 20-lb anterior load as illustrated in Figure 9.

When testing the anesthetized patient, additional care must be taken to adequately stabilize the patella in the femoral trochlea. The lower limbs usually lie in an externally-rotated position in the anesthetized patient. A thigh strap is required to internally rotate the limbs and position the patella anteriorly (Figure 2c). In many patients the knee must be flexed 35–40° to stabilize the patella.[19]

It is important to establish the precision of a testing system prior to utilizing it in decision-making. The manufacturer recommends monthly monitoring of the KT-1000 instrument to confirm accuracy of the load-sensing handle and the displacement sensors. The important indicator of pathology is side-to-side difference. The same machine must be used on both sides to minimize the significance of small calibration errors in the machine itself. The crucial element in the testing process is to duplicate the same testing technique on the second knee that was used on the first knee. Important points are (1) muscle relaxation, (2) similar limb orientation, (3) similar arthrometer placement on the leg, (4) consistent patellar pad pressure technique, (5) establishing the testing reference position, and (6) similar speed of force application. The two great sources of measurement errors with the arthrometer are lack of muscle relaxation and inability to stabilize the patellar sensor pad.

Anterior testing results

Normal subjects   In the published report of A–P displacement testing with the KT-2000,[20] Malcom measured 338 normal subjects (150 females and 188 males) between the ages of 15 and 45 years, and 87 patients with a unilateral ACL-disrupted knee. In the normal population there was no significant difference between age and sex groups. Data of 120 normal subjects tested in our clinic are presented in Table 1. Testing results of normal subjects with the KT-1000

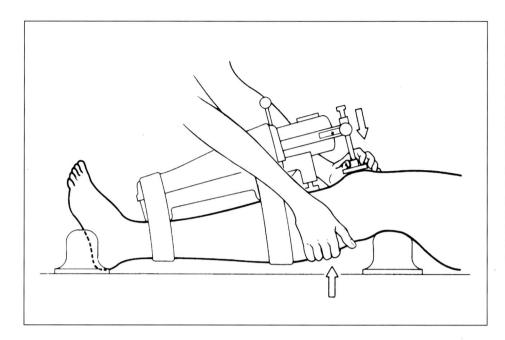

Figure 8

Manual maximum test. The limbs are positioned with the support system, the arthrometer is applied, and the testing reference position is obtained in the standard way. While the patellar sensor pad is stabilized with one hand, the other hand applies a strong anterior displacement force directly to the proximal calf to produce the maximum anterior displacement. Care is taken that the knee is not extended. The tibial displacement is read off the dial.

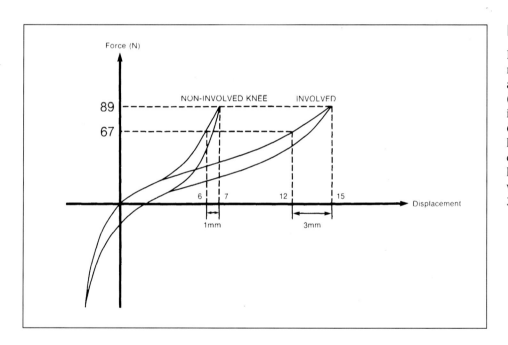

Figure 9

Force-displacement curves of a normal knee (noninvolved) and an anterior cruciate-injured knee (involved). The compliance index is the displacement between the 67-N and 89-N anterior force levels. On this curve, the compliance index for the normal knee is 1 mm and for the knee with an anterior cruciate deficit is 3 mm.

have been reported by Sherman,[21] Daniel,[11] Bach,[22] and Anderson.[23] For all tests reported by these investigators, greater than 95% of normal subjects had a right/left difference of less than 3 mm. We have interpreted a right/left displacement difference of 3 mm in the unilaterally-injured patient on any test as pathologic motion.

To document the test/retest variation by a single skilled examiner, author M.L.S. examined 10 normal subjects on five different days without reference to her previous examinations. The test–retest variations were seldom greater than a millimeter.[24] Wroble[25] reported repeatability studies on six normal subjects.

The mean right/left difference variation was 0.5 mm (89 N) and 0.7 mm (134 N). The 90% confidence limits were 1.6 mm (89 N) and 1.7 mm (134 N). Anderson[23] evaluated 50 normal subjects with five different testing devices: KT-1000 arthrometer, Stryker Knee Laxity Tester (KLT), Acufex Knee Signature System (KSS), Dyonics Dynamic Cruciate Tester (DCT), and Genucom Knee Analysis. All subjects had a right/left variation of less than 3 mm by the KT-1000 and Stryker KLT. One of the patients had a right/left difference of 3 mm or greater with the KSS, 5 mm with the DCT, and 11 mm with the Genucom.

Table 1 Normal A/P displacement measurements.

	Range/low	Range/high	Mean	SD	95% Cut-off
Displacement (n=240)					
20-lb posterior	1	6	2.8	0.9	4.5
20-lb anterior	3	14	7.2	2.0	10
20-lb A–P	5	18	10.0	2.4	12
Manual max anterior	4.5	15	8.6	2.1	12
Quadriceps active displacement	2	12.5	5.7	1.8	9
Right minus left (n=120)					
20-lb posterior	0	2	0	0.7	1.0[a]
20-lb anterior	−0.2	−3.5	−2	1.0	2.0[a]
20-lb A–P	−4	4	0.2	0.9	2.5[a]
Manual max anterior	−4	3	−0.3	1.1	2.0[a]
Quadriceps active displacement	−3	2	−0.4	1.0	2.0[a]

[a] Right/left difference.

Table 2 Unilateral chronic ACL disruption. Injured minus normal displacement difference. Knee flexion angle 20–35°.

	n	Mean	Percent ≥ 3.0 mm
Clinical examination, author			
Test: 20-lb			
Anderson[23]	50	5.1	82
Bach[22]	153	5.1	79
KSD[a]	159	5.4	66
Drez[b]	19	6.3	–
3M LAD[c]	297	6.1	89
Sherman[21]	19	5.1	95
Sommerlath[26]	20	6	85
Test: Manual maximum			
Anderson	50	8.6	100
Bach	153	–	72
KSD	159	8.6	100
Drez	19	7.6	–
3M LAD	297	7.8	96
Test: Quadriceps active			
KSD	159	4.4	72
3M LAD	258	4.4	76
Examination under anesthesia prior to reconstruction			
Test: 20-lb			
KSD	159	5.6	87
3M LAD	297	6.9	96
Test: Manual maximum			
KSD	159	8.9	97
3M LAD	297	8.9	99
Examination under anesthesia after reconstruction			
Test: 20-lb (I–N)[d]			
KSD	223	−1.4	5

[a] Kaiser, San Diego.
[b] Drez, DJ, personal communication.
[c] 3M Multicenter LAD Study.
[d] I–N: involved minus noninvolved.

Table 3 Chronic unilateral ACL disruption, n = 50.

Test	KT-1000	Stryker	DCT	KSS	Genucom
20-lb posterior					
Normal	2.7	2.3	1.9	6.0	
Injured	2.9	2.4	1.7	6.7	
20-lb anterior					
Normal	8.0	6.1	3.7	4.8	9.9
Injured	13.0	10.4	6.9	7.9	13.9
Difference	5.0	4.3	3.2	3.1	4.0
≥ 3 mm	82%	82%	76%	52%	76%
Manual maximum					
Normal	8.2	7.2	5.2	7.2	
Injured	16.8	13.1	11.0	12.7	
Difference	8.6	5.9	5.8	5.5	
≥ 3 mm	100%	92%	86%	82%	

From ref. 23.

Chronic ACL injured patients A number of authors have reported the results of instrumented testing in the unilateral ACL-injured knee with available devices. Some of the reports are presented in Table 2. Anderson[23] evaluated 50 patients with a chronic unilateral ACL disruption with five devices as listed above (Table 3). An injured-minus-normal knee difference of 3 mm or more was defined as pathologic. The measurements were pathologic with an 89-N displacement force in 41 patients with the KT-1000, in 40 with the Stryker KLT, in 34 with the DCT, in 26 with the KSS, and in 37 with the Genucom. The manual maximum test revealed pathologic motion in 50 with the KT-1000, in 46 with the Stryker KLT, in 38 with the DCT, and in 40 with the KSS. Steiner[27] also reported a comparative study of commercially available testing devices. He studied 13 subjects with normal knees and 15 with unilateral chronic ACL disruptions. He reported that the KSS, Stryker KLT, and KT-1000 could identify correctly normal and ACL-injured patients 80–90% of the time. The Genucom was less accurate. Data from our clinic for 159 patients with a unilateral chronic ACL disruption scheduled for ACL reconstructive surgery are presented in Table 4.

Acute ACL disruption We routinely perform KT-1000 measurements in the clinic on patients with suspected ACL disruptions. To allow better stabilization of the patella, we aspirate the knee prior to testing if we estimate that the patient has an effusion of greater than 50 ml. Frequently the examiner must spend a little time coaching the patient to relax and demonstrating that the examination is not going to be painful. Patients who have received an injury to the patella may not tolerate the pressure needed to stabilize the patellar sensor. The normal knee is tested prior to testing the injured knee. In a report from The Hospital for Special Surgery, Bach et al.[22] reported that the clinic measurement of 107 acute ACL disruptions revealed a side-to-side difference of 3 mm or greater in 69% of patients on the 20-lb test and 87% of patients on the manual maximum test. Table 4 presents measurements of 105 consecutive patients tested between October 1982 and June 1986 with an acute ACL disruption who were arthroscoped within 14 days of injury, and had instrumented measurement in the clinic and under anesthesia prior to the arthroscopic examination. The clinical measurements were performed by author M.L.S. and the measurements under anesthesia were performed by the operating surgeon (*n* =15). There were 36 females and 78 males; 55 injured right knees and 59 injured left knees. The mean patient age was 23 years.[3,4,8,10–12,14,15,19,28–45]

We recently added a 30-lb displacement test to our testing routine. This test reveals greater displacement than the 20-lb test, but less than the manual maximum test. If the injured-minus-normal knee displacement difference on any of the four tests routinely performed (20-lb, 30-lb, manual maximum and quadriceps active) is 3 mm or greater, the likelihood of a cruciate ligament disruption is greater than 95%. Both an ACL-injured knee and a PCL-injured knee may result in an increased anterior displacement measured from the supine 30° resting position.[18] An ACL-injured knee will have an increased anterior compliance and a PCL-injured knee will have an increased posterior compliance. The most diagnostic sign of a posterior cruciate ligament disruption is demonstration of posterior sag in 90° of flexion and demonstration of an increased posterior displacement from the anatomic position at or near the quadriceps neutral angle.

Table 4 Anterior displacement measurements.

	Mean	Range	Standard
Acute unilateral ACL disruption (*n*=105)			
89-N (20-lb) test – no anesthesia			
Noninvolved (N)	7.8	3.0–13.0	1.76
Involved (I)	11.5	5.0–18.0	2.59
I minus N	3.6	0.0–13.0	2.12
89-N test – with anesthesia			
Noninvolved (N)	7.3	3.5–13.0	2.04
Involved (I)	11.5	5.0–18.0	2.88
I minus N	4.4	0.0–11.5	2.45
Manual maximum test – no anesthesia			
Noninvolved (N)	9.1	3.5–13.0	1.77
Involved (I)	15.2	10.1–21.0	2.50
I minus N	6.1	1.0–12.0	2.22
Manual maximum test – with anesthesia			
Noninvolved (N)	9.0	3.5–13.0	2.12
Involved (I)	16.3	6.0–20.0	2.83
I minus N	7.3	0.0–11.5	2.48
Quadriceps active test – no anesthesia			
Noninvolved (N)	6.5	1.0–11.0	1.80
Involved (I)	8.5	2.0–20.0	2.45
I minus N	2.0	–3.5– 9.0	2.31
Chronic unilateral ACL disruptions (*n*=159)			
89-N test – no anesthesia			
Noninvolved (N)	7.7	2.5–13.5	1.97
Involved (I)	13.1	4.0–25.0	3.51
I minus N	5.4	0.0–13.5	2.89
89-N test – with anesthesia			
Noninvolved (N)	7.3	3.0–14.0	2.08
Involved (I)	13.1	5.0–23.0	3.40
I minus N	5.9	–1.0–15.0	3.14
Manual maximum test – no anesthesia			
Noninvolved (N)	9.1	4.0–15.0	2.08
Involved (I)	17.7	10.0–28.0	3.94
I minus N	8.6	2.5–20.0	3.28
Manual maximum test – with anesthesia			
Noninvolved (N)	9.3	4.0–15.0	2.32
Involved (I)	18.7	10.0–28.0	3.89
I minus N	9.4	1.0–20.0	3.65
Quadriceps active test – no anesthesia			
Noninvolved (N)	6.4	2.0–13.0	2.37
Involved (I)	10.8	3.0–21.0	3.44
I minus N	4.4	–1.0–16.0	3.04

Evaluation of ACL reconstructive surgery

KT-1000 measurements have been used to document satisfactory graft tensioning at the time of ACL surgery[24,46,47] and to monitor A–P displacement during the early rehabilitation program.[43,48] Numerous authors used KT-1000 measurements as a part of their follow-up documentation system.[24,28–30,33,35,36,39,40,44,50–58] Our preference is to present follow-up data as in Table 5.

Quadriceps active tests

Orthopedic surgeons have routinely evaluated the integrity of knee ligaments by estimating or measuring the amount and direction of motion between the tibia and femur due to manually applied external forces such as drawer tests, varus and valgus stress tests, and pivot shift tests.[34] These are called *passive* tests because the displacing force is applied by the examiner. Another method of assessing ligamentous and capsular integrity is to measure the change in joint position that results from active contraction of the patient's muscles. These are called *active* tests because the patient's muscle contraction provides the joint displacement force.

At full extension, as the patellar tendon runs from the tibial tubercle to the patella, it lies anterior to a reference line drawn perpendicular to the surface of the tibial plateau and passing through the tibial tubercle.[32,34,38,41,42,59,60] As the knee flexes, the femur rolls posteriorly on the tibia guided by the cruciate ligaments.[31]

The orientation of the patellar tendon changes continuously from anterior to posterior relative to the reference line (Figure 10).[37,42,49,60] Thus, the resultant shear force produced by the pull of the patellar tendon on the tibial tubercle also changes from anterior to posterior with increasing flexion angle. The crossover from anterior to posterior shear occurs between 60° and 90° in the normal knee.[42,49,59–61] The angle of flexion at which the crossover occurs in the normal knee is termed the 'quadriceps neutral angle' and is defined as the angle of flexion at which the tibia does not shift anteriorly or posteriorly when the quadriceps is contracted in the normal knee. At this angle, the force in the patellar tendon is parallel to

the reference line, therefore no net shear occurs at the tibiofemoral interface.

At angles less than the quadriceps neutral angle, quadriceps contraction produces anterior movement of the tibia due to an anteriorly angled patellar tendon that may be constrained by the anterior cruciate ligament. Similarly, at angles greater than the quadriceps neutral angle, quadriceps contraction produces backward motion of the tibia resulting from

Table 5 KT-1000 anterior displacement: millimeters injured minus normal SDK79.

	Pre-repair		Post-repair	
	Without anesthesia	*With anesthesia*	*With anesthesia*	*Follow-up[a]*
	20-lb			
n	(*n*=78)	(*n*=77)	(*n*=76)	(*n*=79)
< 3 mm	3 (4%)	9 (12%)	72 (95%)	45 (57%)
3–5 mm	22 (28%)	18 (23%)	3 (4%)	26 (33%)
5.5–7.5 mm	33 (42%)	25 (33%)	1 (1%)	7 (9%)
> 7.5 mm	20 (25%)	25 (32%)	0	1 (1%)
Mean	6.3 mm	6.3 mm	0.0 mm	2.3 mm
	Manual maximum			
n	(*n*=77)	(*n*=77)	(*n*=59)	(*n*=79)
< 3 mm	0	2 (3%)	52 (88%)	20 (25%)
3–5 mm	5 (7%)	4 (5%)	7 (12%)	29 (37%)
5.5–7.5 mm	19 (25%)	20 (26%)	0	23 (29%)
8–10 mm	18 (23%)	15 (20%)	0	4 (5%)
> 10 mm	25 (45%)	36 (47%)	0	3 (4%)
Mean	9.6 mm	9.6 mm	–1.1 mm	4.0 mm
	Quadriceps active			
n	(*n*=77)			(*n*=79)
< 3 mm	15 (20%)			44 (56%)
3–5 mm	26 (35%)			23 (29%)
5.5–7.5 mm	20 (27%)			9 (11%)
> 7.5 mm	14 (18%)			3 (4%)
Mean	4.9 mm			2.3 mm

[a] Mean follow-up 3.2 years; range 2–5 years (ref. 47)

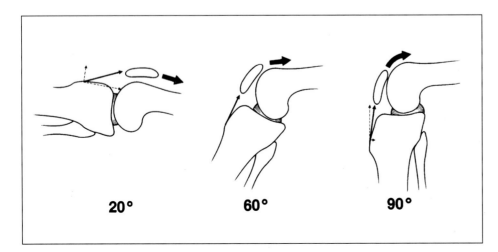

20°   **60°**   **90°**

Figure 10

The patellar tendon force can be resolved into two components: a normal component that is perpendicular to the tibial plateau, and a shear component that is parallel to the tibial plateau. When the patellar tendon is anterior, the shear component tends to slide the tibia forward on the femur; when directed posteriorly, it tends to slide the tibia backwards on the femur.

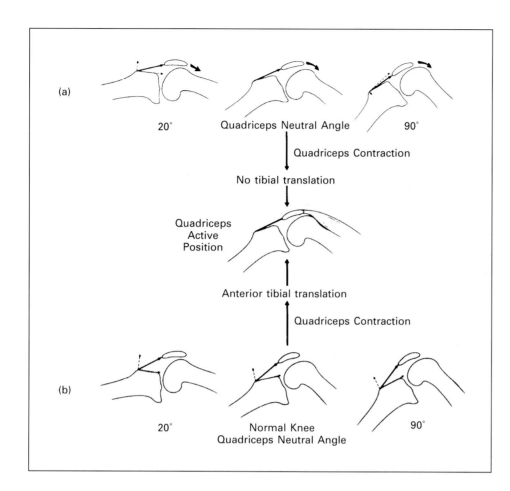

(a)

20°   Quadriceps Neutral Angle   90°

Quadriceps Contraction

No tibial translation

Quadriceps
Active
Position

Anterior tibial translation

Quadriceps Contraction

(b)

20°   Normal Knee   90°
Quadriceps Neutral Angle

Figure 11

At the quadriceps neutral angle, the quadriceps active position (tibial femoral position when the quadriceps is contracted) is independent of the cruciate ligaments. (a) shows the resting position for the normal knee; (b) the resting position for the posterior cruciate ruptured knee.

a posteriorly-angled patellar tendon that may be constrained by the posterior cruciate ligament (Figure 11).

Anterior subluxation of the tibia with contraction of the quadriceps in the anterior cruciate ligament-deficient knee can be documented with the 30° quadriceps active test. The limbs are supported with the thigh support and foot rest as performed for the 30° passive tests. The testing reference position is established and the instrument dial is set at 0. The patient is then asked to gently lift his heel off of the table. The anterior displacement as the heel leaves the table is recorded (Figure 12). Thirty-degree quadriceps active data are presented in Tables 1 and 4.

A posterior cruciate ligament rupture is diagnosed by using the quadriceps active test to demonstrate the posterior tibial subluxation. At 90° of flexion, the patellar tendon in the normal knee is oriented

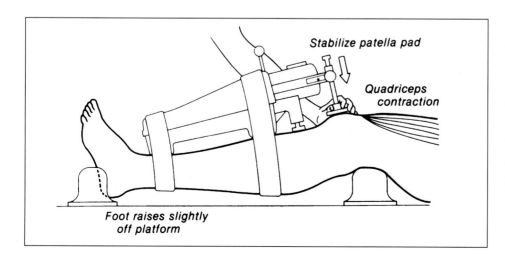

Stabilize patella pad

Quadriceps
contraction

Foot raises slightly
off platform

Figure 12

The thigh is supported in about 30° of flexion. The patellar sensor pad is stabilized and the testing reference position is established by pushing with a 20-lb load posteriorly and then releasing the force. The patient is then asked to 'gently lift her heel off the table.' The anterior displacement as the heel lifts off the table is recorded.

slightly posterior to the reference line, and contraction of the quadriceps results in no movement or a slight posterior shift. If the posterior cruciate ligament is ruptured, the tibia 'sags' into posterior subluxation, and the patellar tendon is then directed anteriorly (Figure 11). Contraction of the quadriceps in the posterior cruciate ligament-deficient knee results in an average anterior shift of the tibia of 6 mm in the chronic PCL-injured knee and 4.2 mm in the acute PCL-injured knee.[18] The test is qualitative. No shift or a slight posterior shift of the tibia on contraction of the quadriceps indicates an intact posterior cruciate ligament, while an anterior shift of the tibia from its 'sagging' position of posterior subluxation indicates a ruptured posterior cruciate ligament.

The quadriceps active test is used to establish the quadriceps neutral position of the knee (the anatomic position) from which anterior and posterior tibial displacement can be observed or measured. This is determined by first locating and measuring the quadriceps neutral angle in the *normal* knee. To determine the quadriceps neutral angle, the patient is placed on the examining table in the supine position with the uninjured knee flexed to about 70°. To facilitate maximum patient muscle relaxation, the examiner supports the limb as shown in Figure 7b. The quadriceps is actively contracted and the tibial motion is observed. The angle of knee flexion is adjusted until there is no observable tibial shift. This is 'the quadriceps neutral angle.' The quadriceps neutral angle ranges from 60° to 90° with a mean of 71°.[18] Having determined the quadriceps neutral angle in the normal knee, the injured knee is then positioned at that angle.

Anterior and posterior passive tibial displacement are measured in the normal knee and in the contralateral-injured knee at the quadriceps neutral angle. The quadriceps is contracted and the amount of forward displacement of the tibia is determined. This distance is added to the measured posterior tibial displacement in the injured knee and subtracted from the measured anterior tibial displacement in the injured knee to reference the measurements to the quadriceps active position (Figure 13 and Table 6). Figures 14a and b present the right/left displacement difference for patients with a posterior cruciate ligament disruption.

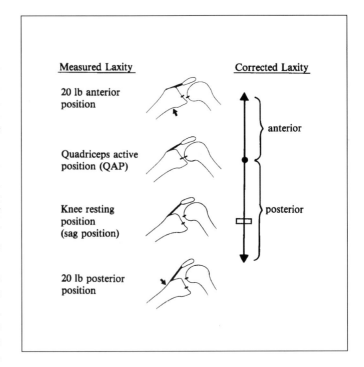

Figure 13

In the injured knee, the measured anterior tibial displacement is the distance from the resting position (rectangle) to the superior arrowhead (10 mm). The measured posterior displacement is from the resting position to the inferior arrowhead (3 mm). With contraction of the quadriceps, the tibia moves forward (5 mm) from the resting position to the quadriceps active position (solid circle). Determinations of the displacement are calculated from the quadriceps active position (corrected displacement) and are shown in Table 6.

Table 6 Determinations of displacement.

	Injured knee Measured laxity	Injured knee Corrected laxity	Normal knee Measured laxity	Injured − normal I−N laxity
20-lb anterior	10	5	4	1
20-lb posterior	3	8	2	6
Quadriceps active displacement	+5		0	

Summary

Instrumented measurements may be used to document anterior–posterior knee motion and to diagnose cruciate ligament disruptions. The test begins with the assessment of posterior tibial sag at 90° of flexion, which indicates a PCL disruption. If the PCL is disrupted, measurements are then performed at the quadriceps neutral angle. If the PCL is intact, measurements are performed at 30° of flexion to evaluate the ACL. Measurements at 30° of flexion are performed with the KT-1000 under five loading conditions, 15-lb, 20-lb, 30-lb, manual maximum, and quadriceps contraction to lift the weight of the leg and testing device. In a unilaterally-injured patient, a right/left difference of <3 mm

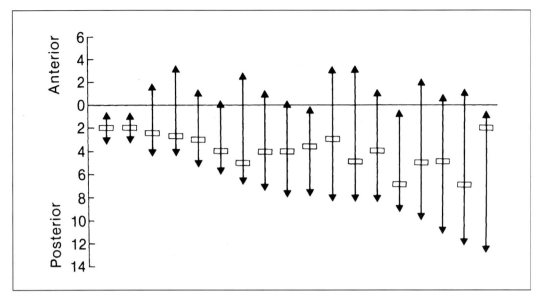

a

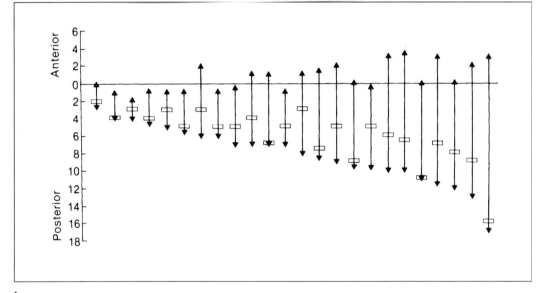

b

Figure 14

Patients with a unilateral PCL disruption. (a) Eighteen patients with an acute PCL disruption. (b) Twenty-four patients with a chronic PCL disruption. Each vertical line represents one patient. The zero mark is the knee neutral position (quadriceps active test position at the quadriceps neutral angle). The rectangle indicates the injured limb resting position, or posterior sag position. Note that in many of the patients there was only a small posterior displacement from the resting position.

is classified as normal motion and a right/left difference on any test of 3 mm or greater is classified as pathologic. To obtain the greatest diagnostic accuracy and testing reproducibility, the patient must be relaxed, the instrument properly positioned, the patellar sensor stabilized against the patella, and the patella positioned in the femoral trochlea. After each test a 20-lb posterior load is applied and released. The dial should then return to the zero resting position to confirm instrument orientation and quadriceps relaxation. It is recommended that physicians, nurses, therapists, and technicians who plan to do instrumented testing receive formal instruction and document their own test/retest reproducibility by testing a number of patients on different days.

References

1. **Shoemaker SC, Daniel DM**, The limits of knee motion, *Knee ligaments: structure, function, injury and repair*, eds Daniel DM, Akeson WH, O'Connor JJ (New York: Raven Press, 1990) 153–161

2. **Sprague RB, Asprey GM**, Photographic method for measuring knee stability: a preliminary report, *Phys Ther* (1965) 45:1055–1058.

3. **Jacobsen K**, Stress radiographical measurement of the antero-posterior, medial and lateral stability of the knee joint, *Acta Orthop Scand* (1976) 47:335–344.

4. **Kennedy JC, Fowler PJ**, Medial and anterior instability of the knee: an anatomical and clinical study using stress machines, *J Bone Joint Surg (Am)* (1971) 53:1257–1270.

5. **Stäubli HU**, Stressradiography—Measurements of knee motion limits, *Knee ligaments: structure, function, injury, and repair*, eds Daniel DM, Akeson WH, O'Connor JJ (New York: Raven Press, 1990) 449–459.

6. **Torzilli PA, Greenberg RL, Hood RW** et al., Measurement of anterior–posterior motion of the knee in injured patients using a biomechanical stress technique, *J Bone Joint Surg (Am)* (1984) 66:1438–1442.

7. **Torzilli PA, Greenberg RL, Insall JN**, An in vivo biomechanical evaluation of anterior–posterior motion of the knee: Roentgenographic measurement technique, stress machine and stable population, *J Bone Joint Surg (Am)* (1981) 63:960–968.

8. **Markolf KL, Graff-Radford A, Amstutz HC**, In vivo knee stability: a quantitative assessment using an instrumented clinical testing apparatus, *J Bone Joint Surg (Am)* (1978) 60:664–674.

9. **Shino K, Inoue M, Horibe S** et al., Measurement of anterior instability of the knee, *J Bone Joint Surg (Br)* (1987) 69:608–613.

10. **Edixhoven P, Huiskes R, DeGraaf R**, et al., Accuracy and reproducibility of instrumented knee-drawer tests, *J Orthop Res* (1987) 5:378–387.

11. **Daniel DM, Stone ML, Sachs R** et al., Instrumented measurement of anterior knee laxity in patients with acute anterior cruciate ligament disruption, *Am J Sports Med* (1985) 13:401–407.

12. **Malcom LL, Daniel DM, Stone ML** et al., The measurement of anterior knee laxity after ACL reconstructive surgery, *Clin Orthop* (1985) 196:35–41.

13. **Bargar WL, Moreland JR, Markolf KL** et al., The effect of tibia–foot rotatory position on the anterior drawer test, *Clin Orthop* (1983) 173:200–203.

14. **Markolf KL, Kochan A, Amstutz HC**, Measurement of knee stiffness and laxity in patients with documented absence of the anterior cruciate ligament, *J Bone Joint Surg (Am)* (1984) 66:242–253.

15. **Nielsen S, Kromann-Andersen C, Rasmussen O** et al., Instability of cadaver knees after transection of capsule and ligaments, *Acta Orthop Scand* (1984) 55:30–34.

16. **Sullivan D, Levy IM, Sheskier S** et al., Medial restraints to anterior–posterior motion of the knee, *J Bone Joint Surg (Am)* (1984) 66:930–936.

17. **Daniel DM, Stone ML**, Instrumented measurement of knee motion, *Knee ligaments: structure, function, injury, and repair*, eds Daniel DM, Akeson WH, O'Connor JJ (New York: Raven Press, 1990) 421–426.

18. **Daniel DM, Stone ML, Barnett P** et al., Use of the quadriceps active test to diagnose posterior cruciate ligament disruption and measure posterior laxity of the knee, *J Bone Joint Surg (Am)* (1988) 70:386–391.

19. **Moore HA, Larson RL**, Posterior cruciate ligament injuries. Results of early surgical repair, *Am J Sports Med* (1980) 8:68–78.

20. **Daniel DM, Malcom LL, Losse G** et al., Instrumented measurement of anterior laxity of the knee, *J Bone Joint Surg (Am)* (1985) 67:720–726.

21. **Sherman OH, Markolf KL, Ferkel RD**, Measurements of anterior laxity in normal and anterior cruciate absent knees with two instrumented test devices, *Clin Orthop* (1987) 215:156–161.

22. **Bach BR, Warren RF, Flynn WM** et al., Arthrometric evaluation of knees that have a torn anterior cruciate ligament, *J Bone Joint Surg (Am)* (1990) 72:1299–1306.

23. **Anderson AF, Snyder RB**, Instrumented evaluation of anterior knee laxity: a comparison of five devices, *Orthop Trans* (1990) 14:586.

24. **Daniel DM, Stone ML**, KT-1000 anterior–posterior displacement measurements, *Knee ligaments: structure, function, injury, and repair*, eds Daniel DM, Akeson WH, O'Connor JJ (New York: Raven Press, 1990) 427–447.

25. **Wroble RR, VanGinkel LA, Grood ES** et al., Repeatability of the KT-1000 arthrometer in a normal population, *Am J Sports Med* (1990) 18:396–399.

26. **Sommerlath K, Gillquist J**, Instrumental testing of sagittal knee laxity in stable and unstable knees. A clinical comparison of simple and computerized devices, *Am J Knee Surg* (1991) 4:70–78.

27. **Steiner ME, Brown C, Zarins B** et al., Measurement of anterior–posterior displacement of the knee, *J Bone Joint Surg (Am)* (1990) 72:1307–1315.

28. **Daniel DM, Woodward EP, Losse GM** et al., The Marshall/MacIntosh anterior cruciate ligament reconstruction with the Kennedy ligament augmentation device: report of the United States clinical trials, *Prosthetic ligament reconstruction of the knee*, ed Friedman MJ, Ferkel RD (Philadelphia: W.B. Saunders, 1988) 71–78.

29. **Engebretsen L, Benum P, Fasting O** et al., A prospective randomized study of three surgical techniques for treatment of acute ruptures of the anterior cruciate ligament, *Am J Sports Med* (1990) 18:585–590.

30. **Glousman R, Shields C, Kerlan R** et al., Gore-Tex prosthetic ligament in anterior cruciate deficient knees, *Am J Sports Med* (1988) 16:321–326.

31. **Goodfellow J, O'Connor J**, The mechanics of the knee and prosthesis design, *J Bone Joint Surg (Br)* (1978) 60:358–369.

32. **Grood ES, Suntay WJ, Noyes FR** et al., Biomechanics of the knee-extension exercise. Effect of cutting the anterior cruciate ligament, *J Bone Joint Surg (Am)* (1984) 66:725–734.

33. **Harter RA, Osternig LR, Singer KM**, Instrumented Lachman tests for the evaluation of anterior laxity after reconstruction of the anterior cruciate ligament, *J Bone Joint Surg (Am)* (1989) 71:975–983.

34. **Henning CE, Lynch MA, Glick KR Jr**, An in vivo strain gage study of elongation of the anterior cruciate ligament, *Am J Sports Med* (1985) 13:22–26.

35. **Higgins RW, Steadman JR**, Anterior cruciate ligament repairs in world class skiers, *Am J Sports Med* (1987) 15:439–447.

36. **Indelicato PA, Pascale MS, Huegel MO**, Early experience with the GORE-TEX polytetrafluoroethylene anterior cruciate ligament prosthesis, *Am J Sports Med* (1989) 17:55–62.

37. **Kapandji, IA**, *The physiology of the joints: annotated diagrams of the mechanics of the human joints*, 2nd edn, trans Honore LH (London: E & S Livingstone, 1974).

38. **Lindahl O, Movin A**, The mechanics of extension of the knee joint, *Acta Orthop Scand* (1967) 38:226–234.

39. **Lipscomb AB, Anderson AF**, Tears of the anterior cruciate in adolescents, *J Bone Joint Surg (Am)* (1986) 68:19–28.

40. **McCarroll JR, Rettig AC, Shelbourne KD**, Anterior cruciate ligament injuries in the young athlete with open physes, *Am J Sports Med* (1988) 16:44–47.

41. **Morrison JB**, Bioengineering analysis of force actions transmitted by the knee joint, *Biomed Eng* (1968) 3:164–170.

42. **Nisell R**, Mechanics of the knee: A study of joint and muscle load with clinical applications, *Acta Orthop Scand (Suppl)* (1985) 216:1–42.

43. **Noyes FR, Mangine RE, Barber S**, Early knee motion after open and arthroscopic anterior cruciate ligament reconstruction, *Am J Sports Med* (1987) 15:149–160.

44. O'Brien SJ, Warren RF, Wickiewicz TL et al., The iliotibial band lateral sling procedure and its effect on the results of anterior cruciate ligament reconstruction, *Am J Sports Med* (1991) 19: 21–25.

45. Anderson AF, Lipscomb AB, Analysis of rehabilitation techniques after anterior cruciate reconstruction, *Am J Sports Med* (1989) 17:154–160.

46. Daniel DM, Stone ML, Case studies, *Knee ligaments: structure, function, injury, and repair*, ed Daniel DM, Akeson WH, O'Connor JJ (New York: Raven Press, 1990) 31–55.

47. Daniel DM, Stone ML, Riehl B, Ligament surgery: The evaluation of results, *Knee ligaments: structure, function, injury, and repair*, ed Daniel DM, Akeson WH, O'Connor JJ (New York: Raven Press, 1990) 521–534.

48. Sachs RA, Reznik A, Daniel DM et al., Complications of knee ligament surgery, *Knee ligaments: structure, function, injury, and repair*, ed Daniel DM, Akeson WH, O'Connor JJ (New York: Raven Press, 1990) 505–520.

49. O'Connor JJ, Goodfellow JW, Young SK et al., Mechanical interactions between the muscles and the cruciate ligaments in the knee, *Trans Orthop Res Soc* (1985) 9:271.

50. Roberts TS, Drez D, McCarthy W et al., Anterior cruciate ligament reconstruction using freeze-dried, ethylene oxide-sterilized, bone–patellar tendon–bone allografts, *Am J Sports Med* (1991) 19:35–41

51. Roth JH, Kennedy JC, Lockstadt H et al., Polypropylene braid augmented and nonaugmented intraarticular anterior cruciate ligament reconstruction, *Am J Sports Med* (1985) 13:321–336.

52. Sgaglione NA, Warren RF, Wickiewicz TL et al., Primary repair with semitendinosus tendon augmentation of acute anterior cruciate ligament injuries, *Am J Sports Med* (1990) 18:64–73.

53. Shelbourne KD, Nitz P, Accelerated rehabilitation after anterior cruciate ligament reconstruction, *Am J Sports Med* (1990) 18:292–299.

54. Shelbourne KD, Whitaker HJ, McCarroll JR et al., Anterior cruciate ligament injury: Evaluation of intraarticular reconstruction of acute tears without repair. Two to seven-year follow-up of 155 athletes, *Am J Sports Med* (1990) 18:484–489.

55. Straub T, Hunter RE, Acute anterior cruciate ligament repair, *Clin Orthop* (1988) 227:238–250.

56. Tibone JE, Antich TJ, A biomechanical analysis of anterior cruciate ligament reconstruction with the patellar tendon—a two-year follow-up, *Am J Sports Med* (1988) 16:332–335.

57. Wainer RA, Clarke TJ, Poehling GG, Arthroscopic reconstruction of the anterior cruciate ligament using allograft tendon, *Arthroscopy* (1988) 4:199–205.

58. Woods GA, Indelicato PA, Prevot TJ, The Gore-Tex anterior cruciate ligament prosthesis: Two versus three year results, *Am J Sports Med* (1991) 19:48–55.

59. Daniel DM, Lawler J, Malcom LL et al., The quadriceps anterior cruciate interaction, *Orthop Trans* (1982) 6:199–200.

60. Smidt GL, Biomechanical analysis of knee flexion and extension, *J Biomech* (1973) 6:79–92.

61. Barnett P, Daniel D, Biden E et al., Posterior cruciate ligament/quadriceps interaction, *Orthop Trans* (1984) 8:258.

6.3   The use of instrumented testing to measure knee displacement

W. Dilworth Cannon, Jr and Joyce M. Vittori

In the late 1970s, several groups of orthopedic surgeons recognized the need to develop a portable and easily used instrument to record knee displacement in the sagittal plane. The ACL Study Group gave encouragement to Larry Malcom and Dale Daniel, as well as one of us (W.D.C.) to develop an arthrometer. Lamoreux in the mid-1970s had independently developed the concept that tibial displacement could be measured through an instrument resting on the patella (assumed to represent the femur) and the tibial tubercle. In 1978, Markolf[1] was able to record sagittal knee displacements in patients seated in a rigid chair. He recorded tibial displacements relative to measurements taken from the patella and tibial tubercle. In 1981, Lamoreux and Cannon independently developed the Knee Laxity Tester (KLT), also known as the Stryker device (manufactured by Orthopaedic Systems, Inc., Hayward, CA, USA). Originally, Malcom and Daniel produced a thigh-mounted device, but converted it soon to a leg-mounted device. Today, this is known as the KT-1000.

From the beginning of 1982 on, all patients presenting in our office with a suspicion of a cruciate ligament tear were tested with the KLT and their data were saved. In an unpublished study, we analyzed a group of 80 patients with documented anterior cruciate ligament (ACL) tears. All 80 patients had been initially examined elsewhere by other physicians. We found that 82.5% of the patients had been incorrectly diagnosed at the time of their first examination. This included a 57% error rate on patients seen by orthopedic surgeons. This high incidence of misdiagnosis would not have occurred if these patients had been tested with an arthrometer when they first sought medical help. In our experience, the accuracy rate in diagnosing an ACL tear with instrumented knee testing exceeds 95%.

Testing technique

We have used the KLT exclusively since its inception to measure anterior–posterior tibial displacement. Patients having ACL reconstruction are tested preoperatively, under anesthesia before and after surgery,

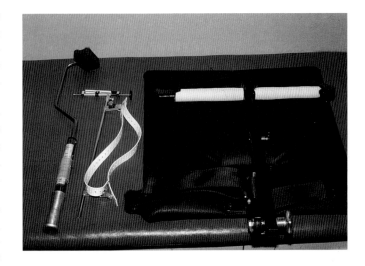

Figure 1

The Knee Laxity Tester consists of a seat support, a measuring device, and a force applicator.

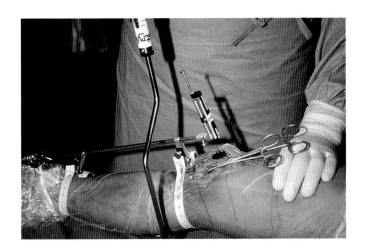

Figure 2

The Knee Laxity Tester can be autoclaved and applied to the leg during surgery. Previously, it was applied to the knee with wounds still open, as shown above. Now, with arthroscopically assisted ACL reconstruction, the device is applied to the knee once incisions are closed, but before dressing application.

and postoperatively at 3 months, 6 months, and annually thereafter. Conservatively treated ACL and PCL deficient patients are also tested at regular intervals to monitor any change in anterior displacement over time.

The unit is a simple apparatus consisting of a seat with a support bar, a measuring device, and a force applicator (Figure 1). Both the measuring device and the force applicator can be autoclaved. The KLT is an invaluable tool in determining intraoperative anterior–posterior displacement of the involved knee after ACL reconstruction but before dressing application (Figure 2). If necessary the graft can be readjusted for optimum results.

Technique for anterior cruciate ligament injuries

Position the seat on an examination table with the leg support extending out from the table. Seat the patient on the device with both ankles on top of the lower crossbar. The knee flexion angle should be between 25° and 35°. If the patient has a flexion contracture or a significant effusion, it should be compensated for by adjusting the support bar to change the flexion angle of the knee. For example, if the patient has a 10° flexion contracture, testing should be done between 35° and 45°.

Affixed to the device are two sets of straps. One set spans the patient's thighs at approximately 2 inches above the patellae before attaching to the seat support. The second set of straps fasten over the ankles to the crossbar. These serve to ensure that both the patient's thighs and ankles are secure and that the flexion angle does not change during testing. This step is, of course, modified when testing a supine patient under anesthesia. Instead of using the support seat, flex the patient's knee to 25–35° and maintain the flexion by placing a roll under the thigh. The patient's ankles can be held down manually, but allow for freedom of rotation.

Apply the calibrated testing instrument to the uninvolved knee first. To facilitate this, twist the patellar button to a horizontal position (Figure 3). Fit the proximal bracket over the most proximal extent of the tibial tubercle. Pull the rubber strap tightly around the calf and fasten it to the other side of the bracket. The strap should fit snugly so that the bracket stays anchored to the tibial tubercle during testing. The distal bracket attaches to the tibia just above the ankle. Cant it laterally so that the axial bar of the instrument parallels the patellar tendon and compensates for the 'Q' angle. Swing the patellar button back to a vertical position. To ensure proper alignment, the patellar button must lie over the middle of the patella. If it is off-center, telescope the patellar button proximally or distally. Once it is in position, tighten it with the thumbscrew. If still not correct, hold the lower

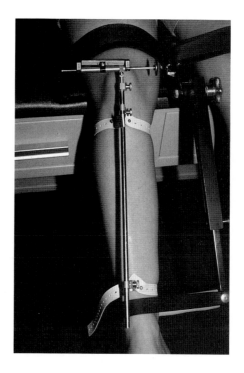

Figure 3

The measuring device is applied to the leg with the patellar button in a horizontal position. The upper and lower brackets are attached. Then the patellar button is placed in a vertical position contacting the middle of the patella.

bracket with one hand while placing the patellar button exactly over the center of the patella with the other hand. Move the lower bracket medially or laterally to center the button on the patella (Figure 4). If the patient has a significant effusion, it is easy to confirm that the patella is contacting the trochlear groove. Push on the patella with the instrument in place. There should be no deflection of the instrument if the patella is well seated. It is not necessary to aspirate the joint before testing.

Patient relaxation is the key to successful KLT testing. To encourage this, have the patient lean back to support the upper body with his or her hands. Oscillate the leg back and forth to be certain that there is no underlying thigh muscle tension.

Right-handed examiners should test both knees while standing to the right side of the patient; left-handed examiners should stand to the left of the patient. With the force applicator, place the groove on the bottom of the black rectangular pad over the crest of the tibia within a centimeter of the proximal bracket. Support the posterior thigh immediately above the knee joint with your left hand. This latter maneuver helps to prevent extension of the knee during force application. Apply a 20-lb (89-N)

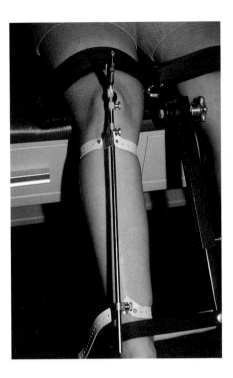

Figure 4

The measuring device is in the proper position prior to beginning force application. Notice the lateral offset of the lower bracket to compensate for the 'Q' angle.

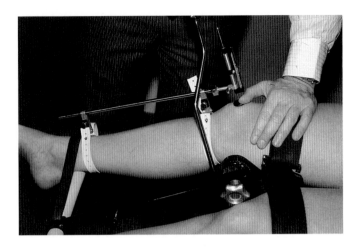

Figure 5

For force application in an anterior direction, the examiner's hand is placed across the upper strap, and the thumb is placed over the patellar button to secure it during testing. Note that the force applicator is always introduced from the medial side of the calf.

posterior force with the force applicator. Do not attempt to read the scale during force application. Next, place the force applicator behind the proximal calf from the *medial* side. The applicator should rest immediately behind the proximal bracket in the middle of the calf. Pull with a 20-lb anterior force. During this maneuver, the examiner should position his or her left hand over the thigh strap with his or her thumb on top of the patellar button (Figure 5). This will stabilize the patellar button during testing. Now record the amount of both anterior and posterior excursion present to the nearest 0.5 mm (Table 1). Do not attempt to read the deflection on the scale *during* force application.

Repeat the testing two more times and average the posterior, anterior, and total excursion scores of the three sets of tests (Table 1). The range for the three numbers in each direction should not exceed 1 mm. If it does, repeat the test until they fall within this range. A low number outside this range usually means that the patient was tense during testing. It is important also to test anterior excursion with a 40-lb (178-N) force. Repeat the test and average the two values (Table 1). Although 40-lb anterior displacement testing is performed preoperatively, it is not repeated until 6 months following ACL reconstruction.

Bilateral knee testing is always done. The only exception is that testing is done with a 20-lb anterior force on the involved knee only, at the end of surgery while the patient is still under anesthesia. Calculate the involved minus uninvolved differences for the categories tested (Table 1).

Several factors may account for absolute anterior–posterior excursion numbers appearing improbably low. Among them are inexperience of the examiner, patient tension, or failure to account for a flexion contracture or a significant effusion. Also, check to see whether the device is mounted incorrectly and determine whether the force application is too distal.

Technique for posterior cruciate ligament injuries

The examiner should do a thorough examination of the knee before KLT testing. This should include an estimate of the degree of posterior subluxation of the tibia. This is done by placing both thumbs at the anterior joint-lines of the knee and palpating the medial and lateral femoral condyles. A subjective grading system can be used to estimate the degree of posterior subluxation in comparison with the control knee. This is done by applying posterior and anterior forces to the proximal tibia in the 90° position. Clancy[2] has devised a system of assessment using this technique that works well in his hands despite being based on a subjective classification system.

Do not test patients with posterior cruciate injuries

Table 1 Sample of Knee Laxity Tester data collected for ACL screening. Twenty-pound testing is done in both anterior and posterior directions between 25 and 35° of flexion, repeated three times and averaged. Forty-pound anterior testing is done twice and averaged. Involved minus uninvolved differences are calculated as shown. Clearly, the left knee of this patient has an ACL tear.

| | Twenty-pound | | | | | |
| | Right knee | | | Left knee | | |
	Post.	Ant.	Total	Post.	Ant.	Total
1.	3.0	4.5	7.5	2.5	10.5	13.0
2.	3.5	5.0	8.5	2.5	11.0	13.5
3.	3.0	5.0	8.0	3.0	11.0	14.0
	3.2	4.8	8.0	2.7	10.8	13.5

Forty-pound

Ant.: 6.0, 6.0 = 6.0   Ant.: 14.5, 14.0 = 14.3

I−U differences

20-lb post.: −0.5 mm   20-lb total.: 5.5 mm
20-lb ant.:   6.0 mm   40-lb ant.:   8.3 mm

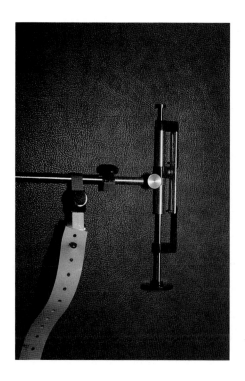

Figure 6

When testing for PCL laxity in the 90° position, in order to maintain proper spring tension of the patellar button, the barrel of the patellar button is slid downward and tightened, as shown in the photograph. Note the usual position of the barrel in Figure 3.

in the Lachman position at 25–35° of flexion. In this position, a PCL deficient patient's knee will experience a drop-back of the tibia secondary to gravity. Applying the anterior forces to the tibia will produce significant excursions, but the starting point will be from the posterior subluxed position, not the neutral position. Therefore, the inexperienced examiner will erroneously interpret the data as an ACL tear rather than a PCL tear. Instead, test suspected PCL deficient patients in the 90° position. Since the hamstrings have an inherent tendency to pull the tibia posteriorly into a subluxed position, a special technique is used to find the neutral position of the tibia relative to the femur. Daniel[3] can be credited with describing the quadriceps active test, by which a quadriceps set will position the tibia from 0 to 2 mm posterior to the neutral position relative to the femur. Daniel flexes the *normal* knee through different positions to find the point of least change with a quadriceps set. He finds that the average position is 71° of flexion and he defines this angle as the quadriceps neutral angle.[3] We have arbitrarily taken 90° as our testing position and find that this position is close enough to Daniel's quadriceps neutral angle.

Therefore, set the seat support at a 90° flexed position. Pull the support forward from the table edge to allow room for the force applicator behind the tibia. Attach the thigh and ankle straps to secure both legs in this position. Apply the KLT to the shank of the leg using the same technique as in the Lachman position, with the exception that the barrel of the spring-loaded plunger and scale should be slid through the retaining bracket and locked with the thumbscrew (Figure 6). (Older KLT models may not have a thumbscrew to allow repositioning of the barrel containing the patellar button. If this is the case, write to the manufacturer and one will be sent to you.) This creates better tension for the patellar button once it is positioned on the patella. The patellar button must be in contact with the patella. In an alternative method, place a 2- or 3-inch roll of Webril underneath the ankle support. This will angle the proximal end of the instrument in a posterior direction and allow contact between the patella and the button. The patient should lean back and relax in the same manner as in the Lachman testing position.

Begin the testing procedure by having the patient do an active quadriceps set. The examiner places his or her hand on the patient's ankle to prevent it from forcibly releasing the Velcro strap. With the patient maintaining a quadriceps contraction, zero the instrument (Figure 7). Then the examiner's hand applies a posteriorly directed force over the tibial tubercle. Ask the patient to relax completely. Take the force applicator in your right hand and place it over the tibial tubercle just below the proximal bracket of the instrument. Release the posteriorly directed force from your hand and simultaneously apply a 20-lb load (Figure 8). While maintaining this load, read the amount of

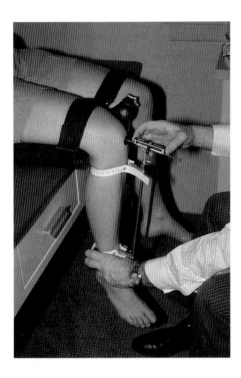

Table 2 Sample of Knee Laxity Tester data collection for PCL screening in the 90° position. Twenty- and forty-pound testing is carried out both anteriorly and posteriorly, and involved minus uninvolved differences are calculated as shown. Clearly, the right knee of this patient has a PCL tear.

Twenty-pound	
Right knee	*Left knee*
Post.: 7.0, 7.0 = 7.0	Post.: 1.0, 1.5 = 1.3
Ant.: 5.5, 5.0 = 5.3	Ant.: 3.5, 4.0 = 3.8
Forty-pound	
Post.: 9.5, 9.0 = 9.3	Post.: 2.0, 2.0 = 2.0
Ant.: 7.0, 6.0 = 6.5	Ant.: 6.0, 6.5 = 6.3
I–U differences	
20-lb post.: 5.7 mm	40-lb post.: 7.3 mm
20-lb ant.: 1.5 mm	40-lb ant.: 0.2 mm

Figure 7

When testing in the 90° position, the quadriceps neutral position is determined by having the patient do a quadriceps set while the instrument is zeroed.

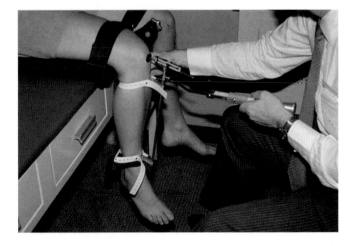

Figure 8

After zeroing the instrument and having the patient relax, 20-lb and 40-lb forces are applied to the tibia in a posterior direction. Displacement measurements are recorded during force application, not when the force is released.

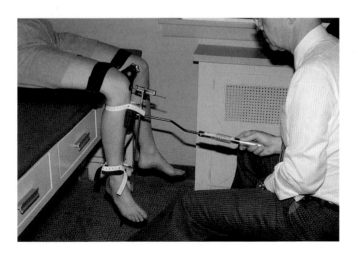

Figure 9

When measuring anterior translation in the 90° position, the instrument is zeroed as shown in Figure 7. An anteriorly directed force is manually applied as the patient simultaneously relaxes in order to prevent posterior subluxation of the tibia. The force applicator is positioned behind the calf from the medial side and gently pulled anteriorly as the examiner's hand is withdrawn. Anterior forces of 20 lb and 40 lb are then applied.

deflection on the scale and memorize it. This is in contrast to the Lachman position where the deflection is not read until the load is released. Increase the load to 40 lb and read the displacement amount while maintaining the load. Record these two figures. Repeat the procedure to obtain a mean value (Table 2).

Have the patient do another quadriceps set and zero the instrument. For measuring anterior translation, place your left hand behind the proximal calf and apply an anteriorly directed force as the patient relaxes. Introducing the force applicator from the medial side, place it behind the proximal calf while maintaining this anteriorly directed force (Figure 9). Apply a 20-lb load while using your left hand to prevent the patient's ankle detaching the distal strap. Read the amount of deflection off the scale while maintaining this 20-lb load. Increase the load to 40 lb and record the amount of deflection (Table 2). Repeat this procedure and take the mean value (Table 2). In a manner identical with testing in the Lachman position, repeat values should fall within a 1 mm range for each deflection series.

Repeat the procedure for the contralateral knee, and calculate the involved-minus-uninvolved differences for 20 lb and 40 lb anterior displacements and 20 lb and 40 lb posterior displacements (Table 2).

Use the same technique in patients presenting with both an anterior and posterior cruciate tear. Define the starting neutral position with the quadriceps active test. Valuable information can be obtained regarding the proportion of anterior and posterior displacement attributable to the anterior and posterior cruciate pathology. A grade 2 ACL tear can be differentiated from a grade 3 posterior cruciate tear in the same patient.

Results

All KLT testing is done by W.D.C. This is to eliminate any potential variations in testing techniques that may occur with different examiners. As Daniel[4] reported in 1986, multiple examiners will produce variability in results. Conversely, if one person does all the testing, there will be a greater consistency in reporting results. Figure 10 demonstrates the consistency of the test–retest variability on one patient tested nine times over a 3-year period by the same examiner.

Displacement means

KLT testing was done in the Lachman position on 50 normal subjects and 94 ACL deficient patients. Anterior, posterior, and total mean displacements with a 20-lb force and anterior displacement with a 40-lb load are illustrated in Figure 11. There is no difference in mean posterior displacement between the normal and ACL groups. Normal subjects tested with a 20-lb and 40-lb anterior load had a mean of 5.3 mm and 6.6 mm, respectively. In contrast, ACL deficient knees had a mean anterior displacement of 11.8 with a 20-lb force and 15.2 with a 40-lb load. Looking at the overall data (Figures 12, 13 and 14) one can see an overlap in anterior displacement scores at 20 lb and 40 lb load and in total sagittal displacement with a 20-lb load. Clearly, absolute values fail to separate completely the ACL population group from the normal group. One reason for this may be the presence of hypermobility in some normal knees. The thumb-to-wrist and elbow hyperextension tests were conducted on the normal subjects in this study. Sixteen of the 50 normal subjects had hypermobile joints. A comparison of these knees (Figure 15) showed that hypermobile knees did have greater anterior and total sagittal displacements than knees that were not hypermobile.

Testing patients with PCL pathology in the 90° position revealed the mean posterior displacements to be 10.2 mm for a 20-lb posteriorly applied load and 10.7 mm for a 40-lb posteriorly applied load. For the normal knee, these values were 2.9 mm and 3.2 mm, respectively. Unfortunately, these figures

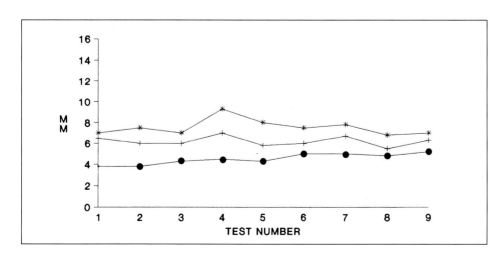

Figure 10

Test–retest variability on one patient's knee tested nine times over a 3-year period by W.D.C. shows excellent consistency of measurements. • posterior 20 lbs; + anterior 20 lbs; * anterior 40 lbs.

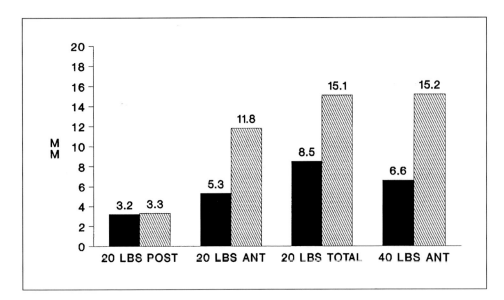

Figure 11

Testing results in the Lachman position on 50 normal (solid) and 94 ACL deficient (shaded) patients. Anterior, posterior, and total mean displacements with a 20-lb force and anterior displacement with a 40-lb load are shown.

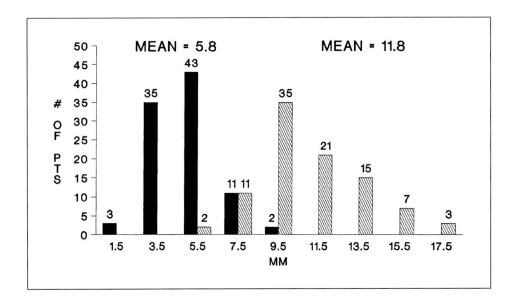

Figure 12

Anterior displacement in 94 ACL deficient knees (shaded) compared to their normal knees (solid) with a 20-lb force. Notice the overlap of the two sets of data.

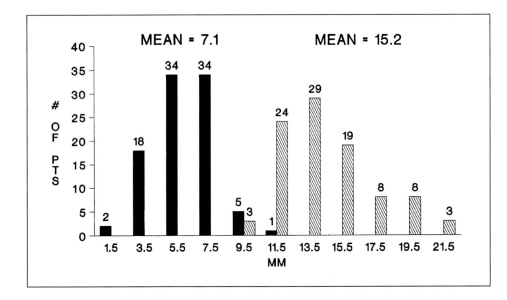

Figure 13

Same testing conditions as in Figure 12, but with a 40-lb anterior force. There is less overlap of the two sets of data.

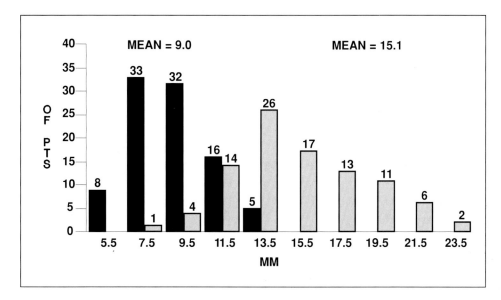

Figure 14

Same testing conditions as in Figures 12 and 13, but the total sagittal anterior–posterior displacement with a 20-lb load is shown. Notice the persisting overlap of the two sets of data.

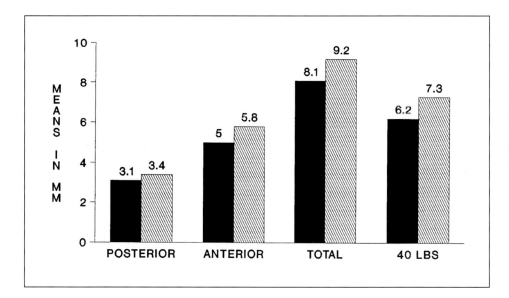

Figure 15

Sixteen hypermobile (shaded) and 34 nonhypermobile (solid) subjects were compared at 20-lb posterior, anterior, and total, and 40-lb anterior force application. The hypermobile subjects had approximately 1 mm more anterior tibial translation than the rest of the subjects.

include some patients who did not have arthroscopy to confirm the presence of a grade 3 PCL tear. This may include some severe grade 2 tears as well.

I−U differences

Involved knee minus uninvolved knee differences (I−U) are more significant than absolute values when measuring knee displacement. Table 3 depicts the mean I−U differences of normal subjects and those with acute and chronic ACL tears. Since its inception, we have been proponents of KLT testing with a 40-lb anterior load. A comparison of the data spread between normal subjects and ACL deficient patients illustrates why it is important. A 20-lb anterior force

Table 3 The means of involved minus uninvolved differences of 20-lb anterior, posterior, total anterior–posterior, and 40-lb anterior testing in normal subjects, acute, and chronic ACL deficient patients.

ACL status	20-lb post. (mm)	20-lb ant. (mm)	20-lb total (mm)	40-lb ant. (mm)
Normal 50 patients	0.8	0.8	1.0	0.7
Acute ACL 26 patients	−0.6	5.5	4.9	7.8
Chronic ACL 68 patients	0.3	6.2	6.6	8.3
Acute/chronic 94 patients	0.1	6.0	6.1	8.1

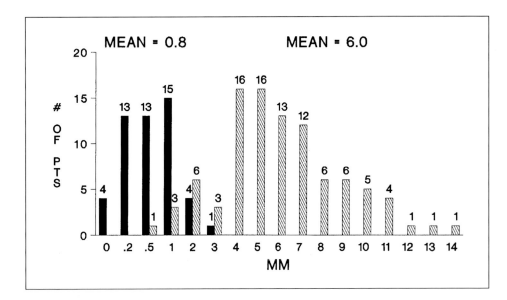

Figure 16

The involved minus uninvolved differences with a 20-lb force are shown in 50 normal subjects (solid) versus 94 ACL deficient patients (shaded). Notice the overlap of data points from the two groups in contrast to that shown in Figure 17.

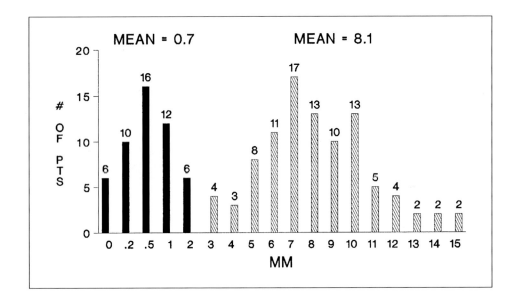

Figure 17

The involved minus uninvolved differences with a 40-lb anterior force in the same two population groups shown in Figure 16. Notice the clear and distinct separation of the two sets of data points, indicating the advantage that 40-lb testing has over 20-lb testing.

produces a mean of 0.8 in normal subjects and 6.0 in ACL deficient patients. Figure 16 breaks these patients down by I−U anterior differences. Note the overlap between the normal and ACL deficient groups. We feel, as Daniel does, that an I−U difference of 3 mm or more is pathognomonic of an ACL tear. Note in Figure 16 that 11% of the ACL deficient patients would have been missed. In contrast to this, testing with a 40-lb load (Figure 17) produces a clear and distinct separation of the two population groups. None of the ACL deficient patients had less than a 3 mm I−U difference. Because of this observation, we have always strongly recommended testing all patients with a 40-lb load. Daniel[5] has reported missing one-third of acute ACL tears when relying solely on 20-lb load testing.

Expressing the results

A mean can give a general picture of the overall results of a series but it will not tell anything about the range of the variables. A series may include several patients with grossly loose knees and some patients with tighter than normal knees. Figure 18 illustrates just such a scenario. Here, four patients have a 4.0 mm anterior displacement at 20 lb and one patient has a very tight knee (−3 mm). The mean for this group is 2.6 mm and the casual reader might construe these results as indicating that all five patients had a good result, whereas none of them did. Taking a mean of the entire group will not reveal the true picture and it is not the best way to express results.

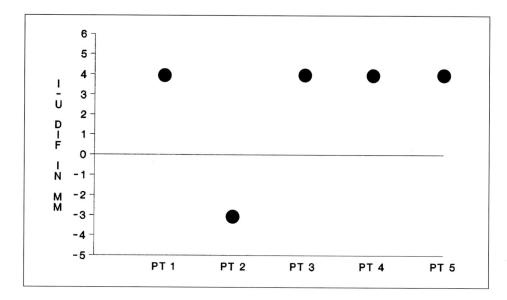

Figure 18

Expressing results as a mean may not give an accurate indication of results. In this example, results of ACL reconstruction, 20 lb anterior force, four patients had an involved minus uninvolved difference of 4 mm and a fifth patient −3 mm, for a mean of 2.6 mm. Although the mean fits into the 'good' category, none of the patients was actually in this category.

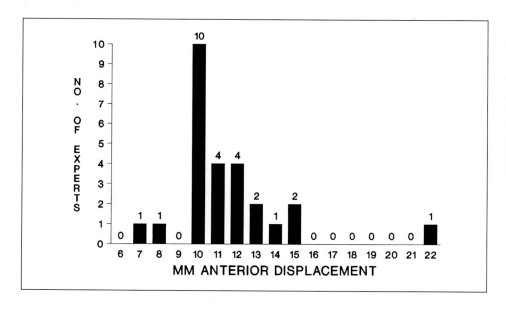

Figure 19

Twenty-six international knee surgeons gave their estimates of the Lachman test in millimeters on a knee model that was preset to have 12 mm of anterior tibial displacement. Although the mean for the group was accurate (11.8), the subjective assessments of these experts were wide-ranging.

In this series, results of ACL reconstruction are classified using the criteria established by Daniel.[6] A result is considered good if the I−U difference was less than 3.0 mm. A fair result is one with an I−U difference greater than 3.0 mm but less than 5.0 mm, and a poor result has a greater than 5.0 mm difference.

A group of 43 ACL reconstructions was followed for 3 or more years. KLT testing with a 20-lb force revealed anterior knee displacement results at 1 year of 84% good, 9% fair, and 7% poor. These results were maintained when the same group was tested again 3 or more years later. This indicates that patients with good results at 1 year's follow-up KLT testing are likely to maintain that result and not loosen with time.

Discussion

Today, orthopedic publications will usually not be accepted without quantification of data from an arthrometer. No longer is it acceptable to publish a paper expressing tibial displacement results as 1+ through 4+. These subjective evaluations are inherently imprecise. In an unpublished study from the ACL Study Group in Zermatt, Switzerland, Stäubli and Cannon used a mannikin knee (developed by Roland Jakob) with preprogrammable tibial displacements that could be dialed in from an opening in the popliteal fossa. Twenty-six international knee surgeons were asked to examine the model knee and estimate the anterior tibial displacement. As illustrated in Figure 19, the subjective assessments of these experts were wide-ranging and largely inaccurate. The mean, however, was close to the amount of actual displacement.

Knee displacement measurements are important for documentation of results. As ACL reconstructive techniques change, it is important to quantitate results to assess whether a change in technique has been beneficial to the patient. For example, we find better results after reconstruction in patients who are less lax going into surgery, who have lower isometry measurements during surgery, and who have tighter graft placement. This information could not be reliably obtained without instrumented knee testing.

Instrumented knee laxity testing is an objective means of evaluating the results of ACL reconstruction, and diagnosing and monitoring the progress of ACL and PCL deficient patients. The availability and reliability of these testers should relegate subjective evaluation and reporting of ligament displacement results to a historical item.

References

1. **Markolf KL, Graff-Radford A, Amstutz HC** et al., In vivo knee stability, *J Bone Joint Surg (Am)* (1978) **60**:664–674.
2. **Clancy WG,** Diagnosis and treatment of posterior cruciate ligament injuries. Instructional Course, American Orthopedic Society for Sports Medicine, Orlando, Florida (10 July 1991).
3. **Daniel DM, Stone ML, Barnett P** et al., Use of the quadriceps active test to diagnose posterior cruciate ligament disruption and measure posterior laxity of the knee, *J Bone Joint Surg (Am)* (1988) **70**:386–391.
4. **Daniel DM, Woodward P, Losse GM** et al., ACL reconstruction with a Kennedy LAD, American Orthopedic Society for Sports Medicine, Sun Valley, Idaho (July 14, 1986).
5. **Daniel DM, Stone ML,** KT-1000 anterior–posterior displacement measurements, *Knee ligaments: structure, function, injury and repair,* ed Daniel DM, Akeson W, O'Connor J (Raven Press: New York, 1990) 427–447.
6. **Daniel DM, Stone ML, Sachs RA,** The classification of anterior displacement measurements, The Department of Orthopedic Surgery, Kaiser Hospital, San Diego and The Division of Orthopedic Surgery, University of California at San Diego (June, 1988).

6.4 The conservative management of the anterior cruciate ligament-deficient knee

Malcolm F. Macnicol

The frequency with which the anterior cruciate ligament is injured, whether in sports or in association with long-bone fractures of the lower limb, has only been widely appreciated over the last two decades. Initially, anteromedial laxity was described and treated as the principal aspect of any resulting disability. It was later realized, with increasing emphasis, that anterolateral tibial subluxation is the pathological component that demands attention.[1]

The anterior cruciate ligament is ruptured by hyperextension of the knee, forced internal rotation of the tibia, and coronal stresses (valgus or varus) combined with deceleration. These mechanisms of injury should be kept in mind when efforts are being made to treat the knee conservatively after the event; physiotherapy attempts to improve hamstring power and thigh muscle tone, while bracing reduces the vectors of force which are normally harnessed by the intact ligament.

Assessment

Undoubtedly the most disabling symptom experienced by the individual convalescing after anterior cruciate ligament rupture is the sensation of giving-way or buckling, induced unexpectedly when the affected knee is rotated when weight bearing. Concordance between this symptom of instability and the pivot shift is high, but the test may be pronounced negative by the inexperienced examiner, or may be guarded against by the patient through protective biceps tone or apprehension. Thus the most valid means of testing for a pivot shift or jerk is under anaesthesia when the thigh muscles are relaxed, and before the application of a tourniquet in those cases where surgery is planned. The Lachman test of anterior and anterolateral laxity, carried out with the knee in 20–30° of flexion, is of adjunctive value and allows the anterior shift of the tibia to be graded as mild, moderate or severe in comparison with the normal leg.

In order to assess the effects of conservative management of cruciate ligament rupture it is important to grade the disability as objectively as possible.

While there is debate about the value of machines for testing knee laxity, the relative precision and re-test reliability afforded by mechanical assessment[2] are to be preferred to clinical perceptions of the Lachman test and pivot shift alone. Admittedly, a commercially available apparatus such as the KT1000 knee laxity recorder is prone to misuse and misinterpretation. But the regular use of recordings of this sort is recommended, if only to ensure that there is a gradual move towards uniformity.

In addition to the problems of assessing anterolateral laxity in the unanaesthetized, but eventually relaxed patient, other factors play a part in determining whether the knee will compensate or remain problematic after conservative management.[3-5] The presence or absence of other injuries is obviously important, none more so than poorly reduced articular fractures of the tibial and femoral condyles. 'Isolated' rupture, or partial bundle tears of the anterior cruciate ligament, may permit a satisfactory restitution of function, but associated tears of the collateral ligaments, posterior cruciate or meniscus may prevent adequate rehabilitation if they heal abnormally or not at all. An exercise programme may also fail in an individual with generalized joint laxity (hypermobility), genu valgum and malrotation of the limb, or with a markedly convex lateral tibial plateau.[6] The greater stability of the medial compartment of the knee partially derives from the concavity of the medial tibial articular surface; increasing convexity of the lateral tibial plateau will lead to a heightened sense of jerk or shift as the femoral condyle moves forcibly over the zenith of the surface.

Gait adaptation

The altered walking pattern which follows ligament injury was clearly shown by Perry and her co-workers[7] when studying the suggested effects of pes anserinus transfer. Gait analysis reveals that stride length, single limb support time and walking velocity are uniformly reduced, and of course these effects may be the product of adaptive changes in locomotion as much as the effects of surgery. The restrictive effect of anterior cruciate rupture was further demonstrated by Berchuck et al.[8] when they assessed kinematic changes in gait resulting from anterior cruciate ligament deficiency. The magnitude of the flexion movement about the knee was appreciably reduced during walking or jogging, in an attempt at 'quadriceps-avoidance'. By this means, anterior subluxation of the proximal tibia, produced by relatively unopposed quadriceps contraction, was largely prevented. Activities employing greater flexion of the knee, such as climbing or descending stairs, were not appreciably different.

It is interesting to note that 25% of the patients investigated by Berchuck et al.[8] did not adopt this quadriceps-avoidance gait. As this group comprised a selected cohort with symptomatic knees, it can be surmised that a proportion of individuals do not require to adapt their walking pattern significantly after anterior cruciate rupture, although increased external rotation of the tibia and greater care during manoeuvres may nevertheless occur instinctively. Further evidence that some patients do not suffer frank episodes of giving-way and lateral joint pain after anterior cruciate ligament rupture also stems from the established fact that arthroscopic inspection occasionally reveals a knee with this pathology but symptoms of a different or lesser kind.

Characterization of the laxity

Before conservative treatment is embarked upon, a baseline of dysfunction should be established. Admittedly, this usually involves little more than the presenting symptoms, physical examination and radiographs in two planes. Yet accurate diagnosis should increasingly include the adjunctive use of magnetic resonance imaging or arthroscopy. Double-contrast arthrography has a lesser role in current investigation. Cineradiography with markers and kinetic/kinematic studies are usually unavailable, and are probably unnecessary when symptoms and the presence of a pivot shift provide graphic proof of decompensation.

However, Gerber and Matter[9] have analysed the knee biomechanically after acute rupture of the anterior cruciate ligament, and after its early repair by primary suture. Using the instant-centre technique Frankel et al.[10] showed that the instant-centre (centrode) remained within the femoral condylar contour when viewed from a standardized lateral projection during movement of the normal knee. When the anterior cruciate ligament was ruptured, the centrode moved anteriorly and inferiorly, below the joint-line, when the knee flexed from 20 to 40°. This abnormality did not correlate completely with the pivot shift sign, which was sometimes negative in these early cases. More significantly, acute repair

failed to abolish the pathological shift of the centrode, confirming the experimental studies of Cabaud et al.[11] who also demonstrated that the progression of degenerative changes was proportional to the length of follow-up after surgical reconstruction as well as the degree of induced joint laxity.

Primary repair of the anterior cruciate ligament has been shown clinically to be unrewarding, at 5 years postoperatively,[12] and therefore autogenous reconstruction is usually recommended, particularly if meniscal pathology is occurring. Sandberg et al.[5] however, confirmed that operative intervention brings its own morbidity and for many surgeons a conservative approach will, at least for the present, remain advisable both clinically and economically unless chronic instability declares itself later.

The Tegner[13] and Lysholm[14] scales are useful indicators of improved function following treatment, as are assessments using the KT1000, the Cybex dynamometer or Kincom apparatus, and dynamic tests such as single hops, repeated squats or bench step-ups, figure-of-eight running and timed side-to-side runs. These tests, modified appropriately, should be repeated after physiotherapy, bracing or surgical reconstruction, although clearly any improvement perceived by the subject will remain the most compelling criterion for patient and therapist alike.

Exercise programme

Before accepting that the anterior cruciate-deficient knee will remain decompensated, it is important to conduct a programme of exercises, preferably under the supervision of a designated physiotherapist (Table 1). Unless medical facilities include the capacity to follow-up all cases with diagnosed, acute ruptures of the ligament, it is usual to find that many patients will refer themselves back for further treatment some time after the initial injury. A referral centre will attract a further proportion of patients with chronic anterior cruciate insufficiency, and many of these will respond to a carefully structured, conservative approach.[15]

In certain instances a surgical approach may be deemed inadvisable (Table 2); more commonly, physiotherapy and bracing are considered to be insufficient or unacceptable by the patient, so that surgery is enlisted at an early or later stage in management, depending in large measure upon the enthusiasm with which the surgeon embraces the surgical option.

The goals of physiotherapy include:

1. A strengthening of hamstring power and tone, reducing the normal predominance of the antigravity quadriceps muscles.
2. Enhanced proprioception, which involves a training in single leg balance and general limb control.

Table 1 Exercise programme to restore power, endurance, movement and proprioception as fully as possible.

Immediate	1	(a)	Ice	
		(b)	Compression	
		(c)	Elevation	
	2	(a)	Gentle active range	
		(b)	Gentle isometric thigh contraction	
	3	(a)	Backshell or brace (20–120° of flexion for 2 weeks)	
		(b)	Protected weight bearing (crutches)	
Subsequent	1	(a)	Isometric exercise[a] at various angles of knee flexion	⎧ for both hamstrings and
		(b)	Isokinetic exercises	⎪ quadriceps, active-assisted (with
		(c)	Isotonic exercises	⎨ springs) progressing to
		(d)	Pes anserinus and other rotational exercises	⎩ increasing load
	2	(a)	Squats: 90°/full	
		(b)	Step ups: forwards / sideways — ⎰ Eyes open ⎱ Eyes closed	
		(c)	Running on spot	
		(d)	Bicycle ergometer	
	3	(a)	Running: straight-line with increasing stride, side-stepping (cutting), figure of eight	
		(b)	Agility (wobble board)	
		(c)	Cross-country running	
		(d)	Sport (graduated return)	

(i) The development of an effusion indicates that rehabilitation is too rapid.
(ii) Rubber plinth or rolled towel can be used as fulcrum when undertaking quadriceps work.
(iii) Always test the patient as fully as possible before permitting a return to sport.
(iv) Ideally the hamstrings should develop 70% of the quadriceps power.

[a] Supine, prone, 'half-long' sitting and upright positions for variety.

Table 2 Conservative approach advisable.

Osteoarthritis radiographically
Persistent pain
Poorly motivated
Poor health
Unrealistic sporting aspirations
Complex knee laxity (multidirectional)

3. Advice about trunk and upper body strength, general fitness and weight control.
4. Education about appropriate sport and an attention to any obviously faulty technique.

Thigh muscle strengthening is ensured by both isometric and isotonic drill. The programme is graduated, avoiding excessive weights and fatigue; sets of exercises and variation in knee flexion and extension disciplines will help to motivate the patient, and much depends upon the ingenuity of the physiotherapist.

The Cybex and Kincom machines can be adjusted to demand increasing work from the patient, and the improvement in thigh muscle power can be plotted accurately. In addition to exercises based upon prone and supine lying, or sitting at the edge of a couch, the use of bench step-ups, jumps, jogging and running figure-of-eight ensure a sense of progress towards the eventual participation in sport. Thigh muscle bulk is used as an indicator of developing power, with intermittent measurements from the Kincom apparatus.

Proprioception is enhanced by wobble board or tilting table exercises. Initially the patient concentrates on simple balance, but later in the programme a second activity, such as catching and throwing a ball, is introduced, while the patient stands on the wobble board or trampette using only the injured leg. Compression bandaging is permissible if this gives confidence and a greater sense of knee control. Strapping with zinc oxide tape is also of value in the early stages of rehabilitation, and can be used to afford patellar support when anterior knee pain is troublesome. When discomfort and insecurity are marked, knee exercises in a warm swimming pool are confidence-boosting and allow measurements which would otherwise prove impossible.

Inevitably, once the stage of supervised physiotherapy and encouragement comes to an end, there is a tendency for the knee to decompensate (Figure 1). The steady deterioration in function that follows conservative treatment can lead to a pessimistic outlook, which may inadvertently affect the attitude of the patient. Yet the long-term effects of cruciate reconstruction are still uncertain, and modification of sporting aspirations, coupled with discipline about continuing the thigh exercises, can certainly deal satisfactorily with a proportion of patients with knee instability.

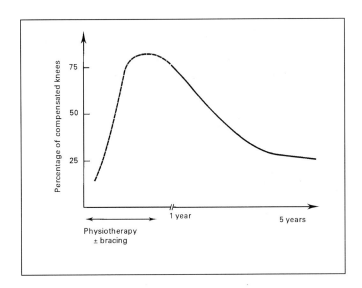

Figure 1

Decompensation of the anterior cruciate-deficient knee with time.

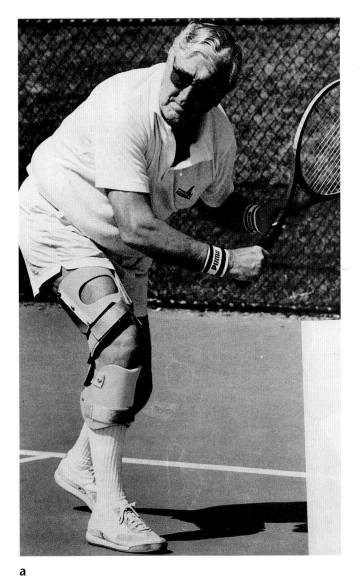

a

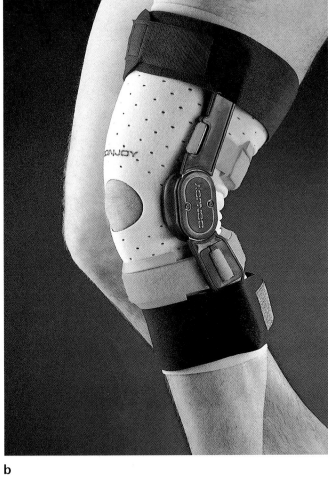

b

Figure 2

Functional knee brace.

Bracing

The value of knee braces for anterior cruciate ligament insufficiency remains a subjective affair dependent to a great extent upon the compliance of the patient. Stark (1850)[16] is reputed to have made the first attempt at bracing, reporting the use of a steel spring for two patients in an Edinburgh journal. A number of contact sports (rugby, soccer, wrestling) rule out the use of braces, but they have proven value in skiing, tennis and squash. The problems inherent in bracing include:

1. Unacceptable weight
2. Awkward design or bulk
3. Too restrictive of flexion or rapid movement
4. Friction over points of contact
5. Loss of position

The efficacy of the brace is significantly reduced by migration of the orthosis, and this remains a significant problem. Custom-made braces are mandatory if migration is to be minimized, particularly in very strenuous activities.

The newer generation of braces, such as the carbon-titanium (CTi) and Don Joy, do not appear to limit function of the normal knee in tests such as sprinting, cutting and vertical jumping (Figure 2), in contrast to earlier reported concern about the inhibiting effect of some braces.[17] Approximately one-half of anterior cruciate-deficient knees are improved by bracing, judged by the protection against episodes of giving-way, swelling and pain. Braces are more effective when there is a combined ligament tear, although excessive rotation is still difficult to prevent.

The use of braces in juvenile sport, and as a prophylactic measure for the normal knee, are controversial topics outside the scope of this contribution. However, it is inconceivable that bracing can ever be looked upon as an entirely innocent or effective protection against injury, and some decrease in performance must be accepted as a rational consequence of this approach. There is also legitimate concern about brace-induced injuries to the opposition.

Conclusion

A successful result from conservative management depends greatly upon the enthusiasm with which physiotherapy and bracing are espoused. Until the longer-term results of anterior cruciate reconstruction are clearly established, it seems appropriate to offer an alternative to surgery, at least initially. If the knee does not compensate sufficiently to contend with sport at the level desired, reconstruction may then be advised. The conservative approach will not have been in vain since the motivation and aspirations of the patient are then known more fully, and the postoperative rehabilitation will be entered into with less trepidation.

References

1. **McDaniel WJ Jr, Dameron TB Jr**, Untreated ruptures of the anterior cruciate ligament: a follow-up study, *J Bone Joint Surg (Am)* (1980) **62**:696–705.
2. **Markolf KL, Kochan A, Amstutz HC**, Measurement of knee stiffness and laxity in patients with documented absence of the anterior cruciate ligament, *J Bone Joint Surg (Am)* (1984) **66**:242–253.
3. **Giove TP, Miller SJ III, Kent BE** et al., Non-operative treatment of the torn anterior cruciate ligament, *J Bone Joint Surg (Am)* (1983) **65**:184–192.
4. **Noyes FR, Matthews DS, Mooar PA** et al., The symptomatic anterior cruciate-deficient knee: Part II. The results of rehabilitation, activity modification and counselling on functional disability, *J Bone Joint Surg (Am)* (1983) **65**:163–174.
5. **Sandberg R, Balkfors B, Nilsson B** et al., Operative versus non-operative treatment of recent injuries to the ligaments of the knee, *J Bone Joint Surg (Am)* (1987) **69**:1120–1126.
6. **Macnicol MF**, The torn anterior cruciate ligament, *J R Coll Surg* (1989) **34**(suppl):4–11.
7. **Perry J, Fox JM, Boitano MA** et al., Functional evaluation of the pes anserinus transfer by electromyography and gait analysis, *J Bone Joint Surg (Am)* (1980) **62**:973–980.
8. **Berchuck M, Andriacchi TP, Bach BR** et al., Gait adaptations by patients who have a deficient anterior cruciate ligament, *J Bone Joint Surg (Am)* (1990) **72**:871–877.
9. **Gerber C, Matter P**, Biomechanical analysis of the knee after rupture of the anterior cruciate ligament and its primary repair: an instant-centre analysis of function, *J Bone Joint Surg (Br)* (1983) **65**:391–399.
10. **Frankel VH, Burstein AH, Brooks DB**, Biomechanics of internal derangement of the knee: pathomechanics as determined by analysis of the instant centres of motion, *J Bone Joint Surg (Am)* (1971) **53**:945–962.
11. **Cabaud HE, Rodkey WG, Feagin JA**, Experimental studies of acute anterior cruciate ligament injury and repair, *Am J Sports Med* (1979) **7**:18–22.
12. **Feagin JA Jr, Curl WW**, Isolated tear of the anterior cruciate ligament: 5 year follow-up study, *Am J Sports Med* (1976) **4**:95–100.
13. **Tegner Y, Lysholm J**, Rating systems in the evaluation of knee ligament injuries, *Clin Orthop* (1985) **198**:43–49.
14. **Lysholm J, Gillquist J**, Evaluation of knee ligament surgery results with special emphasis on use of a scoring scale, *Am J Sports Med* (1982) **10**:150–154.
15. **Macnicol MF, Penny ID, Sheppard L**, The early results of Leeds–Keio anterior cruciate ligament replacement, *J Bone Joint Surg (Br)* (1991) **73**:377–380.
16. **Stark J**, Two cases of rupture of the crucial ligaments of the knee joint, *Edin Med Surg* (1850) **74**:267–271.
17. **Houston ME, Goemans PH**, Leg muscle performance of athletes with and without knee support braces, *Arch Phys Med Rehabil* (1982) **63**:431–432.

6.5   Knee braces

W. Dilworth Cannon, Jr and Joyce M. Vittori

In 1984, The Sports Medicine Committee of the American Academy of Orthopaedic Surgeons (AAOS) classified knee braces into three categories: prophylactic, rehabilitative, and functional.[1] Prophylactic braces are worn to prevent knee injuries or to reduce the severity of injury. Athletes who participate in contact sports are the principal users of these braces. Rehabilitative braces are used to provide protected motion control. Patients who have had ligamentous reconstruction or repair, and those injured but treated nonsurgically are candidates for this type of brace. Functional braces are often prescribed to patients with anterior cruciate ligament (ACL) deficient knees, or to patients who have had previous ACL reconstruction or repair. These braces are designed to prevent giving-way episodes in an ACL deficient knee and to help keep a reconstructed or repaired ACL from rupturing.

Whether designated to be prophylactic, rehabilitative, or functional, there are characteristics that all braces should have in common. Braces should be cost-effective, durable, and comfortable. They should adapt to different leg shapes and sizes and remain in position once applied to the leg. An effective brace will control leg motion without jeopardizing or increasing stress to the unbraced portions of the leg. Ideally, a patient should be able to purchase the brace off-the-shelf. Of these criteria, the adequate control of leg motion is the most difficult to achieve. Ideally, a brace should consider the three rotations and three translations that occur in the knee joint. These are called the six degrees of freedom and consist of flexion and extension, varus and valgus, and internal and external rotations; distraction and compression, medial and lateral, and anterior and posterior translations.

Prophylactic braces

The AAOS[1] defines prophylactic braces as those 'designed to prevent or reduce the severity of knee injuries caused by contact or non-contact forces.' A wide range of claims have been made by various brace manufacturers. Most promise that their device will decrease injuries to the medial collateral ligament (MCL), the ACL, and to the menisci. The idea behind these assertions is that prophylactic braces will disperse and distribute the load of impact away from the knee joint. This eliminates valgus stress as the brace works to increase knee stiffness. Other manufacturers go as far as to profess lateral collateral ligament (LCL) and posterior cruciate ligament (PCL) protection too, by claiming to provide lateral, rotational, anterior and posterior stability.

Some studies have supported the wearing of prophylactic braces by athletes.[2-5] Critics of these studies[6,7] frequently charge bias because follow-up was insufficient and failed to account for alterations in equipment, playing surfaces, rule changes, and modification in coaching techniques. These factors might account for a reduction or increase in the incidence of injury. Also, the number of injuries would naturally fluctuate from year to year with or without the use of prophylactic braces. Therefore, a study would have to be conducted for more than one year to validate any claims of injury reduction.

Other studies[8-10] have shown that prophylactic braces may contribute to an increase in knee injuries. Grace et al.[9] conducted a 2-year study of 579 highschool football players. Single-hinged prophylactic knee braces were worn by 246 players, 83 players wore a double-hinged brace, and 250 athletes were not braced. All groups suffered knee injuries of varying kinds. Still, the single-hinged brace group had a statistically significant higher incidence of injury than the unbraced group. This clearly suggests an adverse effect from wearing this kind of brace. Although not statistically significant, the double-hinged braced group also had more injuries than the unbraced group—evidence that the brace did not prevent injuries. Another finding was an increase in occurrence and severity of foot and ankle problems among the players who wore braces. Grace has speculated that the prophylactic knee brace may cause shifts in stress to the adjacent joints.

It has been suggested[6] that prophylactic braces cause pre-loading to exist in the MCL of athletes who do not have normal valgus alignment. If the brace does not match the athlete's limb alignment exactly, it may pre-load the joint, making it more susceptible to injury. A ligament can only absorb a certain amount of force before it will rupture. Therefore, a pre-loaded ligament will be able to sustain less of a blow than one that is not pre-loaded. After further study, France et al.[11] no longer support this theory. They now believe that the medial side of the knee is pre-loaded naturally in direct proportion to the Q angle of an individual during weight-bearing. The greater the Q angle, the greater the transverse force. Accordingly, an athlete with neutral or varus deformities would not have this pre-loading and may be less likely to sustain an injury of the MCL.

The controversy over the use of prophylactic braces peaked in 1987 when Drez announced the AAOS position that 'So far studies have shown no decrease in the rate of injury for players wearing prophylactic knee braces. Until there are studies to prove otherwise, we cannot say the braces prevent injuries. We cannot recommend their use, especially in preventing the most common type of football injury—tears of the anterior cruciate ligament.'[12]

The debate on prophylactic knee braces will no doubt continue to rage. Nevertheless, to date there has not been sufficient evidence to warrant the expense of outfitting an entire team with two braces for each player. To require a team member to wear a brace that has not proven effective may cause the player harm, and can lead to legal problems for the prescribing physician.

Rehabilitative braces

Joint motion prevents stiffness and damage to the articular cartilage of a rehabilitating knee. The role of the rehabilitative brace is to control the knee joint by allowing protected movement and preventing adverse motion that can be detrimental to healing tissues.

In a cadaver study, Hofmann et al.[13] tested six commercially available rehabilitative braces to determine whether knee stability was enhanced with brace application. ACL and MCL stability was augmented by brace application when compared with the same knee unbraced. Nevertheless, none of the braces tested could reproduce the stability provided by intact ligaments. It should be noted that braces can be fitted tightly to the cadaver limbs as comfort is not a consideration. Tightly constricting a rehabilitating knee may be painful to the patient.

Crawley et al.[14] tested eight rehabilitative braces using a mechanical surrogate of the knee. They found that brace performance was enhanced if 'the straps and bar-shell units interfaced to act as a single unit.' A brace should be stiff and the areas of the bar-shells should be large enough to distribute the load evenly. Distributing the load will help reduce pressure points

and improve control of tibial translation. The study's authors emphasize that rehabilitative braces are probably only effective while the patient is non-weight-bearing or partial weight bearing. These braces are limited in their ability to control the increased translations and rotations of a knee that comprise full weight bearing.

Functional braces

The theory of functional knee bracing is simple: to stabilize the knee and prevent giving-way episodes. In practice, it is an extremely complex goal to achieve. A functional brace should provide stability during activities of daily living and varying athletic activities. It should stabilize the knee of the weekend competitor and the professional athlete. Stabilization should be assured despite the amount of anterior displacement, the presence of defects in other supportive structures of the knee, and the extent of muscular function.[1]

Wojtys et al.[15] tested 14 functional knee braces on six cadaver knees with intact ACLs and MCLs. The braces were tested at 30° and 60° of flexion for displacements of anterior–posterior translation and internal–external rotation. Testing was done in three stages: with the ligaments intact, the ACL cut and the MCL intact; and with both ACL and MCL cut. Force application magnitude was 125 newtons and 12 newtons for the anterior–posterior and internal-external torques, respectively.

The findings showed that the braces were more effective at 60° than at 30° flexion. All of the braces decreased internal–external rotational forces to normal levels in the ACL deficient and MCL intact knees. Unfortunately, even at 60° flexion none of the braces was able to normalize anterior–posterior translation displacements.

In their 1986 study, Beck et al.[16] tested seven brands of functional knee braces on three patients with gross anterior displacement. Instrumented measurements of anterior displacement were conducted using the Medmetric KT-1000 and the Stryker Knee Laxity Tester (KLT). Knees were measured on the KT-1000 and the KLT for anterior and total displacements with a 89-newton (20-lb) force. Maximum anterior drawer and active anterior drawer testing were done with the KT-1000 and 178-newton (40 lb) anterior displacement testing was performed with the KLT. The investigators concluded that 'as forces increase, the effectiveness of the functional knee braces in controlling anterior tibial displacement decreases.' The forces that a knee would experience during intensive physical activity would be greater than those applied for the purposes of this study. The authors were also able to demonstrate anterolateral tibial subluxation in the braced patients when performing Losee testing. This study agrees with others[17-20] that conclude that functional knee bracing may not prevent giving-way episodes even in low-stress situations.

Discussion

Brace application is more an act of faith than of biomechanical engineering. A brace applied around the knee's substantial soft-tissue envelope is an attempt to prevent the bones from abnormal movement that could result in ligamentous injury. This effort may be futile, as even a knee rigidly cast in plaster will have play within the joint,[21] illustrating the difficulty in designing a brace that will allow normal knee movement while curtailing aberrant motion. Whether the brace is prophylactic, rehabilitative, or functional, technology has not sufficiently advanced to the point where a brace can control both rotational instabilities and anterior–posterior translation of the tibia. Given sufficient force, most ligaments will rupture before the brace restraints could come into play.[11,22]

Brace designs might be improved by taking the asymmetry of the knee into consideration. Dye has found that there is a 10-mm medial femoral condylar roll-back during flexion as opposed to a 24-mm lateral femoral condylar roll-back.[23] The hinge mechanisms of a brace should account for this asymmetry.

At present, braces may be providing no better than a 50% reduction in abnormal anterior tibial translations. Some investigators believe[15,20] that many braces serve only as proprioceptive devices that increase tactile sensory input to the brain from the affected knee. They feel that an ace bandage may prove just as effective and more cost-effective than many currently available braces. Nevertheless, in the patient with an acute ACL tear, functional knee bracing is still considered to be an important part of conservative management.

References

1. **American Academy of Orthopaedic Surgeons**, Knee braces, Seminar report, Chairman David Drez (Chicago, 1984).
2. **Anderson G, Zeman SC, Rosenfeld RT**, The Anderson knee stabler, *Phys Sports Med* (1979) 7:125–127.
3. **Hansen BL, Ward JC, Diehl RC**, The preventive use of the Anderson knee stabler in football, *Phys Sports Med* (1985) 13:75–81.
4. **Sitler M, Ryan J, Hopkinson W** et al., The efficacy of a prophylactic knee brace to reduce knee injuries in football. A prospective, randomized study at West Point, *Am J Sports Med* (1990) 18:310–315.
5. **Van Hoeck JE, Brown TD, Brand RA**, A surrogate knee model for dynamic loading studies of prophylactic braces, *Biomechanics in sports: a 1987 update*, ed Redkow ED, Thacker JG, Erdman AG (New York: American Society of Mechanical Engineers, 1987)
6. **Paulos LE, France EP, Rosenberg TD** et al., The biomechanics of lateral knee bracing. Part I: response of the valgus restraints to loading, *Am J Sports Med* (1987) 15:419–429.
7. **Hewson GF, Mendini RA, Wang JB**, Prophylactic knee bracing in college football, *Am J Sports Med* (1986) 14:262–266.
8. **Teitz CC, Hermanson BK, Kronmal RA** et al., Evaluation of the use of braces to prevent injury to the knee in collegiate football players, *J Bone Joint Surg (Am)* (1987) 69:2–9.
9. **Grace TG, Skipper BJ, Newberry JC** et al., Prophylactic knee braces and injury to the lower extremity, *J Bone Joint Surg (Am)* (1988) 70:422–427.
10. **Rovere GD, Haupt HA, Yates CS**, Prophylactic knee bracing in college football, *Am J Sports Med* (1987) 15:111–116.
11. **France EP, Paulos LE, Jajaramon G** et al., The biomechanics of lateral knee bracing. Part II: Impact response of the braced knee, *Am J Sports Med* (1987) 15:430–438.
12. **American Academy of Orthopaedic Surgeons**, A position statement: the use of knee braces (American Academy of Orthopaedic Surgeons, October 1987).
13. **Hofmann AA, Wyatt RWB, Bourne MH** et al., Knee stability in orthotic knee braces, *Am J Sports Med* (1984) 12:371–374.
14. **Crawley PW, France EP, Paulos LE**, Comparison of rehabilitative knee braces, *Am J Sports Med* (1989) 17:141–146.
15. **Wojtys EM, Laubert PV, Samson SY** et al., Use of a knee brace for control of tibial translation and rotation. A comparison, in cadavera, of available models, *J Bone Joint Surg* (1990) 72:1323–1329.
16. **Beck C, Drez D, Young J** et al., Instrumented testing of functional knee braces, *Am J Sports Med* (1986) 14:253–255.
17. **Wojtys EM, Goldstein SA, Redfern M** et al., A biomechanical evaluation of the Lenox Hill knee brace, *Clin Orthop* (1987) 220:179–184.
18. **Mortensen WW, Foreman K, Focht L** et al., An in-vitro study of functional orthoses in the ACL disrupted knee, *Orthop Trans* (1988) 13:520.
19. **Branch T, Hunter R, Reynolds P**, Controlling anterior tibial displacement under static load: a comparison of two braces, *Orthopedics* (1988) 11:1249–1252.
20. **Cook FF, Tibone JE, Redfern FC**, A dynamic analysis of a functional brace for anterior cruciate ligament insufficiency, *Am J Sports Med* (1989) 17:519–524.
21. **Krackow KA, Vetter WL**, Knee motion in a long leg cast, *Am J Sports Med* (1981) 9:233–239.
22. **Pope MH, Johnson RJ, Brown DW**, The role of the musculature in injuries to the medial collateral ligament, *J Bone Joint Surg (Am)* (1979) 61:398–402.
23. **Dye SF, Cannon WD**, Anatomy and biomechanics of the anterior cruciate ligament, *Clin Sports Med* (1988) 7:715–725.

6.6   A combined intra- and extra-articular reconstruction using carbon–Dacron composite prosthesis for chronic anterior cruciate instability: A 2–6-year follow-up study

Dipak V. Patel, Paul M. Aichroth, Cledwyn B. Jones and Jon S. Wand

Rupture of the anterior cruciate ligament (ACL) has been called the 'beginning of the end for the knee'.[1] Significant numbers of patients with chronic ACL deficiency complain of recurrent giving-way, pain and swelling; these symptoms limit sporting activities and eventually interfere with the activities of daily living.

The purpose of this retrospective study was to report a long-term follow-up of a carbon–Dacron composite prosthetic reconstruction and to determine the efficacy of a combined intra- and extra-articular reconstruction.

Materials and methods

Between 1982 and 1986, 53 consecutive operations were performed for chronic ACL deficiency at Westminster Hospital. All procedures were either performed or supervised by the senior author (P.M.A.). Three patients were lost to follow-up, thus leaving 50 available for the review. All patients were examined by one author (D.V.P.), who was not previously known to any of the patients.

There were 41 males and 9 females. The right knee was involved in 27 cases and the left in 23. Their mean age at the time of operation was 28.5 years (range 18 to 50 years). The average duration between the initial injury and the reconstruction was 5.3 years (range 1–16 years). The mean postoperative follow-up was 3.8 years (range 2–6 years).

Mode and mechanism of injury

Soccer and rugby accounted for 60% of the injuries (Figure 1). All 50 patients participated in some previous sport preoperatively but only 33 were involved in contact games. The diagnosis of ACL rupture at the initial presentation was rarely made in this series, agreeing with the findings of Noyes et al.[2] and

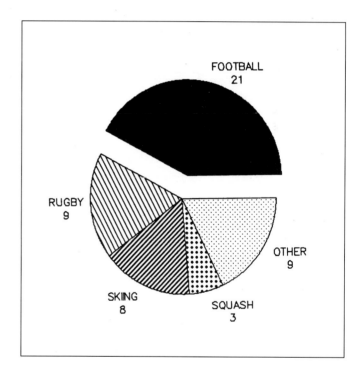

Figure 1

Mode of injury.

Paterson and Trickey.[3] One or more significant re-injuries occurred in 24% of the patients within 2 years of their initial injury.

Indications for surgery and previous surgery

The principal indication was progressive, symptomatic instability in an active, well-motivated young

Table 1 Previous or concurrent surgical intervention.

Procedures	Previous	Concurrent
Arthroscopic partial medial meniscectomy	12	0
Arthroscopic partial lateral meniscectomy	6	0
Open medial meniscectomy	6	0
Open lateral meniscectomy	3	0
Arthroscopic trimming of medial meniscus	0	7
Arthroscopic trimming of lateral meniscus	0	5
MacIntosh procedure	8	42
Medial collateral ligament repair	2	0
Pes anserinus transfer	2	0
Carbon-fibre reconstruction	2	0

individual who failed to improve with physiotherapy, bracing or arthroscopic correction of the meniscal lesion. In addition, those patients who were totally unwilling to modify their sporting lifestyle were also considered.

Twenty-eight patients had undergone previous operations on their knees (Table 1).

Preoperative assessment

All patients had pain, recurrent swelling, giving-way and limitation of knee function (including the activities of daily living or sports). Every patient was subjected to an examination under anaesthetic and arthroscopy prior to the reconstruction.

The Lachman test,[4] the anterior drawer test and the pivot shift sign[5] were graded on a scale of 0 to 3 (zero being regarded as normal). The results of the pre-reconstruction assessment are shown in Figure 2. Eight patients had mild medial collateral ligament laxity and two had an associated posterior cruciate ligament deficiency.

Postoperative assessment

Functional and clinical assessment

The Lysholm scoring system[6] was used to assess the patients' symptoms (Table 2). The clinical assessment was graded as shown in Table 3. A combined score,

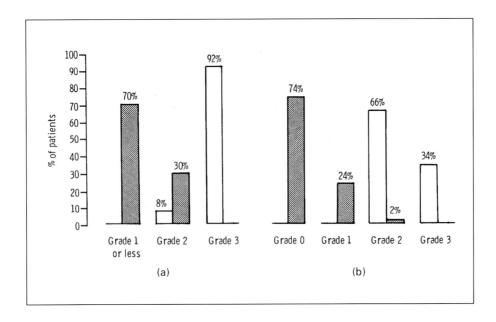

Figure 2

A histogram showing the pre-operative (open) and postoperative (shaded) results of (a) the Lachman and (b) the pivot shift test.

Table 2 The Lysholm Scoring System.[6]

	Points
Limp	
None	5
Slight or periodical	3
Severe and constant	0
Support	
None	5
Stick or crutch needed	3
Weight bearing impossible	0
Stair climbing	
No problem	10
Slightly impaired	6
One step at a time	2
Unable	0
Squatting	
No problem	5
Slightly impaired	4
Not beyond 90° of flexion	2
Unable	0
Walking, running and jumping	
A. *Instability*	
Never giving-way	30
Rarely during athletic or other severe exertion	25
Frequently during athletic or other severe exertion	20
Occasionally in daily activities	10
Often in daily activities	5
With every step	0
B. *Pain*	
None	30
Inconstant and slight during severe exertion	25
Marked on giving-way	20
Marked during severe exertion	15
Marked on or after walking more than 2 km	10
Marked on or after walking less than 2 km	5
Constant and severe	0
C. *Swelling*	
None	10
With giving-way	7
On severe exertion	5
On ordinary exertion	2
Constant	0
Atrophy of thigh	
None	5
1–2 cm	3
>2 cm	0

Table 3 The scoring system for clinical examination at review (maximum points = 50).

	Points allocated
Lachman test	
Grade 0	15
Grade 1	10
Grade 2	5
Grade 3	0
Pivot shift test	
Grade 0	30
Grade 1	20
Grade 2	10
Grade 3	0
Range of movement	
Within 5° of other knee	5
5–10° less than other knee	3
>10° less than other knee	0

with a maximum of 100 points, was calculated for each patient. This was derived from the sum of the Lysholm score (100 points) and the clinical score (50 points) multiplied by 2/3.

Arthroscopic and histopathological assessment

Twenty-two unselected patients underwent 'second-look' arthroscopy at an average of 10.4 months after the reconstruction. The aim was to evaluate the stability of the 'neoligament', and the status of the synovium, menisci and the articular surfaces. An arthroscopic biopsy of the 'neoligament' was undertaken.

Cruciometer assessment

Quantitative evaluation of the Lachman test was made using the Westminster Cruciometer. This device measures the anterior subluxation of the tibia on the femur when an 89-newton force is applied 10 cm distal to the joint-line, countered by an equal force to the patella (Figures 3 and 4).

The carbon–Dacron composite prosthesis

The composite prosthesis consists of a sleeve of specially textured and treated polyester which provides an open network of fibres for tissue in-growth, whilst affording considerable protection for the carbon-fibre core. The carbon fibre is a parallel assembly of 40 000 pure high-strength filaments (Appendix). The prosthesis is provided with a flexible plastic probe and a polyester tape leader loop to aid implantation.

Operative technique

The patient was placed in a supine position with the affected knee flexed to about 90°, over the end of the operating table, with a sandbag placed under the thigh. A high tourniquet was applied following

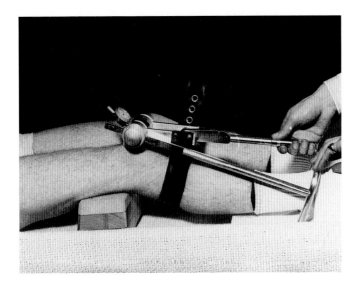

Figure 3

The Westminster Cruciometer has been applied to the leg.

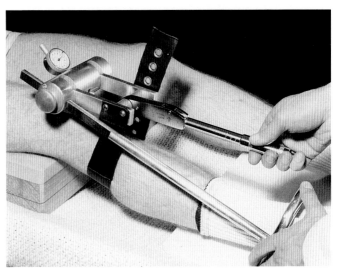

Figure 4

An 89-newton force is applied to the tibia, 10 cm distal to the joint-line. The forward subluxation of the tibia on the femur is recorded on the vernier gauge.

exsanguination. A skin incision was centred over the lateral aspect of the thigh, commencing proximally from a point 10 cm above the supracondylar region, extending distally along the femoral shaft, through the midcondylar point, and terminating at Gerdy's tubercle (Figure 5).

A strip of iliotibial tract (2 cm wide and 18–20 cm long) was raised and detached proximally, remaining attached to Gerdy's tubercle distally (Figure 6). A MacIntosh extra-articular tenodesis was performed with the iliotibial tract passed beneath the fibular collateral ligament, after isolating the latter by extrasynovial dissection. With the knee in flexion and the tibia in 30° of external rotation, the iliotibial tract was kept taut and four Vicryl sutures positioned, but not tied at this stage of the operation (Figure 7).

A drillhole was made in the femoral supracondylar mid-point, emerging posteriorly just above the capsule (Figure 8). The prosthesis was passed through this bony tunnel and a toggle was inserted in the loop. The iliotibial tract was tubulated over a 'T'-shaped cannula using a fine absorbable suture with a continuous, interlocking stitch (Figure 9). The leading loop of the prosthesis was then drawn through the tubulated iliotibial tract and an encircling transfixion suture was taken over the end of the tube and the prosthesis.

Using blunt dissection, the space immediately posterior to the lateral head of the gastrocnemius was exposed. A curved director with a nylon tape was passed through the posterior capsule, into the intercondylar region of the knee joint. A routine medial parapatellar arthrotomy incision was made. The iliotibial tract tube, filled with the prosthesis, was passed 'over the top' of the lateral femoral condyle, through the intercondylar notch, into the knee joint cavity.

Using a tibial drill guide, a tunnel was made through the anteromedial tibia, with consideration of the anatomical insertion of the ACL over the tibial plateau (Figure 10). The proximal end of the tibial tunnel was made smooth using a high-speed burr and a curette. The iliotibial tract tubed prosthesis was then passed through the tibial tunnel and a cortical bone block (2 cm × 1 cm) was raised from the medial aspect of the proximal tibia, just inferior to the exit hole of the tibial tunnel.

The prosthesis was then pulled tight with the tibia in external rotation and drawn posteriorly. The isometricity of the prosthesis was assessed by flexing and extending the knee. At this stage, the four stay-sutures anchoring the iliotibial tract to the fibular collateral ligament were tied. The tubed prosthesis was put into the depression where the bone block was raised, and the bone block was stapled in position with the prosthesis under maximal tension (Figure 11). Suction drainage was employed and the wounds were closed in layers. The operative period was covered with a broad-spectrum antibiotic.

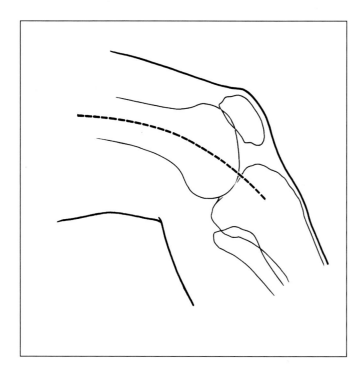

Figure 5

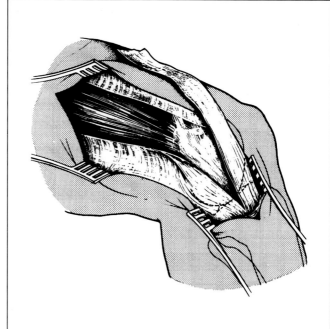

Figure 6

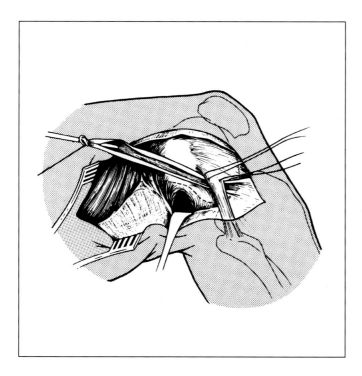

Figure 7

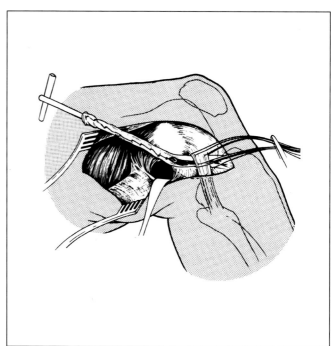

Figure 8

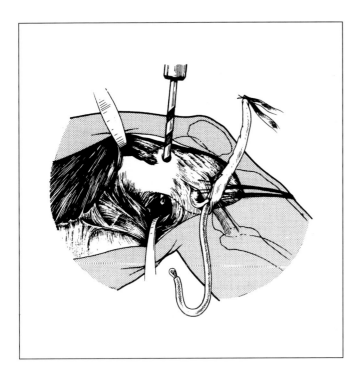

Figure 9

Figure 10

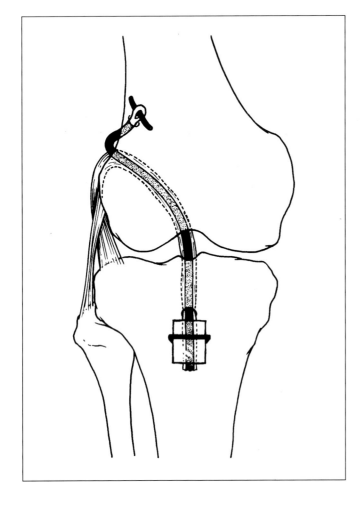

Figure 11

Postoperative management

A well-padded above-knee cast was applied with the knee in 30–40° of flexion and the tibia in external rotation. The patient was mobilized with crutches when comfortable and the plaster cast was maintained for 6 weeks. After plaster removal, the patient was subjected to a well-supervised intensive physiotherapy programme. Between 3 and 6 months, fast walking, jogging and swimming were encouraged. At 6 months, the patient was allowed to participate in mild recreational sporting activities; at 9 months, athletic training began and at 12 months all contact sports were permitted.

Recently, our postoperative management protocol has changed. Now we immediately mobilize the knee from day 1 using a continuous passive mobilization machine. A brace is applied at 5–7 days postoperatively, with the range of movement blocked between 20 and 80°. The brace is discarded after 6 weeks and then a supervised quadriceps rehabilitation is commenced. The patient remains non-weight-bearing while braced. After 6 weeks, full weight bearing is allowed. The rest of the protocol remains the same as mentioned in the previous paragraph.

Results

Functional assessment

Knee pain. At the time of latest review, 27 patients had no pain, 15 complained of an occasional, mild knee pain during severe exertion and 8 had marked pain on giving-way or during severe exertion. None of them had knee pain at rest.

Swelling. Fifteen patients complained of a minor effusion on severe exertion and 2 had a persistent effusion.

Instability. Twenty-seven patients stated that their knee did not give way after surgery. Sixteen patients had occasional giving-way during athletic or other severe exertion and 6 had frequent episodes of giving-way with similar activities. Only one patient complained of an occasional giving-way during daily activities.

Limp. Forty-four patients had no limp and 6 had a slight limp.

Stair climbing. One patient had difficulty in climbing stairs.

Squatting. Eight patients had slight impairment in squatting.

Clinical assessment

The results of the Lachman test, anterior drawer test and the pivot shift test are shown in Figure 2.

Stability. The Lachman test was grade 1 or less than grade 1 in 35 patients and grade 2 in 15 patients. The anterior drawer test was grade 0 in 24 patients, grade 1 in 22 patients and grade 2 in 4 patients. The pivot shift sign was eliminated in 37 patients. Twelve patients had grade 1 pivot shift (glide but no jerk) and one had grade 2 pivot shift with a jerk.

Range of movement. Forty-two patients had a full range of movement (0–140°), 5 had a 10° restriction of terminal flexion and 2 had an extension lag of 10°. One patient had a flexion contracture of 10°.

Thigh atrophy. Quadriceps wasting was less than 1 cm in 5 cases. Forty-three patients had 1–2 cm of wasting and 2 had more than 2 cm of wasting, measured at a point 10 cm above the superior border of the patella.

Cruciometer assessment

The mean cruciometer reading for patients who had been assessed as having a grade 1 or less than grade 1 Lachman test was 4.56 mm (range 3.6–5.6 mm). Patients with grade 2 Lachman test had a mean excursion of 6.62 mm (range 5.8–7.6 mm). There was a highly significant correlation between the Lachman test and the cruciometer reading ($P<0.001$, $r = 0.76$).

Overall score

A score of more than 90 was regarded as excellent, 78–90 as good, 66–77 as fair, and less than 66 was considered a poor result.

The results were excellent in 16 patients, good in 21, fair in 11 and poor in 2. There was a statistically significant correlation between the Lysholm score and the clinical score ($P<0.001$, $r = 0.60$). Patients with a combined intra- and extra-articular reconstruction fared significantly better (Student's *t*-test, $P<0.001$) than those who had had an intra-articular reconstruction alone.

Return to sports

At the time of latest follow-up, 30 patients (60%) were involved in recreational sports and 11 (22%) were actively participating in contact games. The remaining 9 patients had changed their lifestyle and were restricted to the ordinary activities of daily living, and 4 of these were unwilling to expose their symptom-free knees to the risk of further injury. Overall, 32 patients (64%) returned to their previous sporting activities and 13 of them (26%) achieved their pre-injury level of performance.

Complications

There were no deep infections in this series but there was one superficial infection which fully resolved with antibiotics.

The details are shown in Table 4. The prosthesis was completely disrupted in one patient and partially ruptured in two (vide infra).

None of the patients underwent revision of the reconstruction. Two patients had subsequent arthroscopic partial meniscectomy and one had an arthroscopic irrigation and debridement of the knee following partial disruption of the prosthetic ligament.

Table 4 Number of complications in 17 patients.

Rupture of the prosthesis	
Partial	2
Complete	1
Superficial wound infection	1
Persistent effusion	3
Flexion contracture	1
Limitation of terminal flexion	5
Extension lag	2
Tenderness around staple	2
Muscle hernia	3
Total	20

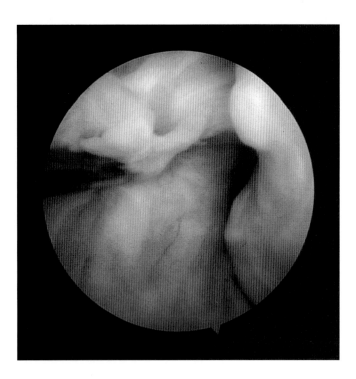

Figure 12

Arthroscopic appearance of the 'neoligament', 6 months after the ACL reconstruction.

Overall patient satisfaction

Twenty-five patients (50%) were delighted with the functional result of their knee reconstruction, 20 (40%) were satisfied and 5 (10%) expressed reservations about the outcome of the procedure.

Arthroscopic and histopathological assessment

Arthroscopic findings in 22 knees at an average of 10.4 months following reconstruction revealed that the prosthesis was stable and well covered by a thick fibrous sheath (Figure 12) in 19 cases. The prosthesis was partially ruptured in two patients (2 and 3 years post-reconstruction) and had completely disrupted in one patient (3 years post-reconstruction). These three patients had undergone reconstruction purely with an intra-articular prosthesis without an additional MacIntosh tenodesis. There were signs of superficial vascularity in all the intact 'neoligaments'.

Arthroscopic biopsy from the fibrous envelope over the iliotibial tract tubed composite prosthesis showed a low-grade synovitis with a mild foreign body giant-cell response. The histological appearance of the 'neoligament' from a patient with a partial rupture of the prosthesis is shown in Figure 13. One section taken from a patient with a complete rupture of the prosthesis showed features of a mixed foreign-fibre granuloma, moderate carbon-fibre deposits along with refractile fragments of Dacron in the subsynovial layer exciting a mild foreign body giant cell and fibrous response (Figure 14).

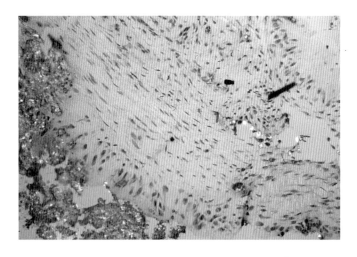

Figure 13

Histology of the 'neoligament' from a patient with an incomplete rupture of the composite prosthesis. It shows granulomatous response to carbon fibre in the synovial membrane, with superficial encrustation of tiny crystals of calcium pyrophosphate as an incidental finding. Haematoxylin and eosin staining, × 63.

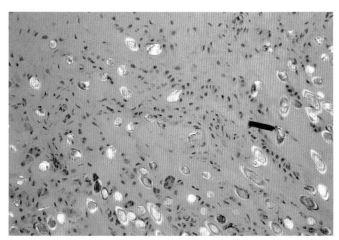

Figure 14

Histology of the 'neoligament' from a patient with a complete rupture of the prosthesis, showing foreign body giant-cell reaction to anisotropic fibres of Dacron and occasional carbon fibres. Haematoxylin and eosin, half-polarized light × 63.

Table 5 Associated pathology: the number of meniscal and articular cartilage lesions at arthroscopy before, during and after reconstruction.

Site of lesion	Before operation	At operation	After operation[a]
Meniscus			
Medial	12	7	1
Lateral	6	5	1
Both	2	1	0
Articular cartilage			
Medial femoral condyle	2	3	1
Lateral femoral condyle	1	2	0
Patella	0	2	1

[a]Only 22 of the 50 patients had a post-reconstruction arthroscopy.

Associated pathology

The incidence of meniscal and articular cartilage lesions found at arthroscopy prior to reconstruction, at the time of operation and after reconstruction is shown in Table 5. The true incidence of meniscal and articular cartilage lesions could not be determined as only 22 patients underwent 'second-look' arthroscopy.

Discussion

There is considerable debate concerning the natural history of ACL rupture and the need for surgical reconstruction.[7-9] Many surgeons feel that with intensive rehabilitation the majority of patients can return to a high level of sporting activities. However, with marked rotatory instability and a pivot shift jerk, it is unlikely that sports requiring control in twisting and cutting will be returned to.

We agree with Noyes et al.[2] that functional deterioration occurs with time. If a patient with marked ACL deficiency continues with a very active sports career, then there is progressive damage to the menisci and the articular surfaces which results in slow onset of osteoarthritis. Hence, knee stabilization is desirable and we have offered this to young, athletically active individuals who wish to return to strenuous sports or to those in whom activities of daily living are altered by their knee instability.

Numerous procedures have been described for the reconstruction of the torn ACL. Various intra-articular techniques substitute portions of the extensor mechanism,[3,10,11] the iliotibial tract,[12,13] the semitendinosus tendon, the gracilis tendon or both. Similarly, numerous lateral extra-articular stabilization procedures have been proposed as a possible solution.[5,14-16]

The MacIntosh extra-articular tenodesis has shown good short-term stability[17] and also recent papers have shown encouraging long-term results.[14,15] However, Ellison[18] reported 55% excellent initial results using a distal iliotibial band transfer, falling off to 44% at 2 years. Kennedy et al.[19] and Andrews[20] both reported a substantial number of their patients with a continued pivot shift jerk following an extra-articular reconstruction for high-performance athletes.

The long-term success of autogenous grafts still remains highly unpredictable. Reconstructive procedures utilizing autogenous tissues often require a prolonged rehabilitation and may have a 30–40% failure rate at 5 years.[21,22] Utilization of autologous ligamentum patellae may weaken the donor site and may lead to functional disability, especially in athletes.[23] Nevertheless, this procedure is popular and the patellar problems may be overstated.

Kennedy et al.[19] showed that in some instances the patellar tendon graft may elongate or fail under low forces or remain in the joint as flimsy, collagenous tissue providing no ligamentous restraint. Johnson et al.[24] reviewed 87 patients treated by a modified Jones procedure at an average follow-up of 7.9 years and found that 67.9% had loss of knee extension which was frequently the cause of an unsatisfactory result.

Filamentous carbon has been studied extensively as a scaffolding material following the pioneer work of Jenkins.[25] Before 1983, carbon-fibre prostheses were used for the reconstruction of chronic ACL instability at Westminster Hospital. However, Aichroth et al.[26] reported that 76.5% of the implants that were passed through a drillhole in the lateral femoral condyle were found to be broken at arthroscopy at a mean of 7 months following surgery, whereas, none of the carbon–Dacron composite prostheses that were routed 'over the top' of the lateral femoral condyle and supplemented with a MacIntosh tenodesis were found to be broken after a mean follow-up of 24 months.

Carbon fibre is brittle and breaks under twisting or angular forces and there are specific stresses at the prosthesis–bone interface. Rushton et al.[27] in a series of 39 patients, questioned the view that carbon fibre was replaced by fibrous tissue to produce a 'neoligament' when used as an intra-articular ligament replacement. They found that carbon fibre had not induced the formation of a 'neoligament' and the prosthesis was merely covered by a thin fibrous sheath. In contrast, the carbon–Dacron composite prosthesis used in the present series showed the formation of a thick fibrous tissue ('neoligament') around the Dacron in 19 of the 22 arthroscopic examinations.

Following animal experimentation, Thomas et al.[28] and Amis et al.[29] demonstrated that Dacron is biocompatible, mechanically strong and exhibits good penetration with fibrous connective tissue. The rationale for covering the central core of carbon fibre with two protective layers (Dacron and the iliotibial tract) was to provide the knee with secure protection from carbon-fibre staining. We have seen severe problems develop when intra-articular carbon fibre alone has been employed, notably carbon-fibre staining of the synovium, articular cartilage and the menisci, which can result in chronic synovitis and effusion.

In our series, it was found that the presence of an iliotibial tract tubulated Dacron coating eliminated the fragmentation and spread of carbon-fibre debris within the joint, provided that the 'neoligament' remained intact. However, it remains uncertain whether this containment of carbon-fibre particles can be attributed specifically to either the Dacron or to the presence of the tube of iliotibial tract.

The additional MacIntosh's extra-articular reinforcement was carried out in 42 of the 50 patients. The other 8 patients had previous, unsuccessful MacIntosh procedures and hence the iliotibial tract could not be utilized. At the time of latest review, the pivot shift test was eliminated in 37 of the 42 patients who had simultaneous MacIntosh procedure and the intra-articular prosthetic replacement.

The poor results in patients who had an intra-articular reconstruction alone may be related to the absence of the additional MacIntosh tenodesis. It is not clear whether the intra-articular prosthetic reconstruction or the MacIntosh procedure was responsible for the excellent or good results.

We preferred the 'over the top' route as it located the prosthesis close to the anatomical origin of the ACL[26,30,31] and allowed the prosthesis to pass over a round, smooth surface. The operative technique described is simple to perform and has produced consistent results. MacDaniel and Dameron[8] noted poor correlation between the knee symptoms and the physical signs. However, in the present series there was a significant correlation between the Lysholm knee score and the clinical stability ($P<0.001$).

Reports in the literature that emphasize return to the sport as an important criterion should be questioned unless they specify the preinjury sport, the postinjury sport and the intensity of sports participation.[32] In our series, 26% of the patients returned to their preinjury level of sporting activities, which compares with Zarins and Rowe,[31] who reported that 35% of the patients were able to return to their preinjury athletic activities, following a combined autogenous intra- and extra-articular reconstruction at an average follow-up of 57 months.

The results of ACL reconstruction with carbon fibre have been discouraging. The failure to induce a 'neoligament'[27] together with the brittle nature of the material[29] has led to early mechanical failure, resulting in chronic synovitis and effusion. In spite of obtaining satisfactory results with a carbon–Dacron composite prosthesis, in the light of the above findings, our practice has since changed and similar consistent results are now being obtained with a prosthesis consisting of Dacron alone.

Summary and conclusions

Fifty patients with chronic symptomatic anterior cruciate insufficiency underwent ligamentous reconstruction using the carbon–Dacron composite prosthesis, which consists of a central core of carbon fibre with an external weave of polyester. In 42 patients, the prosthesis was used as an augmentation within a tube of iliotibial tract, combined with a MacIntosh's extra-articular reconstruction. The prosthetic replacement alone was used in eight patients where there had been a previous extra-articular reconstruction and was associated with only fair results.

The average age of the patients at operation was 28.5 years (range 18–50 years); instability of the knee had been present for a mean of 5.3 years and the average follow-up was 3.8 years (range 2–6 years). The assessment included subjective functional rating (Lysholm knee score) and clinical examination for instability. Thirty-seven patients (74%) had a good or excellent result, 11 (22%) had a fair result and 2 (4%) had a poor result. The Lachman test was grade 1 or less in 35 patients and the pivot shift sign was eliminated in 37 patients. Clinical signs of instability correlated well with the Lysholm knee score ($P<0.001$)

Twenty-two unselected patients (44%) underwent an arthroscopic assessment and biopsy of the 'neoligament' at an average of 10.4 months postoperatively. The prosthesis was found to be stable and well covered by a thick fibrous sheath ('neoligament') in 19 patients. The prosthesis was partially ruptured in two patients and completely disrupted in one. All three ruptures of the prosthetic ligament occurred in patients who did not undergo a simultaneous MacIntosh extra-articular reconstruction.

Thirty-two patients (64%) returned to their previous sports and 13 of them (26%) achieved their pre-injury level of performance. Overall, 45 patients (90%) were pleased or satisfied with the results of their knee reconstruction.

The operative technique described in this review has provided 74% good or excellent results at an average follow-up of 3.8 years. Patients with a combined intra- and extra-articular reconstruction had a significantly better result (P<0.001) than those who had had an intra-articular prosthetic replacement alone. We feel that a combined intra- and extra-articular reconstruction seems to be the current trend in the management of chronic ACL insufficiency. Whether this should be undertaken using the autogenous tissues or with prosthetic ligament augmentation is a matter of personal preference.

Acknowledgments

Our thanks are due to Dina Stanford and the Medical Photography Department at Westminster Hospital for their help with the illustrations.

Appendix: Bio-mechanical data on the carbon–Dacron composite prosthesis

The mechanical strength of the prosthesis relies on the central core of the carbon fibre, and not on the outer covering of the open weave of Dacron. Accordingly, only the carbon fibre component of the prosthesis was tested mechanically.

Number of filaments per tow	40 000
Filament diameter	6.8×10^{-6} m
Tensile strength[a]	0.168 N/decitex
Tow strength[a]	4480 N

[a] Both these tests were conducted at a relative humidity of 60%, at 16°C.

References

1. DeHaven KE, Arthroscopy in the diagnosis and management of the anterior cruciate ligament deficient knee, Clin Orthop (1983) 172:52–56.
2. Noyes FR, Mooar PA, Matthews DS et al., The symptomatic anterior cruciate-deficient knee: Part 1. The long-term functional disability in athletically active individuals, J Bone Joint Surg (Am) (1983) 65:154–162.
3. Paterson FWN, Trickey EL, Anterior cruciate ligament reconstruction using part of the patellar tendon as a free graft, J Bone Joint Surg (Br) (1986) 68:453–457.
4. Torg JS, Conrad W, Kalen V, Clinical diagnosis of anterior cruciate ligament instability in the athlete, Am J Sports Med (1976) 4:84–93.
5. Galway RD, Beaupré A, MacIntosh DL, Pivot shift: a clinical sign of symptomatic anterior cruciate ligament insufficiency, J Bone Joint Surg (Br) (1972) 54:763–764.
6. Lysholm J, Gillquist J, Evaluation of knee ligament surgery results with special emphasis on use of a scoring scale, Am J Sports Med (1982) 10:150–154.
7. Fetto JF, Marshall JL, The natural history and diagnosis of anterior cruciate ligament insufficiency, Clin Orthop (1980) 147:29–38.
8. MacDaniel WJ Jr, Dameron TB Jr, Untreated ruptures of the anterior cruciate ligament: a follow-up study, J Bone Joint Surg (Am) (1980) 62:696–705.
9. Satku K, Kumar VP, Ngoi SS, Anterior cruciate ligament injuries: to counsel or to operate? J Bone Joint Surg (Br) (1986) 68:458–461.
10. Campbell WC, Repair of ligaments of the knee: report of new operation for repair of anterior cruciate ligament, Surg Gynaecol Obstet (1936) 62:964–968.
11. Jones KG, Reconstruction of the anterior cruciate ligament: a technique using the central one-third of the patellar ligament, J Bone Joint Surg (Am) (1963) 45:925–932.
12. Hey Groves EW, The crucial ligaments of the knee joint: their function, rupture and operative treatment of the same, Br J Surg (1920) 7:505–515.
13. Insall JN, Joseph DM, Aglietti P et al., Bone-block iliotibial band transfer for anterior cruciate insufficiency, J Bone Joint Surg (Am) (1981) 63:560–569.
14. Amirault JD, Cameron JC, MacIntosh DL et al., Chronic anterior cruciate ligament deficiency: long-term results of MacIntosh's lateral substitution reconstruction, J Bone Joint Surg (Br) (1988) 70:622–624.
15. Frank C, Jackson RW, Lateral substitution for chronic isolated anterior cruciate ligament deficiency, J Bone Joint Surg (Br) (1988) 70:407–411.
16. Ireland J, Trickey EL, MacIntosh tenodesis for anterolateral instability of the knee, J Bone Joint Surg (Br) (1980) 62:340–345.
17. Bertoia JT, Urovitz EP, Richards RR et al., Anterior cruciate reconstruction using the MacIntosh lateral-substitution over-the-top repair, J Bone Joint Surg (Am) (1985) 67:1183–1188.
18. Ellison AE, Distal iliotibial band transfer for anterolateral rotary instability of the knee, J Bone Joint Surg (Am) (1979) 61:330–337.
19. Kennedy JC, Roth JH, Mendenhall HV et al., Intra-articular replacement in the anterior cruciate ligament deficient knee, Am J Sports Med (1980) 8:1–8.
20. Andrews JR, Sanders R, Morin B, Surgical treatment of anterolateral rotary instability, Am J Sports Med (1985) 13:112–119.
21. Friedman MJ, Sherman OH, Fox JM et al., Autogenic anterior cruciate ligament (ACL) reconstruction of the knee: a review, Clin Orthop (1985) 196:9–14.
22. Odensten M, Lysholm J, Gillquist J, Long-term follow-up study of a distal iliotibial band transfer (DIT) for anterolateral knee instability, Clin Orthop (1983) 176:129–135.
23. Bonamo JJ, Krinick RM, Sporn AA, Rupture of the patellar ligament after use of its central third for anterior cruciate reconstruction: a report of two cases, J Bone Joint Surg (Am) (1984) 66:1294–1297.
24. Johnson RJ, Eriksson E, Haggmark T et al., Five- to ten-year follow-up evaluation after reconstruction of the anterior cruciate ligament, Clin Orthop (1984) 183:122–140.
25. Jenkins DHR, The repair of cruciate ligaments with flexible carbon fibre: a longer term study of the induction of new ligaments and of the fate of the implanted carbon, J Bone Joint Surg (Br) (1978) 60:520–522.

26. **Aichroth PM, Jones CB, Thomas NP**, Carbon fibre and Dacron composites in the prosthetic reconstruction of the anterior cruciate ligament, *J Bone Joint Surg (Br)* (1986) **68**:841.

27. **Rushton N, Dandy DJ, Naylor CPE**, The clinical, arthroscopic and histological findings after replacement of the anterior cruciate ligament with carbon fibre, *J Bone Joint Surg (Br)* (1983) **65**:308–309.

28. **Thomas NP, Turner IG, Jones CB**, Prosthetic anterior cruciate ligaments in the rabbit: a comparison of four types of replacement, *J Bone Joint Surg (Br)* (1987) **69**:312–316.

29. **Amis AA, Kempson SA, Campbell JR** et al., Anterior cruciate ligament replacement: biocompatibility and biomechanics of polyester and carbon fibre in rabbits, *J Bone Joint Surg (Br)* (1988) **70**:628–634.

30. **MacIntosh DL**, The anterior cruciate ligament: 'over-the-top' repair, *J Bone Joint Surg (Br)* (1974) **56**:591.

31. **Zarins B, Rowe CR**, Combined anterior cruciate ligament reconstruction using semitendinosus tendon and iliotibial tract, *J Bone Joint Surg (Am)* (1986) **68**:160–177.

32. **Noyes FR, McGinniss GH, Grood ES**, The variable functional disability of the anterior cruciate ligament-deficient knee, *Orthop Clin North Am* (1985) **16**:47–67.

6.7   Combined intra- and extra-articular reconstruction with Dacron augmentation: operative technique

Paul M. Aichroth

The extra-articular reconstruction of MacIntosh controls anterolateral instability but stretches in time. It is incorporated in this reconstruction and the long strip of iliotibial tract is tubulated and taken over the top of the lateral femoral condyle. The tube then passes through the knee and into a tibial tunnel accurately re-routing this structure. Augmentation of the iliotibial tract with prosthetic material—polyester—is one method of producing a consistent stabilization of the knee over a prolonged period.

The incision

The lateral incision passes superiorly from a point 10 cm above the supracondylar region, laterally along the line of the femoral shaft, through the mid condylar point and finishes inferiorly at Gerdy's tubercle—the prominence on the upper, lateral tibial plateau where the iliotibial tract is inserted. (See Figure 1.)

A strip of iliotibial tract is raised and detached using appropriate skin retraction superiorly. The ribbon of iliotibial tract should be 2–2.5 cm broad and is left inferiorly attached to Gerdy's tubercle. (See Figure 2.)

MacIntosh extra-articular tenodesis

The iliotibial tract passes beneath the lateral collateral ligament. The lateral collateral ligament is isolated anteriorly and posteriorly by extrasynovial dissection and the iliotibial tract is pulled beneath.

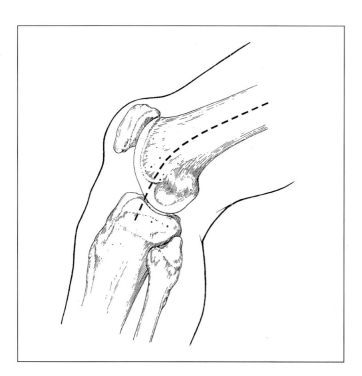

Figure 1

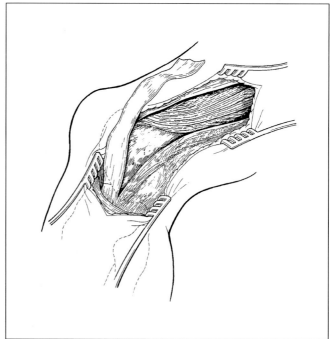

Figure 2

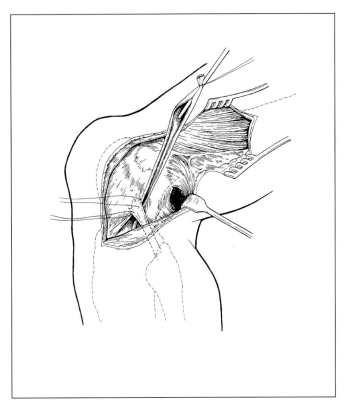

Figure 3

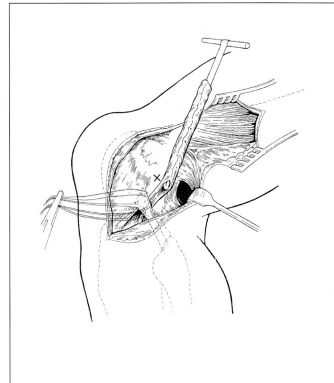

Figure 4

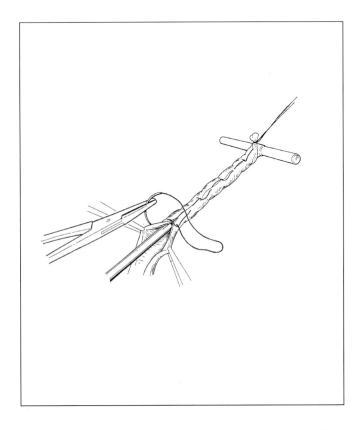

Figure 5

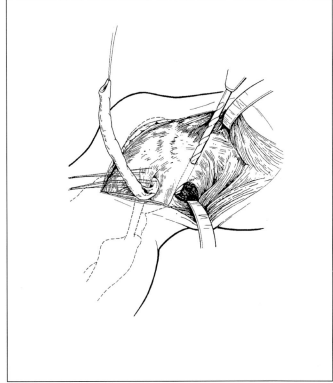

Figure 6

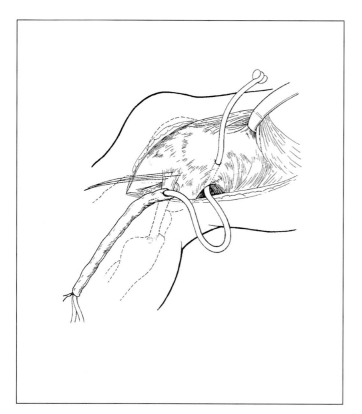

Figure 7

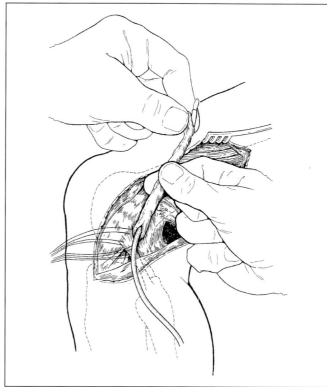

Figure 8

With the knee in flexion and full lateral rotation, the iliotibial tract is tightened and four sutures are positioned to attach it securely to the lateral collateral ligament. It is best to position the sutures at this moment but not to tie them until the later stage. (See Figure 3.)

Tubulation of the iliotibial tract

The iliotibial tract is tubulated from its free end to the point X. This is best undertaken by bringing the two sides of the iliotibial tract over a T-shaped cannula or some other stent. A fine but strong absorbable suture is recommended and a running interlocking stitch has been found preferable. (See Figures 4 and 5.)

A drill hole is made in the supracondylar mid-point emerging just above the capsule at the origin of the lateral gastrocnemius muscle. (See Figure 6.)

The Dacron augmentation is now passed through this bony tunnel and is anchored superiorly with some type of toggle inserted into a loop or alternatively with a staple. (See Figure 7.)

The free end of the Dacron augmentation is now drawn through the iliotibial tract preferably on a 'tendon leader'. The end of the Dacron is now attached to the free end of the iliotibial tract by an encircling stitch so that the tube and prosthesis may be pulled together over the top of the lateral femoral condyle. (See Figure 8.)

Over-the-top route

Attention must now be turned to the dissection of the posterior capsule extending into the intercondylar region. The fibres of the lateral gastrocnemius are identified and dissection continues medially beneath this muscle, exposing the posterior capsule. Using sharp and blunt dissection, the intercondylar region is reached with instruments, keeping close to the posterior capsule. A director is now passed through the intercondylar region and into the knee joint. (See Figure 9.)

The medial dissection

A routine parapatellar arthrotomy is made and extended inferiorly to the medial and inferior aspect of the tibial tubercle.

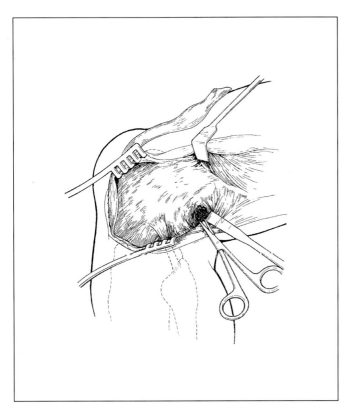

Figure 9

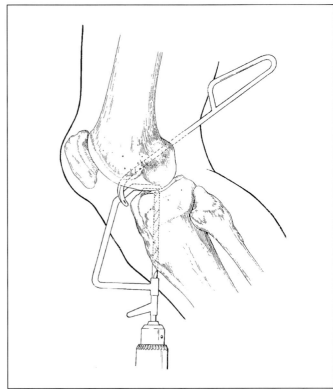

Figure 10

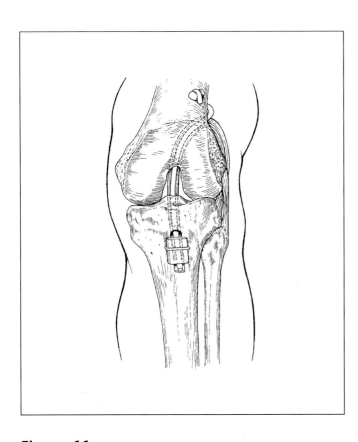

Figure 11

The iliotibial tract tube filled with the prosthesis is now ready to be passed over the top of the lateral femoral condyle, through the intercondylar region and into the knee joint cavity.

Using a tibial drill guide, a hole is made through the anteromedial tibia. Superiorly it emerges at the normal tibial attachment of the anterior cruciate ligament—between and slightly behind the prominence of the anterior tibial spine. The upper end of the tibial hole is champhered, the iliotibial tract tube and Dacron prosthesis is now pulled through the intercondylar region and secondarily pulled through the tibial tunnel to the outside. (See Figure 10.)

Inferior anchorage of the combined 'neoligament'

A bone block of cortical bone 1 x 2 cm in size is raised from the upper medial tibia just below the exit hole of the tibial tunnel.

The combined 'neoligament' is pulled tight with the tibia rotated laterally on the femur and the knee in flexion. The composite is put into the depression where the bone block was raised and the bone block is returned and stapled in position, with the 'neoligament' under tension. The four stay sutures anchoring the iliotibial tract to the lateral collateral ligament are tightened and tied. (See Figure 11.)

The wounds are closed with drainage. The limb is placed on the constant passive motion machine, with a range of movement from 0 to 40° initially. This progressively increases over the next few days to 90° of flexion. A brace is applied maintaining zero to 90° range of motion and the patient remains non-weight-bearing for 6 weeks.

Further rehabilitation

At 6 weeks the brace is removed and walking commences. From 6 to 12 weeks a specific physiotherapy and rehabilitation programme is undertaken with progressive knee movement and strengthening. Increased walking will lead to cycling, swimming and other smooth activities. At 3 months jogging may commence. At the sixth month gentle recreational sports such as tennis re-start. At 9 months all training resumes and competitive sports are undertaken at 1 year.

6.8 A combined intra- and extra-articular reconstruction using polyester augmentation for chronic anterior cruciate instability of the knee

Dipak V. Patel, Paul M. Aichroth and Stuart C. Evans

It is now generally accepted that patients with an anterior cruciate ligament (ACL) deficient knee are at high risk of developing progressive, symptomatic rotatory instability, meniscal tears and early degenerative osteoarthritis.[1-6] This is particularly true for professional or competitive amateur athletes who wish to return to sports at a highly competitive level.[2,7-11]

Numerous extra-articular techniques of ACL reconstruction have been described in the literature and an excellent account of these procedures has been provided by Dr James Arnold in this chapter (contribution 6.9). The MacIntosh extra-articular tenodesis has shown good short-term stability[1,12] and also recent papers have shown encouraging long-term results.[13,14] In contrast, Bray et al.[15] reported that the extra-articular procedures only reinforce the secondary stabilizers of the knee and do not produce long-term functional stability.

Various intra-articular reconstructive procedures using the autografts, allografts or synthetic prostheses have been reported in the management of chronic anterior cruciate deficient knee. An intra-articular reconstruction alone restores the primary ACL deficiency. However, the secondary restraints are usually very lax in chronic situations and, therefore, it was felt that an additional extra-articular reinforcement would be beneficial for long-term stability.

Patients with chronic ACL laxity are frequently ignored or given token conservative treatment in Great Britain for the waiting lists are long and the number of orthopaedic surgeons skilled and interested in the reconstruction is small. In this series, the ACL reconstruction was undertaken for patients with gross symptoms and signs of instability.

Long-term follow-up results of a combined intra- and extra-articular reconstruction using Dacron as an augmentation have not previously been reported. The purpose of this prospective study was to assess the clinical and radiological results of our operative technique and to determine the efficacy of a combined intra- and extra-articular reconstruction using Dacron as an augmentation.

Table 1 Mode of injury.

Mode of injury	Number of patients
Skiing	33
Football and rugby	45
Basketball	1
Netball	2
Volleyball	1
Tennis	3
Squash	2
Cricket	3
Badminton	1
Hockey	1
Water-skiing	1
High jump	1
Gymnasium exercises	1
Table-tennis	1
Road traffic accident	4
Domestic fall	5

Table 2 Previous or concurrent surgical procedures in 48 patients.

Procedures	Previous	Concurrent
Arthroscopic partial medial meniscectomy	21	7
Arthroscopic partial lateral meniscectomy	23	5
Open medial meniscectomy	4	0
Open lateral meniscectomy	1	0
Arthroscopic repair for peripheral detachment of medial meniscus	0	3
Arthroscopic repair for peripheral detachment of lateral meniscus	0	7
Excision of large stub of ACL	7	0
MacIntosh procedure	2	103
Ellison's iliotibial band transfer	1	0
Pes anserinus transfer	2	0
Carbon-fibre reconstruction	2	0
Medial collateral ligament repair	2	0
Excision of osteochondral fragment and curettage of crater in lateral femoral condyle	1	0

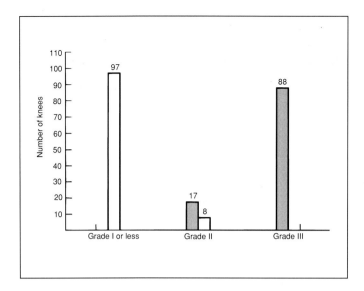

Figure 1

The preoperative (shaded) and postoperative (open) details of the Lachman test.

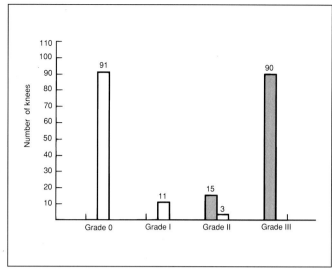

Figure 2

The preoperative (shaded) and postoperative (open) details of the pivot shift sign.

Materials and methods

Between 1985 and 1989, 108 consecutive patients underwent a combined intra- and extra-articular reconstruction using Dacron as an augmentation for chronic ACL deficiency. All procedures were either performed or supervised by the senior author (P.M.A.). Three patients were lost to follow-up, leaving 105 available for detailed clinical, functional and radiological assessment. An independent assessment was carried out by one of the authors (D.V.P.).

There were 72 males and 33 females. Their average age at the time of operation was 27.8 years (range 18–47 years) and the average postoperative follow-up was 57.8 months (range 24–84 months). The average duration between the initial injury and the reconstruction was 47.6 months (range 7–148 months). The right knee was involved in 52 cases and the left in 53.

Mode and mechanism of injury

The mode of injury was football and rugby in 43% of the knees and skiing in 31% (details are given in Table 1). Preoperatively, the majority of the patients participated in either recreational or competitive sports; 47 being involved in contact games such as football and rugby. One or more significant re-injuries occurred in 46% of the patients within 2 years of their initial injury.

Indications for surgery

All patients had an adequate trial of conservative treatment for at least 6–9 months prior to surgery. The indication for surgery was progressive, symptomatic rotatory instability in an active, well-motivated young individual who failed to improve with non-operative measures. In addition, those patients who were reluctant to wear a knee brace or those who were totally unwilling to modify their sporting lifestyle were also considered.

Previous surgery

Forty-eight patients had had previous or concurrent operations on their knees (Table 2).

Preoperative assessment

All patients had pain, recurrent swelling, giving-way and limitation of function (including the activities of daily living or sports). Every patient was subjected to an examination under anaesthetic and arthroscopy prior to the reconstruction. The Lachman test,[16] the anterior drawer test and the pivot shift sign[17] were graded on a scale of 0 to III (0 being regarded as normal) as compared to the opposite uninjured knee. The details of the Lachman test and the pivot shift sign are shown in Figures 1 and 2, respectively. Eighteen patients had an associated mild medial collateral ligament laxity and two had a mild posterior cruciate ligament insufficiency.

The Lysholm-II knee score (Table 3) was used to assess the patients' symptoms. This is basically a modification of the Lysholm score originally described by Lysholm and Gillquist[18] in 1982. The pre-injury and immediate preoperative Tegner activity scales were also recorded as suggested by Tegner and Lysholm.[19]

The mean preoperative Lysholm score was 48.4 points (range 20–76 points). The average pre-injury Tegner activity scale was 6.5 (range 3–10) and the average preoperative Tegner activity level was 3.2 (range 1–7).

Table 3 The Lysholm-II Score

	Points
Limp	
None	5
Slight or periodical	3
Severe and constant	0
Support	
None	5
Stick or crutch needed	2
Weight-bearing impossible	0
Locking	
None	15
Catching sensation, but no locking	10
Locking occasionally	6
Locking frequently	2
Locked joint at examination	0
Instability	
Never	25
Rarely during athletic activities	20
Frequently during athletic activities	15
Occasionally during daily activities	10
Often during daily activities	5
Every step	0
Pain	
None	25
Inconstant and slight during strenuous activities	20
Marked during or after walking >2 km	10
Marked during or after walking <2 km	5
Constant	0
Swelling	
None	10
After strenuous activities	6
After ordinary activities	3
Constant	0
Stairs	
No problem	10
Slight problem	6
One step at a time	3
Impossible	0
Squatting	
No problem	5
Slight problem	4
Not beyond 90° of flexion of the knee	2
Impossible	0

Postoperative assessment

Clinical and functional assessment

The results of the Lachman test, the anterior drawer test and the pivot shift sign were carefully recorded. In addition, the postoperative Lysholm score and the Tegner activity level were documented.

Patients with a score >90 were considered as excellent; 77 to 90 as good; 68 to 76 as fair; and <68 as poor.[20]

Instrumented measurements

Quantitative evaluation of the Lachman test was made using the KT-1000 arthrometer (MEDMetric, San Diego, Calif., USA)[21] An 89-newton force was applied with the knee at 20° ± 5° of flexion. All patients were assessed by one person (D.V.P.) experienced in the use of the KT-1000 arthrometer, thereby eliminating the interobserver error. The measurements were compared with those of the opposite, uninjured side, and side-to-side difference values were calculated.

Statistical analysis

The chi-squared test and Student's *t*-test were used for analysis of the data.

Radiological assessment

Standard anteroposterior, lateral, tunnel and skyline views were obtained in order to record the degenerative changes in the knee.

Arthroscopic and histopathological assessment

Twelve patients had a 'second-look' arthroscopy at an average of 17.6 months (range 6–38 months) after the primary reconstruction. The aim was to evaluate the stability of the 'neoligament' and to ascertain the status of the synovium, the menisci and the articular surfaces.

Factors affecting outcome

Severity of preoperative symptoms
The effect of the severity of preoperative instability was studied by comparing the final outcome in patients who had a preoperative Lysholm score below 60 with that in those who had a score of 60 or above.

There were 85 knees with a preoperative Lysholm score of less than 60 and 20 knees with a score of 60 or above.

Age of the patient
There were 34 patients below the age of 25 years at the time of reconstruction and 71 were aged 25 years or more. The results in these two groups were compared.

Time interval between the injury and operation
Twenty-five patients underwent reconstruction within 24 months of injury and 80 after a delay of 24 months or more. The results in these two groups were compared.

Plaster cast immobilization
The results in the first 62 knees treated by cast immobilization were compared with the remaining 43 knees treated by early mobilization using the continuous passive mobilization (CPM) machine.

The ABC polyester ligament (Surgicraft Ltd, UK)

The pure polyester ligament is manufactured from two mechanically dissimilar fibres of polyester. The ABC unit material is formed from parallel bundles of polyester fibres which are constrained by a partial braid of the second polyester. During the braiding process, the core fibres are disposed into a flat zig-zag configuration. The amount of zig-zag may be varied by adjusting the tension of the core and braid fibres. The zig-zag configuration of the unit material displays a unique biphasic response to loading which protects the implant from plastic deformation. The prosthesis is provided with a flexible plastic probe and a polyester tape leader loop to aid implantation. The ultimate tensile strength is approximately 2950 ± 150 N, a value which is limited by fracture of the filament loops at the point of fixation.

Operative technique

The operative technique of a combined intra- and extra-articular reconstruction using Dacron as an augmentation has been described in detail by Paul M. Aichroth in contribution 6.7.

Postoperative management

In the earlier part of our series, 62 knees were immobilized in an above-knee plaster cast with the knee in 30–40° of flexion and the foot in external rotation. The patient was mobilized with crutches when comfortable and the plaster cast was maintained for 6 weeks. After plaster removal, the patient was subjected to a well-supervised intensive physiotherapy programme.

In the later part of the series, 43 knees were mobilized immediately postoperatively, using the CPM machine. The patient was mobilized non-weight-bearing on crutches when comfortable. Static quadriceps and straight leg raising excercises were encouraged. In the second post-operative week a knee brace was applied. The brace was removed at 6 weeks from the date of operation. The crutches were discarded at 6 weeks and partial weight bearing, followed by full weight bearing was allowed. All patients were subjected to a well-supervised quadriceps and hamstrings rehabilitation programme for the first 6–8 weeks.

Between 3 and 6 months, swimming and cycling were encouraged. At 6 months, the patient was allowed to participate in mild recreational sporting activities; at 9 months, athletic training began and at 12 months all contact sports and skiing were permitted. A Don–Joy knee brace was used for the first season of skiing. The majority of the patients preferred to play recreational or competitive sports without the use of a brace.

Results

Functional assessment

Knee pain
At latest review, 86 patients had no pain, 16 had occasional, mild knee pain during severe exertion, and 3 had mild pain on giving-way. None had knee pain at rest.

Swelling
Seventy-six patients had no swelling, 27 complained of a minor effusion on severe exertion, and 2 had a persistent mild effusion.

Instability
Ninety-four patients stated that their knee did not give way after surgery, 9 patients had occasional giving-way during athletic or other severe exertion, and 2 complained of occasional giving-way during daily activities.

Clinical assessment

Stability
The results of the Lachman test and the pivot shift test are shown in Figures 1 and 2. The Lachman test was grade I or less in 97 knees (92%) and grade II in 8 knees (8%). The pivot shift sign was eliminated in 91 knees (87%); 11 knees (10%) had grade I pivot

Table 4 KT-1000 instrumented testing.

Side-to-side difference[a]	Number of knees	Percentage
≤1.0 mm	52	49.5
1.1–2.0 mm	32	30.5
2.1–3.0 mm	10	9.5
>3.0 mm	11	10.5

[a]At 89 N force with the knee at 20° ± 5° of flexion.

Table 5 Details of Lysholm scores in relation to four factors that could possibly affect the result of reconstruction.

	Mean (range)		Number of patients and percentage of group[a]			
	Pre-op	At follow-up	Excellent >90	Good 77–90	Fair 68–76	Poor <68
Pre-op score						
Below 60 (n=85)	43.4 (20–59)	87.8 (62–100)	44 51.8	25 29.4	14 16.5	2 2.3
Above 60 (n=20)	68.3 (61–76)	89.7 (76–100)	9 45.0	10 50.0	1 5.0	0 —
Age						
Under 25 years (n=34)	48.8 (36–76)	88.9 (68–100)	18 52.9	11 32.4	3 8.8	2 5.9
25 years or over (n=71)	47.6 (20–76)	88.4 (62–100)	35 49.3	24 33.8	12 16.9	0 —
Interval[b]						
Under 24 months (n=25)	44.7 (20–76)	90.7 (62–100)	18 72.0	4 16.0	2 8.0	1 4.0
24 months or over (n=80)	48.6 (43–76)	87.9 (75–100)	35 43.8	31 38.7	13 16.3	1 1.2
Immobilization						
With cast (n=62)	47.2 (39–76)	88.8 (62–100)	31 50.0	21 33.9	8 12.9	2 3.2
No cast (n=43)	49.4 (20–76)	90.6 (69–100)	22 51.2	14 32.5	7 16.3	0 —

[a]Percentages are in italic type.

[b]Interval between initial injury and the operation.

shift (minimal glide but no jerk); and 3 had grade II pivot shift (mild jerk).

Range of movement
One hundred patients had a full range of movement (0–140°); 4 had a 10° restriction of terminal flexion; and one patient had a flexion contracture of 10°.

Thigh atrophy
The quadriceps wasting was measured at a point 10 cm above the superior border of the patella and compared with that of the opposite uninjured knee. The quadriceps wasting was less than 1 cm in 86 cases; 15 patients had 1–2 cm of wasting and 4 had more than 2 cm of wasting.

Radiological assessment

A positive Fairbank sign was seen in 7 knees in the medial compartment and in 9 knees in the lateral compartment. Minimal narrowing of the medial joint space was seen in 3 cases, whereas 4 knees had minimal narrowing of the lateral joint space.

Instrumented measurements

The details of the KT-1000 measurements are shown in Table 4. Ninety-four knees (89.5%) had a side-to-side difference value of 3 mm or less of anterior tibial translation, at the time of latest follow-up.

Results

Based on the Lysholm-II scoring system, 53 patients (51%) had an excellent result, 35 (33%) had a good result, 15 (14%) had a fair result, and 2 (2%) were poor.

Patient satisfaction

Ninety-three patients (88.6%) were pleased or satisfied with the functional result and 12 (11.4%) expressed reservations about the outcome of the procedure.

Return to sports

Fifty-seven patients (54.3%) were involved in recreational sports and 36 (34.3%) were participating in competitive sports (including six international football players, one international cricket player and one international skier). The remaining 12 (11.4%) patients had decreased their sporting activities (9 had changed their lifestyle and 3 were unwilling to subject the symptom-free knee to the risk of further injury).

Overall, 60 patients (57%) returned to their previous sports with pre-injury level of performance, 19 (18%) returned to previous sports with a lower level of performance, and 14 (13%) played different sports.

Factors affecting outcome

Severity of preoperative symptoms
Patients with preoperative Lysholm scores above and below 60 were grouped separately and their results were compared (details in Table 5). There was no significant difference between the postoperative Lysholm scores in the two groups at the final review ($P>0.05$).

Age of the patient
Patients aged 25 years or more at reconstruction had a mean preoperative Lysholm score of 47.6 (range 20–76) as compared to a mean preoperative Lysholm score of 48.8 (range 36–76) in patients aged 25 years or less. There was no significant difference between the Lysholm scores in these two groups at final review ($P >0.05$).

Time interval between the injury and operation
There was no statistically significant difference between the preoperative and postoperative Lysholm scores in those knees reconstructed within 24 months of injury and those reconstructed later. No difference was seen between the age at operation or the length of follow-up in those knees operated within 24 months of injury and those operated after 24 months.

Table 6 Complications.

	Number
Superficial wound infection	0
Deep wound sepsis (requiring removal of Dacron)	2
Persistent mild effusion	2
Flexion contracture	1
Limitation of terminal 10° of flexion	4
Removal of staple	2
Intra-articular adhesions	5
Anterior knee pain	3
Total	19

Plaster cast immobilization
There was no difference between the preoperative and postoperative Lysholm scores, age at operation or the interval between injury and reconstruction in knees treated with or without plaster cast immobilization after operation. Patients in the plaster cast group had a prolonged rehabilitation course as compared to the CPM group.

Complications

The complications encountered are listed in Table 6. Two patients had deep sepsis postoperatively. In both the cases, arthroscopic irrigation was performed and eventually the Dacron prosthesis was removed. No revision of ACL reconstruction has been undertaken for either of these patients and their knees were quiescent when last reviewed.

Five patients required arthroscopic debridement for intra-articular adhesions in the region of the intercondylar notch of the femur.

Manipulation under anaesthetic was undertaken in four patients at an average of 3.3 weeks postoperatively; all these patients were immobilized in a plaster cast following the ACL reconstruction. At latest follow-up, they all had a satisfactory range of movement.

One 41-year-old patient sustained a re-injury to her left knee while skiing 32 months following the primary ACL reconstruction. At 'second-look' arthroscopy, the 'neoligament' was found to be perfectly stable (Figure 3). She had a grade II medial collateral ligament injury which was treated by a knee brace.

Arthroscopic and histopathological assessment

Arthroscopic findings in 12 knees at an average of 17.6 months (range 6–38 months) following reconstruction revealed that the prosthesis was stable and well covered by a thick fibrous sheath (Figure 4) in all 12 cases, with signs of superficial vascularity.

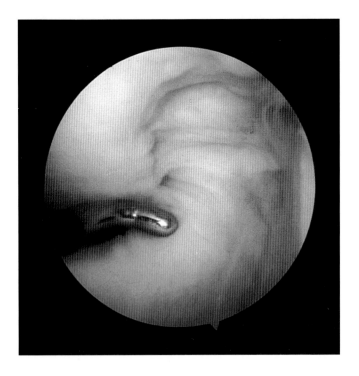

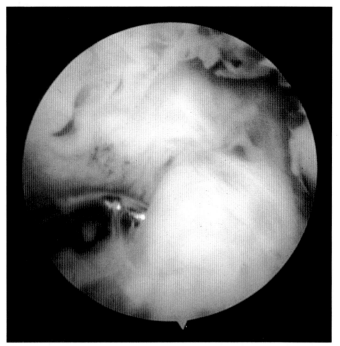

Figure 3

Arthroscopic appearance of the intact 'neoligament' 32 months following the primary ACL reconstruction. This patient had sustained a reinjury to her knee while skiing.

Figure 4

Arthroscopic view of the stable 'neoligament' 6 months following the ACL reconstruction.

Arthroscopic biopsy from the fibrous envelope surrounding the iliotibial tract tubed Dacron prosthesis showed a low-grade synovitis with a mild foreign-body giant-cell response.

Associated pathology

The incidence of meniscal and articular cartilage lesions found at arthroscopy before reconstruction, at the time of operation and after reconstruction is shown in Table 7. The true incidence of meniscal and articular cartilage lesions could not be determined as only 12 patients underwent subsequent arthroscopic assessment.

Discussion

The majority of the orthopaedic surgeons consider the ligamentum patellae as the 'gold standard' for ACL reconstruction. However, the disadvantages of ACL reconstruction using this graft include patellar fracture, avulsion of the patellar tendon, arthrofibrosis with an extension block, patella infera, disturbing patellofemoral crepitus and persistent anterior knee pain. Utilization of autogenous ligamentum patellae may weaken the donor site and may lead to functional disability, especially in athletes.[22]

Johnson et al.[23] reviewed 87 patients treated by a modified Jones procedure at an average follow-up of

Table 7 Associated pathology: the number of meniscal and articular cartilage lesions at arthroscopy before, during and after reconstruction.

Site of lesion	Before operation	At operation[a]	After operation[b]
Meniscus			
Medial	16	8	2
Lateral	15	10	3
Both	9	2	0
Articular cartilage			
Medial femoral condyle	4	2	3
Medial tibial plateau	3	0	0
Lateral femoral condyle	2	3	4
Patella	3	4	3

[a]The changes in the menisci and the articular cartilage were recorded at arthroscopy prior to the reconstruction.
[b]Only 12 of the 105 patients had a 'second-look' arthroscopy.

7.9 years and found that 67.9% had loss of knee extension which was frequently the cause of an unsatisfactory result.

In the past decade, various prosthetic ligaments have been used for the reconstruction of the chronic anterior cruciate deficient knee. The advantages of prosthetic ligament reconstruction include preservation of the biological structures and rapid postoperative rehabilitation provided that the ligament is firmly secured both proximally and distally. Some prostheses, e.g. the Kennedy-LAD (Ligament Augmentation Device) are used as an augmentation to autogenous reconstruction. The Kennedy-LAD consists of a 8-mm braid of polypropylene which acts as a support–reinforcement to the autogenous tissue.

Following animal experimentation, Thomas et al.[24] and Amis et al.[25] demonstrated that Dacron is biocompatible, mechanically strong and exhibits good penetration with fibrous connective tissue. We feel that a pure intra-articular reconstruction using the Dacron prosthesis on its own is not satisfactory. Aichroth et al.[26] reviewed 50 patients who underwent a combined intra- and extra-articular reconstruction using a carbon–Dacron composite prosthesis as an augmentation. In their series, 42 patients had an intra-articular prosthetic reconstruction, supplemented with a MacIntosh extra-articular reinforcement. However, 8 patients had a previous, failed MacIntosh procedure and hence, the iliotibial tract could not be utilized for extra-articular reconstruction. Those patients who had a combined intra- and extra-articular reconstruction fared significantly better than those who had an intra-articular reconstruction alone.

Lukianov et al.[27] reported a multicenter study of 80 patients who underwent ACL reconstruction using the Stryker Dacron ligament. The patient selection was based on a history of a failed autologous reconstruction and/or a failed primary repair of the ACL. The mean follow-up for all patients was 21 months (range 6–42 months). The graft was augmented with autologous tissue in 59 cases and used as a pure prosthesis in the remaining 21 cases. The mean Lysholm score improved from 52 points preoperatively to 82 points postoperatively, and the Tegner activity level improved from 2 to 4. The percentage of a combined excellent/good Lysholm rating increased from 6% preoperatively to 60% at follow-up. The percentage of a negative Lachman test, anterior drawer test and the pivot shift sign was approximately 75% at follow-up. There was no significant difference between the results of augmentation and non-augmentation cases, indicating that the graft acts as a permanent prosthesis rather than as a scaffold.

Recently, Bartolozzi et al.[28] reviewed 53 knees with chronic anterior cruciate instability treated with the Stryker Dacron ligament. In their series, 83% of the knees had excellent or good results on subjective evaluation (based on the degree of patient satisfaction), at an average follow-up of 29 months (range 12–53 months). However, on objective assessment using the 100-point score of the Italian Club for Knee Surgery, only 68.5% of the knees had excellent or good results.

The results of a combined intra- and extra-articular reconstruction using the autogenous tissues has been satisfactory.[2,3,9,11,29,30]

Wilson and Scranton[30] reviewed 30 patients who underwent a combined reconstruction of the ACL, with use of the semitendinosus tendon for the intra-articular portion of the reconstruction and a strip of iliotibial band for the extra-articular reinforcement. In their series, 20% of the patients had an excellent result, 73% had a good result and 7% had a fair result, at an average follow-up of 48 months (range 24–85 months). Twenty-eight of the 30 patients were able to return to full athletic activity, including seven professional football players who all returned to play in the National Football League the following season. Currently, the authors prefer reconstruction with the doubled semitendinosus tendon combined with the modified MacIntosh extra-articular augmentation.

Rackemann et al.[29] reported on 74 patients with isolated chronic anterior cruciate deficiency who were treated using the medial third of the ligamentum patellae as a free graft, supplemented by an extra-articular MacIntosh reconstruction. A satisfactory outcome was found in 93% of the cases at an average follow-up of 70 months.

In our series, 51% of the patients had an excellent result and 33% had a good result at an average follow-up of 58 months. These results are in comparison with other series in which autogenous tissues were utilized for a combined intra- and extra-articular reconstruction.[11,29,30] We noticed that the severity of preoperative symptoms, the age of the patient at operation, the interval between the injury and reconstruction and plaster cast immobilization after operation did not significantly influence the final clinical result. Similar observation has been reported by Rackemann et al.[29]

It is difficult to comment on the status of the 'neoligament' for all patients in our series, as only 12 out of 105 patients had a 'second-look' arthroscopy. We feel that in the absence of clinical symptoms and signs of instability, a routine 'second-look' arthroscopy is not practical. Magnetic resonance imaging (MRI) may be useful for assessment of the 'neoligament'. However, it would be fair to say that MRI is an expensive investigation and certainly cannot be recommended on a routine basis for this purpose.

We believe that the extra-articular reconstruction helps to protect the intra-articular graft. It is not clear whether the intra-articular iliotibial tract tubed prosthetic reconstruction or the MacIntosh procedure was responsible for the excellent or good results. We preferred the 'over-the-top' route as it located the prosthesis close to the anatomical origin of the ACL and allowed the implant to pass over a round, smooth surface.

In our series, 57% of the patients returned to their previous sports with a pre-injury level of performance; 18% returned to pre-injury sports with a reduced intensity level; and 13% played different games. At the time of review, 34.3% of the patients were participating in competitive sports; 54.3% were involved in recreational sports; and 11.4% had decreased their sporting activities.

We believe that a combined intra- and extra-articular reconstruction using Dacron as an augmentation provides excellent stability. This procedure does not interfere with the patellofemoral biomechanics. Further long-term study is required to confirm the longevity of these clinical results.

Summary and conclusions

This is a prospective study of 105 knees with chronic, severe anterior cruciate insufficiency treated by a combined intra- and extra-articular technique using the Surgicraft polyester ligament as an augmentation to the iliotibial tract reconstruction. The prosthesis was placed intra-articularly within a sleeve of iliotibial tract and a MacIntosh type of extra-articular reconstruction was performed. The average age of the patients at the time of operation was 27.8 years (range 18–47 years). The mean interval between the injury and operation was 47.6 months (range 7–148 months). The average follow-up was 57.8 months (range 24–84 months). The mode of injury was football and rugby in 43% of the knees, and skiing in 31%.

All patients were carefully counselled after failed conservative treatment. The mean preoperative Lysholm score was 48.4 (range 20–76), the average pre-injury Tegner activity level was 6.5 (range 3–10), and the average preoperative Tegner activity level was 3.2 (range 1–7).

Patients with a Lysholm score of 91–100 were regarded as excellent; 77–90 as good; 68–76 as fair, and <68 as poor. Eighty-four per cent of the knees had an excellent or good result, 14% had a fair result and 2% were poor. The mean postoperative Lysholm score was 89 (range 62–100) and the mean postoperative Tegner activity level was 6.1 (range 3–10).

Thirty-six patients returned to competitive sports, 57 participated in recreational sports, and 12 had decreased their sporting activities. Overall, 60 patients returned to their previous sports with a pre-injury level of performance, 19 returned to previous sports with a lower level of performance, and 14 played different sports.

Two patients had deep sepsis requiring removal of the Dacron prosthesis. Twelve patients had a 'second-look' arthroscopy at an average of 17.6 months (range 6–38 months) postoperatively, and the 'neoligament' was found to be well-ensheathed and stable in all 12 cases. Eighty-nine per cent of the patients were pleased or satisfied with the result of surgery.

Acknowledgments

The authors thank Dina Stanford for the computer analysis of the data and the Medical Photography Department at Westminster Hospital for their help with the illustrations.

References

1. **Bertoia JT, Urovitz EP, Richards RR** et al., Anterior cruciate reconstruction using the MacIntosh lateral-substitution over-the-top repair, *J Bone Joint Surg (Am)* (1985) **67:**1183–1188.
2. **Clancy WG Jr, Nelson DA, Reider B** et al., Anterior cruciate ligament reconstruction using one-third of the patellar ligament, augmented by extra-articular tendon transfers, *J Bone Joint Surg (Am)* (1982) **64:**352–359.
3. **Fried JA, Bergfeld JA, Weiker G** et al., Anterior cruciate reconstruction using the Jones–Ellison procedure, *J Bone Joint Surg (Am)* (1985) **67:**1029–1033.
4. **McDaniel WJ Jr, Dameron TB Jr,** The untreated anterior cruciate ligament rupture, *Clin Orthop* (1983) **172:**90–92.
5. **Noyes FR, Mooar PA, Matthews DS** et al., The symptomatic anterior cruciate-deficient knee: Part I. The long-term functional disability in athletically active individuals, *J Bone Joint Surg (Am)* (1983) **65:**154–162.
6. **Rovere GD, Adair DM,** Anterior cruciate-deficient knees: a review of the literature, *Am J Sports Med* (1983) **11:**412–419.
7. **Andrews JR, Sanders R,** A 'mini-reconstruction' technique in treating anterolateral rotatory instability (ALRI), *Clin Orthop* (1983) **172:**93–96.
8. **Lambert KL,** Vascularised patellar tendon graft with rigid internal fixation for anterior cruciate ligament insufficiency, *Clin Orthop* (1983) **172:**85–89.
9. **Lipscomb AB, Johnston RK, Snyder RB,** The technique of cruciate ligament reconstruction, *Am J Sports Med* (1981) **9:**77–81.
10. **Noyes FR, Matthews DS, Mooar PA** et al., The symptomatic anterior cruciate-deficient knee: Part II. The results of rehabilitation, activity modification, and counselling on functional disability, *J Bone Joint Surg (Am)* (1983) **65:**163–174.
11. **Zarins B, Rowe CR,** Combined anterior cruciate ligament reconstruction using semitendinosus tendon and iliotibial tract, *J Bone Joint Surg (Am)* (1986) **68:**160–177.
12. **Ireland J, Trickey EL,** MacIntosh tenodesis for anterolateral instability of the knee, *J Bone Joint Surg (Br)* (1980) **62:**340–345.
13. **Amirault JD, Cameron JC, MacIntosh DL** et al., Chronic anterior cruciate ligament deficiency: long-term results of MacIntosh's lateral substitution reconstruction, *J Bone Joint Surg (Br)* (1988) **70:**622–624.
14. **Frank C, Jackson RW,** Lateral substitution for chronic isolated anterior cruciate ligament deficiency, *J Bone Joint Surg (Br)* (1988) **70:**407–411.
15. **Bray RC, Flanagan JP, Dandy DJ,** Reconstruction for chronic anterior cruciate instability: a comparison of two methods after six years, *J Bone Joint Surg (Br)* (1988) **70:**100–105.
16. **Torg JS, Conrad W, Kalen V,** Clinical diagnosis of anterior

cruciate ligament instability in the athlete, *Am J Sports Med* (1976) **4**:84–93.

17. **Galway RD, Beaupré A, MacIntosh DL,** Pivot shift: a clinical sign of symptomatic anterior cruciate ligament insufficiency, *J Bone Joint Surg (Br)* (1972) **54**:763–764.

18. **Lysholm J, Gillquist J,** Evaluation of knee ligament surgery results with special emphasis on use of a scoring scale, *Am J Sports Med* (1982) **10**:150–154.

19. **Tegner Y, Lysholm J,** Rating systems in the evaluation of knee injuries, *Clin Orthop* (1985) **198**:43–49.

20. **Odensten M, Lysholm J, Gillquist J,** Long-term follow-up study of a distal iliotibial band transfer (DIT) for anterolateral knee instability, *Clin Orthop* (1983) **176**:129–135.

21. **Daniel DM, Malcom LL, Losse G** et al., Instrumented measurement of anterior laxity of the knee, *J Bone Joint Surg (Am)* (1985) **67**:720–726.

22. **Bonamo JJ, Krinick RM, Sporn AA,** Rupture of the patellar ligament after use of its central third for anterior cruciate reconstruction: a report of two cases, *J Bone Joint Surg (Am)* (1984) **66**:1294–1297.

23. **Johnson RJ, Eriksson E, Haggmark T** et al., Five- to ten-year follow-up evaluation after reconstruction of the anterior cruciate ligament, *Clin Orthop* (1984) **183**:122–140.

24. **Thomas NP, Turner IG, Jones CB,** Prosthetic anterior cruciate ligaments in the rabbit: a comparison of four types of replacement, *J Bone Joint Surg (Br)* (1987) **69**:312–316.

25. **Amis AA, Kempson SA, Campbell JR** et al., Anterior cruciate ligament replacement: biocompatibility and biomechanics of polyester and carbon fibre in rabbits, *J Bone Joint Surg (Br)* (1988) **70**:628–634.

26. **Aichroth PM, Patel DV, Jones CB** et al., A combined intra- and extra-articular reconstruction using a carbon–Dacron composite prosthesis for chronic anterior cruciate instability, *Int Orthop* (1991) **15**:219–227.

27. **Lukianov AV, Richmond JC, Barrett GR** et al., A multicenter study on the results of anterior cruciate ligament reconstruction using a Dacron ligament prosthesis in 'salvage' cases, *Am J Sports Med* (1989) **17**:380–386.

28. **Bartolozzi P, Salvi M, Velluti C,** Long-term follow-up of 53 cases of chronic lesion of the anterior cruciate ligament treated with an artificial Dacron stryker ligament, *Ital J Orthop Traumatol* (1990) **16**:467–480.

29. **Rackemann S, Robinson A, Dandy DJ,** Reconstruction of the anterior cruciate ligament with an intra-articular patellar tendon graft and an extra-articular tenodesis: results after six years, *J Bone Joint Surg (Br)* (1991) **73**:368–373.

30. **Wilson WJ, Scranton PE,** Combined reconstruction of the anterior cruciate ligament in competitive athletes, *J Bone Joint Surg (Am)* (1990) **72**:742–748.

Further reading

Ellison AE, Distal iliotibial band transfer for anterolateral rotary instability of the knee, *J Bone Joint Surg (Am)* (1979) **61**:330–337.

Fetto JF, Marshall JL, The natural history and diagnosis of anterior cruciate ligament insufficiency, *Clin Orthop* (1980) **147**:29–38.

Friedman MJ, Sherman OH, Fox JM et al., Autogenic anterior cruciate ligament (ACL) reconstruction of the knee: a review, *Clin Orthop* (1985) **196**:9–14.

MacIntosh DL, The anterior cruciate ligament: 'over-the-top' repair, *J Bone Joint Surg (Br)* (1974) **56**:591.

Satku K, Kumar VP, Ngoi SS, Anterior cruciate ligament injuries: to counsel or to operate? *J Bone Joint Surg (Br)* (1986) **68**:458–461.

6.9   Lateral extra-articular reconstruction for the anterior cruciate-deficient knee

James A. Arnold

Extra-articular procedures are divided into three groups: (1) Dynamic procedures rerouting distal advancement of the iliotibial band,[1] (2) proximal realignment of iliotibial band with distal attachment unaltered[2-9] and (3) combined intra-articular and extra-articular reconstructions.[10-14] The primary indication for repairs is functional instability interfering with the patient's desired activity level and failure of conservative management, including activity modification, rehabilitation, and bracing. The patient's needs, including age and activity level, degree of instability—both objectively and subjectively—and associated articular and meniscal pathology are considerations. Sedentary patients may be candidates for a lateral procedure alone. Younger patients may be improved with a lateral tenodesis, as drilling across the femoral or tibial epiphysis may or may not alter the growth plate.[15] Some utilize the reconstruction alone for less active patients with only mild limitation of activities. Actually, combined intra-articular and extra-articular procedures were felt to be advantageous to provide early stability until the intra-articular graft matures and provides a stress sharing function for the intra-articular graft.

Deciding which surgical procedure to use may be difficult.[16]

Biomechanics of lateral reconstructions

The iliotibial tract acts as a reinforcement against anterior subluxation of the lateral tibial plateau. Its fibers parallel the course of the anterior cruciate ligament (ACL) and may be thought of as an extra-articular anterior cruciate ligament that is in better position to resist rotatory movement. The ideal position of a reconstruction to control anterior and posterior excursion of the joint is in the center of the joint. However, in this position the intra-articular placement creates a level arm about the center of rotation that is too short to be truly effective in controlling rotatory movements in those patients with

laxity of lateral restraints. Because of the peripheral location of the extra-articular procedure, it may be more effective in resisting rotatory torques. Andrews and Carson described this event as analogous to turning a steering wheel at the center of the hub versus at the peripheral rim.[16] The axis associated with the pivot shift has been thought to be at the posterior cruciate ligament (PCL);[17] however, Matsumoto[18] found that the axis of the pivot shift is in fact located about the medial collateral ligament (MCL). The articular surface of the lateral tibial plateau was inclined downward and backwards. A compressive force on the lateral tibial plateau produces a force component in the anterior direction and when a valgus torque is applied the lateral tibial plateau is pushed forward. Since the medial plateau is fixed by the tight medial collateral ligament, internal rotation of the tibia results. This torque is mainly resisted by the anterior cruciate at about 30° of flexion and, therefore, the tibia rotates internally about the MCL in that degree of flexion when the ACL is absent. It was believed that rotation after injury of both cruciates was different from rotation after a solitary injury to the anterior cruciate ligament. Division of the PCL has little effect upon tibial movement because the ligament is slack when the tibia is in internal rotation about the MCL. This is because the axis of pivot shift is in fact about the MCL.

Krackow and Brooks[19] studied cadaver knees, locating paired points on the femur and tibia (Figure 1). This was a search for an optimal length in which to select attachment locations better suited for lateral procedures where the distance from the site on the tibia and femur remained constant during the areas of motion in which stability is required. The most ideal sites are a point on the tibia slightly anterior and proximal to Gerdy's tubercle and paired with a femoral attachment high and proximal to the origin of the lateral collateral ligament of the femur. This provides a checkrein with a major restraint to anterior translation from full extension to 45° of flexion. The separation distances between the two attachment points would ideally be the maximum throughout that range of motion where the cycle of

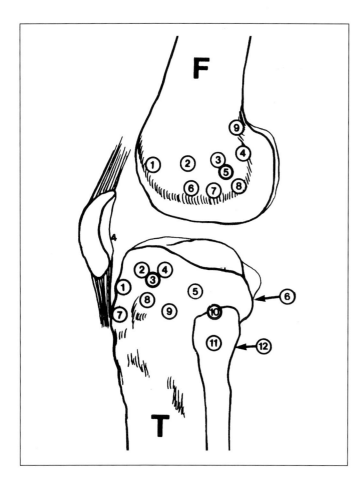

Figure 1

Krackow studied five cadaver knees to predict the behavior of separation distances with various combinations of points on the lateral side of the knee. Attachment of the reconstruction at the proximal anterior tibia near Gerdy's tubercle (point 2 and 3) paired with the more critical femoral attachment high and proximal to the origin of the lateral collateral ligament on the femur (point 9) demonstrated favorable behavior restraining anterior translation and subsequently minimal obligate stretch with full flexion or full extension. (From ref. 19).

new stability is desired. Close attention to detail allows one to approach isometry.

The ideal femoral attachment sites described by Sidles for isometric extra-articular tenodesis were posterior to the lateral epicondyle approximately midway between the epicondyle and articular margin. However, when external rotation was applied, the isometric attachment sites were somewhat more anterior and proximal. If external rotation is induced during the tenodesis, the graft inserted at the latter position may be initially isometric. The graft will become less isometric if subsequent graft stretching relaxes the induced external rotation.[20]

Most of the procedures described in this contribution have their femoral attachment site near the optimal sites described by both Krackow and Sidles.[3,5,7,12,19–21] The less important insertion near Gerdy's tubercle is also the site of tibial attachment of all the above procedures.

Noyes[22] examined the strength of biological implants and felt that an 18-mm wide strip of fascia lata had only 44% of the strength of the anterior cruciate ligament. Yet these studies did not attempt to simulate the direction of forces applied to the iliotibial band with a lateral reconstruction.

Kennedy et al. found the iliotibial tract to exceed the anterior cruciate ligament in strength under equal amount of stress.[23]

History

Lemaire[24] first described a repair to control lateral tibial subluxation utilizing an extra-articular nylon band in an envelope of fascia lata. In 1972, MacIntosh described an iliotibial band tenodesis through the lateral femoral condyle to control anterolateral instability.[8] Ellison[1] described a distal bony elevation of the iliotibial band from Gerdy's tubercle with passage under the fibular collateral ligament to its original base.

Unverferth and Bagenstose[25] (1979) combined the Ellison procedure with anteromedial procedures. Youmans[26] (1978) also used combined medial and lateral reconstructions. Losee[7] (1978) described a lateral tenodesis procedure utilizing a drillhole technique. Andrews[2] (1983) tenodesed the iliotibial band in two bundles to the lateral femoral epicondyle. Fox et al.[4] modified the Ellison procedure by rerouting of the iliotibial band. By early 1980, several other extra-articular reconstructions by themselves were advocated. The biceps tendon has been transferred or advanced to provide an additional dynamic support alone or with a lateral reconstruction.[1,10,27–30]

Repairs

MacIntosh procedure

Galway, Beaupré and MacIntosh[31] described a repair to tighten the iliotibial tract. The functional integrity and tension of the iliotibial tract and tensor fascia lata in the distal part of the knee were supposedly restored.

A long lateral incision follows the lateral line of the thigh distally past the tibial tubercle. A fascia lata strip is prepared with 15 cm × 1.5 cm remaining attached to the lateral tibial tubercle, narrowing to less than 1.0 cm proximally. A small osteoperiosteal flap is cut in the posterior corner of the lateral femoral condyle. A strip of fascia lata is passed through a tunnel beneath the proximal portion of the ligament and brought proximally and looped around a prepared area of the intermuscular septum and pulled as tight as possible with the knee flexed and tibia in full external rotation. The osteoperiosteal flap is sutured over the top of the strip and the lateral ligament is sutured to the strip. Postoperatively, the knee is held in 60° of flexion and the foot is rotated laterally to 30°. Ireland and Trickey[32] reviewed 50 patients who underwent a MacIntosh repair for anterolateral instability of the knee with a mean follow-up of 2¼ years. The repair abolished a positive anterolateral jerk test in 42 out of 50 knees and 37 patients (74%) were involved in some sort of active sport after regaining functional stability. However, 12 of the patients reported injuries after the operation and developed unstable knees.

Ellison procedure

In 1979, Ellison described an operative procedure to prevent anterior subluxation of the proximal end of the tibia with anterolateral rotatory instability of the knee.[1] The procedure was carried out in 18 consecutive patients. Ten had had previous surgery on the involved knee. All patients were unable to participate in their sports prior to reconstruction. The length of follow-up was 31–44 months. Forty-four percent had an excellent result and 39% had a good result. Only 17% of the results were unsatisfactory. The iliotibial band is released distally about 1.5 cm in diameter from Gerdy's tubercle. This is turned up and the fascial strip averaging 1.5 cm in width is shaped with scissors. The broad-based shape is intended to preserve the maximum blood supply to the fascia and the dynamic pull of the tensor fascia lata. The band is passed beneath the lateral collateral ligament. The capsular ligament is reefed beneath the fibular collateral ligament. A bone trough is prepared to receive the distal portion of the transplant. The tunnel beneath fibular collateral ligament must be proximal. The bone plug is anchored in its own bed with a staple and the sutures are placed through the lateral fibers of the patellar tendon. The cam action of the fibular collateral ligament was described as a check-rein on the iliotibial band, limiting anterior excursion of the tibia on the femur.

The tract was also felt to have a dynamic component extending proximally to the tensor fascia lata and gluteus maximus. Although 44% excellent results seems low, the combined excellent and good ratings were 83%. The success rate of 47.5% was greater for cases with combined instability rather than simple anterolateral rotatory instability for an unknown reason.[1]

Teitge and associates[33] described 48 patients who underwent an Ellison distal iliotibial band transfer.

Eighty-seven percent responded that they were improved. Ninety-one percent had a positive jerk test preoperatively but only 46% were positive at follow-up. While 53% reported no episodes of giving way, 28% reported monthly episodes, 9% weekly episodes and 8% daily episodes. Only 15% had no difficulty cutting while 55% had some difficulty and 26% had extreme difficulty or were unable to do so. Ninety-one percent had increased varus instability at follow-up but this did not appear to have clinical significance.

The iliotibial band transfer appears only to function statically. Most patients responded that their knee was 'doing good'; however, the specific functional questions revealed the more true and accurate condition, with a tremendous discrepancy, and it was noted that the group had improved by surgery but certainly not cured by their procedure. Most of these patients, however, had complex lesions with 85% having previous procedures.

Fox and associates[4] reviewed their patients with intra-articular reconstruction and those with a modification of the Ellison procedure. Various superimposed components of knee instability were managed by a variety of methods. Although extra-articular reconstruction seemed to be sufficient for lesser grades of functional disability, those knees with a grade II–III+ instability were felt to require direct anterior cruciate ligament reconstruction in addition to the extra-articular procedure. To enhance the effect of the Ellison procedure, the fascial strip was wrapped around the lateral collateral ligament prior to being re-attached anterior and distal to its previous site.

Kennedy et al.[34] studied 52 knees with the Ellison procedure alone or in combination with other reconstructive procedures. In 28 patients that he evaluated, only 57% had good or excellent results. The pivot shift phenomenon was present in all 28 knees preoperatively and eliminated in only 4 knees at follow-up. The subjective and functional improvement did not seem to correlate with the clinical and radiographic findings. Preferably it was to be used as an adjunctive procedure to other reconstruction procedures in young athletes. It was felt that if the rerouted iliotibial band beneath the fibular collateral ligament extended too far cephalad, the iliotibial band would not have the necessary angulation to make it effective. The thickest portion of the band was selected, leaving a sufficient posterior margin for closure. If the tendon removal was too far posterior, mobilization of the remaining iliotibial tract would not permit closure of the defect. Varus instability could result if the iliotibial tract was rerouted posteriorly at the joint-line and the resulting fascial defect was not closed.[33]

Studies of comparative anatomy and investigation with electrostimulation by Kaplan[35] showed that contraction of the tensor fascia lata muscle with electrical stimulation is not transmitted to the lower part of the structure and that the iliotibial tract acts

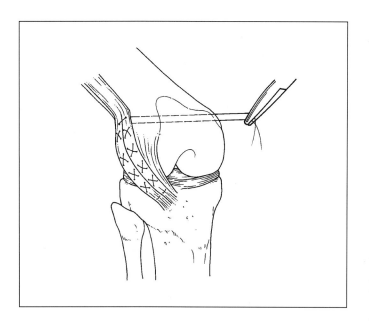

Figure 2

Andrews' mini-reconstruction technique. The iliotibial tract is longitudinally divided with a fiber-splitting incision at the anterior edge of the tract. The iliotibial tract is held against the distal femur by sutures passed through parallel holes and tied medially. A ligament is created to closely proximate the biomechanical function of the anterior cruciate. The posterior bundle is tight in extension. The upper or anterior bundle is more tight in flexion.

as an accessory anterolateral ligament of the knee and not a dynamic structure.

Kennedy's report of the Ellison procedure for control of anterolateral rotatory instability noted that the results were unpredictable and many of those that did not respond well were older or patients with a lengthy interval between the injury and operation.[23]

Andrews' mini-reconstruction (Figure 2)

Andrews[2] (1983) described a 'mini-reconstruction technique' in treating anterolateral rotatory instability (ALRI). He believed that this isolated extra-articular repair was indicated for mild and moderate chronic anterolateral rotatory instability and those patients having meniscal repairs without intra-articular stabilization. It was also used for patients with moderate instability who could not afford the time involved in protecting the biologic incorporation of an intra-articular graft.

The iliotibial tract is split in line of its fibers and the cortex of the femur at the flare of the condyle is 'fishscaled' to promote an osteoblastic response. Bundles of iliotibial band reinforced by Bunnell's stitches of No. 5 nonabsorbable suture are woven into the tract to provide a posterior bundle which is

tighter in extension and near Krackow's point No. 9. This posterior bundle is tighter in extension than the anterior bundle would be in flexion. The sutures are pulled through the femur and tied down medially over a bone bridge with the knee held at 30° of flexion in external tibial rotation. If correct placement has been achieved, the anterior bundle will be relatively tight in flexion and the posterior bundle will be relatively tight in extension.[2] If the iliotibial band tenodesis is not correct, either the drill holes are repositioned or a second attempt at suturing may be required. If it is possible to sublux the tibia or if the lateral pivot shift test is positive, the repair is too loose. Conversely, if the iliotibial tract cannot be pulled against the lateral femur or if the range of motion is not full, the repair is too tight. Once the proper placement is verified, the sutures are tied medially with the knee in approximately 45° of flexion with the tibia externally rotated. The Andrews tenodesis has been used in acute and chronic anterolateral rotatory instability. In 1977, a review of 52 cases with this procedure revealed that objective satisfactory results were obtained in 94% and subjective improvement was noted in 92%.[16]

Losee procedure (Figure 3)

Losee[7] described the 'sling and reef operation' in which a strip of the iliotibial band is used to tenodese the posterolateral corner of the knee. Patients were operated upon from 1971 to 1984, with follow-up from 1 to 6.5 years after the procedure. Good results were noted in 82%. All were satisfied with the procedure and 70% returned to their pre-surgery status. Satisfactory results were noted in all but three knees. Two of the patients rated in the poor category had significant injuries after their surgery. Fifteen of the 50 knees showed a mild degree of laxity. None of the patients had a positive MacIntosh test. In those patients with a notching in the lateral femoral condyle, the fascial repair would not prevent the tibia from subluxing in the notch. Therefore, a surgical repair was not indicated in this group. Progressive arthrosis was felt to be an indication for the procedure as well as a need to eliminate bracing.

A 2.5 cm × 16 cm iliotibial band is dissected proximally and allowed to remain intact distally to Gerdy's tubercle. A tunnel is made through the lateral femoral condyle beneath the lateral epicondyle and the fascial strip is passed through the tunnel. The correct location of the tunnel is determined by trial placement of the strip at various loci on the condyle, just anterior to the fibular collateral ligament. The entrance must be close to the margin of the joint surface and emerges in the substance of the tendon of origin of the lateral head of gastrocnemius. The strip of the iliotibial tract is threaded through the tunnel from front to back and tested, and the anterior

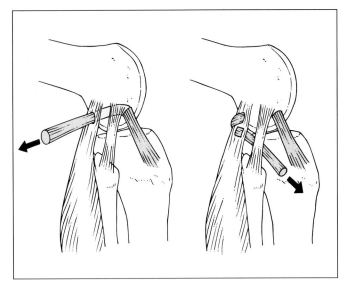

a & b

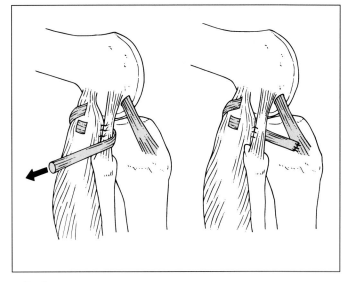

c & d

Figure 3

Losee procedure. (a) A strip of iliotibial band is allowed to remain attached distally to Gerdy's tubercle and passed beneath a tunnel on the lateral femoral condyle near the lateral collateral ligament origin and exiting near the origin of the lateral head of the gastrocnemius. (b) The strip is passed through the gastrocnemius tendon with the fibular collateral ligament. (c) The iliotibial strip is sutured to the lateral collateral ligament and is brought anteriorly. (d) The reflected strip is sutured along its course and attached distally to its origin near Gerdy's tubercle.

translation is evaluated. If laxity is noted, a more horizontal placement of the band beneath the fibular collateral ligament is made and sutured to the periosteum at the points of entrance and exit from the tunnel or sutured to the lateral collateral ligament. The proximal strip then encircles the gastrocnemius tendon at its origin and is sutured to the gastrocnemius and arcuate ligament posterior to the fibular collateral ligament and just above the joint-line. If the tunnel is properly placed, subluxation is eliminated. The knee is also flexed to 90° to make sure that the sling will not pull free. The tibia is held in external rotation and maintained at 45° of flexion. The posterolateral capsule is sutured to the fibular collateral ligament and the strip of fascia lata is carefully sutured to the fibular collateral ligament. Any excess fascia is used to reinforce the repair. A defect in the fascia that persists was noted only to cause a harmless and asymptomatic muscle hernia.

The loop provides a tightening of the posterolateral corner of the knee and draws the gastrocnemius tendon and arcuate ligament anteriorly towards the fibular collateral ligament. The strip is then passed through the previously created bone tunnel from a posterior to anterior direction and then distally beneath the iliotibial tract that is still attached to Gerdy's tubercle. The iliotibial tract may then be brought proximally and sutured under tension to the insertion of the fibular collateral ligament. In review of 25 patients undergoing this lateral procedure for chronic, severe anterolateral instability and with an intra-articular reconstruction, 87% were improved. The lateral pivot shift was eliminated in 100% of cases.

Pivot shift operation

Jackson[5] reviewed 135 patients retrospectively with a maximum follow-up of 12 years. Patients who met the criteria for follow-up had no other ligamentous injuries or previous anterior cruciate reconstructions or combination procedures. Forty patients with major meniscal pathology which could simulate cruciate deficiency were eliminated. A 1.5-cm distally based strip of iliotibial band was passed beneath the lateral collateral ligament in an oblique tunnel and the lateral head of the gastrocnemius, and with the tibia externally rotated it was forwarded distally as a 'return lateral loop.' Eighty-eight percent of the patients reviewed were improved subjectively; 93% of examined patients had no evidence of instability or only objective evidence of minor instability. Twenty-one patients had chondral lesions and most of the unsatisfactory results were in patients with serious chondral lesions. Although some instability persisted with very few 'normalized' knees, it offered low-risk, long-acting improvement in three out of four patients.

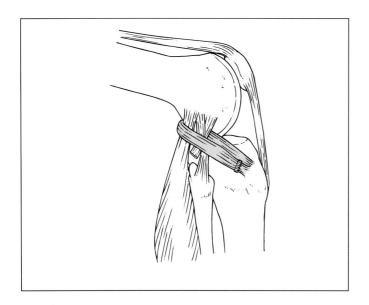

Figure 4

A 1.8 cm × 18 cm strip of iliotibial band is passed beneath the lateral collateral ligament, popliteus tendon and the tendinous origin of the lateral head of the gastrocnemius, then reflected at a site near Krackow's point No. 9 back to an osteoperiosteal flap below Gerdy's tubercle with the foot externally rotated, the knee flexed and tibia in external rotation.

Marder[9] described an extra-articular reconstruction revising a distally based iliotibial band transfer beneath the lateral collateral ligament which is reefed with the tibia externally rotated and a transfer of the iliotibial band is held proximal with the graft secured immediately superior and proximal to the lateral femoral epicondyle with a 6.5-mm AO cancellous screw and washer.

Statistical analysis was provided, but the author felt that there were significant advantages of the extra-articular procedure, with decreased postoperative complication of ankylosis or patellofemoral complaints.

Coker–Arnold technique (Figure 4)

In 1975 Dr Coker developed a modification on MacIntosh's lateral tenodesis and recommended passing the distally based flap beneath the lateral constraints and back to an osteoperiosteal flap near Gerdy's tubercle. Unfortunately, while the authors routinely passed the strip beneath the lateral collateral ligament, popliteus tendon and lateral tendinous origin of the gastrocnemius, they only described passing the strip beneath the lateral collateral ligament and its investing structures.[3,36] An oblique incision is made from Gerdy's tubercle posterior and proximally. A 1.8 cm × 18 cm strip of iliotibial band is dissected proximally from Gerdy's tubercle. A

meniscotome is directed proximally in the plane of the fibers of iliotibial band to define the strip longitudinally and to separate it from the intermuscular septum. A fascial cutting device is used to complete the dissection proximally. It is important to use only the anterior two-thirds of the iliotibial tract with a remaining edge of the very anterior tract, leaving the posterior one-third to provide lateral stability. Resection of Kaplan's fibers (part of the iliotibial tract which blends into the intermuscular septum and inserts on the supracondylar tubercle) is carried out in most of these procedures. The iliotibial band is no longer attached to the femoral condyle. With flexion, the iliotibial tract immediately shifts posteriorly preventing anterior subluxation of the plateau sufficient for a pivot shift sign to occur.[35]

The distally based strip is then passed beneath the lateral collateral ligament, the popliteus tendon and the lateral head of gastrocnemius. Passing the strip beneath the popliteus tendon is quite difficult and requires a long, curved clamp passed distally beneath all three structures. As the strip is reflected around the lateral head of gastrocnemius near its origin it approaches the site as described by Sidles and Krackow.[19,20] It is brought back to an osteoperiosteal flap either anterior or posterior to Gerdy's tubercle and held with a serrated staple with the knee fully flexed and externally rotated. The defect is closed proximally with interrupted sutures. The knee is held in a Velcro-hinged postoperative brace at 50° of flexion. The brace is not removed during the first week. The patient remains non-weight-bearing on two crutches. At the second week, the brace and postoperative dressing are removed and the knee will generally be placed in a sports brace in which there is no contact with the lateral incision, and the brace is extended to 40°. The brace is extended weekly. The brace is gradually extended to 10° at week 6 with full flexion allowed. The brace is then removed when indoors and for sleeping, but is worn otherwise. The patient is able to begin more strenuous activities, such as walking and easy jogging at week 8. Intensive rehabilitation of the lower extremity is carried out. Generally the patients only use the brace for the first few months of competition until they are confident and strong enough to go without it.

Vander Schilden[37] reported on 59 patients followed for 4–9 years utilizing the Coker–Arnold modified MacIntosh extra-articular procedure. Stability and function were evaluated at an average of 70 months utilizing Feagin's subjective evaluation criteria. Over 50% of the patients reported no instability related to activity and average functional rating was 85%, with 100% as normal. Twenty-six patients were evaluated radiographically and by physical examination. Fourteen patients developed mild osteoarthritic changes, two had moderate changes by Fairbank's radiological criteria. On physical examination, 23 patients demonstrated normal range of motion. Three lacked up to 10° of extension. A 1+ drawer or 1+ Lachman's test was present in 23 patients. Two patients had evidence of a pivot shift. Examination of the knee showed no change over an extended period of time. The concurrent degenerative changes were associated with previous meniscectomy and the authors felt that a high percentage of patients had stability and confidence in their knee during demanding situations, whereas this was not the case preoperatively. The procedure was felt to be well designed for anterolateral instability.

Williams[38] reviewed 124 patients with an average follow-up of 20.3 months who underwent the Coker–Arnold procedure. The patients were evaluated preoperatively and postoperatively for ligament laxity utilizing the KT-1000,[39] Lysholm scoring system,[40] and a subjective knee questionnaire developed by Williams.[38] Laxity results indicated preoperatively a right–left difference in anterior displacement (89 N; 20 lb) of 3.7 mm and a postoperative right–left displacement of 1.9 mm. The mean compliance index value was 2.5 mm preoperatively and 1.6 mm postoperatively. The mean preoperative Lysholm function score was 48 points compared to a postoperative score of 88 points.[38] The number did not seem to deteriorate with time.

The prospective study of Taylor et al.[41] with a 17.9-month follow-up of 53 ACL deficient patients with the same procedure had preoperative laxity values of 5.7 mm and an injured–normal laxity difference of 2.9 mm. Follow-up examinations showed that the anterior displacement (89 N; 20 lb) injured–normal difference was 3.1 mm. The mean compliance index values were 2.0 mm preoperatively and 1.4 mm postoperatively. The mean Lysholm score was 86.3. Statistical analysis of data revealed no significance of joint displacement compared to Lysholm function score. On physical examination, 17% showed evidence of a positive pivot shift and 3.8% had mild instability. Seventeen patients indicated that they had returned to prior activity levels; 34 patients indicated that they had mild to moderate problems during their activity participation; 1 patient had severe problems; and 1 patient stopped prior activity but not owing to the injured knee. Fifty-two patients demonstrated a normal range of motion for extension and 30 patients had a range of motion for flexion between 90° and 135° and 23 patients were between 135° and 150° of motion for flexion.

In a retrospective study by McCann et al.,[42] 34 patients undergoing this same procedure were evaluated for subjective improvement and anterior displacement. The average follow-up was 8.6 years. Preoperative laxity and Lysholm scores were not available, but postoperative results indicated a mean right–left anterior displacement (89 N; 20 lb) of 2.2 mm, mean compliance index value of 1.9 mm and a mean Lysholm score of 87.4 (range 70–96). Radiographic evaluation utilizing the criteria established by Fairbank revealed that, for those patients who had a lateral or medial meniscectomy, narrowing plus flattening were the most common changes found in combination. Medial meniscectomy patients had 40% ridging, 30% narrowing, and 13% flattening. Lateral meniscectomy patients revealed 65% ridging, 35% narrowing, and 15% flattening.

Combined repairs

Wilson and Scranton[21] described a combined reconstruction of the anterior cruciate ligament utilizing a semitendinosus for the intra-articular portion of the reconstruction, with a strip of the iliotibial band for the extra-articular augmentation. The clinical, arthrometric and radiographic examination of 32 patients with 2–7 years follow-up showed 6 patients (20%) with an excellent rating, 22 (73%) with a good rating, and 2 (7%) fair. There were no poor results. The lateral extra-articular procedure is similar to that described by Frank and Jackson[5] and also described by Arnold et al.[3] with the iliotibial band passed beneath the lateral collateral ligament and lateral head of gastrocnemius and back to Gerdy's tubercle. Seven professional football players all returned to the National Football League. Four played for an additional 2–7 years and then retired. The other three were still active and functioning at high demand levels. Extra-articular reconstruction was felt to help protect the intra-articular graft during the critical early month of revascularization and the morbidity rate was low as the procedure is presently done arthroscopically assisted. The intra-articular portion is now done arthroscopically assisted.

Combined intra- and extra-articular reconstructions

The rationale for combined intra-articular and extra-articular augmentation is twofold. First, during the initial stages of rehabilitation it may protect the intra-articular repair against the translational forces exerted anteriorly by the extensor mechanism on the tibia. Second, if an extra-articular augmentation is placed isometrically, it may offer lasting capsular stability in the anterolateral region of the capsule and perhaps possibly prolong the ultimate life of the graft. This is yet to be established in the literature.[43]

Clancy and associates[27] described a patellar tendon substitution for the cruciate ligament and extra-articular tendon transfers. A dynamic extra-articular procedure with a transfer of the pes anserinus medially and a transfer of the tendon of the long head of the biceps under the fibular collateral ligament laterally was used to compensate for the stretching of the medial and lateral capsular structures that frequently occurred secondary to insufficiency of the cruciate ligament. Fifty patients were available for personal examinations and none had postoperative episodes of instability. Forty-four had full return to all desired sports activities. Lachman's test was negative in 8 patients, trace-positive in 12, and mildly positive with a hard end-point in 30. Pivot shift was negative in 41 patients, a trace-positive in 8, and mildly positive in 1. The results were graded as excellent in 30 patients, good in 17, and fair in 1 patient, with only 2 failures. The main effect of the biceps tendon transfer as shown by Narechania et al. was noted to enhance its function as a strong flexor and external rotator.[44]

Draganich et al. studied a combination of intra-articular and extra-articular reconstructions with a Müller anterolateral iliotibial band tenodesis.[45]

The Müller lateral reconstruction was modified by using Krackow's point F-9 for the femoral fixation of the tenodesis.[13] This consisted of a Müller anterolateral femorotibial iliotibial band tenodesis and intra-articular reconstruction utilizing the patellar tendon as described by Clancy.[10] The extra-articular reconstruction was found to overconstrain internal tibial rotation of the ACL excised knee between 30° and 90°, while the isolated extra-articular reconstruction did not return normal anterior stability to the ACL deficient knee. It did significantly reduce the anterior laxity of the ACL deficient knee between 30° and 90° of knee flexion. Because the extra-articular reconstruction shared the load and performed with the intra-articular reconstruction as part of the combined procedure, Draganich concluded that it would be useful as an adjunctive procedure in appropriate clinical situations.[45]

The maintenance of normal resting rotatory motion of the tibia was thought to be an important factor in preventing overconstraint of internal rotation. At angles of flexion greater than 15°, the extra-articular reconstruction significantly reduced anterior laxity but this did not return to normal. It shared the anterior load with the intra-articular reconstruction at flexion angles between 19° and 90°.[13]

Drez recommended substitution of the intra-articular cruciate ligament with a free graft. The biceps femoris tendon was passed deep to the fibular collateral ligament to combat the internal medial and lateral capsular laxity and to decrease the load on the intra-articular cruciate substitute. A biceps tendon transfer was used with the medial third of the patellar tendon with a dynamic backup provided by the pes anserinus and biceps tendon.[11]

Zarins and Rowe described a technique of a simultaneous over-the-top transfer of the semitendinosus tendon with a strip of iliotibial tract plus posteromedial and a lateral capsular reefing (Figure 5).[46]

James[12] utilized a lateral extra-articular tenodesis utilizing a strip of iliotibial tract combined with an intra-articular reconstruction of the torn anterior cruciate ligament utilizing a portion of the patellar

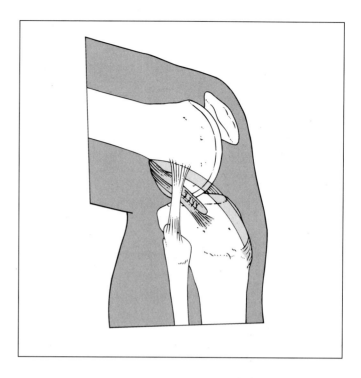

Figure 5

Zarins and Rowe's combined reconstruction utilizing the semitendinosus over the top and repaired to the iliotibial band. Note that this lateral reconstructive procedure, as well as others, has proximal fixation at or near the point on the femur described by Krackow (no. 9).

tendon in the more severe chronic types of anterolateral rotatory instability. He noted that the tenodesis type of procedure was more effective than the dynamic reinforcement. His lateral tenodesis procedure utilizes a strip of the iliotibial band left attached distally to provide a static lateral repair. This procedure is used for more severe forms of chronic anterolateral instability. A 20 cm long × 2–2.5 cm wide strip of iliotibial tract is released proximally and left attached to Gerdy's tubercle and passed through a bony tunnel in the lateral femoral condyle just proximal and anterior to the insertion of the fibular collateral ligament. A soft-tissue tunnel is created through the arcuate ligament, through the gastrocnemius tendon and beneath the fibular collateral ligament. After the bony and soft-tissue tunnels are developed, the iliotibial tract is passed beneath the fibular collateral ligament through the previously created soft-tissue tunnel and the arcuate ligament and gastrocnemius tendon. It is then brought back anteriorly and once again passed through the same passage, forming a loop around the fibular collateral ligament, arcuate ligament, and gastrocnemius tendon. This loop effect provides a tightening of the posterolateral corner of the knee and draws the gastrocnemius tendon and arcuate ligament anteriorly towards the fibular collateral ligament.

Discussion

The use of extra-articular procedures evolved at a time when the available intra-articular reconstructions were not very effective and the surgical community was searching for a method to stabilize the symptomatic ACL deficient knee. Extra-articular lateral reconstructive procedures are designed to strengthen the tissues and align parallel to the intra-articular route of the anterior cruciate ligament. The grafts lie in tissue with a good vascular supply. Lateral extra-articular reconstructions theoretically have a mechanical advantage over intra-articular transfers in possibly preventing anterior subluxation of the lateral tibial plateau by being located farther from the center of rotation, giving them an increased rotational control. The extra-articular procedures do not directly repair the primary lesion causing instability, which of course is the torn anterior cruciate ligament.[47]

The ideal procedure would allow isometric intra-articular replacement of the anterior cruciate to best restore the normal biomechanics, yet many side-effects have been described in intra-articular reconstructions, including patellofemoral pain, restricted motion, extended operative procedure, and failure to provide precise placement of the anterior cruciate graft.[9]

A study group of orthopedic surgeons was challenged in 1989 by the Sports Medicine Society (FSMER) to study the role of lateral procedures. An extended review was carried out by 24 orthopedic surgeons and it was noted that there is only a limited role for primary extra-articular augmentations and they should only be utilized in selective patients. Some lateral procedures have been noted to stretch with time. They may appear tight at the time of surgery but if the F-9 position is not of the proximal fixation site the natural kinematics try to become re-established. Several clinical series have suggested that it is not necessary to use an extra-articular lateral tenodesis as a supplement to the intra-articular reconstruction and noted that these may add to the morbidity problem.[48]

Dr Robert Jackson was a member of the FSMER group and has noted that the indications for this procedure are (1) young patients with proven instability, (2) isolated partial anterior cruciate ligament tears, (3) isolated total anterior cruciate tears, (4) combined lesion if secondary pathology is repairable.[49] Various factors seem to be related to the final outcome of the lateral tenodesis repair, including meniscectomy, pre-operative KT-1000 values, degenerative changes, and importantly, the posterior inclination of the lateral tibial plateau.

Further studies may show that those knees with less convex lateral tibial plateaux may provide more stability and be more reliably suited to a lateral tenodesis. Superiority of one of the many extra-articular repairs over another has not been established as no comparative studies have been performed.

References

1. **Ellison AE,** Distal iliotibial-band transfer for anterolateral rotatory instability of the knee, *J Bone Joint Surg (Am)* (1979) **61:** 330–337.
2. **Andrews JR, Sanders R,** A 'mini-reconstruction' technique in treating anterolateral rotatory instability (ALRI), *Clin Orthop* (1983) **172:** 93–96.
3. **Arnold JA, Coker TP, Heaton LM** et al., Natural history of anterior cruciate tears, *Am J Sports Med* (1979) **7:** 305–313.
4. **Fox JM, Blazina ME, Del Pizzo W** et al., Extra-articular stabilization of the knee joint for anterior instability, *Clin Orthop* (1980) **147:** 56–61.
5. **Frank C, Jackson RW,** Lateral substitution for chronic isolated anterior cruciate ligament deficiency, *J Bone Joint Surg (Br)* (1988) **70:** 407–411.
6. **Hanks GA, Joyner DM, Kalenak A,** Anterolateral rotatory instability of the knee: An analysis of the Ellison procedure, *Am J Sports Med* (1981) **9:** 225–232.
7. **Losee RE, Johnson TR, Southwick WD,** Anterior subluxation of the lateral tibial plateau: A diagnostic test and operative repair, *J Bone Joint Surg (Am)* (1978) **60:** 1015–1030.
8. **MacIntosh DL, Darby TA,** Lateral substitution reconstruction, *J Bone Joint Surg (Br)* (1976) **58:** 142.
9. **Marder RA,** Lateral extra-articular reconstruction for anterolateral rotatory instability of the knee, *Operative orthopaedics,* Vol. 3, ed Chapman MW (Philadelphia: JB Lippincott, 1988).
10. **Clancy WG Jr,** Anterior cruciate ligament functional instability: A static intra-articular and dynamic extra-articular procedure, *Clin Orthop* (1983) **172:** 102–106.
11. **Drez D Jr,** Modified Eriksson procedure for chronic anterior cruciate instability, *Orthopaedics* (1978) **1:** 30–36.
12. **James SL,** Knee ligament reconstruction, *Surgery of the musculoskeletal system* ed Evarts, CM (New York: Churchill Livingstone, 1983) 67–87.
13. **Müller W.** In: *The knee: Form, function and ligament reconstruction* (New York: Springer-Verlag, 1983) 253–257.
14. **Zarins B,** Combined intra-articular and extra-articular reconstructions for anterior tibial subluxation, *Orthop Clin North Am* (1985) **16:** 223–226.
15. **Lipscomb AB, Anderson AF,** Tears of the anterior cruciate ligament in adolescents, *J Bone Joint Surg (Am)* (1986) **68:** 19–28.
16. **Andrews JR, Carson WG Jr,** The role of extra-articular anterior cruciate ligament stabilization, *The anterior cruciate deficient knee: New concepts in ligament repair,* ed Jackson DW, Drez D, Jr (St Louis: CV Mosby, 1987) 168–192.
17. **Hughston JC, Andrews JR, Cross MJ** et al., (A): Classification of knee ligament instabilities, Part I—The medial compartment and cruciate ligaments, *J Bone Joint Surg (Am)* (1976) **58:** 159–172.
18. **Matsumoto H,** Mechanism of the pivot shift, *J Bone Joint Surg (Br)* (1990) **72:** 816–821.
19. **Krackow KA, Brooks RL,** Optimization of knee ligament position for lateral extra-articular reconstruction, *Am J Sports Med* (1983) **11:** 293–302.
20. **Sidles JA, Larson RV, Garbini JL** et al., Ligament length relationships in the moving knee, *J Orthop Res* (1988) **6:** 593–610.
21. **Wilson WJ, Scranton PE,** Combined reconstruction of the anterior cruciate ligament in competitive athletics, *J Bone Joint Surg (Am)* (1990) **72:** 742–748.
22. **Noyes FR, Butler DL, Grood ES** et al., Biomechanical analysis of human ligament grafts used in knee-ligament repairs and reconstruction, *J Bone Joint Surg (Am)* (1984) **66:** 344–352.
23. **Kennedy JC, Stuart R, Walker DM,** Anterolateral rotatory instability of the knee joint, *J Bone Joint Surg (Am)* (1978) **60:** 1031–1039.
24. **Lemaire M,** Ruptures anciennes du ligament croise antérieur du genou, *J Chir* (1967) **93:** 311–320.

25. Unverferth LJ, Bagenstose JE, Extra-articular reconstructive surgery for combined anterolateral anteromedial rotatory instability, *Am J Sports Med* (1979) **7**: 34–39.
26. Youmans WT, The so-called 'isolated' anterior cruciate ligament tear or anterior cruciate ligament syndrome: a report of 32 cases with some observation on treatment and its effect on results, *Am J Sports Med* (1978) **6**: 26–30.
27. Clancy WG Jr, Narechania RG, Rosenberg TD et al., Anterior and posterior cruciate ligament reconstruction in Rhesus monkeys: A histological, microangiographic and biomechanical analysis, *J Bone Joint Surg (Am)* (1981) **63**: 1270–1284.
28. Ellison AE, The pathogenesis and treatment of anterolateral rotatory instability, *Clin Orthop* (1980) **147**: 51–55.
29. Marshall JL, Girgis FG, Zelko RR, The biceps femoris tendon and its functional significance, *J Bone Joint Surg (Am)* (1972) **54**: 1444–1450.
30. Torg JS, Cooley L, Anterior cruciate ligament substitution utilizing fibular head osteotomy with lateral collateral ligament and biceps tendon advancement techniques, *Orthop Trans* (1983) **7**: 485.
31. Galway RD, Beaupré A, MacIntosh DL, Pivot shift: A clinical sign of symptomatic anterior cruciate insufficiency, *J Bone Joint Surg (Br)* (1972) **54**: 763–764.
32. Ireland J, Trickey EL, MacIntosh tenodesis for anterolateral instability of the knee, *J Bone Joint Surg (Br)* (1980) **62**: 340–345.
33. Teitge RA, Indelicato PN, Distal iliotibial band transfer for anterolateral rotatory instability: A progress report, *Orthop Trans* (1978) **2**: 24.
34. Kennedy JD, Roth JH, Mendenhall HV et al., Presidential Address. Intra-articular replacement in the anterior cruciate ligament deficient knee, *Am J Sports Med* (1980) **8**: 1–8.
35. Kaplan EB, Some aspects of functional anatomy of the human knee joint, *Clin Orthop* (1962) **23**: 18–29.
36. Arnold JA, A lateral extra-articular tenodesis for anterior cruciate ligament deficiency of the knee, *Orthop Clin North Am* (1985) **16**: 213–222.
37. Vander Schilden JL, personal communication presented to the Anterior Cruciate Study Group, 1990.
38. Williams T, Arnold JA, Subjective rating scale for the anterior cruciate deficient knee, unpublished study, 1988.
39. Daniel DM, Stone ML, Sachs R et al., Instrumented measurement of anterior knee laxity in patients with acute anterior cruciate ligament disruption, *Am J Sports Med* (1985) **13**: 401–407.
40. Lysholm J, Gillquist J, Evaluation of knee ligament surgery results with special emphasis on use of a scoring scale, *Am J Sports Med* (1982) **10**: 150–154.
41. Taylor M, Arnold JA, Williams T et al., personal communication, 1990.
42. McCann B, Arnold JA, Williams TK, A retrospective study of lateral tenodesis procedure: an 8.6 year follow-up, personal communication (1989).
43. Wilcox PG, Jackson DW, Factors affecting choices of anterior cruciate ligament surgery, *The anterior cruciate deficient knee: New concepts in ligament repair,* ed Jackson DW, Drez D, Jr (St. Louis: CV Mosby, 1987) 127–141.
44. Narechania RG, Clancy WG Jr, Brannan R, Biomechanical aspects of biceps tendon transfer, Read at the Annual Meeting of the Society of Biomechanics, Ann Arbor, MI, October 1978.
45. Draganich LF, Reider B, Ling M et al., An in vitro study of an intra-articular and extra-articular reconstruction in the anterior cruciate ligament deficient knee, *Am J Sports Med* (1990) **18**: 262–266.
46. Zarins B, Rowe CR, Anterior cruciate ligament reconstruction using semitendinosus tendon and iliotibial tract, *Orthop Trans* (1980) **4**: 291. (Presented at the Annual Meeting of American Academy of Orthopedic Surgeons, Atlanta, Georgia, January 1980.)
47. Carson WG Jr, Extra-articular reconstruction of the anterior cruciate ligament: Lateral procedures, *Orthop Clin North Am* (1985) **16**: 191–211.
48. Singer KM, Management of anterior cruciate ligament injuries—A symposium, *Contemp Orthop* (1990) **21**: 393–424.
49. Bergfield J, Sports Medicine Meeting, Sun Valley, Idaho, July 1990.

Further reading

Andrews JR, Sanders RA, Morin B, Surgical treatment of anterolateral rotatory instability: A follow-up study, *Am J Sports Med* (1985) **13**: 112–119.

Arnoczky SP, Tarvin GB, Marshall JL, Anterior cruciate ligament replacement using patellar tendon: An evaluation of graft revascularization in the dog, *J Bone Joint Surg (Am)* (1982) **64**: 217–224.

Burnett QM II, Fowler PJ, Reconstruction of the anterior cruciate ligament: Historical overview, *Orthop Clin North Am* (1985) **16**: 143–157.

Butler DL, Noyes FR, Grood ES, Ligamentous restraints to anterior–posterior drawer in the human knee: A biomechanical study, *J Bone Joint Surg (Am)* (1980) **62**: 259–270.

Chiroff RT, Experimental replacement of the anterior cruciate ligament: A histological and microradiographic study, *J Bone Joint Surg (Am)* (1975) **57**: 1124–1127.

Cubbins WR, Calahan JJ, Scuderi CS, Cruciate ligaments: A resumé of operative attacks and the results obtained, *Am J Surg* (1939) **43**: 481–485.

DeHaven KE, Acute ligament injuries and dislocations, *Surgery of the musculoskeletal system,* ed Evarts CM (New York: Churchill Livingstone, 1983) Vol. 3, section 7, 5–30.

Fetto JF, Marshall JL, The natural history and diagnosis of anterior cruciate ligament insufficiency, *Clin Orthop* (1980) **147**: 29–38.

Fleming RE, Blatz DJ, McCarroll JR, Lateral reconstruction for anterolateral instability of the knee, *Am J Sports Med* (1983) **11**: 303–307.

Galway R, Lateral pivot shift injury of the knee, *J Bone Joint Surg (Br)* (1971) **53**: 772–773.

Galway HR, MacIntosh DL, The lateral pivot shift: A symptom and sign of anterior cruciate ligament insufficiency, *Clin Orthop* (1980) **147**: 45–50.

Giove TP, Miller SJ III, Kent BE et al., Non-operative treatment of the torn anterior cruciate ligament, *J Bone Joint Surg (Am)* (1983) **65**: 184–192.

Graf B, Biomechanics of the anterior cruciate ligament, *The anterior cruciate deficient knee: New concepts in ligament repair,* ed Jackson DW, Drez D, Jr (St. Louis: CV Mosby, 1987) 55–71.

Jackson RW, Anterior cruciate ligament injuries, *Arthroscopy: Diagnostic and surgical practice,* ed Cassalls SW (Philadelphia: Lea and Febiger, 1984) 52–63.

Jackson DW, Drez D, Jr, (eds) *The anterior cruciate deficient knee: New concepts in ligament repair* (St. Louis: CV Mosby, 1987) 154–167.

Kostuik JP, Anterior cruciate reconstruction by the MacIntosh techniques, *J Bone Joint Surg (Br)* (1977) **59**: 511.

Larson RL, Combined instabilities of the knee, *Clin Orthop* (1980) **147**: 68–75.

McLeod WD, Biomechanics and function of the secondary restraints to the anterior cruciate ligament, *Orthop Clin North Am* (1985) **16**: 165–170.

Norwood LA, Treatment of acute anterolateral rotatory instability, *Orthop Clin North Am* (1985) **16**: 127.

6.10 Anterior cruciate ligament reconstruction using allogeneic tendon

Konsei Shino

Anterior cruciate ligament (ACL) injuries, if left untreated, often produce significant disability in athletically active populations. As the injured ligament rarely heals as the result of any type of conservative treatment, various autogenous reconstructions using tendons or fasciae around the knee have been used, since their immunogenicity is virtually non-existent and graft incorporation is thus expected to be feasible. However, the functional amount of tissue available for those procedures is limited by the risk of creating a defect at the donor site, which may result in functional disability.[1] Furthermore, individual variations in anatomical structures such as patella baja, a thin fascia or hypoplastic hamstring tendons occasionally make it difficult to perform autogenous reconstructions with thick collagenous tissue.

Although an artificial ligament made of synthetic materials appears to offer some potential advantages, the currently available ligaments have not yet demonstrated any long-term success for athletically-active patients.

It would therefore be highly advantageous if allogeneic tissue could be used to reconstruct the ACL.

There are some reports on successful clinical use of freeze-dried allogeneic soft tissues for the treatment of various soft-tissue lesions in the musculoskeletal system.[2,3] Their patients showed no graft rejection, while improved movement and/or relief of pain were usually attained. At re-operation the allograft was found to be completely reorganized as a viable tissue. Furthermore, successful use of allograft tendons in reconstructive procedures for the hand was also reported by several authors, though their treatment and preservation techniques varied.[4-6]

Therefore, use of allogeneic tissues for ACL reconstruction is considered to be one of the most reasonable approaches to treat patients with ACL deficiency.

Experimental studies on allograft ACL reconstructions

Webster and Werner (1983) reported preliminary canine experimental results in which the ACLs were reconstructed with freeze-dried allogeneic flexor tendons. They sacrificed the dogs at 8 months post-implantation, and found that all ACL grafts were intact and repopulated by host cells without any evidence of rejection. They also found that the mean ultimate load of the allografts was 29% of that of the control ACLs (Table 1).[7]

The present author and his colleagues produced the first comprehensive report focusing on ACL allografts in a canine model. They replaced the ACLs using a fresh-frozen patellar tendon without bone at either

Table 1 ACL allograft ultimate load, experimental/control (%).

Investigator	Tissue used to replace ACL	Experimental animal	Weeks post-op			
			6–8	12–16	24–40	52–
Webster (1983)[7]	Digital flexor tendon	Dog	–	–	29	–
Shino (1984)[8]	Free patellar tendon	Dog	–	–	35	36
Curtis (1985)[9]	Fascia lata	Dog	15	17	63	–
Nikolaou (1986)[11]	Bone–ACL–bone	Dog	50*	66*	90*	88*
Vasseur (1987)[12]	Bone–ACL–bone	Dog	–	–	14	–
Jackson (1987)[33]	Bone–ACL–bone	Goat	–	–	–	25

*The values for the controls (96.0~183.9N) were significantly lower than those in other studies.

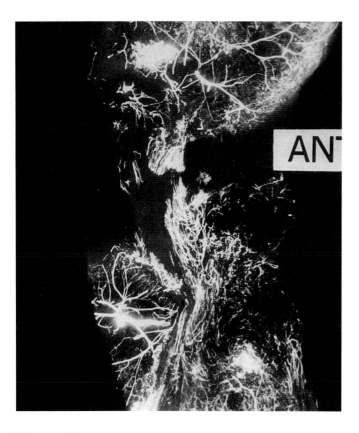

Figure 1

A microangiogram of the ACL allograft at 3 weeks. Note that over half of the graft was already revascularized, and that the anterodistal part was apparently hypervascular, suggesting the importance of the infrapatellar fat pad as a source of blood vessels. (From ref. 8.)

end.[8] Microangiographically, the allografts were entirely revascularized by 6 weeks post-implantation, and had developed an intrinsic vascular pattern similar to that of a normal ACL by 52 weeks (Figure 1). Histologically, the allografts had undergone fragmentation of collagen bundles in the initial necrotic phase, revascularization and then remodeling, and later regained a fibrous framework similar to that of a normal ACL, as in the case of an autograft (Figure 2). Furthermore, most of the graft–bone junction showed columnation of fibrocartilage (Figure 3). There was no evidence of immunological rejection at any time. Biomechanically, the mean maximum tensile load on the ACL replacements at 30 weeks was approximately 30% of that of the control ligaments, whether they were allografts or autografts. There were no significant differences in the biomechanical properties at 30 weeks and at 52 weeks (Table 1).

A similar canine study, this time replacing the ACL with a freeze-dried fascia lata allograft, was undertaken by Curtis, DeLee and Drez (1985).[9]

Arnoczky, Warren and Ashlock (1986) used fresh and fresh-frozen patellar tendon allografts with bone blocks on each end to replace the ACL in canines.[10] They found that marked inflammatory reaction was noticed in the fresh allografts, characterized by perivascular cuffing and lymphocytic invasion in contrast to the frozen allografts.

Similar allograft studies using bone–ACL–bone allografts as substitutes for ACLs were undertaken in a canine model.[11,12] These studies have failed to prove advantage of bone–ACL–bone allografts over bone-

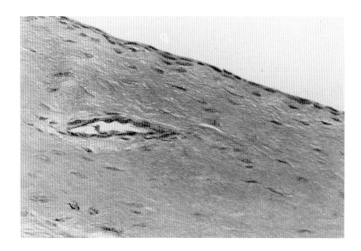

Figure 2

Photomicrograph of an allograft at 52 weeks. Note that both the cells and the collagen bundles were arranged longitudinally, suggesting maturity of the ligament. Hematoxylin and eosin, ×50.

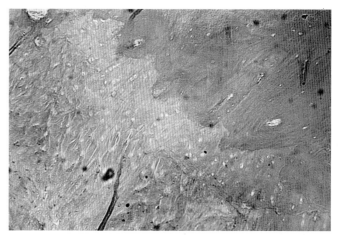

Figure 3

Photomicrograph of an allograft at 52 weeks showing the graft–bone junction. Note columnation of fibrocartilage. Hematoxylin and eosin, ×16.5.

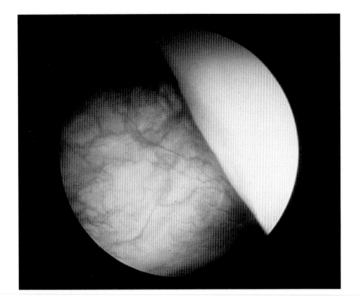

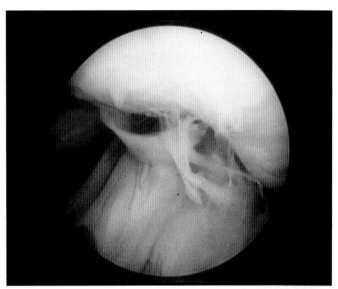

Figure 4

Arthroscopic appearance through the anterolateral portal of a human ACL allograft of the left knee at 6 months post-implantation. Note that the graft is covered with a thin, homogeneous synovial membrane that has many capillaries. (From ref. 15.)

Figure 5

Arthroscopic appearance through the anterolateral portal of a human ACL allograft of the left knee at 12 months post-implantation. Note that the graft is thick and taut. Also note that a hypovascular mid-zone like that in a normal ACL is seen.

free tendon allografts in terms of revascularization and remodeling processes, restored mechanical strength, or immune responses.

Clinical studies on allograft ACL reconstruction

The present author's earliest clinical trial using fresh-frozen bone-free tendons without secondary sterilization

Long-term clinical results

The present author and colleagues (1990) reported the long-term results of their first series of patients who had undergone ACL reconstruction because of chronic unilateral ACL insufficiency using fresh-frozen free allogeneic tendons such as Achilles, tibialis and/or peroneus tendons without any secondary sterilization.[13] The study covered 84 of 106 patients who had undergone the reconstruction with the open technique through drillholes between 1981 and 1985. The average follow-up period was 57 months with a range from 36 to 90 months. The subjective and functional results were rated excellent or good in 94%; the retear rate was 3%. Instrumented

laxity measurement with a 'Knee Instability Tester' showed 88% of the patients had less than 3 mm left–right difference in anterior laxity at 200 newtons anterior force.[14] Direct observation during 'second-look' arthroscopy revealed that the allografts were elaborately remodeled, viable and taut.[15] There were no signs or symptoms of immunological rejection at any time. Additional extra-articular procedures consisting of both pes anserinus transfer on the medial and iliotibial band reinforcement on the lateral side had no favorable effect on the results.

In vivo graft evaluations

Since we started the clinical trials in 1981, one of the most major concerns for the author has been how the transplanted allografts are remodeled or survive inside the human knee joint. Therefore, we have been trying to perform 'second-look' arthroscopy as frequently as possible during removal of graft-fixation hardware. This enables us not only to observe the grafts directly and measure their surface blood flow by laser Doppler flowmetry, but also to examine their microstructures by taking biopsies.

The present author has performed approximately 200 'second-look' arthroscopies at 6 weeks to 89 months after allograft ACL reconstruction. The results are summarized as follows.

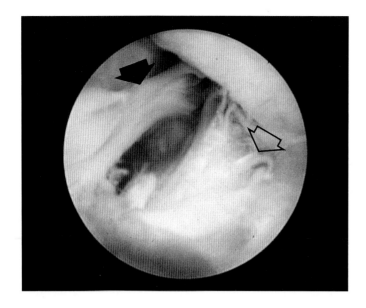

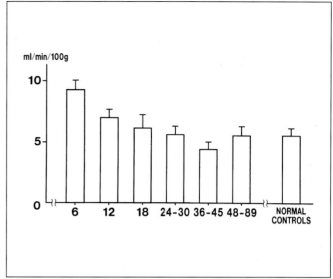

Figure 6

Arthroscopic appearance through the anterolateral portal of a human ACL allograft of the left knee at 52 months post-implantation. Note the fragmented necrotic portion in the anterolateral part (open arrow). Also note the regenerated ligamentum mucosum (solid arrow).

Figure 7

Diagram showing surface blood flows of human ACL allografts with laser Doppler flowmetry for various postoperative periods. Note that the surface blood flow declines with time from 6 months post-implantation onward, reaches a plateau by 12 months and maintains a level equivalent to that of normal ACLs thereafter.

Arthroscopic appearance

By 6 weeks, the graft was covered with a thick hypervascular synovial sheath which mainly originated from the infrapatellar fat pad (Shino et al., 1988).[15] The synovial sheath covering the graft became thinner and the superficial hypervascularity subsided with time. Around 6 months, the grafts were covered with a thin synovial sheath and appeared to consist of longitudinally oriented thick bundles of fibers (Figure 4). At 11–12 months, the grafts closely resembled the normal ACL (Figure 5). Relative hypovascularity was noted in the mid-zone, and hypervascularity in either the proximal third or in the distal third. Over the next few years, the grafts appeared similar to the 11- to 12-month-old grafts, and had not deteriorated at all.

A small number of the grafts showed fragmented necrosis which failed to be incorporated into the recipient tissues in the anterolateral part (Figure 6).[16] This may be attributed either to minor graft impingement on the notch or to stress shielding due to uneven stress inside the thicker graft. However, no abnormal laxity or insufficiency of the graft was noted as the other major parts of the graft appeared viable and taut.

Blood flow measurement

In the 6-month-old grafts, the surface blood flow was 9.3 ± 0.8 (mean $\pm$ SD) ml/min per 100 g, which was significantly higher than that for the normal control ACLs (5.3 ± 0.6 ml/min per 100 g). In the 12-month-old grafts, the value was 7.0 ± 0.7, and in the 18-month grafts, 6.1 ± 0.7. For 24–30-, 36–45- and 48–89-month-old grafts, the respective blood flow values were 5.5 ± 0.8, 4.3 ± 0.6, and 5.2 ± 0.7 ml/min per 100 g. In summary, the surface blood flow of the allografts declined with time from 6 months post-surgery onward, reached a plateau by 12 months, and maintained a level equivalent to that of the normal ACLs thereafter (Figure 7).[17]

Light-microscopic evaluation

Six-month-old taut grafts had single or multiple layers of synovial lining cells on the surface and many fibroblasts with spindle-shaped nuclei in the substance. Though a crimp pattern suggesting regular arrangement of collagen bundles was already noticeable in the substance, the cellularity was significantly higher (Figure 8). In 12-month-old taut grafts, there was no thickening of the synovial covering, as was seen in most of the 6-month-old specimens. In the substance, there were relatively many longitudinally-aligned fibroblasts with spindle-shaped nuclei. Cellularity was still significantly high (Figure 9). In 18-month-old taut grafts, hypercellularity, which was commonly seen in the specimens in the earlier phases, had subsided and showed normocellularity, and a crimp pattern was also noted. These findings

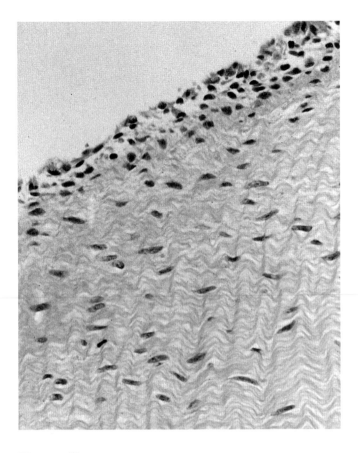

Figure 8

Photomicrograph of a taut human ACL allograft at 6 months post-implantation. Note its surface is covered with a thick synovial sheath. Also note that it already has longitudinally aligned collagen bundles as shown by their crimp pattern and that its cellularity is significantly higher. Hematoxylin and eosin, ×75. (From ref. 15.)

suggest taut grafts reach stability at 18 months, as the specimens from the taut grafts at 24–89 months closely resembled those at 18 months (Figure 10).

On the other hand, a specimen from one lax graft showed obvious hypercellularity of its substance with randomly shaped nuclei and randomly oriented collagen bundles (Figure 11).[15]

Collagen fibril evaluation with electron microscopy

In 3-month-old specimens, frequency distribution of collagen fibrils was slightly bimodal. Though small-diameter fibrils (30–80 nm) were predominantly seen, there was a small number of large-diameter fibrils (90–120 nm) which accounted for the bimodal distribution (Figure 12).

In biopsies at 6 months, the collagen fibril profile was almost unimodal and the peak of the fibril diameter was at 60 nm. Large fibrils with a peak diameter of 110 nm occurred much less frequently than in 3-month-old specimens (Figure 13).

In biopsies at 12 months, most of the collagen fibrils belonged to small-diameter groups (<80 nm), resulting in the unimodal pattern of the collagen profile. The almost complete disappearance of the larger fibrils was most characteristic in this stage of the grafts (Figure 14). In specimens older than 12 months, collagen fibril profiles were equivalent to those seen in the 12-month-old allografts.[18]

The following conclusions can be drawn from these graft evaluation studies:

1. ACL allografts survive as viable ligaments inside the human knee joint for a long time.

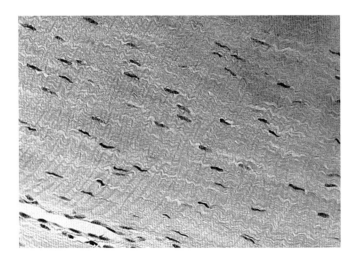

Figure 9

Photomicrograph of a taut human ACL allograft at 12 months post-implantation. Note that it has longitudinally aligned collagen bundles as shown by their crimp pattern and that its cellularity is still a little higher. Hematoxylin and eosin, ×55.

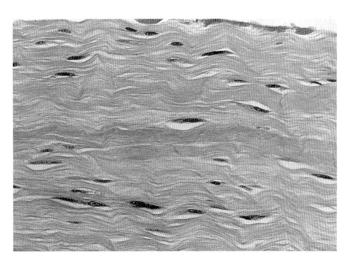

Figure 10

Photomicrograph of a taut human ACL allograft at 24 months post-implantation. Note its normal cellularity and the longitudinally-oriented collagen bundles. Hematoxylin and eosin, ×55. (From ref. 15.)

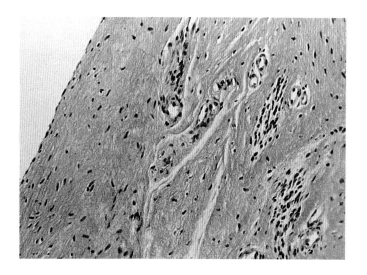

Figure 11

Photomicrograph of a lax human ACL allograft at 36 months post-implantation. Note that it consists of amorphous hypercellular and hypervascular scar tissue. Hematoxylin and eosin, ×55. (From ref. 15.)

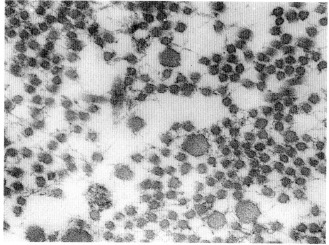

Figure 12

Electron micrograph of a 3-month-old ACL allograft biopsy (×40 000). Note that small-diameter fibrils (30–80 nm) are predominant, and that there is a small number of large-diameter fibrils (90–140 nm), accounting for the bimodal distribution.

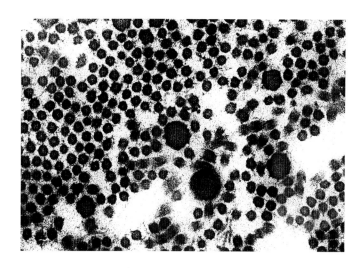

Figure 13

Electron micrograph of a 6-month-old ACL allograft biopsy (×40 000). Small-diameter fibrils (30–80 nm) are predominantly seen. Also note that there is an even smaller number of large-diameter fibrils (90–140 nm).

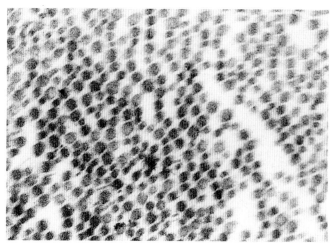

Figure 14

Electron micrograph of a typical 12-month-old ACL allograft biopsy (×40 000). Small-diameter fibrils (30–80 nm) are predominantly seen, while there are almost none of large-diameter fibrils (90–140 nm).

2. After 6 months post-implantation, the allografts do not degrade biologically over time.
3. The allografts are stabilized in the microstructure around 12 months post-implantation.
4. The allografts do not reattain the microstructure of the original allograft or to that of the normal ACL.

Studies in the United States

Allograft treated with freeze-drying and ethylene oxide sterilization

Paulos et al. (1988) found that approximately 15% of the patients who had undergone ACL reconstruction with freeze-dried, ethylene oxide-sterilized bone–patellar tendon–bone allograft showed an acute synovial reaction manifested by swelling and pain 5–18 months postoperatively.[19] Furthermore, from 9 to 24 months they encountered a late, gradual failure manifesting itself as an increase in laxity in a significant number of their patients. They concluded that foreign-body-type response elicited by ethylene glycol residues in the graft tissue was the major reason for the reaction.

Pinkowski et al. (1989) tested, with the lymphocyte blast transformation technique, eight patients who had undergone ACL reconstruction with bone–patellar tendon–bone allograft treated with freeze-drying and ethylene oxide.[20] They found that half of the patients scored positive in the test, and concluded that immunologic reaction to the ethylene oxide-treated allograft consisting of lymphocyte stimulation both in the synovial fluid and in the peripheral blood tissue does occur.

Grafts without secondary sterilization

Wainer, Clarke and Poehling (1988) reported 1–2-year results for their 23 patients who underwent ACL reconstruction with freeze-dried allografts in which the flexor hallucis longus, the posterior tibialis, and the toe flexors were most commonly utilized. Neither deep infection nor signs of graft rejection, such as fever, persistent effusion or erythema were found in their series.[21] They reported success for 22 of 23 patients. Similar preliminary results for the allograft reconstructions with freeze-dried Achilles tendon were reported by Leavitt (1987), and by Malek and Fields (1987).[22,23]

Manning et al. (1989) reported 2–5-year follow-up results for ACL reconstruction with freeze-dried fascia lata or Achilles tendon allograft without secondary sterilization.[24] They found satisfactory results for 90% of their 60 patients, and there were no infections or rejections.

Indelicato et al. (1990) reported their 24–36-month results for ACL reconstruction with bone–patellar tendon–bone allografts, which were tested by either freeze-drying (Group 1, $n=14$) or freezing and thawing (Group 2, $n=27$) without any secondary sterilization.[25] Of Group 1, 79% were rated satisfactory and 93% of Group 2. Instrumented laxity measurement with the KT-1000 arthrometer at an anterior force of 89 newtons revealed that the mean left–right difference in anterior laxity was 1.2 mm for Group 1 compared with 0.9 mm for Group 2. They concluded that there was a marked improvement in both groups relative to overall subjective and objective results, and that there was no clinical evidence of rejection phenomena in either group. Furthermore, they stated that the fresh-frozen graft recipients were doing slightly better than those who received a freeze-dried allograft.

These reports closely coincide with the present author's results, suggesting the following criteria for successful allograft ACL reconstruction:

1. The allogeneic thick tendons or fascia, whether connected to bone blocks or not, should be harvested from sterile donors under sterile conditions.
2. The grafts should be either kept frozen at below –70°C for at least several days before use or freeze-drying.
3. There seems to be some evidence that fresh-frozen grafts are slightly superior to freeze-dried ones. It should be kept in mind that pharmaceutical companies use freeze-drying techniques to preserve antigens for immunology. On the other hand, it is generally known that the freezing and thawing technique has been utilized among biochemists to extract the cell components, in which major histocompatibility antigens reside, from tissues.

The present author's current approach for a patient with an ACL deficient knee

Patient selection

For chronic cases, our first criterion for allograft ACL reconstruction is the presence of functional instability during daily activities or during recreational sports. A further requirement is a positive Lachman sign. If the patients are recreational athletes not involved in collision sports or sports requiring special agility, they are recommended to undergo a vigorous rehabilitation program including activity modification as well as muscle drills in which hamstring-strengthening exercises are emphasized. They are taught how to land from a jump, how to turn, and how to avoid sudden stops. If the patients show little improvement with this conservative treatment for at least 3 months, then reconstruction is indicated. If the patient is a competitive athlete in collision or high-agility sports and strongly wishes to return to the pre-injury level of sports, reconstruction is indicated as early as possible.

For acute cases, the procedure is indicated only if patients are very eager to return to their original sports involving agility and/or collision. Furthermore, preoperative effusion is not contraindication for allograft reconstruction.

The present author believes that there are no particular contraindications for allograft reconstruction when compared with autogenous procedures, and that high-performance athletes are the most appropriate candidates for this procedure.

Donor selection and graft procurement

To avoid transmission of disease such as AIDS, donors should be thoroughly screened by family interviews, and their blood should be tested for the HIV antibody with the ELISA test. Donors who have suffered from a viral disease such as Creutzfeld–Jacob disease, multiple sclerosis, hepatitis or liver cirrhosis should not be utilized.

It is our belief that grafts for ACL substitutes procured from aged donors are not significantly inferior to those procured from younger donors in terms of the remodeling process, as experimental studies have pointed out that the original grafts initially suffer from fragmentation of the collagen bundles but that it is followed by a remodeling process by invading cells and vessels from the recipients.

Thick tendons such as the Achilles, tibialis anterior or posterior, peroneus, or toe flexor are procured from a cadaver or an amputated limb with standard sterile techniques, put into separate sterile, airtight tubes, and then stored in a deep freeze at below –70°C. The frozen state should be maintained for several days before clinical use.

Graft preparation

Immediately before the operation, the freeze-stored allogeneic tendon is rapidly thawed in room-temperature saline for several minutes, and shaped to 8–9 mm in diameter and to at least 6.5 cm in length by dividing or bundling. Then 3 to 4 thick polyester sutures (No. 2 or No. 1) are placed in each end of the graft (Figure 15).

No matching of any type of antigens between donors and recipient is required.

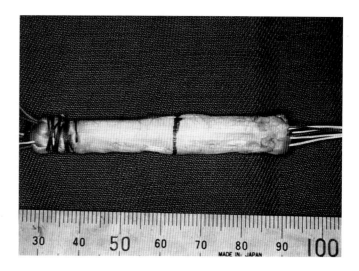

Figure 15

Reconstituted human ACL allograft immediately before use. Note the center line, which makes it easy to monitor position of the graft during the arthroscopic procedure.

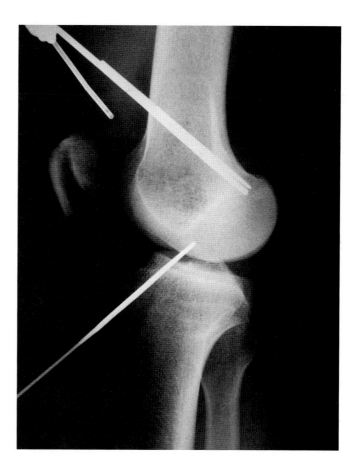

Figure 16

Lateral radiograph with the knee extended to reconfirm position of the tips of the guidewires. This also tells us whether the graft impinges on the top of the intercondylar notch.

Surgical technique

Our earlier experience has shown that there is no need for extra-articular augmentations for ACL reconstruction. Therefore, it was reasonable to switch from an open to an arthroscopic technique to minimize surgical invasion and postoperative morbidity.

At the time of reconstruction, with the patient supine, the knee is kept flexed at 90° using a foot holder. Three arthroscopic portals, i.e. anteromedial, anterolateral and central (transpatellar tendon) are always utilized. After dividing the ligamentum mucosum, the tibial and femoral stumps of the original ACL are excised, whether the ACL injury is chronic or acute, for arthroscopic visualization of the anatomic ACL attachments. At this stage, partial excision of the hypertrophic fat pad may occasionally be required. A 2.2-mm Kirschner wire is inserted from the lateral femoral cortex to the superoposterior portion of the femoral ACL attachment site with the aid of a femoral aimer, part of the Acufex drill guide system. A tibial aimer is used to insert another guidewire from the anteromedial aspect of the tibia to the point just medial to the center of the tibial ACL attachment site. A lateral radiograph with the knee fully extended is then taken to reconfirm the positioning of the tips of the guidewires (Figure 16). If the guidewires are located incorrectly, then a third or fourth wire is introduced to attain to the correct position. The guidewires are then overdrilled with an 8–9 mm cannulated reamer according to size of the graft. After chamfering the sharp edges of the drill-holes, an 8-mm artificial ligament made of Dacron or Gortex smoother is introduced to check for graft impingement on the intercondylar notch and for isometricity throughout the range of motion. Notchplasty is frequently added if the graft impinges on the superior and/or lateral wall of the notch. Finally, the graft is introduced and length pattern of the graft is directly measured with a tension isometer, to facilitate safer postoperative range of motion exercises. Then the graft is fixed by tying the sutures over buttons or around screws under tension at an appropriate knee flexion angle determined by the measured length pattern (Figure 17).

If meniscal tears occur in combination, they should be repaired or treated with partial meniscectomy prior to ACL reconstruction. If there are combined ligamentous injuries in the medial or in the lateral aspect, they should be corrected with the reefing technique or with tendon grafting.

Postoperative protocol

No postoperative immunodepressants or steroids are required. It is essential that the rehabilitation protocol be individualized on the basis of associated

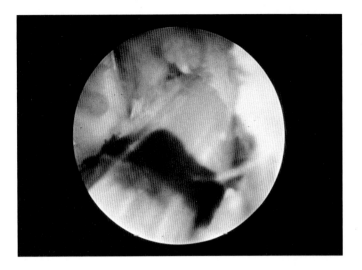

Figure 17

Arthroscopic appearance through the anterolateral portal of a human ACL allograft immediately after implantation. Note the center line of the graft.

ligamentous injuries, meniscal tears or variations in the length pattern of the graft throughout the range of motion. With this in mind, the knee is immobilized at 0–10° of flexion for a few days. Partial weight bearing is allowed at 4 weeks, followed by full weight bearing at around 6 weeks. Jogging is recommended at around 5 months. Return to strenuous activity is not allowed until 9–10 months postoperatively.

From our canine experimental study, it is assumed to take approximately 4–6 weeks for the graft to unite to the bone. For this reason, the range of motion exercises during the first 6 weeks after surgery should be individualized according to the length pattern of the graft. In most cases, the patient may not be allowed to extend the knee beyond 5° of flexion during the first 4 weeks, since intraoperative isometry measurements show that most grafts stretch 1–2 mm during passive extension from 5° flexion to full extension.

Preliminary results

Quantitative laxity measurements with our knee instability tester have revealed that 90% of our cases showed a difference in anterior laxity at 200 newton anterior force of less than 3 mm between postoperative and control knees, though long-term follow-up results are not available at the time of writing. The subjective and functional results based on Hughston-modified criteria have also shown a success rate of over 90%.

Complications and their treatments

The present author has not encountered any complications specific to allograft ACL reconstruction either locally or systemically. The following complications described are those which may take place in ACL reconstructions using autogenous grafts.

Fragmentation of the allografts

Some grafts may show fragmented necrosis of the anterolateral or midlateral part at the time of 'second-look' arthroscopy (6% in our early series) (Figure 6). However, further observation always shows that the central and anteromedial parts (two-thirds or more of the cross-sectional area) are viable and, therefore, functional. This partial necrosis may be attributed either to stress shielding of the involved part or to minor impingement against the anterolateral portion of the intercondylar notch due to insufficient notch plasty. Some of these patients may complain of a catching sensation, though most of them do not. Arthroscopic debridement of necrotic tissue is very effective for such symptoms.

Graft rupture

The results of our earliest clinical practice showed a retear rate of 3%.[13] As the series included a less active population as well, the incidence was not so high. However, the more active in athletics the patients are postoperatively, the higher the incidence of graft rupture that can be expected. In our total series of patients, the incidence of graft rupture was almost the same as that of subsequent ACL tear in the contralateral knee. There were no spontaneous ruptures without a significant traumatic episode.

In our series, most of the patients with graft rupture were treated with a second replacement using allogeneic tendon, and then resumed their sports activity.

Infection

We have not so far encountered any deep infection. The reason may be that fresh-frozen allografts show a greater affinity to the human body than any synthetic materials.

However, if deep infection occurs, it should be treated with irrigation of saline with antibiotics added after removal of the graft.

Effusion

We have not encountered any persistent effusion. If such a complication should occur with the use of a fresh-frozen graft, the cause should be sought in other complications such as infection or degenerative changes on the articular surfaces.

Effusion should be treated with aspiration. If the culture of the aspirated joint fluid proves to be negative, then the effusion may subside spontaneously without any particular treatment.

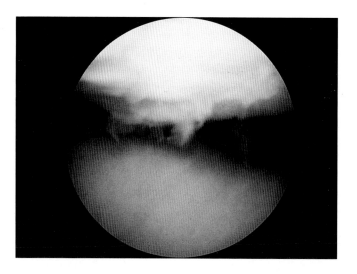

Figure 18

Arthroscopic view of fibrillation on the articular surface of the patella after ACL reconstruction, which is commonly seen postoperatively regardless of whether the graft is allogeneic or autogenous.

Degenerative changes on the articular surface of the patellofemoral joint

Patellar pain or anterior knee pain has not been common in our series. However, 'second-look' arthroscopy occasionally revealed significant degenerative changes on the articular surface of the patella even for patients who had not complained of such pain (Figure 18). Though the causes and clinical significance of these lesions are still unclear, our current study has suggested patellar tendon graft procurement, arthrotomy and notch plasty as the most probable areas producing risk factors. To minimize the risk of this unfavorable complication, either procurement of the patellar tendon graft or arthrotomy may have to be avoided, or notch plasty should be less frequently combined.

Stiffness

Stiffness is the most serious complication in knee ligament surgery. Though we are now applying a relatively aggressive postoperative rehabilitation protocol, a few of the patients still experience difficulty in regaining motion. If the patients fail to regain the full range of motion by 8 weeks postoperatively, the earliest possible manipulation under anesthesia is indicated. We believe this type of salvaging technique is most effective when it is performed early enough.

It should be kept in mind that acutely treated patients are more likely to be affected by stiffness than chronically treated ones. The reconstruction may be postponed until intraarticular hemosiderin synovitis secondary to hemarthrosis subsides. However, it should also be remembered that the healing rate in the case of meniscal repair less than 8 weeks after injury is significantly better than for repair more than 8 weeks afterward.[26] Therefore, the acute knee should be operated on either within a few days after injury when the hemosiderin synovitis has not yet been established, or several weeks afterwards when it has subsided.

Disease transmission

The risk of transmission of communicable disease such as AIDS can be reduced by screening donors but not completely eliminated, as the current tests for AIDS virus may not detect HIV antibodies for 6–12 weeks after initial contamination. With the current multifactorial screening process, however, the risk of AIDS-virus transmission by bone allograft is estimated to be less than one in a million in the USA, which is considered to be much lower than most other risks associated with surgical procedures.[27]

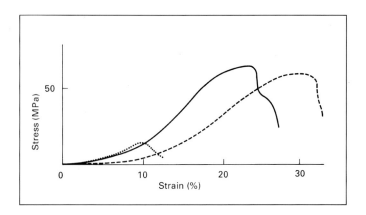

Figure 19

Stress vs. strain curves showing the effect of gamma-irradiation on the mechanical properties of the tendons. Solid line, control tendons; dots, gamma-irradiated tendons after solvent treatment; broken line, solvent-treated tendons after gamma-irradiation. Note marked deterioration of the mechanical properties of the gamma-irradiated tendons after solvent treatment.

Future directions

Graft collection

It is not difficult to obtain good allograft tendons from suitable donors where organ transplantations are frequently performed. Twenty or more tendon allografts for ACL reconstruction can be harvested from one donor, and can be stored for years until safety of the donor is confirmed.

Otherwise, it is necessary to establish a tissue bank with strict control of donor selection, tissue procurement, and storage.

Secondary sterilization

Treatment with ethylene oxide gas is not recommended for sterilization of tendons or ligaments because of its unfavorable side-effects, as demonstrated by studies in the United States.

Irradiation

Secondary sterilization techniques other than ethylene oxide treatment have been considered with the spread of AIDS virus infection. One of the simplest approaches to minimize the risk should be use of irradiation, as 2 Mrads has been shown in vitro to kill the AIDS virus in contaminated tissues.

Biomechanically, Butler et al. (1987) found that 1.95 Mrad gamma-irradiation did not cause significant deterioration of the mechanical properties of frozen fascia-lata.[28] Gibbons et al. (1989) demonstrated that a higher dose of irradiation (i.e. 3 Mrads) produced a significant deterioration of the mechanical properties of frozen goat bone–patellar tendon–bone specimens.[29] However, Haut and Powlison (1989) found 2 Mrads of irradiation to cause a significant deterioration of the mechanical properties of human patellar tendon allografts (25% in ultimate strength).[30] They also found that 2 Mrads of irradiation applied to freeze-dried allografts caused marked decrease in the strength of the grafts (75% in ultimate strength). Furthermore, Siegel and Larkin (1989) found that 2 Mrads irradiation caused an increase of creep characteristic of the Achilles tendon, and recommended pretensioning of the tissue for 5 minutes with a tensile force of 15 lb (67 newtons) immediately before clinical use.[31]

Biological effects of irradiation on the remodeling process of the allograft have not been studied yet. However, we can reasonably expect that irradiation does not produce any toxic residues in the graft, unlike treatment with ethylene oxide gas.

Bone–patellar tendon–bone and Achilles tendon allografts stored in a deep freeze and treated with gamma irradiation have been in clinical use for years in Cincinnati, Ohio, USA.[32]

Though 2 Mrads of gamma irradiation may be used to decrease risk of transmission of viral infection, it should be realized that such irradiation cannot entirely eliminate risk. Donor selection is essential for safe, successful allograft ACL reconstruction.

Solvent treatment

Organic solvents (e.g. acetone) are known to be effective in devitalizing viruses by melting the fat in the superficial membrane. A German company (Pfrimmer-Viggo, GmbH, Erlangen) has been producing human dura mater and fascia lata since 1985. As the treatment does not cause significant decrease in the mechanical properties of the tendons, the allograft tendons treated by the solvent should be better than those treated by freeze-drying in terms of toxic effect on viruses (Figure 19). The company and the present author are now collaborating to develop solvent-dried human allogeneic tendon products (tibialis anterior tendon, Achilles tendon, bone–patellar tendon–bone) for ligament reconstruction.

References

1. **Bonamo JJ, Krinick RM, Sporn AA,** Rupture of the patellar ligament after use of its central third for anterior cruciate reconstruction, *J Bone Joint Surg (Am)* (1984) **66**: 1294–1297.
2. **Neviaser JS, Neviaser RJ, Neviaser TJ,** The repair of chronic massive ruptures of the rotator cuff of the shoulder by use of a freeze-dried rotator cuff, *J Bone Joint Surg (Am)* (1978) **60**: 681–684.
3. **Bright RW, Green WT,** Freeze-dried fascia lata allografts: a review of 47 cases, *J Paediatr Orthop* (1981) **1**: 13–22.
4. **Peacock EE Jr,** Morphology of homologous and heterologous tendon grafts, *Surg, Gynaecol Obstet* (1959) **109**: 735–742.
5. **Peacock EE Jr, Petty J,** Antigenicity of tendon, *Surg, Gynaecol Obstet* (1960) **110**: 187–192.
6. **Iselin M, De La Plaza R, Flores A,** Surgical use of homologous tendon grafts preserved in Cialit, *Plastic Reconstruc Surg* (1963) **32**: 401–413.
7. **Webster DA, Werner FW,** Freeze-dried flexor tendons in anterior cruciate ligament reconstruction, *Clin Orthop* (1983) **181**: 238–243.
8. **Shino K, Kawasaki T, Hirose H** et al., Replacement of the anterior cruciate ligament by an allogeneic tendon graft: an experimental study in the dog, *J Bone Joint Surg (Br)* (1984) **66**: 672–681.
9. **Curtis RJ, DeLee JC, Drez DJ,** Reconstruction of the anterior cruciate ligament with freeze-dried fascia lata allografts in dogs: A preliminary report, *Am J Sports Med* (1985) **13**: 408–414.
10. **Arnoczky SP, Warren RF, Ashlock MA,** Replacement of the anterior cruciate ligament using a patellar tendon allograft, *J Bone Joint Surg (Am)* (1986) **68**: 376–385.
11. **Nikolaou PK, Seaber AV, Glisson RR** et al., Anterior cruciate ligament allograft transplantation: long-term function, histology, revascularization and operative technique, *Am J Sports Med* (1986) **14**: 348–360.
12. **Vasseur PB, Rodrigo JJ, Stevenson S** et al., Replacement of the anterior cruciate ligament with a bone–ligament–bone anterior cruciate ligament allograft in dogs, *Clin Orthop* (1987) **219**: 268–277.
13. **Shino K, Inoue M, Horibe S** et al., Reconstruction of the anterior cruciate ligament using allogeneic tendon: Long-term follow-up, *Am J Sports Med* (1990) **18**: 457–465.
14. **Shino K, Inoue M, Horibe S** et al., Measurement of anterior instability of the knee: a new apparatus for clinical testing, *J Bone Joint Surg (Br)* (1987) **69**: 608–613.
15. **Shino K, Inoue M, Horibe S** et al., Maturation of allograft tendons transplanted into the knee: an arthroscopic and histological study, *J Bone Joint Surg (Br)* (1988) **70**: 556–560.
16. **Shino K, Inoue, M, Nakamura H** et al., Arthroscopic follow-up of anterior cruciate ligament reconstruction using allogeneic tendon, *Arthroscopy* (1989) **5**: 165–171.
17. **Shino K, Inoue M, Horibe S** et al., Surface blood flow and histology of human anterior cruciate ligament allografts, *Arthroscopy* (1991) **7**: 171–176.
18. **Shino K, Oakes BW, Inoue M** et al., Human ACL graft: Collagen fibril populations studied as a function of age of the graft. *Trans Orthop Res Soc* (1990) **15**: 520.
19. **Paulos LE, Rosenberg TD, Gurley WD,** Anterior cruciate ligament allografts, *Prosthetic ligament reconstruction of the knee* ed Friedman MJ, Ferkel RD (Philadelphia: WB Saunders, 1988) 186–192.
20. **Pinkowski JL, Reiman PR, Chen S-L,** Human lymphocyte reaction to freeze-dried allograft and xenograft ligamentous tissue, *Am J Sports Med* (1989) **17**: 595–600.
21. **Wainer RA, Clarke TJ, Poehling GG,** Arthroscopic reconstruction of the anterior cruciate ligament using allograft tendon, *Arthroscopy* (1988) **4**: 199–205.
22. **Leavitt RL,** Allograft reconstruction of the anterior cruciate ligament, *Proceedings of Triennial Scientific Meeting of the International Arthroscopy Association (Sydney, Australia, 1987)* 63–64.
23. **Malek MM, Fields RH,** Arthroscopic reconstruction of anterior cruciate deficient knee using Achilles tendon allograft, *Proceedings of 5th Congress of the International Society of the Knee* (Sydney, Australia, 1987) 73–74.
24. **Manning JB, Meyers JF, Caspari RB** et al., Arthroscopic intra-articular reconstruction of the anterior cruciate ligament using lyophilized allograft ligament substitute, Paper presented at the 56th Annual Meeting of the American Academy of Orthopaedic Surgeons (Las Vegas, Nevada, USA, 1989).
25. **Indelicato PA, Bittar ES, Prevot TJ** et al., Clinical comparison of freeze-dried and fresh frozen patellar tendon allografts for anterior cruciate ligament reconstruction of the knee. *Am J Sports Med* (1990) **18**: 335–342.
26. **Henning CE, Lynch MA, Yearout KM** et al., Arthroscopic meniscal repair using an exogenous fibrin clot, *Clin Orthop* (1990) **252**: 64–72.
27. **Buck BE, Malinin TI, Brown MD,** Bone transplantation and human immunodeficiency virus: An estimate of risk of acquired immunodeficiency syndrome (AIDS). *Clin Orthop* (1989) **240**: 129–136.
28. **Butler DL, Noyes FR, Walz KA** et al., Biomechanics of human knee ligament allograft treatment, *Trans Orthop Res Soc* (1987) **12**: 128.
29. **Gibbons MJ, Butler DL, Grood ES** et al., Dose-dependent effects of gamma irradiation of the material properties of frozen bone–patellar tendon–bone allografts, *Trans Orthop Res Soc* (1989) **14**: 513.
30. **Haut RC, Powlison AC,** Order of irradiation and lyophilization on the strength of patellar tendon allografts, *Trans Orthop Res Soc* (1989) **14**: 514.
31. **Siegel MG, Larkin JL,** Evaluation of creep elongation in irradiated soft tissue allograft, Paper presented at the 56th Annual Meeting of the American Academy of Orthopaedic Surgeons (Las Vegas, Nevada, USA, 1989).
32. **Noyes FR, Barber SD, Mangine RE,** Bone–patellar ligament–bone and fascia lata allografts for reconstruction of the anterior cruciate ligament, *J Bone Joint Surg (Am)* (1990) **72**: 1125–1136.
33. **Jackson DW, Grood ES, Arnoczky SP** et al., Freeze dried anterior cruciate ligament allografts. Preliminary studies in a goat model, *Am J Sports Med* (1987) **15**: 295–303.

6.11 Reconstruction of chronic anterior cruciate deficiency with the Leeds–Keio prosthesis

Roger B. Smith

Rupture of the anterior cruciate ligament can lead to a mechanically unstable knee with progressive degenerative changes as demonstrated in both animal studies and clinical practice.[1-3] Other studies have claimed favourable results from non-operative management and suggested that complete loss of the anterior cruciate ligament may be compatible with a high level of athletic performance.[4,5] Reports vary in specific detail, but there is now a general consensus that, if untreated, the affected knee is subjected to recurrent episodes of clinical and subclinical rotatory instability resulting in progressive functional deterioration,[6] meniscal injury, and joint degeneration.[7-10]

The well-established techniques of reconstruction using local autogenous tissues have been reassessed in view of their often complicated procedures, damage to normal structures, the difficulties in fixation and variable long-term results. The extra-articular tenodesis as described by MacIntosh[11] suffers deteriorating results with time.[12] The patellar tendon substitution first described by Campbell[13] and popularized by Jones[14] has proved to be a useful technique in the hands of experienced surgeons, but many patients do not regain full extension, and after a period of time the results do not bear close examination.[15-17]

Carbon fibre, the synthetic substitute in use for the longest period, has not lived up to its initial expectations. It does not induce the formation of new collagen but merely becomes covered in a thin fibrous sheath and does not bond to bone.[18] A significant proportion of patients develop pain, effusions and synovial thickening due to carbon-fibre fragmentation within the joint.[19,20]

It was with this background that Seedhom, Senior Lecturer, and Fujikawa, Visiting Fellow from Keio University, Tokyo, at the Department of Rheumatism Research in the University of Leeds developed their open-weave polyester prosthesis. This device has similar biomechanical properties to the natural ACL,[21] and has been shown to induce fibrous tissue and the formation of new collagen, both in the experimental model of immature pigs and from clinical biopsy. A unique method of long-term fixation using bone dowels within the tubular part of the open-weave prosthesis shows experimental and clinical evidence of sound ingrowth.[22]

Patients and method

The patients in this series all presented with knee instability. Referral patterns show roughly equal numbers from the Accident and Emergency department, general practitioners and orthopaedic surgeons. This last group is now an increasing source of referral.

Patients complained of their knees giving way on walking or light sporting activities. In addition, most complained of pain and swelling. All exhibited a significant anterior drawer sign with the knee at 20° of flexion, and a positive pivot shift or jerk test preoperatively.[23-25] Arthroscopy was performed together with examination under anaesthesia, and meniscal tears were treated arthroscopically. If physiotherapy to develop hamstring and quadriceps strength failed to produce an improvement in clinical stability, then reconstruction was advised.

Operative technique

(1) We use an extended medial parapatellar incision, dividing the expansion of vastus medialis to allow lateral displacement of the patella. This gives good exposure of the subcutaneous upper surface of the tibia, the intercondylar region and the lateral femoral condyle. Any remaining avascular anterior cruciate ligament is resected and sufficient tissue is removed to allow vision to the most posterior part of the lateral wall of the intercondylar notch. Care is taken not to damage the blood supply to the posterior cruciate ligament, leaving its investing synovium intact.

(2) The site of the femoral tunnel in the intercondylar notch on the medial aspect of the lateral

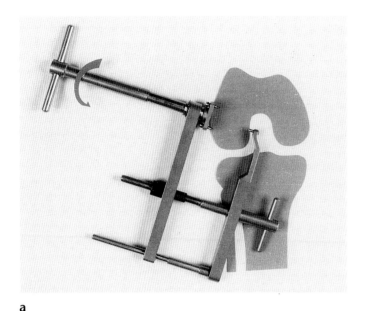

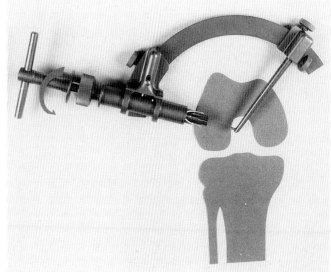

a   b

Figure 1

(a) Mark I jig in use up to mid-1989 with bone plug cutter in position on diagrammatic representation of the knee. (b) Mark II jig in use from mid-1989 shown diagrammatically with bone plug cutter in position.

femoral condyle is then identified and marked with a bone awl. It should lie at the most superior and posterior part of the original anterior cruciate attachment. If this is not clear then the back of the condyle is identified with a dissector and the bone awl located 3–4 mm anterior to the posterior edge in the most superior part of the notch.

(3) The jig is then positioned with the point in the intercondylar notch at the prepared mark. After tightening, the femoral bone plug is cut with the reamer (Figure 1).

(4) The plug is removed with the extractor and the guide sleeve is inserted, through which a 6-mm drill bit is inserted and a tunnel is drilled into the intercondylar region. Care is taken to protect the posterior cruciate ligament and the articular surface. The drill emerges at the femoral attachment previously marked. The anterior edge of the intercondylar origin of the tunnel is smoothed with a curette.

(5) The next stage is to prepare the tibial tunnel. The guide point is made with a bone awl at the most anteromedial aspect of the anterior cruciate ligament attachment. This lies just posterior to the anterior horn of the medial meniscus and transverse ligament and adjacent to the articular surface of the medial tibial plateau. The same sequence of procedures is used to create a bone plug and shouldered tunnel on the tibial side (Figure 2).

(6) A nylon tape is passed through the tibial and femoral tunnels using a blunt probe from below upwards and clamped at either end with the knee in 30° of flexion. Flexion and extension of the knee will then test whether the placement is isometric; any movement of the tape within the tunnels means this is not so. The most frequent error is that the femoral tunnel emerges too anteriorly. Under these circumstances it may be possible to create a more posterior tunnel by repositioning the jig within the notch and angling the drill bit more posteriorly to create a separate exit. If there is still instability on anterior drawer and jerk testing with the tape clamped, or if isometricity is not total, then it is usually necessary to use a long ligament with an extra-articular component.

(7) If the instability is fully controlled and the placing is isometric, then a short prosthesis is used. The device, encased in a protective polythene sheath, is passed upward through the tibial and femoral tunnels. The sheath is gradually withdrawn inferiorly from over the femoral section to allow the bone plug to be inserted into the open pocket of the ligament. A firm downward tension is usually sufficient to seat the bone plug firmly against the shoulders of the tunnel (Figure 3).

(8) Fixation techniques at the upper end have improved with the development of the system. Initially, no upper fixation was used other than the pressure of the closed end of the tube of the ligament against the bone plug. However, it was noted that the bone plug could partially collapse after a period of

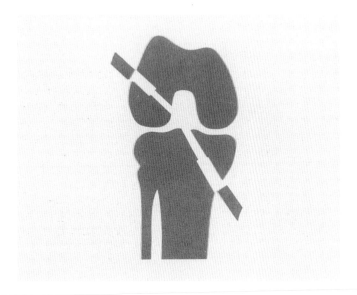

Figure 2

Diagrammatic representation of shouldered bone tunnels with bone plugs.

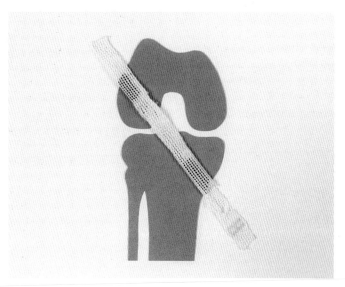

Figure 3

Diagrammatic representation of prosthesis through the tunnels and across the knee with bone plugs within the weave.

immobility and this could lead to loosening of the ligament. The next development was to introduce a barbed staple through the double-weave section of the ligament. In 1988, double stapling was used in order to confer greater mechanical security, and in 1990 a buckle/staple device was introduced with enhanced mechanical stability. The prosthesis is then sutured back on itself and into the surrounding tissue. Long-term stability develops when the bone plug, within the prosthesis, is secured through the prosthesis to the surrounding bone by fibrous or bony ingrowth.

(9) Maintaining tension in the line of the prosthesis, the tibial bone plug is inserted using the barrel and plunger introducer (Figure 4). The prosthesis is tightened at between 30° and 50°, at which point it is most relaxed. The bone plug is tapped home, maintaining the tension, and a single staple is used to secure the prosthesis to the tibia. The same modifications with double stapling and the staple/buckle were introduced over the last few years. The prosthesis is then sutured back onto itself. If a long prosthesis is selected, this passes from the emerging tunnel on the lateral femoral condyle extra-articularly to Gerdy's tubercle and then through a further bone tunnel to the medial tibial surface. This enables both ends of the ligament to be stapled together or independently.

(10) Secure closure of the capsule, in particular the vastus medialis expansion, is extremely important in order to prevent lateral tracking of the patella. After

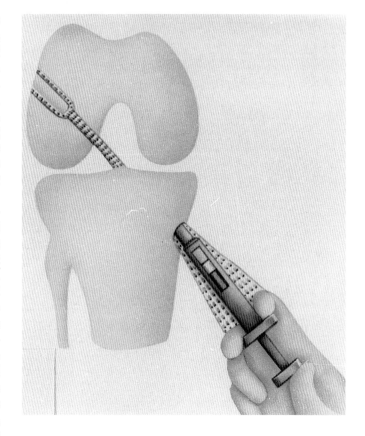

Figure 4

Diagrammatic representation of insertion of lower bone plug with the introducer.

wound closure the knee is immobilized in a full-leg cast, including the foot, in external rotation with the knee flexed 30–50°. Two weeks postoperatively, the plaster is changed when the sutures are removed and at 6 weeks a hinged knee brace is applied, blocking the last 10° of extension. With the introduction of more biomechanically sound methods of fixation, the time in plaster has been progressively reduced and we are now running a prospective trial between plaster fixation and immediate continuous passive motion and bracing. At 6 weeks, physiotherapy is commenced with progressive active and passive movements, and partial weight bearing is allowed. At 12 weeks, the brace is removed and more vigorous rehabilitation is continued. Full weight bearing is permitted and the patient is advised against all sports for 6 months and against contact sports for 12 months.

Results

From June 1982 to November 1989, 66 patients were operated upon, 56 men and 10 women. All suffered chronic anterior cruciate instability unresponsive to conservative therapy. All operations have been performed by or under the supervision of the author. Follow-up was 1.8–7.5 years with a mean of 3.2 years. The age at the time of surgery ranged from 15 to 47 years with a mean of 27.5 years. Reviews have been carried out by Registrars. An attempt was made to recall all the patients and a data base was set up. The assessment involved a scoring system after Lysholm,[26] preoperative and postoperative assessment of the anterior drawer at 20° flexion (Lachman), and the pivot shift test. In addition a Stryker laxometer has been available since 1986. Testing was performed by a single observer in 1990 and results were compared in appropriate cases with the assessments performed in 1987.

Fifty-two patients attended the follow-up clinics and a further 8 patients returned questionnaires, leaving 6 patients who did not reply and whom we could not contact. This gives a 91% follow-up.

The mode of injury was as follows: soccer (29); rugby (Union/League/American) (9); fall/industrial (10); racquet sport/running (8); skiing (5); and RTA (5).

Previous surgery had been carried out in several cases: meniscectomies (17); collateral repairs (2); and anterior cruciate repairs (2).

Operations performed

The operation consisted of insertion of a short ligament in 49 patients and a long ligament in 17 patients. Other procedures performed include medial capsule advancement and pes anserinus transfer, meniscectomy and patellar realignment.

Assessment

Subjective score

The Lysholm scoring of 60 patients who were seen or who returned questionnaires shows a preoperative range of 23–86 with an average of 60. The postoperative range is 32–100 with an average of 89 (Figure 5). These results are highly significant when analysed using the Wilcoxon Signed Rank test ($P<0.05$).

Objective clinical measurements

The Lachman test was positive in all cases preoperatively. Postoperatively the number of positive Lachman tests is reduced (Figure 6). Preoperatively all

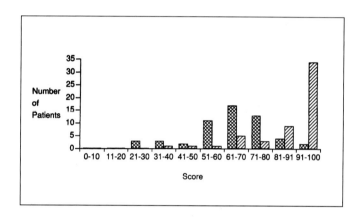

Figure 5

Lysholm preoperative (crossed) and postoperative (lined) scores for 60 patients.

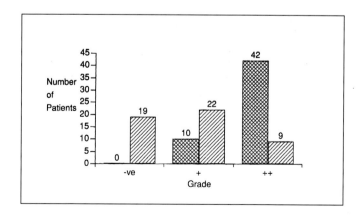

Figure 6

Lachman test results: preoperative (crossed) and postoperative (lined) scores.

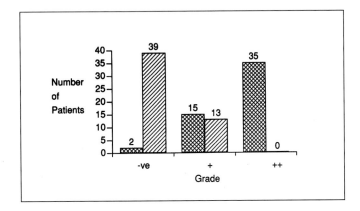

Figure 7

Pivot shift test results: preoperative (crossed) and postoperative (lined) scores.

patients but two (both with previous ACL surgery and global laxity) had a positive pivot shift test. Postoperatively the pivot shift was eliminated in 39 of the 52 cases, leaving a positive test in 13 (Figure 7). Most of these had been examined under anaesthetic because of some persisting clinical instability but by no means all had disabling symptoms.

Laxometer measurement

Some doubt has been cast upon various laxometers, but with a single observer using a standardized technique we found that results were reliable to within ±2 mm. This conformed to more recent observations by Steiner.[27] We looked at two groups of patients:

(A) Recent group. We have been able to perform a preoperative and postoperative laxometer measurement on 28 patients. Mean laxometer reading preoperatively was 8.8 mm and postoperatively was 6.6 mm. The mean follow-up was 2.5 years.

(B) Early group. This group had been tested in 1987 and again in 1989/90. There were 24 patients in this group. The mean laxometer reading in 1987 was 4.8 mm and in 1989/90 was 6.7 mm. Only five of these patients showed a deterioration of greater than 3 mm. These, however, did not have a significant decrease in their Lysholm scoring between the two assessments. There is no statistical correlation between residual Lachman anterior drawer or laxometer reading and the Lysholm score. There is a statistical correlation between those patients with a negative pivot shift and those with a higher Lysholm score.

Loss of movement occurred in several cases: extension loss $N = 2$ (mean 2.5°); flexion loss $N = 30$; intra-articular $N = 22$ (mean loss 6°); and extra-articular $N = 8$ (mean loss 10°).

Complications

Complications were as follows: septic arthritis (1); symptomatic loosening (including 4 revisions and 1 arthrodesis of the knee) (6); implant rupture (1 with synovitis) (2); thromboembolism (non-fatal) (3); patellofemoral pain (3); progressive arthritis (total knee replacement) (1); and lateral popliteal nerve palsy (recovering) (1).

The patient who suffered septic arthritis was the first in the series. He was treated by thorough washout of the knee and continuous irrigation with antibiotics and in fact made an excellent recovery. We were able to leave prosthesis in place. He was able to return to competitive football and squash.

The majority with loosening suffered one or more episodes of twisting or sudden strain in the few weeks following removal of the brace. In one of the patients, posterior and lateral instability was also present. Revision with posterior and lateral reconstruction was performed, without success, and arthrodesis was ultimately performed.

Patellofemoral pain is not often a significant problem provided secure wound closure has been performed. Two patients have required patella re-alignment.

Of the patients who suffered a rupture, both went back to contact sports, one to Rugby League and the other to Association Football. In both, meniscal damage was also sustained. One of these has been revised. Both have retired from professional sports.

Discussion

The anterior cruciate ligament is a complex structure with at least two distinct fibre bundles[28,29] and an extensive attachment to both femur and tibia. A single articular band cannot fully reproduce the natural structure, but if correctly positioned in the 'isometric' position it can contribute sufficiently to the stability of the knee to eliminate the jerk and pivot shift. We believe that it is this mechanism which causes the progressive meniscal and articular damage that leads to osteoarthritis in the anterior cruciate deficient knee.

In order to achieve and maintain the stability, prosthetic material should match as closely as possible the histological properties of the natural ligament. The breaking strain of this prosthesis is approximately 2000 newtons, which compares favourably with the natural ligament, whose breaking strain varies from 1730 newtons in cadaver specimens from young subjects to 740 newtons in specimens from elderly subjects.[30] The fatigue life of the ligament has been tested by soft clamping over 63 million cycles. After this period the breaking strain of the prosthesis is still around 1300 newtons.[21]

Biological as well as mechanical compatibility is also vital. Polyester material has been used in thousands of arterial grafts and found to be highly biologically compatible. The Leeds–Keio prosthesis has now been implanted into over 5000 subjects with an incidence of synovitis of under 1% in a recent European study.[31] In the present series, the only patients who showed synovitis were one patient in whom the ligament ruptured after several further injuries, and another patient who had had previous anterior cruciate reconstruction some 10 years previously and pre-existing synovitis. Twenty-two prosthesis in this series were examined arthroscopically or during further surgical procedures. All showed infiltrating fibrous tissue with a covering of synovial tissue around the prosthesis. This was confirmed histologically. Four cases underwent revision and one case was biopsied. The collagen appears to be in the line of the polyester fibres, but we have no evidence that this increases the strength of the 'neoligament'. We believed that accurate placement of the prosthesis, by good vision and access to the intercondylar notch is fundamental for stability. Whether this is achieved through a medial parapatellar incision or arthroscopically through separate femoral and tibial approaches is the choice of the surgeon. The majority of patients in this series had a wide exposure through an extended medial parapatellar incision, but we are now using more limited approaches including arthroscopic implantation. There is little point in leaving avascular remnants of the anterior cruciate ligament and sufficient synovium needs to be resected to allow access to the back of the intercondylar notch, but not to deprive the area of all vascularity, which is important in fibrous ingrowth.

The fixation of the device, both long- and short-term, is of vital importance in the maintenance of improved stability. The bone plug technique does confer long-term secure biological fixation, as shown in the initial experimental work in immature pigs and subsequently in biopsy specimens from patients who have had revision surgery. Even in patients who had loosening at one stage, there is excellent fibrous growth in and around the bone plug, although we do not have a great deal of histological evidence that there is direct bone contact through the weave of the ligament as was shown in experimental animals. However, we believe that fibrous ingrowth through the polyester within the bone tunnel is sufficient to produce stability. In order to protect the placement of the prosthesis within the bone tunnels around the bone plug it is important to have secure short-term fixation. In the early patients in this series, single staples were used. Biomechanical strength of this is insufficient to allow any form of early mobilization and we protected our patients for 6 weeks in a cast. Even when the cast was removed, during rehabilitation in the brace and afterwards, the knee was still vulnerable to sudden injury and we have had a number of loosenings from simple falls or vigorous exercise. The double-stapling technique confers extra stability. The most recent innovation, the buckle/staple, has even greater resistance against being dislodged. We modified the technique as we became aware of loosening in the early stages and the more secure fixation techniques are allowing us to mobilize our patients with confidence at a much earlier stage.

The overall results in this series compare favourably with other series of cruciate reconstruction using both autogenous materials,[12,17,32] and prosthetic substitutes.[19,20,33,34] The technique described in this contribution avoids the problems associated with stretching of autogenous materials and damage to normal structures, which can have complications such as patellar tendon rupture, patellofemoral problems and stiffness of the knee. In addition, we avoid synovitis associated with Gore-Tex.[34]

We now have follow-ups which extend up to 8 years. Many of the original patients are still indulging in vigorous sporting activity without clinical deterioration. There have, however, been a number of patients with increased loosening in reviews over a period of time. These patients have instability only on clinical testing, either by Lachman test or the laxometer, but there is no concomitant reduction in their Lysholm scoring or function. These patients do appear to have reduced their level of sporting performance. There has been a report of patients with Leeds–Keio prostheses who underwent arthroscopy showing a high incidence of loosening and rupture in the early stages.[35] This may be due to the inadequate short-term fixation, which is certainly our experience in some of the patients in this series; early rupture without significant trauma may be due to incorrect placement of the prosthesis. We are continuing to study this group and are using the prosthesis in some acute repairs, in multicomplex injuries and in posterior cruciate reconstructions. For patients with a high expectation of return to contact sports, an intra-articular prosthesis alone is probably insufficient. In these patients, we feel, an extra-articular component is required, although in many cases there will be a sacrifice of full flexion.

In summary, we have presented the results of a group of 66 patients with a Leeds–Keio implantation for chronic anterior cruciate insufficiency. We were able to follow up 91% of the patients. The complication rate is relatively low and the main concern has been the number of patients who had rupture or loosening. The overall results have been encouraging, 78% showing good or excellent results with Lysholm scores of over 84. The clinical instability in the form of the pivot shift test has been completely eliminated in 75% of the series and the majority of the improvements have been maintained after sequential testing.

Acknowledgment

I should like to thank Registrars Fergal Monsell for preparation of much of the data, and David Shaw and Steve McLoughlin who carried out much of the assessment. Thanks are also due to the Department of Medical Illustration at the Royal Preston Hospital for preparation of the illustrations and my secretary, Miss H. Rylance, for the manuscript.

Mr Monsell's post is partly supported by a grant from Howmedica.

References

1. **Bohr H**, Experimental osteoarthritis in the rabbit knee joint, *Acta Orthop Scand* (1976) **47**: 558–565.

2. **Marshall JL, Olsson SE**, Instability of the knee: a long-term experimental study in dogs, *J Bone Joint Surg (Am)* (1971) **53**: 1561–1570.

3. **Marshall JL, Rubin RM, Wang JB** et al., The anterior cruciate ligament: The diagnosis and treatment of its injuries and their serious prognostic implications, *Orthop Rev* (1978) **7**: 35–46.

4. **Hughston JC, Barrett GR**, Acute anteromedial rotatory instability: long-term results of surgical repair, *J Bone Joint Surg (Am)* (1983) **65**: 145–153.

5. **McDaniel WJ Jr, Dameron TB Jr**, Untreated ruptures of the anterior cruciate ligament: a follow-up study, *J Bone Joint Surg (Am)* (1980) **62**: 696–705.

6. **Noyes FR, Mooar PA, Matthews DS** et al., The symptomatic anterior cruciate-deficient knee. Part I: the long-term functional disability in athletically active individuals, *J Bone Joint Surg (Am)* (1983) **65**: 154–162.

7. **Giove TP, Miller SJ III, Kent BE** et al., Non-operative treatment of the torn anterior cruciate ligament, *J Bone Joint Surg (Am)* (1983) **65**: 184–192.

8. **Feagin JA Jr, Curl WW**, Isolated tear of the anterior cruciate ligament: 5-year follow-up study, *Am J Sports Med* (1976) **4**: 95–100.

9. **Noyes FR, Matthews DS, Mooar PA** et al., The symptomatic anterior cruciate-deficient knee. Part II: the results of rehabilitation, activity modification and counselling on functional disability. *J Bone Joint Surg (Am)* (1983) **65**: 163–174.

10. **Satku K, Kumar VP, Ngoi SS**, Anterior cruciate ligament injuries: To counsel or to operate?, *J Bone Joint Surg (Br)* (1986) **68**: 458–461.

11. **MacIntosh DL, Darby TA**, Lateral substitution reconstruction, *J Bone Joint Surg (Br)* (1976) **58**: 142.

12. **Bray RC, Flanagan JP, Dandy DJ**, Reconstruction for chronic anterior cruciate instability: a comparison of two methods after six years, *J Bone Joint Surg (Br)* (1988) **70**: 100–105.

13. **Campbell WC**, Repair of ligaments of the knee: report of new operation for repair of anterior cruciate ligament, *Surg Gynaecol Obstet* (1936) **62**: 964–968.

14. **Jones KG**, Reconstruction of the anterior cruciate ligament: a technique using the central one-third of the patellar ligament, *J Bone Joint Surg (Am)* (1963) **45**: 925–932.

15. **Bonamo JJ, Krinick RM, Sporn AA**, Rupture of the patellar ligament after use of its central third for anterior cruciate reconstruction: a report of two cases, *J Bone Joint Surg (Am)* (1984) **66**: 1294–1297.

16. **Johnson RJ, Eriksson E, Haggmark T** et al., Five- to ten-year follow-up evaluation after reconstruction of the anterior cruciate ligament, *Clin Orthop* (1984) **183**: 122–140.

17. **Paterson FWN, Trickey EL**, Anterior cruciate ligament reconstruction using part of the patellar tendon as a free graft, *J Bone Joint Surg (Br)* (1986) **68**: 453–457.

18. **Rushton N, Dandy DJ, Naylor CPE**, The clinical, arthroscopic and histological findings after replacement of the anterior cruciate ligament with carbon-fibre, *J Bone Joint Surg (Br)* (1983) **65**: 308–309.

19. **Harilainen A, Myllynen P**, Treatment of fresh tears of the anterior cruciate ligament: a comparison of primary suture and augmentation with carbon fibre, *Injury* (1987) **18**: 396–400.

20. **King JB, Bulstrode CJK**, Extra-articular carbon fibre at the knee, *J Bone Joint Surg (Br)* (1985) **67**: 156–157.

21. **Seedhom BB**, The Leeds–Keio ligament: biomechanics. In *Prosthetic ligament reconstruction of the knee*, ed Friedman MJ, Ferkel RD (Philadelphia: WB Saunders, 1988), 118–131.

22. **Fujikawa K, Iseki F, Seedhom BB**, Arthroscopy after anterior cruciate reconstruction with the Leeds–Keio ligament, *J Bone Joint Surg (Br)* (1989) **71**: 566–570.

23. **Galway RD, Beaupré A, MacIntosh DL**, Pivot shift: a clinical sign of symptomatic anterior cruciate insufficiency, *J Bone Joint Surg (Br)* (1972) **54**: 763–764.

24. **Losee RE, Johnson TR, Southwick WO**, Anterior subluxation of the lateral tibial plateau: a diagnostic test and operative repair, *J Bone Joint Surg (Am)* (1978) **60**: 1015–1030.

25. **Slocum DB, Larson RL**, Rotatory instability of the knee: Its pathogenesis and a clinical test to demonstrate its presence, *J Bone Joint Surg (Am)* (1968) **50**: 211–225.

26. **Lysholm J, Gillquist J**, Evaluation of knee ligament surgery results with special emphasis on use of a scoring scale, *Am J Sports Med* (1982) **10**: 150–154.

27. **Steiner ME, Brown C, Zarins B** et al., Measurement of anterior–posterior displacement of the knee, *J Bone Joint Surg (Am)* (1990) **72**: 1307–1315.

28. **Girgis FG, Marshall JL, Al Monajem ARS**, The cruciate ligaments of the knee joint: anatomical, functional and experimental analysis, *Clin Orthop* (1975) **106**: 216–231.

29. **Norwood LA, Cross MJ**, Anterior cruciate ligament: functional anatomy of its bundles in rotatory instabilities, *Am J Sports Med* (1979) **7**: 23–26.

30. **Noyes FR, DeLucas JL, Torvik PJ**, Biomechanics of anterior cruciate ligament failure: an analysis of strain-rate sensitivity and mechanisms of failure in primates, *J Bone Joint Surg (Am)* (1974) **56**: 236–253.

31. **Seedhom BB, Bowes M**, European surgical questionnaire, unpublished data (1989).

32. **Clancy WG Jr, Ray JM, Zoltan DJ**, Acute tears of the anterior cruciate ligament: surgical versus conservative treatment, *J Bone Joint Surg (Am)* (1988) **70**: 1483–1488.

33. **Jenkins DHR**, The repair of cruciate ligaments with flexible carbon fibre: a longer term study of the induction of new ligaments and of the fate of the implanted carbon, *J Bone Joint Surg (Br)* (1978) **60**: 520–522.

34. **Dahlstedt L, Dalén N, Jonsson U**, Gore-Tex prosthetic ligament versus Kennedy Ligament Augmentation device in anterior cruciate ligament reconstruction: a prospective randomized 3-year follow-up of 41 cases, *Acta Orthop Scand* (1990) **61**: 217–224.

35. **Macnicol MF, Penny ID, Sheppard K**, Early results of Leeds–Keio anterior cruciate ligament replacement, *J Bone Joint Surg (Br)* (1991) **73**: 377–380.

6.12   The ABC ligament for chronic anterior cruciate ligament insufficiency

Angus E. Strover

Other scaffold-type ligament replacements

Autogenous grafts

Autogenous tissue as a material for reconstruction of ligaments in chronically unstable knees is attractive as a totally biocompatible material. However, the harvesting of autogenous grafts can constitute a major drawback of the operation where perfectly competent musculotendinous structures such as the iliotibial tract, the hamstring tendons or part of the patellar tendon are compromised, leading to a significant number of cosmetic and functional complications.[1-9] Revision procedures are then made more difficult and damaging, firstly by the fact that important secondary stabilizing structures have been either weakened or lost, and secondly by the scarification of the donor sites which are unable to yield a second crop of autogenous grafting material. This leads to more difficult surgery and the likelihood of a second-rate result in the revision procedure.

Patellar tendon grafts—the 'gold standard'?

At the time of harvest, most autogenous grafts do not possess the tensile strength of the natural anterior cruciate ligament (ACL) which they are replacing. The central third of the patellar tendon with its attached bony insertions does appear to perform better than the normal anterior cruciate ligament during tensile testing in vitro.[10] The donor site appears to regenerate satisfactorily in most patients and the graft itself revascularizes to produce a structure almost identical in appearance to the original anterior cruciate ligament.[11] Patellar tendon grafting has, therefore, recently been regarded as the 'gold standard'[12] for its mechanical strength, biological acceptance and clinical results.

In vitro tensile testing of the graft, however, does not adequately reproduce the shear stresses and angular forces encountered during flexion and extension in vivo,[13] and this would seem to throw doubt on the actual mechanical adequacy of the patellar tendon graft. Also the fibres of the patellar tendon graft in general run parallel, unlike the fibre bundles of the normal anterior cruciate ligament. Therefore, in vivo it may well be that the tensile properties of the patellar tendon graft are much reduced.

Furthermore, the transplanted autogenous patellar tendon graft initially undergoes a process of ischaemic necrosis, revascularization and proliferation,[11] during which time there is a drop in its tensile strength. These processes are followed by remodelling, when the graft regains some of its lost strength,[14] but it is dubious whether the grafted anterior cruciate ligament ever totally regains its original tensile strength.[15]

Morbidity of graft harvest

Complications of patellar tendon reconstruction include persistent flexion contracture of the knee,[13] postoperative fracture of the patella,[16] avulsion of the patella tendon from the inferior pole of the patella,[17] weakness of the quadriceps mechanism and poor hop function,[13,18] patellar tendon discomfort and patellofemoral pain,[18] infrapatellar contracture or secondary patella baja.[19,20]

Although postoperative flexion contracture and joint stiffness in autogenous repairs have been reduced during the past 5 years with improved postoperative mobilization,[21,22] occasionally manipulations under anaesthesia, arthroscopic release of adhesions and open surgery have been necessary following autogenous grafting.[13,19,23-25] The complication of peripatellar pain, which can be very disabling, is particularly disturbing.

The 'gold standard' patellar tendon reconstruction of the anterior cruciate ligament is, therefore, not without its hazards. In particular, the morbidity of graft harvest and the necessary postoperative reduction of mobilization continue to reduce the number of excellent results and to make revision of the failed operations problematic.

Human allografts

The use of fresh allografts has recently shown promising results,[26] but the problem of possible inoculation of the recipient with the HIV organism, although remote, has yet to be solved before this technique can be utilized in all countries.

The search for a better operation and a source of donor or prosthetic material that will adequately substitute for the original anterior cruciate ligament and allow patients to return to normal physical activities at their original level of involvement is an ongoing quest of orthopaedic surgeons and sportsmen alike.

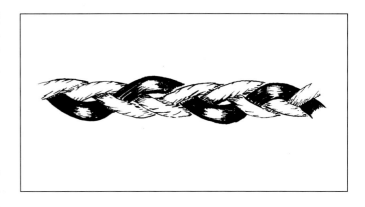

Figure 1

Zig-zag composite assembly of carbon and polyester yarns.

Choice of synthetic materials for the ABC ligament

Carbon fibres

Carbon fibre had shown promising results in animal experimentation and in early clinical results, particularly in the extra-articular situation.[27–31] Biocompatibility studies and histological studies in man[30,32] corroborated the animal experiments in that fibroblasts were shown to use the carbon filaments as a scaffold, producing collagen fibres orientated in the direction of these filaments. In subsequent clinical use of carbon fibre,[33–36] it became obvious that carbon fibres suffered from the disadvantages of their extreme stiffness and the fact that they have little resilience to shear forces.[37,38] Fragmentation of the fibres within the knee joint led to unsightly staining of the synovium, with a variable degree of foreign body reaction. To some extent, poor results could be put down to a failure of surgical technique, and it was shown that successful results using carbon-fibre implants could be achieved by careful attendance to the operative technique.[39] Nevertheless, disillusionment with carbon fibre as a material for the synthetic reconstruction of the anterior cruciate ligament became general.

Polyester fibres

Polyesters are in common usage in surgery[40–43] and indeed one study has indicated that the fibrous tissue

ingrowth into a scaffold of polyester fibres could be better than that induced by carbon.[44]

In the form of sutures[45] and vascular prostheses[46–49] polyester has been well documented over the past 35 years and clinical experience has shown its efficacy and safety in this respect.[49–52] In particular, the durability of Dacron vascular grafts, their relative tissue inertness and the ability of the knitted material to encourage both endothelial tissue and adventitial fibrous tissue around the graft make it attractive as a material for use as fibrous tissue scaffolds for the anterior cruciate ligament.[46]

Disadvantages of polyester fibres are to be found in terms of their mechanical creep under tensile load.[38]

Combination of carbon and polyester fibres

It seemed logical to combine the relatively good properties of polyester fibres in terms of durability, biocompatibility and long-term clinical experience with the good properties of carbon in terms of its stiffness and tissue induction to produce an improved biological scaffold. The disadvantages of the polyester fibres in terms of mechanical creep under tensile load could in theory be counterbalanced by the complete lack of creep of the stiff carbon fibres if the two sets of fibres were combined.

After some experimentation, a composite assembly was discovered in which carbon fibres were interwoven with polyester fibres in a type of plaited arrangement (Figure 1), the so-called zig-zag configuration.[53]

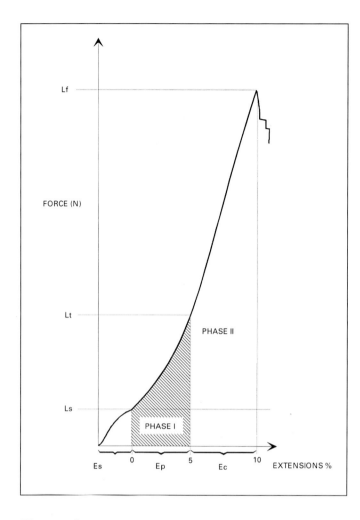

Figure 2

Representative force–extension curve for the ABC zig-zag material, showing the biphasic response to tensile loading. Es, extension due to settling of the yarns; Ep, extension mostly involving polyester fibres; Ec, extension mostly involving carbon. Ls, settle point; Lt, transition point; Lf, failure point. (Adapted with permission from data supplied by the Quality Control Dept., Surgicraft Limited, Redditch, UK.)

Tensile testing of the ABC material

The biphasic response to tensile loading

The zig-zag composite material was tested by tensile loading and found to have a biphasic response in which load was first taken by the polyester fibres, which extended until the carbon fibres straightened out. The overall stiffness of the material then increased dramatically as the carbon took its share of the load. In the first phase the characteristics of the load–extension curve were predominantly those of the polyester fibres, whereas in the second phase the stiffer carbon fibres played the predominant role (Figure 2).[54]

Achievement of true mechanical compatibility

By adjustment of the relative tensions of the carbon and polyester fibres, it became clear that the desired stiffness of the assembly could be engineered to produce mechanical characteristics remarkably similar to those shown by Butler and co-workers[55] for normal human knee ligaments.

This is perhaps not surprising when it is recognized that natural tendons and ligaments are made up of a tissue of collagen and elastin fibres. Collagen fibres, which are very stiff, are naturally crimped in their native state. Elastin fibres, on the other hand, are highly extensible and exhibit elastic behaviour well beyond that of the collagen. During the first phase of extension under load both the crimped collagen and the elastin fibres allow extension to occur in an approximately elastic manner. The crimp of the collagen is then straightened out and the second phase of the load–extension curve is almost linear up to the

Table 1 Summary of histological and strength findings related to the ABC ligament replacement in vivo, goat studies (not placed retrosynovially). (After ref. 59.)

	Instant	6 months	12 months
Synovial tissue		Carbon staining	Mild synovitis
Intra-articular tissue		Good soft tissue ingrowth	Two ruptures, soft tissue ingrowth
Intra-osseous tissue*		Bone and soft tissue around outer sheath	Similar to observations at 6 months
Breaking load ABC (N)	979±183	726±335	1134±83

* Interosseous sections—new bone was seen to have formed in a ring around the implant but was separated from the ligament replacement by a layer of fibroblastic tissue. No attempt by this tissue to penetrate the periphery.

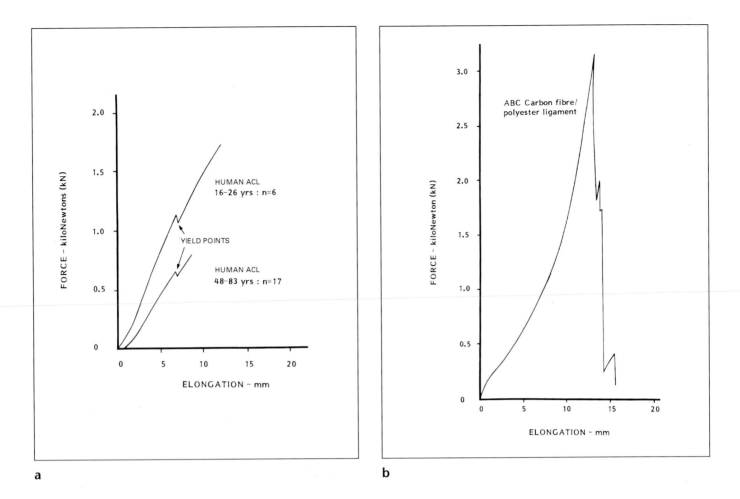

a

b

Figure 3

(a) Average force–extension curves of human anterior cruciate ligaments. (After ref. 56.) (b) Actual force–extension curve of a 15.5 cm ABC carbon fibre/polyester ligament.

point of failure (Figure 3a),[56] just as in the load–extension curve displayed by the carbon/polyester ABC ligament (Figure 3b).[57,58]

The theoretical advantages of implanting a biological scaffold that is biomechanically compatible with naturally occurring ligament tissue have obvious attractions. An early form of this material was made into a prosthetic anterior cruciate ligament for goats and implanted in a controlled trial comparing it with three other types of currently used ligament.[59] The results (Table 1) showed that the ABC material exhibited both an exuberant ingrowth of tissue over a period of months and an increase in its mechanical strength with the passage of time.

Design of the ABC prosthetic ligaments

Using the ABC material, definitive ligament implants were designed for the medial collateral, lateral collat-

eral and cruciate ligaments, all retaining the same general principles: (a) an open region of unconstrained strands of unit material designed to allow the ingrowth of fibrous tissue and (b) terminal loops where the strands of unit material are constrained by overbraiding with polyester yarn (Figure 4).

The anterior and posterior cruciate ligaments were designed to be exactly the same size. On the basis of published data for the tensile strength of cruciate ligaments,[55,56] a safety factor of approximately 2 was decided upon, with the ultimate tensile strength chosen being 3000 newtons for the cruciate ligament implants, 1200 and 600 newtons for the medial and lateral collateral ligaments, respectively.

Attachment to bone

Osseous attachment or ingrowth into carbon and polyester fibres has not been shown in the human or animal experiments using the ABC ligament.[36,58] The aim of the ABC procedure is to create a *fibrous attach-*

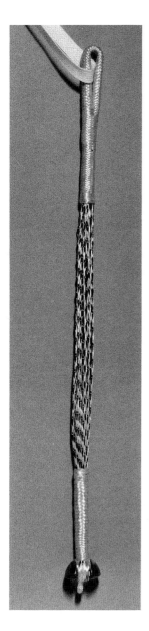

Figure 4

ABC ligament structure. Open section in middle and overbraiding at end towards terminal loops.

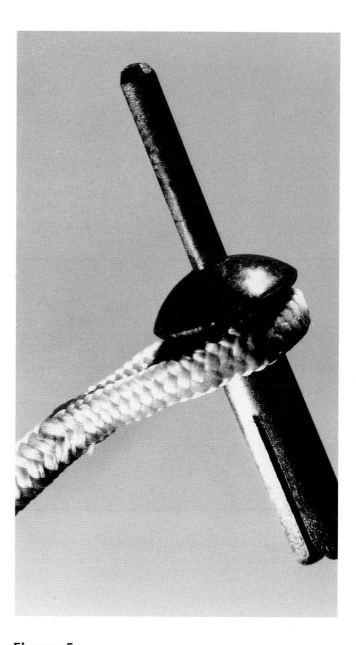

Figure 5

Polysulphone/carbon composite bollard placed into loop of ABC ligament.

ment to bone. The actual attachment of the ingrowth fibrous tissue and the artificial fibres of the scaffold should be to the original bony attachment of the natural ligament itself. It was, therefore, decided to manufacture the double-looped ligament longer than the natural ligament, with the unconstrained active scaffolding area only in the region of the reconstructed ligament and with the loops attached to bone well beyond this (Figures 4 and 7).

It was decided to avoid the use of metallic staples as anchorage devices to bone, partly because of the danger of creating electrochemical reactions between the metal and the carbon fibres, and partly to avoid the hazard of breaking the fibres by creating stress risers. The loops on the implants were therefore designed to be used with bollards[60-62] made from a polysulphone–carbon composite (Figure 5). In the cruciate ligament implants, a polysulphone button was attached to one loop to anchor the implant into the mouth of the tibial drillhole.

Polysulphone had been chosen as a plastic with excellent biomechanical properties for use in bone[63] and extensive experience had been gained with the use of composite carbon and polysulphone devices in the reconstruction of cruciate ligaments with carbon fibres.[60-62]

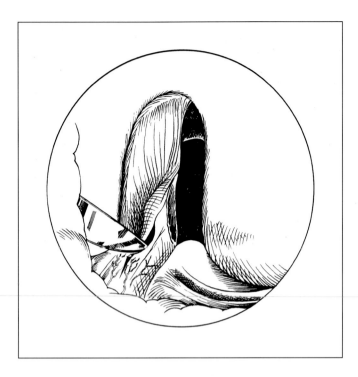

Figure 6

Intact synovium with torn cruciate ligament showing splitting of remnant for retrosynovial placement of ABC anterior cruciate ligament.

Surgical principles for implantation

The important principles for the implantation of the ABC ligament in the human were decided to be the following: (1) the retrosynovial principle; (2) the central to posterior position of the tibial drillhole; (3) the 'straight-through' route with the knee in full extension; (4) avoidance of abrasion or breakage of the synthetic material on sharp edges or corners; (5) the 'over-the-top route'; (6) attention to size and shape of the intercondylar notch; and (7) tensioning of the ligament with the knee in 20° of flexion.

The retrosynovial principle

The cruciate ligaments, although intra-articular, are retrosynovial or extrasynovial structures and are almost entirely dependent for their neurovascular support on the popliteal vessels and nerves. Very little of their biological support comes from their attachment areas to bone. It is logical, therefore, when using a biological scaffold replacement for cruciate ligaments to place the scaffold material where it is most able to be invaded by healing fibrovascular tissue. To this end, the following surgi-

cal principles were decided upon depending upon the extent of the cruciate ligament remnant.

Intact synovium covering torn or ruptured ligament

The intercondylar synovium should be split and the synthetic ligament placed posterior to the intercondylar synovial face. In order to gain access to this position, the intercondylar synovium should be split vertically (Figure 6), taking care to preserve the intact posterior cruciate ligament, and the probe of a jig should be placed through the split on to the bone of the interspinous fossa of the tibia. A guide wire is then brought through the tibia accurately into the middle of the interspinous region and the artificial ligament will subsequently be placed in the retrosynovial tissues, rather than within the synovial cavity of the knee.

Tibial remnant

Whenever possible, the tibial remnant of the anterior cruciate ligament should be preserved and used as a biological augmentation for the artificial ligament. It may be split by sharp dissection, bringing the drillhole into the middle of the split. Alternatively, the drillhole should be placed posterior to the bulk of the remnant, which will ensure adequate biological cover for the biological scaffold.

Absence of tibial remnant

When the cruciate ligament has been removed from its tibial attachment and there is no remnant in this area, the interspinous fossa is covered by a tongue of synovial tissue. Splitting this synovial remnant and continuing the split superiorly to include the intercondylar synovium overlying the posterior cruciate ligament will usually give adequate biological cover.

No remnant or synovium after removal of tibial spines

Where excessive bone has developed by encroachment of the tibial spines, these should be removed by osteotomy, in which case no biological remnant, either synovial or ligamentous, remains in this area. It may be necessary to steal some of the intercondylar synovium from the medial side overlying the posterior cruciate ligament. In a few cases, even this may prove to be difficult and a free graft of fat and synovium is taken from the retropatellar fat pad and lightly sutured into position to cover the ligament.

The central to posterior position of the tibial drillhole

The position of the tibial drillhole within the interspinous fossa was chosen to be central and posterior rather than anteromedial for the following reasons:

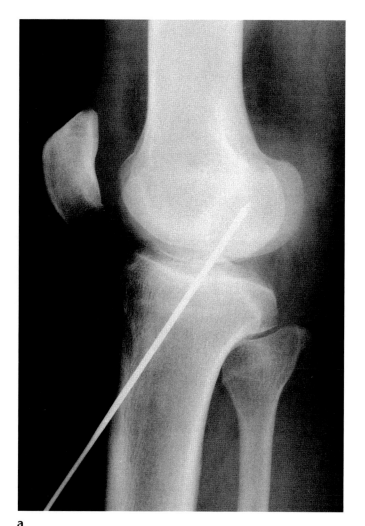

a

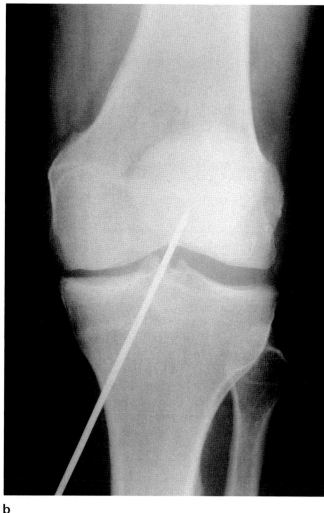

b

Figure 7

(a) Lateral and (b) anteroposterior radiographs of the knee demonstrating 'straight through' positioning of tibial guide-wire in extension.

(a) In full extension the anterior edge of the inter-condylar notch reaches the position of the tibial spines and, indeed, may abut on them in this position. In order to avoid impingement and damage to the synthetic ligament, it is important to position it out of harm's way.

(b) The biological reasons for this position are mentioned above—the retrosynovial principle.

(c) The anterior cruciate ligament is attached to the tibia by an area which measures approximately 17 mm in length by 11 mm in width.[64] It tends to be pear-shaped with the stem of the pear anteriorly. A 6-mm drillhole for the artificial ligament placed in the widest area of this attachment is easily accommodated and occupies approximately one-tenth of the total area.

The 'straight-through' position in full extension

It was decided to choose a route through the knee in the extended position for the following anatomical and biomechanical reasons:

(a) Most weight-bearing activity in the human knee takes place in the first 20° of flexion.

(b) In about 20° of flexion, the restraint supplied by the anterior cruciate ligament has its maximum importance. In the cruciate deficient knee, it is in this position that the collateral ligament and the posterior capsule are in a state of relative laxity, allowing the tibia to translate forward maximally.

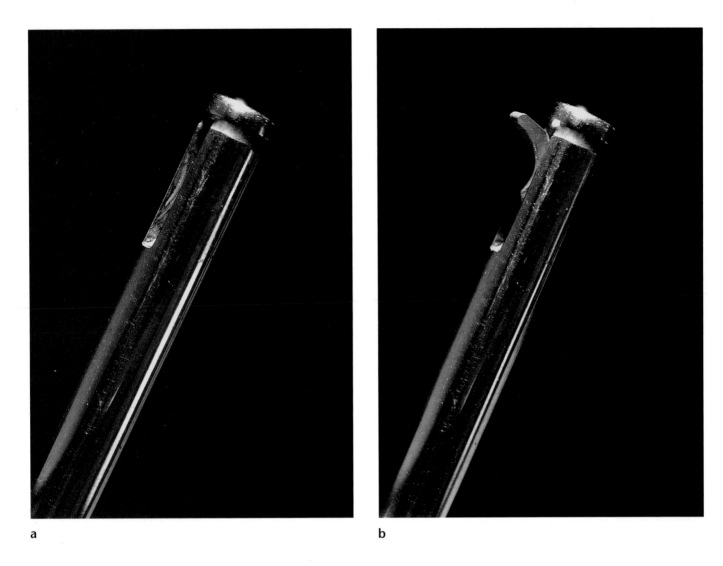

a   b

Figure 8

ABC back radius cutter. (a) Blade retracted, (b) blade protruded.

(c) In anterior cruciate insufficiency, the disabling pivot shift phenomenon occurs within the first 20° of flexion.[65]

(d) The angulation of the main body of the anterior cruciate ligament to the tibial plateau corresponds to the angle made by the roof of the intercondylar notch when the knee is placed in full extension.

The angulation of the drillhole through the tibial head was, therefore, chosen to coincide with the angle of the anterior cruciate ligament in the sagittal, transverse and coronal planes with *the knee in the position of full extension*, and a jig was made to place a guidewire for a drillhole in this position (Figure 7).

Avoidance of fibre abrasion or breakage on drillholes

Abrasion or breakage of artificial fibres on the internal edges of the drillholes has already been identified as a major problem in the survival of scaffold-type grafts.[62] The naturally occurring anterior cruciate ligament attachment to bone by Sharpey's fibres and by an intermediate zone of fibrocartilage[66] cannot be mimicked by the bony attachment of the artificial scaffold-type ligament.

By appearing through a drillhole in tibia, there is a permanent danger of creating areas of high stress at the edges of the hole that may break the artificial fibres while under tension during movements of the knee.

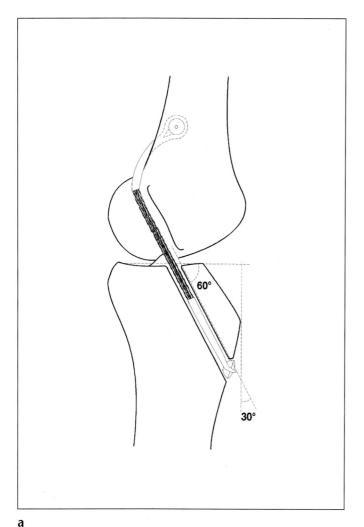

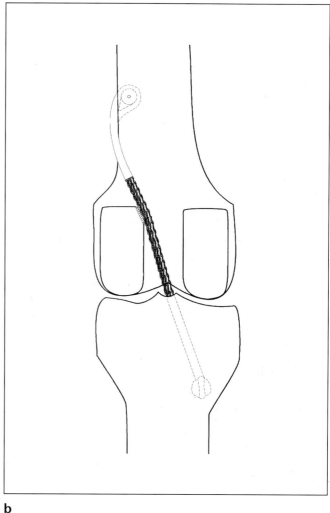

a   b

Figure 9

'Straight through' route of ABC ligament: (a) lateral and (b) posteroanterior views.

This problem has been addressed by the use of a radius cutter (Figure 8) which has a retractable curved blade. The instrument is passed through the tibial drillhole with the blade in the retracted position. Once through the hole, the blade is protruded and the edge of the hole is carved into a smooth, curved shape.

This instrument had already been introduced and tried in the use of carbon fibre implants[39,62] with some measure of success, but it remains difficult to use effectively and depends upon the manual skill of the surgeon to adequately remove the sharp edge of the drillhole.

The 'over-the-top' route

The 'over-the-top' route was chosen for attachment of the ligament to the femur in preference to the percondylar route via a hole in the lateral femoral condyle for the following reasons:

(a) Most importantly, it was decided to avoid the danger of fibre breakage on the edges of a second drillhole.

(b) The 'straight-through' principle in full extension would be more closely complied with by the use of the 'over-the-top' route.

(c) The operative technique in drilling a hole through the femoral condyle is subject to variation between surgeons, and it was thought that the 'over-the-top' route would lead to more consistency in this respect.

(d) The use of the 'over-the-top' route always ensures full flexion of the knee. In other words, no limitation of flexion can be caused by an overtightened restraint, as it is maximally loose in flexion and tightens in full extension.

The direction of the 'over-the-top' route was modified so that the ligament passed behind the lateral supracondylar ridge of the femur in an almost axial direction to be anchored onto the cortical bone on the lateral aspect of the femoral shaft (Figure 9).

A rasp was designed to take off any sharp edges around the 'over-the-top' route, and at the same time to remove any periosteum and soft tissue intervening between the implant and the bone; this also recesses the implant slightly into the lateral supracondylar ridge. The final route of the implant was then seen to be straight through the knee in both AP and lateral views (Figure 9).

Attention to the size and shape of the intercondylar notch

Osteophytic encroachment causing irregularity and narrowing of the intercondylar notch is well known[64] and constitutes a danger to both autogenous and artificial ligament replacements. In the chronic ACL deficient knee, the size of the notch is often severely reduced and inadequate to accommodate both the posterior cruciate and a reconstructed anterior cruciate ligament.

Although the position of the tibial drillhole is designed to avoid impingement on the anterior edge of the intercondylar notch, this in itself is not always sufficient and the notch requires enlargement both superiorly and laterally. This procedure should leave the notch large enough to accept the ABC ligament; the side-walls and edges of the notch should be regular and rounded-off where appropriate.

To test the direction and positioning of the drillhole in the intercondylar notch, a blunt-ended instrument, the T-bar, was designed to be passed up the tibial drill hole. Its position in relation to the walls and roof of the intercondylar notch and to the posterior cruciate ligament with the knee in full extension gives a clear idea of the space available for the ABC ligament. With the T-bar in place, the knee is put through a range of movements. If the T-bar is found to be abutting on the lateral superior edges of the notch, either the notch can be increased in size by notchplasty using osteotomes and burrs or the tibial drillhole can be made again. The instruments were designed so that they could be used by arthroscopic control as well as the open technique.

Tensioning the ligament with the knee in 20° of flexion

The tibial end of the ABC ligament is first anchored either by the attached button or by a bollard (on request from the manufacturers) situated 1 cm distally to the entrance of the tibial drillhole. The positioning of the bollard anchorage on the femur is chosen using a centre punch in the proximal loop of the implant.

Final tensioning of the ligament is performed manually with the knee in approximately 20° of flexion and the foot externally rotated. A bollard hole is drilled in the chosen anchorage position of the femur and the bollard is positioned through the ABC ligament loop into the anchorage hole while the knee is checked for full extension.

Approximately 5° of flexion deformity at the time of operation is acceptable, as our experience has been that this will stretch out. It the ligament has been anchored in a position of excessive tightness, however, the unexpanded bollard may be simply removed, and a separate drillhole made in the femoral cortex slightly more distally and more anteriorly may be chosen. The system lends itself to precise adjustment and precise positioning of the ligament at operation.

Principles of postoperative treatment

The main concern in the postoperative period is to establish the following:

1. Incorporation of the scaffold material with protective fibrovascular tissue.
2. Avoidance of breakage of artificial fibres on the edges of the drillhole in the tibia and around the 'over-the-top' route.
3. Establishment of relatively early motion of the knee and avoidance of excessive disuse atrophy of muscle and bones.
4. The avoidance of reduced range of movement, either in flexion or extension, due to cicatricial adhesions.

The postoperative regime for the ABC ligament has been modified empirically by the users. The author has chosen to immobilize the knee in full extension while allowing full weight bearing for the first 6 postoperative weeks. Others[67] have chosen to allow the patient immediate free motion with restricted weight bearing for 3 weeks, after which full weight bearing is permitted.

Physiotherapy in both instances is directed towards gaining a full range of knee movement within the first 12 weeks after the operation. In the 5 years' usage of the ABC ligament the postoperative treatment of patients appear to have made little significant difference to the results and complications.

Results

Results to date from more than one clinical study show that at least within the first 2–5 years, 70% of patients return to sporting activity.[68] Of these, approximately 67% return to their original level and 33% to a lower level of sporting activity. This compares favourably with other methods of reconstruction, but long-term follow-up is required to see whether these results deteriorate after 5 years. Reported complications have been surprisingly few, and in the series reported by Rees et al.[69] out of 45 cases a small number of complications were documented arthroscopically and histologically (Tables 2, 3, 4).

It is important to note that stiffness is not a major feature of these cases and in practically all cases a full range of movement was obtained. All these cases were operated upon using the arthrotomy technique as the results in arthroscopic introduction of ABC ligament have not yet been analysed.

Table 2 Complications of anterior cruciate ligament reconstruction using ABC carbon fibre/polyester ligament demonstrated during arthroscopic examination. (280 ligaments implanted in 268 knees; 49 post-operative arthroscopic examinations in 45 knees, average follow-up 18 months, range 6–47 months.) The reason for arthroscopy. (After ref. 69.)

Routine arthroscopy	13
Recurrence of instability	19
Locking	6
Pain	5
Stiffness	4
Persistent swelling	1
Stretched ligaments*	9

*Tightened-up stretching due to creep; problem solved since 1988, as ligament is now pre-stressed.

Table 3 Arthroscopic findings. (After ref. 69.)

Synovitis	5
Coverage	
fully covered	18
partial	19
largely uncovered	2
ruptured, varying coverage	10
Meniscal tears	7

Table 4 Histological findings. (After ref. 69.)

Foreign-body giant cell reaction to particulate polyester or carbon	26
No evidence of inflammation	10
Non-specific chronic inflammation no different from pre-op unstable knee	13

Failure of the ABC ligament

Mechanical failure of the fabric of the ABC ligament has occurred in approximately 10% of cases[70] and in practically all of these cases the failure occurred at the level of the tibial drillhole.[71] Failed specimens have been retrieved from several sources and an analysis of the mode of failure of the material[71] has shown the following important features:

1. Gross specimens practically without exception show an exuberant ingrowth of fibrovascular tissue within the region of the intercondylar notch and around the 'over-the-top' route. Some specimens have more than doubled their diameter and, therefore, increased their cross-sectional diameter by a factor of 4. Histological studies have shown an exuberant ingrowth of fibrovascular tissue between both the carbon and polyester fibres, but more significantly between the individual units of composite material (Figure 10).[70]

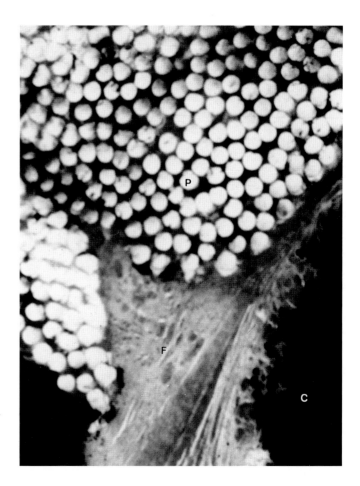

Figure 10

Histology showing growth of fibrovascular tissue (F) between both carbon (C) and polyester (P) fibres and between individual units of composite material. (After ref. 70.)

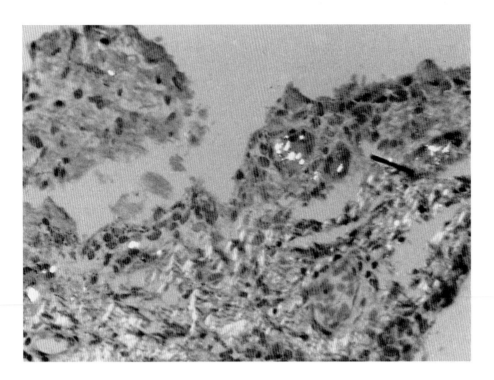

Figure 11

Histology showing synovium with increase of inflammatory cells stimulated by fragments of carbon and polyester. Note the intracellular polyester fragments in foreign-body giant cells and macrophages.

2. The synovium in failed cases has shown a variable degree of synovitis with the presence of histiocytes, macrophages and foreign-body giant cells which appear to be stimulated by the appearance of fragments of carbon and polyester. In some of the macrophages, intracellular debris can be clearly seen (Figure 11).

The individual reaction to the presence of the foreign material appears to vary from individual to individual and also within separate specimens. In general, however, it appears that neither the polyester fibres nor the carbon fibres are inert and this foreign-body response may be implicated in both the beneficial and adverse features of the histological findings.

While the fibrous tissue ingrowth into the material is encouraging for the possible long-term survival of the material in the artificial ligament, the synovial reaction to the products of abrasion and breakage are an obvious cause for concern. On the other hand, both Rees et al.[69] and Strover et al.[70] have shown that where no breakage has occurred and where the ligament has been macroscopically completely covered by synovium at arthroscopy, no foreign-body response in the synovium has been seen in biopsy specimens.

Ultramicroscopic analysis of failed specimens

The polyester fibres of failed ABC ligaments have lent themselves to analysis using scanning electron microscopy at the region of failure.[71] The appearance of the broken ends of the polyester fibres gives evidence of the mechanism by which failure has occurred. Several mechanisms of failure have been elucidated:

1. Early failures show signs of crushing and flattening (Figure 12a), with longitudinal splitting and fragmentation. One fibre becomes a set of multiple fibrils (Figure 12b).
2. Failures due to fatigue show damage in two forms, separately or in combination: (a) kink bands due to strand rotating against another and (b) transverse splits from biaxial rotational fatigue (Figure 12c).
3. Traumatic failure has been seen in one case only as a result of a rugby tackle. SEM studies show a clean break (Figure 12d).

Clean-cut division of the fibres as might have been expected from sharp spicules of bone or abrasion on

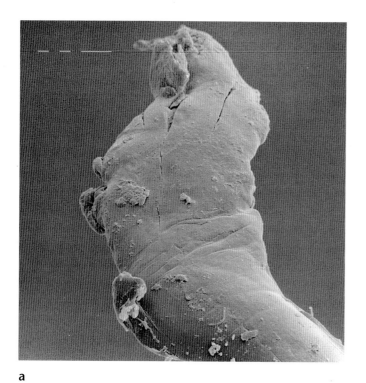

a

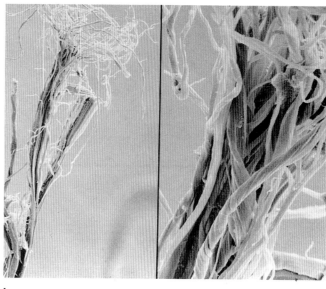

b

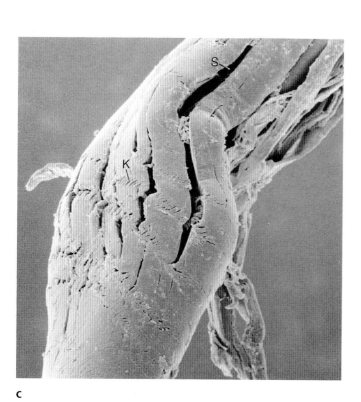

c

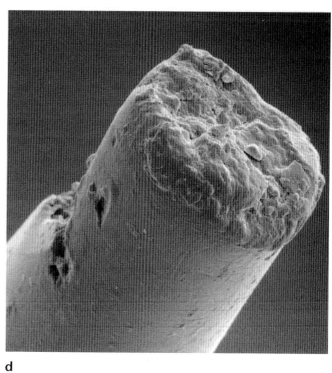

d

Figure 12

Scanning electron micrographs: (a) crushed end of polyester fibre; (b) fibrillated end to fibre; (c) fatigue-damaged kink bands (K) and splits (S); (d) tensile break. (Courtesy of Mr A.R.M. McLeod, Department of Textiles, University of Manchester Institute of Science and Technology, Manchester, UK.)

bony trabeculae has not been a feature in the failure of these specimens.

Anchorage failure

The bollard has been the most successful anchorage and has not been a cause of failure in any of the 150 cases followed from 2 to 5 years by Rees et al.[69] There have been a number of reported cases, however, where the tibial button has pulled into the upper end of the tibia. This has occurred in one of my patients with excessively osteoporotic bone and in another in whom early, very active mobilization took place. The implication is that the button is a weaker system of anchorage than the bollard and, indeed, in vitro testing has confirmed this.[72] This problem has been addressed by the making of double-bollard implants. In vitro testing of this system showed greatly improved tensile strength in comparison with the button fixation.

MRI scanning studies

New evidence from magnetic resonance imaging (MRI)[73] has shown that there appears to be more than one reason for failure of the ABC ligament in the intercondylar region.

1. The anterior positioning of the drillhole. Sagittal cuts through the ligament show quite clearly that, where the drillhole is placed too anteriorly, the impingement of intercondylar notch in full extension has precipitated failure (Figure 13). In a successful case, the straight-through positioning well posterior to the roof of the notch has avoided this problem (Figure 14).
2. The posterior edge of the tibial drillhole is apparently the other source of failure (Figure 13). This evidence correlates with the findings of McLeod et al.[71] and the evidence suggests that an improved and enlarged radius cutter is important as a future development for the ABC ligament.
3. It may be that tissue ingrowth into and between the fibres of the ABC ligament could produce a problem on the edges of the tibial drillhole by virtue of the increase in diameter of the ligament at this site. Plain radiographs and MRI scans have shown that the fibrous tissue ingrowth into the ABC ligament greatly enlarges the cross-sectional diameter of the tibial drillhole. This in itself may cause problems at the exit point of the tibial drill hole. It appears that the cancellous bone becomes eroded by the expanding ligament, leaving a sharp edge of subchondral bone which in itself may create a new hazard to the survival of the ligament.

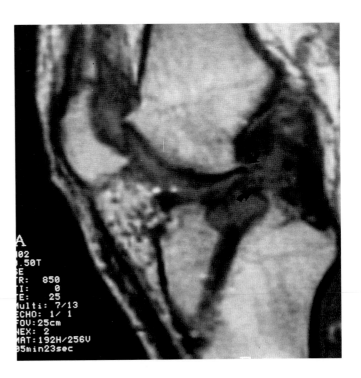

Figure 13

MRI sagittal section showing (arrows) impingement failure of ABC anterior cruciate ligament by intercondylar notch in full extension.

The problem of synovitis

Independent studies have shown that, where the ABC ligament has failed, the fragments of fibres, both polyester and carbon, have been associated with a foreign-body response and a variable degree of synovitis in the knee joint.[69,74] Although in most cases the synovitis appears to be mild and unassociated with symptoms of persistent effusion, in two cases referred to the author the damaged ligaments have caused an aggressive synovitis with persistent painful effusion. In both cases the ligaments were damaged and not broken but required removal on the grounds of persistent effusion. Neither of these cases has elected to undergo revision to an autogenous ACL substitute as both are apparently managing tolerably well without further operation.

In several patients, mild effusion at the time of increased activity at approximately 3 months after the operation have settled following a period of rest and anti-inflammatory drugs.

'Second-look' arthroscopies have been useful in the author's hands, not only in monitoring the survival of the ligament scaffold but also in assessing either the improvement or deterioration of osteochondral defects, meniscal lesions, etc. Although the incidence

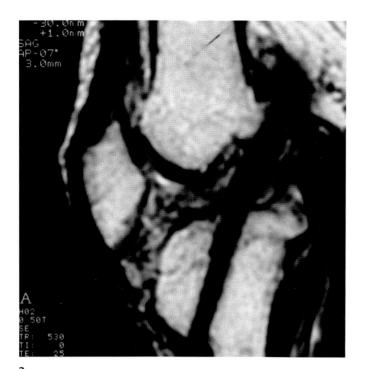

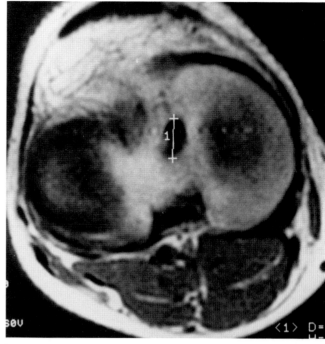

a   b

Figure 14

MRI scans, successful case, after 2 years: (a) sagittal and (b) coronal horizontal sections. Note especially the increased diameter of the ligament due to tissue ingrowth in the intercondylar region.

of subsequent meniscal tears in Rees's series has not been shown to be high, in two of my 5-year follow-up cases who have returned to sporting activity at their original levels, both have had subsequent meniscal tears on two occasions each. In these two cases, it was possible to monitor progress of degenerative changes which were present at the time of operation and in neither case was there any severe progression of these changes. Both these cases have maintained stability and their levels of sporting activity during the last 5 years.

Conclusions

The main advantages in the clinical use of the ABC scaffold type of artificial ligament are to be found in its long-term survival, its relative lack of associated complication, the absence of donor-site problems and its ability to be revised successfully in the case of failure. Results to date show that its use compares favourably with those of patellar-tendon grafts in the numbers of patients returning to sporting activities.

The main disadvantages lie in the fact that artificial fibres are not inert, and are fragile within the

hostile and physically demanding implantation site in the intercondylar region of the knee. At best, they are tolerated by the host with a relatively benign fibrovascular response, resulting in a strong composite structure of artificial fibres and scar tissue which is able to withstand the demands of sporting activity for at least 5 years. At worst, the fibres of the ABC ligament occasionally elicit a foreign-body reaction and synovitis which settles only after removal of the ligament. Mechanical failure of the ligament occurs almost exclusively at the site of the tibial drillhole and careful analysis of these failures suggests that the problem is largely one of surgical technique.

References

1. **Jones KG,** Reconstruction of the anterior cruciate ligament: A technique using the central one-third of the patellar ligament, *J Bone Joint Surg (Am)* (1963) **45:** 925–932.
2. **Brostrom L, Gillquist J, Liljedahl SO** et al., Behandling av inveterad ruptur av framre kors bandet, *Svenska Läkartidn* (1968) **64:** 449.
3. **Gillquist J, Liljedahl SO, Lindvall N,** Reconstruction for old rupture of the anterior cruciate ligament: A follow-up study, *Injury* (1971) **2:** 271–278.

4. Cho KO, Reconstruction of the anterior cruciate ligament by semitendinosus tenodesis, *J Bone Joint Surg (Am)* (1975) **57**: 608–612.

5. Lindemann K, Über den plastischen Ersatz der Kreutzbänder durch gestielte Sehnenverpflanzung, *Z Orthop* (1950) **79**: 316–334.

6. Hey Groves EW, The crucial ligaments of the knee joint: Their function, rupture and the operative treatment of the same, *Br J Surg* (1920) **7**: 505–515.

7. O'Donoghue DH, A method for replacement of the anterior cruciate ligament of the knee: Report of 20 cases, *J Bone Joint Surg (Am)* (1963) **45**: 905–924.

8. Lindström N, Cruciate ligament plastics with meniscus, *Acta Orthop Scand* (1959) **29**: 150–151.

9. Marshall JL, Reconstruction of functioning anterior cruciate ligament: Preliminary report using quadriceps tendon, *Orthop Rev* (1979) **8**: 49–55.

10. Noyes FR, Butler DL, Grood ES et al., Biomechanical analysis of human ligament grafts used in knee ligament repairs and reconstructions, *J Bone Joint Surg (Am)* (1984) **66**: 344–352.

11. Arnoczky SP, Tarvin GB, Marshall JL, Anterior cruciate ligament replacement using patellar tendon: An evaluation of graft revascularization in the dog, *J Bone Joint Surg (Am)* (1982) **64**: 217–224.

12. Eriksson E, personal communication, 1990.

13. Sachs RA, Reznik A, Daniel DM et al., Complications of knee ligament surgery, *Knee ligaments: structure, function, injury and repair*, ed Daniel DM, Akeson W, O'Connor J (New York: Raven Press, 1990) 505–520.

14. Kondo M, An experimental study on reconstructive surgery of the anterior cruciate ligament, *J Jpn Orthop Assoc* (1979) **53**: 521–533.

15. Woo SL-Y, Adams J, The tensile properties of human anterior cruciate ligament (ACL) and ACL graft tissues, *Knee ligaments: structure, function, injury and repair*, ed Daniel DM, Akeson W, O'Connor J (New York: Raven Press, 1990) 279–289.

16. McCarroll JR, Fracture of the patella during a golf swing following reconstruction of the anterior cruciate ligament: A case report, *Am J Sports Med* (1983) **11**: 26–27.

17. Bonamo JJ, Krinick RM, Sporn AA, Rupture of the patellar ligament after use of its central third for anterior cruciate reconstruction: A report of two cases, *J Bone Joint Surg (Am)* (1984) **66**: 1294–1297.

18. Huegel M, Indelicato P, Trends in rehabilitation following anterior cruciate ligament reconstruction, *Clin Sports Med* (1988) **7**: 801–811.

19. Paulos LE, Rosenberg TD, Drawbert J et al., Infrapatellar contracture syndrome: An unrecognised cause of knee stiffness with patellar entrapment and patella infera, *Am J Sports Med* (1987) **15**: 331–341.

20. Sachs RA, Daniel DM, Stone ML et al., Patellofemoral problems after anterior cruciate ligament reconstruction, *Am J Sports Med* (1989) **17**: 760–765.

21. Noyes FR, Mangine RE, Barber S, Early knee motion after open and arthroscopic anterior cruciate ligament reconstruction, *Am J Sports Med* (1987) **15**: 149–160.

22. Noyes FR, Butler DL, Paulos LE et al., Intra-articular cruciate ligament reconstruction. I: Perspectives on graft strength, vascularization and immediate motion after replacement, *Clin Orthop* (1983) **172**: 71–77.

23. Parisien JS, The role of arthroscopy in the treatment of postoperative fibroarthrosis of the knee joint, *Clin Orthop* (1988) **229**: 185–192.

24. Sprague NF III, O'Connor RL, Fox JM, Arthroscopic treatment of post-operative knee fibroarthrosis, *Clin Orthop* (1982) **166**: 165–172.

25. Nicoll EA, Quadricepsplasty, *J Bone Joint Surg (Br)* (1963) **45**: 483–490.

26. Shino K, Inoue M, Horibe S et al., Maturation of allograft tendons transplanted into the knee: An arthroscopic and histological study, *J Bone Joint Surg (Br)* (1988) **70**: 556–560.

27. Forster IW, A study of the mechanism by which carbon fibre acts as a tendon prosthesis, *J Bone Joint Surg (Br)* (1976) **58**: 376.

28. Jenkins DHR, Carbon fibre as a prosthetic implant material in orthopaedics, *J Bone Joint Surg (Br)* (1976) **58**: 253.

29. Jenkins DHR, Forster IW, McKibbin B et al., Induction of tendon and ligament formation by carbon implants, *J Bone Joint Surg (Br)* (1977) **59**: 53–57.

30. Wolter D, Biocompatibility of carbon fibre and carbon fibre microparticles, *Aktuelle Problems im Chirurgie und Orthopädie*, No. 26: Alloplastic Ligament Replacement, ed Burri C and Claes L (Bern: Hans Huber, 1983) 28–36.

31. Alexander H, Parsons JR et al., Anterior cruciate ligament replacement with filamentous carbon, *Trans Ann Meet Orthop Res Soc* (1982) **7**: 45.

32. Kramer B, King RE, The histological appearance of carbon fibre implants and neo-ligament in man, *South Afr Med J* (1983) **63**: 113–115.

33. Jenkins DHR, McKibbin B, The role of flexible carbon-fibre implants as tendon and ligament substitutes in clinical practice: a preliminary report, *J Bone Joint Surg (Br)* (1980) **62**: 497–499.

34. Weiss AB, Alexander H, Parsons JR, Ligament replacement with absorbable polymercarbon fibre scaffolds: early clinical experience, *Trans Ann Meet Soc Biomater* (1983) **6**: 54.

35. Rusch RM, Integraft anterior cruciate ligament reconstruction, *Prosthetic ligament reconstruction of the knee*, ed Friedman MJ and Ferkel RD (Philadelphia: WB Saunders 1988) 52–58.

36. Rushton N, Dandy DJ, Naylor CPE, The clinical, arthroscopic and histological findings after replacement of the anterior cruciate ligament with carbon-fibre, *J Bone Joint Surg (Br)* (1983) **65**: 308–309.

37. Bokros JC, Carbon biomedical devices, *Carbon* (1977) **15**: 355–371.

38. Claes L, Neugebauer R, Mechanical properties of ligament replacement with carbon fibres, *Aktuelle Problems im Chirurgie und Orthopädie*, No. 26: Alloplastic Ligament Replacement, ed Burri C and Claes L (Bern: Hans Huber, 1983) 58–62.

39. Strover AE, Firer P, The use of carbon fibre implants in anterior cruciate ligament surgery, *Clin Orthop* (1985) **196**: 88–98.

40. Park JP, Arnold JA, Coker TP et al., Treatment of acromioclavicular separations: A retrospective study, *Am J Sports Med* (1980) **8**: 251–256.

41. Frazier CH, Tendon repairs with Dacron vascular graft suture: a follow-up report, *Orthopaedics* (1981) **4**: 539–540.

42. Kappakas GS, McMaster JH, Repair of acromioclavicular separation using a Dacron prosthesis graft, *Clin Orthop* (1978) **131**: 247–251.

43. King RN, McKenna GB, Statton WO, Novel uses of fibres as tendons and bones, *J Appl Polymer Sci: Appl Polymer Symp* (1977) **31**: 335–350.

44. Amis AA, Campbell JR, Kempson SA et al., Comparison of the structure of neotendons induced by implantation of carbon or polyester fibres, *J Bone Joint Surg (Br)* (1984) **66**: 131–139.

45. Latimer EO, Werr JA, Clinical experience with Dacron as a non-absorbable suture material, *Surg Gynecol Obstet* (1961) **112**: 373–374.

46. Deterling RA Jr, Bhonslay SB, Evaluation of synthetic materials and fabrics suitable for blood vessel replacement, *Surgery* (1955) **38**: 71–89.

47. Creech O, Vascular prostheses: Report of the committee for the study of vascular prostheses of the Society for Vascular Surgery, *Surgery* (1957) **41**: 62–80.

48. Harrison JH, Synthetic materials as vascular prostheses, *Am J Surg* (1958) **95**: 3–24.

49. De Bakey ME, Cooley DA, Crawford ES, Clinical application of a new flexible knitted Dacron arterial substitute, *Arch Surg* (1958) **77**: 713–728.

50. De Bakey ME, Jordan GL, Abbott JP, The fate of Dacron vascular grafts, *Arch Surg* (1964) **89**: 757–782.

51. **Hall CW, Liotta D, Ghidoni JJ**, Velour fabrics applied to medicine, *J Biomed Mater Res* (1967) **1**: 179–196.

52. **Mitchell RS, Milleo DC, Billingham MB**, Comprehensive assessment of the safety, durability, clinical performance and healing characteristics for a double velour knitted Dacron arterial prosthesis, *Vasc Surg* (1980) **14**: 197–212.

53. **Moorse DJ, Strover AE**, Zig-zag sutures etc. UK Patent No. 8414344 (June 1984).

54. **Wrzesien A**, *Development of carbon fibre polyester composite ligaments*, (Manchester: Shirley Institute, 1984).

55. **Butler DL, Kay MD, Stouffer DC**, Comparison of material properties in fascicle-bone units from human patellar tendon and knee ligaments, *J Biomech* (1986) **19**: 425–432.

56. **Noyes FR, Grood ES**, The strength of the anterior cruciate ligament in humans and rhesus monkeys: Age-related and species-related changes, *J Bone Joint Surg (Am)* (1976) **58**: 1074–1082.

57. **Strover AE, Hughes F, O'Brien T** et al., Mechanical properties of the ABC carbon and polyester fibre anterior cruciate ligament, *Inst Mech Eng* (1989) **c384/064**: 97–102.

58. **Hughes F**, *Report on testing of carbon/polyester cruciate ligament to establish production pre-loading, effect of reducing overbraiding and effects of washing*, Technical documentation (Surgicraft Limited, 1987).

59. **Turner IG, Thomas NP**, Comparative analysis of four types of synthetic anterior cruciate ligament replacement in the goat: in vivo histological and mechanical findings, *Biomaterials* (1990) **11**: 321–329.

60. **Hunt MS, Mundell PJ, Strover AE**, UK patent No. 2084468B (1981).

61. **Hunt MS**, An introduction to the use of carbon fibre reinforced composite materials for surgical implants, *Council for Scientific and Industrial Research Report* ME 1689 (Pretoria: South Africa, 1981) 1–24.

62. **Strover AE**, Technical advances in the reconstruction of knee ligaments using carbon fibre, *Aktuelle Problems im Chirurgie und Orthopädie*, No. 26: Alloplastic Ligament Replacement, ed Burri C and Claes L (Bern: Hans Huber, 1983) 127–134.

63. **Spector M, Michno MJ, Smarook WH**, A high modulus polymer for porous orthopaedic implants: Biomechanical compatibility of porous implants, *J Biomed Mater Res* (1978) **12**: 665–677.

64. **Odensten M, Gillquist J**, Functional anatomy of the anterior cruciate ligament and a rationale for reconstruction, *J Bone Joint Surg (Am)* (1985) **67**: 257–262.

65. **Slocum DB, Larson RL**, Rotatory instability of the knee: Its pathogenesis and a clinical test to demonstrate its presence, *J Bone Joint Surg (Am)* (1968) **50**: 211–225.

66. **Arnoczky SP**, Anatomy of the anterior cruciate ligament, *Clin Orthop* (1983) **172**: 19–25.

67. **Barba L**, Utilisation du ligament ABC dans les ruptures récentes du ligament croise antérieur, *3ᵉ journée sur les ligaments ABC* (April 1990).

68. **Markolf KL, Kochan A, Amstutz HC**, Measurement of knee stiffness and laxity in patients with documented absence of the anterior cruciate ligament, *J Bone Joint Surg (Am)* (1984) **66**: 242–253.

69. **Rees A, Mowbray M, Strover AE**, Arthroscopic and histological findings in the knee joint following reconstruction of the anterior cruciate ligament with the ABC polyester/carbon fibre prosthesis, *Am J Sports Med*, in press.

70. **Strover AE, Vaishya R, Darby A**, Are prosthetic ligaments inert? *Abstracts—5th General Meeting, Société Internationale de recherche en orthopédique et de traumatologie*, Montreal (1990).

71. **McLeod A, Strover AE, Cardama F** et al., Prosthetic anterior cruciate ligament devices, biomechanics, failure modes and surgical implications, *Proceedings 1st International Conference on Textiles in Medicine and Surgery*, UMIST, Manchester (1989).

72. **O'Brien T, McLeod A, Cooke W** et al., Successes and failures following 5 years of clinical experience with the Surgicraft ABC prosthetic anterior cruciate ligament, *Third Journal of the ABC Ligament* (April 1990).

73. **Pullicino V**, personal communication.

74. **Strover AE, Mowbray MAS, Shafighian B** et al., Tissue ingrowth into a prosthetic knee ligament: The role of surgical technique, *J Jpn Orthop Assoc* (1988) **62**: S588–589.

Further reading

Daniel DM, Woodward EP, Losse GM et al., The Marshall/MacIntosh anterior cruciate ligament reconstruction with the Kennedy ligament augmentation device: report of the United States clinical trials, *Prosthetic ligament reconstruction of the knee*, ed Friedman MJ, Ferkel RD (Philadelphia: WB Saunders, 1988) 71–78.

Insall J, A midline approach to the knee, *J Bone Joint Surg (Am)* (1971) **53**: 1584–1586.

Losee RE, Johnson TR, Southwick WO, Anterior subluxation of the lateral tibial plateau: a diagnostic test and operative repair, *J Bone Joint Surg (Am)* (1978) **60**: 1015–1030.

McIntosh D, Acute tears of the anterior cruciate ligament: over-the-top repair, Presented at the Annual Meeting of the AAOS, Dallas, Texas (1974).

Sullivan D, Levy IM, Sheskier S et al., Medial restraints to anterior–posterior motion of the knee, *J Bone Joint Surg (Am)* (1984) **66**: 930–936.

Woo SL-Y, Hollis JM, Roux RD et al., Effects of knee flexion on the structural properties of the rabbit femur–anterior cruciate ligament–tibia complex (FATC), *J Biomech* (1987) **20**: 557–563.

6.13   Gore-Tex prosthetic ligament in anterior cruciate-deficient knees

Peter A. Indelicato and Howard R. Brown

Rupture of the anterior cruciate ligament (ACL) is recognized as a major knee injury that often results in functional impairment. Many aspects in the treatment of the ACL deficient knee remain controversial. Surgical reconstructions using patellar autografts have gained acceptance with their high success rates at 5–10-year follow-up evaluations.[1-4] Possibly owing to even higher expectations from ligament reconstruction, the prosthetic ligament has increased in its popularity in ACL reconstructive procedures in the past 5 years.[1,3,5-7] The development of a synthetic substitute for the ACL has many advantages either alone or in comparison with autogenous tissue. These advantages, such as availability, ease of storage, avoidance of sacrifice of normal tissue and immediate fixation to allow early motion followed by aggressive rehabilitation are important, even intoxicating, when dealing with a young athlete interested in returning quickly to competitive sports.

In addition to the advantages mentioned above, the ideal prosthetic ligament would approximate the biomechanical features of a normal ACL and be compatible with intra-articular placement along with other soft tissues.[8] With the increasing concern over HIV or other viral transmission, a synthetic substitute has a comforting lack of risk in these regards. The Gore-Tex polytetrafluoroethylene (PTFE) ligament is designed to serve as a 'permanent' replacement for the ACL deficient knee. Although early results using the Gore-Tex prosthesis were good,[9,10] the long-term success of this device appears to depend upon the technique of implantation and the structural properties of the prosthesis.[8,11]

Synthetic ACL substitutes fall into one of three general categories. Grafts that permanently replace the ACL, those that act as a stent or augmentation device, and those that act as a scaffold that allows for ingrowth of collagenous materials. The implantable device should be technically feasible and reproducible. It should be capable of producing the desired clinical result in both the short and long terms. With implantation in the nonathlete, the prosthesis should allow return to activities of daily living with few or no limitations. Athletes should be able to return to sports at a level comparable to their pre-injury state.

A failure in the prosthetic device should not preclude further reconstruction of the knee because of its tissue-sparing aspects.

Human implantation

The US Food and Drugs Administration (FDA) governs the marketing and regulation of medical devices in the United States. It requires stringent evidence of the safety and effectiveness of all biomedical implants distributed or imported within the United States and is responsible for protecting the public from faulty or fraudulent device use or marketing.

Before a device that is implanted into humans can be marketed in the USA, the manufacturer must first obtain a Pre-market Approval Application (PMA). Approval of this status by the proper FDA division requires review of preclinical studies, which includes in vitro biological testing, mechanical testing and in vivo animal studies. Device manufacturers can then apply for Investigational Device Exemption (IDE), which allows them to conduct clinical trials. Once all the evidence is accumulated, the device panel can either reject or approve the PMA and allow public use.[8]

Currently, there are three 'permanent' or true prosthetic ACLs available for use in the United States that have FDA approval. The Gore-Tex PTFE Ligament (WL Gore & Associates, Flagstaff, AZ), the Stryker Dacron Graft (Stryker-Meadox Dacron, Meadox Medicals, Inc., Oakland, NJ) and the Swiss Polyethylene Ligament. Richards' Polyethylene Ligament (Richards, Memphis, TN) has IDE and is undergoing clinical trials. This chapter will be limited to reviewing the indications, technique and long-term results of prosthetic ligament replacement using the Gore-Tex prosthesis.

Gore-Tex ligament

The Gore-Tex ligament, made of a continuous strand of expanded PTFE woven into loops and plaited into

Table 1 Biomechanical data on human ACL and Gore-Tex prosthesis

Material	Synthetic type	Load to failure (N)	Stiffness (kN/m)	Creep (% change in length)	Strain at yielding (%)
Human ACL[a]	Autogenous	1725 ± 270	182 ± 56	—	25.5 ± 8
Gore-Tex (PTFE)[b]	Prosthesis	4830 ± 280	322	4% (285 N, 300 × 10^6)	2–5

[a]Refs. 13, 14.
[b]Refs. 15, 16.

a 3-bundle braid, was given IDE in October 1982 and became commercially available with FDA approval in October 1986. The FDA approved this device for use as a replacement for the ACL of the knee with a previously failed intra-articular autogenous ACL reconstruction. It is not approved for primary reconstructions in the ACL deficient knee. The Gore-Tex prosthesis has been implanted in more than 18 000 cases worldwide since 1982.[12]

Butler et al.[13] estimated loads of 210 newtons on the human ACL with level walking, rising to 630 newtons while jogging. The normal ACL will undergo up to 14% elongation during flexion and extension without any permanent deformation and can elongate up to 25% before any plastic deformation occurs.[14] Synthetic ACL substitutes have attempted to match the biomechanical and kinetic properties of the normal ACL.

Pure PTFE is the most inert polymer known and is not subject to biochemical degradation.[15,16] The device is designed to be placed in the 'over-the-top' position on the femur and through a tibial tunnel. It has eyelets at each end for screw fixation to the femur and tibia, which allows early motion with this prosthesis. The Gore-Tex prosthesis functions as a true prosthesis, although it frequently becomes covered with a synovial-like sheath intra-articularly.[6] Bone ingrowth occurs readily and its bone tunnel fixation compares favorably with that of other prostheses.[17] Biomechanically, the Gore-Tex ligament is stronger, yet stiffer, than the human ACL. Noyes et al.[14] have analyzed the human ACL in vitro with the following parameters: ultimate tensile strength (load to failure), yield load (load at which plastic deformation occurs), strain at that load, creep (change in length after multiple cyclic loads) and stiffness (a measure of elasticity of the material) among other properties.[13,14] Bolton and Bruchman[15,16] have tested the Gore-Tex prosthesis for these parameters. As shown in Table 1, the Gore-Tex ligament has higher strength than the human ACL (4830 ± 280 N vs. 1725 ± 270 N) and is stiffer (322 kN/m vs. 182 ±

56 kN/m). Its strain at yielding was only 2–5%, compared with 25.5 ± 8% for the human ACL. The Gore-Tex ligament is braided and thus capable of creep. Under loading of 285 N for 300 × 10^6 cycles, it showed a 4% creep.

Materials and methods

From November 1983 to May 1985, we implanted the Gore-Tex prosthesis in 41 patients, none of which had any significant associated medial or lateral instability. The mean age of the patients was 25 years and 85% of the patients had injured their knees as a result of a sports-related accident. Our 2-year postoperative review included 39 (98%) of these patients and identified four failures or ruptures of their prosthesis at that time.[10] Of 35 'successful' patients, 29 (83%) had subsequent follow-up at a minimum of 3 years (Group A).[11]

To better evaluate the prosthesis, the patients were divided into two clinical categories of injury at the time of implantation: acute and chronic. Reconstructions performed during the acute stage took place within 6 weeks of the original injury. Those performed later than 6 weeks were considered chronic. There were 5 acute and 28 chronic patients.

For comparison purposes, Group A was separated into subgroups. Subgroup A-S consisted of 22 patients who were classified as having successful results at their last examination (minimum 3-year follow-up) and Subgroup A-F with the remaining 7 patients classified as failures.

The patient population consisted of 8 patients who had no previous knee surgery, 10 patients with previously performed medial meniscectomy, and 6 patients who had lateral meniscectomies. Two patients had undergone a previous extra-articular reconstruction and two had intra-articular reconstruction attempts.

Surgical technique

The surgical procedure included an examination of the knee under anesthesia, diagnostic arthroscopy with appropriate meniscal surgery, followed by a miniarthrotomy and implantation of the appropriate-sized Gore-Tex prosthesis. Access to the intercondylar notch was achieved through a 3-cm medial parapatellar arthrotomy incision. Ten (34%) of the 29 patients had a wide anterior and posterior notchplasty performed during the operative procedure. The importance of an adequate anterior and posterior notchplasty was not appreciated until later in the clinical investigation. Thus, many of our patients did not undergo a wide notchplasty. At the time of implantation, 10 patients (34%) underwent a partial medial meniscectomy, 9 patients (31%) underwent a partial lateral meniscectomy, and 1 patient (3%) underwent partial medial and lateral meniscectomies. Two additional patients (7%) underwent a peripheral repair of a torn meniscus. None of the patients in our series underwent an associated extra-articular 'back-up' procedure.

Rehabilitation

All patients were started on an identical rehabilitation program immediately after surgery. The program emphasized unrestricted early active motion and aggressive strengthening exercises aimed equally at the quadriceps and hamstring muscle groups. All patients were ambulating without crutches 3 weeks after surgery.

Patient evaluation method

Only those patients who returned for follow-up examination were included in the data base. Several measures of outcome were defined and used to evaluate the patients' knee function. These measures were divided into two categories: subjective and objective results.

The subjective results include the following categories:

(A) *Overall evaluation.* Each patient was asked whether the knee was 'normal,' 'improved,' 'unchanged,' or 'worse' compared to before implantation.
(B) *Giving-way.* The functional stability of the reconstructed knee relative to their activity level was evaluated. Available responses were 'none,' 'sensation of giving-way' and 'actual giving-way.'
(C) *Return to athletics.* The patients were asked whether they were able to return to the level of athletics they were engaged in prior to the injury. Choices were 'nonathlete,' 'yes' or 'no.'

(D) *Pain.* Patients were asked to evaluate the presence of pain in the following categories: 'none,' 'mild,' 'moderate' and 'severe.' They were also questioned as to whether the pain was related to activities.
(E) *Swelling.* The presence of joint swelling was evaluated as 'none,' 'slight' and 'marked.' In addition, patients were asked to decide whether swelling was activity-related or not.
(F) *Lysholm knee score.* In this subjective evaluation system, rating and points were established in eight categories. A 'normal' knee received a total of 100 points. The pre-established categories were 'instability' (25), 'pain' (25), 'locking' (15), 'swelling' (10), need of 'support' for ambulation (5), 'limp' (5) and difficulties with 'stairs' (10) or 'squatting' (5).[18]

The objective results included anterior drawer test, Lachman test and pivot shift test. The first two tests were noted 0, 1+, 2+, 3+ based on the degree of abnormal excursion compared to the uninjured knee (0 = no detectable difference, 1+ = 0–5 mm difference, 2+ = 5–10 mm difference, 3+ = >10 mm difference). The pivot shift was graded as 'absent,' 'trace positive' (gentle slide) and 'present' (gross pivot).

In addition, objective testing also consisted of performance using instrumented testing. *KT-1000 arthrometer:* An experienced examiner used the KT-1000 device both pre- and post-reconstruction. The laxity was measured at 30° of flexion with 89 N (20 lb) of passive force applied to the tibia. *Genucom laxity testing:* The Genucom testing was not done on all patients preoperatively, but was done on all patients during the postoperative follow-up examination by a certified tester, measuring the displacement created with 28 lb (125 N) of passive force at 30° of knee flexion.

Each patient was further evaluated postoperatively by using a Modified Hughston Knee Evaluation Form.[19] The patients' clinical performances were rated in three categories: subjective, objective, and functional. Each of these categories was rated 'excellent,' 'good,' 'fair,' and 'poor.' A 'combined' score was then determined by combining all these results into a final score. In this 'combined' score, the result could only be as good as the 'lowest' score in any of the separate categories.

Failures

The patients were classified as failed based upon one of the following criteria. (A) A complete tear of the prosthesis seen at arthroscopy. (B) A partial tear of the prosthesis seen at arthroscopy and one of the following: (1) Lysholm Knee Score less than 75; (2) KT-1000 injured-to-uninjured difference greater than 4 mm; (3) positive pivot shift. (C) In the absence of arthroscopic data on integrity of the prosthesis, any two of the three criteria listed in (B).

The criteria for failure were applied to each patient at each follow-up examination. When a patient was considered a failure by the preceding criteria, the result could not be reversed on the basis of a subsequent examination.

Complications

The complications are divided into two categories: major and minor. The major complications were those that obviously influenced the ultimate outcome of the operation (i.e., rupture of the device, infection). The minor complications were those that did not appear to influence the final outcome of the operation (i.e., effusion, removal of painful fixation screws).

Results

Group A, consisting of the 29 successful patients, had a mean follow-up of 48 months. These 29 patients plus the four failures identified at the 2-year examination allowed a minimum 3 years of follow-up on 33 of the original 41 patients (80%) undergoing Gore-Tex PTFE ligament reconstruction.

There were no statistically significant differences in sex, age, 'acute'/'chronic' status, side of reconstruction, or any of the preoperative subjective or objective findings between any of the groups at either the 2-year or 3-year minimum follow-up studies.[20] Subgroups A-S (successful) and A-F (failures) also had no significant statistical difference between any of the preoperative subjective or objective findings.

A comparison was then made to detect whether any difference existed, either subjective or objective, between Subgroups A-S (successful) and A-F (failures) when they presented for their 2-year follow-up examination. At that time, in Subgroup A-S, 21 patients had no subjective symptoms of giving-way and 1 patient had 'sensation' of giving-way. In Subgroup A-F, there was no sensation of giving-way in 4 patients, 2 patients had 'sensation' of giving way and 1 had 'actual' giving-way. This was statistically significant (P=0.009). At the 2-year postoperative examination, the mean Lysholm score was 97 for Subgroup A-S and 89 in Subgroup A-F (P=0.07). Functional instability as measured by the instability portion of the Lysholm score was significantly greater in Subgroup A-F (P=0.007).

The only statistically significant objective findings at the 2-year examination between Subgroups A-S and A-F was the anterior drawer sign. This revealed more laxity in Subgroup A-F (P=0.05).

The Modified Hughston Knee Score in Group A revealed 83% with Good or Excellent results at the 2-year examination. This decreased to 66% Good or Excellent results at the 3-year follow-up (P=0.16).

There was no significant difference in any of the subjective or objective findings in Subgroup A-S between the 2-year and 3-year examinations.

There were numerous significant (P<0.05) changes in Subgroup A-F when comparing their early and late follow-up data. These included more subjective symptoms of swelling, pain and instability; lower Lysholm and Modified Hughston Knee Scores; and more laxity in the anterior drawer test, Lachman and pivot shift tests.

A more comprehensive evaluation of the entire cohort of patients (n=39) was performed in several areas including failures, notchplasty, survival analysis and arthroscopic examination.

Failures After the initial 4 failures, there were 7 more, for an overall failure rate of 33% (11 of 33). The only statistically significant differences between the failure group and Subgroup A-S were preoperative symptoms of swelling (P=0.01). Specifically, the failure group had 3 patients with no swelling, 2 patients with slight swelling related to activity, 4 patients with marked swelling unrelated to activity, and 2 patients with slight swelling unrelated to activity. Subgroup A-S had 11 patients with no swelling and 11 patients with slight swelling related to activity.

Although not statistically significant (P=0.08), all of the failures were from 'chronic' ACL deficient knees, while Subgroup A-S consisted of a mixture of 5 'acute' and 17 'chronic' cases.

Three of the 11 failures occurred after a specific traumatic event. The mean time to failure was 32 months post-implantation.

Notchplasty The possible need to decompress the intercondylar notch did not become apparent until the study was more than half complete. Twenty-five patients did not have a notchplasty, while 14 patients did. There were no statistically significant differences between these two groups.

Nine failures occurred in the non-notchplasty group (36%). Three were due to trauma and 6 due to attrition. There were two failures in the notchplasty group (14%). Both of these were attritional failures that occurred at 39 and 48 months post-implantation. However, as mentioned above, the failure rate in the non-notchplasty group was not significantly different from the notchplasty group (P=0.16). Survival curve analysis with Kaplan–Meier techniques[21] revealed a survival rate at 48 months of 79% in the non-notchplasty group and 89% in the notchplasty group. Again, this was not statistically significant (P=0.58).

Survival analysis Survival analysis was performed on the entire group of 39 patients using the

Kaplan–Meier survival curve. Sixty-four percent of the failures occurred between 24 and 50 months post-reconstruction, suggesting a continued attritional failure of the prosthetic ligament. There was an 82% probability of survival at 48 months post-implantation and a 44% probability of survival of the prosthesis at 62 months post-implantation.

Arthroscopy   Sixteen of the original 39 patients had arthroscopic evaluation post-implantation. Three complete tears and 9 partial tears of the prosthesis were identified. Of the nine partial tears, 3 progressed to failure with a mean time to failure of 12 months. However, 6 did not progress to failure with a mean follow-up of 48 months. Of the partial tears that had not failed, there was no significant degradation between their 2-year and their last follow-up examination.

Complications

There was one immediate postoperative infection, which was treated with lavage and partial synovectomy. This patient had salvage of the prosthesis and has had no recurrence of the infection to date. The knee is stable with a good clinical result. Adding to this major complication were the 11 prosthesis failures.

The most frequent major complication was the appearance of sterile effusions. Prior to the 2-year examination, 10 patients had at least one episode of a sterile effusion. There were only two patients with an episode of a sterile effusion after the 2-year examination. One was a recurrent effusion and the other was a new onset of a sterile effusion. Thus, a total of 11 of 39 patients (28%) had at least one episode of sterile effusion. Five of these patients had recurrent episodes.

Five of the 39 patients had removal of painful fixation screws. There were no cases of phlebitis, fractures through screw holes, or neurological complications.

Discussion

In evaluation of a prosthetic implant, the results must always be evaluated as a factor of time, since failure is very likely to occur at some point. Therefore, as one would expect, our 3-year follow-up shows some deterioration in results when comparing to the 2-year data. Although the group analysis provided a characterization of a suspected deterioration in subjective and objective findings over time, as evidenced by the increase in number of failures, there was no statistical significance. This does not support the idea that there is a slow deterioration in the examination until

failure occurs. Rather, it seems more consistent with a subclinical deterioration until a critical event occurs that results in obvious clinical failure. Another explanation would be that our examination is not sensitive or specific enough to detect this suspected deterioration.

Our only significant finding prior to implantation that appeared to predispose to failure was increased preoperative symptoms of knee swelling. In addition, two possible 'predictors' of failure at the 2-year examination may be subjective symptoms of 'giving-way,' and an increased anterior drawer sign in 90° of flexion. These were the only significant findings between Subgroup A-S (successful) and Subgroup A-F (failures) at the 2-year examination. Although not quite statistically significant, all of the failures to date have had 'chronic' ACL insufficiency. This would correlate with lax secondary restraints and increased symptoms of giving-way and swelling and an increased anterior drawer sign.

Three of the failures had a traumatic event associated with failure of the prosthetic device. Aside from these, the mode of device failure was likely to be one of attrition secondary to abrasion against the intercondylar notch.

Olson et al.[22] showed that wear particles generated from artificial ligaments may have the potential to induce osteoarthritis through their biochemical activation of synoviocytes and chondrocytes. The most common minor complication in our series was sterile effusions. All of the patients responded favorably to aspiration, temporary immobilization, and a short course of oral nonsteroidal anti-inflammatory medications. Arthroscopy was performed in 7 of these patients. Only 1 patient had a completely intact implant. In the other patients, there was some structural damage to the prosthesis. Synovial biopsy revealed probable PTFE particles in 3 of these 6 patients.

Survival analysis is a well-accepted and useful technique used in the evaluation of prosthetic total joint arthroplasty.[21] The technique appears well-suited for this situation as well. However, the value of survival analysis depends upon the definition of failure and the extent of follow-up. In our series, there were only 6 patients (18%) with 60-month or longer follow-up. This may not be a sufficient number of patients to place heavy emphasis on the 44% survival rate at 62 months. On the other hand, with 64% of the patients having at least 48 months follow-up, the 82% survival figure seems reliable. However, we are concerned about the continued downward trend of the survival curve. Therefore, we would reserve judgment as to the extent of long-term survivability of the Gore-Tex prosthesis used in our profile of patients until better long-term follow-up is available.

The value of a complete notchplasty may not be known until further long-term follow-up is available. Despite the small amount of evidence suggesting that abrasion in the notch may be a cause of failure, there was no statistically significant difference in the failure rate, or the survival curves, between those patients who underwent a notchplasty and those who did not. This may yet be explained by the fact that the degree of notchplasty was still inadequate.

The majority of complications in our study can be described as technique-related. The device seems to be very sensitive to bony edges or ridges. As stated previously, the importance of an adequate decompression of the anterior and posterior intercondylar notch was not realized until this study was almost complete in relation to implantation. As a result, only one patient had what we now consider an adequate anterior and posterior notchplasty. Although not statistically significant in terms of abrasion, the failures can be explained by this reason alone. Over the past 5 years, the implantation technique always included an aggressive decompression of the intercondylar notch. In addition, instrumentation has been developed to help smooth any sharp ridges or edges with which the prosthesis may come into contact, thus further minimizing the risk of abrasion.

Early experience with the prosthesis revealed a gradual increase in laxity as measured with instrumented arthrometers.[23] Possible explanations for this included reorientation of the strands or settling of the prosthesis within the tunnels.[23,24] Consequently, the manufacturer recommends pretensioning of the ligament by pulling it taut for 20 cycles prior to implantation.[25] Our current technique uses a tensiometer to accurately measure the amount of tension at the time of implantation and screw fixation. This may prevent a recurrence of laxity resulting from 'nesting' of the prosthesis or soft-tissue interposition.

Although the 3-year complication rate is a cause for concern, subjectively the majority of the patients still appear to be reasonably satisfied with the results. At a minimum of 3 years follow-up, 87% thought that their knee was either 'normal' or definitely 'improved' from its preoperative condition. In addition, 85% of the patients had either the sensation of giving-way or actual buckling of their knee preoperatively, but only 29% of these patients had the same sensation post-implantation. These results correspond to those of other studies.[14,25] However, a more critical scale (Modified Hughston Knee Score) found a 'combined' score of only 66% with 'good' or 'excellent' results at this follow-up. The Lysholm Knee Score[18] did not significantly deteriorate between the 2-year and 3-year study (92 to 90 points).

Conclusion

Although the results at 2 years' follow-up were satisfactory, they tend to deteriorate with time. Three possible 'predictors' of failure at later follow-up were identified: preoperative subjective symptoms of swelling, subjective symptoms of giving-way at 2 years, and an increased anterior drawer sign at 2 years. The device is very technique-sensitive with respect to the sharp edges that exist in the tunnel exits and the intercondylar notch. With this in mind, better design and instrumentation are likely to improve the performance of this implant. However, a minimum 5-year follow-up should allow a more accurate comparison of the Gore-Tex prosthesis with other biological and synthetic substitutes used in treating ACL insufficiency of the knee. Currently, we can only recommend prosthetic ACL implantation in the low-demand patient who has a functionally unstable knee, mild to moderate ACL insufficiency (not severe), and minimal degenerative changes, and who has failed a biological reconstruction attempt.

References

1. **Gillquist J, Lukianov A,** A recent survey of treatment results for anterior cruciate ligament insufficiency, Abstract, 5th International Conference, Advances in Cruciate Ligament Reconstruction of the Knee: Prosthetic vs Autogenous. Palm Springs, CA, 4–6 March 1988.

2. **Johnson RJ, Eriksson E, Haggmark T** et al., Five- to ten-year follow-up evaluation after reconstruction of the anterior cruciate ligament, *Clin Orthop* (1984) **183**: 122–140.

3. **Pattee GA, Friedman MJ,** A review of autogenous intra-articular reconstruction of the anterior cruciate ligament, *Prosthetic ligament reconstruction of the knee*, ed Friedman MJ, Ferkel RD (Philadelphia: WB Saunders, 1988) 22–28.

4. **Sandberg R, Balkfors B,** Reconstruction of the anterior cruciate ligament: A five-year follow-up of 89 patients, *Acta Orthop Scand* (1988) **59**: 288–293.

5. **Ahlfeld SK, Larson RL, Collins HR,** Anterior cruciate reconstruction in the chronically unstable knee using an expanded polytetrafluoroethylene (PTFE) prosthetic ligament, *Am J Sports Med* (1987) **15**: 326–330.

6. **Ferkel RD, Fox JM, Wood D** et al., Arthroscopic 'second-look' at the GORE-TEX ligament, *Am J Sports Med* (1989) **17**: 147–153.

7. **Lukianov AV, Richmond JC, Barrett GR** et al., A multicenter study on the results of anterior cruciate ligament reconstruction using a Dacron ligament prosthesis in 'salvage' cases, *Am J Sports Med* (1989) **17**: 380–386.

8. **McFarland EG, Indelicato PA,** The development of anterior ligament prostheses—Implications for treatment of sports people, *Sports Med* (1990) **10**: 405–413.

9. **Glousman R, Shields C Jr, Kerlan R** et al., GORE-TEX prosthetic ligament in anterior cruciate deficient knees, *Am J Sports Med* (1988) **16**: 321–326.

10. **Indelicato PA, Pascale MS, Huegel MO,** Early experience with the GORE-TEX polytetrafluoroethylene anterior cruciate ligament prosthesis, *Am J Sports Med* (1989) **17**: 55–62.

11. **Woods GA, Indelicato PA, Prevot TJ,** The GORE-TEX anterior cruciate ligament prosthesis—Two versus three year results. *Am J Sports Med* (1991) **19**: 48–55.

12. **Schepsis AA, Greenleaf J,** Prosthetic materials for anterior cruciate ligament reconstruction, *Orthop Rev* (1990) **19**: 984–991.

13. **Butler DL, Grood ES, Noyes FR** et al., On the interpretation of our anterior cruciate ligament data, *Clin Orthop* (1985) **196**: 26–34.

14. **Noyes FR, Butler DL, Grood ES** et al., Biomechanical analysis of human ligament grafts used in knee ligament repairs and reconstructions, *J Bone Joint Surg (Am)* (1984) **66**: 344–352.

15. **Bolton CW, Bruchman B**, Mechanical and biological properties of the GORE-TEX expanded polytetrafluoroethylene (PTFE) prosthetic ligament, *Aktuel Probl Chir Orthop* (1983) **26**: 40–51.

16. **Bolton CW, Bruchman WC**, The GORE-TEX expanded polytetrafluoroethylene prosthetic ligament: An in vitro and in vivo evaluation, *Clin Orthop* (1985) **196**: 202–213.

17. **Arnoczky SP, Torzilli PA, Warren RF** et al., Biological fixation ligament prosthesis and augmentations, *Trans Orthop Res Soc* (Feb 1986) 241.

18. **Tegner Y, Lysholm J**, Rating systems in the evaluation of knee ligament injuries, *Cruciate ligament injuries in the knee: Evaluation and rehabilitation* (Linköping: Linköping University Medical Dissertations, 1985) 203: 39–47.

19. **Hughston JC, Barrett GR**, Acute anteromedial rotatory instability: Long-term results of surgical repair, *J Bone Joint Surg (Am)* (1983) **65**: 145–153.

20. **Rimm AA, Hartz AJ, Kalbfleisch JH** et al., *Basic biostatistics in medicine and epidemiology* (New York: ACC Prentice-Hall, 1980) 310–311.

21. **Cornell CN, Ranawat CS**, Survivorship analysis of total hip replacements, *J Bone Joint Surg (Am)* (1986) **68**: 1430–1434.

22. **Olson EJ, Kang JD, Fu FH** et al., The biochemical and histological effects of artificial ligament wear particles: In vitro and in vivo studies, *Orthop Trans* (1989) **13**: 56–57.

23. **More RC, Markolf KL**, Measurement of stability of the knee and ligament force after implantation of a synthetic anterior cruciate ligament: In vitro measurement, *J Bone Joint Surg (Am)* (1988) **70**: 1020–1031.

24. **Markolf KL, Pattee GA, Strum GM** et al., Instrumented measurements of laxity in patients who have a GORE-TEX anterior cruciate ligament substitute, *J Bone Joint Surg (Am)* (1989) **71**: 887–893.

25. **Collins HR**, US experience with GORE-TEX reconstruction of the anterior cruciate ligament, *Prosthetic ligament reconstruction of the knee*, ed Friedman MJ, Ferkel RD (Philadelphia: WB Saunders, 1988) 156–164.

6.14　Complications of synthetic knee ligaments: intra-articular wear particles

Freddie H. Fu and Eric J. Olson

Clinical problem

While it has become established that patients who have symptomatic instability due to anterior cruciate ligament (ACL) laxity are candidates for ligament reconstruction, the search continues for the ideal replacement material. Many surgeons consider harvesting the central-third of a patient's own bone–patellar tendon–bone (B-PT-B) complex to be the 'gold standard' for ACL reconstruction. Nevertheless, there are problems with autografts. A long incision is required over a patient's patellar tendon. This region is often quite painful during the immediate postoperative period. Additionally, in patients with patellofemoral symptoms prior to reconstruction, autograft harvest frequently aggravates their patellar complaints, and is thus less satisfactory. In patients who are older than 40 years, the patellar-tendon complex becomes weaker,[1] and is less suitable for use in ACL reconstruction.

Consequently, surgeons have looked to artificial anterior cruciate ligaments in hopes that they would prove an attractive alternative to autograft reconstruction. Specific advantages of synthetic ligaments include the ability to preserve a patient's own healthy, uninvolved tissues. Artificial ligaments are available if a patient's autogenous tissue has been previously used and has subsequently gone on to fail. In many cases, the use of synthetics is technically less demanding than autograft harvest and implantation. Additionally, a frequently stated advantage of artificial ligaments is their ability to offer immediate postoperative stability. Patients may be pushed more aggressively during their initial rehabilitation because the synthetic ligament does not go through a period of relative weakness. Autografts lose strength during the first 6 months after implantation, during the synovial revascularization period of graft maturation.[2] Furthermore, B-PT-B autografts have bone plugs on their ends which must heal to the bone tunnel that surrounds them, a process which requires approximately 6 weeks. With artificial ligaments there are no fears of disrupting bone–bone healing, which provides some surgeons with more confidence to push their patients early.

While these theoretical considerations spurred the development of artificial ligaments, more recent experience by Shelbourne and others has demonstrated that autograft patients could be pushed more aggressively than had been previously believed, with more rapid return of range of motion and no increased short-term ligament laxity.[3]

A brief history of synthetic ligaments

A variety of anterior cruciate ligament replacement devices have been tried in the past. Beginning with wire loops and the fascia lata in the early twentieth century, surgeons have sought suitable materials for ACL reconstruction.[4] These may be divided into (1) the true *prostheses*, which are permanent and immediate replacements of the anterior cruciate ligament, which do not rely upon intra-articular tissue ingrowth for their strength; (2) *scaffolds*, which are designed to provide a lattice upon which new host tissue may theoretically grow; and (3) *mechanical augmentation devices*, which are designed to protect autogenous reconstruction tissue from breakage during the early implantation period. In theory, these augmentation devices progressively load-share with the autogenous tissue, and eventually the autogenous tissue takes over the tensile demands of the ACL construct.[5]

Prior to a ligament being available for marketing in the United States, it must be approved by the Food and Drug Administration (FDA). This agency's responsibility is to determine whether implant devices are both safe and effective. Towards this end, in September 1987 the FDA published the 'Guidance Document for the Preparation of the Investigational Device Exemptions (IDE) and Premarket Approval Applications for Intra-articular Prosthetic Knee Ligament Devices.'[6] Manufacturers of synthetic ligaments must first present data from in vitro and animal studies, which support the safety of their device. They may then be granted an IDE, which allows them to perform controlled clinical trials with the ligament, with 2- to 5-year follow-up. The results of these clinical trials are then presented to a panel of orthopedists and scientists who advise the FDA whether the ligament should be approved for general marketing in the USA.

If premarket approval (PMA) is obtained, the ligament is 'released' and may be marketed to the public for use in the FDA's approved indications. While manufacturers may not advertise the use of the ligament for indications not included in the PMA, it is not illegal for surgeons to prescribe the ligament for use in their individual patients, regardless of the FDA's 'approved' indications. Consequently, once a ligament has been approved, a wide variety of use patterns develop.

Three synthetic ligaments have been approved in the United States; the Gore-Tex polytetrafluoroethylene (PTFE) braid ligament was approved in October 1986; the Meadox-Stryker Dacron (polyester) ligament was approved in January 1989. Both of these were approved for patients who have had at least one failed autogenous, intra-articular reconstruction of their ACL, so-called 'salvage' cases. The Kennedy LAD (polypropylene) ligament was approved in November 1986. The LAD was approved for the augmentation of the relatively weak prepatellar periosteum and adjacent quadriceps and patellar tendon, a technique which had been originally described by Marshall and MacIntosh, in an 'over-the-top' anterior cruciate ligament reconstruction.[7] The Kennedy LAD is also under investigation for use with a variety of other materials such as semitendinosus.

Reported clinical complications

The total joint experience with wear debris

Charnley had early clinical experience with the potentially devastating complications arising from wear debris generated by the deterioration of orthopedic implants.[8,9] The relatively soft Teflon first used in his acetabular components led to caseous necrosis around the hip joint, with severe inflammation, pain, prosthesis loosening and rapid clinical failure. The use of silastic implants in load-bearing locations such as the elbow and wrist has had similar difficulties owing to wear particle-induced 'silicone synovitis.'[10–12] Carbon implanted tibial trays have also resulted in severe wear debris problems in total knee replacements. More recently, clinical failures due to polyethylene wear debris have been reported in total hip and total knee replacements.[13–17]

Artificial ligaments and wear debris

Clinically, Roth has reported significant synovitis resulting in the need for graft removal 15 months following standard placement of a Kennedy LAD.[18] Del Pizzo recently reported 2-year minimum follow-up on 269 of 721 patients who had the LAD used to augment a variety of autogenous tissues. He found infection in 10 patients, culture-negative effusions in 28, and rupture in 10.[19]

Glousman et al. found that 4 of 82 patients who had Gore-Tex ligament implantation developed persistent sterile effusions. One of these patients required graft removal. Four other patients had complete graft rupture between the seventh and tenth postoperative months, and small wear particles were found in the area of synovial inflammation.[20]

More recently, Indelicato et al. presented 2-year follow-up on 39 Gore-Tex ligament recipients. A total of 23 episodes of sterile effusions were seen in 9 of these patients. The authors found definite arthroscopic evidence of strand breakage in 7 of those 39. Chronic inflammatory tissue with multinucleated giant cells were seen around small (<50 μm) particles in 3 of 6 patients who had synovial biopsies performed.[21] Paulos reported higher effusion rates as follow-up was increased. In his 188 patients followed an average of 4 years, effusions occurred in 34%, with ligament rupture in 12%.[22]

In a particularly difficult group of patients, Lukianov et al. reported that 2 of 41 patients who had 'salvage' reconstruction of their ACL with the Stryker-Meadox Dacron prosthesis developed significant synovitis. One of these cases required graft removal and was found to have failed intra-articularly. The other case had intercondylar impingement. No synovial biopsies were reported.[23] Gillquist found increasing Stryker-Meadox Dacron ligament rupture rates over time in his Swedish population: by 4 years, 23% of the implants had failed.[24]

Many of the synthetic ligaments which the FDA has rejected have induced similar, undesirable intra-articular responses. A number of investigators have reported clinical failures following xenograft implantation. The xenograft ligament was formed by preparing a bovine foreleg tendon with glutaraldehyde. While glutaraldehyde treatment decreased the xenograft's immunogenicity and increased its strength through collagen crosslinking, the trace amounts of glutaraldehyde remaining in the device and its wear debris contributed to the adverse clinical outcomes reported.[25,26] Corroborating the inflammatory effect of even small dosages of glutaraldehyde was the work performed by Harner et al., who demonstrated that trace amounts of Cidex, a 2% glutaraldehyde solution used to sterilize arthroscopic equipment, could induce gross, diffuse synovitis in a rabbit model in vivo.[27]

Filamentous carbon fiber reconstruction of the anterior cruciate ligament was popular in the early 1980s, but had problems with excess breakdown when used intra-articularly, owing to fiber brittleness. Rushton et al. reported that 10 of 39 patients required arthroscopic examination to evaluate persistently painful synovitis between 12 and 30 months after carbon ACL implantation.[28] Although Parsons et al. found that injection of carbon wear particles into rabbits produced only a mild synovitis,[29] other investigators found scarce tissue ingrowth into the carbon, and adverse joint reactions if the tow of carbon fibers was disrupted.[30]

Bone–patellar tendon–bone allografts have been implanted as biological ligament replacements. While these are composed of human tissue, rather than synthetic polymers, allografts have also had clinically adverse outcomes due to wear debris. Jackson reported an 'applesauce-like' reaction in the knees of 7 of 109 patients who underwent ACL reconstruction using allografts which had been secondarily sterilized with ethylene oxide.[31] These patients had persistent effusions, with collagenous particulate and inflammatory cells seen on joint aspiration. Arthroscopy demonstrated disruption of the allograft's collagen fibers, and synovial biopsies revealed a chronic inflammatory process. Gas chromatography demonstrated that ethylene chlorohydrin, a breakdown product of ethylene oxide, was present in elevated levels in the synovium and graft material of patients who had this applesauce reaction. Complete removal of the allograft allowed the synovitis to resolve. Lonnie Paulos, David Drez, and others have reported similar experiences with ethylene oxide-sterilized allografts (personal communication).[32]

Investigations with wear particles

Technique of wear-particle formation

The synthetic polymers used to produce artificial ligaments are deliberately chosen for their ability to resist wear. Consequently, producing experimentally useful quantities of wear particles from these materials is inherently difficult. In the orthopedic laboratory at the University of Pittsburgh, we developed techniques for the production of debris which closely resembled the wear debris recovered from clinical failures and synovial biopsies in humans.

Each ligament was first minced into small pieces and placed into a grinding tube along with a steel cylinder. The grinding tube was inserted into a liquid nitrogen-cooled freezer-mill at −197°C, which made the ligament materials brittle and thus susceptible to grinding. The freezer-mill magnetically shuttled the steel cylinder between metallic end plugs on the grinding cylinder and shattered the frozen ligament pieces into small particles. This particulate material was then examined under a microscope to determine its size and shape, and confirm that its distribution matched the best available clinical data.[33]

In vitro effects of wear particles

Initial in vitro work with this ligament debris involved testing seven materials: human patellar tendon allograft, Stryker-Meadox Dacron, Kennedy LAD (polypropylene), Gore-Tex (PTFE), Versigraft filamentous carbon, Leeds–Keio (polyester), and the xenograft ligament. A line of rabbit synovial cells (HIG-82)[34] was exposed to varying doses of wear particles generated from each of the seven ligaments.[35] After 72 hours of contact with wear particles, the synovial cells were induced to produce statistically significant quantities of several enzymes capable of digesting articular cartilage and periarticular tissues. These enzymes are found in elevated levels in joints with osteoarthritis and rheumatoid arthritis.[36] Specifically, carbon and xenograft induced significantly greater quantities of the neutral proteinases, collagenase, gelatinase and stromelysin than the other five ligaments tested.

Additionally, the synoviocytes produced interleukin-1 (IL-1) following phagocytosis of ligament wear debris.[35] IL-1 is a powerful modulator of chondrocyte metabolism. It decreases the chondrocyte's production of cartilage-maintaining proteoglycans, and induces the chondrocyte's own production of neutral proteinases, which can digest the cartilage around the chondrocyte.[37,38] Other studies in this cell line have shown that activation of the cells causes production of prostaglandin E_2.[39] Through these mechanisms, artificial ligaments, rather than preserving joint function, may form wear particles which initiate a biochemical chain of events, potentially leading to the destruction of the joint into which they are placed.

Allograft preservation methods and wear-particle reactivity

In a related study, further synovial cell work has been performed to study the effects of different preservation methods of anterior cruciate ligament allografts. Silvaggio et al. compared deep-frozen anterior cruciate ligament allografts with those that were freeze-dried and then secondarily sterilized with ethylene oxide.[40] Significantly increased levels of IL-1 and neutral proteinases were induced by wear particles from ligaments which had been secondarily sterilized with the ethylene oxide, when compared with those which had been deep-frozen. This demonstrated that the method of preservation was significant in terms of allograft's ability to be compatible in the synovial environment.

Moreover, this work may help explain the 'applesauce' phenomenon reported by Jackson and others in failed ethylene oxide-sterilized allografts.[31] Abrasion and impingement of the allograft produced wear particles, which were taken up by the knee's synovial lining. The trace amounts of ethylene chlorohydrin, the ethylene oxide breakdown product which Jackson reported measuring in his patient's synovium, may have initiated the vigorous synovial response he observed. In our experiments, the phagocytosis wear particles of the ethylene oxide-sterilized grafts caused IL-1 production. In addition to its effect on chondrocytes, IL-1 is a powerful recruiter of this type of inflammatory cells and can cause bone resorption, which Jackson reported finding in his 'applesauce' knees.[41]

Immunohistochemistry of wear particles

Newer work in our laboratory has studied the immunohistochemistry of wear-particle debris. In general, phagocytosis leads to synoviocyte activation.[42] Therefore, small particles (i.e., those less than 30 µm) may be more reactive than large particles, because they are more easily phagocytosed and, therefore, more prone to induce synoviocyte activation. However, fluorescently labeled anticollagenase antibody studies have shown that large (>50 µm) Dacron particles were also able to induce HIG-82 synoviocyte activation, without being phagocytosed (Olson et al.[33] and Greis PE, Georgescu HI, Fu FH et al., in preparation). Therefore, more work is needed to characterize the effects of particle shape as well as surface properties on synoviocyte activation.

In vivo effects of wear debris

Our laboratory has also conducted in-vivo work on the effects of synthetic ligament wear debris.[35] Twenty-eight rabbits had 5 mg (1 mg/kg) of particles from one of seven ligament types injected into their right knees, and were followed for 14 weeks. Histological analysis showed that small accumulations of the polymeric wear debris induced macrophage accumulation around the particles. Multinucleated giant cells were seen around collections of small debris or if the individual particles were too large to be phagocytosed. Carbon induced a distinct histologic response: subsynovial hyperplasia, with less inflammatory infiltrate. Incorporation of carbon into the articular cartilage surface of one animal was seen. In general, the greater the amount of debris in a given area, the greater was the amount of histologic reaction.

Increased synovial fluid was seen in 4 of 14 rabbit knees injected with wear particles, but only one of the control knees. Whether wear particles are responsible for the production of the sterile effusions seen in 5–20% of patients who undergo synthetic ligament ACL reconstruction remains uncertain. Given the biochemical effects of the particles, however, it is prudent for surgeons to utilize ligament materials whose debris is minimally reactive, and to use surgical techniques which decrease the risk of abrasion, impingement and wear debris formation.

Future directions

More investigation is needed into the long-term effects of a bolus of wear particles, which occurs clinically when there is a sudden failure of a synthetic anterior cruciate ligament. These 'acute failure' results should be compared with the response produced from a slow 'chronic' abrasion of a ligament over time, which produces progressive shedding of ligamentous debris into the joint. We currently have insufficient knowledge about the time-course of synovial cell activation in vivo, and the resulting histologic changes. In-vivo immunohistochemical techniques should be used to study the periarticular tissues of animals which have received wear-particle injections. These experiments could determine the relative role of the synovial lining versus the subsequently recruited inflammatory cells in mediating the foreign-body response which synthetic ligament debris engenders. On the basis of these studies, it is hoped that safer and more effective prosthetic ligaments may eventually be developed and marketed. In the meantime, synthetic ligaments should be used with caution.

References

1. **Noyes FR, Butler DL, Grood ES** et al., Biomechanical analysis of human ligament grafts used in knee ligament repairs and reconstructions. *J Bone Joint Surg (Am)* (1984) **66**: 344–352.
2. **Clancy WG Jr, Narechenia RG, Rosenberg TD** et al., Anterior and posterior cruciate ligament reconstruction in rhesus monkeys: A histological, microangiographic and biomechanical analysis, *J Bone Joint Surg (Am)* (1981) **63**: 1270–1284.
3. **Shelbourne KD, Nitz P,** Accelerated rehabilitation after anterior cruciate ligament reconstruction, *Am J Sports Med* (1990) **18**: 292–299.
4. **Pattee GA, Snyder SJ,** Prosthetic reconstruction of the anterior cruciate ligament: historical overview, *Prosthetic ligament reconstruction of the knee*, ed Friedman MJ, Ferkel RD (Philadelphia: WB Saunders, 1988) 29–33.
5. **Fu FH, Greis PE,** Prosthetic replacement of anterior cruciate ligament: review of current clinical applications, *Perspect Orthop Surg* (1990) **1**: 23–40.
6. **US Food and Drugs Administration,** Division of Surgical and Rehabilitation Devices, *Guidance document for the preparation of investigational device exemptions and premarket approval for intra-articular prosthetic knee ligament devices* (US Government Printing Office, Bethesda, 1987) 1–54.
7. **Marshall JL, Warren RF, Wickiewicz TL** et al., The anterior cruciate ligament: a technique of repair and reconstruction, *Clin Orthop* (1979) **143**: 97–106.
8. **Charnley J, Kamangar A, Longfield MD,** The optimum size of prosthetic heads in relation to the wear of plastic sockets in total replacement of the hip, *Med Biol Eng* (1969) **7**: 31–39.

9. **Charnley J**, *Low friction arthroplasty of the hip: Theory and practice* (New York: Springer-Verlag, 1979) 6–7.

10. **Worsing RA Jr, Engber WD, Lange TA**, Reactive synovitis from particulate silastic, *J Bone Joint Surg (Am)* (1982) **64**: 581–585.

11. **Gordon M, Bullough PG**, Synovial and osseous inflammation in failed silicone-rubber prostheses: a report of six cases, *J Bone Joint Surg (Am)* (1982) **64**: 574–580.

12. **Wroblewski BM**, Wear and loosening of the socket in the Charnley low-friction arthroplasty, *Orthop Clin North Am* (1988) **19**: 627–630.

13. **Buchhorn GA**, Willert HG, Effects of plastic wear particles on tissue, *Biocompatibility of orthopedic implants*, ed Williams DF (Boca Raton: CRC Press, 1982) 249–267.

14. **Eftekhar NS, Doty SB, Johnstone AD** et al., Prosthetic synovitis, *Hip* (1985) **1**: 169–183.

15. **Landy MM, Walker PS**, Wear of ultra-high-molecular-weight polyethylene components of 90 retrieved knee prostheses, *J Arthroplasty* (1988) **3** (suppl.) S73–S85.

16. **Mathiesen EB, Lindgren JU, Reinholt FP** et al., Tissue reactions in wear products from polyacetal (Delrin) and UHMW polyethylene in total hip replacement, *J Biomed Mater Res* (1987) **21**: 459–466.

17. **Pazzaglia UE, Dell'Orbo C, Wilkinson MJ**, The foreign body reaction in total hip arthroplasties: a correlated light-microscopy, SEM, and TEM study, *Arch Orthop Trauma Surg* (1987) **106**: 209–219.

18. **Roth JH, Shkrum MJ, Bray RC**, Synovial reaction associated with disruption of polypropylene braid-augmented intra-articular anterior cruciate ligament reconstruction: a case report, *Am J Sports Med* (1988) **16**: 301–305.

19. **Del Pizzo W**, US experience with Kennedy LAD, *Proceedings of the Seventh Annual International Symposium on Advances in Cruciate Ligament Reconstruction of the Knee: Autogenous vs Prosthetic* (Palm Desert, CA, March 1990) 90–96.

20. **Glousman R, Shields C, Kerlan R** et al., Gore-Tex prosthetic ligament in anterior cruciate deficient knees, *Am J Sports Med* (1988) **16**: 321–326.

21. **Indelicato PA, Pascale MS, Huegel MO**, Early experience with the GORE-TEX polytetrafluoroethylene anterior cruciate ligament prosthesis, *Am J Sports Med* (1989) **17**: 55–62.

22. **Paulos LE, Rosenberg TD, Grewe SR** et al., The GORE-TEX anterior cruciate ligament prosthesis: a long-term follow-up, AAOS 57th Annual Meeting (New Orleans, 8–13 February 1990).

23. **Lukianov AV, Richmond JC, Barrett GR** et al., A multicenter study on the results of anterior cruciate ligament reconstruction using a Dacron ligament prosthesis in 'salvage' cases. *Am J Sports Med* (1989) **17**: 380–386.

24. **Gillquist J**, Stryker Dacron ligament: Techniques and results, *Proceedings of the Seventh Annual International Symposium on Advances in Cruciate Ligament Reconstruction of the Knee: Autogenous vs Prosthetic* (Palm Desert, CA, March 1990) 106–116.

25. **Allen PR, Amis AA, Jones MM** et al., Evaluation of preserved bovine tendon xenografts: a histological, biomechanical and clinical study, *Biomaterials* (1987) **8**: 146–152.

26. **Van Steensel CJ, Schreuder O, Van Den Bosch BF** et al., Failure of anterior cruciate-ligament reconstruction using tendon xenograft, *J Bone Joint Surg (Am)* (1987) **69**: 860–864.

27. **Harner CD, Fu FH, Mason GC** et al., Cidex-induced synovitis, *Am J Sports Med* (1989) **17**: 96–102.

28. **Rushton N, Dandy DJ, Naylor CPE**, The clinical, arthroscopic and histological findings after replacement of the anterior cruciate ligament with carbon-fibre, *J Bone Joint Surg (Br)* (1983) **65**: 308–309.

29. **Parsons JR, Bhayani S, Alexander H** et al., Carbon fibre debris within the synovial joint: a time-dependent mechanical and histologic study, *Clin Orthop* (1985) **196**: 69–76.

30. **Mäkisalo S, Skutnabb K, Holmström T** et al., Reconstruction of anterior cruciate ligament with carbon fibre: an experimental study on pigs, *Am J Sports Med* (1988) **16**: 589–593.

31. **Jackson DW, Windler GE, Simon TM**, Intra-articular reaction associated with the use of freeze-dried, ethylene oxide-sterilized bone–patellar tendon–bone allografts in the reconstruction of the anterior cruciate ligament, *Am J Sports Med* (1990) **18**: 1–11.

32. **Roberts TS** et al., Anterior cruciate reconstruction using freeze-dried ethylene oxide sterilized bone–patellar tendon–bone allografts: two year results in 35 patients, AAOS 56th Annual Meeting (Las Vegas, Nevada, February, 1989).

33. **Olson EJ, Greis PE, Georgescu HI** et al., Wear particle production and the effect of particle size on synovial cell activation, *Pittsburgh Orthop J* (1990) **1**: 48–52.

34. **Georgescu HI, Mendelow D, Evans CH**, HIG-82: an established cell line from rabbit periarticular soft tissue, which retains the 'activatable' phenotype, *In Vitro Cell Develop Biol*, (1988) **24**: 1015–1022.

35. **Olson EJ, Kang JD, Fu FH** et al., The biochemical and histological effects of artificial ligament wear particles: in vitro and in vivo studies, *Am J Sports Med* (1988) **16**: 558–570.

36. **Martel-Pelletier J, Cloutier JM, Pelletier JP**, Neutral proteinases in human osteoarthritic synovium, *Arthritis Rheum* (1986) **29**: 1112–1121.

37. **Evans CH, Georgescu HI, Mendelow D** et al., Modulation of chondrocyte metabolism by cytokines produced by a synovial cell line, *Development and diseases of cartilage and bone matrix*, ed Sen A, Thornhill T (New York: Alan Liss, 1987) 319–329.

38. **Dingle JT, Page Thomas DP, Hazleman B**, The role of cytokines in arthritic diseases: in vitro and in vivo measurements of cartilage degradation, *Int J Tissue React* (1987) **9**: 349–354.

39. **Baratz ME**, Synovial cell activation by interleukin-1: a characterization of the response and a search for possible second messengers (Master's thesis, University of Pittsburgh, 1987).

40. **Silvaggio V, Fu FH, Georgescu HI** et al., The induction of interleukin-1 by freeze-dried ethylene oxide treated bone–patellar tendon–bone allograft wear particles: an in vitro study, *Trans Orthop Res Soc* (1991) (in press).

41. **Gowen M, Wood DD, Ihrie EJ** et al., An interleukin-1 like factor stimulates bone resorption in vitro, *Nature* (1983) **306**: 378–380.

42. **Werb Z, Reynolds JJ**, Stimulation by endocytosis of the secretion of collagenase and neutral proteinase from rabbit synovial fibroblasts, *J Exp Med* (1974) **140**: 1482–1497.

Posterior cruciate ligament injury

7.1 Posterior cruciate ligament insufficiency of the knee: An overview

Zaid Al-Duri, Dipak V. Patel and Paul M. Aichroth

Posterior cruciate ligament insufficiency has received increasing attention in the literature in view of the important role the posterior cruciate ligament plays in knee biomechanics and function.

Incidence

The incidence of acute posterior cruciate ligament rupture has varied in the literature as the methods of evaluation have steadily improved from solely clinical methods, later to be supplemented by arthroscopy and with eventually the addition of magnetic resonance imaging to the armamentarium helping to document posterior cruciate ligament tears more efficiently. O'Donoghue,[1] put the incidence at 3.4% whilst Clendenin et al.[2] put it at 20%. The effect of posterior cruciate ligament rupture on knee function is variable. The reason for the variability is the way in which knee function has been viewed, in that unless the posterior cruciate ligament is considered as a member of a team it is inevitable that other supportive tissue is given less consideration, leading to inadequate appraisal of the deficit and subsequent underestimation of the size of the problem.

The natural history

It is important to mention here that the majority of the following discussion refers to the mid-substance tears of the posterior cruciate ligament as there is very little disagreement, if any, on the necessity of reattachment of the avulsed tibial bony attachment of the posterior cruciate ligament.

The first question to be addressed here is conservative versus operative treatment. The conclusion of many authors is that the majority of athletes with isolated posterior cruciate ligament rupture who maintain strength in the musculature return to sports without functional disability; hence the importance of an invasive quadriceps exercising programme.[4-8] However, there are some reservations towards some posterior cruciate ligament-deficient knees; for example, for posterior instability that is greater than 15 mm and that does not decrease with internal rotation of the tibia or if a 5-15 mm posterior instability is associated with other major ligamentous instability, then surgical intervention is advised.

On the other hand, there are advocates of surgical intervention as a primary procedure on the grounds that unless such early intervention is implemented then knee function will not be at its best[1,9,10] and that there will be increasing likelihood of the development of degenerative arthritis that is directly proportional to the length of delay in instituting the operative treatment.[11]

Another important question is the claim of secondary degenerative arthritis subsequent to a posterior cruciate ligament rupture and the related factors. Whilst some authorities have implicated delay of the instigation of the operative treatment with the development of osteoarthritis,[11,12] others have found no relation between the length of the follow-up and the severity of arthritis in the conservatively treated group.[5] Some even implicate operative treatment in the development of arthritis and have reported a higher percentage of arthritis in the surgically treated group of patients when compared to the conservatively treated ones.[13]

It is suggested that should arthritis develop then it is the medial joint compartment that suffers most.[5,11] Torg et al.[14] disagree with the suggestion that the medial joint compartment is the one mainly involved. Degenerative knee changes have been correlated to the type of instability of the involved knee. In general those with unidirectional instability had far fewer degenerative changes on their radiographs than those with multidirectional instability.[14]

Whilst it has been generally agreed that there is no correlation between the amount of instability and clinical results, Torg et al.[14] correlated functional results and the radiographic changes in the posterior cruciate ligament-deficient knee. Few degenerative changes were found in patients with good or excellent functional results; however, of those with fair or poor ratings approximately 50% exhibited moderate degenerative changes.

In conclusion, although the natural history is important, it is the functional deficit in the individual case that is the determinant of surgical consideration because of the lack of correlation between the function and the clinically demonstrable laxity. Many authorities believe, and the authors agree, that the available surgical treatment does not bring the posterior cruciate ligament-deficient athlete to his formal level of athletic capability.[4,7,8]

Mechanism

Posterior cruciate ligament injuries are associated mainly with motor vehicular accidents[7,9,10,38,39] and athletic activity.[5,6] Mechanisms of posterior cruciate ligament ruptures include a blow to the uppermost part of the tibia with the knee flexed. Hyperflexion injury is another mechanism (Figures 1 and 2). A fall on a flexed knee with the foot plantar flexed is another[16] (Figure 3).

Types of posterior cruciate ligament ruptures

Posterior cruciate ligament rupture could occur at mid-substance or at its bony attachment (tibia or femur) with or without bony fragmentation. Trickey[9] believes the highest incidence of posterior cruciate ligament rupture to be an avulsion of a tibial fragment. Insall[17] reported an incidence of 35% proximal ruptures, 35% midportion ruptures and 30% distal-third ruptures.

Diagnosis of a posterior cruciate ligament insufficiency

A careful history with particular emphasis on the mechanism of the injury is important. Symptoms are variable with a posterior cruciate ligament-deficient knee, and not all posterior cruciate ligament-deficient knees are symptomatic. Symptoms include pain on coming downstairs or on changing direction during running. Such pain can also occur on squatting, prior to or after exercise, and on walking long distances. Other symptoms include giving way, locking, recurrent swelling, intermittent clicking and stiffness related to prolonged sitting.

Clinical examination for a posterior cruciate ligament deficiency should be part of a systematic examination of the knee joint as a whole. Bruising can give an idea of the direction of the impact. Of particular importance is the so-called 'neutral point' or the 'resting position' of the knee joint. This represents an angle of flexion in the normal knee joint

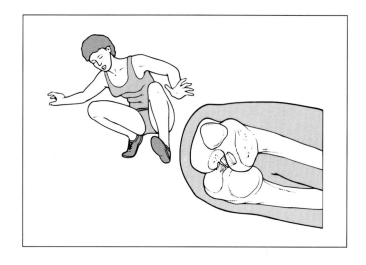

Figure 1

Hyperflexion injury causing a posterior cruciate ligament rupture (after ref. 6).

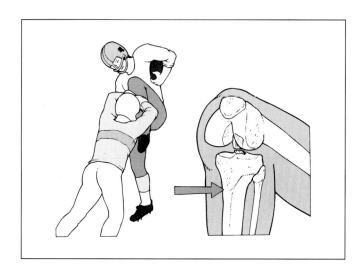

Figure 2

Pretibial trauma to the hyperflexed knee leading to a posterior cruciate ligament rupture (after ref. 6).

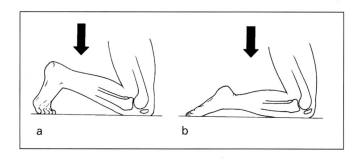

Figure 3

(a) The impact of a fall is on the patellofemoral joint if the foot is dorsiflexed. (b) If the foot is plantar flexed, then it is the front of the tibia that receives the impact (after ref. 16).

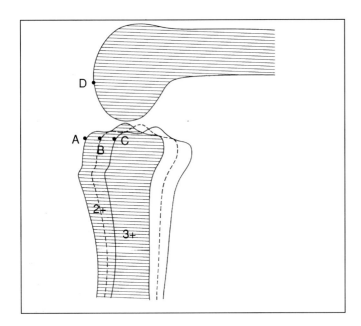

Figure 4

With the knee flexed to 90° the anterior tibial plateau should have an 8–10 mm step off (A). If the posterior cruciate ligament is insufficient, there should be a complete loss of this step off and the anterior aspect of the tibial plateau (B), should be flush with the medial and lateral femoral condyles (D). This should be considered a 2+ drawer. If the anterior tibial plateau (C) is displaced posterior to the anterior of the femoral condyles (D), this should be considered a 3+ posterior drawer (after ref. 16).

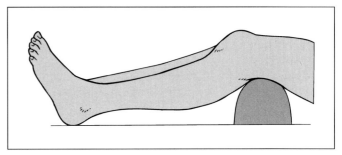

Figure 5

The gravity sign, i.e. drop back of the tibia on the femur near extension (after ref. 21).

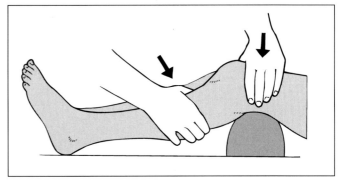

Figure 6

The posterior drawer test performed near extension (after ref. 21).

where tension on the patellar tendon through an active quadriceps contraction does not result in an anterior or posterior tibial translation.[3,8,18-21]

One of the signs of posterior cruciate ligament rupture is the drop back of the tibia on the femur. Clancy[16] defined the relation of the tibia to the femur by considering the anterior tibial plateau in the normal knee to have an approximate 10-mm step off the anterior femur (Figure 4). The back drop of the tibia on the femur is examined with the patient lying supine, the hips flexed to 45°, and the knees either flexed to 90° or held at near extension[21] (Figure 5).

The posterior drawer test has been described as the classic sign for posterior cruciate ligament disruption.[10] Whilst this test is classically performed with the patient lying supine, the hips flexed to 45° and the knees at 90°, Stäubli and Jakob[21] described performing the test near extension (Figure 6). A variation of the posterior drawer test whereby the patient is examined prone has been described by Whipple.[8] This test is very sensitive in discriminating a true straight posterior instability from a posterior rotatory instability. The posterior drawer test can be performed with the tibia in neutral rotation as well as in internal rotation; this will help differentiate a posterior cruciate ligament rupture from that associated with posterolateral rotatory instability.[22] Posterior drawer test may be negative despite an acute posterior cruciate ligament tear. Hughston[23] believes that in such cases there is a coexisting medial and posteromedial structures rupture and that the arcuate complex prevents posterior displacement. Clancy[16] disputes the validity of the posterior drawer test in internal rotation in patients with isolated posterior cruciate ligament ruptures. He believes that the ligaments of Humphry and Wrisberg are rarely injured in isolated posterior cruciate ligament ruptures and so nullify the test.

Daniel et al.[19] described the 'quadriceps active test'. This is an active test in that the subject's muscle contraction, namely quadriceps, results in anterior translation of the tibia on the femur in the posterior cruciate ligament-injured patient. This test can be performed with the knee in 90° of flexion (Figure 7) or with the knee near extension[21] (Figure 8).

Another dynamic test is the 'dynamic posterior shift test'.[25] It is performed to assess both posterior instability and posterolateral rotatory instability.

Jakob and Stäubli[26] described the 'reverse pivot shift test' for diagnosing posterolateral rotatory instability. It is analogous to the pivot shift test, indicating reduction of the posterior subluxation of the lateral tibial plateau. This test is clinically significant only when it is positive on one side and also reproduces the painful subluxation phenomenon that is described by the patient.[27]

Hughston et al.[22] described two tests for the diagnosis of posterolateral rotatory instability commonly associated with a posterior cruciate ligament rupture. These are the 'posterolateral drawer test' (Figure 9) and the 'external rotation recurvatum test' (Figure 10). In posterolateral rotatory instability (PLRI), the arcuate complex of the knee joint is stretched and so the lateral tibial plateau rotates posteriorly (subluxes) and externally around an intact posterior cruciate ligament to an increased extent. Feagin[28] performs the soft posterolateral drawer test' with the patient sitting and the knee flexed to about 60°.

Another test is the 'reversed Lachman test', which is not specific for an isolated posterior cruciate ligament rupture.[27] Feagin[28] performs the reversed Lachman test with the patient prone.

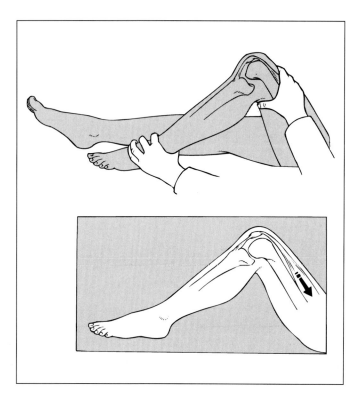

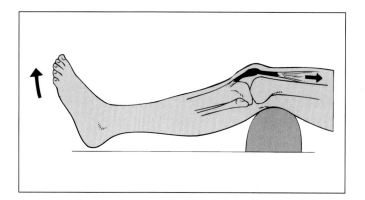

Figure 7

The 90° quadriceps active test (after ref. 24).

Figure 8

Quadriceps active test with the knee near extension (after ref. 21).

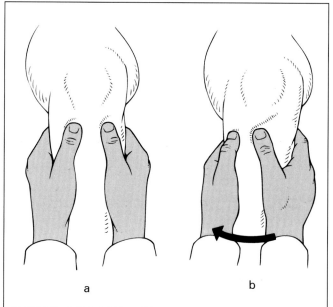

Figure 9

The posterolateral drawer test: (a) starting position for the test; (b) positive test with posterior and external rotation of the lateral tibial condyle (after ref. 22).

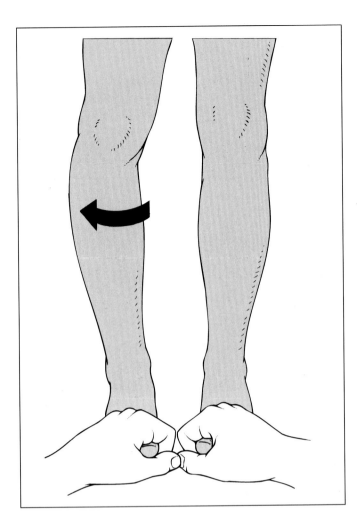

Figure 10

External rotation recurvatum test demonstrating the posterolateral rotatory instability in the right knee with relative tibia vara (after ref. 22).

An interesting observation is that 60% of patients with posterolateral instability can produce a voluntary positive posterolateral drawer test by muscular contraction.[29] These patients appear to have the ability to contract muscles such as the popliteus and the biceps femoris selectively.

Aids to diagnosis of the posterior cruciate ligament-injured knee

Plain radiography

Plain radiography is helpful in demonstrating the avulsion of the posterior cruciate ligament insertion with a bony fragment. If there is a high index of suspicion and the anteroposterior view is not helpful,

then oblique views of the knee will be helpful in demonstrating the avulsion.

Stress radiography allows the plain radiography a more defined role. The principle of stress radiography is to apply a certain amount of force to the front of the tibia, displacing it posteriorly in relation to the femur whilst a lateral plain film of the knee is taken. The lateral film can be taken with both the hips and knees flexed to 90°[16] or it can be done with the knee near extension[21] (Figures 11 and 12). The application of such stress radiography is not difficult (Figures 13–16). The role of stress radiography in quantifying lateral and medial rotatory displacements is limited.

Arthrography

Arthrography is not very helpful in delineating a posterior cruciate ligament rupture, yet it may be helpful in showing associated lesions of the anterior cruciate ligament, menisci or the capsule.

Arthroscopy

The role of arthroscopy in diagnosing posterior cruciate ligament rupture is controversial. If arthroscopy is performed for an acute knee injury, it should be performed by an experienced surgeon with a particular interest in knee surgery. DeHaven[30] emphasized the importance of arthroscopy in the acutely injured knee when he followed up 113 athletes with acute knee injuries and found lesions of surgical significance in 90% of them. Lysholm and Gillquist[31] believe that the incidence of posterior cruciate ligament rupture is understated in the literature owing to the infrequent use of arthroscopy in diagnosing the posterior cruciate ligament rupture.

Computerized tomography

Computerized tomography is not used commonly in diagnosing posterior cruciate ligament tears. However, Golimbu et al.[32] reported on its use in posterior cruciate ligament tears, stating that it reveals the entire posterior cruciate ligament thickness and can be used in acute knee injuries as well.

Magnetic resonance imaging

Complete tears of the posterior cruciate ligament are readily identifiable on both T_1 and T_2 weighted spin-echo images (Figure 17). Incomplete tears of the posterior cruciate ligament are also readily detected as areas of increased signal intensity within the substance of the low-signal intensity ligament.

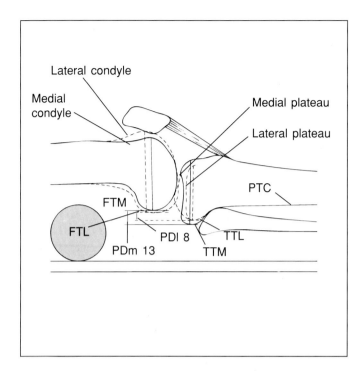

Figure 11

Diagram of a posterior stress radiograph. Lines parallel to the posterior tibial cortex (PTC) are drawn tangential to the most posterior contour of the medial (FTM) and lateral (FTL) femoral condyles and the medial (TTM) and lateral (TTL) tibial plateaux. The distance between those tangential lines are measured directly on the radiograph. In this knee, the posterior displacement of the lateral tibial plateau was 8 mm and of the medial tibial plateau 13 mm, showing both posterior translation and internal rotation, representing posterior cruciate ligament rupture with damage to posteromedial structures (after ref. 21).

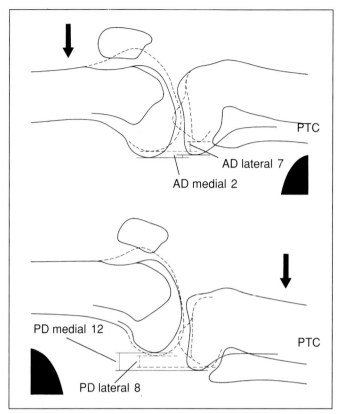

Figure 12

Top: Diagram showing the anterior displacement of the medial and lateral tibial plateau in a knee with intact posterior cruciate ligament. Anterior displacement of the lateral plateau was 7 mm, that of the medial plateau was 2 mm. This is normal anterior joint play. AD = anterior displacement. *Bottom:* Diagram showing posterior displacement of the tibial plateau in a knee with a posterior cruciate ligament injury. Posterior displacement of the medial tibial plateau was 12 mm and that of the lateral tibial plateau 8 mm. This represents a posteromedial subluxation due to injuries to the posterior cruciate ligament and posteromedial structures. PD = posterior displacement. (After ref. 21.)

Treatment of the posterior cruciate ligament-deficient knee

Avulsion of the tibial attachment of the posterior cruciate ligament

There is a general consensus that a bone fragment that has been avulsed should be fixed back into its bed as soon as feasible, preferably within the first week. Trickey[9] stressed that surgical repair after 3 weeks was not worthwhile, whilst Torisu[33] had excellent results when the surgery was performed within 7 weeks of the injury.

Mid-substance tears of the posterior cruciate ligament

The indications for surgical treatment here are primarily in the young athlete who places a high demand on his knee, or in the mid-substance posterior cruciate ligament tear that is associated with other knee ligament injuries, or gross rotational instabilities, especially the posterolateral variety usually associated with posterior cruciate ligament rupture. For the average individual, an intensive physical therapy programme of quadriceps strengthening for a period of at least 6–9 months is advised. Only in

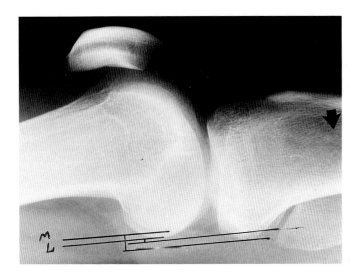

Figure 13

Stress radiograph showing (arrow) posterior displacement of the right tibia on the femur (posterior cruciate ligament intact knee). PD lateral = 1.0 mm. PD medial = 6.5 mm. Note: mean medial and lateral compartment displacement in a normal knee is 3.7 ± 2.1 mm. Mean medial and lateral compartment displacement in a posterior cruciate-deficient knee is 10.4 ±2.4 mm. (PD = posterior displacement.)

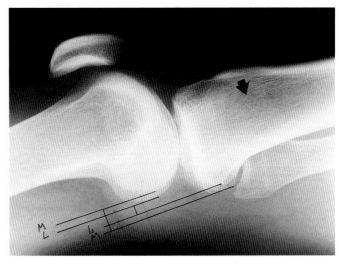

Figure 14

Stress radiograph showing (arrow) posterior displacement of the left tibia on the femur (posterior cruciate ligament-deficient knee). PD lateral = 5.0 mm. PD medial = 12.0 mm. (PD = posterior displacement.)

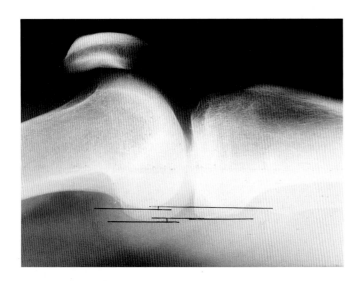

Figure 15

Stress radiograph showing (arrow) anterior displacement of the right tibia on the femur. AD lateral = 1.5 mm. AD medial = 2.0 mm. (AD = anterior displacement.)

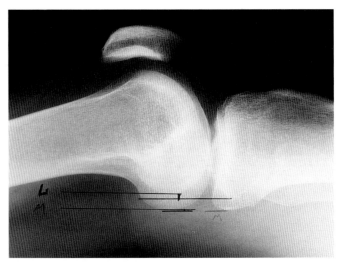

Figure 16

Stress radiograph showing (arrow) anterior displacement of the left tibia on the femur. AD lateral = 2.5 mm. AD medial = 0.5 mm. (AD = anterior displacement.)

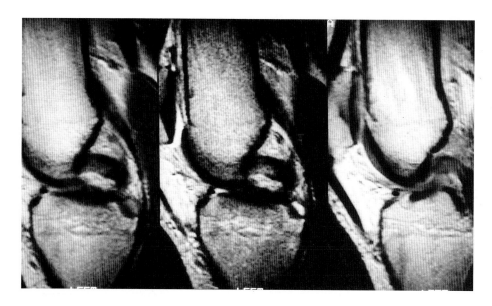

Figure 17

MRI of the left knee showing a tear of the posterior cruciate ligament near its femoral attachment (courtesy of Peter Renton).

those in whom a residual functional deficit persists that interferes either with their activities of daily living or their aspirations, is surgery considered.

Surgical treatment options include primary repair, primary repair with augmentation, and primary reconstruction. The authors believe that primary repair is inadequate. Many, therefore, perform primary repair with augmentation using other tissues, such as the medial head of the gastrocnemius[2] or a free graft of one-third of the patellar tendon;[11] others use the semitendinosus.[34]

For primary reconstruction of the acutely ruptured posterior cruciate ligament without attempting repair, any one of the procedures designed for the reconstruction of the chronically ruptured posterior cruciate ligament can be employed. The authors currently use the combined tendons of the semitendinosus and gracilis for the reconstruction of the acutely ruptured posterior cruciate ligament.

Treatment of the chronically ruptured posterior cruciate ligament

Two broad categories of substitutes are available for the reconstruction of the chronically ruptured posterior cruciate ligament: autogenous tissues and prosthetic ligaments. Many types of autogenous tissues have been used. The semitendinosus and gracilis tendons have been used separately or in combination.[35,37,38] Wirth and Jager[39] described a 'dynamic double tendon replacement' of the posterior cruciate ligament using both of these muscles (Figure 18).

The medial head of the gastrocnemius can be used by detaching its femoral attachment[40] or it can be detached from the femur with a bone block[7] to gain length and improve anchorage.

Barfod[41] described the use of the popliteus tendon which was later recommended by McCormick.[42] Tillberg[43] described the use of either meniscus for the posterior cruciate ligament reconstruction. Southmayd et al.[44] used the semimembranosus for posterior cruciate ligament reconstruction. The patellar tendon has been used by Clancy et al.[11] and recommended by Sisk.[36] Eriksson et al.[45] use the patellar tendon as well in what they call the 'reversed Jones procedure'.

Either prosthetic material can be used as an extension to autogenous material to gain length and better anchorage, such as the proplast used by Woods et al.[15] with the medial head of the gastrocnemius, or the prosthetic ligament can be used as a strut providing stability until maturity of the reconstructed body tissues.[46] Finally, the prosthetic material can be used alone as a posterior cruciate ligament replacement, in which case it is best used as a salvage procedure in a

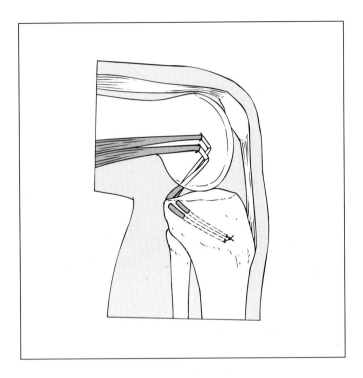

Figure 18

'Dynamic double tendon replacement' using the tendons of the semitendinosus and gracilis (after ref. 39).

failed posterior cruciate ligament reconstruction.[47] The authors recommend reconstruction of the chronically ruptured posterior cruciate ligament in the individual who has had an adequate trial of conservative treatment and yet continues to have recurrent swelling, giving way and inability to perform daily activities, and the individual with an associated posterolateral rotatory instability.

PLRI and PLI

Posterolateral rotatory instability (PLRI) is a clinical entity describing rotation of the lateral tibial plateau both posteriorly and externally around an intact posterior cruciate ligament to an increased extent (i.e. subluxing) due to stretching or damage to the arcuate complex. This complex consists of the arcuate ligament, the fibular collateral ligament, the popliteus muscle and the lateral head of the gastrocnemius.[22] The symptoms of PLRI are often misleading:

the primary symptom is medial joint pain; the next most frequent symptom is an inability to push off.[48]

Posterolateral instability (PLI) is one of the most disabling ligamentous lesions and is different from PLRI. With PLI there is a combined injury of both the posterior cruciate ligament and the posterolateral structures, i.e. the arcuate complex.[29,49] With PLI the proximal tibia moves posteriorly without initial tibial rotation, followed by external rotation of the tibia as the posterior subluxation increases at time of the posterior drawer test. Müller[50] considers PLI as a severe form of PLRI.

We believe that PLRI occurs more frequently than assumed with posterior cruciate ligament injuries, that it needs to be addressed more frequently both diagnostically and therapeutically and that it may well be the reason why the results of the operative treatment of the chronic posterior cruciate ligament injury are not universally satisfactory.

Discussion

We believe that the so-called isolated posterior cruciate ligament injury can be very deceptive and that recurrence of the symptoms is frequently associated with PLRI that has not been addressed. Since the posterior cruciate ligament provides some 95% of the total restraining force of the posterior tibia on the femur,[51] it follows that a truly isolated posterior cruciate ligament injury can only occur if the posterior cruciate ligament is avulsed from its attachment.

It is worthwhile noticing that whereas the 'resting position' is important in appreciating displacement in the anteroposterior plane, it is the posterior cruciate ligament that is very important in interpreting the rotational instabilities occurring in the knee joint and, therefore, it follows that PLI must be an advanced form of the PLRI. Owing to the strength and location of the posterior cruciate ligament, it follows that a substance tear is most probably associated with stretch to the secondary restraints and hence a rotational element of instability.

References

1. **O'Donoghue DH,** An analysis of end results of surgical treatment of major injuries to the ligaments of the knee, *J Bone Joint Surg (Am)* (1955) **37:** 1–13.
2. **Clendenin, MB, DeLee JC, Heckman JD,** Interstitial tears of the posterior cruciate ligament of the knee, *Orthopaedics* (1980) **3**(8): 764–772.
3. **Kapandji IA,** The knee. *The physiology of the joints,* 5th edn, vol 2, ed Kapandji IA (Edinburgh: Churchill Livingstone, 1987).
4. **Cain TE, Schwab GH,** Performance of an athlete with straight posterior knee instability, *Am J Sports Med* (1981) **9**(4): 203–208.

5. Parolie JM, Bergfeld JA, Long term results of non-operative treatment of isolated posterior cruciate ligament injuries in the athlete, *Am J Sports Med* (1986) **14**(1): 35–38.

6. Fowler PJ, Messieh SS, Isolated posterior cruciate ligament injuries in athletes, *Am J Sports Med* (1987) **15**(6): 553–557.

7. Insall JN, Hood RW, Bone-block transfer of the medial head of the gastrocnemius for posterior cruciate insufficiency, *J Bone Joint Surg (Am)* (1982) **64**: 691–699.

8. In: Allen WC, Henstorf JE, Knee ligament reconstruction. *Surgery of the musculoskeletal system*, 2nd edn, vol. 4, ed. Evarts CM (New York: Churchill Livingstone, 1990) 3331–3347.

9. Trickey EL, Rupture of the posterior cruciate ligament of the knee, *J Bone Joint Surg (Br)* (1968) **50**: 334–341.

10. Trickey EL, Injuries to the posterior cruciate ligament: Diagnosis and treatment of early injuries and reconstruction of late instability, *Clin Orthop* (1980) **147**: 76–81.

11. Clancy WG Jr, Shelbourne KD, Zoellner GB et al., Treatment of the knee joint instability secondary to rupture of the posterior cruciate ligament: Report of a new procedure, *J Bone Joint Surg (Am)* (1983) **65** (3): 310–322.

12. Kennedy JC, Roth JH, Walder DM, Posterior cruciate ligament injuries, *Orthop Dig* (1979) **2**: 19–31.

13. Tibone JE, Antich TJ, Perry J et al., Functional analysis of untreated and reconstructed posterior cruciate ligament injuries, *Am J Sports Med* (1988) **16**(3): 217–223.

14. Torg JS, Barton TM, Pavlov H et al., Natural history of the posterior cruciate ligament-deficient knee, *Clin Orthop* (1989) **246**: 208–216.

15. Woods GW, Homsy CA, Prewitt JM et al., Proplast leader for use in cruciate ligament reconstruction, *Am J Sports Med* (1979) **7**(6): 314–340.

16. Clancy WG Jr, Repair and reconstruction of the posterior cruciate ligament. *Operative orthopaedics*, vol. 3, ed. Chapman MW, Madison M (Philadelphia: Lippincott, 1988) 1651–1653.

17. Insall JN, Chronic instability of the knee, *Surgery of the knee*, ed. Insall JN (New York: Churchill Livingstone, 1984) 292.

18. Insall JN, Chronic instability of the knee, *Surgery of the knee*. ed. Insall JN (New York: Churchill Livingstone, 1984) 296.

19. Daniel D, Malcom L, Stone ML, Quantification of knee stability and function, *Contemp Orthop* (1982) **5**(1):83.

20. Podesta L, Sherman MF, Bonamo JR et al., Rationale and protocol for postoperative anterior cruciate ligament rehabilitation, *Clin Orthop* (1990) **257**: 262-273.

21. Stäubli HU, Jakob RP, Posterior instability of the knee near extension: A clinical and stress radiographic analysis of acute injuries of the posterior cruciate ligament, *J Bone Joint Surg (Br)* (1990) **72**: 225–230.

22. Hughston JC, Bowden JA, Andrews JR et al., Acute tears of the posterior cruciate ligament: Results of operative treatment, *J Bone Joint Surg (Am)* (1980) **62**: 438–450.

23. Hughston JC, The absent posterior drawer test in some acute posterior cruciate ligament tears of the knee, *Am J Sports Med* (1988) **16**: 39–43.

24. Daniel DM, Stone ML, Barrett P et al., Use of the quadriceps active test to diagnose posterior cruciate ligament disruption and measure posterior laxity of the knee, *J Bone Joint Surg (Am)* (1988) **70**(3): 386–391.

25. Shelbourne KD, Benedict F, McCarroll JR et al., Dynamic posterior shift test: An adjuvant in evaluation of posterior tibial subluxation, *Am J Sports Med* (1989) **17**(2): 275–277.

26. Jakob R, Stäubli HU, The reversed pivot shift sign — a new diagnostic aid for posterolateral rotatory instability of the knee. Its distinction from the true pivot shift sign, *Orthop Trans* (1981) **5**: 487.

27. Strobel M, Stedtfeld HW, Evaluation of the ligaments. *Diagnostic evaluation of the knee*, ed Strobel M, Stedtfeld HW (Berlin: Springer-Verlag, 1990) 139.

28. Feagin JA, Principles of diagnosis and treatment. *The crucial ligaments: Diagnosis and treatment of ligamentous injuries about the knee*, ed Feagin JA (New York: Churchill Livingstone, 1988) 3–136.

29. Shino K, Horibe S, Ono K, The voluntarily evoked posterolateral drawer sign in the knee with posterolateral instability, *Clin Orthop* (1987) **215**: 179-186.

30. DeHaven KE, Diagnosis of acute knee injuries with haemarthrosis, *Am J Sports Med* (1980) **8**: 9–14.

31. Lysholm J, Gillquist J, Arthroscopic examination of the posterior cruciate ligament, *J Bone Joint Surg (Am)* (1981) **63**: 363–366.

32. Golimbu C, Firooznia H, Raffi M et al., Computerised tomography of the posterior cruciate ligament,*Comput Radiol* (1982) **6**: 233.

33. Torisu T, Avulsion fracture of the tibial attachment of the posterior cruciate ligament: Indications and results of delayed repair, *Clin Orthop* (1979) **143**: 107–114.

34. DeHaven KE, Acute ligament injuries and dislocations. *Surgery of the musculoskeletal system*, ed Evarts CM, 2nd edn, vol. 4 (New York: Churchill Livingstone, 1990) 3265–3274.

35. Hey Groves EW, The crucial ligaments of the knee joint: Their function, rupture, and the operative treatment of the same, *Br J Surg* (1919) **7**: 505–515.

36. Sisk TD, Knee injuries, *Campbell's operative orthopaedics*, 7th edn, vol 3 (St Louis: CV Mosby, 1987) 2371–2372.

37. Kennedy JC, Grainger RW, The posterior cruciate ligament, *J Trauma* (1967) **7**: 367–377.

38. Lipscomb AB, Johnston RK, Snyder RB, The technique of cruciate ligament reconstruction, *Am J Sports Med* (1981) **9**: 77–81.

39 Wirth CJ, Jager M, Dynamic double tendon replacement of the posterior cruciate ligament, *Am J Sports Med* (1984) **12**(1): 39–43.

40. Hughston JC, Degenhardt TC, Reconstruction of the posterior cruciate ligament, *Clin Orthop* (1982) **164**: 59–77.

41. Barfod B, Posterior cruciate ligament reconstruction by transposition of the popliteal tendon, *Acta Orthop Scand* (1971) **42**(5): 438.

42. McCormick WC, Bagg RJ, Kennedy CW Jr et al., Reconstruction of the posterior cruciate ligament: preliminary report of a new procedure, *Clin Orthop* (1976) **118**: 30–34.

43. Tillberg B, The late repair of torn cruciate ligaments using menisci, *J Bone Joint Surg (Br)* (1977) **59**: 15–19.

44. Southmayd WW, Rubin BD, Reconstruction of the posterior cruciate ligament using the semimembranosus tendon, *Clin Orthop* (1980) **150**: 196–197.

45. Eriksson E, Häggmark T, Johnson RJ, Reconstruction of the posterior cruciate ligament, *Orthopaedics* (1986) **9**: 217–220.

46. James SL, Woods GW, Homsy CA et al., Cruciate ligament stents in reconstruction of the unstable knee. A preliminary report, *Clin Orthop* (1979) **143**: 90–96.

47. Van Loon T, Van Dijk CN, Marti RK, The placement of a Gore-Tex prosthetic ligament in posterior cruciate deficient knees as a salvage procedure, ESKA abstract book, June 25–30 (1990) 148.

48. Hughston JC, Jacobson KE, Surgical treatment of posterolateral rotatory instability of the knee, *Operative Orthopaedics*, ed. Chapman MW (Philadelphia: JB Lippincott, 1988) 1669.

49. Trillat A, Posterolateral instability. *Late reconstruction of injured ligaments of the knee*, ed Schulitz KP, Krahl H, Stein WH (New York: Springer-Verlag, 1978). 99–105.

50. Müller W, *The knee — Form, function, and ligament reconstruction* (New York: Springer-Verlag, 1983) 140.

51. Butler DL, Noyes FR, Grood ES, Ligamentous restraints to anterior–posterior drawer in the human knee: A biomechanical study, *J Bone Joint Surg (Am)* (1980) **62**: 259–270.

7.2 Acute posterior cruciate ligament tears—diagnosis and management

Roland P. Jakob

Incidence

Among knee ligament injuries the incidence of posterior cruciate ligament involvement is relatively small. In our University Department, out of 10 knees with pathology of the cruciate ligaments we would observe 8 with anterior cruciate ligament (ACL) and 2 with posterior cruciate ligament (PCL) instability. One knee would have both anterior and posterior instability, i.e be of 'mixed' type. In a ski injury population this is even smaller, with 1 PCL in 9 ACL tears. In an athletic injury clinic with a predominance for football or soccer lesions, 3–4 out of 10 cruciate tears will be associated with PCL damage. In a trauma center with a high number of severe lower extremity fractures, the incidence of PCL tear is high as compared to the ACL (3–4 in 10). However, many of those go initially or permanently undiagnosed.

Mechanism of injury

The isolated PCL tear results from an anterior blow to the tibia with the knee in some flexion; in combined PCL and ACL injuries it becomes difficult to discern specific injury patterns.

Anatomy and biomechanics

The strength of the PCL and its central position in the knee joint underline its relevance as the primary restraining pillar. Alone it can absorb more than 90% of the posteriorly directed forces. In resisting valgus and varus forces it works in concert with the postero-medial and posterolateral capsule and the collateral ligaments.[1] Its central function as the axis of rotation has been described by Hughston as serving as the basis for the classification system of rotational instabilities.[2] Both the anterior (Humphry) and posterior (Wrisberg) meniscofemoral ligaments reinforce the PCL. Their presence is inconstant but they are usually observed in association with each other. According to the direction of force, an isolated tear of the PCL may be associated with lesions of the posterolateral corner or (rarely) the posteromedial corner. Angular forces directed predominantly in the frontal plane (varus or valgus) will lead to a complete rupture of the collateral ligament and the posterior capsule with PCL and ACL involvement.

Natural history

The untreated isolated tear of the PCL is initially well tolerated since it does not lead to the phenomenon of subluxational buckling of the knee as a tear of the ACL does. Nevertheless, various factors explain why an important proportion of patients develop pain and discomfort from femoropatellar and medial femoro-tibial compartment overload following a PCL tear. The tibia subluxates posteriorly in the swing phase of gait and is reduced during stance phase by quadriceps contraction. If this reduction is incomplete, the joint will be submitted to unphysiological shear forces. The posterior displacement of the tibia beneath the femur also results in higher femoropatellar pressure.

With loss of PCL function the secondary restraints will loosen, leading to a loss of lateral femorotibial coaptation. Since 60% of the load passes medial to the tibial eminence during the one-leg standing phase, the lateral structures (arcuate complex) are loose and more weight is shifted medially, with development of chondral damage and medial osteoarthrosis.

The loosening of the medial secondary restraints is less of a problem. The more complex the injury and the more marked the peripheral (mainly lateral) involvement, the more rapidly will this process take place. The clinical signs will accordingly be more marked. The AP translation in the lateral compartment is definitely more marked (2 cm or more) than in the medial, and the center of rotation is shifted more towards the medial side with more congruous joint anatomy. Thus PCL damage tends to stretch the arcuate complex, which allows the lower leg to externally rotate and fall in posterolateral subluxation.

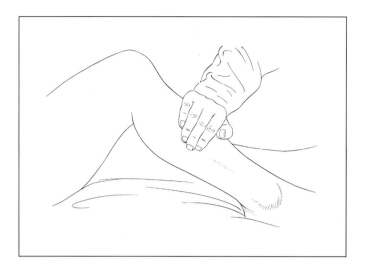

Figure 1

Posterior drawer test in rotation.

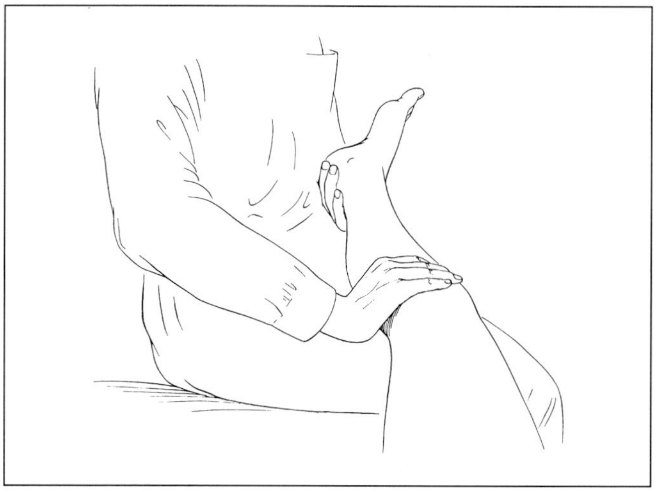

Figure 2

Testing for varus laxity is best performed with the patient's knee on the examiner's leg.

Diagnosis and clinical signs

The knee with a fresh, isolated PCL tear often does not show much intra-articular effusion, owing to the PCL being partially extra-articular. This allows leakage of the effusion into the popliteal fossa and the calf. Inspection may reveal skin contusions in the anterior half of the proximal tibia. When examining the knee for presence of PCL plus posterolateral or posteromedial involvement, one attempts to guide the knee on the path of its greatest laxity, allowing it to fall into the extreme position of the envelope of motion.[3] Thus the tests should be done in an unconstrained manner; however, quantification may be facilitated by using some degree of rotational constraint.

The most common sign, obvious and easy to recognize, is the *posterior sag sign*. It is detected by comparison of the anterior profile of the proximal tibia to the contralateral side with both knees in 70–80° of flexion. Owing to gravity the tibia falls posteriorly, with the thigh resting on a support to relax the quadriceps muscle. Slight pressure on the proximal tibia will lead to the *posterior drawer sign*, the classic and most commonly used sign, obvious and easy to recognize.[2] This is elicited in various positions of rotation of the lower leg. In neutral rotation, the isolated PCL tear is depicted with a 1–2+ posterior drawer. This is unchanged in external rotation, but disappears in internal rotation. The extent of posterior translation of the tibial tuberosity can be quantified in 1+ (3–5 mm), 2+ (6–10 mm) or 3+ (over 10 mm) increments—though more commonly we now use estimates in millimetres in analogy to instrumented laxity measurement, which is important for therapeutic decision making.

When performing this test one faces the difficulty of determination of the neutral or 0 point of the tibia to the femur in the sagittal plane. Owing to the spontaneous posterior subluxation, the tibia has to be reduced by pulling it in a forward direction. At this time anterior insufficiency has to be ruled out by comparing the contour of the tibial tuberosity and the amount of step off to the other side. With a competent ACL the posterior displacement can now be measured by pushing the tibia posteriorly (Figure 1).

The next important diagnostic element is the comparison of the *end point quality* when performing the posterior drawer test at flexion at 80° and 25°. This end point can be estimated as *firm, marginal or absent*. We have repeatedly observed that, despite an increased posterior translation of 10 mm, the posterior end point at 80° of flexion was still firm. In contrast the end point could be absent at 25° of flexion. We therefore advise checking for end point quality in the near-extended position (25°), since an osseous contact between the eminence or the concavity of the medial compartment and the femur while eliciting the posterior drawer manoeuvre at 90° gives a false impression. Estimating the extent of displacement in the 90° flexed position, however, results in a more accurate picture of the true PCL weakness than estimates in near-extended position.[4] The posterior translation as detected in the posterior sag sign can be measured by palpating and estimating the *step off* in millimetres at the anterior joint-line medially and laterally to the patellar ligament.

Posterolateral instability

If the posterolateral subluxation is definitely more marked in external rotation, a lesion of the arcuate complex is suspected. When this completely reduces in internal rotation it is most likely that the meniscofemoral and meniscotibial ligaments are still intact.[5]

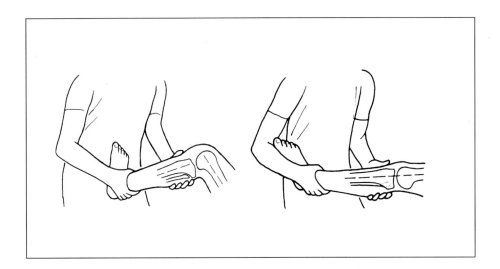

Figure 3

Reversed pivot shift test.

However, we believe that the tibia winds up the medial collateral ligament, bringing the knee into a reduced position. When the posterior drawer is absent in flexion and posterolateral rotation is marked in near extended position, this implies more of a peripheral posterolateral lesion.[6]

Posteromedial instability is present whenever internal rotation causes the posteromedial corner to subluxate posteriorly—a rare clinical situation.

Varus laxity: Posterior–posterolateral instability may be associated with varus laxity, which is tested with the knee in flexion of 20° and in full extension. When varus laxity is present in full extension, and is associated with posterior–posterolateral instability, marked deficiency of the arcuate complex is the cause. When varus laxity is present in the 20° flexion position, it points to an isolated lateral collateral ligament injury (Figure 2).

Valgus laxity: When the medial joint can be opened in slight flexion of 20° but not in full extension, an isolated MCL tear is present; valgus laxity in full extension signals an MCL tear with a tear of the posteromedial capsule and the PCL.

A number of other clinical signs point to the association of PCL damage and posterolateral rotatory instability. One relevant finding supporting the suspicion of chronic posterolateral rotational instability (PLRI) is the observation that practically all patients suffering from a severe instability of this type show a constant tendency to walk with their involved tibia and *foot in marked internal rotation*. In this position the patient is at decreased risk of taking an unguarded step with his knee giving way. Active internal rotational force against resistance is markedly decreased. Another important finding which substantiates the presence of chronic PLRI is *recurvatum* of the involved knee when standing and a positive

external rotation recurvatum test. In this test the knee will go into relative hyperextension at the lateral side when both legs are lifted up by the heels. The tibia will at the same time externally rotate, the tibial tuberosity moving to the lateral side. The medial side of the knee will reveal an apparent *bow leg deformity*.[2] We have found this sign to be of significance only in those cases where, besides the chronic PLRI, we also detected a concomitant weakness of the function of the ACL. This reflects the pathomechanical behaviour of the knee under hyperextension: the ACL is tethered in Grant's notch at the intercondylar fossa and ruptures *before* lesions of the PCL occur. In the cadaver knee when the posterior cruciate ligament and the arcuate complex are sectioned, there results no increased recurvatum as long as the ACL and the posteromedial capsule (which act as a barrier against hyperextension) are left intact. Likewise in fresh posterolateral injuries there is usually no recurvatum detectable.

Finally, there is an important dynamic sign present in PLRI which reflects the mechanism of the giving-way episodes. This is the so-called *reversed pivot shift* (RPS).[7] This phenomenon may be difficult to distinguish from a true pivot shift sign and may confuse the examiner. To check for this sign the patient is placed supine on the examining table (Figure 3). To test the right knee the examiner faces the patient and lifts the foot by the heel with his right hand resting the leg against his waist. The left hand supports the lateral side of the calf with the thumb on the proximal fibula. The knee is moved several times through a full range of motion to decrease muscular resistance. Then the examiner bends the knee to 70–80° of flexion. In this position external rotation of the foot and the lower leg causes the lateral tibial plateau to subluxate posteriorly in relation to the lateral femoral condyle. This is visualized as a posterior sag of the proximal tibia. The knee is now allowed to straighten using nothing more than the weight of the leg. When the examiner leans slightly against the foot, an axial load is transmitted through the leg and a valgus stress is applied to the knee. The iliac crest is used as a fulcrum. As the knee approaches 20° before full extension, one can feel and observe the lateral tibial plateau moving anteriorly with a jerk-like shift. It moves from a position of posterior subluxation and external rotation into a position of reduction and neutral rotation. The test is even more pertinent if it reproduces the patient's symptoms of his *knee giving way*. The intensity of the finding of subluxation and reduction, and the patient's reaction to it, depend on the degree of instability, the skill with which the examiner performs the test and the patient's ability to relax his muscles. The anatomical deficiency producing this sign is complex. In cadaver experiments with sequential sectioning, the sign could be attributed to the intactness of the popliteus tendon and muscle. It is definitely more prominent when the associated structures of the arcuate complex are sectioned and the PCL is absent.

Besides the actual traumatic lesion, other poorly understood factors seem to play a role. These include constitutional joint laxity, geometry of the lateral compartment, convexity of the lateral tibial plateau and hyperextension of the knee. It was observed and mentioned in the initial description of the RPS sign that it can be positive in both knees at a moderate degree without any previous history of injury.[7,8] We estimate the incidence of these physiological reversed pivot shifts to be about one-quarter of the normal population. This is important, since we have observed that in chronic anterior instability patients with a 1+ reversed pivot shift on the other side tend to have a global residual laxity that is more marked. This may also influence the results of the ACL reconstruction in that residual laxity of +3 mm Lachman compared to the opposite side may already lead to a grade I pivot shift (slide, trace), as if the reversed pivot shift adds to the increased anterior translation. In a knee with an absent reversed shift this would not be the case. Although we do not yet understand the significance of a 1+ pivot shift after ACL reconstruction, since these patients are without symptoms and function well, it is well worth recognizing and recording it.

The distinction between a true pivot shift and reversed pivot shift that has a component of posterior laxity may be difficult for the unexperienced examiner. As a rule, marked internal rotation of the tibia on the femur will cause the reversed pivot shift to disappear, while increasing a true pivot shift.

As for the true pivot shift, we grade RPS as follows: The 1+ RPS sign is insignificant when present in both knees. When associated with an anterior laxity it will unfavorably enlarge the sagittal play. A 2+ RPS

demonstrates the situation where the sign is found only in the involved damaged knee with other signs of PLRI present and the opposite knee showing absolutely no constitutional laxity. We talk about a 3+ RPS when this is associated with true posterior cruciate laxity as detected with a posterior drawer sign in neutral rotation of the tibia and when this sign reproduces the patient's symptom.

Radiological diagnosis

Plain radiographs may reveal an avulsion of the tibial attachment on the lateral view. In injuries combined with severe varus trauma to the lateral side, an osseous avulsion of the biceps tendon of the fibular head or a rare osseous avulsion of the iliotibial tract underlines the severity of the injury. The Segond fracture, an avulsion of the anterolateral capsule with a small piece of bone from the margin of the tibia, suggests an ACL injury.[9,10] Examination under anesthesia is often extremely helpful in these situations, though in cases of combined instabilities it is quite difficult to determine the neutral point between anterior and posterior displacement. In these situations, stress radiography is the only way to demonstrate the direction and degree of instability in both the frontal and sagittal planes. For practical purposes the examination is done in the near-extended position.

Treatment options

Compared to the treatment of anterior cruciate ligament tears, the results of treatment for PCL tears are somewhat frustrating. This is due to various reasons, among which the following are the most important.

Theoretically, revascularization of a sutured PCL or an autologous graft should be more favorable than of an ACL. The ACL is exposed to the synovial fluid and reaches soft-tissue contact only at the side where it is lying in close relationship to the PCL. This also explains how the ACL in a proximal tear falls on the PCL, and, thanks to an immediate vascular connection, scars down in a few weeks creating a type of spontaneous pseudohealing.[11] The PCL is closer to the posterior capsule and can be reached more easily by vessels from the neighbouring tissue. During the phase of revascularization (which for the ACL lasts up to 5 months) the ligament tends to elongate when it is mechanically loaded. This is even more of a problem for the PCL which, owing to the force of gravity, is constantly exposed to a force tending to separate origin and insertion of the ligament.

Furthermore, the results of an untreated complex tear (with involvement of the posteromedial and posterolateral structures) are poor when surgery addresses the PCL alone. On the other hand, when reconstruction of the peripheral structures, which act in synergism with the PCL, is performed without the PCL, they may also stretch out.

Braces to prevent posterior subluxation are inefficient. Attempts to stabilize the knee operatively have met with limited success. Skeletal fixation using an olecranization nail from the patella to the tibia and creating an anterior buttress is hazardous for the femoropatellar joint. They furthermore allow a range of motion of only 10–60° because with greater flexion there may be a posteriorly directed force on the tibia.

Indications for surgery in a fresh PCL tear

Isolated tear

Experience with the relatively benign course after partial, isolated rupture of the PCL has led to the following recommendations. They are based on the amount of posterior translation. Surgery is indicated when clinically, and with confirmation on stress radiographs at 25° of flexion, the posterior translation exceeds 8–10 mm side-to-side difference compared to the uninvolved side. Partial tears, or PCL tears where the ligaments of Wrisberg and Humphry remain intact, will produce smaller translations. The preservation of some ligamentous fibers will most likely prevent an initial instability from becoming worse.

If a diagnosis is in doubt, stress radiographs are taken under anesthesia prior to an arthroscopic evaluation.

Tibial spine avulsion

The osseous tibial spine avulsion justifies, whenever a clear-cut fragment is present, a posterior approach as recommended by Trickey[12] and refixation with screws and washers. Sometimes there are several fragments of the tibial spine that need to be put back using a washer and screw fixation. When entering between the two heads of the gastrocnemius muscles, great care has to be taken not to injure its vascular and nervous supply. If high neurovascular branches prevent an easy approach we do not hesitate to enter inferior to these branches either on the medial or preferably on the lateral side. This facilitates the surgery markedly. The oblique popliteal ligament (the connection between the semimembranosus insertion medially and the arcuate ligament laterally) covers the posterior approach to the intercondylar fossa. It is divided initially internal to the midline, then sutured after the repair.

Ligamentous tear

When radiological signs of an osseous fragment are absent, arthroscopic evaluation will allow easy evaluation of the site of the anatomical lesion. With a proximal tear of the PCL or a subperiosteal avulsion of the femur, the prognosis is relatively good thanks to the obvious facility of the repair. Owing to the previously mentioned factor of elongation of a repair, we augment such a lesion with the semitendinosus tendon and reinforce it with a small synthetic ligament augmentation device (Prolad, Protek Company) with loops on either side for screw fixation. An arthroscopically assisted placement of the tibial tunnel is recommended. Using an aiming device entered through the posteromedial portal, and not through the poorly visualized intercondylar fossa, placement of the tibial tunnel is facilitated. Open retrieval of the semitendinosus tendon is best. This can be done by using a tendon stripper that detaches it proximally at the musculotendinous junction. The tendon is left attached distally and is guided from its distal tibial insertion through the tibial tunnel in a posterior direction. It is then brought back up into the notch and guided through a tunnel in the medial condyle. The synthetic ligament is fed through the same tunnels and fixed proximally and distally with screws and special grommets. The femoral screw will incorporate the fixation of the semitendinosus tendon, the ligament augmentation device and the sutures of the stump of the ligament. When drilling the femoral tunnel, care has to be taken not to place it too anterior in the notch. The ideal insertion of the ligament is observed when the tunnel is at about 1 cm posterior to the cartilaginous margin superomedially in the fossa.

With a midsubstance tear of the PCL, or as more commonly observed a distal rupture, there often remains little or no tissue in which to place sutures. In such a situation (unfortunately the most common one) a formal bone–patellar ligament–bone graft reconstruction is utilized. Since arthroscopically it is difficult to drill the tibial tunnel from anteriorly with incorrect exit points being selected and to feed the ligament through the tunnels starting from a tibial or a femoral direction, the surgery is divided into two phases. Augmentation with a synthetic device is the only way to avoid stretching of the graft and permanent elongation. To avoid fragmentation, disintegration and debris formation of the synthetic ligament, the augmentation device is buried within the ligament (the 'hot-dog technique').[13] From an anteromedial arthrotomy the composite graft is first passed through the medial condyle and fixed together with the artificial stint outside the condyle, and the tibial bone block, armoured by the other loop of the Prolad, is provisionally stored in the back of the intercondylar notch and the wound is closed. Either in the same session or 10 days later the tibial bone block is retrieved through a posterior approach as described and anchored with a screw in a trough at the posterior tibial metaphysis, thus avoiding malplacement and kinking at the graft. This makes up for more extensive surgery; it is, however, worth it (Figure 4). The LAD is tightened on a separate screw at 50 N, the autograft at 25 N, which requires a special instrument. Needless to say, the arthroscope helps to detect meniscal pathology that needs resection or suturing at the same time, although this is extremely rare with an isolated tear of the PCL.

Combined injuries

Whenever a fresh PCL tear is combined with a tear of the ACL, reinforcement using either the semitendinosus for the PCL and the patellar ligament for the ACL, or vice versa, sometimes harvesting the patellar ligament from the opposite side plus synthetic augmentation with a LAD, will make this reconstruction a major procedure. Tightening of the sutures and the ligaments is best performed with the knee in full extension since it may be difficult to find the neutral point in combined ACL–PCL lesion. In full extension the tibia is well reduced; in a flexed position it is difficult to know where the tibia stands. An intraoperative lateral radiograph, however, should confirm the proper relationship of the tibia to the femur.

The better the central pillar is repaired, the less needs to be done for the peripheral lesions provided that they are fresh. This is now established for those lesions that are combined with a tear of the ACL. In PCL injuries, we believe that an anatomical repair of the peripheral lesions is justified, mainly posterolateral injuries. They would be approached through a lateral incision entering anteriorly and posteriorly through the iliotibial tract. There the exposure will reveal the rupture of the popliteus tendon. This is sutured or reinserted in a transosseous manner. If a distal avulsion of the tendon is observed it is best left in position, or the tendon remaining at its proximal attachment may be used to reinforce the lateral collateral ligament. Unfortunately, the suturing of the torn LCL is useless owing to the lack of ligament substance. The posterolateral capsule is carefully sutured. An avulsion of the biceps tendon is refixed. In the presence of associated damage to the peroneal nerve, it can be exposed through the same incision for prognostic purposes.

Lesions of the posteromedial capsule are sutured similarly.

Aftertreatment

The aftertreatment unfortunately is much more difficult than with the ACL tear. As previously outlined, there is a risk of stretching the graft during revascu-

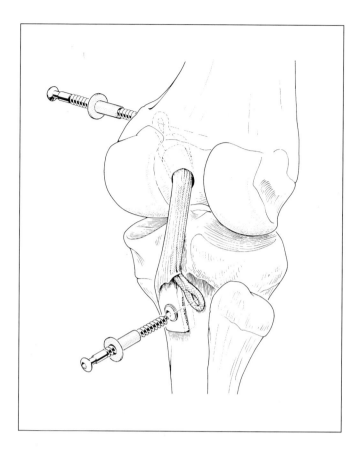

Figure 4

Posterior approach for tibial fixation of bone block.

larization. The synthetic augmentation device acts as an internal splint and has become a prerequisite for achievement of an acceptable result that justifies the surgery. It is obvious that the LAD needs to be fixed on either side and prestretched to at least 50 N because of stress elongation of the synthetic material.

The patient is allowed full range of motion, especially full extension; quadriceps strengthening is enhanced from the beginning. If the knee does not reach 90° of flexion within 6 weeks, a careful manipulation under anesthesia should be performed because of the risk of permanent loss of flexion. Increased weight bearing is allowed depending on the muscular control of the knee and is usually complete after 8 weeks. A return to sports is not allowed before 8–10 months.

The success of a repair depends on the accuracy of graft placement, the quality of the repair and reconstruction, and the patient's successful guidance through the rehabilitation programme. The following complications are observed. *Stiffness:* loss of flexion is more prominent than loss of extension since we immediately begin with full extension. Unfortunately, fear of graft stretching makes the surgeon withhold full range of motion. Since late complaints after a repair are more directed to a loss of motion than to a slight residual laxity, regaining full activity should be emphasized. *Stretching of the graft:* in the past PCL reconstructions were unfortunately complicated by a marked loss of stability. The resulting values were more than half the initial ones. With augmentation, the quality of the results has definitely improved, in both the acute and the chronic situation. *Osteoarthrosis:* An unisometric graft may lead to a loss of function and recurrence of instability and thus be a factor in cartilage degeneration due to increased contact pressure on the cartilage or disturbed kinematics of the knee with secondary meniscal entrapment. However, late meniscal pathology has been rare and osteoarthritic degeneration is more connected to the lack of initial conservation of meniscal tissue or to loss of lateral ligamentous coaptation with load shift to the medial compartment—all factors that need to be taken care of when the necessity of an immediate repair is evaluated.

Chronic lesion

The treatment of chronic instability is less gratifying owing to lack of repair response of the peripheral capsular and ligamentous tissues. The surgical considerations for reconstruction of the PCL are no different from the acute situation one regarding the type of reconstruction. The techniques for reconstruction of the peripheral structures, however, are more complicated.

References

1. **Butler DL, Noyes FR, Grood ES**, Ligamentous restraints to anterior–posterior drawer in the human knee: a biomechanical study, *J Bone Joint Surg (Am)* (1980) **62**: 259–270.
2. **Hughston JC, Norwood LA Jr**, The posterolateral drawer test and external rotation recurvatum test for posterolateral rotatory instability of the knee, *Clin Orthop* (1980) **147**: 82–87.
3. **Noyes FR, Grood ES, Suntay WJ** et al., The three dimensional laxity of the anterior cruciate deficient knee as determined by clinical laxity tests, *Iowa Orthop J* (1983) **3**: 32.
4. **Fukubayashi T, Torzilli PA, Sherman MF** et al., An in vitro biomechanical evaluation of anterior–posterior motion of the knee: tibial displacement, rotation and torque, *J Bone Joint Surg (Am)* (1982) **64**: 258–264.
5. **Clancy WG Jr, Shelbourne KD, Zoellner GB** et al., Treatment of knee joint instability secondary to rupture of the posterior cruciate ligament: report of a new procedure, *J Bone Joint Surg (Am)* (1983) **65**: 310–322.
6. **Gollehon DL, Torzilli PA, Warren RF**, The role of the posterolateral and cruciate ligaments in the stability of the human knee: A biomechanical study, *J Bone Joint Surg (Am)* (1987) **69**: 233–242.
7. **Jakob RP, Hassler H, Stäubli HU**, Observations on rotatory instability of the lateral compartment of the knee: Experimental studies on the functional anatomy and the pathomechanism of the true and the reversed pivot shift sign, *Acta Orthop Scand* (1981) **52**, Suppl 191.
8. **Cooper DE**, Tests for posterolateral instability of the knee in normal subjects: results of examination under anaesthesia, *J Bone Joint Surg (Am)* (1991) **73**: 30–36.
9. **Segond P**, Recherches cliniques et expérimentales sur les épanchements sanguins du genou par entorse, *Progr Med* (1879) **7**: 297–299, 319–321, 340–341, 379–381, 400–401, 419–421.
10. **Woods GW, Stanley RF, Tullos HS**, Lateral capsular sign: x-ray clue to a significant knee instability, *Am J Sports Med* (1979) **7**: 27–33.
11. **Wittek A**, Ueber Verletzungen der Kreuzbänder des Kniegelenks, *Dtsch Z Chir* (1927) **200**: 491–515.
12. **Trickey EL**, Rupture of the posterior cruciate ligament of the knee, *J Bone Joint Surg (Br)* (1968) **50**: 334–341.
13. **Gächter A**, Plastik aus einem transligamentären Zugang, *Kniegelenk und Kreuzbänder*, ed. Jakob RP, Stäubli HU (Berlin: Springer-Verlag, 1990) 393–398.

7.3   Chronic posterolateral knee instability

Brian Casey

Chronic posterolateral knee instability is a complex problem made more difficult by highly variable normal anatomy and the multiple structures involved. The instability is rare in isolation[1] and is most commonly associated with chronic anterior cruciate ligament loss and anterolateral instability but is more severe when accompanied by posterior cruciate and/or lateral ligamentous damage. Discussion of the topic in the English literature is sparse[2,3] with greater recognition in the European literature.[4–7] There are many unsolved problems in both diagnosis and management. The discussion below outlines the evolution of my thoughts and experience up to 1990 following a special interest in the topic for more than 10 years.

Clinical considerations

Anterior cruciate deficiency may be associated with chronic posterolateral instability of the knee. Postero-lateral structures may be damaged together with the anterior cruciate ligament acutely in an external rotation or hyperextension knee injury. In the chronic phase, a slow stretching of the posterolateral structures may occur with repeated episodes of pivot shift instability.[8] Damage may occur iatrogenically in poorly executed ligament surgery, particularly extra-articular stabilization for the pivot shift. The patients have usually sustained their injury from sport and expect to return to a high level of participation. If significant posterolateral instability is present and not corrected, the patient may have objectively an excellent result as measured by the Lachman test or KT1000, but subjectively the knee will still feel unstable.

The standard pivot shift described by MacIntosh is present with the tibia in internal rotation.[9] In some patients the shift becomes more severe with external rotation. For this to happen there must be additional damage to secondary restraints either on the postero-medial corner producing associated anteromedial instability or on the posterolateral corner producing posterolateral instability, or both may be present. In more severe cases there is a separate excessive posterolateral glide that the patient can identify as a different feeling from that of their pivot shift instability. Jakob[5] has used the term 'reverse pivot shift' for this type of instability. It typically occurs close to full extension and is a posterior subluxation of the tibia that occurs as the knee unlocks from the fully extended position or reduces as full extension is approached.

A patient with instability in both internal and external rotation of the tibia is much more disabled than one with a simple pivot shift occurring only in internal rotation. Such patients are more likely to require surgery, since there is no position of leg and foot rotation where the knee will remain stable under load.

Separating the relative amount of posterolateral instability when anterolateral instability is also present is difficult, as assessment of the neutral position becomes somewhat subjective. Grood[10] has shown that posterolateral laxity is maximum with the knee flexed at 30°. At this angle, there is maximal expression of posterolateral damage with least super-imposition of any associated damage to the posterior cruciate ligament. This test can be combined with the Lachman test as a reverse Lachman test. Normally at 30° flexion there is a step of 0.5 cm from the femoral condyle to the anterior margin of the tibial plateau. The step must be compared between the two knees and also the medial and lateral plateaux must be compared, with and without a posterior force applied to the particular tibial plateau. The two limbs are also compared with maximum external rotation of the tibiae. The step from femoral condyle to tibia normally increases to 1 cm at 80–90° flexion.[11] It is checked in neutral, internal and external rotation with and without posterior force applied.

Clinically isolated posterolateral instability is detected at 30° flexion and there is no increase of posterior subluxation of the lateral plateau at 80–90° flexion. If the latter is present, it indicates posterior cruciate damage which is confirmed by the presence of posterior drawer in neutral rotation at the same angle. This is more useful to me than the postero-lateral drawer test of Hughston,[12] which relies on observations at 80° only. Clancy[11] has observed that the ligaments of Humphry and Wrisberg may prevent backward displacement of the tibia in internal rotation at 80°, giving a false impression of posterolateral instability by Hughston's test. Clinically, static testing at 80–90° gives more easily detectable information about the posterior cruciate ligament, which also is in agreement with the laboratory studies of Grood.[10] When anterior cruciate laxity is also present, the active quadriceps drawer test[13] is especially useful. With the knee flexed to 80° and the leg in neutral rotation, posterior force is applied to the upper tibia. If with quadriceps contraction the tibia moves forward there is posterior cruciate damage. The neutral point is the position of the tibia with quadriceps contracted. If passive forward movement of the tibia can be produced beyond this point, anterior cruciate damage must also be present.

Another static test is the external rotation recurvatum test described by Hughston.[12] This test is useful when positive and indicates a severe degree of posterolateral and deep posterior damage. It will frequently be negative in patients who are nevertheless troubled by posterolateral instability. Stäubli[14] did not find it positive in any of 24 patients with acute posterior instability examined under anaesthesia, although 17 patients gave a positive test for reverse pivot shift.

Instability as described above refers to static testing to determine a degree of pathological laxity in the affected ligamentous structures. To be certain that the pathological laxity detected is a source of symptomatic instability to the patient, dynamic tests are needed that reproduce the instability feeling in a way patients can recognize as being similar to their own problem. If such test is too painful, the patient's muscle will spasm, particularly the hamstrings, making further examination of that patient's knee instability impossible. I have developed a method of testing that avoids major discomfort to the patient and allows testing to be repeated and graded for severity. The method is usable to separate posterolateral and anterolateral instability and to quantitate each. The key principle is appropriate posturing of the patient's lower limb such that the abnormal glide of subluxation/reduction can be produced and felt by the examiner with one hand palpating and applying minimal force around the joint-line.

The detailed 'glide test' method is as follows. The patient's foot and ankle of the involved side are locked between the examiner's elbow and trunk leaving the hands free (Figure 1). To examine the patient's left knee, the left foot and ankle are gripped between the examiner's left elbow and trunk at and above the iliac crest. The elbow controls valgus and axial compression force at the knee, and trunk movements control knee flexion and extension. The left hand supports and grips the patient's left leg, controlling anteroposterior force and applying tibial rotation as desired. The right hand has the thumb applied to the posterolateral aspect of the fibular

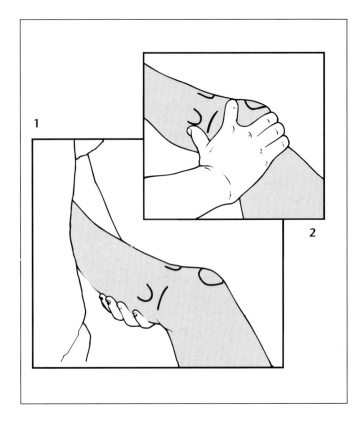

Figure 1

Starting position for 'glide test' with patient's ankle locked against examiner's trunk by the elbow.

Figure 2

'Glide test' seeking abnormal translation of the lateral tibial plateau.

head with the fingers on the joint-line, patella and lower femur (Figure 2). For posterolateral instability I start with the knee fully extended without valgus but with an external rotation force applied. The knee is flexed gradually, seeking a point where the thumb can rotate the tibia forwards. In some patients the lateral tibial plateau drops back excessively (subluxes) as full extension is lost. At around 20° off full extension, a point is found where a free forwards/backwards glide of the lateral tibial plateau can be achieved by the examiner's thumb. It can be quantified by the index finger palpating on the joint-line. For this test to be regarded as positive clinically for discrete posterolateral instability:

1. The patient must recognize the sensation so produced as being similar to that felt when the knee is unstable during activity.
2. The examiner must feel by palpation of the joint-line that the lateral tibial plateau is abnormally *posterior* relative to the femur.

The posterior translation of the lateral tibial plateau will be increased and the subluxation/reduction glide will be more easily detectable if there is posterior cruciate ligament damage associated with the posterolateral instability.

To look for coexistent anterolateral instability I commence with the knee flexed 50° and gradually extend, applying valgus and internal rotation together with anterior pressure to the upper tibia, feeling with the thumb behind the fibula head for uncontrolled forward subluxation occurring at around 35°. As before, the patient is asked whether they recognize the abnormal shift so produced and the index finger palpates the joint-line. The test can be repeated with variable force and variable rotation of the tibia without too much discomfort to the patient. The extent of the glide or shift is compared with the tibia in external and in internal rotation. Posterior and anterior subluxation of the lateral plateau may either occur in the patient at different degrees of knee flexion, with the posterior subluxation usually occurring when the knee is more extended, provided the posterior cruciate ligament is intact, or the knee may swing from a position of posterior subluxation to that of anterior subluxation at the same angle of knee flexion. Careful palpation of the joint-line is critical for accurate differentiation. If the patient is uncertain whether a particular test position reproduces the instability feeling, the test can be repeated with greater axial force applied to approximate more closely to the weight-bearing situation.

In a few patients, the tibia moves obliquely anteromedial from the posterolateral subluxed position without any rotation. This appears to correlate with the acute injury pattern produced by direct force on to the upper anteromedial tibia described by DeLee.[1]

The test must be compared with the opposite side, particularly if the patient is uncertain as to whether the test really reproduces the feeling of his or her instability. False positive results may occur especially in the patient with hyperlax tissues. The normal mobility of the lateral compartment is high when compared to the stability of the normal medial compartment. A degree of mobility that is abnormal for one patient may be normal for another of elastic tissue type. When true posterolateral instability occurs in a patient with hyperelastic tissues, surgical correction is difficult, with an increased risk of stretching of tissues and return of instability. Such patients should probably be restricted from very high demand sporting activities even if the knee is initially stable post-surgery. I find the best prognostic indicator for this type of tissue type is the ability to hyperflex the normal knee excessively for the age of the patient. For patients under 25 years old, this equates with the ability to bring the heel less than 10 cm from the greater trochanter. This test is a better indicator of knee ligament hyperlaxity than the presence of knee hyperextension or any of the finger hyperlaxity tests.

Another dynamic test for posterolateral instability is the reverse pivot shift described by Jakob.[5] In this test, the tibia is kept externally rotated as the knee is extended from a position of 70–80° of flexion. The initially posteriorly subluxed lateral tibial plateau reduces at around 20° of flexion, and this can be felt to occur by the examiner. This test is probably less sensitive than the 'glide test', particularly where the posterior cruciate ligament is intact. It is also more uncomfortable for the patient. It is of note that Jakob looked at a control group of 100 soldiers of a mountain infantry regiment. A bilateral reverse pivot shift sign was found in three soldiers, none of whom complained of knee problems. In another eight, a slightly positive test occurred bilaterally. Six of the 11 were considered to have some constitutional ligamentous laxity. For either of these dynamic tests of posterolateral instability to be regarded as positive, it is thus essential that the test produces discomfort and reproduces a feeling of instability that the patient can recognize. Shelbourne et al.[15] have recently described a further dynamic test for reduction of the posteriorly subluxed tibia but do not mention patient recognition of the test feeling.

The notes of a group of 57 consecutive patients coming to surgery for chronic anterolateral instability were reviewed in 1984. Thirty of those patients had their anterolateral instability present in both internal and external rotation of the tibia. In 10 of these, there was an additional separately identifiable shift of posterior subluxation of the lateral tibial plateau occurring with the knee close to full extension and a separate 'glide test' feeling was identified by the patient. Three of these 10 patients identified the posterolateral instability as their dominant instability. Two of the three had partial damage to both cruciate ligaments.

Posterolateral instability associated with lateral and/or posterior ligamentous damage

In this group of patients the degree of instability is usually severe. It may follow sporting injuries but frequently occurs after motorcycle accidents or in pedestrians hit by motor vehicles. Whilst soft-tissue reefing procedures are usually adequate for patients in the group described above, in this group more extensive procedures are required. The notes of a group of 19 consecutive patients seen in 1987–1988 and judged clinically to require more than simple reefing procedures for their posterolateral instability were reviewed. At arthroscopy, 3 had been noted to have total loss of the posterior cruciate ligament while 11 had partial posterior cruciate damage. Of the remaining 5 with intact posterior cruciate ligaments, all had had unsuccessful procedures of the extra-articular type for anterolateral instability. Fourteen had anterior cruciate loss with associated anterolateral instability, worse with external rotation of the tibia. Six of the 19 were hyperlax ligament type as judged from excessive knee hyperflexion. Four had a significant varus laxity associated with a bony varus limb alignment.

The assessment of *partial* posterior cruciate ligament injuries is difficult. This is particularly so if there is associated anterior cruciate ligament damage such that the neutral position anteroposteriorly is hard to define. In addition to clinical testing, much information can be gained from arthroscopy in spite of the synovial cover of the ligament. The bulk is probed. It is often reduced near the front of the notch in partial lesions. The ligaments of Humphry and Wrisberg are inspected and probed. If the anterior cruciate is torn, the bulk may best be seen in the 'figure 4' position. The posterior cruciate is probed with and without posterior force and with internal and external rotation. Even if in continuity, there is considerable damage if it does not become taut with internal rotation and with posterior drawer. In contrast to chronic tears of the anterior cruciate, it does not usually disappear when damaged but remains as relatively thick scar tissue.[17] The 70° arthroscope passed through the intercondylar notch allows direct view of the ligament.[18]

In patients coming to surgery for chronic posterior cruciate deficiency, Clancy had 5 of 13 with posterolateral instability.[11] Hughston did not mention posterior cruciate injuries in his series of 141 knees undergoing surgery directed at chronic arcuate complex injuries.[2] For acute posterior cruciate injuries the reported incidence of associated posterolateral instability ranges from 1 in 10[11] to 13 in 40.[16]

The state of the posterior cruciate has major significance in both evaluation and management. When it is intact, posterolateral instability presents clinically as increased posterior translation of the lateral tibial plateau without drop-back of the medial tibial plateau—a rotary instability—and surgical procedures are directed to the posterolateral peripheral structures. With associated increasing posterior cruciate laxity, there is a continuum of increasing posterior subluxation or translation of the lateral tibial plateau accompanied by some degree of posterior subluxation of the medial plateau. The subluxation involves both external rotation and posterior translation of the tibia.

Surgical procedures must also address the posterior cruciate ligament and/or posteromedial structures.

Associated varus laxity requires careful evaluation avoiding any distortion by tibial rotation. Using the position for the start of the 'glide test' (see Figure 1), the patient's lower leg and ankle are locked against the examiner's pelvis and trunk by his elbow, preventing tibial rotation and leaving the hands free to assess exactly what is happening at the knee joint-line as varus and valgus forces are applied. Testing at 15 and 30° knee flexion assesses the midlateral structures: lateral collateral ligament, popliteal fibular ligament, anterolateral femorotibial ligament and iliotibial tract. At 30°, an intact iliotibial tract may mask deeper damage (such as popliteofibular, arcuate complex). Excess varus at 0° indicates damage more posteriorly in the popliteal arcuate structures, deep capsule and posterior cruciate ligament.

Where there is varus laxity present greater than on the opposite side, any tendency for varus thrust on walking or for varus bone alignment must be carefully assessed, including use of standardized long weight-bearing radiographs. Soft-tissue reconstructive procedures alone are doomed to failure where there is significant varus bone alignment or varus thrust while walking.

In summary, combined with the 'glide test' the following static tests are recommended for clinical posterolateral assessment in the chronic knee:

1. Posterolateral (PL) instability. Posterior subluxation of the lateral tibial plateau at 30° knee flexion.
2. Posterior cruciate (PC) instability. Posterior subluxation of the tibia in neutral rotation at 80° knee flexion.
3. Combined instability (PL/PC). Increase in lateral plateau subluxation (from that in 1 or 2) with tibia in external rotation at 80° knee flexion.
4. Varus instability. Lateral joint opening with neutral tibial rotation at 15 and 30° knee flexion.
5. Tissue hyperelasticity. Heel–trochanter distance with knee hyperflexed.

Management

Conservative management with quadriceps and popliteus strengthening exercises is of use with or without surgical treatment and may avoid the need for surgery, particularly in patients with a naturally valgus knee.

Prior to reconstruction, examination under anaesthesia and arthroscopy are needed. The degree of tibial subluxation associated with each instability is assessed with the muscles relaxed. A complete arthroscopy, where posterolateral instability is present, includes special attention to the posterior cruciate ligament as previously discussed, the popliteus tendon and the lateral meniscus attachments. If the popliteus is lax to probing, can the site of damage be visualized? Is it in the joint or more distal? If the lateral meniscus is intact but hypermobile to probing, is there damage to the meniscotibial ligament at the front or back of the popliteal recess that needs repair?

For very mild degrees of posterolateral instability associated with anterior cruciate loss, replacement of the anterior cruciate ligament alone may correct the instability. It can be observed at surgery that, with external tibial rotation, the graft locks into the anterolateral corner of the intercondylar notch of the femur. More usually, capsular procedures are required with the cruciate reconstruction. Lateral dissection should carefully protect and preserve the anterolateral femorotibial ligament.[8]

I reinforce my intra-articular anterior cruciate replacement with a 1 cm distally based strip of the central fibres of the iliotibial tract, leaving the anterolateral femorotibial ligament intact deep and attaching to the posterior of the tract. The strip is passed under the popliteus tendon and then the lateral collateral ligament before being brought back more superficially towards Gerdy's tubercle. It is sutured with minimal tension to itself with the leg in neutral rotation to act as a check rein against excess anterior movement of the lateral tibial plateau. This strip is also sutured to the femur as it turns around behind the collateral ligament origin, if necessary picking up some of the tendinous origin of the arcuate ligament and lateral head of gastrocnemius. Inferiorly closer to joint-line, the arcuate ligament and the lateral part of the fascia that covers popliteus and blends laterally with joint capsule are sutured onto the inferior margin of this strip as it turns around the collateral ligament. The arcuate tightening so produced may be considerable and must be checked to avoid any block to terminal extension.

If the iliotibial tract is not used in this manner, the arcuate popliteal tissues can be sutured to the middle-third capsular ligament, the sutures passing deep to the lateral collateral ligament. There is a huge anatomical variation in the development of the arcuate and popliteal tissues, so that the amount of tightening must be individually judged for every patient. The original tissues are much better developed in patients with genetic varus.

The biceps femoris tendon has a complicated insertion with anterior extensions both superficial and deep towards Gerdy's anterolateral tubercle and the fascia over the anterolateral aspect of the upper tibia.[19] Surgically these superficial and deep fibres anterior to the collateral ligament may be detached as a flap that is swung forwards, enlarging the inverted V in the insertion of the biceps at the fibular head. The flap is sutured to the soft tissues on the front of the iliotibial tract (Figure 3). Moving the attachment from Gerdy's tubercle reduces the backward pull of the biceps directly on to the tibia

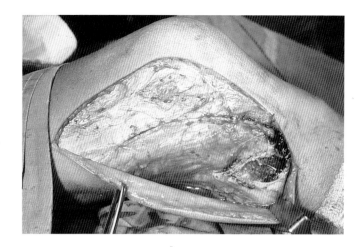

Figure 3

Lateral side of right knee showing advancement of the anterior part of biceps insertion from Gerdy's tubercle together with lateral patellar release.

and spreads it more anteriorly onto the anterior knee tissues. The anterolateral femorotibial ligament inserting into the more posterior fibres of the iliotibial tract is advanced and tightened, since the posterior part of the iliotibial tract is advanced with the anterior biceps where the two blend together. The exact dissection of the biceps varies because of the individual variability in the development of the superficial and deep lamina of insertion.

For more severe posterolateral instability, I have tried in 15 patients in 1984–1985 the 'popliteal bypass' procedure using the biceps femoris tendon.[8] The tendon is left attached to the fibular head and then dissected out from the muscle belly. It is fixed to the posterolateral corner of the tibia and threaded up through the posterolateral capsule and attached to the femur close to the popliteus origin. In my hands the procedure was not satisfactory in correcting posterolateral instability and I no longer use it. It stretched or failed in less than a year in 12 patients and stretched subsequently in the remaining three. In three that came to revision, the femoral attachment was attenuated and minimally functional. This appeared to be due to failure to obtain a solid attachment to the bone of the lateral femoral condyle, perhaps aggravated by the graft placement being bone-to-bone but not strictly isometric. Müller (personal communication, 1988) has informed me that he has ceased using this procedure.

Since 1986, for these more severe cases of posterolateral instability I have used a ligament augmentation device (LAD) to reinforce the lateral capsular structures and reduce the mobility of the lateral compartment. Originally the LAD was attached to the

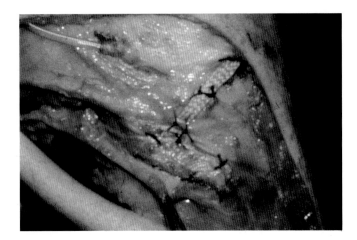

Figure 4

Lateral side of right knee showing ligament augmentation device threaded through lateral capsular tissues extending from patellar tendon to the popliteal fibrous connections deep to biceps femoris and the head of fibula via the posterior superior tibiofibular ligament.

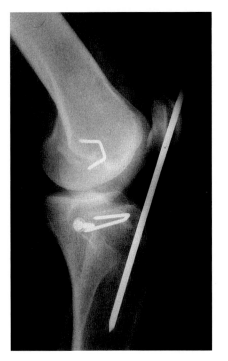

Figure 5

Patellotibial pin producing olecranization to prevent drop-back of upper tibia.

patellar tendon adjacent to its site of insertion into the patella laterally. It was also sutured into the adjacent deep fibrofatty tissue. From there it was passed back inferiorly and posteriorly, being threaded in and out of the capsular tissues and under the lateral collateral ligament close to the head of the fibula. The end was stitched to the posterosuperior tibiofibular ligament and adjacent capsular tissues. This included some of the insertions of the popliteus complex (Figure 4). While the LAD is being sutured, the leg is kept in full internal rotation. In the original concept the LAD was both a static stabilizer against posterior subluxation of the lateral tibial plateau and also tensioned the lateral structures further with quadriceps contraction. If the patient has reasonable tissue, it will reduce posterior subluxation of the lateral tibial plateau by 5–10 mm.

The procedure was carried out in 19 patients between September 1986 and January 1989. It was associated with other procedures for ligamentous problems in most patients so that it is difficult to state precisely how much the LAD contributed. Of these first 19 patients reviewed at an average of 1 year post-surgery, 5 had no residual posterolateral instability. Ten had a mild residual instability to clinical testing; however, they were not complaining of functional instability.

At the posterior or distal end a partial, lateral popliteal nerve palsy was produced in one patient by the hard tip of the LAD. It is essential to bury this tip and suture it firmly away from the nerve.

Although a lateral retinacular release was performed in all patients, two had problems with patellar tracking, one requiring more distal repositioning of the patellar-tendon end of the LAD. The tracking of the patella is checked carefully at arthroscopy prior to reconstruction and, if there is any lateral subluxation tendency, the anterior attachment of the LAD is placed only to the front of the iliotibial tract.

As a result of this experience, the concept of the function of the LAD was modified, increasing emphasis on static stabilization against posterior sag of the lateral tibial plateau. Anteriorly, it is now sutured 1 cm below the patella. In the functional instability position close to full extension, it acts as an extra-articular posterior cruciate ligament running from the fibula head via the posterior superior tibiofibular ligament to the anterior soft tissues that ensheath the lower femur (see Figure 4).

Secondly, with increasing realization of the importance of the complex fibromuscular popliteus system,[6] I now tension this system laterally to the posterior end of the LAD, using heavy (No 5) nonabsorbable deep transverse sutures. Bousquet et al.[4] and

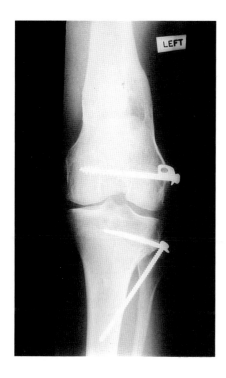

Figure 6

Radiograph following upper tibial osteotomy and biceps femoris advancement.

Pasquali-Lasagni[20] have described techniques to re-tension the chronically lax popliteus tendon using a strip of the tendinous part of the biceps femoris, left attached to the fibular epiphysis, while Pasquali-Lasagni[6] may use semitendinosus as a distally based tenodesis to replace the popliteus tendon and its long distal fibrous lamina.

Posterolateral instability is further complicated if there is posterior cruciate damage and particularly if in addition there is extensive posterior capsular damage and a positive external rotation recurvatum test. The long-term results of posterior cruciate reconstruction are not sufficiently reliable to justify reconstruction where part of the posterior cruciate only has been lost and posterior drawer is less than 2+. With total posterior cruciate loss combined with posterolateral instability, I have used the patellar tendon middle 40% with bone blocks on each end to replace the posterior cruciate ligament.[11] This improves but does not reliably eliminate posterior drop-back. The use of a patellotibial pin (olecranization) (Müller,W, personal communication, 1986) has been helpful to protect the graft in the early phases (Figure 5). A 4-mm Steinman pin (AO) is drilled through the patella and into the proximal tibia with the tibia held forwards to its normal position. The pin is threaded at its proximal end so that it grips the proximal patellar cortex and does not track. It has a cutaway of three flat surfaces on the proximal 1 cm to allow a small section (5 mm long) left protruding from the patella to be grasped with a drill chuck for easy removal. The protruding proximal end is thus short enough to be underneath the skin and fascia and avoid causing skin irritation.

The bone blocks of the posterior cruciate graft are placed in position prior to patellar pin insertion but they are not fixed until the knee is stabilized by the pin. This same technique is useful for acute knees with massive ligamentous damage, allowing the knee to remain stable whilst repair of soft tissues is carried out. It is apparent that the patella held by this pin cannot track anatomically in the femoral groove throughout a full range of knee flexion. I have viewed the tracking arthroscopically in three patients and there is a definite distortion of trochlear cartilage adjacent to a point pressure site of the patella as the knee is flexed beyond 60–70°. I therefore insert the pin with the knee flexed to 30° and allow motion of only 10–50° for the period of 3–6 weeks during which the pin is left in situ.

With a severe chronic posterolateral instability, the posterior capsular structures will be stretched, involving not only the popliteus arcuate system but also the semimembranosus system, especially the oblique popliteal ligament. On the lateral side at the back the superior part of the popliteus system can be tightened from its deep surface as described by Hughston.[2] Rather than take a bone block off the lateral femoral condyle, I prefer to tighten these structures from the posterior or superficial aspect using heavy non-absorbable sutures that take purchase via a tunnel drilled in the lower femur just proximal to the lateral gastrocnemius origin. Medially the oblique popliteal ligament and posterior oblique ligament are tensioned onto the main semimembranosus tendon with sutures placed at or below the joint line and as horizontal as technically possible. Occasionally, the posteromedial capsule is retensioned on to bone at the back of the medial tibial plateau.

Varus instability is often associated with posterolateral instability in these more severe cases. If the patient has a varus thrust on walking or a varus bone alignment associated, an upper tibial lateral closing wedge osteotomy is necessary prior to or at the same time as any soft-tissue procedure, otherwise the latter is doomed to stretch. I prefer the technique of osteotomy described by Burkhart (personal communication, 1986). Great care must be taken to bend and not break the medial cortex of the tibia as the osteotomy wedge is taken. Subsequently, excellent compression and stability are obtained using a transverse flattened semitubular AO plate in the proximal epiphysis plus a single long screw into the anterior cortex of the tibia (Figure 6). If the osteotomy is firm, reconstruction can be carried out at the same time and the knee carefully mobilized postoperatively.

The treatment of associated soft-tissue varus has been a major difficulty. Additionally to the lateral collateral ligament, stability is contributed to by the femoral-to-fibula popliteus fibres as well as the iliotibial tract, and on its deep posterior aspect the antero-lateral femorotibial ligament.[8] In the mid-1980s, I tried to re-tension the collateral ligament by taking it off the femur with a bone block and then re-sinking it deeper into the same hole to achieve isometric retensioning. I found that the healing of the attachment back onto the femur was unreliable, often becoming attenuated. I had similar experience endeavouring to retension the popliteus at its femoral attachment in a similar manner. This experience contrasted with my results for the corresponding procedure for the medial ligament onto the medial femoral condyle, where retensioning worked well.

Clancy[21] has described a procedure that he claims will simultaneously correct posterolateral and varus instability. The biceps tendon is mobilized anteriorly in continuity and the anterolateral femorotibial ligament is divided. A screw is inserted across the femur from the lateral femoral epicondyle immediately adjacent to the lateral ligament attachment (see Figure 6) and the tendon is advanced anteriorly so that it turns around this screw. A trough is created in the lateral femoral condyle proximal to the screw to try to get attachment of the tendon to bone. At operation, the biceps tendon is under extreme tension as it turns around this screw in the lateral epicondyle. I performed this procedure in 9 patients during 1987–1988. Varus laxity has returned to some degree in all patients, mild and currently asymptomatic in 4 but sufficiently severe in 5 to require further procedures. An upper tibial lateral closing wedge osteotomy was performed to reduce lateral soft-tissue load in 2 patients in whom it had not been done previously at the time of initial biceps rerouting. This has provided some symptomatic benefit. Difficulty was also encountered due to prominence of the screw on the lateral femoral condyle, which contributed to screw removal in 3 patients. I have now discontinued the use of this procedure.

It is important to address the individual components of the patient's problem. It is difficult to assess the separate contribution of each of these elements in the final result, be it good, fair or poor. The LAD appears a useful adjunct, improving posterolateral instability by one or two grades, but alone it is not enough for the more severe instabilities where the challenge is to more adequately tension the popliteus. For posterior cruciate reconstruction, use of patellar tendon protected by a patellotibial pin seems the most reliable procedure currently available. A lateral closing wedge osteotomy is essential when posterolateral instability is associated with varus thrust or varus bone alignment. Although osteotomy takes much strain off the lateral soft tissues and considerably improves many patients, reliable correction of varus soft tissue instability remains a major challenge.

References

1. **DeLee JC, Riley MB, Rockwood CA Jr,** Acute posterolateral rotatory instability of the knee, *Am J Sports Med* (1983) **11**(4): 199–207.

2. **Hughston JC, Jacobson KE,** Chronic posterolateral rotatory instability of the knee, *J Bone Joint Surg (Am)* (1985) **67**: 351–359.

3. **Fleming RE Jr, Blatz DJ, McCarroll JR,** Posterior problems in the knee: posterior cruciate insufficiency and postero-lateral rotatory insufficiency, *Am J Sports Med* (1981) 9(2): 107–113.

4. **Bousquet G, Charmion L, Passot JP** et al., Stabilisation du condyle externe du genou dans les laxités antérieures chroniques: importance du muscle poplite, *Rev Chir Orthop* (1986) 72(6): 427–434.

5. **Jakob RP, Hassler H, Stäubli H-U,** Observations on rotatory instability of the lateral compartment of the knee: experimental studies on the functional anatomy and the pathomechanism of the true and the reversed pivot shift sign. *Acta Orthop Scand* (1981) **52** (suppl. 191): 1–32.

6. **Pasquali-Lasagni M,** *Le lassita rotatorie postero-laterali del ginocchio: monograph,* Latina, Italy. Istituto Chirurgico Ortopedico Traumatologico, 1988).

7. **Trillat A,** Posterolateral instability, *Late reconstructions of injured ligaments of the knee,* ed Schultiz KP, Krahl H, Stein WH (Berlin: Springer-Verlag, 1978) 99–105.

8. **Müller W,** *The knee: form, function and ligament reconstruction* (New York: Springer Verlag, 1983).

9. **Galway RD, Beaupré A, MacIntosh DL,** Pivot shift: a clinical sign of symptomatic anterior cruciate insufficiency, *J Bone Joint Surg (Br)* (1972) **54**: 763–764.

10. **Grood ES, Stowers SF, Noyes FR,** Limits of movement in the human knee: effect of sectioning the posterior cruciate ligament and posterolateral structures, *J Bone Joint Surg (Am)* (1988) **70**: 88–97.

11. **Clancy WG Jr, Shelbourne KD, Zoellner GB** et al., Treatment of knee joint instability secondary to rupture of the posterior cruciate ligament: report of a new procedure, *J Bone Joint Surg (Am)* (1983) **65**: 310–322.

12. **Hughston JC, Norwood LA Jr,** The posterolateral drawer test and external rotational recurvatum test for posterolateral rotatory instability of the knee, *Clin Orthop* (1980) **147**: 82–87.

13. **Daniel DM, Stone ML, Barnett P** et al., Use of the quadriceps active test to diagnose posterior cruciate-ligament disruption and measure posterior laxity of the knee, *J Bone Joint Surg (Am)* (1988) **70**: 386–391.

14. **Stäubli H-U, Jakob RP,** Posterior instability of the knee near extension: a clinical and stress radiographic analysis of acute injuries of the posterior cruciate ligament, *J Bone Joint Surg (Br)* (1990) **72**: 225–230.

15. **Shelbourne KD, Benedict F, McCarroll JR** et al., Dynamic posterior shift test: an adjuvant in evaluation of posterior tibial subluxation, *Am J Sports Med* (1989) **17**(2): 275–277.

16. **Baker CL Jr, Norwood LA, Hughston JC,** Acute posterolateral rotatory instability of the knee. *J Bone Joint Surg (Am)* (1983) **65**: 614–618.

17. **Shino K, Horibe S, Ono K,** The voluntarily evoked posterolateral drawer sign in the knee with posterolateral instability, *Clin Orthop* (1987) **215**: 179–186.

18. **Lysholm J, Gillquist J,** Arthroscopic examination of the posterior cruciate ligament, *J Bone Joint Surg (Am)* (1981) **63**: 363–366.

19. **Marshall JL, Girgis FG, Zelko RR,** The biceps femoris tendon and its functional significance, *J Bone Joint Surg (Am)* (1972) **54**: 1444–1450.

20. **Pasquali-Lasagni M,** La tenodesi poplitea nel trattamento delle lassita postero-laterali del ginocchio, *Il Ginocchio* (1988) 7.

21. **Clancy WG Jr,** Repair and reconstruction of the posterior cruciate ligament, *Chapman's operative orthopaedics,* ed. Chapman MW (Philadelphia: Lippincott, 1988) 1651–1665.

7.4 Gore-Tex prosthetic ligament reconstruction for chronic posterior cruciate instability of the knee

Dipak V. Patel, Zaid Al-Duri and Paul M. Aichroth

The purpose of this contribution is to describe our experience with the use of Gore-Tex prosthesis in the reconstruction of the posterior cruciate ligament. The study is a prospective one and the authors aimed at attempting to answer a few questions such as the possibility of reconstruction of the posterior cruciate ligament using the Gore-Tex as a prosthetic ligament replacement, assessing the adequacy of the use of such ligament alone without or with associated procedures, the possible use of a reproducible documentation method, and the reasons why some posterior cruciate ligament insufficiencies require surgery.

Nine patients (10 knees) underwent Gore-Tex reconstruction for chronic posterior cruciate ligament insufficiency. There were 6 males and 3 females. The mean age at the time of operation was 29.2 years (range 23–38 years). The average follow-up was 39.7 months (range 27–60 months). The mean interval between the injury and the operation was 6.4 years (range 2–16 years). Road traffic accident was the cause of the injury in 6 patients and contact sports in 3.

Since it is the policy of the authors to allow an adequate trial of conservative treatment (at least 6–9 months) to all patients with mid-substance posterior cruciate ligament tears, it follows that only those who fail to respond to such measures are possible candidates for surgery. All the patients in this study fall in this group.

Associated ligament injuries included:

Medial collateral ligament	1 knee.
Lateral collateral ligament	2 knees.
Anterior cruciate ligament	1 knee.
No associated ligament injury	6 knees.

Five patients had previous operations on their knees as follows:

Arthroscopic excision and trimming of degenerative posterior horn of the medial meniscus: 1 patient.

Arthroscopic trimming of the posterior horn of the lateral meniscus: 1 patient.

McIntosh procedure for a concomitant anterior cruciate ligament injury: 1 patient.

Medial collateral ligament repair: 1 patient.

Fibular collateral ligament reconstruction using the iliotibial tract: 1 patient.

The diagnosis of the chronic posterior cruciate rupture is based on a careful history-taking with a particular stress on the mechanism of the injury. It is always very useful to assess the pre-injury activity status of the individual, to have some idea about the patient's aims, expectations and expected performance. All such data should be carefully correlated to post-injury status.

Examination of the patient was performed in the clinic and a systematic method of clinical recording was used (see below). The clinical examination is not always accepted (to its full extent) by the patient in the outpatient department and so examination under anaesthesia was performed in all patients, combined with arthroscopy to confirm the diagnosis and exclude meniscal lesions and to assess the state of the articular cartilage of the joint.

Routine plain radiographs in the anteroposterior, lateral, skyline and intercondylar planes were performed. Stress radiography can be used to demonstrate relative displacement of the tibia on the femur; however, the authors did not use it routinely. Magnetic resonance imaging displays the posterior cruciate lesion very neatly but it was not available routinely for our study.

It was important to use a reproducible, reliable assessment method. The patients in this series had been assessed using the Lysholm II score (emphasizing evaluation of instability symptoms)[1] and the Tegner activity scale (which is a functional assessment of the disability).[2] It was clear, therefore, that a clinical grading assessment was required as well so as to correlate to other scores. Such a clinical assessment was performed mostly by examination under anaesthesia and included the following tests:

Sagging of the proximal tibia: the estimation of the amount of sagging is based on the grading of Clancy.[3]

Posterior drawer test: graded as 1, 2 or 3 depending on the amount of posterior displacement (5, 10, or 15 mm).

The reverse pivot shift test: as described by Jakob et al.[4]

The range of movement: compared to the range of movement of the contralateral uninvolved knee in unilateral cases.

The reverse pivot shift test is actually a grading of posterolateral rotatory instability, which is the commonest rotatory instability type associated with posterior cruciate ligament insufficiency. The clinical grading was based on awarding various points to a total of 100 as follows:

Sagging of the proximal tibia:
Grade 0   30 points
Grade 1   20 points
Grade 2   10 points
Grade 3   0 points

Posterior drawer test:
Grade 0   30 points
Grade 1   20 points
Grade 2   10 points
Grade 3   0 points

Reverse pivot shift test:
Grade 0   30 points
Grade 1   20 points
Grade 2   10 points
Grade 3   0 points

Range of movement:
Within 5° of the other knee   10 points
5–10° less than the other knee   5 points
10° less than the other knee   0 points

The authors felt that by combining the points of the Lysholm II score and the clinical evaluation score and dividing the total number by 2, a better, more accurate figure is produced than either of the two scoring systems alone. The final result of the total scoring is then seen as follows:

>90 points   excellent
75–90 points   good
60–74 points   fair
<60 points   poor.

Whilst all scoring systems are dependent on the surgeon's judgment and are not precision systems, they still provide a method of correlation and allow reproducibility. The same system was applied both pre- and post-operatively. Two patients had a 'second-look' arthroscopy, post-operatively; one of them subsequently underwent reconstruction for lateral collateral ligament instability using the iliotibial tract.

The patients' evaluation of the overall result of operative treatment was documented. A patient's reply fell into one of three categories:

Pleased: If the patient can go back to a level of activity as near as possible to the pre-injury level.
Satisfied: If the patient can carry out his daily activities and participate in some recreational sports.
Dissatisfied: If the patient can only just manage some daily activities, has changed job because of disability, and can do no sports.

Indications for surgery

Patients with persistent pain, recurrent swelling, giving way and significant restriction of the activities of daily living despite adequate conservative treatment were considered suitable for reconstruction. The primary aim of the operation was to enable the patient to perform routine daily activities more efficiently rather than to return to competitive sports.

Operative technique

The patient was placed in a supine position with the affected limb flexed at the knee joint and externally rotated at the hip joint to allow access to the posteromedial aspect of the knee joint. A high tourniquet was applied following exsanguination. A longitudinal incision was employed as shown in Figure 1. The medial hamstring tendons were dissected and the semimembranosus tendon was divided transversely near its insertion, allowing easier access to the popliteal fossa (Figure 2). The origin of the medial head of the gastrocnemius was then partially divided near its femoral attachment and the muscle belly was retracted laterally (Figure 3).

The popliteal vessels were now visualized in the popliteal fat and areolar tissue. The middle genicular and the superior medial genicular vessels were carefully identified, ligated and divided. Once these vascular leashes were cut, the popliteal vascular bundle could be retracted laterally. The posterior capsule was divided longitudinally in the intercondylar region. Some of the proximal border fibres of the popliteus muscle may obstruct the upper tibia at this site, and they should be stripped with a periosteal elevator (Figure 4).

Using a fine guide-wire and a cannulated drill, a tunnel was made in the proximal tibia with the exit point just at the anatomical attachment of the poste-

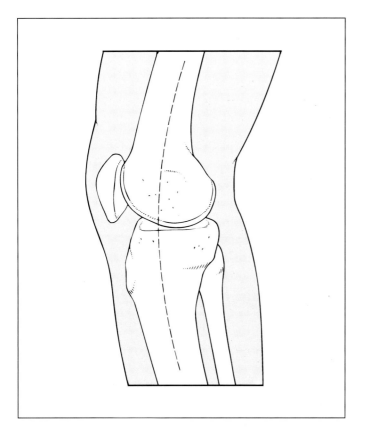

Figure 1

A longitudinal incision is taken.

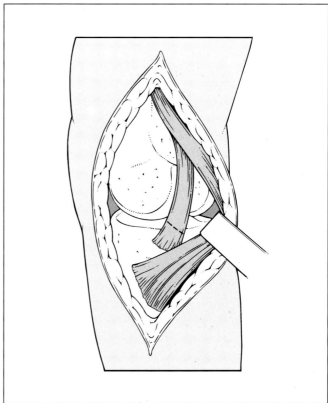

Figure 2

The semimembranosus tendon is divided near its insertion, allowing easier access to the popliteal fossa.

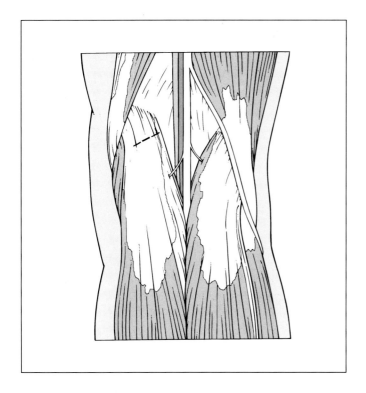

Figure 3

The origin of the medial head of the gastrocnemius is partially divided near its femoral attachment.

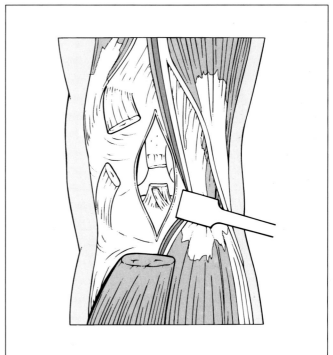

Figure 4

The popliteal vascular bundle is gently retracted laterally. The posterior capsule in the intercondylar region is divided vertically in the midline.

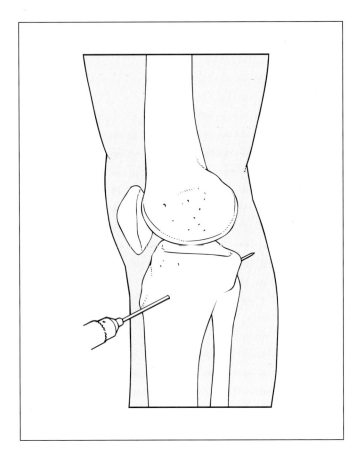

Figure 5

A tunnel is made in the proximal tibia, using a fine guide-wire and a cannulated drill.

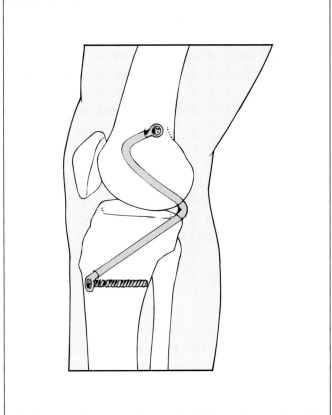

a

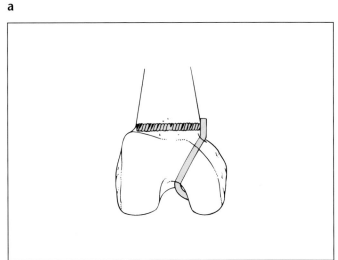

b

Figure 6

Diagrams showing the route of the Gore-Tex prosthetic ligament. The proximal and the distal ends of the prosthesis are fixed using screws.

rior cruciate ligament (PCL) in the intercondylar region (Figure 5). A long nylon tape was taken up through this tunnel and into the knee joint cavity with the help of an appropriate guide. Through a medial parapatellar incision, the joint was opened and the tape was picked up at this site. The site of the PCL attachment on the lateral surface of the medial femoral condyle was identified. A tunnel was made in the medial femoral condyle using a fine guide-wire and a cannulated drill. The tunnel should emerge at the apex of the intercondylar region at 1.30 p.m. in the right knee and 11.30 a.m. in the left knee. The nylon tape was then brought through this tunnel and measurements were made to calculate the length of the prosthesis.

The bony tunnels were made smooth using a high speed burr. The Gore-Tex prosthesis was passed through the femoral tunnel and fixed to the medial supracondylar region of the femur with a screw. The prosthesis was maximally tensioned with the tibia drawn anteriorly and the knee in 20° of flexion. The prosthetic ligament was secured to the proximal, anteromedial aspect of the tibia with a screw (Figure 6).

The wound was closed in layers with two redivac drains, and a compressive dressing was applied.

Postoperative management

A continuous passive mobilization machine was used after 48 hours. The patient was mobilized with crutches when comfortable. Partial weight-bearing was encouraged from the second postoperative week. A well-supervised intensive physiotherapy programme was started to rehabilitate the quadriceps to the maximum. The patient was allowed to return to mild recreational sporting activities between 6 and 9 months. Contact sports and skiing were permitted after 12 months. All patients were given a broad-spectrum antibiotic 24 hours prior to surgery and continued postoperatively for 7–10 days.

Results

The results of this study can easily be summarized (Table 1).

Table 1 Results of preoperative and postoperative testing.

Patient	Lysholm scores		Clinical scores		Tegner scale		Combined scores	
	Pre	Post	Pre	Post	Pre	Post	Pre	Post
1	34	81	30	60	1	4	32	71
2	44	85	15	65	1	4	30	75
3	33	84	15	65	2	3	24	75
4	58	80	5	55	1	2	32	68
5	43	59	0	40	1	1	22	50
6	45	83	5	80	2	6	25	82
7	57	85	40	80	2	7	49	83
8	60	76	20	70	2	7	40	73
9	56	82	25	70	2	5	41	76
10	46	80	0	50	1	4	23	65

It is worth noting that the results of the combined scoring show that all knees were in a 'poor' condition preoperatively.

Posterolateral rotatory instability (PLRI) is the most common rotatory instability associated with a chronic posterior cruciate ligament rupture. As stated before, the PLRI was clinically assessed by grading the reverse pivot shift test. Preoperative grading included:

PLRI	Number of knees
Grade 0	2
Grade 1	2
Grade 2	3
Grade 3	3

Of the two knees with a Grade (0) PLRI, one was a rugby injury whilst the other had an associated lateral collateral ligament injury which obviated preoperative detection of PLRI. Therefore, it is reasonable to assume that all knees except one had an associated PLRI.

As far as complications are concerned, none of the patients had wound infection, haemarthrosis or wound dehiscence.

The final evaluation of the postoperative results was:

Excellent	0%
Good	50%
Fair	40%
Poor	10%

As far as the satisfaction rating of the patient is concerned, there were 45% pleased; 27% satisfied; 18% dissatisfied.

Discussion

As can be seen, the results of posterior cruciate reconstruction are not especially encouraging. It is important to try to evaluate the posterior cruciate ligament instability in relation to the secondary restraints. Therefore, a serious attempt must be made to differentiate the isolated posterior cruciate ligament lesion from that associated with PLRI. This may not be straightforward but is a very worthwhile endeavour.

In our series, only 5 out of 10 patients had satisfactory (good) results. Retrospective analysis confirms that we had not dealt with PLRI adequately; therefore, we recommend that the posterolateral structures should be stabilized when necessary using the iliotibial band. The ruptured posterior cruciate ligament may be simultaneously reconstructed using autogenous tissue (such as the semitendinosus and gracilis tendons) either by an open or arthroscopically assisted technique. It is advised at this stage that the Gore-Tex reconstruction be used as a salvage procedure for the failed posterior cruciate reconstruction. We feel that chronic PLRI is poorly addressed as far as its clinical diagnosis and subsequent management is concerned.

References

1. **Torg JS, Conrad W, Kalen V,** Clinical diagnosis of anterior cruciate ligament instability in the athlete, *Am J Sports Med* (1976) **4:** 84–91.
2. **Tegner Y, Lysholm J,** Rating systems in the evaluation of knee ligament injuries, *Clin Orthop* (1985) **198:** 43–49.
3. **Clancy Jr WG,** Repair and reconstruction of the posterior cruciate ligament, *Operative orthopaedics,* vol. 3, ed Chapman MW (Philadelphia: Lippincott, 1988) 1651–1653.
4. **Jakob RP, Hassler H, Stäubli H-U,** Observations on rotatory instability of the lateral compartment of the knee: experimental studies on the functional anatomy and the pathomechanism of the true and the reversed pivot shift sign, *Acta Orthop Scand* (1981) **52** (suppl. 191): 1–32.

7.5 Chronic posterior cruciate ligament instability

Lonnie E. Paulos and Jon K. Nisbet

The chronic posterior cruciate ligament (PCL) deficient knee presents a different constellation of problems from the acute injury. In athletes especially, isolated PCL ruptures may function well and remain asymptomatic, only to be diagnosed during preseason physical examinations. Those patients who seek medical care for complaints from a chronic PCL deficient knee have often suffered concurrent or subsequent injuries. The secondary restraints may have begun to fail, or the late sequelae of arthrosis and patellofemoral chondrosis may be generating their own symptoms separate from those referable to the PCL instability.

As with acute injuries, both symptomatology and treatment vary with the site of PCL injury and the presence of ligamentous laxity. We must consider the chronic bony avulsion a separate entity just as the isolated PCL injury must be considered separate from the multiple ligament injured knee.

Chronic posterior cruciate tibial avulsion fracture

In 1968, Trickey[1] reported a series of acute (all less than 2 weeks from injury) tibial PCL avulsions. He demonstrated the superiority of open reduction and internal fixation (ORIF) over cast immobilization. He stated that 'surgical repair after 3 weeks is usually not worthwhile.' Meyers[2] reported obtaining 'good functional capacity' from two knees that underwent ORIF at 3 and 7 months. Torisu[3] reported on eight patients treated similarly, all more than 3 weeks after injury. He found that his results were better in the subacute group (3–7 weeks) than in the more chronic group (11 weeks to 30 years). He noted that surgery eliminated the pain and swelling associated with motion but was complicated by some cases of restricted flexion and extension. This is undoubtedly due to the contraction of the torn PCL stump preventing accurate reduction or presenting an overtensioned but anatomic repair.

While anatomic reduction and internal fixation is widely accepted[4] for acute repairs, its applicability to chronic PCL avulsions has limitations. Through 6 to 8 weeks, repair can be successful. At the completion of the procedure the leg must be taken through a full range of motion and the repair observed. If after reduction the knee will not fully extend or flex, a surgical reconstruction should be considered. This step is predicated on the presence of significant laxity and applicable symptomatology.

The posterior approach as described by Abbott and Carpenter[5] and later by Trickey[1] is adequate and acceptable for the isolated repair. It is not acceptable nor extensile for concurrent medial or lateral ligament reconstruction.[6] Additionally, arthroscopic diagnosis[7] with attention to meniscal and cartilage pathology must precede repositioning for a posterior approach. The posterior approach is only correct after thorough examination and arthroscopy have ruled out any associated pathology.

A method of arthroscopically controlled percutaneous fixation has recently been described by Martinez-Moreno.[8] A clamping apparatus holds the avulsion in position while an anterior-to-posterior lag screw is applied. This technique does not allow for use of a washer posteriorly and requires considerable technical expertise and equipment.

The natural history of the chronic PCL deficient knee

The natural history of the chronic PCL deficient knee depends greatly on the presence of associated injuries, rotational and straight ligamentous laxities, meniscal tears, and articular cartilage damage. The incidence of these confounding factors depends on the mechanism of injury. Athletic endeavours are less likely to produce associated injuries than motor vehicle injuries or falls, and thus have an improved prognosis. Additionally, greater motivation in the athlete during rehabilitation may contribute to an improved prognosis.[9] The ability to achieve improved quadriceps strength has been correlated with overall result.[10]

Published reports[10–12] on isolated chronic PCL deficiency indicate pain to be present in 34–71% after a minimum 2-year follow-up. This pain is

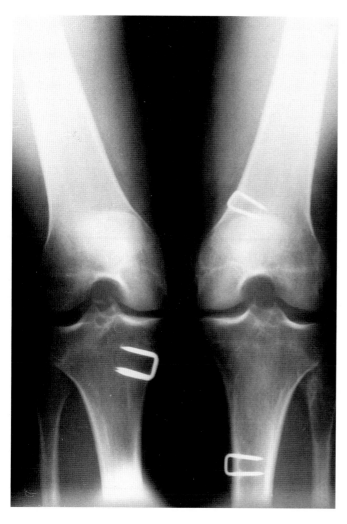

Figure 1

Left knee shows early medial compartment degenerative changes after posterior cruciate ligament reconstruction.

changes. He also documented a strong correlation between the time from injury and the presence of moderate or severe chondrosis in the medial compartment (2/31 with less than a 2-year interval, 5/7 with 2–4-year interval, 9/10 with more than a 4-year interval). These patients were preselected by ongoing symptoms during rehabilitation, but these findings held for both isolated PCL injuries and combined ligament injuries. It may be inferred that those patients with chronic complaints have a progression of intra-articular degenerative changes with time.

Patients with associated ligamentous instabilities follow yet more stormy courses; however, many of their symptoms may be referable to the associated pathology.[15] These concurrent ligamentous, meniscal, and chondral injuries may prevent the patient from adequately achieving quadriceps rehabilitation, or may create functional instability or pain on their own. In addition, degenerative radiographic changes and patellofemoral disease occur more frequently in multiple ligament injured patients than in isolated PCL injuries.[15]

Review of chronic PCL surgical reconstructions

Robson[16] performed the first attempt at PCL repair in 1903. In 1917, HeyGroves and Lond[17] described the first graft reconstruction of the PCL. They rerouted semitendinosus and gracilis tendons through a femoral tunnel and sewed them to tibial periosteum posteriorly. This was modified in 1927 by Gallie and LeMesurier.[18] By leaving semitendinosus and gracilis attached distally, they created both tibial and femoral tunnels for a more anatomic routing, and secured the proximal end of the tendons to the medial femoral condyle near the medial collateral ligament. This technique or a similar modification was used by most surgeons until the mid-1960s,[19] but literature documenting their results remained lacking.

Other structures described for PCL reconstruction include the medial meniscus,[20] the lateral meniscus,[21] the biceps femoris,[22] the popliteal tendon,[23] and the semimembranosus.[24] Reports of critical analyses of these techniques are also lacking.

In 1969, Jack Hughston reported on use of the medial head of the gastrocnemius tendon for PCL reconstruction.[25] He originally describes the technique as a two-stage reconstruction. Initially there is the transfer of the proximal tendon end to the medial femoral condyle. Next the tendon is severed at the musculotendinous junction, and tacked down to the fovea of the posterior tibia to create a static restraint. The 1-year delay was expected to allow growth of an intra-articular blood supply for the graft. His reports of the results of the first stage of the procedure were so gratifying that the second stage was unnecessary.[26] He theorized that the

described as mild, and occasional or infrequent, occurring with long walks and descending stairs. Swelling occurs in 16–20% of isolated chronic PCL injuries, and is associated with activity and is infrequent. Giving-way occurs in 20–45% but is a less dramatic sensation than that seen with ACL injuries. This sensation of instability is prevalent when walking over uneven ground and descending stairs. Participation in sports after aggressive quadriceps rehabilitation ranges from 68% to 100%[10,13] at 2 years but decreases with time. Radiographic changes of degenerative joint disease are reported in as many as 36%.[10] These changes are more likely to occur in the medial compartment (Figure 1) and in the patellofemoral articulation.

Clancy et al. in 1983[14] demonstrated that radiographic changes correlate poorly (31%) with arthroscopic documentation of chondral degenerative dynamic function of the first-stage operation is to activate a tibial support to prevent posterior sag or drawer when the foot is passively dorsiflexed or actively plantar-flexed against resistance. Thus, it actively stabilizes the knee during weight bearing. The objective results belie the lack of static restraint, as posterior sag and drawer, while reduced, remained apparent in almost all knees. Similar reports on this technique by Kennedy and Galpin[27] and Insall and Hood[28] described modifications to overcome the frequently short length of tendon by use of polypropylene braided leader or bone block, respectively. These authors also performed only the first stage and noted little or no objective improvement, albeit promising subjective improvement.

A recent report by Roth and Bray[29] critically reviewed their results using this method. They found similarly dismal static stability and a disappointing subjective improvement in just 69%. Of the patients, 90% still had pain and 59% had continued instability. Those patients who had concurrent associated surgery produced a statistically significant improvement in subjective result compared to those undergoing PCL reconstruction alone. Roth and Bray theorized that the associated procedures may have skewed the results in previous studies and that the gastrocnemius medial head transfer contributed little to the patients' improvement. Among other condemning results were significant patellofemoral, quadriceps, and hamstring weakness at an average of 53 months after surgery. This was more severe than in a group of controls managed nonoperatively with rehabilitation. The patients also felt that their knees were worsening with time. There have been no long-term studies demonstrating a halt in the progression of osteoarthritis after this or any other procedure.

The most promising reconstruction reported to date is that of Clancy et al. in 1983, using middle-third patellar bone–tendon–bone graft, secured in bony femoral and tibial tunnels.[14] They report on 13 chronic patients with a minimum 2-year follow-up. All were subjectively better, with the sag and posterior drawers graded zero or 1+ in all 13. Overall, 11 of 13 were rated excellent or good on subjective and objective grounds. This study demonstrated that an anatomic reconstruction with a strong graft could achieve a high standard of both objective and subjective results. It currently represents the 'gold standard' for repairs reported in the literature.

Reconstruction of the PCL using prosthetic ligament substitutes has been performed with early good results. The strength of the graft and ability to tension the reconstruction more easily allows for the elimination of posterior sag and an early return to full motion and aggressive rehabilitation. Unfortunately, as demonstrated in prosthetic ACL reconstructions, the graft is unable to withstand the variations in applied stress. It is doomed to fatigue and eventual rupture since no remodeling can occur.

In our own series of patients undergoing PCL reconstruction, 13 had a Gore-Tex ligament. Over a 2-year period, 50% had failed by objective criteria (equal to preoperative laxity), but only 20% by subjective criteria. A good subjective response despite a poor objective grade is usually associated with a reduction in associated patholaxities and a firm posterior drawer end-point. Despite acceptable subjective results, we cannot recommend current prosthetic designs for PCL reconstruction.

Authors' indications for PCL reconstruction

1. Combined ligamentous instability with at least grade II PCL laxity.

   A. Straight lateral or posterolateral rotational laxity.
   B. Straight medial or posteromedial rotational laxity.
   C. Knee dislocation or near dislocation (ACL, PCL, and a collateral with or without rotational laxities).

2. 'Isolated' straight posterior instability in patients who have failed a conservative quadriceps-emphasizing rehabilitation program of 12 months' duration.

3. Chronic contracted avulsion that meets one of the above two conditions and, upon exposure, cannot stretch to be replaced in its bony bed, or after ORIF will not stretch to allow full range of motion.

Posterolateral and true lateral instability of at least a grade II commonly accompanies a PCL rupture. In patients with varus mechanical axis (as measured on long-cassette weight-bearing radiographic view) or with demonstrable varus thrust in walking, it is prudent to offer reconstruction in two stages. First, with valgus producing high tibial osteotomy, and second, with PCL reconstruction if symptoms continue. On occasion, the osteotomy alone will eliminate the symptoms of instability caused by the straight lateral or posterolateral corner laxity and subsequent PCL reconstruction will not be necessary.

Posteromedial rotational or straight medial laxity can undergo medial repair, advancement, or reefing. Use the medial approach to the tibial attachment of the PCL[6] instead of the standard lateral approach.

Knee dislocations generally produce more stable and functional results with acute repair or reconstruction but suffer from stiffness that may complicate early surgery in the face of such massive trauma. When, for vascular, neurologic, or skin contamination reasons, surgery must be delayed beyond 1 week, begin motion and regain motor function and tone. Use a hinged brace and protected weight bearing for

12–16 weeks. Often, what initially was three or four major ligament ruptures will settle and scar into one or two predominant instabilities that can be handled electively. This course has enabled older patients with a greater risk of stiffness and less functional demand to have less surgical reconstruction.

Also, when faced with multiple ligamentous instability acutely, one must be vigilant to avoid capsular leakage during arthroscopy. There is a risk of compartment syndrome developing.

Several authors suggest reconstruction for an isolated PCL injury with greater than 10 mm[19] or greater than 15 mm[10] of laxity noted in the posterior drawer at 80–90° of knee flexion. We believe it is rare to have such significant straight posterior laxity and no concurrent associated injury. We rely in these instances on a clinical posterior drawer performed at 20–30° of knee flexion.[30] If large posterior displacements over 10 mm are identified near full extension, then the secondary restraints and posterior capsule must be injured or stretched out. This suggests a poor prognosis in our hands. This would constitute a relative indication for surgery.

Special considerations

Isometry

Sophisticated isometry studies have tried to identify the position of an isometric band of PCL during normal knee kinematics. These studies are conducted with the ACL and PCL intact. A computerized six-degree-of-freedom instrumented spatial linkage monitors the femoral and tibial insertions of the intact ligament during motion. Grood demonstrated that different portions of the PCL were tight at different ranges of flexion and that no single band could be truly isometric.[31] This sort of analysis cannot be conducted effectively in a PCL deficient knee as the tibia will sag back if the PCL is lax. This creates abnormal kinematics and sabotages all attempts at supine isometry. As a result, intra-operative isometry is unreliable. Instead, anatomic landmarks must guide tunnel placement until development of a reliable method for determining isometry.

Graft choice

The significant bulk and strength of the native PCL, and the presence of tension in some parts of the ligament throughout the range of knee flexion, create great demands on a graft. A large, strong graft must be used and secured solidly on both ends to allow early motion and rehabilitation to prevent disuse atrophy. The lessons learned from the success of quadriceps strengthening regimens in the isolated

PCL injury suggest that risking weakness in the extensor mechanism may further compromise the quality of result. The prevalence of concurrent ACL and posteromedial or posterolateral laxities requiring reconstruction puts a premium on preserving autogenous tissue and finding alternate sources of graft tissue.

We currently prefer allograft Achilles or patellar tendon with adjacent bone blocks to allow secure fixation. Using allograft allows 12–13 mm ligament harvest and sufficient bone for fixation without risk of further weakening to the extensor mechanism and delaying rehabilitation. The patient must understand the potential risk of disease transmission inherent with allograft usage. Other options include ipsilateral or contralateral bone–tendon–bone patellar tendon graft or semitendinosus and gracilis harvest. Supplementation of these tissues with an adjacent prosthetic ligament (as a stent or affixed on both ends) yields more confidence in early motion and resistive exercise protocols.[32] It also allows for the complete elimination of the posterior sag and drawer. It probably functions only on a short-term basis, sharing the load with the adjacent ligament graft. Although we cannot strongly recommend the use of a ligament augmentation device at this time, we are encouraged by the results so far.

Postoperative immobilization and protection

The benefits of early motion and specific muscle strengthening are well documented. Use of a femoral–tibial transfixion pin or patellar olecranization maintains the anterior position of the tibia in the early postoperative weeks. It increases the incidence of patellar entrapment and patellofemoral chondrosis and infection. There is also a risk of pin breakage and the need to subject the patient to an extraction procedure. We emphasize the use of sturdy graft material and strong fixation so that a simple postoperative hinged brace may be used to control progression of range of motion without fear of overstressing the graft and creating a posterior sag. An initial 3–4-week period of immobilization can safely be employed when reconstructing multiple ligaments.

Graft position

Grood,[31] as well as others, has shown the femoral attachment to be the more sensitive determinant of graft function (Figure 2). Medial–lateral variations in the tibial tunnel site lead to fewer significant alterations in isometry. Additionally, the PCL has been described as consisting of an anterolateral and posteromedial bundle. The anterolateral bundle has the greater bulk and strength and tightens in flexion, while the posteromedial bundle tightens in extension. Although isometry studies reveal no single band to be isometric, they do suggest a greater mechanical leverage for the anterolateral band in elimination of posterior sag and drawer in the flexed position. In extension, secondary restraints contribute signifi-cantly to resistance to the posterior drawer and corner reconstructions do contribute to extension stability. We emphasize reconstruction of the strong anterolateral band. Also, placement of the tibial attachment site slightly more laterally reinforces posterolateral stability, which is important to overall results.

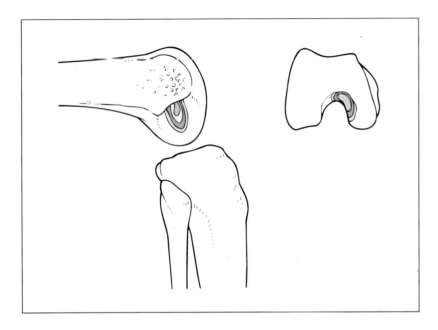

Figure 2

Isometric map as determined from intact cadaver knees.

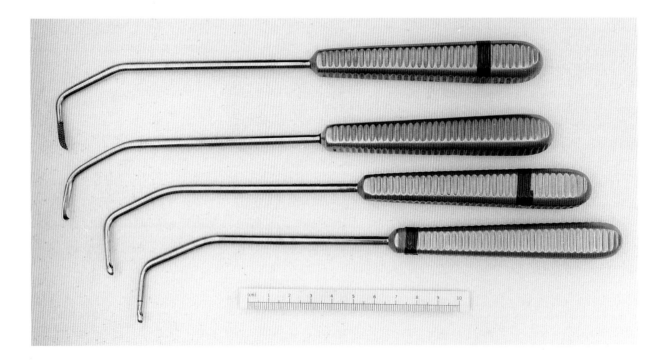

Figure 3

The posterior tibial attachment site is prepared with specially-designed reverse cutting knives, curettes, and rasps through the anteromedial portal.

Arthroscopically assisted PCL reconstruction technique[33]

Complete a diagnostic arthroscopy. View the PCL both from the anterolateral and from the postero-medial portals.[7] Perform a posterior drawer test and probe the PCL during visualization. This may demonstrate a deficient PCL still contained within its sheath, as is often the case. Overhanging osteophytes may be removed from the femoral condyles and notch, but a notchplasty is not necessary.

With the arthroscope anterolateral, place the series of reverse cutting knives, curettes, and rasps (Figure 3) along the course of the PCL to prepare the tibial attachment site. Confirm their positions by placing the arthroscope posteromedially. The proper tibial site is 10 mm below the joint-line (Figure 4). Extra effort must be made to clear a spot inferiorly enough for the placement of the drill-guide.

In patients undergoing concurrent posterolateral corner reconstructions or lateral meniscal repair, create an extra-articular approach laterally. This allows for placement of a finger in the proper tibial attachment site. This access augments the safety of the tibial tunnel drilling procedure until facility with an entirely arthroscopic site determination is gained. Make a 3-cm longitudinal skin incision just posterior to the lateral collateral ligament at the joint-line. Develop it through the iliotibial band expansion anterior to the biceps femoris. Remember that the peroneal nerve lies just posterior to and beneath the biceps femoris, so the interval must be accurately determined anterior to this tendon. After penetrating the first layer,[34] dissect between the lateral head of the gastrocnemius and the popliteus tendon to allow passage of an index finger behind the tibia and just below the joint-line. Palpate for the posterior slope of the median eminence. Follow it inferiorly to the angular prominence of the posterior tibial tubercle, slightly lateral of midline and covered by the popliteus muscle. Move further medially until you feel a soft depression known as the tibial fovea. On the medial side of the fovea is a bony prominence. This soft fovea defines the attachment limits, medially and laterally, of the PCL.

Position the index finger in the fovea. At the inferior end of its soft contents, position the tibial tunnel drill-guide through the anteromedial portal at its inferior and lateral extent (Figure 5). Place the guide-pin from the anterolateral tibia at an angle of 45° to the plateau surface. This will require elevation of some anterior compartment musculature from the tibia. The guide-pin enters the anterior tibia below the level of the tibial tubercle, approximately 10 mm distal to the joint-line. Bring the pin to the posterior cortex but not through it. Obtain anterior–posterior and lateral radiographs to confirm the positions. If correctly positioned, a cannulated 11-mm drill passes over the guide-pin and drills two-thirds of the way

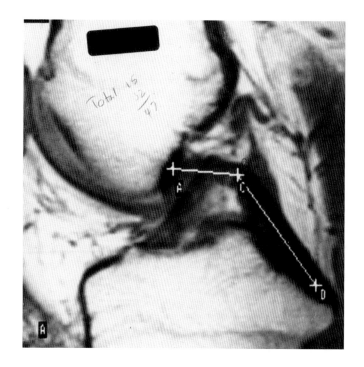

Figure 4

A sagittal cut magnetic resonance image of the knee shows the posterior cruciate ligament running from A–C–D. The tibial attachment at D is positioned about 1 cm below the joint-line.

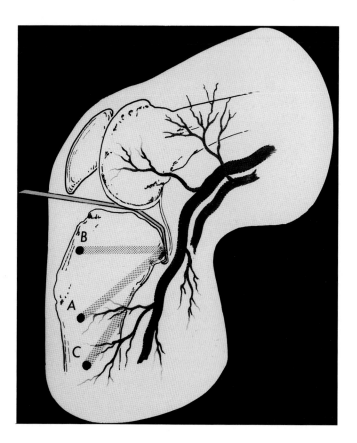

Figure 5

The tibial guide hooks over the posterior lip of the tibia at the fovea.

through to the posterior cortex (Figure 6). *Remove* the guide pin and drill the last third. This is to prevent the inadvertent spinning of the pin through the cortex and into the popliteal vessels and nerve. Rasp the posterior cortex edges smooth. Insert the knife anteromedially over the eminence. Cut posteroinferiorly until arthroscopic irrigant flows out through the tibial tunnel, signifying a completed pathway through the overlying soft tissue.

The femoral tunnel preparation begins with passage of an arthroscopic knife through the anteromedial portal into the notch to clear the PCL remnant from the medial wall. Pass a calibrated probe through the anteromedial portal and position it parallel to the superomedial wall of the notch at 10 o'clock or 2 o'clock (with the knee flexed 70°) (Figure 7). Mark a point 8 mm proximal from the chondral border and secure the femoral drill-guide tip.

With the knee flexed 90°, make a longitudinal skin incision about halfway between the medial pole of the patella and the medial epicondyle. The 3-cm incision ends inferiorly over the chondral border of the medial femoral condyle (Figure 8). Retract the vastus medialis obliquus superiorly and dissect through the capsule and synovium down to bone. The proper external guide-pin drilling position is about 10 mm from the chondral border and just proximal to a line from the epicondyle to the mid-patella. Position the pin and drill into the notch. If necessary, remeasure and adjust the external and internal bone entry points. The direction of the pin is posteroinferior, away from the arthroscope. Create the femoral tunnel with a cannulated drill and rasp the internal edges.

Since we began using Achilles tendon allografts for our reconstructions, we have employed a femoral wedge fit for the bone block proximally and use no metallic fixation. This requires the creation of sequential step-drilling in the femoral tunnel. Fashion a tapered allograft bone plug of similar dimensions and of 25-mm length for impaction into this tunnel. Interference screw fixation with a short

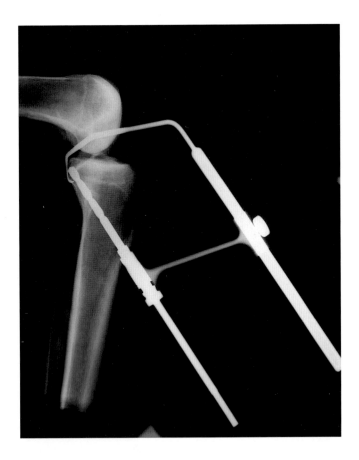

Figure 6

AP and lateral views show proper placement of the tibial guide pin for the posterior cruciate ligament tibial tunnel. With the tibial drill-guide in place, the cannulated drill is passed in two-thirds of the distance towards the posterior cortex. The guide-pin is then removed prior to completion of the tibial tunnel drilling.

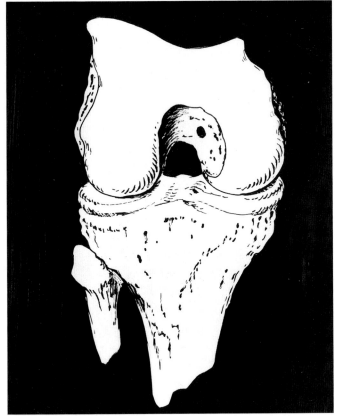

Figure 7

The position of the femoral drill-guide point is 8 mm proximal to the chondral margin and at 10 o'clock or 2 o'clock.

length of screw also works well with a cylindrical femoral tunnel (for use with patellar tendon autograft or allograft).

To ease the graft from the femoral to the tibial tunnel, pass a dilator through the tunnels to enlarge the aperture in the posterior capsule near the tibial tunnel exit. The dilator consists of detachable bullets on a chain of progressively increasing diameters (Figure 9). Pass it from the femoral to tibial tunnels. After the final bullet dilates the soft tissue at the posterior capsule to 10 mm, it will pull the tibial end of the graft through the capsule and into position within the tunnel.

To pass the dilator chain with graft attached, a wire (18-gauge, bent in half with the blunt end curved up slightly) is passed through the tibial tunnel to the region of the posterior capsule. If finger access to the fovea is available, manipulate the wire forward into the notch. Grasp it and redirect it out the femoral tunnel (Figure 10). Without finger access to the fovea, this passage may be hampered by the prominence of capsular soft tissue or by the cramped quarters within the notch. This may complicate the manipulation of the arthroscope and grasper from anterior portals. Make this maneuver considerably easier by placing the arthroscope through the medial femoral condylar bone tunnel and directing the 30° lens postero-inferiorly. This aims the arthroscope inferiorly where

the wire emerges from the tunnel. It also frees the anterior portals so that a grasper and a second probe may be used to simultaneously sweep the soft tissue aside (or elevate the posterior capsule) and grasp the emerging wire.

Pass the wire retrograde from the tibial tunnel to the femoral tunnel. Pull the dilator and graft into

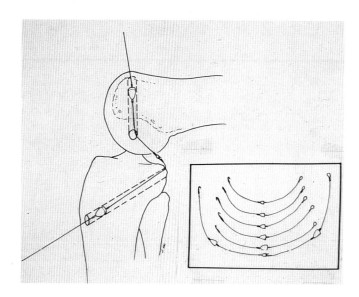

Figure 9

Progressive soft-tissue dilator.

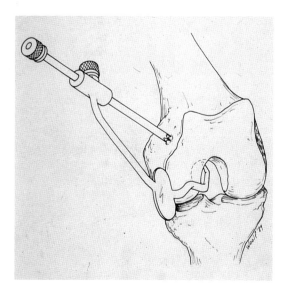

Figure 8

The external entrance for the guide-pin in the femoral tunnel is midway between the epicondyle and the medial pole of the patella and just proximal to a line connecting these two landmarks.

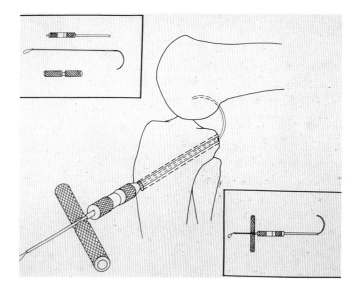

Figure 10

A curved and bent wire is passed up through the tibial tunnel and grasped to allow passage anteriorly and superiorly out of the femoral tunnel.

position antegrade. If employing a bone–tendon–bone patellar graft, use a short 20-mm length of bone block for the distal tunnel. This allows manipulation of the block into the tibial tunnel at a sharp angle. Finger access to the fovea also helps considerably here. Unfortunately, the bone–tendon–bone patellar tendon construction will not be long enough to bring the distal end of the graft into view to perform interference screw application in the tibial tunnel. To accomplish this, use a cannulated interference screw. Insert the 30° arthroscope into the tibial tunnel alongside the tensioning suture secured to the graft. While visualizing through the tibial tunnel, pass a guide-wire alongside the arthroscope to the proper side of the bone block and remove the scope. Thread the interference screw along the wire and secure it between the tunnel wall and bone block. A short screw must be used and its position must again be checked with the arthroscope to ensure that it is inserted far enough. This screw will be so deep within bone that it will never be available for removal if revision is required. It may be prudent to tie the bone block leader sutures over a post or button. This fixation however, compromises early motion.

These problems can be overcome by use of a prosthetic stent or an allograft Achilles tendon, both of which ensure adequate length for staple or screw-and-washer fixation to the anterior tibia. Perform this fixation with the knee flexed 30°. Apply maximal tension to the graft through the tibial end and do an anterior drawer test to reduce the posterior sag fully. A full range of motion must be documented after fixation, but before closure. View the graft again arthroscopically while slowly flexing the knee from 20° to 100°. Gradual tightening should occur with increasing flexion and no impingement on the medial femoral condyle.

Prepare the Achilles allograft with a 25-mm long bone block proximally, which tapers from 11 mm to 13 mm. The tendon itself should pass through a 10-mm sizer. Secure the distal suture leader to the graft starting about 7 cm from the bone block with a Krackow-type locked-weave stitch for several centimeters. Follow this with a tight Roman-sandal weave to the far distal tip and tie the suture to secure the weave.

Rehabilitation

The physical therapy regimen is shown in Figure 11. It requires non-weight-bearing for 12 weeks with partial weight bearing and use of crutches through 16 weeks. Patients wear a postoperative hinged brace for the first 16 weeks. Thereafter, patients wear a functional PCL brace for 1 year. Begin progressive range of motion exercises on postoperative week three. Isometrics and neuromuscular stimulation begin immediately. Progressive resistance exericses (PREs) begin at the time of mobilization, at 3 weeks. Prolonged weight bearing and brace protection are designed to reduce the forces on the repair secondary to lateral joint distraction that occurs with weight bearing.

Clinical impressions

We are presently comparing our PCL reconstruction results, using fresh-frozen Achilles tendon allograft with and without the ligament augmentation device (LAD-3M Company). Compilation of the results has not been completed. Nevertheless, it is our impression that the ligament augmentation device does improve the overall long-term stability results of our chronic PCL reconstructions.

Using our present reconstructive techniques, the 90° posterior drawer is reduced by at least 5–6 mm approximately 80% of the time. The posterior drawer, however, is not eliminated. In contrast, there is significant reduction and sometimes obliteration of the posterior drawer at 20° of knee flexion. By objective criteria, we would consider this result a good or excellent rating. Patients' subjective evaluations parallel our static results, both at 2- and at 4-year follow-up.

We find that results diminish in patients who are failures by objective criteria but who were successes by subjective criteria, within the 2–4-year follow-up interval. These patients tend to develop more pain, particularly in the patello-femoral joint and medial compartment as follow-up time progresses.

As mentioned previously, a firm end-point to posterior drawer appears to correlate positively with a good subjective result. Also, reduction of varus laxity, and posterolateral laxity, correlates highly with both static and subjective results.

Finally, those patients presenting for PCL reconstructive procedures who demonstrate significant patellofemoral pain and arthrosis are poor candidates for reconstructive surgery. Over 60% of those presenting with these types of symptoms prior to reconstruction continued to have equal or more severe complaints when seen at both short- and long-term follow-up. A patient presenting for PCL reconstruction because of significant patellofemoral complaints should be discouraged from undergoing this type of procedure. The use of allograft tissues in patients with significant patellofemoral disease has significantly reduced the complaints referable to the patellofemoral joint, but does not eliminate the risk.

In our experience, those patients who have PCL reconstruction early after their injury, and prior to the development of patellofemoral arthrosis or loss of menisci, have a greater chance of success than those presenting late. Also, when secondary and other primary restraint damage is demonstrable at the time

LONNIE E. PAULOS, M.D.

Patient: _____ Date: _____

Surgical Procedure: __POSTERIOR CRUCIATE RECONSTRUCTION_____ Date: _____

Physical Therapist: _____ POW = Post Operative Week

PHASE I — IMMOBILITY AND BRACING
Brace locked at __15__° until __6__ POW; Unlock brace to prescribed angles for ROM exercises only on __1&2__ POW

☐ Leave unlocked; Ext. stop __10__°   Flex stop __60__°   on __6__ POW

Sleep without brace on __10__ POW;   Shower without brace on __6__ POW

Use functional brace (Donjoy) on __16__ POW for ambulation and exercise until __52__ POW; then exercise only Donjoy PCL Brace or Orthotist made Brace

PHASE II — RANGE OF MOTION (ROM)
Begin Passive ROM on __1__ POW from __0__° extension to __40__° flexion;

Increase __0__° extension and __10__° flexion per week beginning on __6__ POW For 2 wk only then lock at 10° for 4 wks.

☐ May increase PROM PRN

Begin Active ROM on __1__ POW from __0__° extension to __40__° flexion;

Increase __0__° extension and __10__° flexion per week beginning on __6__ POW

☐ May increase AROM PRN

PHASE III — PROGRESSIVE WEIGHT BEARING
Begin weight bearing on __12__ POW; Start with __25__% body weight and increase __25__% per week,

then: ☒ Keep on one crutch (75% body weight) until notified;   ☐ Wean from crutches as tolerated Total 16 weeks on Crutches

PHASE IV — ISOMETRICS
☒ Quad/Hamstring Isometrics;   ☒ Spectrum Isometrics;   ☐ PNF Isometrics

☒ Straight leg raises;   ☒ May use weight to __10__ lbs. placed   ☐ proximally   ☒ distally on tibia

☒ Patella glides & tilts __3__ times/day

☐ TENS

☒ Neuromuscular Stimulation: ☐ Hamstrings   ☒ Quadriceps

Frequency __3__/day;   Duration __2__ hrs/session __6__ weeks Until Active Quadriceps Contraction

PHASE V — ISOTONIC PROGRESSIVE RESISTANCE EXERCISES (PRE)
Knee extension prohibited until __6__: POW;   ☐ Indefinitely

Knee flexion prohibited until _____ POW;   ☒ Indefinitely

Knee Extension PRE: ☒ Increase PRN; Increase to _____ lbs.; from __0__° extension to __70__° flexion until __26__ POW;

then advance PRN; No limits on weight from __0__° extension to __40__° flexion

Knee Flexion PRE: ☐ Increase PRN; Increase to _____ lbs.; from _____° extension to _____° flexion until _____ POW;

then advance PRN; No limits on weight from _____° extension to _____° flexion

Leg Press PRE: ☒ Increase PRN; Increase to ____ lbs.; from __0__° extension to __70__° flexion until after __6__ POW;

then advance PRN; No limits on weight from __0__° extension to __40__° flexion

☒ Must wear brace during PREs;   Prone PREs until __16__ POW;   Eccentric only until _____ POW

PHASE VI — FUNCTIONAL EXERCISES
Start program on __12__ POW;   Restrict ROM to __10__° extension to __90__° flexion until __52__ POW

☐ Full PNF program;   PNF isotonics prohibited until _____ POW

Minisquats __20__ POW;   Sports cord __12__ POW;   Pogo ball/stick __none__ POW;

Trampoline __48__ POW;   Balance Board __26__ POW

Begin stationary cycling on __12__ POW;   Outdoor biking on __asap__ POW knee flexion at least 110°

Level ground only until __24__ POW;   Adjust seat: ☒ High   ☐ Low;   ☐ Patellar restraint

Begin swimming on __8__ POW;   ☒ Straight   ☐ Bent Leg Kicks Only;   Pool jogging __36__ POW

Stationary track _____ POW;   Rowing _____ POW;   Nordic Track __36__ POW

PHASE VII — ISOKINETICS
☐ Prohibited indefinitely

Start on __36__ POW;   Pad Placement: ☐ High tibia ☒ Low tibia;   Body position: ☒ Sitting ☐ Prone

☒ ROM restriction: High speed performance from __0__° to __90__° flexion

Low speed performance from _____° to _____° flexion

☐ Use patellar restraining brace;   ☒ Must wear functional brace

☐ Burn outs OK;   ☒ High speed only

PHASE VIII — RETURN TO SPORTS
Run with stretch cords _____ POW;   ☐ Wear functional brace

Begin progressive running on _____ POW up to _____ miles/session; _____ sessions/week

Level ground only until _____ POW;   Progressive sprints on _____ POW;

Progressive cutting on _____ POW;   Progressive jumping on _____ POW

Anticipated return to sports on _____ POW;   ☐ Needs strength evaluation prior to return

Sports restriction: _____

Comments: _____

Figure 11

A standard rehabilitation protocol for use with posterior cruciate ligament reconstruction.

of surgery, these structures should be reconstructed or repaired simultaneously to ensure more consistent results. Early range of motion in association with prolonged weight bearing appears to improve the overall surgical results.

References

1. Trickey EL, Rupture of the posterior cruciate ligament of the knee, *J Bone Joint Surg (Br)* (1968) **50**: 334–341.
2. Meyers MH, Isolated avulsion of the tibial attachment of the posterior cruciate ligament of the knee, *J Bone Joint Surg (Am)* (1975) **57**: 669–672.
3. Torisu T, Avulsion fracture of the tibial attachment of the posterior cruciate ligament: Indications and results of delayed repair, *Clin Orthop* (1979) **143**: 107–114.
4. Satku K, Chew CN, Seow H, Posterior cruciate ligament injuries, *Acta Orthop Scand* (1984) **55**: 26–29.
5. Abbott LC, Carpenter WF, Surgical approaches to the knee joint, *J Bone Joint Surg* (1945) **27**: 277–310.
6. Levy IM, Riederman R, Warren RF, An anteromedial approach to the posterior cruciate ligament, *Clin Orthop* (1984) **190**: 174–181.
7. Lysholm J, Gillquist J, Arthroscopic examination of the posterior cruciate ligament, *J Bone Joint Surg (Am)* (1981) **63**: 363–366.
8. Martinez-Moreno JL, Blanco-Blanco E, Avulsion fractures of the posterior cruciate ligaments of the knee: An experimental percutaneous rigid fixation technique under arthroscopic control, *Clin Orthop* (1988) **237**: 204–208.
9. Cross MJ, Powell JF, Long-term follow-up of posterior cruciate ligament rupture: a study of 116 cases, *Am J Sports Med* (1984) **12**: 292–297.
10. Parolie JM, Bergfeld JA, Long-term results of non-operative treatment of isolated posterior cruciate ligament injuries in the athlete, *Am J Sports Med* (1986) **14**: 35–38.
11. Dandy DJ, Pusey RJ, The long-term results of untreated tears of the posterior cruciate ligament, *J Bone Joint Surg (Br)* (1982) **64**: 92–94.
12. Hirshman HP, Daniel DM, Miyasaka K, The fate of unoperated knee ligament injuries, *Knee ligaments: structure, function, injury and repair,* ed. Daniel D, Akeson W, O'Connor J (Raven Press: New York, 1990) 481–503.
13. Fowler PJ, Messieh SS, Isolated posterior cruciate ligament injuries in athletes, *Am J Sports Med* (1987) **15**: 553–557.
14. Clancy WG, Shelbourne KD, Zoellner GB et al., Treatment of the knee joint instability secondary to rupture of the posterior cruciate ligament: Report of a new procedure, *J Bone Joint Surg (Am)* (1983) **65**: 310–322.
15. Torg JS, Barton TM, Pavlov H et al., Natural history of the posterior cruciate ligament-deficient knee, *Clin Orthop* (1989) **246**: 208–216.
16. Robson AWM, Ruptured crucial ligaments and their repair by operation, *Ann Surg* (1903) **37**: 716–718.
17. HeyGroves EW, Lond MS, Operation for the repair of the crucial ligaments, *Lancet* (1917) **2**: 674–675.
18. Gallie WE, LeMesurier AB, The repair of injuries to the posterior crucial ligament of the knee joint, *Ann Surg* (1927) **85**: 592–598.
19. Trickey EL, Injuries to the posterior cruciate ligament: diagnosis and treatment of early injuries and reconstruction of late instability, *Clin Orthop* (1980) **147**: 76–81.
20. Collins HR, Hughston JC, DeHaven KE et al., The meniscus as a cruciate ligament substitute, *Am J Sports Med* (1974) **2**: 11–21.
21. Tillberg B, The late repair of torn cruciate ligaments using menisci, *J Bone Joint Surg (Br)* (1977) **59**: 15–19.
22. Cubbins WR, Callahan JJ, Scuderi CS, Cruciate ligaments: A resume of operative attacks and results obtained, *Am J Surg* (1939) **43**: 481–485.
23. McCormick WC, Bagg RJ, Kennedy CW et al., Reconstruction of the posterior cruciate ligament, *Clin Orthop* (1976) **118**: 30–34.
24. Southmayd WW, Rubin BD, Reconstruction of the posterior cruciate ligament using the semimembranosus tendon, *Clin Orthop* (1980) **150**: 196–199.
25. Hughston JC, The posterior cruciate ligament in knee joint stability, *J Bone Joint Surg (Am)* (1969) **51**: 1045–1046.
26. Hughston JC, Degenhardt TC, Reconstruction of the posterior cruciate ligament, *Clin Orthop* (1982) **164**: 59–77.
27. Kennedy JC, Galpin RD, The use of the medial head of the gastrocnemius muscle in the posterior cruciate deficient knee: Indications, technique, results, *Am J Sports Med* (1982) **10**: 63–74.
28. Insall JN, Hood RW, Bone-block transfer of the medial head of the gastrocnemius for posterior cruciate insufficiency, *J Bone Joint Surg (Am)* (1982) **64**: 691–699.
29. Roth JH, Bray RC, Best TM et al., Posterior cruciate ligament reconstruction by transfer of the medial gastrocnemius tendon, *Am J Sports Med* (1988) **16**: 21–28.
30. Stäubli HU, Jakob RP, Posterior instability of the knee near extension: A clinical and stress radiographic analysis of acute injuries of the posterior cruciate ligament, *J Bone Joint Surg (Br)* (1990) **72**: 225–230.
31. Grood ES, Hefzy MS, Lindenfeld TN, Factors affecting the region of most isometric femoral attachments. Part I: The posterior cruciate ligament, *Am J Sports Med* (1989) **17**: 197–207.
32. Barrett GR, Savoie FH, Operative management of acute posterior cruciate ligament injuries with associated pathology: long-term results, *Orthopedics* (1991) **14**: 687–692.
33. The Acufex posterior cruciate ligament guide set is employed in this technique description. The set includes a technique synopsis and a video demonstration.
34. Seebacher JR, Inglis AE, Marshall JL et al., The structure of the posterolateral aspect of the knee, *J Bone Joint Surg (Am)* (1982) **64**: 536–541.

8

Patellofemoral joint disorders

8.1   Dislocation and subluxation of the patella: An overview

Paul M. Aichroth and Zaid Al-Duri

Classification

The classification of patellar subluxation and dislocation is by no means an easy task. Review of the literature shows that not only are the different entities seldom defined accurately but at times these entities are synonymously described.

For instance, subluxation refers to partial lateral displacement of the patella early in the process of knee flexion. Fulkerson and Hungerford[1] stressed the fact that subluxation is different from the permanent lateral patellar tracking that some patients may have owing to lateral tilt of the patella. They emphasize that subluxation can occur with or without tilt and tilt with or without subluxation.

Lateral patellar subluxations

Lateral patellar subluxations are of the following types.

Recurrent subluxation may either be minor, reflecting mild incongruence between the patellar articular surface and the femoral trochlea, or major when it is closely related to recurrent dislocation. Recurrent major subluxation tends to occur at the beginning of flexion or semiflexion and may be associated with patella alta.[1]

With habitual subluxation the patellar displacement occurs at every knee movement.[2]

With permanent lateral subluxation there is persistent subluxation through 90° or more of knee flexion with little tendency towards recentring of the patella with progressive flexion and there is almost always associated tilt.[1]

Subluxation in extension is uncommon[2] and will be considered separately.

Medial patellar subluxations

This condition may occur following operations for the realignment of the extensor mechanism, including arthroscopic lateral release. Arthroscopic release of the vastus lateralis followed by early lateral movement of the knee frequently results in retraction and atrophy of this muscle with a subsequent medial subluxation of the patella.[3] Treatment is difficult and Hughston and Deese[3] found the retraction of vastus lateralis too severe to allow mobilization and advancement. Fulkerson and Hungerford[1] advised reattachment of vastus lateralis to establish normal tracking.

Dislocations of the patella

Definitions are again required. *Habitual dislocation* refers to the patella deviating from the normal tracking on every occasion that the knee flexes or extends.[2,4,5] Habitual dislocation has been used synonymously with recurrent dislocation.[1] They prefer to call it 'acquired permanent dislocation'. Others have diagnosed habitual dislocation when the patella could be reduced in extension but dislocated every time the knee was flexed.[6]

Permanent dislocation means that the patella is no longer in contact with the articular cartilage of the distal femur throughout the full range of flexion. On extension, the patella may return towards, or nearly to, the midline, but on flexion the patella always returns to the lateral surface of the lateral femoral condyle.[1] There are two forms of permanent dislocation: congenital and acquired.

Persistent dislocation of the patella is essentially the same. In such a condition, the patella remains dislocated through the whole range of knee movement in both flexion and extension.[2]

Congenital dislocation of the patella refers to an irreducible dislocation present since birth and associated with a lateral position of the entire quadriceps mechanism.[4,6] The congenital form is believed to occur either in utero or at birth and there may be a hereditary predisposition.[1]

It seems that permanent and persistent dislocations are used synonymously.

Medial dislocation is exceedingly uncommon and may occur as a result of overcorrection of the lateral dislocation.[2]

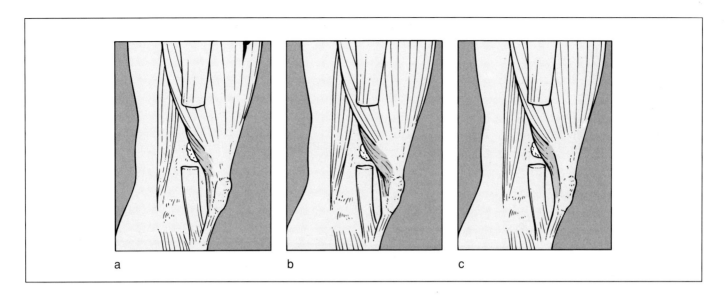

Figure 1

Patterns of insertion of vastus lateralis and its obliquus subdivision (after ref. 11).

Traumatic dislocation of the patella tends to be mostly lateral. However, it can be intra-articular,[7] superior,[8,9] or medial.[10]

Anatomy

This section is not intended to give a detailed account of the anatomy of the patellofemoral joint. The intention is to shed light on some of the relevant and interesting findings that are related to the aetiology of dislocation and subluxation of the patella.

The extensor mechanism takes the shortest course between its origin and its insertion and this results in the patella being pulled laterally. There are anatomical features which are responsible for active and passive stabilization of the patella, such as the sulcus between the femoral condyles and the vastus medialis obliquus, which tend to balance the tendency of the rectus femoris and vastus lateralis to displace the patella laterally.[2] Therefore, in a normal knee, the stability of the patella depends to some extent on the relative prominence of the lateral femoral condyle and the lower oblique fibres of the vastus medialis. When the knee is flexed from the extended position, the normal quadriceps tendon has an excursion of 2–3 cm. In cases of contracture of the extensor mechanism, there is loss of excursion of the quadriceps tendon and the extensor mechanism has to slip over the lateral femoral condyle for full knee flexion to be achieved.[6]

Hallisey et al.[11] gave an interesting account of the vastus lateralis part of the quadriceps muscle. The anatomy of the junction of the vastus lateralis and the patella is important for an understanding of the stability of the knee joint. They described the vastus lateralis obliquus portion of the vastus lateralis muscle and stressed that the vastus lateralis obliquus muscle in particular creates an important lateral force-vector on the patella. Not all of the fibres of the vastus lateralis muscle arise from the femur, as some of the lower fibres, including those of the vastus lateralis obliquus muscle, originate from the lateral intermuscular septum. The origin of the vastus lateralis obliquus muscle appears to be consistent as it originates beneath the main muscle belly of the vastus lateralis and then circles inferiorly and anteriorly to its insertion. Three distinct anatomical patterns in the insertion of the vastus lateralis obliquus were delineated. (1) It inserts obliquely into the vastus lateralis portion of the quadriceps tendon. A distinct plane of fatty tissue separates the body of vastus lateralis obliquus from the vastus lateralis muscle (Figure 1a). (2) It does not join the quadriceps tendon but may cross inferiorly to interdigitate with the superficial oblique fibres of the lateral retinaculum (Figure 1b). (3) The pattern of insertion is related to the fibres of the vastus lateralis muscle which does not always travel completely over the patella to join the patellar tendon. Some tendon fibres of the vastus lateralis may interdigitate with the superficial oblique fibres of the lateral retinaculum, thus receiving the vastus lateralis obliquus muscle without contributing to the patellar tendon (Figure 1c).

It is clear, therefore, that the lateral retinaculum cannot be considered static, since it receives the tendinous insertions of the vastus lateralis and the vastus lateralis obliquus.

Regarding the trochlear surface of the femur, it seems that there is no universal agreement as to what constitutes normal anatomy of the anterior-femoral surface. However, the average depth of the patellar groove or sulcus is 5.2 mm, and the average height of the lateral femoral condyle above the medial is 4.5 mm. Wide variations from this norm are seen; occasionally a sulcus measures as much as 10 mm in depth and the anterior aspect of the femur may be flat or slightly convex.[12] Damage to the patellar cartilage occurs more frequently than in any other cartilaginous area in the body and this may be related to this variation. It is also of interest to note that the length of the articular surface of the patella measured at operation is almost always 3.5 cm regardless of the shape or size of the individual.[13]

The quadriceps (Q) angle is measured by drawing an imaginary line connecting the centre of the patella and the anterior superior iliac spine to produce a surface marking that approximates the line of pull of the quadriceps tendon.[14,15] Others have drawn this line between the centre of the femoral shaft and the centre of the patella.[16] The direction of the patellar tendon is indicated by a second line drawn from the centre of the patella to the centre of the tibial tubercle. The intersection of these two imaginary lines forms the Q angle. Various suggestions have been made as to what constitutes a normal Q angle. Insall[15] states that in the normal knee this measures 15°, and that an angle exceeding 20° is considered unequivocally abnormal. Chen and Ramanathan[14] consider the normal Q angle to be 14°; subsequently readings above 14° are considered abnormal.

It is true that the valgus vector may increase with an increase in the Q angle; however, the valgus angle (which is independent of the position of the patella) does not correlate directly with the Q angle. That is why genu valgum is not altered by realignment of the patella, whereas the Q angle is.[16] The Q angle is increased in genu valgum, femoral and tibial torsion, and in outward rotation of the tibia during extension and flexion of the knee.[17]

The Q angle is related to the position of the patella as well as that of the tibial tubercle. The position of the patella is variable depending on the angle of flexion or extension plus the condition of the patellar stabilizers. The tibial tubercle may have a static position in the sagittal plane but it certainly moves in the horizontal plane owing to the tibial rotation relative to the femur in the final few degrees of extension in the so-called 'screw-home movement'. That ultimately means that the tibial tubercle changes position in the horizontal plane in flexion and extension. It thus becomes a dynamic rather than the static angle that many mention. It is best to correlate the Q angle on the involved knee to that of the contralateral knee in unilateral patellofemoral involvement. In cases of bilateral patellofemoral involvements, one is obliged to refer to the so-called normal values.

Aetiological factors in patellar subluxation and dislocation

Whilst it is true that the aetiology of patellar subluxation and dislocation remains unknown, there has been considerable progress in understanding the various aetiological factors that may contribute to such an event. Recurrent dislocation and subluxation is usually the result of a minor injury superimposed upon some mechanical abnormality which allows recurrent and then possibly habitual dislocation.[2]

In a review by Aichroth[2] of children's knees in which a lateral patellar dislocation occurred recurrently or habitually, the following associated abnormalities were noted in 35 patients (6 with bilateral dislocations, 41 knees assessed):

Congenital lax ligaments	11 patients
Valgus knees	4 patients
Congenital dislocation of the hip	3 patients
Spastic hemiparesis	2 patients
Marfan's syndrome	1 patient
Ehlers–Danlos syndrome	1 patient
Turner's syndrome	1 patient
Peroneal muscular atrophy	1 patient

Soft-tissue abnormalities

Cash and Hughston[18] believe that a patellar dislocation in a knee without a congenital deficit of the extensor mechanism is rare.

Ligamentous laxity

Recurrent and habitual dislocation or subluxation has been associated with ligamentous laxity.[1,2,5,10,17,19–21] Patients with generalized joint laxity thus constitute a subgroup in whom dislocation of the patella may be one of many expressions of a systemic disorder of connective tissue.[17] A higher incidence of the recurrent dislocation of the patella is present in children with generalized ligamentous laxity, such as osteogenesis imperfecta, arachnodactyly, or Ehlers–Danlos syndrome.[2,10] The laxity may be either generalized or that of the medial retinaculum alone.[5]

Abnormalities of the extensor expansion and the iliotibial band

The iliotibial band may be abnormally attached to the lateral side of the patella and the lateral patellar expansion pulls the bone towards the lateral side.[2,10] Contracture of the lateral patellar tissue is a definite pathogenic factor in recurrent subluxation and dislocation of the patella. The vastus lateralis may be contracted, hypertrophied, and inserted low.[10,11] Tight and/or abnormal fascial bands of the vastus lateralis has been reported too.[1,5,19]

Muscular or developmental defects

Floyd et al.[20] reported on 12 patients with recurrent dislocation of the patella. Eleven of the 12 patients had joint hypermobility. Muscle biopsies were taken from 8 of the 9 patients surgically treated. They propose that there is an association between hypermobility and recurrent dislocation of the patella. Their preliminary findings suggest that there may be a primary muscular defect in many cases of recurrent patellar dislocation.

Sharma[22] feels that recurrent, habitual and congenital dislocations are expressions of varying grades of the same aetiology; all of them being due to a developmental defect.

Muscle imbalance

There may be an imbalance between the vastus medialis and the vastus lateralis, producing a bow-stringing effect on the patella.[5] Atrophy, weakness, or high oblique insertion of the vastus medialis is a factor in most patients.[10] The orientation of the vastus lateralis and vastus lateralis obliquus can definitely be a factor.[1,10,11]

Soft-tissue damage following injury

Major damage to the medial patellar retinaculum and the medial side of the patellar tendon may occur in severe traumatic dislocation of the patella. The patellar tendon may be avulsed from the tibial tuberosity and there may also be a fracture through the medial side of the tuberosity. This is likely to be followed by recurrent dislocation if operative repair is not undertaken.[2,10]

Bony abnormalities

Genu valgum

Genu valgum is a rare cause of recurrent dislocation or subluxation of the patella. Bizou[23] reported five recurrent dislocations treated by supracondylar osteotomy for correction of genu valgum.

External tibial torsion

Despite the likelihood of predisposition with increased external tibial torsion, no statistically significant series has shown it.[10]

Lateral location of the tibial tuberosity

This has been thought an important factor by Trillat et al.[24] It is difficult to measure and may be associated with external tibial torsion.[2,10] Brattström[25] could find no statistical significance between the degree of external tibial torsion in his patients with recurrent dislocation of the patellae and in a control group. Heywood[26] reported only two examples in his series of 54 cases.

Femoral anteversion

Femoral anteversion occurring in congenital dislocation of the hip does seem to be associated in some children with recurrent dislocation of the patella.[2] Excessive femoral anteversion, on the other hand, is claimed to interfere with patellar alignment only if progressive compensatory external tibial torsion is involved.[10]

Abnormalities of the femoral sulcus and condyles

The lateral femoral condyle is normally more prominent than the medial. When the patella dislocates recurrently, the lateral condyle has been said to be underdeveloped and is lower than usual. Brattström[25] used a precise radiological technique for assessing this trochlear abnormality in 131 patients with recurrent dislocation of the patella and compared them with 200 normal controls. He felt that the most important factor in patients with recurrent dislocation of the patella was an abnormality of the trochlea and suggested that the change in the trochlear angle figure was due to a decrease in the depth of the sulcus rather than a decrease in the prominence of the lateral femoral condyle.

Dysplasia of the femoral sulcus has been reported as a factor contributing to acute and recurrent patellar dislocation.[21,27] This leads to increased shallowness of the trochlea, i.e. abnormally high sulcus angle.[10] Dysplasia of the lateral femoral condyle is a contributing factor too.[19]

Variations in the shape of the patella

Wiberg[28] recognized three types of patellar shape:

Type I: Both facets are of the same size with both medial and lateral articular facets being concave (10%).

Type II: The medial facet is smaller with the lateral facet concave and the medial slightly convex (65%).

Type III: The medial facet is small and convex (25%). This type may have a greater tendency to recurrent dislocation.

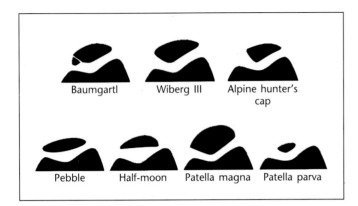

Figure 2

Dysplastic patellae: variations in form (after ref. 1).

Ficat[29] stressed the importance of skyline views of the patella in 30°, 60° and 90° of flexion and introduced another classification of patellar shape which was based on the angle which the two patellar facets made with each other (the normal angle being 120–140°). The groups described were:

1. A pebble-shaped patella in which the angle was greater than 140°.
2. Wiberg type III patella, in which this angle measures 90–100°.
3. A hemipatella with one articular facet (alpine-hunter's cap deformity) in which the angle is 90°.
4. A patella in the form of a half-moon with a very acute angle. Ficat considered that this type was most commonly present in persistent dislocation of the patella.

Fulkerson and Hungerford[1] gave a detailed account of patellar dysplasias (Figure 2).

Although the absence of the patella has been reported without related musculoskeletal abnormalities, it is most commonly found in the nail–patella syndrome.

Patella alta

It is still not known whether patella alta is an inherited or an acquired trait. It is said, however, that the overgrowth that occurs during the growth spurt can lead to patella alta in some individuals.[30] Others believe that it is the increased tension on the patellar ligament that results in its greater length.[1]

There is little doubt that a high patella is an important factor in recurrent patellar dislocation or subluxation.[1,2,5,10,19,20,27] If there is a high-riding patella the

buttressing effect of the lateral femoral condyle will be lost. Similarly, a congenital hypoplasia and flattening of the lateral femoral condyle will have the same effect as that of patella alta.[10]

There are several ways of assessing patellar height, which have their own advantages and disadvantages:

1. Blumensaat's lines indicate the correct position of the patella when flexed to 30°.
2. Insall's method of assessment is commonly used but may be inaccurate in the presence of Osgood–Schlatter's or Sinding–Larsen's disease.
3. Blackburne's method is probably the most reliable and can be easily made on a lateral view of the knee with the joint flexed 30°.

Traumatic dislocation

Most patients describe an injury as the cause of the first dislocation. The most common mechanisms of injury were twisting, valgus stress, or a direct blow to the knees.[2,18] A direct blow to the patella, however, is not as common as the twisting injuries and is also associated more with the rare intra-articular and superior patellar dislocations.[7–9]

Vainionpää et al.[27] reviewed 55 cases of acute patellar dislocation. It occurred in the following activities: athletic performance (56.4% of cases); leisure (32.7% of cases); at work (11% of cases). The mode of injury in the same series included: indirect force, 83.6% of cases; direct force, 11% of cases; uncertain, 5.5%.

Cash and Hughston[18] reviewed 100 patients (103 knees) with acute patellar dislocation. Activities most often associated with the injury were sporting ones involving football, falls, basketball, baseball, and softball. The most common mechanisms of injury were twisting, valgus stress, or a direct blow to the knees.

Jackson[5] stated that acute dislocations occur most commonly during adolescence when the knee gives way without warning. Usually a valgus/external rotation force was the precipitating factor. Direct trauma to the knee cap is an uncommon cause.

The effect of patellar dislocation is well exemplified by the findings of Vainionpää et al.[27] In a series of 55 patients with acute patellar dislocation, the operative findings were: haemarthrosis in 55 cases; rupture of the medial retinaculum in 54 cases; stretch of the medial retinaculum in 1 case; medial marginal fracture of the patella in 23 cases; intra-articular fracture of the patella in 3 cases; fracture of the lateral femoral condyle in 3 cases; partial detachment of the patellar tendon in 1 case.

Articular cartilage breakdown is common following blunt trauma, with or without fracture. It is important for the clinician to recognize when a patient has articular degeneration related to trauma as opposed to malalignment. In the former, treatment should be directed to the articular surface itself, and procedures such as lateral retinacular release generally are not helpful. Lateral release should not be the treatment of choice for patients with blunt articular injury to the patella and subsequent arthrosis.[1]

Treatment of acute patellar dislocation

Fulkerson and Hungerford[1] stress the role of *non-operative treatment in patellar subluxation* as follows: Medial quadriceps strengthening and taping to hold the patella medially may be helpful. Patellar cut-out braces may add some feeling of security. Orthotics may improve lower extremity alignment and diminish valgus thrust at the knee, thereby reducing the risk of patellar dislocation or symptoms of subluxation. The response to non-operative treatment is dependent, to some extent, on the degree of patellar subluxation. Most patients with symptomatic minor subluxation will improve or become asymptomatic with non-operative treatment. Some patients with major or permanent subluxation also respond remarkably well to non-operative treatment. Should disabling symptoms and significant activity limitation persist after non-operative treatment, then surgery is indicated.

Stressing the important role of *non-operative treatment in acute patellar dislocations*, Hughston and Walsh[31] emphasized that it is exceedingly rare for them to proceed with surgical treatment without a concentrated attempt at non-operative treatment. Patients with acute patellar dislocations are treated by cast immobilization with a foam-rubber pad over the vastus medialis obliquus followed by rehabilitation programme (straight leg raising exercises, hamstring stretches where indicated, and elastic knee sleeve with a lateral felt pad). Fulkerson and Hungerford[1] stated that if the treating physician is confident that there is no major articular fragment displacement, and if the patella can be reduced well into the trochlea and maintained there, a period of 6 weeks immobilization may restore adequate stability. Non-operative treatment will give satisfactory results, particularly when there is no pre-existing congenital abnormality of the extensor mechanism. They advise that major reconstructions should generally be avoided immediately after an acute dislocation. They recommend selective arthroscopy to aid in the diagnosis of osteochondral fragments avulsion, to allow for a selective lateral retinacular release, and to help in simple replacement of osteochondral fragments.

The standard treatment of the uncomplicated cases is conservative. However, following acute dislocations, recurrent dislocation is the rule and there are those who favour immediate repair following acute dislocation. If treated conservatively, the chances of a further dislocation have been estimated by Heywood[26] to be 85%.[5]

Larsen and Lauridsen,[32] in assessing the value of conservative treatment of patellar dislocation, reviewed 79 knees with a diagnosis of patellar dislocation. There were 44 females and 27 males. Median age among females was 18.1 years (range 6–52 years) and among males was 19.3 years (range 12–44 years). The mean follow-up period was 5 years and 11 months (range 1–31 years). They concluded that conservative treatment of patellar dislocation cannot sufficiently re-establish stability in the patellofemoral joint. They recommend conservative treatment of the primary dislocation, with special emphasis on re-education of the quadriceps muscle, but redislocation should be treated more aggressively with operation.

Several alternatives are available to treat acute patellar dislocation. Cash and Hughston[18] stated that early surgical repair has been recommended by many surgeons on the grounds that there is continuing disability and a lack of pain relief following non-operative treatment. They reviewed 100 individuals (103 knees) who had an acute patellar dislocation, i.e. in whom there had been no previous dislocation or subluxation, and who were treated within 14 days of the original injury. The patients had no concomitant ligamentous injuries, long bone fractures or other injuries. One of three methods of treatment was used:

1. Immobilization and exercise (74 knees) was undertaken if there was no osteochondral fracture, or when the surgeon preferred.
2. Arthroscopy (13 knees) was undertaken in some patients within 14 days of the dislocation if there was suspicion of a large osteochondral fracture or associated intra-articular pathology.
3. Surgical repair (16 knees) was undertaken if there was suspicion of intra-articular pathology or there was a palpable defect in the insertion of the vastus medialis obliquus.

Vainionpää et al.[27] performed medial reefing and lateral release in 54 out of 55 patients. Five cases redislocated and these were treated by the Hauser operation.

Tachdjian[10] advised that the acute dislocations associated with osteochondral fractures require surgical treatment. The fragment was removed or reattached (if large and in the weight-bearing area) and torn soft tissues were repaired.

Fulkerson's approach to acute patellar dislocation is that if there is evidence of an osteochondral fragment, arthroscopy is performed. If the fragment is less than 1 cm in diameter, it is removed arthroscopically. If it is larger, then a limited arthrotomy is performed for fixation. Lateral release can be performed arthroscopically if indicated in patients with patellar tilt. If an arthrotomy for fixation of the osteochondral fragment is performed, a limited lateral arthrotomy may be utilized for the lateral release. If acute dislocation of the patella has been the result of direct trauma without underlying malalignment, there is no reason to perform a lateral release.

Intra-articular dislocation of the patella

Murakami[7] described intra-articular dislocations of the patella as of two types: horizontal and vertical. The horizontal type is more common than the vertical type but both types are rare. In the horizontal type, the patella dislocates and rotates around its horizontal axis. Such rotation most often detaches the upper pole of the patella from the quadriceps tendon, causing it to be trapped within the joint, with the articular surface facing inferiorly. In the vertical variety, the patella rotates on its vertical axis, with the patellar edge lying in the notch and the articular surface facing medially or laterally. The mechanism tends to be a direct impact on the knee cap. Whilst the majority of the cases might require surgical reduction, some might reduce by closed methods and therefore each case may be treated individually.

Superior dislocation of the patella

Superior dislocation of the patella is a very rare type of patellar dislocation, with the total number of reported cases being four.[8] The patella tends to lie higher than its normal location with no palpable gap or tenderness along the patellar tendon, hence the importance of differentiating it from a ruptured patellar tendon.[9]

The mechanism of injury in all cases appears to be a posteriorly directed blow on the anterior surface of the patella,[8] possibly accompanied by a sudden quadriceps contraction.[9] Such a dislocation appears to occur in a knee with osteophytosis of the inferior pole of the patella and anterior surface of the femoral condyles which causes the knee cap to become locked in its elevated position after the impact. Hence it is not a dislocation of the young person. The dislocation is simple to reduce by closed means,[8,9] but recurrence may be an indication for surgical excision of the osteophytes.[9]

Recurrent dislocation of the patella

Recurrent dislocation of the patella is more common in girls, perhaps because of greater ligamentous laxity[2] or anatomic predisposition.[21] The various reports substantiating this claim are as follows. Chrisman et al.[33]: In a study of 87 knees with recurrent patellar dislocation [age range 9–43 years], there were 47 recurrent dislocations in females and 40 in males. Dandy and Griffiths:[19] In reviewing 35 patients with recurrent dislocation of the patella, there were 25 females and 10 males. Vainionpää et al.:[27] Of 55 adolescent to adult patients, there were 62% females. Scuderi et al.[34] reviewed 52 patients with patellar dislocation or subluxation. There were 25 females and 27 male patients. Fulkerson and Hungerford[1] stated that there is a female predominance varying from 1.5:1 to as high as 5:1.

Cash and Hughston[18] are not in agreement with the principle of female predominance in recurrent dislocation. In a review series of acute patellar dislocation of 100 patients (103 knees), the dislocation occurred more frequently in athletic males (70 patients) than females (30 patients). The average age at injury was 21.7 years (range 9–72 years).

A clear family history may be obtained[2,10] and approximately one-third of the cases are bilateral. If the dislocation remains unilateral then the incidence is equal between right and left knees. The most common age of onset of the condition is between 15 and 17 years in girls and a year or two later in boys.[1,2,5]

Whether the patella dislocates or subluxes recurrently is a question of degree. The subluxing patella rides on the lateral femoral condyle and almost dislocates. The subluxation may be considered minor to major depending upon the degree of the lateral movement without full dislocation. All the aetiological factors mentioned previously apply here.[2]

Clinical features of recurrent dislocation

'The experience of dislocating a patella is quite impressive to the patient, and usually the patient is aware that something very significant has occurred.'[1] A few patients may never dislocate or sublux their patella again after a traumatic dislocation, but the number is small and Heywood[26] has indicated a figure of 15%. Most patients have a further dislocation of the patella with much less violence and eventually only minor twists or strains produce the displacement and cause a feeling of insecurity which manifests as 'the knee giving way'. The typical patient is a short, young, obese female with patellar malalignment and ligamentous laxity, but patellar dislocation occurs fairly frequently in vigorous young athletes, male or female.[1]

Recurrence of the dislocation of the patella tends to be rare under the age of 15 years[18] and the incidence tends to decrease after the age of 26 years, although some patients continue to have a recurrence later in life.[2] The decreased incidence with increasing age may be due to decrease of athletic activities.

Physical signs

In the acute stage the knee is flexed owing to painful hamstring spasm and the femoral condyles appear prominent; the patella may be felt laterally. There may be some tenderness medially and this may lead to the incorrect diagnosis of a torn meniscus.

If the patient presents several hours later with the dislocation reduced then the haemarthrosis is rarely under tension; the patella is hypermobile laterally and may easily be redislocated if the patient would allow. The most pathognomonic sign is tenderness along the medial border of the patella, which testifies to the torn medial parapatellar structures.[1]

After several dislocations, the most important sign is that described by Fairbank[35] and Apley[36] and is appropriately called the 'apprehension sign'. An attempt is made to displace the patella laterally, but this is clearly painful and is resisted by the patient whose apprehension is obvious. Fulkerson and Hungerford,[1] whilst acknowledging the significance of the apprehension sign in recurrent dislocation of the patella, believe that it is not constant. Hughston and Deese[3] stress the importance of diagnosing lateral patellar subluxation and dislocation based on the actual passive subluxation of the patella rather than on the basis of the apprehension test, which is not an objective evidence of lateral patellar subluxation.

An abnormality of movement of the patella may also be noted. This by definition implies that the instability is a dynamic one and therefore the knees are to be examined in motion. The knees are flexed with the patient sitting at the edge of the examination couch, and as the knee is slowly extended by the patient the patella jumps medially as full extension is reached. It should be noted, however, that when recurrent subluxation of the patella is due to patella alta, the patella will be displaced laterally with the knee in extension owing to loss of the buttress of the lateral femoral condyle. Attempting to push the patella medially with the knee in extension may impart a sense of lateral tautness.[10]

One must remember the substantial articular injury that can occur at the time of dislocation of the patella. Thus, a loose body may be palpated and this is due to an osteochondral fracture in the acute stage. To diagnose it, arthroscopy becomes the cornerstone of decision-making in this regard.[1]

Investigations of patellar subluxation and dislocation

The purpose of radiographic evaluation is to try to establish the criteria for malalignment, reveal associated osteochondral fragments, check for loose bodies, and interpret the significance of calcifications once found. Some of these lesions may be caused by the

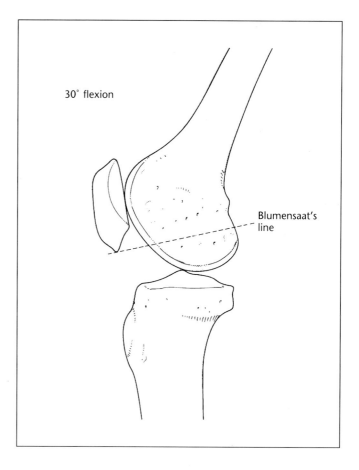

Figure 3

Blumensaat's line projecting anteriorly from the intercondylar notch to the lower pole of the patella.

dislocation of the patella; others could be the sequelae of the event.

Radiography

Standard anteroposterior (AP)

Weight-bearing views should be taken if degenerative changes are present. Rotation of the limb must be controlled. It is said that turning the feet to straight AP alignment may introduce internal rotation and distort patellar alignment.[1]

Lateral views

Lateral views are of particular value in evaluating the height of the patella. The most popular methods include the following:

(1) Blumensaat's line. The lower pole of the patella should lie on a line projected anteriorly from the

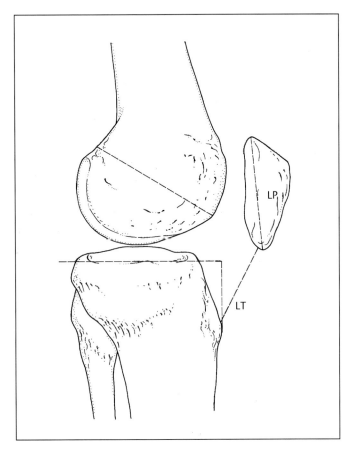

Figure 4

The Insall–Salvati index = LT/LP; where LT is the patellar tendon length and LP is the patellar length.

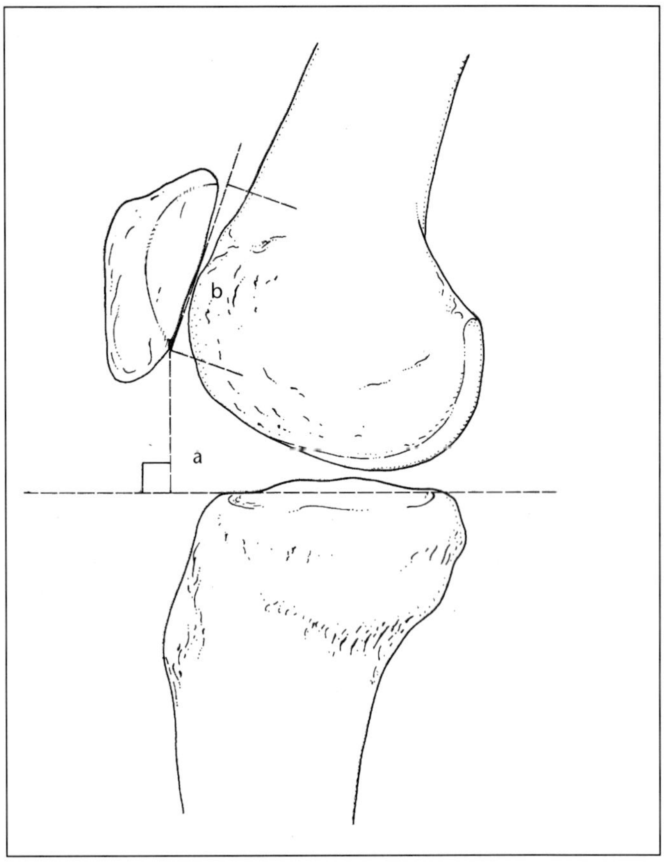

Figure 5

The Blackburne–Peel index: a/b = 0.8 in normal knees.

intercondylar notch in a 30° flexed knee on the lateral radiograph. Therefore, elevation of the lower pole of the patella above that line is regarded as patella alta[37] (Figure 3).

(2) The Insall–Salvati index. Unlike the Blumensaat line, this method does not depend on the exact positioning of the knee.[1] It depends on determining the ratio of the length of the patellar ligament (from the inferior pole of the patella to the tibial tubercle) to the length of the patella (the greatest diagonal length of the patella). The average value of the ratio was 1.02, with a mean standard deviation of 0.13,[15] so the normal value is 1.20 (Figure 4).

(3) Blackburne and Peel[38] criticized the Insall–Salvati index on the grounds that the inferior pole of the patella may be of varying lengths, while it is the position of the articular surface that is of greatest significance; also, the position of the tibial tubercle may be difficult to depict in disorders such as Osgood–Schlatter's disease. It is interesting here to note that Hughston, on measuring the length of the articular surface of the patella intraoperatively,

commented that the length of this surface of the patella is almost always 3.5 cm regardless of the shape or size of the patella.[13]

A new ratio was accordingly proposed between the length of the articular surface of the patella and the distance between the tibial articular surface and the patellar articular surface. This ratio is 0.8 in normal knees that are flexed to 30° (Figure 5).

Axial views

Axial views are also called tangential, sunrise, or skyline views. They are very important in giving specific information about the patellofemoral joint. Unfortunately, they either tend to be omitted by many or, when requested, are inaccurately executed. This is one area where standardization is a must. The most popular methods of doing these views are those described by Laurin et al.[39] and Merchant et al.[40]

In the Laurin et al.[39] method, the knee is in 20° of flexion. The beam is directed parallel to the anterior

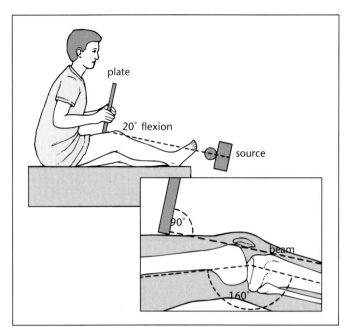

border of the tibia and to the longitudinal axis of the patella (Figure 6). Laurin et al. showed that the patella is settled in the trochlea by 20° of knee flexion in 97% of normal individuals.[39] Fulkerson and Hungerford stated that the Laurin view is difficult to obtain but is helpful in detecting patients with more subtle tracking abnormalities as well as those with severe patellar tilt, subluxation, or dislocation.[1] The lateral patellofemoral angle and the patellofemoral index are estimated as in Figure 6. The patellofemoral index represents the ratio between the thickness of the medial patellofemoral interspace and that of the lateral patellofemoral interspace. It is 1.6 or less in normal individuals and more than 1.6 in 93% of patients with chondromalacia.

a

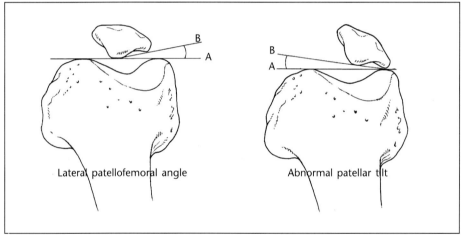

b

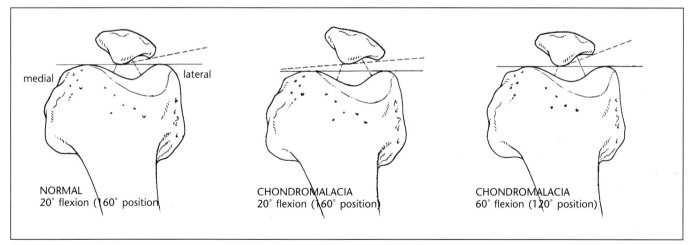

c

Figure 6

(a) The Laurin method. (b) In the normal knee the angle between line A and line B opens laterally (the lateral patellofemoral angle). In recurrent subluxation, the angle opens medially. (c) The patellofemoral index is the ratio of the thickness of the medial patellofemoral interspace to the lateral patellofemoral interspace. The medial patellofemoral interspace is equal to, or slightly less than, the lateral patellofemoral interspace. In normal individuals, it is 1.6. At 20° of flexion, patients with chondromalacia will reveal their tilt.

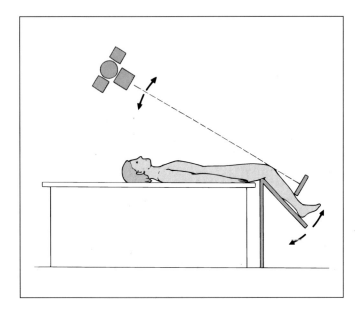

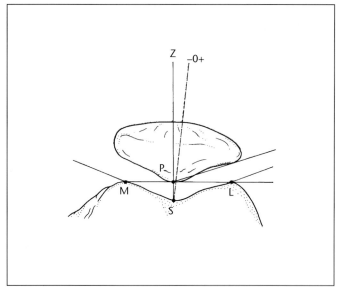

Figure 7

Merchant's radiographic technique for the axial view of the patellofemoral joint.

Figure 8

Measurement of the sulcus and congruence angles of Merchant. S=sulcus, M=medial femoral condyle, L=lateral femoral condyle. P=patellar crest. Line SO=reference line. MSL=sulcus angle=137°±6°. ZSO=congruence angle= –8°±6°.

In the Merchant et al. method, the knee is flexed at 45° over the end of the table and the X-ray tube is angled 30° from the horizontal[40] (Figure 7). The sulcus and congruence angles are measured (Figure 8). Merchant's technique is reproducible and provides an excellent overview of the patellofemoral congruence.[1]

In trauma, the modalities mentioned so far do not necessarily have a direct application. Vainionpää et al. reported on 55 patients with acute patellar dislocation.[27] Before operation lateral patellar displacement, as assessed on tangential radiographs taken at 20° of knee flexion, was significantly more frequent in the injured than in control knees. After operation, radiographic alignment of the patella was normal; this was still true in 90% of cases at 2 years follow-up. They found no difference in the shape of the patella between the injured and control knees by Wiberg's classification. They consider that an abnormal patellofemoral angle is not a reliable radiological sign of patellar instability in acute dislocation since the patellofemoral angle was abnormally open on the medial side in only 34% of injured knees. They noted that the Q angle measurement is not reliable in acute dislocation of the patella. The conclusion was that the stability of the patella could not be reliably estimated in tangential views taken with the knee in 20° of flexion; false negative findings were numerous.

In the lateral view, patella alta was observed in 15 injured knees and in 12 unaffected ones. However, the position of the patella in the knee joint measured according to Insall and Salvati[41] is less reliable in the injured knee with haemarthrosis than in the intact one. The rupture of the medial retinaculum may allow the patella to turn so that its upper pole is located laterally. In addition, effusion raises the patella and medial subcutaneous haematoma pushes it again more laterally. Therefore, the measured diagonal length of the patella is shorter than the true length.

Computed tomography

Computed tomography (CT) offers, apart from the usual details of patellar morphology, invaluable information about patellofemoral alignment. Fulkerson and Hungerford[1] believe that CT scanning provides sequential images at any degree of knee flexion using the midtransverse patella as a stable plane of reference.

CT may show signs of a patella that is slow to centralize in the trochlea with notable subluxation on 10° and 20° flexion tomographic cuts. This may be important information in the patient who has failed conservative treatment, because such patients may have considerable functional instability with athletic activities despite normal standard radiographs at 45° knee flexion. CT scanning may be very helpful also in determining whether there is tilt associated with subluxation.[1] Some believe that, despite its accuracy, its routine use is not recommended because of the cost and the exposure to irradiation.[10]

Inoue et al.[42] stressed the value of CT scanning in malalignment of the patella. Fifty patients who had patellar subluxation and 30 control subjects were examined using axial radiographs of the patellofemoral joint that were made with the knee joint in full extension. They stated that both normal and subluxating patellae usually tilt laterally when the knee approached full extension. The phenomenon of an increase in the lateral patellar tilt as the knee is extended should be considered as a typical finding in patients with patellar subluxation. Inoue et al. considered the patella that increased in its lateral tilt with flexion to be an unusual variety. They highlighted the role of CT scanning in patients with subluxing patella as follows.

(1) The difference in the amount of tilt between the control subjects and the patients who had patellar subluxation doubled when computed tomographic imaging was used, compared with that found on the axial radiographs made with the knee in 30° of flexion. Therefore, they concluded that there is a type of patellar subluxation in which the abnormal patellar tilt can be detected only with CT. Without CT, the diagnosis of this type of patellar subluxation is difficult or impossible, because the symptoms are indefinite and there are no objective signs. Therefore, when axial radiographs of the patellofemoral joint show no abnormal findings in a patient who has persistent pain in the anterior aspect of the knee, computed tomography examination is highly recommended.

(2) CT is more useful in the detection of attenuation of the supporting soft tissues medial to the patella, such as the medial retinaculum and the vastus medialis.

(3) CT is very helpful in assessing rotational deformities of the lower limb if serial scans were made at the level of the hip, knee, and ankle.

Malghem and Maldague[43] agree with Inoue et al.[42] on the value of CT scanning in diagnosing subluxation of the patella. However, they stress that the sensitivity of the conventional axial radiograph with the knee in 30° of flexion can be greatly enhanced if lateral rotation is applied to the leg during exposure by turning the leg outward manually while maintaining the knee within the beam axis. They assessed 27 knees that had been operated on for recurrent dislocation or subluxation of the patella. The preoperative patellar instability was depicted in all of the knees on the 30° lateral rotation axial radiograph, whereas it was demonstrated in only 7 knees (26%) on a routine axial radiograph. In the same group, in 13 contralateral knees that were not operated on, subluxation of the patella was demonstrated in 10 knees on the 30° lateral rotation axial radiograph, but in only 3 knees on the routine axial radiograph.

Magnetic resonance imaging

While magnetic resonance imaging (MRI) is the most effective non-invasive modality currently available for viewing patellar articular cartilage, it is believed that at this stage MRI offers little beyond CT for patellar tracking.[1] On the other hand, Kujala et al.[21] used magnetic resonance imaging to analyse the patellofemoral relationship during the first 30° of knee flexion in women with recurrent dislocation of the patella.

On the basis of logistic regression analysis the sulcus angle at 10° of knee flexion was the most diagnostic feature, indicating that there was an anatomical predisposition to recurrent dislocation and that pathological patellar tracking starts from the beginning of flexion. Traditional skyline radiographic films taken at 25–35° of knee flexion clearly miss diagnostically important information.

In a study employing MRI, Kujala et al.[21] showed that the patella normally lies in a lateral and tilted position in knee extension and undergoes medialization during the first 30° of flexion. In this study, the authors produced an axial image through the centre of the patellar articular cartilage and considered that this gave the most accurate information regarding condylar support for the patella at different angles. They stated that Fulkerson et al.[44] had used the posterior femoral condyles for reference when measuring patellar tilt, but Kujala et al. measured the indices from axial images with reference to the anterior femoral condyles. At the beginning of flexion the patella normally lies laterally in a somewhat tilted position; it moves to a congruent position during the first 30° of knee flexion. In patients with recurrent dislocation, tilting and lateralization are more obvious than in normal knees, the difference being most evident at the beginning of flexion. Other interesting findings include the following. (a) In 38% of the dislocating knees the sulcus angle was actually convex. (b) Seventy-seven per cent of the dislocating patellofemoral joints were congruent at 30° knee flexion but the difference between the groups was greater during the beginning of flexion.

In the acute traumatic patellar dislocation, CT or MRI examinations are not usually necessary. Certainly, if meniscal or cruciate ligament damage is suspected, then MRI may be helpful.[1]

Treatment of recurrent patellar dislocation and patellar instability

An attempt must be made to realign the extensor mechanism—including the patella—and to stabilize it. The stabilization depends upon many factors as described above, and if there is substantial dysplasia of the femoral sulcus then centralization of the patella may be difficult or even impossible.

Many procedures have been described for realignment and stabilization which suggest that there is no one adequate procedure for all. Houkom[45] stated that 'the treatment of recurrent dislocation of the patella has been a fertile field for the growth and development of the surgical ingenuity'. This summarizes the present position after 150 years of surgical effort.

Bony operations

(a) Transfer of the tibial tuberosity was described by Hauser[46] and modified by Smillie.[47] (b) Raising of the lateral femoral condyle after osteotomy and insertion of a graft as described by Albee.[48] (c) Maquet's operation, in which the tibial tuberosity is elevated forwards.[49] (d) A femoral osteotomy. If a valgus deformity is associated with recurrent dislocation of the patella, the possibility of realignment by supracondylar osteotomy must be considered. (e) Patellectomy. The extensor apparatus may still subluxate or dislocate after patellectomy. West and Soto-Hall[50] added advancement of the vastus medialis to the patella to control this possibility (Figure 9).

Soft-tissue operations

Simple lateral retinacular release

Lateral retinacular release was undertaken as an open or a limited open procedure with excellent to good results in 75–85% of cases.[10] The lateral release may be performed arthroscopically. It is effective and allows visualization of the patellar tracking and associated pathology.[10,51] Its scars are minimal. An arthroscopically assisted closed lateral release either using a Mayo scissors[52] or a Smillie meniscotome may be undertaken.[14,52] Full arthroscopic inspection is performed before proceeding to exclude any other pathology such as chondromalacia. It has been suggested that if the lateral release is performed extrasynovially then excessive bleeding is avoided.[14]

Whether lateral retinacular release should be performed by the closed arthroscopic or the open methods is by no means a settled issue. Hallisey et al.[11] argue that releasing the vastus lateralis obliquus tendon, as well as the entire lateral retinaculum, is important when performing a lateral release or patellofemoral realignment. Since the orientation of the vastus lateralis obliquus muscle is such that it must exert significant dynamic force on the patella, they believe that freeing these fibres will allow the quadriceps complex to shift its vector of pull medially, resulting in slightly improved patellofemoral alignment and in the elimination or reduction of pain that originates in the lateral retinaculum. Fulkerson and Hungerford[1] perform the lateral retinacular release through a small 3–4-cm incision

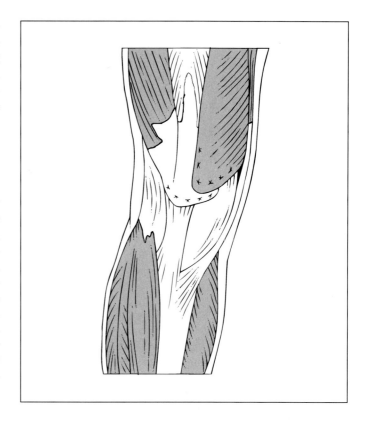

Figure 9

West and Soto-Hall's tendon transposition after patellectomy. The vastus medialis is freed and transferred laterally and distally to partially cover the defect left by excising the patella.

immediately adjacent to the lateral patella. The lateral retinaculum and synovium are incised under direct vision and the vastus lateralis obliquus of Hallisey is released with Mayo scissors along the fatty plane that separates it from the main vastus lateralis tendon.

A review of the indications for lateral release in the literature

Tachdjian[10] stated his indications for a lateral retinacular release, which include: a history of chronic intermittent anterior knee pain aggravated by physical activities that involve flexion and extension, failure of response to an adequate trial of conservative treatment, typical physical findings of lateral patellar subluxation due to lateral parapatellar soft-tissue contracture, radiographic confirmation of lateral patellar subluxation or tilting and arthroscopic determination of lateral patellar subluxation and compression. He stressed that simple clinical demonstration of lateral subluxation of the patella is not an indication for diagnostic arthroscopy and lateral release.

In the report by Dandy and Griffiths,[19] indications for lateral retinacular release in recurrent patellar dislocation include all patients who had at least three complete lateral dislocations of the patella; the patella had been felt or seen to lie on the lateral aspect of the femur, and all patients had some conservative treatment including physiotherapy before operation.

Fulkerson and Hungerford[1] advise that lateral release becomes particularly desirable in the patient with tilt and subluxation because the tilt component may respond particularly well to lateral release. Whilst these authors state that most patients with patellar subluxation improve after lateral retinacular release alone, as confirmed by observation and CT, Hughston and Deese[3] express their doubts of the effect of lateral retinacular release in cases of lateral subluxation alone.

The results of lateral retinacular release in the literature

Chen and Ramanathan[14] reviewed 39 patients who had closed lateral retinacular release of the patella performed for recurrent dislocation or subluxation or for acute dislocation of the patella. The average age was 20 years (range 13–35 years). The average follow-up was 6 years (range 3.33–9.11 years). The results of this procedure were as good as those after more major procedures. In a small number of patients a second operation such as tibial tubercle transfer or patellectomy may be necessary, especially in patients with an underlying congenital abnormality; but in many patients this type of major surgery has proved unnecessary.

Bigos and McBride[53] performed isolated lateral retinacular release on 102 knees in 76 patients. Diagnoses included chondromalacia patellae, patellar compression syndrome, and subluxation and dislocation of the patella. Patients reported that their symptoms improved after isolated lateral retinacular release in 95 of 102 knees. At follow-up evaluation (mean 14.5 months after surgery), independent observers found no recurrence of dislocation in the 23 knees having had frank dislocations before surgery. In 71% of the knees with limitation of activity before surgery, unlimited activity was tolerated after isolated lateral retinacular release. Hypothetically, lateral retinacular release decreases the work load of an overpowered or weakened vastus medialis obliquus muscle.

Henry et al.[52] reviewed 100 knees with patellofemoral subluxation that underwent lateral retinacular release in a closed arthroscopically assisted fashion. There were 57 females and 39 males with an average age of 28 years (range 10–59 years). The follow-up averaged 34 months (range 24–72 months). They considered the lateral release accomplished when the patella could be tilted to 90° medially and called it the 'turnip' sign. They stated that good results were obtained in 88% of the involved knees. All symptom parameters improved, but stability improved the most. This improvement paralleled a study of open reconstructions that the authors had reported previously. The failure rate was 12% [10 of those patients improved after a patellofemoral reconstruction was performed as described by Hughston].[54] The return rate of the patients to their previous sports was 81%. The authors considered reconstruction to be a good salvage procedure.

Dandy and Griffiths[19] reviewed 41 knees (35 patients) after lateral retinacular release for recurrent dislocation of the patella and graded the results according to the criteria of Crosby and Insall[55] The average age at operation was 20.5 years (range 8–40 years). The mean follow-up length was 48.4 months (range 12–96 months). There were no dislocations after the operation in 68% of the knees. Less satisfactory results were seen in patients with subluxation of the patella on extension of the knee and in those cases with generalized ligamentous laxity. A characteristic, previously unreported patellar surface lesion was seen in 19.5% of the cases. It consisted of parallel longitudinal striations that extended obliquely through the articular surface to give a characteristic appearance of interleaved strips. When the knees which showed subluxation of the patella on extension of the knee and patients with generalized ligamentous laxity were excluded from the calculations, 97% of their patients had an excellent or good result. The authors recommend open or arthroscopic lateral retinacular release.

Contraindication to lateral retinacular release

Contraindications include the following.

1. Marked ligamentous laxity,[19] especially when associated with recurrent dislocation due to patella alta.[10,56]
2. Patellae that dislocate on flexion and sublux on extension.[5,19]
3. Advanced degenerative osteoarthritis of the patellofemoral joint.[10]
4. That group of patients with severe recurrent dislocation of the patella, with multiple adverse factors such as an abnormal Q angle, deficient vastus medialis obliquus, and a shallow sulcus angle.[56]

Lateral release is frequently combined with other procedures as part of the method to realign the whole extensor apparatus.

Complications of lateral retinacular release

Henry et al.[52] commented that it is the impression among some orthopaedic surgeons that lateral release is an innocuous procedure. In their series, they found a 13% complication rate, consisting mostly of haematomas (9%) and reflex sympathetic dystrophy (4%). There was no infection.

Complications of lateral retinacular release were reported by Hughston and Deese[3] and include:

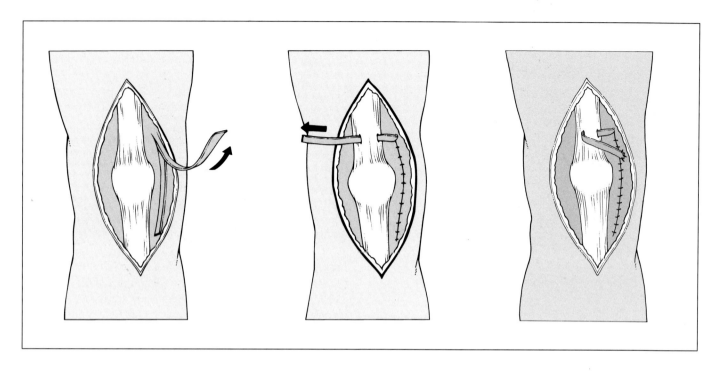

Figure 10

Campbell's operation. The strip of fascia medially has been freed and left attached proximally. It is then pulled laterally through the quadriceps tendon and back on itself to act as a sling which is attached medially.

1. Haemarthrosis.
2. Reflex sympathetic dystrophy.
3. Quadriceps tendon rupture (one reported case).
4. Medial subluxation of the patella. In a review of 60 failed lateral retinacular releases for a presumed diagnosis of lateral patellar subluxation or dislocation, 30 knees developed medial patellar subluxation following arthroscopic lateral retinacular release. Eighteen of these 30 knees had only lateral retinacular release, whilst the remainder underwent additional varying types and numbers of operations in an attempt to resolve the disability. One of the reasons for this complication appears to be the subsequent severe atrophy and retraction of the vastus lateralis.

Fulkerson and Hungerford[1] reported haemarthrosis as the most common complication. However, they incise both the lateral retinaculum and synovium.

Fascioplasty

Campbell's procedure is the most commonly undertaken (Figure 10).[57] An attempt has been made over the years to graft skin, nylon and other materials to reinforce the medial structures. These procedures, however, have had dubious success.[1,2] The Campbell operation may be done as the only corrective measure or in conjunction with other operations, especially the distal realignment of the quadriceps mechanism.[58]

Patellar ligament procedures

Goldthwait[59] and Roux[60] both described splitting of the patellar tendon with detachment of the lateral half from the tibial tuberosity (Figure 11). This part of the tendon is then re-routed beneath the intact medial part and sutured to the medial capsule.[2] The procedure may be modified as shown in Figure 12.

Fulkerson and Hungerford[1] stated that the Goldthwait procedure has never gained widespread popularity and carries some risk of adversely affecting patellar contact pressure distribution by pulling down the lateral facet. Hughston criticized the operation, saying that it does not correct patella alta; he also described traumatic rupture of the remaining half of the patellar tendon.[13]

The Roux–Goldthwait operation is usually combined with other procedures for realigning the extensor mechanism. The procedure is best avoided in vigorous and active patients with strong, well-developed quadriceps. Bowker and Thompson[61] reported a high failure rate with this procedure.[58]

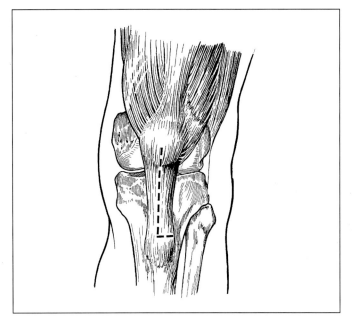

a

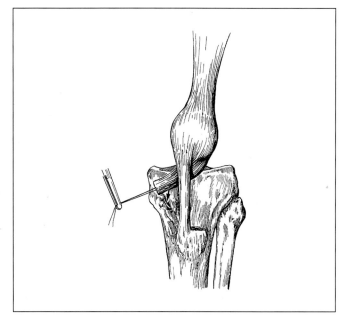

b

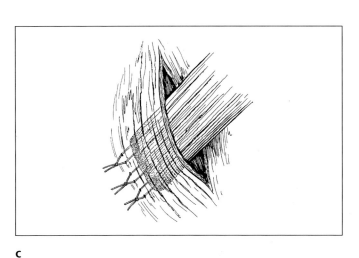

c

Figure 11

The Roux–Goldthwait operation.

Figure 12

Aichroth's modification of the Roux–Goldthwait procedure.

A very interesting study is that by Chrisman et al.,[33] who compared the results of the Roux–Goldthwait procedure with that of the Hauser operation. Eighty-seven knees in 75 patients (age range 9–43 years) with recurrent dislocations of the patella were operated on using either the Roux–Goldthwait procedure or the Hauser procedure and followed up for 4–12 years (average 7.7 years). In 10 patients less than 15 years of age, the Roux–Goldthwait operation was per-formed. No Hauser procedure was done on patients younger than the age of 15 years. Forty-seven knees had the Hauser procedure and 40 knees the Roux–Goldthwait procedure. In both the Hauser and Roux–Goldthwait procedures, the lateral capsule was widely released and the medial capsule was overlapped by at least 1 cm. Prior to the reefing, the joint was explored from the medial side.

Results of the Hauser procedure (47 knees) were:

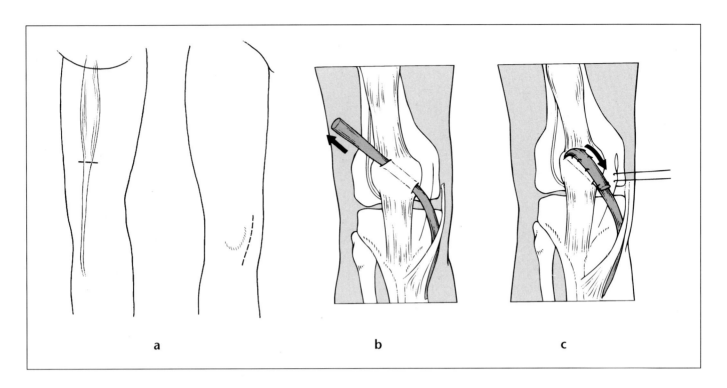

a   b   c

Figure 13

The Galeazzi semitendinosus tendon transfer. It provides medial patellar support in the skeletally immature patient, especially in those with permanent patellar subluxation (after ref. 63).

Excellent	55% of knees.
Good	17% of knees.
Fair	6% of knees.
Poor	21% of knees.

Those of the Roux–Goldthwait procedure (40 knees) were:

Excellent	70% of knees.
Good	23% of knees.
Fair	0%.
Poor	8% of knees.

The intra-articular findings of torn menisci, loose bodies and chondromalacia for which excision, or shaving and drilling were done did not prove to be predictors of unsatisfactory results. It would appear that while both procedures produce high rates of acceptable results (Hauser 72%, Roux–Goldthwait 93%), the Roux–Goldthwait repair had considerably fewer complications. Also, severe degenerative changes were present in six cases, five of which had the Hauser repair and one the Roux–Goldthwait repair. It is apparently easier to overcorrect with the Hauser procedure than the Roux–Goldthwait.

Templeman and McBeath,[62] reporting on two cases of medial overcorrection of the patella following the Roux–Goldthwait procedure, advise on the impor-tance of assessing patellar tracking dynamically in the operating theatre by performing surgery under local anaesthesia supplemented with intravenous sedation.

Tendon and muscle transfers

Gracilis, semitendinosus and sartorius have all been used independently or together to act as a medial tendon transfer to stabilize the patella. Tendon trans-fers were first described by Galeazzi.[63] Semitendinosus tendon transfer has gained popularity after Baker et al.[64] described excellent results in 81% of their series of 53 patients (Figure 13). There have been multiple methods of attachment of the medial tendons to the patella: Max Lange[65] (Figure 14a); McCarroll and Schwartzmann[66] (Figure 14b), and Lexer[67] (Figure 14c).

Baksi[68] described the transfer of the lower pes anser-inus with good results. Crosby and Insall[55] described medial capsulorrhaphy with advancement of the vastus medialis as an important part of many surgi-cal techniques. This is particularly true in skeletally immature patients.

The gracilis, semitendinosus and sartorius can be used to produce dynamic or static effects: when the tendon is inserted from above, it is designed to act dynamically; when from below as a tenodesis effect.[1]

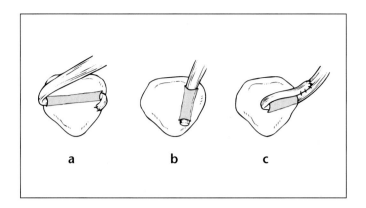

Figure 14

(a) The semitendinosus tendon is brought through a transverse patellar tunnel from the lateral to the medial side.[65] (b) The semitendinosus tendon is attached by passage through a vertical medial tunnel.[66] (c) Lexer's[67] method of attachment of the semimembranosus tendon.

The main indications for semitendinosus tenodesis for recurrent subluxation of the patellofemoral joint are subluxation or dislocation associated with a high-riding patella and when there is marked generalized ligamentous hyperlaxity that is familial or as in Down's syndrome, Ehlers–Danlos syndrome or Marfan's syndrome.[10]

Hall et al.[69] presented the results of semitendinosus tenodesis performed on 26 knees (3 congenitally dislocated patellae, 14 frank dislocations, 9 recurrent subluxations) with a mean age of 14.5 years (range 4–30 years) and followed up for an average of 43 months (range 1–6.5 years). In analysing the results, the following factors were considered:

(1) Duration of preoperative symptoms. There were 87% excellent and good results compared with 13% fair and poor results in those patients with less than 2 years' duration, whereas there were only 27% excellent and good results in those patients with symptoms of 2 years duration or longer.

(2) Excessive ligament laxity. Despite the poor results in the ligamentously lax patients, this procedure may serve to buy time and preserve growth plates until such time as bony realignment is indicated.

(3) The addition of the Roux–Goldthwait procedure did not significantly affect the overall result:

Roux–Goldthwait + semitendinosus tenodesis:
    Excellent and good results: 63%.
    Fair and poor results: 37%.
Semitendinosus tenodesis:
    Excellent and good results: 57%.
    Fair and poor results: 43%.

The major influence on the functional end result is the condition of the articular surface of the patella at the time of surgery. The duration of postoperative symptoms adversely affects the end result of the operation and therefore opening of the joint at the time of surgery is important.

Fulkerson and Hungerford[1] described the procedure by Krogius[70] which is popular in Europe. A strip of

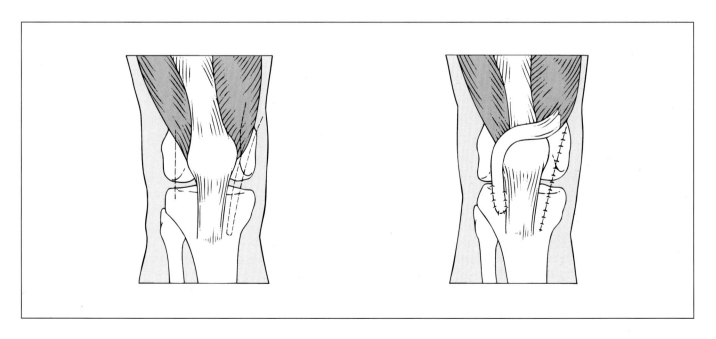

Figure 15

Krogius technique for patellar stabilization.

medial capsule with the attachment of the vastus medialis is developed, creating a medial defect. A lateral retinacular release is then carried out and the medial defect is closed. The myofascial strip that has been developed is then sutured into the lateral defect that has been created by medial plication (Figure 15). It is the opinion of Fulkerson and Hungerford that lateral retinacular release with medial imbrication without excision of any medial capsule has proved to be satisfactory in the majority of the skeletally immature patients.[1] Henrik Bauer et al.[71] reviewed 33 patients with recurrent dislocation of the patella who were treated with Krogius tenoplasty and followed up for 3 years. There were 8 males with an average age at first dislocation of 18 years (range 10–29 years) and 25 females with an average age at the first dislocation of 12 years (range 3–30 years). The average number of years between the first dislocation and surgery was 4 years for the females and 10 years for the males. In 14 of 34 operated knees, dislocations had recurred. Most of the recurrences were found in patients with generalized joint laxity, whereas only 1 of 9 knees with only a high Insall index had redislocated.

Patients with generalized joint laxity should not be treated with the Krogius tenoplasty as the sole procedure. These authors also found that scars after surgical treatment of recurrent patellar and shoulder dislocations are wide in patients with generalized joint laxity. They reflect abnormal connective tissues, and recurrences were most common in patients with wide scars.

Capsulorrhaphy

Capsulorrhaphy consists of simple release of the lateral retinaculum and imbrication of the medial retinaculum. Here it is important that the lateral release is adequately done, i.e. extending from the tibial tubercle across the entire lateral retinaculum and releasing the vastus lateralis obliquus.[10]

Scuderi et al.[34] reviewed the results of lateral release and proximal realignment of the patella in 60 knees (52 patients) with dislocation or subluxation of the patella. Their operation entailed a medial parapatellar capsular incision extending from the upper edge of vastus medialis into the quadriceps tendon, around the patella, and down to the tibial tubercle. Also, a lateral retinacular release extending through the synovial membrane and into the vastus lateralis was performed before the medial imbrication. The patients' average age was 22.1 years (range 11–37 years). The average follow-up duration was 3.5 years (range 2–9 years). At the follow-up, 80.8% of the patients had a good or excellent result; only one patient had redislocation of the patella. The differences in the results correlated statistically with age and sex in that the older patients had poorer results and the male patients better results. The results were

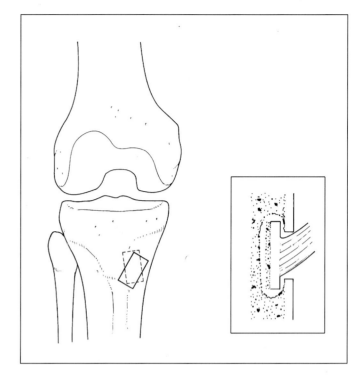

Figure 16

Smillie's modification of the Hauser's tibial tuberosity transfer. The rectangle of bone with the attached patellar tendon is locked beneath the cortex by rotation.

not affected by the grade of chondromalacia that was present at the time of operation. Centralizing the patella, as evidenced by the Merchant views, yielded the most favourable results.

Transfer of the tibial tuberosity

Although Roux in 1888 first described successful medial transfer of the tuberosity to the medial side in one case,[60] it was not until 1938 that Hauser[46] reported a small series and so popularized the procedure. The tibial tuberosity with the patellar tendon was detached, transferred medially and fixed in position with a screw. Smillie[72] modified the technique and used an ingenious method of fixation of the tibial fragment in which the bony fragment was locked beneath the cortical bone of the tibia (Figure 16). The short-term results have been good, but longer follow-up has shown that patellofemoral osteoarthritis frequently follows this procedure.[55,73,74] There is no doubt that downward transposition of the tibial tuberosity produces tightness of the patellar tendon and increased patellofemoral osteoarthritis; Smillie's modification produces a similar effect. Hughston[13] advised that the Hauser operation produces too much displacement medially, distally and posteriorly in comparison to the original anterior insertion of the tibial ridge. Fulkerson and Hungerford[1] stated emphatically that posterior placement of the tibial tubercle has no place in the management of the patella with incipient or apparent patellar arthrosis.

Tachdjian[10] stated that when there is patella alta with increased Q angle, the proximal tibial tubercle is transferred medially and distally to realign the quadriceps pull. However, the hazards of the procedure are stressed, especially in children and adolescents with open physes and apophyses because such a procedure will lead to growth arrest of the anterior portion of the proximal tibial epiphysis, resulting in a genu recurvatum. Another hazard is the distal migration of the patella with the tibial tubercle, causing patellofemoral incongruity and early degenerative arthritis. Add to that the fact that medial transfer of the tibial tubercle will often produce excessive lateral rotation of the tibia. A very serious complication of this procedure is the development of anterior compartment syndrome. Tachdjian[10] quoted Wall (1979) who reviewed a series of 11 patients who had the Hauser operation, and reported two above-knee amputations secondary to muscle necrosis.

Barbari et al.[75] reviewed the results of the Hauser operation performed in 34 women and 20 men, median age 18 years (average 3–55 years). At the average time of 8 years follow-up (range 3–32 years) after the operation, 57 knees had normal or almost normal patellar stability, but only 26 knees were free from pain. Only 16 knees had normal patellar stability and were without pain. Patellar arthrosis had developed in 16 knees and femorotibial arthrosis in 23 knees. Eleven patients operated on before the age of 15 years showed varying grades of axial deformity of the proximal tibia. Some of the complications of the Hauser procedure included one deep infection with septic arthritis and the final outcome was an above-knee amputation 6 years after the primary procedure. Peroneal nerve palsy developed in three cases, with full recovery in only one case. Two patients with Down's syndrome were not improved by the procedure. These authors quoted Dugdale and Renshaw,[76] mentioning that patellar instability, although frequent in this group, is rarely disabling and does not require surgical correction in most cases. They concluded that the use of Hauser's operation is still associated with a relatively high complication rate and should be limited to severe cases of patellar instability.

Noll et al.[77] described a procedure for distal realignment of the extensor mechanism based on the principles of Hauser and Maquet. The technique includes a lateral retinacular release approximately 3 cm above the upper pole of the patella. Moving then to the tibial tubercle, a bone block 3 cm long, 1.5 cm wide and 1.25 cm deep is prepared. A new bed is then made medial to the site of origin of the bone block. The proximal end of the new bed is flush with cortex and becomes deeper more distally, so that when the bone block is placed on it, it sits completely proud proximally. The bone block is fixed in its new position using a 6.5-mm cancellous AO screw. Their indications for surgery were patellofemoral pain due to malalignment of the extensor mechanism which is unresponsive to conservative treatment, recurrent subluxation or dislocation of the patella, patients who had had a previous patellectomy with subsequent lateral subluxation of the patellar tendon associated with pain, and finally as a prerequisite for this procedure the Q angle should be 20° or more.

Using their own technique modified from the Hauser and Maquet operations, they corrected malalignment of the quadriceps mechanism in 17 knees (16 patients). The average age of the patients was 29 years. The follow-up period was 1–4 years. Eighty-five per cent of the patients had excellent to good results. The only complication was a stress fracture which developed in one of the bone blocks.

Fielding et al.[78] in a long-term follow-up study, reported on tibial tubercle transfer. They recommended that in patients with patella alta the tibial tubercle should be transplanted medially ¾ inch and distally ½ inch. They reviewed 214 patients with an average postoperative follow-up of 3.5 years (range 6 months to 21 years). The results were as follows:

Good or excellent results (normal extremities with minimal or no symptoms), 157 patients.
Fair results (mild to moderate pain and some residual patellar instability, not preventing normal activity), 29 patients.
Failures, 28 patients.

Retrospective analysis by the same authors of 23 children with 37 transfers performed at the age of 11 years or younger, all followed until they were adults (at an average of 6 years) showed that:

1. The epiphyseal extension in the tibial tubercle was damaged because it was included in the transferred tibial tubercle.
2. The tubercle failed to develop in the transplanted position and the attachment of the patella migrated up the tibia as the tibia increased in length.
3. No tendon was lengthened and no patella was pulled down.
4. Over the years the patella conformed to the shape of the underlying femur.
5. There were two instances of recurvatum due to damage to the proximal tibial epiphysis.

Trillat et al.[24] used a technique with a cancellous screw to fix the tibial tuberosity, which is tilted and swung over to the medial side. Medialization of the extensor apparatus may, however, sometimes be inadequate with this method.[2] The Trillat procedure forms the basis of realigning a chronically dislocating extensor mechanism, particularly when the lateral trochlea is deficient.[1]

Combined procedures

Any single procedure will not be appropriate for all types of recurrent patellar dislocation and combinations of different methods are frequently necessary. Careful assessment of the cause and type of malalignment will indicate the best operation for any particular patient. Examination under anaesthesia will allow assessment of the degree of capsular laxity. Arthroscopy is important to exclude associated meniscal tears and it is also helpful in evaluating the state of the patellar and femoral articular surfaces.

Chrisman et al.[33] quoted Smith, in reviewing the results of the various operations for recurrent lateral dislocations of the patella at the Campbell clinic, mentioning that there were essentially three options for operative treatment: realignment of the patellar tendon, release of the lateral capsule and reefing or advancement of the medial expansion. One or two of these procedures, done by whatever technique, might be adequate for a mild case, but all three were necessary for the severe cases of dislocation. Chrisman et al. recommend all three procedures in every instance to obtain the best possible result.[33]

Merchant prefers Insall's proximal realignment if the vastus medialis is deficient proximally.[56] Abraham et al. reported on Insall's proximal realignment for disorders of the patella.[79] In Insall's procedure, the lateral retinacular incision detaches the vastus lateralis insertion from the quadriceps tendon. The medial retinacular tissue is cut along the medial border of the tendon. A tube is then formed by suturing the vastus medialis muscle complex to the lateral border of the quadriceps mechanism. Insall et al.[15] considers failure to release the vastus lateralis from the quadriceps tendon as a common fault. Abraham et al. believe that this very step of release of the vastus lateralis from the quadriceps body would significantly weaken the quadriceps complex.[79]

For distal realignment, Merchant believes that surgery must not involve bone until after maturity, to avoid epiphyseal damage;[56] therefore, he advises the Roux–Goldthwait or other soft-tissue procedures. After maturity, he believes that the tibial tubercle should never be moved posteriorly while it is being moved medially; thus the Elmslie–Trillat procedure is advised.[1,56] The Elmslie–Trillat procedure includes a lateral retinacular release and a medial shift of the tibial tubercle with screw fixation.

Wootton et al.[80] reviewed 68 knees retrospectively that were treated by proximal and distal reconstruction of the extensor mechanism as described by Trillat[24] for patellofemoral malalignment. The diagnoses included 45 knees with recurrent patellar

dislocation, 18 knees with recurrent subluxation (of these, 2 knees had congenital subluxation occurring in flexion) and there was one case of nail–patella syndrome. The follow-up was for an average of 56 months following the surgical procedure. The results were excellent in 48 knees (71%), good in 12 (17%) and poor in 8 (12%). In no patient had there been any further episodes of dislocation. Their conclusion was that the Trillat procedure is a straightforward procedure producing consistent correction of the patellofemoral instability with low morbidity. Their complications, however, included:

Superficial wound infection:	1 patient.
Removal of a painful staple:	1 patient.
Wound haematoma:	2 patients.
Manipulation under anaesthesia:	8 patients.
Partial rupture of the patellar tendon 2 years post-operatively:	1 patient.

Hughston[13] commented on proximal reconstructions in general, stating that the patellofemoral joint has a dynamic and not a static stability; therefore, various fascial reconstruction are doomed to failure. Accordingly, he releases the lateral retinaculum, the vastus lateralis, and the vastus medialis. They are then rearranged until a centralized pull on the patella is achieved, as evidenced by smooth tracking and good stability during flexion and extension.

Hughston and Walsh[31] reviewed 364 knees (304 patients) with symptomatic, disabling patellar subluxation between the years 1950 and 1975 that had proximal and distal reconstruction of the extensor mechanism for patellar subluxation. Proximal extensor reconstruction was always done, as was arthrotomy and correction of intra-articular pathology. Distal reconstruction, i.e. patellar tendon transplantation, was undertaken in the skeletally mature patients with Q angles greater than 10°. Chondrectomy was performed in cases of associated chondromalacia patellae.

Over 90% of the athletes had returned to what they considered normal performance. Using a critical method of strict grading in which only a perfectly normal knee was considered an excellent result, they reported the following subjective results: excellent, 22%; good, 49%; fair, 22%; poor, 7%. Objective results were as follows: excellent, 23%; good, 43%; fair, 26%; poor, 8%.

Cerullo et al.[81] reviewed 116 patients who underwent extensor mechanism reconstruction for extensor mechanism malalignment associated with a dislocating, subluxing, or painful patella. Ninety-four returned at follow-up 3–11 years after surgery. All patients were treated conservatively for 6–9 months before the decision on surgical treatment. The surgical procedures included (1) proximal and distal reconstruction according to the procedures of Hughston[82] and Trillat et al.[24] in 70% of the cases;

(2) only proximal reconstruction according to Hughston in 30% of cases.

Distal reconstruction with a medial transposition of the anterior tibial tubercle was performed when the knee had an increased Q angle in individuals with closed growth plates. In three patients with open growth plates, distal reconstruction was performed using Goldthwait's technique. The treatment results were evaluated subjectively (the patients rated themselves on the basis of swelling, pain, symptoms of instability, and limitation of activity) and objectively (according to range of motion, pain, effusion, quadriceps atrophy, and passive patellar mobility). The results were as follows: (a) Dislocating patellae: all the patients had excellent or good subjective and objective results. (b) Subluxing patellae: 81% of the patients had excellent or good subjective results and 97.6% had excellent or good objective results. (c) Stable or mildly unstable patellae: only 50% of the patients had satisfactory (excellent or good) subjective results and 59% had satisfactory objective results.

On comparing the results of the combined proximal and distal realignment to that of proximal realignment alone they advise that:

1. Reconstruction undertaken proximally only retains its therapeutic validity when the Q angle does not exceed 15° in females or 12° in males.
2. There was no substantial difference between the combined reconstruction procedure of the extensor mechanism compared to that of proximal realignment procedures when performed for subluxating patellae.
3. In the patients with a stable or mildly unstable patella, proximal reconstruction was the more efficacious method. In dealing with these patients who normally complain of anterior knee pain, it is better to employ conservative treatment since the pathological basis of the clinical syndrome is still obscure.

Dandy and Griffiths[19] discussed the merits of lateral release as a simple, effective non-traumatic procedure. They described the complications that can occur with the more elaborate operations such as proximal and distal realignments: osteoarthritis of the patellofemoral joint; loss of flexion; tenderness over staple or screw fixation; detachment of the patellar tendon; genu recurvatum after distal realignment before closure of the upper tibial physis.

Malalignments are best demonstrated dynamically, i.e. with the patient flexing and extending his or her knees. Templeman and McBeath[62] advise on the importance of assessing patellar tracking dynamically in the operating theatre by performing the surgery under local anaesthesia supplemented by intravenous sedation. Fulkerson and Hungerford[1] described femoral nerve stimulation by a percutaneous electrode to help the surgeon to assess patellar tracking under anaesthesia.

Habitual dislocation

This occurs with the knee in either flexion or extension. The patella dislocates at every flexion and extension movement.[2] We have seen an increasing number of patients with habitual dislocation, particularly in extension, and it seems the more one looks for this condition the more it is found. McKeever[83] stated that dislocation in extension did not occur despite its being described by Mayer[84] and Daunegger[85] as the most usual form. Habitual dislocation in extension has, therefore, been observed for a very long time.

Factors which allow the habitual dislocation to occur are:

1. Rotation of the knee at full extension produces external rotation of the tibia in a final screw-home mechanism.
2. Genu recurvatum unloads the patellofemoral joint and allows more patellar laxity.
3. Patella alta is common in this condition so that the patella lies above the femoral condylar sulcus.
4. Dysplasias of the femoral condyles and the patella may be present.

Bergman and Williams[4] stated that habitual dislocation of the patella in flexion implies that dislocation occurs every time the knee is flexed. The habitual displacement which is lateral is painless in marked contrast to recurrent dislocation which occurs as isolated episodes, often in response to trauma. They reported on 43 knees (35 patients) with habitual dislocation of the patella in flexion. The possible aetiological factors were:

1. A history of multiple intramuscular injections in the neonatal period in 8 patients (the most common injections were those of antibiotics such as chloramphenicol, penicillin, and streptomycin).
2. A family history of dislocation in 10 patients. A number of untreated affected parents were also examined and they all had significant disability consisting of a flexion deformity of the knee and marked patellofemoral arthritis. One patient had quadriceps fibrosis of the opposite side without patellar dislocation.
3. Associated congenital anomalies existed in 7 patients, including bilateral congenital talipes equinovarus, idiopathic infantile scoliosis, congenital scoliosis, bilateral absent fibula and kyphotic tibia, discoid lateral meniscus, Down's syndrome, hypoplastic thumb, undescended testicles, and Hirschsprung disease.

Sharma[22] commented upon habitual dislocation of the patella and stated that it may be regarded as being the result of fibrosis following injections and that this is the commonest cause in India. The author feels that habitual, recurrent and congenital dislocation are expressions of varying grades of the same aetiology, all of them being due to a developmental defect.

Fulkerson and Hungerford[1] prefer to use the term 'acquired permanent dislocation' for what is generally called habitual dislocation. They mention that progressive quadriceps fibrosis has been implicated. Some believe that this fibrosis is of congenital dysplastic origin similar to club foot, arthrogryposis, or congenital torticollis. However, in most cases one can obtain a history of multiple intramuscular injections. Whatever the origin, only the vastus lateralis, intermedius, and rarely the rectus femoris have been reported to be involved. The tethering then inevitably produces a lateral vector. Where the medial tissues hold, a progressive limitation of flexion occurs. When the medial soft-tissue structure gives way, permanent dislocation of the patella results.

Gao et al.[6] in discussing the aetiology of congenital dislocation of the patella and habitual dislocation of the patella gave the following facts: the underlying pathology in both habitual and congenital patellar dislocations is contracture of the quadriceps mechanism, which was more severe in congenital dislocation of the patella. The short quadriceps tendon is permanently dislocated laterally, thus exerting a lateral pull on the tibia which results in a valgus and external rotation deformity. As the quadriceps tendon is behind the axis of the knee, it also causes the flexion deformity of the knee. In habitual patellar dislocation the same pathology is noted, but the extent of contracture is less and the clinical manifestation is delayed. In both congenital patellar dislocation and habitual patellar dislocation, due to the contracture of the extensor mechanism, there is loss of excursion of the quadriceps tendon, and the extensor mechanism has to slip over the lateral femoral condyle for full knee flexion to be achieved.

Bergman and Williams[4] described quadricepsplasty as the operative treatment in habitual dislocation of the patella. They operated on 43 knees. The average age at presentation was 9 years (range 3–15 years). In principle, the tight lateral bands are released from the patella and the incision is continued proximally, lateral to the rectus femoris tendon, thus fully releasing vastus lateralis. Vastus intermedius is inspected and divided if tight. When necessary, rectus femoris is lengthened by extending the medial release proximally, medial to the rectus tendon and dividing rectus femoris at its musculotendinous junction. The knee is then flexed, lengthening the rectus femoris. Vastus medialis and vastus lateralis are sutured to each other and to the rectus femoris tendon in its lengthened position. If lateral dislocation is still not controlled, a medial advancement of vastus medialis, medial plication and patellar tendon transfer using soft-tissue technique is added.

Forty-three patients were operated upon. The details were:

Division of the lateral bands plus lengthening of the rectus femoris, 16% of cases.
Medial plication, 16%.
Advancement of the vastus medialis, 44%.
Patellar tendon transfer, 14%.
Sartorius transfer, 5%.

The operative findings were:

Vastus lateralis bands, 72%.
Abnormal iliotibial band attachment to the patella, 58%.
Rectus femoris contractures, 42%.
Vastus intermedius contractures, 16%.
Tight vastus medialis in one knee.

The results were:

Normal function, 79%.
A history of occasional giving way, 14%.
Patellofemoral pain, 7%.

Gao et al.[6] reported that, whilst complete release and realignment of the extensor mechanism is applicable in most cases of congenital dislocation of the patella, the treatment of habitual dislocation must be individualized.

Persistent or permanent dislocation of the patella

The patella remains dislocated through the whole range of knee movement in both flexion and extension.[2] Fulkerson and Hungerford[1] use the term permanent dislocation to mean that dislocation in which the patella is no longer in contact with the articular cartilage of the distal femur throughout the full range of flexion. On extension the patella may track towards or nearly to the midline but returns to the lateral surface of the lateral femoral condyle on flexion. Jackson noted that the patella is usually hypoplastic and the trochlear groove absent.[5] The condyles are dysmorphic and on occasions the medial condyle is completely obscured by an enlarged and thickened medial plica. The menisci may be absent or discoid. The same author has seen a case of permanent patellar dislocation associated with a fixed flexion deformity of the knee and congenital absence of the anterior cruciate ligament.[5] Two forms of permanent dislocation are described: congenital and acquired.

Congenital permanent dislocation

This is a rare condition described by Green and Waugh.[86] They pointed out that the diagnosis is usually made rather late.[2] A flexion contracture of the knee is present from birth and this persists. Fulkerson and Hungerford[1] believe that the cause of this dislocation may be an anomalous insertion of fibrous tissue into the lateral patella, an abnormal band of fascia lata to the patella, or an abnormal fibrous band appearing to arise from vastus lateralis. Gao et al.[6] stated that:

> Several aetiologies for congenital dislocation of the patella have been proposed such as intrauterine trauma, increase in internal rotation of the distal femur, and failure of internal rotation of the myotome, which contains the quadriceps femoris and the patella. The pathogenesis in these cases is conjectural, but it may be similar to that of congenital torticollis. The quadriceps muscles become fibrotic and contracted very early in intrauterine life or in the neonatal period due either to trauma or to an infarct. The muscles, then, are not in a position to rotate with the femur or to keep pace with the growth of the bones. The flexion deformity of the knee and the valgus and external rotation deformity of the leg are secondary to the contracture of the quadriceps. There may also be a hereditary predisposition.

The same authors believe that the permanent pull of the extensor mechanism in its abnormal position results in a valgus and external rotation deformity of the tibia.

Acquired permanent dislocation

Hněvkovský[87] described a condition of progressive quadriceps fibrosis in a small series. His cases showed progressive contracture of the quadriceps leading to persistent dislocation of the patella. Neonatal injections of antibiotics into the lateral thigh region and vastus lateralis muscle in particular may produce contractures of the lateral quadriceps. The injections are usually given for respiratory infections in the neonatal period and progressive contracture of the vastus lateralis ensues.[88]

The senior author reviewed 12 children who presented with persistent patellar dislocations. The following causes were suggested:

Nail–patella syndrome, 3 patients.
Neonatal injections into the thigh which produced a vastus lateralis contracture, 3 patients.
Gross congenital ligamentous laxity, 2 patients.
Significant trauma, 1 patient.
Congenital dislocation of the patella, 1 patient.

Treatment of persistent dislocation

The length of the extensor apparatus may be very short when the patella has been persistently dis-located. The femoral condylar sulcus may also be flat, or even convex, which may make successful repositioning of the patella impossible. Gao et al.[6] remarked that the same pathology is noted in congenital dislocation of the patella as in habitual dislocation, but in the latter the extent of contracture is less and the clinical manifestation is delayed. They reviewed 35 patients with congenital dislocation of the patella and habitual dislocations. Their intra-operative findings to varying degrees were:

1. Contracture and fibrosis of the quadriceps, mainly the vastus lateralis.
2. Contracture of the iliotibial band, preventing reduction of the dislocated patella.
3. Contracture of the lateral capsule and laxity of the medial capsule.
4. Loose and atrophic vastus medialis.
5. More lateral insertion of the patellar tendon.
6. External rotation of the tibia and a valgus deformity of the knee.
7. Smaller patella with decreased patellar ridge, and a flat articular surface of the femur with a shallow intercondylar groove.

The lateral release must be extensive and all abnormal bands anchoring the patella laterally are divided. It is usually necessary to cut across the fibrotic lower end of the vastus lateralis as far as the border of the vastus intermedius. This type of extensive release will usually allow the patella to be centralized.[2] If the knee will still not flex owing to shortening of the remaining quadriceps muscle and tendon, the adhesions between the vastus lateralis, the vastus intermedius and the rectus femoris are freed. If flexion is still limited with the patella centrally placed, then a Z or V–Y lengthening of the rectus femoris is done. Gao et al.[6] performed similar steps; however, for the restricted flexion after patellar centralization, they would release the vastus intermedius. A Roux–Goldthwait type half-patellar tendon transfer is also recommended once the patella is centralized.[2,6]

References

1. **Fulkerson JP, Hungerford DS**, *Disorders of the patellofemoral joint*, 2nd edn (Baltimore: Williams and Wilkins, 1990) 124–169.
2. **Aichroth PM**, Dislocation of the patella, *Surgery of the knee joint*, ed Jackson JP, Waugh W (London: Chapman and Hall, 1984) 192–209.
3. **Hughston JC, Deese M**, Medial subluxation of the patella as a complication of lateral retinacular release, *Am J Sports Med* (1988) 16(4): 383–388.
4. **Bergman NR, Williams PF**, Habitual dislocation of the patella in flexion, *J Bone Joint Surg (Br)* (1988) 70: 415–419.
5. **Jackson AM**, The knee and leg. *Orthopaedics in infancy and childhood* 2nd edn, ed Lloyd Roberts GC, Fixen J (London: Butterworth Heinemann, 1990) 1761–1778.

6. Gao G-X, Lee EH, Bose K, Surgical management of congenital and habitual dislocation of the patella, *J Pediatr Orthop* (1990) 10(2): 255–260.

7. Murakami Y, Intra-articular dislocation of the patella: A case report, *Clin Orthop* (1982) 171: 137–139.

8. Fridén T, A case of superior dislocation of the patella, *Acta Orthop Scand* (1987) 58: 429–430.

9. Hanspal RS, Superior dislocation of the patella, *Injury* (1985) 16: 487–488.

10. Tachdjian MO, *Pediatric orthopedics*, vol 2, 2nd edn (Philadelphia: W.B. Saunders, 1990) 1551–1582.

11. Hallisey MJ, Doherty N, Bennett WF et al. Anatomy of the junction of the vastus lateralis tendon and the patella, *J Bone Joint Surg (Am)* (1987) 69: 545–549.

12. Casscells SW, The arthroscope in the diagnosis of disorders of the patellofemoral joint, *Clin Orthop* (1979) 144: 45–50.

13. Hughston JC, Patellar subluxation, *Clin Sports Med* (1989) 8(2): 153–161.

14. Chen SC, Ramanathan EBS, The treatment of patellar instability by lateral release, *J Bone Joint Surg (Br)* (1984) 66: 344–348.

15. Insall JN, Disorders of the patella, *Surgery of the knee*, ed Insall JN (New York: Churchill Livingstone, 1984) 195.

16. Fondren FB, Goldner JL, Bassett FH III, Recurrent dislocation of the patella treated by the modified Roux–Goldthwait procedure, *J Bone Joint Surg (Am)* (1985) 67: 993–1005.

17. Runow A, The dislocating patella: Etiology and prognosis in relation to generalized joint laxity and anatomy of the patellar articulation, *Acta Orthop Scand* (1983), suppl 201: 1–53.

18. Cash JD, Hughston JC, Treatment of acute patellar dislocation, *Am J Sports Med* (1988) 16(3): 244–249.

19. Dandy DJ, Griffiths D, Lateral release for recurrent dislocation of the patella, *J Bone Joint Surg (Br)* (1989) 71: 121–125.

20. Floyd A, Phillips P, Khan MRH et al., Recurrent dislocation of the patella: Histochemical and electromyographic evidence of primary muscle pathology, *J Bone Joint Surg (Br)* (1987) 69: 790–793.

21. Kujala UM, Österman K, Kormano M, et al., Patellofemoral relationships in recurrent patellar dislocation, *J Bone Joint Surg (Br)* (1989) 71: 788–792.

22. Sharma SV, Habitual dislocation of the patella, *Int Orthop* (1990) 14(1): 21–23.

23. Bizou H, Contribution à l'étude des desequilibres de l'appareil extenseur du genou dans le plan frontal (Thesis, Toulouse, 1966).

24. Trillat A, Dejour H, Couette A, Diagnostic et traitement des subluxations recidivantes de la rotule, *Rev Chir Orthop* (1964) 50: 813–824.

25. Brattström H, Shape of the intercondylar groove normally and in recurrent dislocation of patella, *Acta Orthop Scand* (1964), suppl. 68: 134–148.

26. Heywood AWB, Recurrent dislocation of the patella, *J Bone Joint Surg (Br)* (1961) 43: 508–517.

27. Vainionpää S, Laasonen E, Pätiälä H et al., Acute dislocation of the patella: Clinical, radiographic and operative findings in 64 consecutive cases, *Acta Orthop Scand* (1986) 57: 331–333.

28. Wiberg G, Roentgenographic and anatomic studies on the femoropatellar joint: with special reference to chondromalacia patellae, *Acta Orthop Scand* (1941) 12: 319–410.

29. Ficat P, *Pathologie femoro-patellaire* (Paris: Masson, 1970).

30. Micheli LJ, Slater JA, Woods E et al., Patella alta and the adolescent growth spurt, *Clin Orthop* (1986) 213: 159–162.

31. Hughston JC, Walsh WM, Proximal and distal reconstruction of the extensor mechanism for patellar subluxation, *Clin Orthop* (1979) 144: 36–42.

32. Larsen E, Lauridsen F, Conservative treatment of patellar dislocations. Influence of evident factors on the tendency to redislocation and the therapeutic result, *Clin Orthop* (1982) 171: 131–136.

33. Chrisman OD, Snook GA, Wilson TC, A long-term prospective study of the Hauser and Roux–Goldthwait procedures for recurrent patellar dislocation, *Clin Orthop* (1979) 144: 27–30.

34. Scuderi G, Cuomo F, Scott WN, Lateral release and proximal realignment for patellar subluxation and dislocation, *J Bone Joint Surg (Am)* (1988) 70: 856–861.

35. Fairbank HAT, Internal derangement of the knee in children, *Proc R Soc Med* (1937) 3: 11.

36. Apley AG, The diagnosis of meniscus injuries, *J Bone Joint Surg (Am)* (1947) 29: 78–84.

37. Blumensaat C, Die Lageabweichungen und Verrenkungen der Kniescheibe, *Ergeb Chir Orthop* (1938) 31: 149–223.

38. Blackburne JS, Peel TE, A new method of measuring patellar height, *J Bone Joint Surg (Br)* (1977) 59: 241–242.

39. Laurin CA, Dussault R, Levesque HP, The tangential x-ray investigation of the patellofemoral joint: X-ray technique, diagnostic criteria and their interpretation, *Clin Orthop* (1979) 144: 16–26.

40. Merchant AC, Mercer RL, Jacobsen RH et al., Roentgenographic analysis of patellofemoral congruence, *J Bone Joint Surg (Am)* (1974) 56: 1391–1396.

41. Insall J, Salvati E, Patella position in the normal knee joint, *Radiology* (1971) 101: 101–104.

42. Inoue M, Shino K, Hirose H et al., Subluxation of the patella: Computed tomography analysis of patellofemoral congruence, *J Bone Joint Surg (Am)* (1988) 70: 1331–1337.

43. Malghem J, Maldague B, Subluxation of the patella: Computed tomography analysis of patellofemoral congruence (letter: comment), *J Bone Joint Surg (Am)* (1989) 71: 1575–1576.

44. Fulkerson JP, Schutzer SF, Ramsby GR et al., Computerized tomography of the patellofemoral joint before and after lateral release or realignment, *Arthroscopy* (1987) 3: 19–24.

45. Houkom SS, Recurrent dislocation of patella, *Arch Surg (Chicago)* (1942) 44: 1026.

46. Hauser EDW, Total tendon transplant for slipping patella, *Surg Gynaecol Obstet* (1938) 66: 199–214.

47. Smillie IS, *Injuries of the knee joint* (London: E & S Livingstone, 1946).

48. Albee FH, *Orthopedic and reconstructive surgery* (Philadelphia: W.B. Saunders, 1919).

49. Maquet P, Advancement of the tibial tuberosity, *Clin Orthop* (1976) 115: 225.

50. West FE, Soto-Hall R, Recurrent dislocation of the patella in the adult, *J Bone Joint Surg (Am)* (1958) 40: 386–394.

51. Sojbjerg JO, Lauritzen J, Hvid I et al., Arthroscopic determination of patellofemoral malalignment. *Clin Orthop* (1987) 215: 243–247.

52. Henry JH, Goletz TH, Williamson B, Lateral retinacular release in patellofemoral subluxation: Indications, results, and comparison to open patellofemoral reconstruction, *Am J Sports Med* (1986) 14(2): 121–129.

53. Bigos SJ, McBride GG, The isolated lateral retinacular release in the treatment of patellofemoral disorders, *Clin Orthop* (1984) 186: 75–80.

54. Hughston JC, Subluxation of the patella, *J Bone Joint Surg (Am)* (1968) 50: 1003–1026.

55. Crosby EB, Insall J, Recurrent dislocation of the patella. Relation of treatment to osteoarthritis, *J Bone Joint Surg (Am)* (1976) 58: 9–13.

56. Merchant AC, Patellofemoral disorders, *Operative orthopaedics*, vol 3, ed Chapman MW (Philadelphia: JB Lippincott, 1988) 1699–1707.

57. Campbell WC, Arthroplasty of the knee: Report on cases, *Am J Orthop Surg* (1921) 14: 430.

58. Freeman III BL, Recurrent dislocations, *Campbell's operative orthopaedics*, 7th edn, ed Crenshaw AH (St Louis: CV Mosby, 1987) 2173–2184.

59. Goldthwait JE, Slipping or recurrent dislocation of the patella: with the report of eleven cases, *Boston Med Surg J* (1904) 150: 169–174.

60. Roux C, Luxation habituelle de la rotule: Traitement opératoire. *Rev Chir Paris* (1888) 8: 682–689.

61. **Bowker JH, Thompson EB,** Surgical treatment of recurrent dislocation of the patella, *J Bone Joint Surg (Am)* (1964) **46:** 1451–1461.

62. **Templeman D, McBeath A,** Iatrogenic patellar malalignment following the Roux–Goldthwait procedure, corrected by dynamic intraoperative realignment, *J Bone Joint Surg (Am)* (1986) **68:** 1096–1098.

63. **Galeazzi R,** Nuove applicazione del trapianto muscolare e tendino (XII Congresso della Società Italiana de Ortopedia), *Arch Ortop* (1922) 38.

64. **Baker RH, Carroll N, Dewar FP et al.,** The semitendinosus tenodesis for recurrent dislocation of the patella, *J Bone Joint Surg (Br)* (1972) **54:** 103–109.

65. **Lange M,** *Orthopädisch Chirurgische* (Munich: JB Bergmann, 1951).

66. **McCarroll HR, Schwartzmann JR,** Lateral dislocation of the patella, *J Bone Joint Surg* (1945) **27:** 446–452.

67. **Lexer E,** *Wiederherstellung chirurgie,* 2nd edn, Vol II (Leipzig: Ambrosias Barth, 1931) 822.

68. **Baksi DP,** Restoration of dynamic stability of the patella by pes anserinus transposition, *J Bone Joint Surg (Br)* (1981) **63:** 399–403.

69. **Hall JE, Micheli LJ, McManama GB,** Semitendinosus tenodesis for recurrent subluxation or dislocation of the patella, *Clin Orthop* (1979) **144:** 31–35.

70. **Krogius A,** Zur operativen Behandlung der habituellen luxation der Kniescheibe, *Zentralbl Chir* (1904) **31:** 254.

71. **Henrik Bauer FC, Wredmark T, Isberg B,** Krogius tenoplasty for recurrent dislocation of the patella, *Acta Orthop Scand* (1984) **55:** 267–269.

72. **Smillie IS,** *Diseases of the knee joint* (Edinburgh: Churchill Livingstone, 1974).

73. **Loff P, Friedebold G,** Die habituelle patellar luxation als pararthrotische deformit, *Ergeb Chir* (1969) **52:** 60.

74. **Macnab I,** Recurrent dislocation of the patella, *J Bone Joint Surg (Am)* (1952) **34:** 957–967.

75. **Barbari S, Raugstad TS, Lichtenberg N et al.,** The Hauser operation for patellar dislocation, *Acta Orthop Scand* (1990) **61**(1): 32–35.

76. **Dugdale TW, Renshaw TS,** Instability of the patellofemoral joint in Down syndrome, *J Bone Joint Surg (Am)* (1986) **68:** 405–413.

77. **Noll BJ, Ben-Itzhak I, Rossouw P,** Modified technique for tibial tubercle elevation with realignment for patellofemoral pain: A preliminary report, *Clin Orthop* (1988) **234:** 178–182.

78. **Fielding JW, Liebler WA, Krishne Urs ND et al.,** Tibial tubercle transfer, *Clin Orthop* (1979) **144:** 43–44.

79. **Abraham E, Washington E, Huang TL,** Insall proximal realignment for disorders of the patella, *Clin Orthop* (1988) **248:** 61–65.

80. **Wootton JR, Cross MJ, Wood DG,** Patellofemoral malalignment: a report of 68 cases treated by proximal and distal patellofemoral reconstruction, *Injury* (1990) **21:** 169–173.

81. **Cerullo G, Puddu G, Conteduca F et al.,** Evaluation of the results of extensor mechanism reconstruction, *Am J Sports Med* (1988) **16**(2): 93–96.

82. **Hughston JC,** Reconstruction of the extensor mechanism for subluxating patella, *J Sports Med* (1972) **1:** 6–13.

83. **McKeever DC,** Recurrent dislocation of the patella, *Clin Orthop* (1954) **3:** 55–60.

84. **Mayer HN,** Congenital absence or delayed development of the patella, *Lancet* (1897) **2:** 1384–1385.

85. **Daunegger C,** Versuche und Stucken über die Luxation des Patellae (Diss. Zürich, 1880).

86. **Green JP, Waugh W,** Congenital lateral dislocation of the patella. *J Bone Joint Surg (Br)* (1968) **50:** 285–289.

87. **Hněvkovský O,** Progressive fibrosis of the vastus intermedius muscle in children, *J Bone Joint Surg (Br)* (1961) **43:** 318–325.

88. **Lloyd-Roberts GC, Thomas TG,** The etiology of quadriceps contracture in children, *J Bone Joint Surg (Br)* (1964) **46:** 498–502.

8.2 Radiologic evaluation of the patellofemoral joint

Alan C. Merchant

The single most important fact to remember concerning radiologic evaluation of the patellofemoral joint is that radiographs only serve as adjuncts to a careful history and physical examination. Certainly, they are very important adjuncts, sometimes even surprising adjuncts, but they must be used in context with all the rest of the clinical data to arrive at a correct diagnosis, appropriate differential diagnosis, and reasonable treatment plan. In many areas of Orthopedics these radiologic techniques are so accurate and helpful that it is tempting to 'cheat' on the histories and physical examinations. Patellofemoral disorders is not one of these areas.

For example, if an axial-view radiograph of the patellofemoral joint depicts a chronically subluxed patella, that finding only supplies a possible diagnosis. A careful history will detect the presence or absence of episodic collapse, the presence of which would indicate a recurrent dislocation of the patella. Furthermore, the radiograph will not show the cause or causes of the chronic patellar subluxation: a tight lateral retinaculum, a deficient vastus medialis obliquus, an increased quadriceps angle, or any combination of the three. Without this information an appropriate treatment plan and reasonably accurate prognosis cannot be developed.

Given these natural limitations of radiologic studies, and assuming that a proper history and physical examination have been done, they do represent the most logical, cost-effective, and productive next step that is available for evaluating the patellofemoral joint.

Ordering proper radiographs of the knee

It is axiomatic that radiographs, and all laboratory and ancillary tests for that matter, should be ordered to produce the highest yield of positive results in order to be most helpful and cost-effective. Because radiographs show a two-dimensional image of a three-dimensional part of the anatomy, a minimum of two views should be ordered. In the knee these are the anterior–posterior (AP) and lateral views. Furthermore, local custom, who is ordering the study, and certainly economics, all play a part in determining what views of the knee are 'routine'.

For instance, in my geographic area, if a private primary physician orders 'X-ray, Right Knee' from the radiologist, three views will be taken as the routine study: AP, lateral, and tunnel. If, however, he works in the largest health maintenance organization (HMO) locally, only AP and lateral views will be taken. All these images will be depicted on 8-in. × 10-in. films. Neither of these approaches strikes me as cost-effective or productive from the patient's point of view. First, I would recommend using the next larger size of film (10-in. × 12-in.) for the AP and lateral exposures. This increase will add very little to the overall cost of the procedure, but will depict more of the femur and tibia, thus reducing the chance of missing a possible nearby osseous lesion that could be the true cause of the patient's symptoms.

Perhaps more important is the fact that both these 'routine' protocols do not address the most common complaint our patients have, namely anterior knee pain and dysfunction.[1-3] Therefore, the yield of positive results will be disproportionately low. The tunnel view is best at depicting loose bodies and osteochondritis dissecans, which are far less frequent than patellofemoral problems. For these reasons the most cost-effective and productive routine protocol for radiographs of the knee is: AP, lateral, and axial (patellofemoral) views.

An orthopedist ordering radiographs after the history and physical examination has the added advantage of being able to be even more selective and precise in the choices of additional views than the family or emergency-room physician. If the orthopedist is examining a teenager with a history of deep aching and locking, a tunnel view would be important to show a loose body or osteochondritis dissecans. If the patient is middle-aged or older, the recumbent AP view should be omitted in favor of a full weight-bearing AP view in which the patient stands with all his or her weight on one leg and the

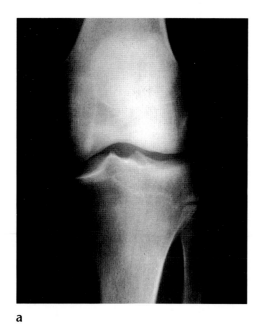
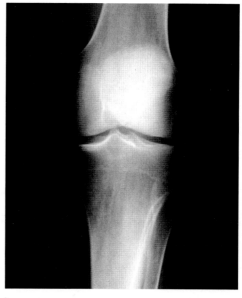

a   b

Figure 1

(a) Anterior–posterior radiograph of a knee, showing lateral displacement of the patella on the distal femur. Note the normal relationship of the proximal tibia and fibula. (b) Anterior–posterior radiograph of a normal knee, showing false lateral displacement of the patella on the femur due to a 10° external rotation positioning error. Note the abnormal relationship of the proximal tibia and fibula.

exposure is made on a long film (14-in. × 17-in.). The extra weight will frequently show earlier and more minor changes of joint-space narrowing and the long film allows assessment of varus or valgus alignment. The 45° flexion posterior–anterior weight-bearing view advocated by Rosenberg et al.[4] can be selected in addition. It is said to be more accurate, more sensitive, and more specific in assessing significant articular cartilage loss in the medial and lateral compartments of the knee than the AP extension weight-bearing radiograph. Varus and valgus stress films can be added when appropriate and indicated.

The anterior–posterior view

The initial assessment of the size, shape, and position of the patella relative to the femur is made on the AP view. Normally the patella lies centered on the femoral condyles with its lower pole at or near the joint-line. Lateral displacement indicates lateral subluxation of the patella. However, external rotation of the entire limb during the exposure could give the false appearance of a lateral displacement. One should assess the proximal tibiofemoral relationship in order to be sure the film is a true AP view (Figure 1). A hypoplastic or bipartite patella can also be seen on this view.

The lateral view

The lateral projection can also provide a clue to lateral subluxation of the patella. If the two femoral condyles are superimposed in a true lateral position, a subluxed patella will sometimes appear thickened front to back. This appearance is caused by the patella rotating on its vertical axis as it subluxes over the lateral femoral condyle. This presents an oblique view of the patella on a lateral view of the knee, making it appear thicker than normal. I call this the 'thick patella sign' (Figure 2).

The lateral radiograph also gives the best clinical assessment of the position of the patella above or below its normal location on the lower end of the femur, patella alta or patella infera. Insall and Salvati[5] have shown that the length of the patellar tendon, measured from the lower pole of the patella to the tibial tubercle, should equal the vertical height of the patella, plus or minus 20%. In some instances, such as a hypoplastic patella or a patella with an elongated lower pole, this measurement can be misleading. Other measurements[6,7] are perhaps more accurate, but from a clinical viewpoint the relative vertical position of the patella assumes importance only when its deviation from normal is large. Therefore, because the Insall and Salvati technique is both quick and sufficiently accurate clinically, it has become the most useful assessment of patella alta and infera.

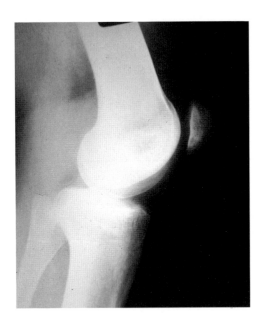

Figure 2

A true lateral radiograph of a knee with lateral patellar subluxation, demonstrating a 'thick patella sign.'

The axial view

There is no doubt that an accurate axial ('skyline') view of the knee gives the most information about the patellofemoral joint. Because anterior knee pain and dysfunction is the most common complaint of patients with knee problems, an axial view must be part of any routine radiographic examination of the knee. Even if the final diagnosis is not related to the patellofemoral joint, the clinician should have a physical and radiographic assessment of the extensor mechanism before starting any treatment program for the knee. It has been estimated that about 20% of the general population have asymptomatic and unrecognized abnormalities of the patellofemoral joints.[8] If these patients are unwittingly given vigorous and forceful resistive knee extension exercises on an isokinetic machine, or isotonically with free weights, either by the doctor or the physical therapist, the patellar articular cartilage can be quickly overloaded and permanently damaged.

Axial patellofemoral radiographic techniques

Proper interpretation of the axial view demands that the radiologist and orthopedist know which technique was used by the technician. Many terms

have been applied to this view such as 'skyline,' 'sunset,' 'sunrise,' 'mountain,' and 'tangential,' but to avoid confusion the most accurate term—axial view—should be used. Many different techniques for taking the axial-view radiograph have been described. Table 1 depicts those most commonly used.

The Settegast technique (Table 1, A) has several disadvantages. Because this exposure is made with the knee acutely flexed, the position is frequently too painful for the patient with a recent injury or a swollen knee. Furthermore, the flexion will reduce patellae that are subluxed with the knee more extended. Finally, it does not demonstrate the trochlea and the patella's relationship to it.

The popular modified-Jaroschy technique (Table 1, B) flexes the knees 60°, but this is still too much and will reduce many otherwise subluxed patellae back into the groove. There is also a distortion of the image caused by the central X-ray beam striking the film plane at a 45° angle. This exaggerates the depth of the sulcus as well as the height of the patella. Therefore, a truly shallow sulcus will appear normal in this view unless the clinician knows what a 'normal' modified-Jaroschy view should look like.

To capture the most information from the axial view, the technician must adhere to several important criteria. The central X-ray beam should be perpendicular to the film plane to avoid image distortion. The knees should be flexed 30–45°. This not only shows the trochlea at a point where most recurrent dislocations occur, but also avoids passive reduction of an otherwise subluxed patella. The X-ray tube should be about 2 m from the knee to minimize the distortion of magnification and parallax. By exposing both knees on one film, comparisons can easily be made. Strapping the legs and knees together will not only prevent external rotation of the limbs, which can simulate a low lateral condyle, but also will allow the patient to relax. Contraction of the quadriceps will reduce a subluxed patella.

We prefer the technique shown in Table 1, D. Because most patellar subluxations will be demonstrated on an axial view taken with the knees flexed 45°, and this degree of flexion makes the exposure simple for the technician, we use the 45° view for the initial exposure. However, there are some mild subluxations that will appear on a 30° flexion view but not on the 45° view (Figure 3). Therefore, assuming that the history and physical examination indicates a patellofemoral problem, I use the following guidelines to save the technician's time and effort. If the patient is thin, a 45° view and a 30° view are ordered at the same time. If the patient is heavy, muscular, or stocky, the 30° view will be more difficult, if not impossible, for the technician to obtain and so the 45° view is ordered first. If it demonstrates the pathology, no further studies are necessary; but if it does not, the patient is returned for the 30° flexion view, which will sometimes be rewarding.

Table 1 Axial patellofemoral radiographic techniques.

	Technique	Comments
	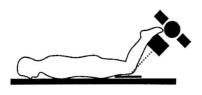	1. Acutely flexed position is too painful for recently injured or swollen knees. 2. Position reduces subluxed patellae, causing false negative images.
A.	Settegast[9]	
	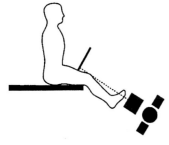	1. X-ray beam not perpendicular to film distorts the image; shallow trochleas appear normal. 2. 60° knee flexion reduces many subluxed patellae, causing false negative images.
B.	Jaroschy[10]	
	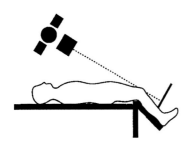	1. Accurate, undistorted image. 2. Knee flexion can be varied. 3. Increased radiation exposure.
C.	Ficat[11]	
		1. Accurate, undistorted image. 2. Knee flexion can be varied. 3. Decreased radiation exposure.
D.	Merchant[12]	
	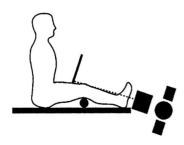	1. Accurate, undistorted image. 2. 20° knee flexion difficult to image. 3. Increased radiation exposure.
E.	Labelle[13]	

From ref. 8 with permission.

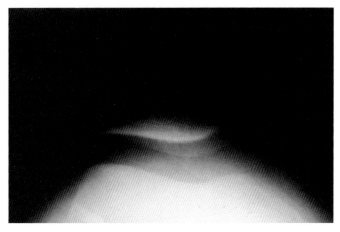
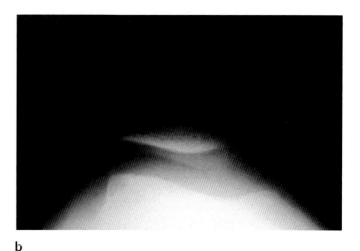

a   b

Figure 3

(a) Axial radiograph of a patellofemoral joint taken at 45° of knee flexion, depicting a congruent relationship. (b) Axial radiograph of the same knee taken at 30° of flexion, showing lateral patellar subluxation.

Obtaining a useful exposure of an axial view at knee flexion angles less than 30° (Table 1, E) has proven so technically difficult and time-consuming that we no longer attempt it.

On occasion, the articular surface of the patella will appear blurred or indistinct on the axial view. This occurs when the X-ray beam is not parallel to the articular surface of the patella. Sometimes the technician can correct the exposure by moving the X-ray tube up or down to make the central X-ray beam parallel to the articular surface of the patella, using the palpable anterior surface as a guide. However, there are patients in whom the patella is positioned so low (patella infera) that the articular surface is nearly parallel with the long axis of the tibia and in whom a perfect axial view of the patellofemoral joint cannot be obtained.

Evaluation of axial patellofemoral radiographs

The interpretation of axial patellofemoral radiographs is usually not difficult. Bipartite patellae and fractures are easily seen. An avulsion fracture from the medial edge of the patella serves as mute evidence of a previous dislocation (Figure 4). The more subtle changes in perpendicular trabecular alignment and sclerotic density in the subchondral bone of the lateral patellar facet can provide radiologic confirmation for a diagnosis of a lateral patellar compression syndrome[14] (Figure 5). A traction spur at the lateral margin of the

patella supports the same diagnosis and indicates hypertrophy and excessive tightness of the lateral retinaculum. Patellofemoral osteoarthritis is easily seen, with its joint-space narrowing, subchondral sclerosis, marginal osteophytes, and almost always lateral subluxation of the patella (Figure 6). In the advanced case of reflex sympathetic dystrophy, unilateral severe osteopenia of the patella is seen. Certainly, any osseous lesions that are common to all joints can be seen as well, such as neoplasms, osteomyelitis, and osteochondritis dissecans.

Assessment of patellofemoral congruence

An accurate axial view will provide the best information with which to evaluate patellofemoral congruence. However, one must be careful when defining this term and assigning clinical significance to it. If the patella is incongruent with the trochlea, it will either tilt or sublux laterally. (Medial subluxation can occur, but I have never seen it without iatrogenic excessive medial transfer of the tibial tubercle.) Tilt and subluxation are different from one another and must be defined. Tilt is rotation of the patella around its longitudinal axis, usually laterally, in relationship to the trochlea. Subluxation starts as a lateral translation of the patella out of the femoral sulcus, but as it rides up and over the convex contour of the lateral femoral condyle, it must tilt laterally as well. Thus it is a combination of lateral translation and tilt, and

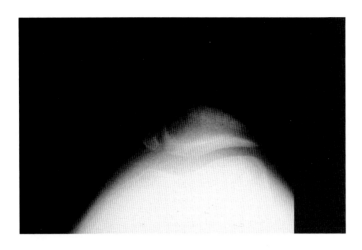

Figure 4

Axial radiograph demonstrating an old avulsion fracture of the medial edge of the patella which is pathognomonic of a prior lateral patellar dislocation.

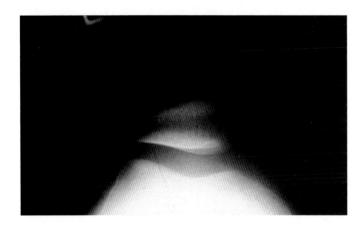

Figure 5

Axial radiograph with perpendicular trabecular pattern and sclerosis of the subchondral bone of the lateral patellar facet. These findings are typical of a lateral patellar compression syndrome.

the amount of tilt will depend upon the shape of the lateral femoral condyle. If the contour is relatively flat or dysplastic, the patellar tilt will be relatively small; if it is more normal, then the degree of tilt will be greater. Tilt can occur without subluxation when a tight lateral retinaculum holds the lateral patella down and the medial side lifts off.

The sulcus angle

There are several measurements of patellofemoral congruence and dysplasia that have proven clinically useful. Brattström,[15] in an elegant radiographic study of the distal end of the femur, demonstrated that the depth of the trochlea had an excellent correlation with dysplasia and recurrent dislocation. He called this the 'sulcus angle' (Table 2, A). His findings indicated that the shallow sulcus found in patellofemoral dysplasias was not due to a decrease in height or size of the lateral and medial condyles, but rather to a relative raising of the sulcus bottom.

His normal values for the sulcus angle, a mean of 138° with a standard deviation of 6°, have been confirmed repeatedly. This measurement correlates well with patellar instabilities: the greater the angle, the greater the dysplasia and the more severe the recurrent or chronic dislocation of the patella (Figure 7).

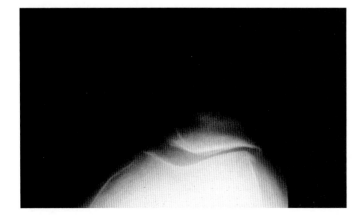

Figure 6

Axial radiograph with chronic subluxation of the patella and secondary patellofemoral osteoarthritis.

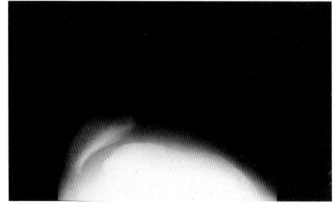

Figure 7

Axial radiograph of the left knee of an 11-year-old girl with severe patellofemoral dysplasia and chronic dislocation of the patella.

Table 2 Radiographic measurements of patellofemoral congruence.

A. SULCUS ANGLE
    The angle is formed by the condyles
    and the sulcus.[15]
    Mean = 138°; SD = 6°.
    Correlates well with instability.

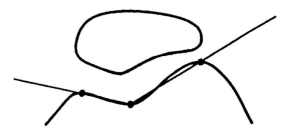

B. CONGRUENCE ANGLE
    A zero reference line bisects the sulcus angle; the
    angular distance of the articular ridge from that
    line is the congruence angle.[12]
    Mean = –6°; SD = 6°.[17]
    Measures subluxation.

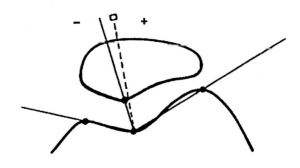

C. LATERAL PATELLOFEMORAL ANGLE
    The angle between the intercondylar line and the
    lateral facet.[16]
    It should open laterally.
    Measures tilt with subluxation.

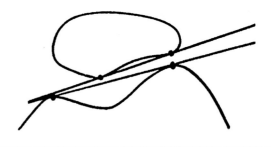

D. PATELLOFEMORAL INDEX
    M = the closest distance between the articular ridge
    and the medial condyle; L = the closest distance
    between the lateral facet and condyle.
    Ratio M/L = 1.6 or less.[16]
    Measures tilt and subluxation.

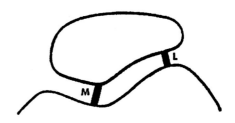

(From Merchant AC, Patellofemoral disorders: biomechanics, diagnosis, and nonoperative treatment, *Operative arthroscopy*, ed McGinty JB (New York: Raven Press, 1991) 261–275. Used with permission.)

The lateral patellofemoral angle

Several measurements of patellofemoral congruence have been described. Laurin et al.[16] developed the lateral patellofemoral angle (Table 2, C). The angle made by the intercondylar line and the lateral patellar facet normally opens laterally. If these lines become parallel or open medially, a diagnosis of chronic subluxation or recurrent dislocation of the patella is suggested. It is a measure of tilt with subluxation.

The patellofemoral index

The patellofemoral index was also described by Laurin and his co-workers[16] (Table 2, D) as an even more sensitive measurement of incongruence or tilt and subluxation. This index compares the closest distance of the lateral facet with that of the medial facet expressed as a ratio. Normally the ratio should be no greater than 1.6.

The congruence angle

In 1974, we defined the congruence angle to measure the degree of patellar subluxation[12] (Table 2, B). It measures the angular distance between the articular ridge of the patella and a reference line that bisects the sulcus angle. The mean congruence angle in our normal control group was –6° with a standard deviation of 11°. Nine years later, Aglietti et al.[17] repeated our work using a different control group, and found a very similar mean of –8°, but their standard deviation was only half as large at 6°. This smaller standard deviation is significant because it makes the range of normal values smaller, so that there will be less overlap between normal and abnormal groups of subjects. This makes the test more clinically useful.

A careful evaluation of the control groups within these two independent studies reveals an important difference. In selecting our 'normal' controls we somewhat naively assumed that anyone who had no history of knee complaints, problems, or injuries could be considered normal. The later group of investigators not only eliminated those subjects who had a history of knee problems but also those with abnormalities of the extensor mechanism on physical examination. Thus I believe their standard deviation to be more accurate than ours.

Interestingly, when their standard deviation of 6° was applied to our original control group, we found that approximately 20% of our asymptomatic 'normals' actually had radiographic evidence of patellofemoral incongruence. This serendipitous finding gives an excellent indication of just how prevalent patellofemoral dysplasia is in the general asymptomatic population. The reason why this group does not have symptoms is not difficult to discover. Symptoms sufficient for the patient to seek help depend upon an inverse relationship between the severity of the anatomic defect and that individual's activity level. Those with mild patellofemoral dysplasia become symptomatic only after strenuous and prolonged use or later in life, while those with severe abnormalities cross the symptomatic threshold at a younger age merely with activities of daily living.

Perhaps the most important concept to understand concerning these radiographic measurements of patellofemoral congruence is that they are not absolute and will not provide a diagnosis or treatment plan by themselves. They must be placed in context with a careful history and a detailed physical examination of the extensor mechanism. Certainly, they can be very helpful in establishing guidelines between normal and abnormal, in assessing the amount of postoperative change, and comparing different forms of treatment in follow-up studies. These radiographic measurements are on a continuously variable scale from normal to abnormal, and their plots will depict the usual bell-shaped curves with some overlap between normal and abnormal. If a particular patient's measurement just exceeds twice the standard deviation, it only indicates that there is a 95% chance that this patient is abnormal. It is just one more clue to the diagnosis and an aid in developing a treatment plan to correct the abnormal pathomechanics involved.

It is interesting to note that of all these radiographic measurements of patellofemoral abnormality, the congruence angle provides the least overlap between known normal and abnormal populations. Dzioba[18] has taken a more basic approach, using no measurements but merely assessing each axial-view radiograph as congruent (normal) or not congruent (abnormal) by its visual appearance. He found that this method provided a very good correlation between congruent radiographic appearance and successful postoperative outcome.

Other patellofemoral imaging techniques

The advent of computed tomography (CT scans) and magnetic resonance imaging (MRI) has provided additional methods for examining the skeleton and its soft-tissue attachments. With specific reference to the extensor mechanism, these techniques can examine the patellofemoral relationships within the last few degrees of extension, from 20° to 0°, which is not possible with the axial radiographic views.

In full extension, the normal patella rests in a central position superior to the trochlea. With flexion, the patella first engages the lateral condyle at about 20°. As more flexion occurs, the articular ridge centralizes within the trochlea at approximately 30–45°. CT scans have been used to depict the patellofemoral relationships within these last few degrees of extension.[19,20]

Clinically, however, it is the position of the patella relative to the trochlea during its dynamic excursion in active flexion and extension that is most important. Does it remain lateral as flexion exceeds 30°— chronically subluxed? Or does the patella suddenly shift medially as soon as it engages the trochlea during initial flexion, and then in terminal extension does it again shift laterally as it leaves the confines of the trochlea—a 'J sign'? If the goal is to determine the position of the patella in relation to the trochlea during these last few degrees of extension, then a careful physical examination, to test the tightness of the lateral retinaculum and check for a 'J sign,' correlated with routine axial views, will usually provide the same information as a CT scan and at a fraction of the cost. Obviously there are those complex cases of extensor mechanism pathomechanics, or when considering revision surgery, in which the clinician can use all available data. Then the use of CT scans, MRI, and even cineradiography of the patellofemoral joint can be most useful.

References

1. **Hughston JC, Walsh WM, Puddu G**, *Patellar subluxation and dislocation* (Philadelphia: WB Saunders, 1984) 14–17.
2. **Liebler WA**, Treatment of patellar lesions for instability, a perplexing problem, *Orthop Rev* (1974) 6: 25–37.
3. **Whitman PA, Melvin M, Nicholas JA**, Common problems seen in a sports injury clinic, *Phys Sports Med* (1981) 9: 105–110.
4. **Rosenberg TD, Paulos LE, Parker RD et al.**, The forty-five-degree, posteroanterior flexion weight-bearing radiograph of the knee, *J Bone Joint Surg (Am)* (1988) 70: 1479–1483.
5. **Insall J, Salvati E**, Patella position in the normal knee joint, *Radiology* (1971) 101: 101–104.
6. **Blackburne, JS and Peel TE**, A new method of measuring patellar height, *J Bone Joint Surg (Br)* (1977) 59B: 241–242.
7. **Norman O, Egund N, Ekelund L et al.**, The vertical position of the patella, *Acta Orthop Scand* (1983) 54: 908–913.
8. **Merchant AC**, Patellofemoral malalignment and instabilities, *Articular cartilage and knee joint function: basic science and arthroscopy*, ed Ewing JW (New York: Raven Press, 1989) 79–91.
9. **Settegast**, Typische Roentgenbilder von normalen Menschen, *Lehmanns Med Atlantan* (1921) 5: 211.
10. **Jaroschy**, Die diagnostische Verwertbarkeit der Patellaraufnahmen, *Fortschr Roentgenstr* (1924) 31: 781.
11. **Ficat P, Phillipe J, Bizou H**, Le défile fémoro-patellaire, *Rev Med Toulouse* (1970) 6: 241–244.
12. **Merchant AC, Mercer RL, Jacobsen RH et al.**, Roentgenographic analysis of patellofemoral congruence, *J Bone Joint Surg (Am)* (1974) 56: 1391–1396.
13. **Labelle M, Piedes JP, Levesque HP et al.**, Evaluation de la position rotulienne en incidence radiographique tangentielle, *Union Med Can* (1976) 105: 870.
14. **Ficat P, Ficat C, Bailleux A**, Syndrome d'hyperpression externe de la rotule (S.H.P.E.), *Rev Chir Orthop* (1975) 61: 39–59.
15. **Brattström H**, Shape of the intercondylar groove normally and in recurrent dislocation of the patella; a clinical and x-ray anatomical investigation, *Acta Orthop Scand (Suppl)* (1964) 68: 1–148.
16. **Laurin CA, Dussault R, Levesque HP**, The tangential x-ray investigation of the patellofemoral joint, *Clin Orthop* (1979) 144: 16–26.
17. **Aglietti P, Insall JN, Cerulli G**, Patellar pain and incongruence, *Clin Orthop* (1983) 176: 217–224.
18. **Dzioba RB**, Diagnostic arthroscopy and longitudinal open lateral release. A four year follow-up study to determine predictors of surgical outcome, *Am J Sports Med* (1990) 18: 343–348.
19. **Schutzer SF, Ramsby GR, Fulkerson JP**, The evaluation of patellofemoral pain using computerized tomography, *Clin Orthop* (1986) 204: 286–293.
20. **Fulkerson JP, Schutzer SF, Ramsby GR et al.**, Computerized tomography of the patellofemoral joint before and after lateral release or realignment, *Arthroscopy* (1987) 3: 19–24.

8.3   Patellar malalignment

John P. Fulkerson

In order to understand patellar malalignment, this contribution will emphasize those patellar alignment disorders which lead to displacement of the patella from its normal course in the femoral trochlea (sulcus), resulting in chronic pain or instability. Either such patients have congenital malalignment of the patella or there must be trauma to the extensor mechanism such that the patella is dislodged from its normal pattern of alignment within the femoral groove causing pain or instability. To understand these problems, one must recognize that (1) the patella may go from a pattern of normal alignment to being forcibly displaced out of the trochlea by external forces; (2) it may track normally with day-to-day functional loading but may be 'subluxable' with extremes of lower extremity rotation;[1] (3) it may track in a slightly abnormal way such that the patella is displaced or tilted from the femoral trochlea during normal functional activity but is thereby subject to further displacement with extremes of rotation such that pain or feelings of instability may ensue; or (4) the patella may be chronically dislocated such that it never is in the femoral trochlea at all.

Historically, attention has been directed primarily at patellar subluxation with little regard for tilt. Laurin,[2] however, described the lateral patellofemoral angle as an indicator of tilt. Distinguishing tilt and subluxation is imperative in understanding the pathomechanics of patellar malalignment.[1] It is important for the reader to recognize that patellar 'tilt' may or may not be associated with patellar instability (subluxation). There are patients who have subluxation with absolutely no evidence of patellar tilt, just as there are patients with patellar tilt who have absolutely no subluxation. Chronic patellar tilt is worrisome since it may lead ultimately to the excessive lateral pressure syndrome (ELPS).[3] Lateral facet arthrosis is most often associated with patellar tilt, with *or without* subluxation. Indeed, there are patients with subluxation alone, for example the adolescent with patellar instability whose patella is freely mobile medially and laterally with the patella tracking too far laterally but with no evidence of tilt and therefore, no excess of lateral facet pressure. In such cases, there is often little or no evidence of articular cartilage damage at the time of surgery.

In order to understand the array of patellar instability problems, it is imperative that the student of patellofemoral disorders pay close attention to the exact configuration of patellar malalignment and associated articular lesions. These problems are static and dynamic, involving complex motion of the knee joint, and have challenged the diagnostic skills of orthopedic surgeons since before the time of Ambroise Paré! Newer imaging techniques and research studies have begun to clarify the nature of these problems and lend a scientific basis to what was previously a disorder often treated by empirical methods.

Clinical evaluation and classification

As published by Fulkerson and Hungerford,[4] alignment disorders of the patellofemoral joint may be classified, taking into account each specific alignment pattern and degree of articular degeneration (Table 1). Through careful clinical examination, using diagnostic tests including evaluation of retinacular tightness,[5-8] the clinician can gain significant insight into the nature of each patellar alignment disorder. It is not enough to flex or extend the knee with pressure on the patella to see whether there is crepitation. Crepitation may be significant in causing pain of an articular nature; however, alignment disorders can cause significant abnormal stress on peripatellar retinacular and tendinous supports leading to retinacular fibroneuropathy,[9,10] patellar tendonitis, plical irritation, and other soft-tissue pain problems in the anterior knee. The examining physician must recognize these associated problems in fully evaluating patients with patellofemoral pain.

Full clinical evaluation of the patient with patellar instability must emphasize careful soft-tissue palpation around the patella, including the patellar tendon, distal quadriceps, and retinaculum both medially and laterally. After testing for retinacular tightness (Figure 1) and checking the patient's passive patellar tilt[5-8] and medial/lateral glide[6-8] (play) the examiner should observe patellar 'tracking' to see

Table 1 Fulkerson–Schutzer classification of patellar alignment and articular degeneration.

A. Fulkerson–Schutzer classification of patients with patellofemoral pain

Type I (A) Patellar subluxation, with no articular lesion
         (B) Patellar subluxation with grade 1–2 chondromalacia
         (C) Patellar subluxation with grade 3–4 arthrosis
         (D) Patellar subluxation with a history of dislocation and minimal or no chondromalacia
         (E) Patellar subluxation with a history of dislocation, with grade 3–4 arthrosis
Type II (A) Patellar tilt and subluxation with no articular lesion
          (B) Patellar tilt and subluxation with grade 1–2 chondromalacia
          (C) Patellar tilt and subluxation with grade 3–4 arthrosis
Type III (A) Patellar tilt with no articular lesion
           (B) Patellar tilt with grade 1–2 chondromalacia
           (C) Patellar tilt with grade 3–4 arthrosis
Type IV (A) No malalignment and no articular lesion
          (B) No malalignment and grade 1–2 chondromalacia
          (C) No malalignment and grade 3–4 arthrosis

B. Treatment recommendations (failed conservative treatment and intolerable patellofemoral pain or instability *not* complicated by reflex sympathetic dystrophy)

Type I (A and B) Lateral retinacular release (VMO advancement if necessary) and Trillat procedure
            (C) Lateral retinacular release and possible anteromedial tibial tubercle transfer
            (D) Acute dislocation – selective arthroscopy and reconstruction of osteochondral damage; consider lateral retinacular release; delay reconstruction. Recurrent dislocation – lateral retinacular release and Trillat procedure
            (E) Lateral retinacular release and anteromedial tibial tubercle transfer
Type II (A and B) Lateral retinacular release and possible Trillat procedure
             (C) Lateral retinacular release, careful debridement, and anteromedial tibial tubercle transfer
Type III (A and B) Lateral retinacular release
              (C) Lateral retinacular release, careful debridement, and anteromedial tibial tubercle transfer
Type IV (A) Continue nonoperative treatment; look for another pain source
            (B) Consider arthroscopic debridement of grade 2 lesion
            (C) Arthroscopic debridement and possible tibial tubercle anteriorization – 15 mm in severe cases

From ref. 4.

whether the patella falls accurately into the sulcus upon flexion of the knee and whether the patella appears to remain tilted on range of motion. The quadriceps (Q) angle, as noted by Insall,[11] may be helpful, but does not, in itself, assure that there is, or is not, patellar malalignment. The Q angle is most helpful when evaluated at neutral flexion/extension, 30° knee flexion, 60° knee flexion, and 90° knee flexion. Most important, however, is that the patella tracks appropriately within the femoral sulcus, regardless of the Q angle. When the patella does *not* track appropriately, the Q angle becomes more important, because an abnormally high Q angle may be one of several factors leading to abnormal tracking of the patella and it may give one target for correcting inappropriate alignment. The patient should be evaluated in a standing position by looking at overall alignment factors such as knee valgus, pronation of the foot and ankle, femoral anteversion, torsional abnormalities around the hip, or any other alignment factor that might distort patellar tracking during normal function. Finally, excessive tightness of the hamstrings or quadriceps should be noted, as these may also aggravate an extensor mechanism

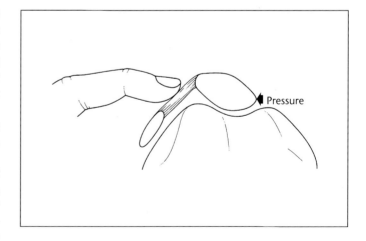

Figure 1

The lateral retinaculum should be examined carefully for tenderness, excessive tightness and restriction of lateral facet elevation. This illustration shows normal mobility of the lateral patella. Normally, the lateral facet is not tethered by the lateral retinaculum and the lateral patella may be elevated above the medial patella (from Fulkerson J, Awareness of the lateral retinaculum in evaluating patellofemoral pain, *Am J Sports Med* (1982) **10:** 147).

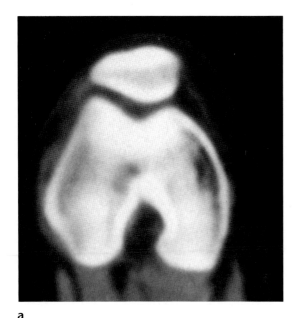

a

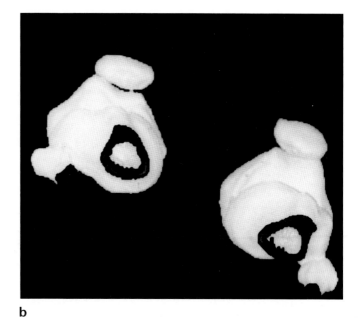

b

Figure 2

(a) Computed tomographic (CT) image of the patellofemoral joint at the mid-patellar transverse plane. Since there is no image overlap, it is possible to define precisely what one is looking at. The mid-patellar transverse plane correlates well with the articulating surface of the patella in early knee flexion. (b) Three-dimensional CT offers the capability of sectioning the patella at any level using the computer.

alignment problem. Detection of specific tightness or lower extremity alignment abnormality may enable the physician to prescribe simple exercises, stretching, or orthotics and thereby give relief after a single visit.

Radiographic studies will normally include an axial radiograph. The Laurin[2] view with the knee flexed 20° is sensitive for picking up subtle disorders which might not be detected upon further knee flexion. The Merchant[12] view (mountain view) with the knee flexed 45° and the x-ray beam angled 30° is also helpful as a basic screening axial radiograph. However, with the knee flexed 45°, more subtle alignment abnormalities may be missed. None the less, if a Merchant or Laurin view is positive, it is helpful in establishing an appropriate treatment protocol. The majority of patients require nothing more than an appropriate, well performed axial radiograph.

When surgery becomes more likely, one may wish to obtain tomographic views of the patellofemoral joint in order to gain insight into a specific alignment disorder. Tomographic imaging through the mid-patellar transverse articulating plane is, perhaps, most accurate in detecting specific alignment patterns. Unfortunately, such studies require a great deal of technical care and poorly done tomographic studies are not helpful. Consequently, if one wishes to proceed with patellofemoral tomography, strict adherence to established protocols[4] is imperative. Computed tomography (CT) is readily available at our institution and is less expensive than magnetic resonance imaging (MRI), although MRI can also provide excellent tomographic images of the patellofemoral joint as long as images are taken in normal standing alignment through the mid-patellar transverse plane. Mid-patellar transverse tomographic images are most helpful with the knee flexed 15° and 30° (Figure 2). According to studies by Schutzer et al.,[13] the patella should enter the femoral sulcus by 10° knee flexion and should remain there with a congruence angle (mid-transverse patella) of 0° in a normal population. Furthermore, there should be no tilt of the patella (with a lower limit of 12–14° patellar tilt in asymptomatic age-matched controls) when the knee is flexed. Looking at these indices, the examiner should be able to appropriately classify each patient with regard to subluxation and tilt (see Table 1).

Table 2 Noyes classification of articular cartilage lesions

Surface description	Extent of involvement	Diameter (mm)	Location	Degree of knee flexion
1. Cartilage surface intact	A. Definite softening with some resilience remaining	<10 ≤15 ≤20	*Patella* A. Proximal 1/3 Middle 1/3 Distal 1/3	Degree of knee flexion where the lesion is in weight-bearing contact (e.g. 20–45°)
	B. Extensive softening with loss of resilience (deformation)	≤25 >25	B. Odd facet Middle facet Lateral facet	
2. Cartilage surface damaged: cracks, fissures, fibrillation, or fragmentation	A. <1/2 thickness B. ≥1/2 thickness		*Trochlea* Medial femoral condyle (a) Anterior 1/3 (b) Middle 1/3 (c) Posterior 1/3	
3. Bone exposed	A. Bone surface intact B. Bone surface cavitation		Lateral femoral condyle (a) Anterior 1/3 (b) Middle 1/3 (c) Posterior 1/3 Medial tibial condyle (a) Anterior 1/3 (b) Middle 1/3 (c) Posterior 1/3 Lateral tibial condyle (a) Anterior 1/3 (b) Middle 1/3 (c) Posterior 1/3	

From ref. 14.

Finally, at the time of surgery, an even greater understanding of the specific alignment and articular disorder is necessary. At this point, an *arthroscopy* will give the best possible access to location and characterization of articular lesions. The arthroscopist may use distal or proximal portals, but usually a combination of both approaches is most helpful in thoroughly understanding the articular condition of a patella. *When arthroscopy of the patellofemoral joint is performed, the specific size, nature, and location of each articular lesion should be carefully noted in the operation report.* The Noyes classification[14] is most helpful in defining specific lesions. The Outerbridge classification[15] is simpler and notes specifically the size and fibrillation of each articular lesion in a more general way. We have found the Outerbridge classification consistently helpful, easy to remember, and widely accepted. To have a thorough grasp of each lesion, one may wish to use both the Noyes and Outerbridge classifications (Tables 2 and 3).

With the information obtained through careful clinical examination, appropriate radiographic studies, and arthroscopy, the examiner will be able to make the best possible determination of appropriate treatment. In short, one should choose treatment methods for the anterior knee that are specific to correcting a defined mechanical disorder. Specific indications for procedures will be discussed later.

Malalignment patterns

Tilt alone

Many patients with patellofemoral pain have mild tilt that may not be detected on routine axial radiographs. When a patient presents with anterior knee

Table 3 Outerbridge classification

Grade 1	Articular cartilage softening only
Grade 2	Articular cartilage fibrillation less than ½ inch in diameter
Grade 3	Articular cartilage fibrillation greater than ½ inch in diameter
Grade 4	Erosion of articular cartilage with exposed bone

From ref. 15.

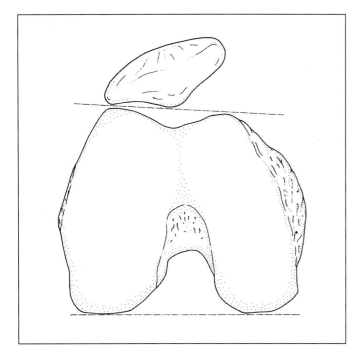

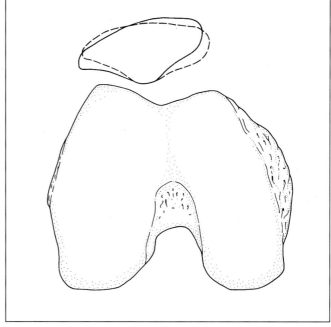

Figure 3

Patellar tilt without subluxation. Note that the tilting patella may appear congruent if the apex of the patella remains at the mid-sulcus level. It is important to detect whether there is tilt, either alone or in association with subluxation.

Figure 4

Subluxation may occur with (Type II, solid line) or without (Type I, dotted line) associated tilt, but most patients with patellar subluxation have some tilting of the patella. One should note whether there is subluxation with no tilt, mild tilt, moderate tilt, or severe tilt.

pain and no preceding history of injury or instability, the examiner should consider the possibility of chronic patellar tilt (Figure 3).

Patellar tilt is often detected at the time of initial clinical examination and is usually associated with adaptive tightness of the lateral peripatellar retinaculum. The examiner should palpate the peripatellar retinaculum for evidence of tightness[5] with particular attention to the lateral retinaculum (Figure 1). Tenderness of the lateral retinaculum, related to the chronic retinacular tightness, is common. The examiner should determine whether patellar tilt is correctable passively by raising the lateral facet with the patella held in the sulcus.[5-8]

Appropriate radiographic studies will often show patellar tilt, particularly axial views with limited knee flexion (Laurin view) and tomographic views through the mid-patellar transverse plane. A patellar tilt angle (lateral patellar facet relative to the posterior femoral condyle line as determined on a 10–20° knee flexion, mid-patellar transverse tomographic image) of less than 12–14° indicates significant patellar tilt.[4]

Patellar tilt may respond to nonoperative treatment including stretching of the lateral retinaculum, quadriceps strengthening, and patellar taping[6] or bracing. It is safest to avoid heavy loads against the patella in strengthening the quadriceps. Low-speed isokinetic training may cause damage to an already vulnerable patella.

In those patients who do not respond to nonoperative treatment, lateral retinacular release is a good procedure for relieving patellar tilt. If there is minimal articular damage at the time of release, most patients will do well. If, however, there is patellar arthrosis associated with tilt, it may be necessary to unload the defective articular surface using tibial tubercle anteriorization[16] or anteromedialization.[17,18] In short, one must design the treatment to correct or unload the specific lesions found by clinical, radiographic, and arthroscopic study.

Subluxation alone

This alignment pattern usually causes a sense of instability and sometimes uncomfortable feelings of patellar displacement that may impair the patient's ability in sports and daily activities. When evaluation indicates that there is excessive lateral glide (play) of the patella without tilt, nonoperative treatment such as bracing, taping, vastus medialis strengthening, orthotics as indicated, and modification of activities will succeed in managing most patients. Typically, subluxation alone is not associated with as much articular disruption as in those patients who have subluxation and tilt (Figure 4).

In those patients who do not respond to nonoperative care, realignment may be necessary. Simple lateral release may give adequate relief; however, our study of CT scans before and after lateral release in patients with subluxation showed that there is not consistent realignment of the subluxed patella using lateral release alone.[19] Consequently, the surgeon must be aware that medial imbrication or tibial tubercle transfer may be necessary in addition to the lateral release in some patients. Logically, medial displacement of the tibial tubercle is one of the most appropriate ways to control recurrent or persistent subluxation (as opposed to tilt), since medial imbrication suffers the risk of stretching out if the vector of strain on the patella is chronically in a lateral direction.

Subluxation or dislocation caused by specific trauma (without pre-existing malalignment)

When one who has no predisposition to lateral displacement of the patella sustains a traumatic blow causing the patella to subluxate or dislocate, there may be articular injury from the blow itself or from re-entry of a displaced patella into the sulcus with a shearing effect on the medial patellar facet or lateral trochlea. In such patients, treatment may be directed most appropriately toward restoration of displaced osteochondral fragments, removal of useless loose bodies, and restoration of satisfactory patellar alignment through splinting to allow healing of disrupted medial structure. Restoration of major articular fragments is most important in the acute period after injury. In such patients, when this treatment does not give sufficient restoration of patellar stability, and if there is recurrent instability, particularly recurrent dislocation, medial imbrication to restore medial support for the patella may be necessary. In such patients, if there has been adaptive lateral retinacular shortening because of chronic lateralization of the patella from the traumatic event, lateral release may also be necessary in order to allow the patella to fall back into the sulcus with medial repair. It is most important in such patients not to overdo this surgery, so that the patella is not made prone to medial subluxation. The logic in most patients is to restore a normally aligned patellofemoral joint, repairing osteochondral and soft tissues when damage is too severe to allow adequate healing with nonoperative management.

Subluxation and tilt

When there is tilt associated with subluxation, nonoperative treatment may be more difficult and attention will need to be directed to stretching tight lateral retinacular structures. The majority of these patients may be managed with nonoperative measures including bracing, taping, vastus medialis strengthening, reassurance, and orthotics as indicated.

In those patients who have recurrent patellar instability with subluxation and tilt, lateral retinacular release may remove the tilt component and potentially render the patient symptom-free, but the surgeon must be aware that there is some risk of leaving a residual subluxation, as lateral release is not consistently effective in relieving subluxation.[19] In this situation, the operating surgeon should do the lateral retinacular release and then treat the patient as he would a patient with subluxation alone if this is noted at the time of surgery (see section on *subluxation alone*). One must be particularly aware, however, that chronic tilt may accelerate arthrosis, and additional treatment, possibly including anteromedialization of the tibial tubercle, may be helpful in selected patients when lateral facet or distal medial facet arthrosis have become troublesome[4] (Figure 5).

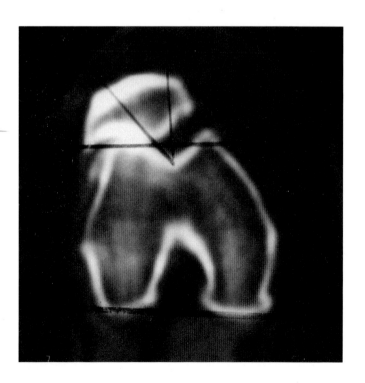

Figure 5

When the lateral patellar facet or distal medial facet is grossly degenerated, lateral release alone may not be sufficient to provide sustained relief of pain in many patients.

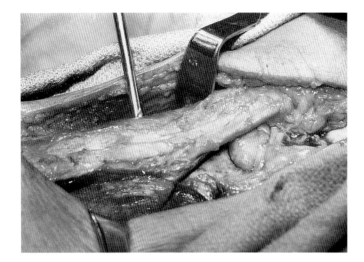
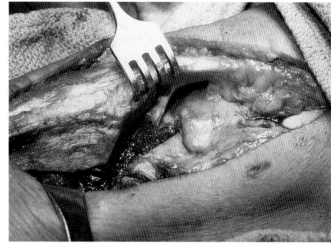

a   b

Figure 6

Anteromedial tibial tubercle transfer provides relief of lateral and distal medial facet contact pressure when these areas are arthritic. It is most beneficial when there is good proximal medial facet articular cartilage. (a) before; (b) after transfer (lateral view).

Permanent dislocation

At the time of initial evaluation, a small number of patients may have complete and permanent dislocation of the patella. Often this is associated with congenital or traumatic dysplasia of the extensor mechanism and trochlea. Surprisingly, some such patients function extremely well and may require only symptomatic treatment, physical therapy or reassurance. None the less, when permanent patellar dislocation leads to chronic pain or instability, realignment may be necessary.

The surgeon must be very cautious in planning surgery for the patient with permanent patellar dislocation. The following factors must be considered. (1) The extensor mechanism will be relatively short, so that knee flexion will be difficult following reduction of the patella into the trochlea. (2) The patella and extensor mechanism may be strikingly dysplastic. (3) Soft-tissue surgery alone will probably be inadequate in most patients.

For the patient with chronic complete patellar dislocation, the author prefers to use the Trillat procedure[20] with a generous block of the tibial tubercle to allow substantial tibial tubercle medialization as needed in these patients. One should view the entire extensor mechanism at the time of surgery in order to evaluate specific dysplasias and allow adequate revision as necessary. Patellar anlage may be 'splayed' across the anterior knee, leaving only a small button of bone for a patella. Substantial medial imbrication or even a V–Y plasty of the quadriceps tendon proxi-

mal to the patella may be necessary in order to maintain reduction of the patella in the trochlea. The end result, using soft-tissue and bony surgery, should be a congruent patellofemoral joint with no tendency to dislocate or significantly limit knee flexion on the operating room table at the conclusion of surgery.

Summary

Accurate treatment of patients with patellar malalignment requires (1) precise clinical evaluation with differentiation of soft-tissue/retinacular pain from articular pain, and careful appraisal of the specific alignment pattern; (2) appropriate and carefully performed radiographic studies; and (3) characterization and localization of articular lesions using arthroscopy when nonoperative treatment fails and surgical correction is necessary.

Classification of patients with patellofemoral pain and malalignment will enable the clinician to direct treatment – either nonoperative or operative – such that specific mechanical disorders are corrected. Simple nonoperative treatment such as exercise, stretching and orthotics is all that is necessary in most patients. Sometimes, patellar taping and bracing will be helpful when there is a defined malalignment.

Surgical treatment may be necessary for some patients with more advanced malalignment and intractable pain. No surgical treatment should be undertaken until there is an appreciation of (1) whether there is tilt, subluxation, or both; (2) the location and extent of patellar and trochlear articular lesions; and (3) failure of a well-constructed nonoperative treatment program.

Lateral retinacular release is most appropriate to relieve chronic patellar tilt when there is little or no articular cartilage breakdown. When there is lateral facet or distal medial facet patellar arthrosis, anteromedial tibial tubercle transfer (Figure 6) may be necessary to unload the defective areas and correct chronic patellar tilt, particularly if there is mild subluxation also. On the other hand, lateral release is not consistently effective for correcting subluxation. In such patients, if there are persistent problems of subluxation or dislocation, medial transfer of the tibial tubercle (Trillat procedure) may be necessary in the skeletally mature patient, or medial imbrication in the skeletally immature patient.

In general, patients respond favorably to treatment of patellofemoral pain when the clinical examination is careful, radiographs are accurate, articular lesions are localized, and the resulting treatment plan is logical.

Acknowledgment

The author thanks Mrs Susan Philo for help in preparing the manuscript.

References

1. **Fulkerson JP, Shea KP**, Current concepts review: Disorders of patellofemoral alignment, *J Bone Joint Surg (Am)* (1990) **72:** 1424–1429.
2. **Laurin CA, Dussault R, Levesque HP**, The tangential x-ray investigation of the patellofemoral joint: X-ray technique, diagnostic criteria and their interpretation, *Clin Orthop* (1979) **144:** 16–26.
3. **Ficat P, Ficat C, Bailleux A**, Syndrome d'hyperpression externe de la rotule: son intérêt pour la connaissance de l'arthrose (SHPE), *Rev Chir Orthop* (1975) **61:** 39–59.
4. **Fulkerson J, Hungerford D**, *Disorders of the patellofemoral joint*, 2nd edn (Baltimore: Williams and Wilkins, 1990).
5. **Fulkerson JP**, Awareness of the retinaculum in evaluating patellofemoral pain, *Am J Sports Med* (1982) **10:** 147–149.
6. **McConnell J**, The management of chondromalacia patellae: a long-term solution, *Aust J Physiother* (1986) **32:** 215–220.
7. **Ficat P, Hungerford D**, *Disorders of the patellofemoral joint* (Baltimore: Williams and Wilkins, 1977).
8. **Kolowich P, Paulos L, Rosenberg T et al.**, Lateral release of the patella: indications and contra-indications, *Am J Sports Med* (1990) **18:** 359–365.
9. **Fulkerson JP, Tennant R, Jaivin JS et al.**, Histologic evidence of retinacular nerve injury associated with patellofemoral malalignment, *Clin Orthop* (1985) **197:** 196–205.
10. **Fujimoto A, Mori Y, Iino H et al.**, Lateral release for excessive lateral pressure syndrome, Read at the Annual Meeting of the Western Pacific Orthopaedic Association, Singapore, November, 1989.
11. **Insall JN**, Patella pain syndromes and chondromalacia patellae, *Instruct Course Lect AAOS* (1981) **30:** 342–356.
12. **Merchant AC, Mercer RL, Jacobsen RH et al.**, Roentgenographic analysis of patellofemoral congruence, *J Bone Joint Surg (Am)* (1974) **56:** 1391–1396.
13. **Schutzer SF, Ramsby GR, Fulkerson JP**, Computed tomographic classification of patellofemoral pain patients, *Orthop Clin North Am* (1986) **17:** 235–248.
14. **Noyes FR, Stabler CL**, A system for grading articular cartilage lesions at arthroscopy, *Am J Sports Med* (1989) **17:** 505–513.
15. **Outerbridge RE**, The etiology of chondromalacia patellae, *J Bone Joint Surg (Br)* (1961) **43:** 752–757.
16. **Maquet P**, Advancement of the tibial tuberosity, *Clin Orthop* (1976) **115:** 225–230.
17. **Fulkerson JP**, Anteromedialization of the tibial tuberosity for patellofemoral malalignment, *Clin Orthop* (1983) **177:** 176–181.
18. **Fulkerson JP, Becker GJ, Meaney JA et al.**, Anteromedial tibial tubercle transfer without bone graft, *Am J Sports Med* (1990) **18:** 490–497.
19. **Fulkerson JP, Schutzer SF, Ramsby GR et al.**, Computerized tomography of the patellofemoral joint before and after lateral release or realignment, *Arthroscopy* (1987) **3:** 19–24.
20. **Cox JS**, An evaluation of the Roux–Elmslie–Trillat procedure for knee extensor realignment, *Am J Sports Med* (1982) **10:** 303–310.

8.4   Radiographic criteria for assessing the patellofemoral joint on axial radiographs

Carroll A. Laurin and David Zukor

Objective assessment of patellofemoral alignment requires a consistent radiographic technique and specific measurement criteria. This contribution is an attempt to standardize the evaluation of the patellofemoral joint when visualized on axial radiographs. Correct positioning of the patient and the radiographic equipment are essential (Figure 1).

Positioning of the patient (Figure 1a)

Since it is relatively easy to manually tilt a normal patella within the femoral groove, the patella must not be submitted to any pressure while the radiograph is being taken. The patella should not be compressed by the weight of the leg, as would happen when the patient was prone; hence the patient must be supine or seated, with the patella topmost.

Positioning of the knee (Figure 1a)

It is vital to assess patellar tracking at the precise moment (which varies from patient to patient) when the patella enters the femoral groove, usually as the knee is flexed from 20° to 40°. Once the patella is in the groove (i.e., when the knee is flexed beyond 45°), the tension on the knee extensor mechanism will inevitably normalize the position of the patella within the groove, even in the presence of a clinically unstable patella. Hence skyline views of the patellofemoral compartment (i.e., when the knee is flexed more than 90°) are useless in assessing patellofemoral tracking, since one is then visualizing the relationship between the distal portion of the femoral condyles (rather than the femoral groove) and the patella. Furthermore, although the 'skyline' radiograph incidence may be useful for visualizing the distal patellofemoral joint, it is not adequate for assessing patellofemoral tracking, since the extensor mechanism is then passively under tension.

For similar reasons, the extensor mechanism must not be under active tension (i.e., active quadriceps contraction), since this will also normalize or 'center' the patella and may give a false radiographic image of normal patellar tracking. Hence, the knee should rest on a special, adjustable support (with an incor-

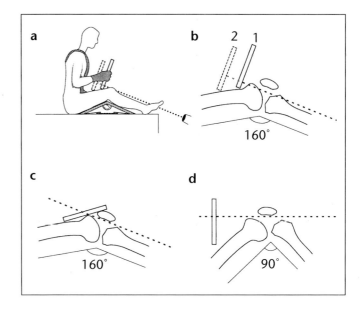

Figure 1

Axial radiography of the patellofemoral joint: Correct positioning of the patient, the knee, the plate, and the radiography machine. (a) Note the lead gloves and apron, the goniometer, and the special rest to sequentially position the knee in 20°, 30°, and 40° of knee flexion. The X-ray beam is parallel to the anterior border of the tibia and to the patellofemoral joint-line; the film cassette is at 90° to the X-ray beam and to the patellofemoral joint. (b) If the patellofemoral joint appears low on the plate (1), the plate is moved proximally and pushed firmly against the femur (2). The orientation of the plate and the position of the knee are unchanged. (c) Incorrect positioning of the plate, i.e., parallel to the femur rather than at 90° to the X-ray beam. (d) Incorrect position of the knee, i.e., flexed more than 40°.

porated goniometer) to ensure correct positioning of the knee, as radiographs are taken in the 20°, 30°, 40° positions while the quadriceps is relaxed.

Conversely, CT scans of the patellofemoral compartment in complete knee extension, i.e., 0° position, may show a laterally displaced patella which tracks normally at 30°, hence providing false CT images of patellar malalignment.

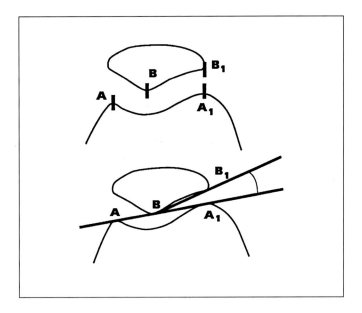

Figure 2

Patellofemoral angle: Points A and A_1 correspond to the summits of the femoral condyles, while points B and B_1 correspond to the limits of the lateral patellar facet. The patellofemoral angle is above line A–A_1, and is formed by the junction of points A and A_1, and B with B_1.

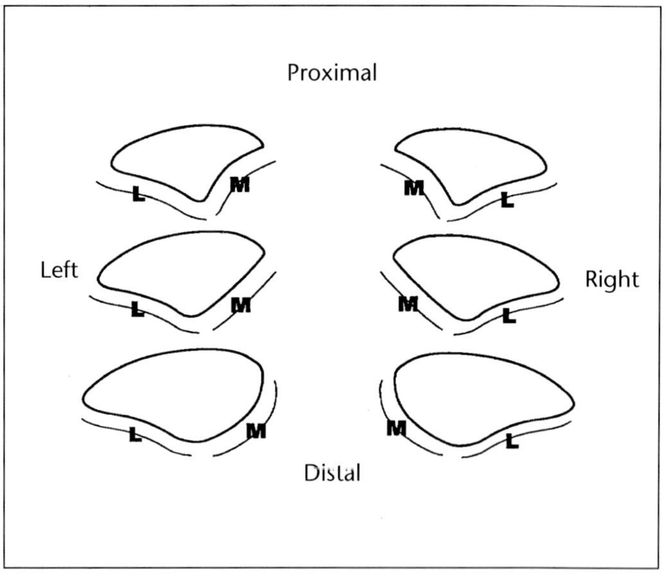

Figure 3

Medial and lateral patellar facets: Coronal section of right and left patellae of the same individual; note that the shape of the medial facet changes while the shape of the lateral facet remains constant; hence reference to the lateral facet as a reliable patellar landmark.

Positioning of X-ray beam and radiographic plate (Figures 1b,c,d)

Once one has positioned the knee correctly, it is equally important to standardize the position of the X-ray beam and radiographic plate. As for the radiological visualization of any joint, the X-ray beam must be parallel to the patellofemoral joint-line while the plate should be at 90° to the joint-line and to the X-ray beam.

Using the above technique, the patellofemoral joint will necessarily appear at the bottom of the plate (Figure 1b). If, as frequently happens, the patellofemoral joint is incompletely visualized, because it is too low on the radiographic plate, one must not make either of two incorrect adjustments. The first is to 'raise' the position of the patellofemoral joint on the plate by flattening the plate on the thighs (Figure 1c); this will distort the contour of the patellofemoral joint since the plate is then not at 90° to the joint-line. The other, incorrect adjustment (Figure 1d) is to

flex the knees further, which could give a false normal radiographic image of patellofemoral tracking.

If the patellofemoral joint is too low on the plate (Figure 1b) and is not well visualized, the orientation of the plate should not be modified and the knee should not be flexed beyond 40°; rather, while the plate is maintained at 90° to the X-ray beam, it is mobilized proximally and pushed vertically in a downward direction, i.e., towards the floor (Figure 1b). Since it is easier to compress the plate against the soft quadriceps muscle (rather than against the bony tibial crest), the plate is best held proximal to the knee by the patient (wearing lead gloves and apron). It is then relatively easy to position the radiography machine, between the feet, with the X-ray beam directed proximally, parallel to the tibial axis.

It is admittedly possible also to position the machine proximal to the knees and to direct the X-ray beam distally, but a special plate holder is then necessary and adjustments of the plate position can be more tedious.

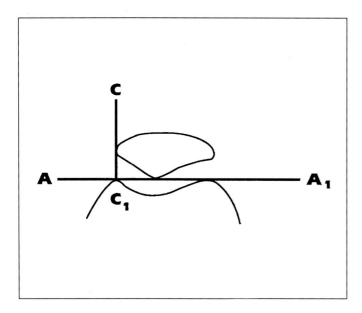

Figure 4

Medial patellofemoral line: Line A–A$_1$ joins the summits of the femoral condyles. The medial patellofemoral line (C–C$_1$) starts at the apex of the medial femoral condyle and is perpendicular to line A–A$_1$.

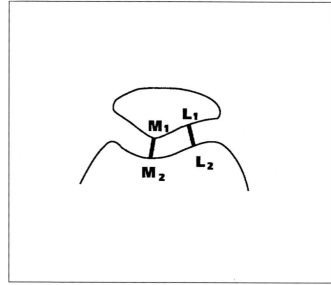

Figure 5

Patellofemoral index (M/L). The patellofemoral index (M/L) is the ratio between the thickness of the medial patellofemoral compartment (M$_1$–M$_2$) and the thickness of the lateral patellofemoral compartment (L$_1$–L$_2$). M$_1$ is the lateral limit of the medial patellar facet and corresponds to the junction of the medial and lateral patellar facets; M$_2$ is that point on the medial femoral condyle which is closest to M$_1$. Point L$_1$ is the mid-point of the lateral patellar facet; L$_2$ is that point on the lateral femoral condyle which is closest to L$_1$.

Objective criteria for the assessment of axial patellofemoral radiographs

The proposed measurement criteria for assessment of axial radiographs of the patellofemoral joint are the patellofemoral angle, the medial patellofemoral line, and the patellofemoral index.

The patellofemoral angle (Figure 2)

The patellofemoral angle (the angle between the patella and the femoral groove, Figure 2) is formed by the junction of two lines, one drawn along the summits on the femoral condyles (A–A$_1$), the other on the patella (B–B$_1$). Line A–A$_1$ is simply drawn along the summits of both femoral condyles.

Since the shape of the medial patellar facet is inconsistent (as illustrated by coronal cuts of the same patella at different levels) (Figure 3), and indeed changes from patient to patient (these changes in the shape of the medial facet are the basis of the Wiberg classification of patellar shapes), the medial patellar facet is not a reliable reference point for the patella. Line B–B$_1$, is therefore drawn by joining the limits of the lateral patellar facet (the only constant landmark on the articular surface of the patella).

The angle *above* line A–A$_1$, formed at the junction of lines A–A$_1$ and B–B$_1$, is the patellofemoral angle (Figure 2).

The medial patellofemoral line (Figure 4)

The medial patellofemoral line is a radiological criterion for assessment of side-to-side displacement (i.e., translation rather than tilt) of the patella. Line A–A$_1$ is drawn as for the patellofemoral angle. Line C–C$_1$ starts at the apex of the medial femoral condyle and is perpendicular to line A–A$_1$.

It will be noted that the apex of the proximal portion of the medial femoral condyle (i.e., the portion that is usually visualized when the axial radiograph is taken in the 30° position, as the patella enters the femoral groove) has a sharp contour, unlike the more distal portion of the medial femoral condyle (visualized as the knee is flexed more), which has a more rounded contour. Hence, the sharp contour of the medial femoral condyle is a useful indicator, confirming that axial radiographs were indeed taken in the correct, 30° position.

Patellofemoral index (M/L) (Figure 5)

The patellofemoral index is the ratio between the thickness of the medial patellofemoral compartment (M_1–M_2) and the thickness of the lateral patellofemoral compartment (L_1–L_2).

Point M_1 is the lateral limit of the medial patellar facet and corresponds to the junction of the medial and lateral patellar facets. Point M_2 is that portion of the medial femoral condyle which is closest to point M_1. Point L_1 is the mid-point of the lateral patellar facet. Point L_2 is that portion of the lateral femoral condyle that is closest to L_1.

Significance of the patellofemoral angle, the medial patellofemoral line and the patellofemoral index (Figure 6a,b,c)

Patellofemoral angle (Figure 6a)

The advantage of the patellofemoral angle is that no measurement of the angle is necessary since, although there is considerable variation of the patellofemoral angle in normal individuals (Figure 6a(I,II)) it is always open laterally. If the angle is open medially (Figure 6a(IV)), the patient can be assumed to have a dislocating or unstable patella.

Occasionally, lines A–A_1, and B–B_1, do not form an angle and are parallel to one another (Figure 6a(III)). This may be noted in instances of a clinically stable patella or in patients with mild patellar malalignment (which can also be recognized by referring to the patellofemoral index, M/L).

Although parallel A–A_1 and B–B_1 lines are sometimes seen in normal individuals, the absence of a normal patellofemoral angle (i.e., open laterally) usually signifies an unstable patella.

Medial patellofemoral line (Figure 6b)

In normal individuals, and in 50% of patients with a dislocating patella, the medial patellofemoral line

(C–C_1) will touch the patella (Figure 6b(I,II)). In the remaining 50% of patients with a dislocating patella (Figure 6b(III)) (always with a reverse patellofemoral angle), the patella is lateral to the medial patellofemoral line (a consideration to keep in mind when surgically correcting a dislocating patella).

Patellofemoral index (M/L) (Figure 6c)

The patellofemoral index is an attempt to assess the relative thicknesses of the medial and lateral patellofemoral compartments. As in any normal joint (e.g., the ankle or the tibiofemoral joint), the medial and lateral halves of the normal patellofemoral joint are equal; hence the normal patellofemoral index (M/L) equals 1 (Figure 5; Figure 6c(I)).

The patellofemoral index may be abnormal, i.e., greater than 1, if there is an increase in measurement M (as in instances of an unstable patella) (Figure 6c(II,III)) or if there is a decrease in measurement L (as in instances of lateral compartment syndrome or patellofemoral osteoarthritis) (Figure 6c(IV)).

Patellar contour

Wiberg distinguished four types of patellae, depending on the changing contour of the medial patellar facet: Type I, the medial patellar facet is convex; Type II, the medial patellar facet is concave but smaller than the lateral patellar facet; Type III, the medial patellar facet is concave and of similar size as the lateral patellar facet; Type IV, the medial facet is vertical, i.e., a unifacet patella.

The incidence of Type I, II, or III patellae is roughly the same in patients with patellar malalignment syndromes and in the control population. The unifacet patella (Type IV), however, is noted in 8% of the patient population but is never seen in individuals with normally tracking patellae. In other words, the unifacet patella is rarely seen; but, when present, it can be assumed almost always to track abnormally and/or contribute to the presenting knee complaints.

Discussion

Patellar malalignment is undoubtedly a factor in the pathogenesis of patellar instability and anterior knee pain syndromes; consistent, objective radiological assessment of patellar position is therefore essential.

An abnormal, reversed, patellofemoral angle is noted in most patients with a dislocating patella (Figures 6a(IV), 6b(II,III) and 6c(III)).

Parallel patellar lines are occasionally seen in normal patients but are mostly noted in patients with a subluxing patella (Figure 6a(III)).

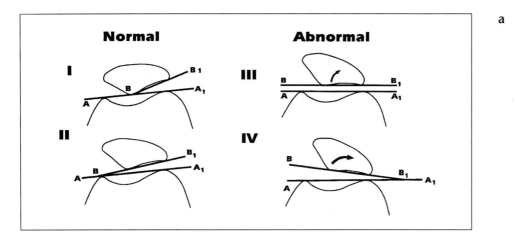

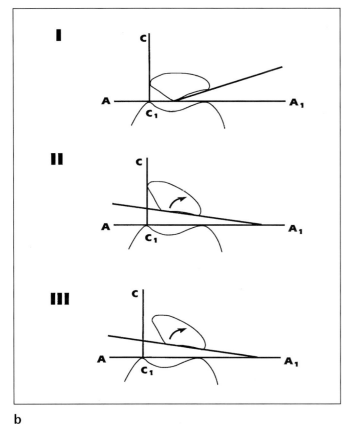

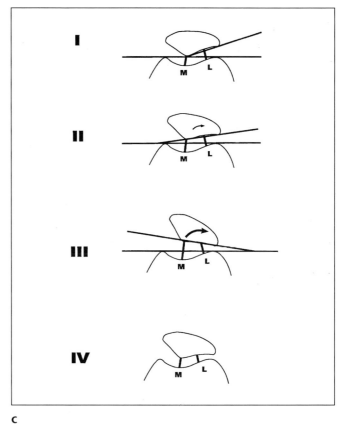

b   c

Figure 6

(a) Significance of the patellofemoral angles. The normal patellofemoral angle varies but is always open laterally (I,II). Occasionally the A–A_1, and B–B_1 lines are parallel (III). This is seen in normal individuals and in patients with mild patellar malalignment. In the presence of gross patellar instability there is a patellar tilt and the patellofemoral angle is then reversed and open medially (IV).

(b) Significance of the medial patellofemoral line. In normal individuals (I), and in 50% of patients with a dislocating patella (II) (with a patellofemoral angle that is open medially), there is no lateral patellar displacement and part of the patella touches the medial patellofemoral line (C–C_1). In the remaining 50% of patients with a dislocating patella (III), the patella is lateral to line C–C_1, thus documenting lateral patellar displacement in association with a patellar tilt.

(c) Normal and abnormal patellofemoral index (M/L). (I) The normal patellofemoral index normally corresponds to a value of 1, since the thicknesses of both patellofemoral compartments (medial and lateral) are equal: $M/L = 1$. (II) In instances of mild patellar tilt, the patellofemoral angle may still be normal, but there is sufficient tilt of the patella to increase measurement M, thus making the patellofemoral index abnormal; i.e., it measures more than 1. (III) In instances of an obvious, or gross, patellar tilt, the patellofemoral angle is abnormal, i.e., reversed and open medially. Measurement M is then much greater than measurement L; hence, a grossly abnormal patellofemoral index, i.e., measuring more than 1. (IV) In instances of lateral compartment patellofemoral osteoarthritis, the patellofemoral index is also abnormal, i.e., more than 1, because measurement L has decreased.

Lateral patellar displacement is noted in 50% of patients with a dislocating patella (Figure 6b(III)).

In normal individuals, the thickness of the medial and lateral patellofemoral compartment is the same; hence a normal patellofemoral index (M/L) of 1 (Figure 5, Figure 6c(I)). An abnormal patellofemoral index (M/L) is a reliable radiographic sign of patellofemoral osteoarthritis (Figure 6c(IV)) (i.e., the patellofemoral index measures more than 1, because of a decrease in measurement L) and reflects the loss of thickness of the lateral patellofemoral compartment.

The patellofemoral index may also be abnormal (i.e., measure more than 1, because of an increase in measurement M) and yet be associated with a normal patellofemoral angle (Figure 6c(II)). This probably reflects minor degrees of patellar malalignment, which may be insufficient to cause instability, but is sufficient to cause patellar pain, i.e., a lateral patellar syndrome.

An abnormal patellofemoral index is also noted in instances of gross patellar tilting (Figure 6c(III)), i.e., a dislocating patella. However, recurrent dislocation of the patella is more easily recognized by referring to the patellofemoral angle, which is easier to draw and conceptualize (even without actually drawing the angle on the radiograph).

No reference has been made to radiographic findings associated with chondromalacia since the term should probably be avoided as a diagnosis. Chondromalacia is not a diagnosis; the term refers to a pathological finding (which need not be symptomatic) or to a clinical symptom (e.g., patellar pain) which may be due to a variety of causes (e.g., degenerative, inflammatory, post-traumatic, or chronic malalignment).

In order to evolve a better understanding of the pathogenesis of patellar lesions and 'patellar' pain, accurate radiographic assessment of the axial view patellofemoral joint is crucial. The patellofemoral angle, the medial patellofemoral line, and the patellofemoral index are proposed as objective and reproducible measurements of axial radiographs of the patellofemoral joint.

Acknowledgment

The authors acknowledge the expert work of the artist, David Rolling.

8.5   Factors in patellar instability

Henri Dejour, Philippe Neyret and Gilles Walch

In the study of patellofemoral pathology, the problem of terminology arises, in particular regarding the notion of instability. This is fundamental by definition in the problem of the mechanical instability of the knee. In other words, we need to know whether the patella can become dislocated or not.

If the patella is or has already been dislocated, we use the term 'objective patellar instability' (OPI). In the opposite case, clinical analysis is insufficient to confirm that the patella is truly unstable, and thus we use the term 'subjective patellar instability' (SPI), i.e. the feeling the patient has that the knee is not firm, that it will 'give way'. SPI may be a tendency to subluxation but may equally be something else: amyotrophy of the quadriceps, chondromalacia through direct blow, etc.

Patellofemoral pathology is dominated by the question whether there is or is not a tendency to kneecap luxation. Clinical analysis is unable to answer this question. We shall attempt to show that whenever a patella becomes dislocated or has a tendency to do so, it presents well-defined morphological characteristics, and that if these are absent the likelihood of kneecap luxation is very slight, even negligible.

We compared two populations that were clinically very distinct from each other:

1. Patients having had at least one indisputable luxation of the patella (eliminating those patients with a permanent or habitual luxation) – 143 knees.
2. Control patients free of any kneecap pathology – 190 knees.

Radiological examinations included:

1. Strict profile view of each knee in 30° of flexion.
2. An axial view of the patella in 30° of flexion, the two knees being radiographed simultaneously.
3. A CT scan of the lower limbs. This is done with the subject in dorsal decubitus, feet in 15° lateral rotation, with plantar weight bearing. After performing a tomogram, the examination consists of taking five sections passing through (a) the hip; (b) the trochlea (the correct level of

the section is the one where the intercondylar groove has the form of a Roman arch); in the case of a high kneecap, a supplementary image should be obtained passing through the middle of the patella; (c) the superior tibial epiphysis; (d) the anterior tibial tuberosity; (e) the ankle.

The scanner enables several parameters to be measured, including the tibial tuberosity–trochlear groove (TT–TG, Figure 10) and the patellar tilt (Figure 6).

In the second part of this contribution, and with the aid of this analysis grid, we shall study a third population presenting with clinical patellar signs (pain, subjective instability) but without any history of luxation. We shall see that in 12% of cases the same morphological characteristics are found in this population as in the population where at least one luxation had occurred. This group, designated potential patellar instability (PPI), is of particular interest as, on the one hand, it may account for the lateral patellofemoral osteoarthritis observed around the age of 50 years and, on the other, it opens up reasoned therapeutic perspectives.

Definition of the factors of patellar instability

Dysplasia of the trochlea

The strict profile (lateral) view of the knee in 30° of flexion enables one to detect a dysplasia of the trochlea,[1,2] It is from this incidence that one can best judge the morphology of the trochlea for the simple reason that the morphological anomaly is situated very high. This is the most discriminant criterion; we can state with 97% reliability that there is no recurrent luxation with trochlear dysplasia. To study this point, we employed three parameters: the intersection sign; the trochlear boss; and the trochlear depth.

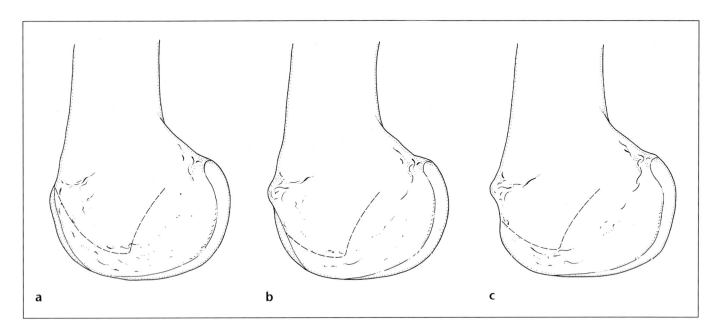

a   b   c

Figure 1

The intersection of the line of the bottom of the trochlea with the two condyles allows the determination of a typology of dysplasia (a, Type 1; b, Type II; c, Type III), minor in Type I, major in Type III.

The intersection sign

The profile view of a normal knee reveals the existence of three contours at the level of the trochlea (Figure 1). The two most anterior curves correspond to the contours of the medial and lateral *verges* of the trochlea. The medial condyle is recognizable by its notch, which is more anterior and less pronounced than that of the lateral condyle. The third curve, posterior to the other two, corresponds to the line of the groove of the trochlea. It continues towards the back by the Blumensaat line delineating the intercondylar notch. In normal conditions, the line of the groove of the trochlea remains parallel to the trochlear *verges* (Figures 1 and 2). Sometimes, the line of the groove of the trochlea crosses the medial condyle, which means that the trochlea no longer has a medial side; in other cases, there is no intersection with the lateral condyle, which means that the trochlea still has a lateral side. When the line of

the bottom crosses the lateral condyle, this means that from this point onwards the trochlea is completely flat – this is what we term the 'intersection sign'. Very often this intersection, if there is one, is marked by a tiny spiculum that we call the 'recentering beak'. This intersection does not depend on the rotation of the epiphysis; it is there whatever the rotation may be. We consider this intersection sign to be of great importance; in the normal population it is present in only 2% of cases, whereas in objective patellar instabilities it is present in 96% of the cases. The dysplasia is all the greater as the intersection occurs early.

It is thus possible to establish a typology of trochleas. Type I minor dysplasia is when the intersection occurs in the mid-part (12%). Beyond the intersection, there is a line which joins the anterior edge of the lateral condyle, the anterior edge of the medial condyle and the line of the bottom of the trochlea. In type II dysplasia (intermediate form), the most frequent (59%), the medial condyle–lateral condyle intersection occurs at a different level; the trochlea is flat but still has a certain lateral slope which resists luxation of the patella (Figure 1).

The trochlear boss

This parameter allows the position of the groove of the trochlea to be located and quantified in relation

Table 1 The intersection sign and the type of trochlea according to their clinical characteristics.

No. of knees (OPI)	No intersection sign	Type I	Type II	Type III
143	4%	27%	43%	26%

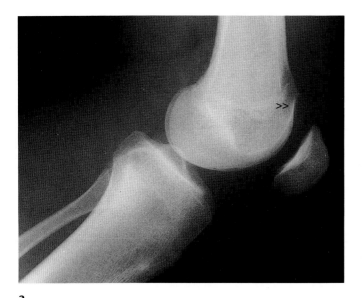

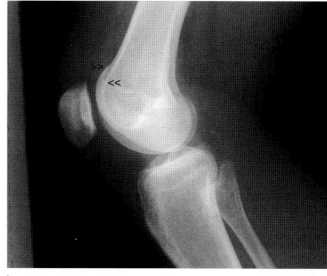

a   b

Figure 2

(a) Type III trochlear dysplasia. Nineteen-year-old male patient with objective patellar instability. The intersection of the line of the bottom of the trochlea with the condyles occurs very low down (>>) and the upper part of the trochlea is flat. (b) Type II dysplasia. Twenty-eight-year-old woman with objective patellar instability. The intersection occurs first with the medial condyle (<<) then with the lateral condyle (>>).

to the anterior cortical margin of the femur. To measure it, we trace three straight lines (Figure 3):

1. The line X tangent to the last 10 cm of the anterior cortex of the femur.
2. The line Y tangent to the last 10 cm of the posterior cortex of the femur.
3. The line Z which joins the summit of the femoral condyles towards the back at the most anterior point of the line of the bottom of the trochlea.

The trochlear boss is the distance B–C, it may be interpreted in two ways: by direct reading—it is the distance in millimetres between the points B and C; or by relating it to the size of the inferior epiphysis of the femur—as the ratio BC × 100/AD (Figure 3). Whatever the measurement, the boss may be positive, nil or negative. The result expressed as a ratio seems more sensitive and more precise. However, direct reading in millimetres conserves the advantage of being easier to use in routine practice, which is why we have adopted it. The boss is negative, close to 0, in the control series, whereas it is distinctly positive in the case of objective patellar instability. The boss increases according to the type of trochlea in the latter population. There is a significant difference ($P < 0.05$) between type I and type III trochleas. Lastly, the existence of a threshold value allows one to distinguish between the pathological population (OPI) and the control

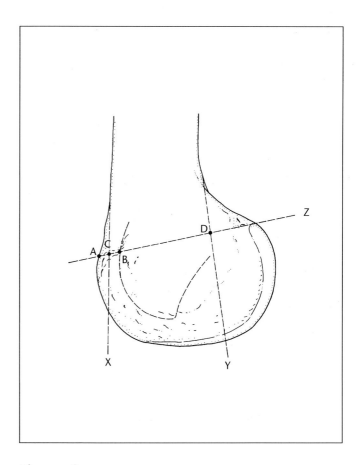

Figure 3

Measurement of the trochlear boss.

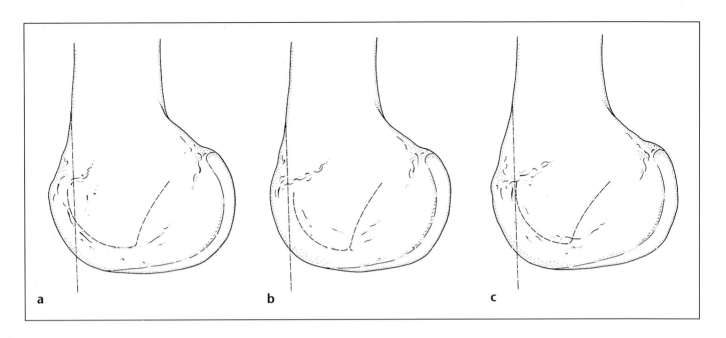

Figure 4

The boss may be positive (a), negative (b) or nil (c).

population. The threshold value of the boss is 3 mm (ratio of 7.5).

From Tables 2 and 3 it can be seen that, at least theoretically, the boss is of importance; when the trochlea is hollow the value is negative; the more the trochlea is dysplasic, the more positive is the value. This indicates that the trochlear dysplasia (flat trochlea) is in some way linked to bony filling of the groove of the trochlea. The trochlea is then situated like a superstructure above the anterior cortex of the femur, on one hand creating a springboard favourable to luxation and on the other hand increasing the patellofemoral forces by an anti-Maquet effect. This should be taken into account in explaining the patellofemoral osteoarthritis. In patellofemoral osteoarthritis where a history of luxation is common (40%), the boss is significantly elevated even in patients who have never had a luxation (2.2 mm);[3] this would appear to demonstrate that there is a direct affiliation between objective patellar instability and lateral patellofemoral osteoarthritis (Figure 4).

The trochlear depth

This parameter was first studied on axial views at 30° of flexion through the trochlear angle.[2] Brattström[4] was the first to point out the interest of the profile view in analysing this feature. We have adopted a new method for quantifying this parameter (Figure 5). We trace the perpendicular to the line Y at the summit of the femoral condyles to the back, then we lower it by 15° to the bottom. It will intersect successively the line of the bottom of the trochlea and the contour of the trochlear verges. The depth of the trochlea, measured at 15°, is equal to the distance in millimetres between the line of the bottom of the trochlea and the most anterior contour. We thus have an intermediate measurement between the

Table 2 Trochlear bosses, pathological threshold value (in mm).

	≥3 mm	<3 mm
OPI (n = 143)	66%	34%
Controls (n = 30)	6.5%	93.5%

Table 3 Trochlear boss results according to group (control vs OPI).

	Control	OPI
Value in millimetres (BC)	−0.8 ± 2.9	3.2 ± 2.4
	P = 0.0001	
Value as a ratio (BC/AD)	−2.6 ± 8.5	8.4 ± 6.2
	P = 0.0001	

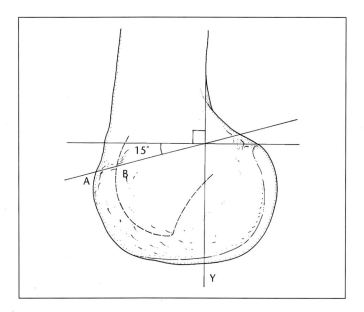

Figure 5

Measurement of the depth of the trochlea.

all patients are included in the OPI group; nevertheless, in 80% of the cases, the trochlear angle at 30° appears normal (<145°), even for recurrent luxations.

Dysplasia of the quadriceps

This can be seen from two very distinct elements:

The short quadriceps

This is the fundamental factor encountered in cases of permanent or habitual luxations, of which it would appear to be the main cause. To realign the patella and restore the knee's normal flexion, it is absolutely necessary to disinsert totally the quadriceps, according to Judet,[5] i.e. to 'lengthen' the muscle. Minor forms of short quadriceps may occur.

Dysplasia of the vastus medialis (VM)

This has been especially studied by Hughston[6] and Insall.[7] The vastus medialis obliquus (VMO), the lowermost part of the VM, appears inserted at a distance from the patella and its fibres remain strictly vertical. It therefore cannot play a role in patellar stabilization. This dysplasia is undeniable but its evaluation is highly subjective and it is impossible to measure. We attempted to determine it objectively by direct observation on a CT scan section passing through the summit of the patella, where the VMO is situated. A filiform insertion is often found representing a long insertion tendon and not a muscle body, which would suggest a dysplasia of the muscle insertion. However, CT scans are difficult to interpret. Further, there is nothing to prove that the dysplasia is not more complex, and we are in favour of the hypothesis of a dysplasia associating an impairment of the VM with hypertonia, a retraction of the VM.

A study of the patellar tilt in extension as observed on CT scans, with relaxed quadriceps, led us to envisage another hypothesis: that this patellar tilt is the expression, the reflection of the dysplasia of the quadriceps. We shall provide support for this hypothesis by drawing on CT scans performed before and after operation. The patellar tilt in extension is the angle formed by the transverse axis of the patella and the plane of the posterior condyles. This tilt should be measured at the level of the intercondylar groove, when it has the aspect of a regular Roman arch. This measurement, made with the quadriceps relaxed, is reliable, reproducible and constant for a given knee, even over several examinations. The contraction of the quadriceps increases the tilt by 5–10°, but this measurement can be very variable between two successive examinations. During the patellar tilt in extension, in the OPI group (mean = 31.5°) and in the control group

shallowest trochlear depth (intersection) and that measured at 30° of flexion.

The trochlear depth is an indication of the shallowness of the trochlear groove. It is a quantitative criterion of trochlear dysplasia. The trochlear groove of the knees belonging to the OPI group is almost 4 times more shallow on average than that of the control knees. The difference is significant (P <0.0001). This factor allows us to obtain a quantitative evaluation of trochlear dysplasia (Tables 4 and 5).

The trochlear angle measured on axial radiographs at 30° of flexion is the classical measurement of interest but is inadequate. Above 145° of trochlear angle

Table 4 Depth of the trochlea (mm) at 15° according to group (control vs OPI).

Control	OPI
7.8 ± 1.6	2.3 ± 1.8
$P = 0.0001$	

Table 5 Depth of trochlea, pathological threshold value

	≤4 mm	>4 mm
OPI ($n = 138$)	85%	15%
Control ($n = 30$)	3%	97%

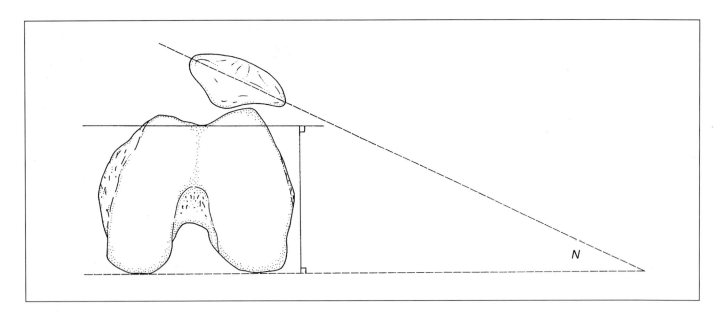

Figure 6

The patellar tilt is defined by the transverse axis of the patella and the posterior bicondylar plane ($N<20°$).

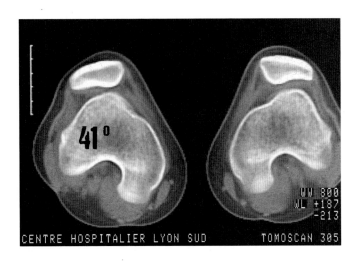

Figure 7

Nineteen-year-old female patient who has had several luxations of the patella: the patellar tilt is 41°.

Table 6 Patellar tilt (degrees) according to group (control vs OPI).

Control	OPI
10.8 ± 5.4	31.5 ± 9.4
	$P < 0.05$

Table 7 Patellar tilt, pathological threshold value

	$\geqslant 20°$	$<20°$
OPI ($n = 93$)	90%	10%
Control ($n = 27$)	3%	97%

(mean = 10°) the values are highly significantly different (Table 6). The threshold beyond which the value is pathological is 20° of patellar tilt. Beyond 20°, there is thus an anomaly, which we found in 90% of OPI. The specificity was increased when the mean patellar tilt was measured with quadriceps contracted; with the quadriceps relaxed, the threshold still remained at 20° (Figures 6 and 7) (Table 7).

Therapeutic procedures allow the origin of this tilt to be determined: sectioning of the lateral retinaculum does not modify it; suturing of the medial capsule does not modify it; medialization of the anterior tibial tuberosity diminishes it, without ever completely abolishing it. In such cases, the therapeutic procedure is therefore not physiological.

The only procedure able to perfectly correct the patellar tilt is plasty of the vastus medialis. We perform an Insall type of plasty; thus, it is perfectly possible to horizontalize the patella and sometimes, even if the end of the vastus medialis is oversectioned, to obtain a medial tilt. However, it cannot be claimed that this is a perfectly physiological procedure as, in these cases of horizontalization of the patella, the contraction of the quadriceps does not increase the tilt as in normal subjects. For this reason we consider that the dysplasia of the quadriceps is not limited to an abnormality of the vastus medialis.

The height of the patella (Figures 8 and 9)

This is very difficult to measure, and the reliability of the measurement is still unsatisfactory. We have used the index of Caton[8] and Deschamps:[9] this is the ratio

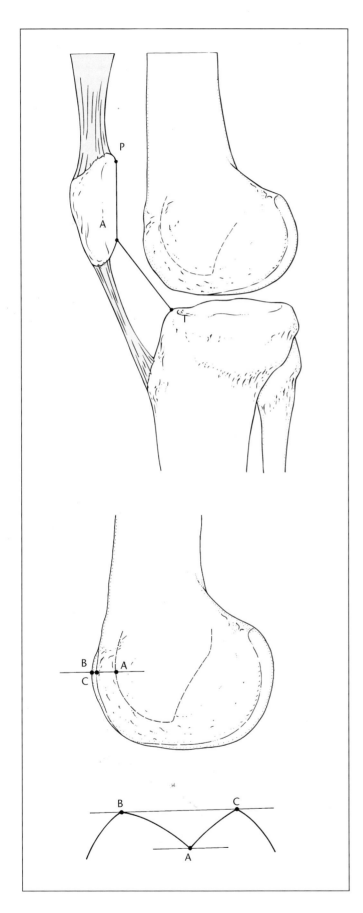

Figure 8

The patellar height is defined by the relation AT/AP: the normal value is between 0.8 and 1.2.

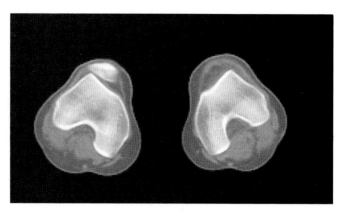

Figure 9

Thirty-one-year-old woman with record of patellar luxations: left, the patella is high as shown by the absence of the patella on the left of the CT scan and the patellar index (41/33 = 1.24), which is abnormally high.

between the distance of the lower edge of the patellar joint surface to the upper edge of the tibial plateau and the length of the patellar articular surface. The control subjects have a mean index of 0.95, whereas in the OPI group the mean is 1.12. There is a significant difference between these two groups: we speak of high patella when the patellar index is greater than 1.12; this factor has considerable significance, since we do not find a high patella in the control subjects, whereas it occurs in 24% of the OPI group. It may thus be said that if the index is 1.2, the patella is high. This essential factor is found most often in postoperative relapses when the surgeon has overlooked this correction.

It is to be noted that in these high patellae, we almost always observed a stiffness of the anterior part of the quadriceps. This sign is demonstrated by attempting to obtain, with the hip in extension, a complete flexion of the knee; the heel remains at a distance from the buttock. It may be that the high patella is a minor form of quadriceps contracture.

The excessive TT–TG (Figure 10)

Albert Trillat[11] had insisted on the importance of the baionnette, i.e. the angle formed by the patellar tendon and the implantation of the anterior tibial tuberosity. This obliquity of the patellar tendon, which is one of the elements of the Q angle, is a long-established factor in subluxation whose consequent therapeutic indication is medialization of the anterior tibial tuberosity. This procedure proved very efficacious against patellar luxations, but at the expense of a medial patellofemoral conflict when the medialization was excessive.

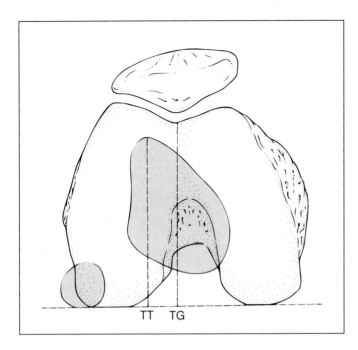

Figure 10

Measurement of the TT–TG: a value greater than 20 mm is pathological.

Goutalier and Bernageau[12] have refined this concept and made it radiographically measurable. The TT–TG, measured by scanner, is obtained by the superimposition of the femoral section passing through the upper portion of the trochlea, on the tibial section passing through the anterior tibial tuberosity. The groove of the trochlea and the middle part of the tibial tuberosity are lowered perpendicularly on the posterior bicondylar line where the TT–TG is measured in millimetres. This measure

Table 8 TT–TG, results (mm) according to group (control vs OPI).

Control	OPI
12.7 ± 3.4	19.8 ± 6
P = 0.0002	

Table 9 TT–TG, pathological threshold value

	≥20 mm	<20 mm
OPI (n = 143)	56%	44%
Control (n = 27)	3.5%	96.5%

expresses the resultant of the lateral implantation of the anterior tibial tuberosity on the tibia and of the lateral rotation of the knee. In the case of a highly dysplastic trochlea, the bottom of the trochlea may be difficult to determine. The TT–TG was measured with the knee in extension. In the control subjects it is on average 12.7 mm, whereas in the OPI group it measures an average of 19.8 mm (Table 8). There is a statistically significant difference between these two groups (by definition, measurement of the TT–TG includes the rotation in the knee; in fact this rotation is not a very specific factor, unlike the TT–TG) (Table 9).

Secondary factors

Secondary factors also appear to be very different in the control group and the OPI group. We have retained three secondary factors:

1. Genu valgum: this is present in 23% of the cases in the control population as against 46% in the OPI population.
2. The mean femoral anteversion, whose value is 15° in the control population and 21° in the OPI population.
3. The recurvatum, whose mean value is 1.7° in the control population and 4° in the OPI group.

All these figures are statistically very different in the two populations.

Luxating dysplasia of the patella

Armed with these criteria, we were able to analyse all the cases presenting with patellofemoral pathology. We found that in patellofemoral pathology it is possible to isolate a very characteristic group, i.e. objective patellar instability. In all cases the patella had been luxated once or several times. In this OPI group there are a certain number of morphological abnormalities as mentioned above. A fundamental factor is dysplasia of the trochlea, and a high-sited patella. The secondary factors genu valgum, femoral anteversion and recurvatum must also be assessed.

In cases of OPI, several factors are present: almost always dysplasia of the trochlea. In addition, one or more main factors are encountered, but not necessarily all of them. We have found these same morphological abnormalities to be more marked in some cases of permanent or habitual luxations.

In addition to this easily identifiable population (12% of the subjects have had one or more luxations), there are patients who present with a patellofemoral symptomatology without history of true luxation.

With the criteria that we have defined, we analysed all the cases presenting a pathology with history of true luxation. Two distinct populations can be defined:

1. Where one factor is present, such as dysplasia of the trochlea.
2. Where there is no known morphological abnormality. This is known as 'painful patellar syndrome'.

Thus, we can say that in patellofemoral pathology it is possible to isolate a very characteristic population where there is luxation and dysplasia of the trochlea. This population is quite unlike the overall population of painful patellar syndrome, where there is no patellar instability in the mechanical sense of the term. It is interesting to note that these patellar syndromes are comparable to the control subjects.

In conclusion, we have been able to establish the following classification:

1. Luxation dysplasia of the patella with following three forms:
   (a) Major patellar instability
   (b) Objective patellar instability
   (c) Potential patellar instability.
   Certain aetiological data are of interest: the frequency of family cases (10%), as well as the age at which problems commence. The mean age is 10.5 years in the case of objective patellar instability and 27 years in the case of potential patellar instability.
2. Painful patellar syndromes.

Surgical treatment of patellar instability

Surgical treatment is often indicated, especially when the patients are young. Certainly, diligent re-education and the wearing of a knee support may improve the patient's comfort temporarily. Although re-education may be very efficacious where there is atrophy of the quadriceps, it can never compensate a true dysplasia of the quadriceps with a high patella and an excessive TT–TG. The correction of structural defects, if possible before the cartilage damage, will prevent or delay the onset of patellofemoral osteoarthritis. Our opinion is that one should operate systematically in any true objective patellar instability once dysplasia of the trochlea with clinical symptoms is established.

There is no 'miracle' operation applicable to all cases. It is indispensable to carry out a complete examination of the knee, with strict profile radiography at 30° of flexion, axial view at 30° of flexion and,

in particular, CT scan following the strict protocol to calculate the TT–TG and the patellar tilt.

It may be said that in patellar instability surgical treatment is 'à la carte'. The anatomical defects must be treated as they are discovered. Sectioning of lateral retinaculum should be undertaken systematically, but this is never sufficient in itself. Another necessary procedure is to recentre the patella. A high patella (patellar index greater than 1.2) necessitates lowering of the patella so that the patellar instability is brought to a value of 1.

The presence of an excessive TT–TG (greater than 20 mm) requires a medialization so that the TT–TG is reduced to 10 mm (below this the risk of hypercorrection is very high). A patellar tilt greater than 20° requires an Insall type plasty of the vastus internus.

The problem of dysplasia of the trochlea

The most commonly observed defect is the filling in of the upper portion of the trochlea, but it is also the most difficult to correct. For flat, convex trochleas, trochleoplasty hollowing[1] is logical but technically difficult to perform, and its outcome will depend on the shape of the patella, which is difficult to analyse with precision. The flat trochlea often but not always corresponds to a flat patella. Here, trochleoplasty would not be a logical procedure.

If correction of subluxation factors is perfect, there will still be a trochlea that remains dysplastic. This no doubt accounts for our results. With the treatment proposed, it can be said that our results of stability correction are excellent, giving over 90% perfectly stable patellae. On the other hand, our results are not so good regarding the problem of pain and resumption of sports activities. Certainly, the presence of cartilaginous lesions of patellar chondromalacia have their role to play. However, for us this problem is not as important as the persistence of the trochlear dysplasia. The complete disappearance of pain is observed in 60% of the cases and resumption of normal sports activities in only 40% of the cases.

Complementary surgical procedures may be necessary, essentially for pronounced dysplasias. In such cases, we have seen that it is sometimes necessary to disinsert the quadriceps, using the technique of Judet.[5]

In cases of very large trochlear dysplasia, it is possible to perform a trochleoplasty by superolateral verge heightening.[13] This is not a physiological procedure but it may prove efficacious, raising the lateral slope of the trochlea to counter the luxation irrespective of the shape of the patella.

Similarly, in very marked type III trochleas, when the patella has a tendency to subluxate even in flexion at 30°, it may be useful to perform what we call a low plasty, i.e. a transfer of the sartorius muscle and the semitendinosus tendon to the inferior portion of the patella. This transfer results in a very efficacious tenodesis in flexion, thereby providing some support to the medial aileron of the patella.

It is only in very rare cases that we perform femoral osteotomies, whether of high derotation type or of the distal femoral variety, to correct an excessive valgus.

References

1. Dejour H, Walch G, Neyret Ph et al., La dysplasie de la trochlée fémorale, *Rev Chir Orthop* (1990) 76: 45–54.
2. Maldague B, Malghem J, Apport du cliché de profil du genou dans le dépistage des instabilités rotuliennes, *Rev Chir Orthop* (1985) 71 (suppl. II): 5–13.
3. Dejour H, Walch G, La pathologie fémoro-patellaire, 6ème Journées Lyonnaises de Chirurgie du Genou, Lyon, 1987.
4. Brattström H, Shape of the intercondylar groove normally and in recurrent dislocation of patella: A clinical and X-ray anatomical investigation, *Acta Orthop Scand* (1964) suppl. 68: 1–148.
5. Judet J, Judet H, L'allongement du vaste externe dans les luxations et subluxations de la rotule, *Nouv Press Med* (1975) 4 (22).
6. Hughston JC, Walsh WM, Puddu G, Patellar subluxation and dislocation (Philadelphia: WB Saunders, 1984).
7. Insall J, Bullough PG, Burnstein AH, Proximal "tube" realignment of the patella for chondromalacia patellae, *Clin Orthop* (1979) 144: 63–69.
8. Caton J, Les ruptures du système extenseur du genou (Diss., Lyon, 1979).
9. Deschamps G, Les rotules basses. Etude étiopathologique clinique et propositions thérapeutiques (Diss., Lyon, 1981).
10. Levigne C, Chirurgie itérative des instabilités rotuliennes et syndrome rotuliens douloureux (Diss., Lyon, 1988).
11. Trillat A, Dejour H, Couette A, Diagnostic et traitement des subluxations récidivantes de la rotule, *Rev Chir Orthop* (1964) 50: 813–824.
12. Goutalier D, Bernageau J, Lecudonnec B, Mesure de l'écart tubérosité tibiale antérieure—gorge de la trochlée: TA–GT, *Rev Chir Orthop* (1978) 64: 423–428.
13. Albee FH, The bone graft wedge in the treatment of habitual dislocation of the patella, *Med Rec* (1915) 88: 257–259.

9

Chondral and osteochondral lesions

9.1   Osteochondritis dissecans of the knee: An overview

Paul M. Aichroth and Dipak V. Patel

The term osteochondritis dissecans (OCD) was first used by König in 1887.[1] He claimed that loose bodies in the knee joints of young individuals had three causes: (1) severe trauma; (2) less severe trauma causing contusion and necrosis; and (3) minimal trauma acting on an underlying lesion—for which he coined the term 'osteochondritis dissecans'. König had an ear for a euphonious title, as pointed out by Barrie.[2] The name was misleading as osteochondritis suggests an inflammatory condition. However, despite much dispute the title is still being used universally.

Osteochondritis dissecans is a condition characterized by separation of a segment of articular cartilage together with subchondral bone, either completely or partially, from the joint surface. It most commonly involves the knee joint but the lesion has also been reported in the elbow (capitellum), ankle (dome of the talus) and femoral head.[3] In the knee, the femoral condyles are usually affected. The lesion is often unilateral, but symmetrical and bilateral lesions are sometimes encountered in clinical practice. The fragment may stay in its crater, remaining silent clinically, or alternatively may produce symptoms of pain, intermittent swelling, joint irritability, and giving way or locking.

Historical review and aetiological factors

Loose bodies in joints were first recognized by Ambroise Paré in 1558, who must be credited not only for the first recognition of the disease but also for the first reported case of the surgical removal of a loose body from the knee joint.[4,5] Monroe in 1726 found a pea-sized arthrophyte which originated from the lateral femoral condyle during a cadaveric examination. He assumed that the origin of the loose body was trauma.[4]

Although numerous articles have been written about OCD, its precise aetiology still remains controversial. Multiple theories have been proposed.

Trauma theory

In 1870, Sir James Paget gave a classic account of OCD.[6] He had two patients in whom he thought that trauma was the predisposing factor. As mentioned previously, König was the first to use the term osteochondritis dissecans and he believed the cause of this 'dissection' to be traumatic.[1] Since then, various authors have agreed with them.[7-13] Fairbank suggested that impingement of the anterior tibial spine against the lateral aspect of the medial femoral condyle during the last few degrees of knee extension may be responsible.[8] His concept was later supported by Smillie.[12,14]

Rosenberg examined osteochondral fractures in 15 subjects and concluded that non-union of undisplaced osteochondral fractures appears radiologically and microscopically indistinguishable from OCD.[15] Aichroth, while reviewing 100 patients with OCD found that trauma was an important aetiological factor.[7] In his series, a history of significant trauma was obtained in 46% of the patients. He suggested that the pathogenesis of OCD is an ununited osteochondral or subchondral fracture.

Various experimental studies also support the clinical impression that trauma is the aetiology of OCD.[16-19] Rehbein subjected dogs' knees to repeated minor trauma, thereby producing lesions that were radiologically and histologically similar to OCD.[18]

Langenskiöld and later Tallqvist excised portions of the epiphyseal cartilage in the knees of young rabbits.[17,19] The fragments were left attached by a bridge of synovial tissue in the intercondylar notch. It was noted that the fragments developed a bony nucleus resembling osteochondritis. Langenskiöld concluded that OCD may be caused by a cartilage fracture in childhood. Aichroth conducted a similar study using adult New Zealand White rabbits and showed that undisplaced but stable osteochondral fractures resembled OCD in the human both radiographically and histologically.[16]

Milgram examined the specimens from 50 operated cases of OCD of the distal femur.[20] On histological analysis, he found that 24 specimens showed no attached subchondral osseous fragments, whilst the remaining 26 did. This led him to believe that the defect was not at the subchondral bone level as postulated by Axhausen,[21] Green and Banks[22] and Chiroff and Cooke.[23] On the basis of pathological findings, Milgram suggested trauma as the possible aetiological factor.

Recently, Anderson et al.[24] agreed with the consensus of the literature that the aetiology of OCD, in the classic site on the medial femoral condyle, is trauma. They believed that a subchondral fracture is the precursor to OCD.

Cahill et al. suggested that juvenile OCD lesions are stress fractures of the subchondral bone resulting from the cumulative stresses of exercise.[25]

A history of previous knee injury (usually of minimal to moderate degree) has been reported in approximately 40% of the patients with OCD.[4,7,9,22,23,26–30] In contrast, Carroll and Mubarak, while reviewing 75 patients with OCD, found no relation between OCD and trauma, patellar dislocations or hypertrophic tibial spines.[31]

However, the incidence of bilateral lesions cannot be explained solely on the basis of trauma. Clearly, some other factors (not yet known) must be responsible.

Ischaemia theory

Some authors have postulated that OCD results from an interruption of blood flow which causes ischaemic necrosis and eventual sequestration of the subchondral bone and articular cartilage. Koch in 1879 performed a series of experiments on bone necrosis and reported that articular bone infarction with loose body formation was the result of obstruction of the entire capillary bed of the area concerned.[32]

Axhausen suggested that an embolus of tubercle bacilli blocked the blood supply.[21] Rieger[33] implicated fat emboli, whereas Watson-Jones[34] suggested that OCD in multiple sites in the adolescents was due to bone infarcts caused by the clumping of the red blood cells.

Enneking noted that the subchondral bone has a vascular arcade similar to that of the bowel mesentery, which has poor anastomosis with the surrounding arterioles.[35] Additional trauma can lead to fracture of the articular cartilage and detachment of the fragment. In contrast, Rogers and Gladstone found that there is a rich blood supply to the distal femur, with numerous anastomoses in the cancellous bone.[36] They concluded that ischaemia was unlikely to be the aetiological factor of OCD.

Ficat et al. performed bone marrow pressure studies in patients with OCD and osteonecrosis and revealed that all their patients had high marrow pressure, which they felt signified vascular obstruction.[37]

Other theories

Various other factors have been suggested as to the aetiology of OCD. These include abnormalities of ossification of the epiphyseal cartilage,[38,39] hereditary influences and generalized disorders such as epiphyseal

dysplasia multiplex and Fröhlich's syndrome.[14,40–42]

Several papers have reported on the familial incidence of OCD.[43–49] However, Petrie revealed no definite genetic aetiology associated with OCD.[50] He examined first- and second-degree relatives of 34 patients with OCD and found that only one had OCD. It seems that heredity has very little, if any, relationship with OCD other than a rare familial form described by Clanton and DeLee.[51] None the less, there are a few reported associations of OCD with dwarfism,[52] tibia vara[53] and Legg–Calve–Perthes' disease,[54] which would support the genetic theory in isolated cases.

In conclusion, the aetiology of OCD still remains uncertain. Further experimental and clinical research is needed to resolve the continuing controversy.

Clinical features and diagnosis of osteochondritis dissecans

Lindén studied the incidence of OCD in the city of Malmö (Sweden) and estimated that 15–21 cases per 100 000 knees had OCD.[55] He concluded that at least 4% of all cases of primary gonarthrosis in men were caused by OCD earlier in life. Recently, Federico et al. (1990) reported an incidence of 3–6 per 10 000 in adults.[56]

Osteochondritis dissecans commonly occurs in children and adolescents between 10 and 20 years of age. The condition is more prevalent in boys than in girls. Green and Banks reported that the condition is common in children over the age of 4 years.[22] In Clanton and DeLee's series, two groups of patients were encountered: one of children under the age of 15 years and the other of adults up to the age of 50 years.[51]

The condition predominantly affects the lateral aspect of the medial femoral condyle. The lateral femoral condyle is involved in approximately 15–20% of all the affected knees.[7,9,22,55] The lesion can also affect the trochlea of the femur, an unusual site. An excellent account of OCD involving the trochlea is given by Smith.[57]

The symptoms of OCD of the knee are often vague and intermittent. The patient presents with low-grade pain, recurrent swelling, joint irritability, and giving way or locking. The clinical signs may be inconclusive. Examination findings include localized tenderness over the affected area, effusion, quadriceps atrophy, crepitus, restriction of knee movement, and sometimes a positive Wilson's sign (pain with extension of the knee and internal rotation of tibia).[58] On rare occasions, a detached loose body may be palpated in the knee joint.

The plain radiographs usually show a well-circumscribed fragment of subchondral bone which is demarcated from the surrounding femoral condyle by

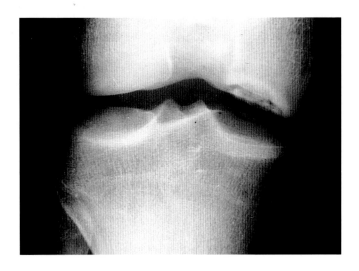

Figure 1

Radiograph showing osteochondritis dissecans involving the medial femoral condyle in a 22-year-old male patient.

a radiolucent crescent-shaped line (Figure 1). The affected bone may appear denser than the surrounding parent bone. As the fragment gradually separates, a crater or depression may be seen.

The topographic location and size of the lesion must be meticulously recorded. It should also be stated whether the weight-bearing or non-weight-bearing area of the femoral articular surface is affected. The radiographs in Figure 2 show a massive OCD defect affecting the weight-bearing surface of the medial femoral condyle in an 18-year-old male patient.

Radioisotope bone scan, tomography, computed tomographic (CT) scan and magnetic resonance imaging (MRI) are useful for the evaluation of this lesion.

Cahill et al. concluded that radioisotope bone scan is the most sensitive diagnostic procedure for monitoring the clinical course of juvenile OCD.[25] It is often also useful in determining the need for operative intervention, especially in patients with large and undisplaced lesions.[59,60]

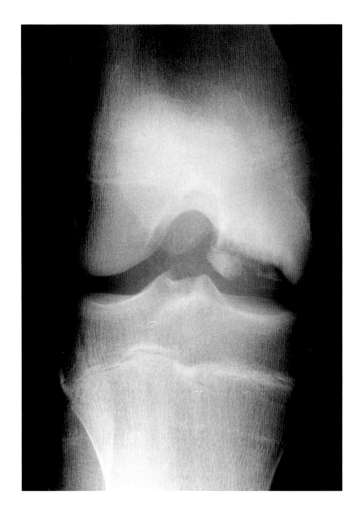

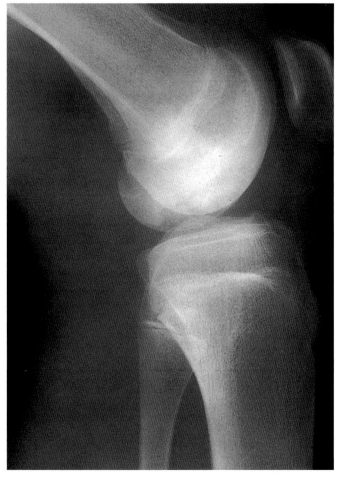

Figure 2

Radiographs showing a massive osteochondritis dissecans defect involving the weight-bearing surface of the medial femoral condyle in an 18-year-old male patient.

McCullough et al. reported the preliminary results of dynamic bone scintigraphy in OCD.[61] They studied 18 patients, 11 of whom had OCD. The diagnosis rate was 29% with static scintigraphy and this improved to 57% when dynamic flow studies were used. A positive pattern in the dynamic study together with plain radiographs and static scintigraphs raised the specificity to 100% and the sensitivity to 90%. However, a prospective clinical study involving a larger number of patients is required before definite conclusions can be drawn.

Tomography and CT scans provide architectural description of the lesion but do not provide an index of spontaneous healing potential.[56] Magnetic resonance imaging holds considerable promise as a more sensitive technique for early diagnosis of OCD of the knee. MRI appears to be the investigation of choice to follow sequentially the healing process and revascularization of OCD lesion, and is also useful in assessing the status of the articular cartilage.[62] However, Anderson et al. reported that the status of the articular cartilage, as demonstrated by MRI, could not be correlated with the degree of degenerative changes or the results of surgery.[24]

With recent advances in both arthroscopic technique and instrumentation, the diagnosis and management of this disorder has undergone considerable evolution. Arthroscopic assessment is helpful for diagnostic confirmation and staging of the lesion. The most important advantage of arthroscopy is that it can be used therapeutically to treat the OCD lesion. Moreover, the healing response of the disease process can also be monitored by percutaneous visualization. One can argue that the same objective may be achieved by a non-invasive technique such as MRI, and thus spare the patient from undergoing arthroscopy.

Osteochondritis dissecans must be differentiated from osteonecrosis and osteochondral fracture of the femoral condyles. Bradley and Dandy reviewed lesions of the femoral condyles in 5000 consecutive arthroscopies and were able to distinguish the characteristics of developing and late osteochondritis dissecans, acute and old osteochondral fractures, chondral separations, chondral flaps and idiopathic osteonecrosis.[63]

Osteochondral fractures at the knee

Osteochondral fractures of any part of the articular surface of the knee may occur in a variety of traumatic incidents. Direct blows, ligament ruptures and patellar dislocations are frequently responsible. Matthewson and Dandy pointed out that indirect violence and especially pivoting on an extending knee produces shearing forces severe enough to avulse segments of articular cartilage and subchondral bone.[64] The lateral femoral condyle is especially involved with an osteochondral fracture after this type of sports injury.

Osteochondral fractures of the patella have been recognized since the beginning of this century; Milgram was the first to describe the tangential osteochondral fracture so characteristic of a patellar dislocation.[65]

Kennedy et al. classified two groups: (1) exogenous fractures resulting from direct injury, and (2) endogenous fractures resulting from combined rotatory and compression forces.[66] These workers found clinical examples where fractures of most areas of both condyles were present with separation of a fragment. They further studied these endogenous fractures, setting up experiments in the cadaveric knee joint in which strong axial compression and rotatory forces were applied. They found that certain osteochondral fractures of the weight-bearing surface could be produced by this method.

In clinical practice, osteochondral fractures of the medial and lateral condylar weight-bearing surfaces may be sustained by rotatory forces on the flexed knee as in football and skiing injuries. A direct shearing force on the anterior surface of the medial condyle may occur in a fall on the flexed knee, and a direct shearing force on the lateral condyle may be sustained by a kick on the outside of the knee.

It has been pointed out by Landells[67] and Rosenberg[15] that adult articular cartilage tears at the junction between the calcified and uncalcified zones. The immature adolescent cartilage does not have this calcified zone, hence the shearing forces are transmitted to the subchondral bone; it is here that osteochondral fractures occur. Clinically, the osteochondral fracture is nearly always confined to adolescence. O'Donoghue believed that there is no real difference between an osteochondral fracture and OCD.[68]

Experimental osteochondral fractures in animals

Aichroth studied the natural history of experimental osteochondral fractures of various types in an attempt to relate these fractures to the clinical disease.[16] Sixty adult New Zealand White rabbits were used. A knee arthrotomy was undertaken under general anaesthesia and various osteochondral cuts were made into the medial femoral condyle (Figure 3).

In 31 animals the fragments were fully separated from the joint surface. In Group I, the fragments were cut in such a way that they remained unstable and would shift on joint movement. In Group II, the fragments were cut in such a way that when they were replaced in their crater they remained in situ, well embedded and fairly stable. In Group III, the fragments were returned to their crater and internally fixed with fine stainless steel pins.

In 29 animals fractures were made through the femoral condyle. In Group IV, a substantial intercondylar bridge was left. In Group V, a minimal inter-condylar bridge of bone remained, leaving a bridge that was unstable and that usually broke when the animals were exercised.

The union and non-union rates in each group were noted. In Group I, in which the fragment was shifting, most fragments remained ununited. In Group II, in which there was a more stable fragment in situ, 8 of the 13 animals' fragments united. In those in which internal fixation pins stabilized the fragments, all united rapidly. In Group V, the medial femoral condylar cut was made, leaving only a minimal bridge of intercondylar bone. This bridge proved unstable and 8 of the 17 united, with 9 remaining ununited.

To summarize these results, osteochondral fractures which were cut in such a way that shift occurred progressed to a non-union state. Those adequately fixed did unite. Non-union of an osteochondral fragment was characterized by a necrotic osseous portion with viable cartilage. The junctional zone between the crater and the fragment contained much fibrous tissue and fibrocartilaginous material. The appearance of the ununited osteochondral fragment was similar to that in OCD in the human.

Treatment

It is generally agreed that the management of OCD depends on skeletal maturity and the stage of the lesion. It is imperative that healing is obtained prior to the epiphyseal closure.

Management of juvenile osteochondritis dissecans

Lindén studied the natural history of juvenile osteochondritis dissecans (JOCD).[27] He reviewed 23 joints (open physis) at an average follow-up of 33 years after the time of diagnosis, and commented that 'there were no complications later in life which could with certainty be referred to osteochondritis dissecans'. He concluded that secondary gonarthrosis usually does not develop in patients with a diagnosis of JOCD irrespective of the treatment. However, one must point out that the mean age of these patients at the time of review was 45.5 years, and many of them had not attained an age at which secondary degenerative changes are likely to occur.

Spontaneous healing of JOCD lesions is reported by various authors.[22,69–71] However, not all lesions of JOCD heal spontaneously, as shown by others.[7,25,39,60,72] Large, detached lesions often lead to non-union and therefore require surgical intervention.[59,73]

Cahill and Berg observed that if the fragment of JOCD does not heal before skeletal maturity (that is, before closure of physis), its natural history resembles that of the adult with OCD, and may have a poor overall prognosis.[60] They suggested that radioisotope bone scan is useful to determine the healing response and possible surgical intervention.

The management of JOCD is controversial. Conservative measures include immobilization or restricted activity.[9,51,74] Green and Banks reported a series of children treated by non-weight-bearing and immobilization, and found that the lesions healed in 17 out of

	Group 1	Group 2	Group 3	Group 4	Group 5
	SHIFTING	STABLE	PINNED	BRIDGED	UNSTABLE BRIDGE
Animals	8	13	10	12	17
Fragments united	1	8	10	12	8
Fragments not united	7	5	0	0	9

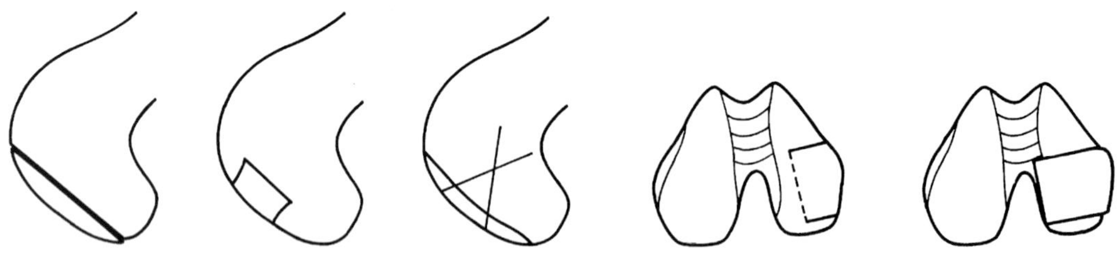

60 Animals — 31 Fragments / 29 Fragments

Figure 3

The experimental plan. Osteochondral fractures in animals (From Aichroth P, Osteochondral fractures and their relationship to osteochondritis dissecans of the knee: an experimental study in animals, *J Bone Joint Surg (Br)* (1971) **53**: 448–454, reproduced with kind permission).

18 cases in an average of 4 months.[22] Smillie suggested that immobilization should not exceed 16 weeks for undisplaced lesions in patients under 15 years of age.[75] Later, Salter and Field[76] and Hughston et al.[72] demonstrated the deleterious effects of prolonged immobilization, including knee stiffness, quadriceps atrophy and possible cartilage degeneration.

We believe that immobilization should be kept to a minimum and reserved only for acute painful situations. Once the child is comfortable, quadriceps rehabilitation should be commenced. Some authors prefer activity modification, but this may be impractical in a child. If the symptoms do not subside within 8–10 weeks and if the bone scan or MRI provides evidence of decreased healing, then arthroscopic assessment should be undertaken. We share the opinion with Anderson et al.[24] that a more aggressive surgical intervention should be undertaken if the conservative measures fail in a child who is approaching skeletal maturity.

If the fragment is found detached from its crater and may have been a loose body for some time, then this loose fragment should be removed at arthroscopy or via arthrotomy in difficult situations. If the fragment is mobile in its crater, then arthroscopic assessment of the lesion must be undertaken to ascertain the stability of the fragment. If the fragment is shown to be tightly in situ, the lesion may be left alone and the patient treated conservatively as outlined previously.

Some surgeons feel that the symptomatic stable fragment should be drilled in an effort to increase the vascularity of the non-union. There has not been a controlled trial of drilling to determine its efficacy, and the author assessed a small series of similar stable fragments—some drilled and some left alone. There was no real difference in the outcome of the two groups, as some lesions united and some loosened in both treatment programmes.

Numerous surgical procedures have been advocated for the management of persistently symptomatic lesions. These include drilling, pinning or screw fixation, bone grafting or excision of the unstable fragment with or without curettage of the crater.

Smillie recommended open drilling of the lesion in children if healing is not adequate by 4 months.[75] With the advent of arthroscopy, percutaneous drilling has become possible. Various authors have claimed good or excellent results with arthroscopic drilling.[51,73,77–79]

Bradley and Dandy[77] in their series of 10 children with classical lesions of OCD treated by arthroscopic drilling noticed significant pain relief within one week of surgery. The lesion had healed radiologically within 12 months in 9 out of 11 knees.

Replacement and fixation of a loose fragment

An acute osteochondral fracture with a substantial portion of bone that fits accurately into the crater from which it was detached may be replaced and internally fixed with success. It must be emphasized that it is the acute osteochondral fracture that may be treated in this way, and the results of this type of reattachment are usually excellent.

The reattachment of a chronic OCD loose body is a different matter, as the osseous fragment is always covered by fibrous tissue or by a hyperplastic hyaline cartilage. When the fibrous or cartilaginous tissue is removed, the bony apposition is less accurate and the fragment may fit poorly into its crater. The fit can be improved by curettage of the crater to remove all the fibrocartilaginous material present and adding bone graft.

Smillie successfully treated 10 patients with screw or pin fixation.[75] Bone pegs have also been used for fixation of the fragment.[28,29,80–84] Lipscomb et al. used Kirschner wires to fix loose fragments in 8 knees.[85] They stressed the importance of removing the fibrous tissue from the base of the crater and drilling the subchondral bone to improve vascularity. They used cancellous bone graft before replacing and pinning the fragment.

Hughston et al. fixed large fragments in nine cases using bent Kirschner wires, which can be removed percutaneously.[72] They felt that the results of replacement and fixation were superior to excision of the fragment.

Johnson et al. reviewed 29 patients (32 knees) with OCD who underwent arthroscopic compression screw fixation.[26] Results were excellent or good for 88% of the knees at an average follow-up of 3.5 years (range 2–6 years). The procedure is technically demanding and requires considerable experience and expertise. The results are excellent at this relatively early stage and we feel that this must be the treatment of choice where the fragment is large and replacement is possible.

The Herbert screw has also been recommended for securing the OCD fragment under arthroscopic control.[86,87] This is certainly an attractive concept that may be useful for unstable OCD fragments that are not completely detached from the femoral condyles. In Thomson's series, 16 of the 18 lesions united as determined by radiographs.[87] The follow-up was short and was reported as 4–28 months.

Bone grafting with or without pinning has been used with varying success.[24,88,89]

Excision of the fragment

Excision of the unstable fragment is suggested by various authors.[7,90,91] Excision of the fragment should be undertaken if the lesion is small, if it is impossible to fix the fragment internally owing to its mechanical characteristics, or if the defect contains multiple small broken fragments. The arthroscopic appearance of a massive defect affecting the medial femoral condyle in a 17-year-old girl is shown in Figure 4.

The crater should be curetted down to bleeding subchondral bone. This is undertaken with an arthroscopic curette and rongeurs and should then be completed with the powered instruments, including the burr (Figures 5 and 6). The edges of the crater should be cut cleanly to make absolutely certain that there are no loose osteochondral fragments at this site.

There appears to be no need to immobilize the patient postoperatively and normal function and weight bearing is to be encouraged. We advocate a 'second-look' arthroscopy at approximately 6 months to make sure that the fibrocartilaginous covering is satisfactory and the edges of the crater are smooth and require no further trimming.

The appearance of the crater filled with reparative fibrocartilage is usually satisfactory by 6–9 months (Figure 7). Although the fibrocartilaginous material is soft, it is stable on the osseous bed beneath and by 18 months the thickness of the fibrocartilage may be remarkable. The appearance of the crater filled with reparative fibrocartilage at 12 months in a 17-year-old boy is shown in Figure 8.

It should be noted that most knees affected by OCD in which a loose body has been shed demonstrate an obvious defect on the condylar surface from which the fragment came. However, in some knees examined radiologically or by arthroscopy, the site of separation cannot be detected and the weight-bearing surfaces – the classic site – and the retropatellar region all appear pristine. The quality of resurfacing of the OCD defect has been so good in these cases that the examiner cannot determine the original site of the lesion. The defect fills with fibrous tissue and fibrocartilaginous material that appears smooth and seems to be of good weight-bearing quality.

The quality and quantity of repair in fibrocartilage depend upon the depth of the crater and its size.[92] Experiments in large animals confirm that articular cartilage has very limited capacity of repair if the defect is of partial thickness. Full-thickness defects are replaced by a major ingrowth of vascularized connective tissue, with the primitive stem cells from which it arises being the mesenchymal cells of the exposed bone.[92] The completeness of repair, however, seems to depend upon the size of the osteochondral defect. Poor quality and quantity of repair material in the defect will have an increasingly deleterious effect on the articular cartilage on the opposite side of the joint.

Recently, Homminga et al. treated 30 chondral lesions of the knee using an autogenous strip of costal perichondrium, which was fixed to the subchondral bone with Tissucol (human fibrin glue).[93] Three of these lesions were from OCD which had been treated unsuccessfully by arthroscopic drilling. They concluded that perichondral grafting of cartilage defects of the knee gives excellent results, but long-term follow-up studies with a large number of patients are needed.

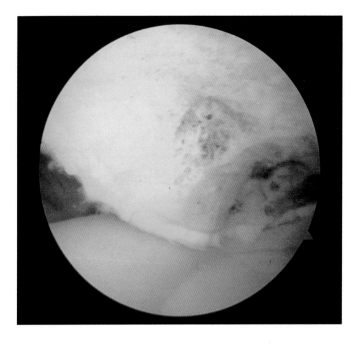

Figure 4

Arthroscopic view of a massive defect affecting the medial femoral condyle in a 17-year-old girl.

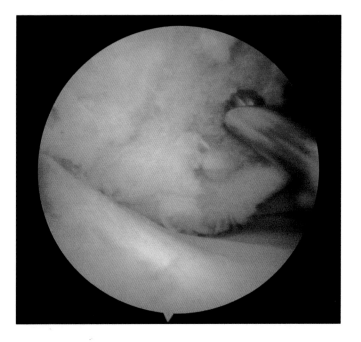

Figure 5

Arthroscopic appearance of a large osteochondritis dissecans defect involving the medial femoral condyle in a 12-year-old male patient. The base of the crater is debrided down to bleeding subchondral bone using an arthroscopic burr.

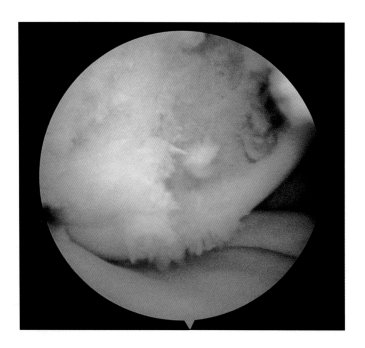

Figure 6

Arthroscopic view of the same lesion (Figure 5) after debridement and burring.

Osteochondral allografts

The incomplete repair of large defects has stimulated much research into the possibility of replacement with autografts and allografts. Bentley has shown that grafts of chondrocytes isolated from epiphyseal growth plates will allow rapid resurfacing of small defects with good-quality hyaline cartilage.[94] This research continues. Much work in both small animals and sheep has shown that shell allografts of articular hyaline cartilage and subchondral bone will produce satisfactory resurfacing and union of the graft if fixation is perfect.

Gross and Langer extended this line of research to the human and are now regularly replacing the knee hemijoint with cadaveric block allografts with good early results.[95]

Adult osteochondritis dissecans

The natural history of adult osteochondritis dissecans (AOCD) has been reported by Lindén.[27] He reviewed 40 patients (average age at diagnosis 29.4 years) over a 32.5-year mean follow-up period. An additional eight adults were included in the radiographic evaluation. All patients were treated conservatively. In his series, 79% of the patients showed evidence of gonarthrosis about 10 years earlier in life than

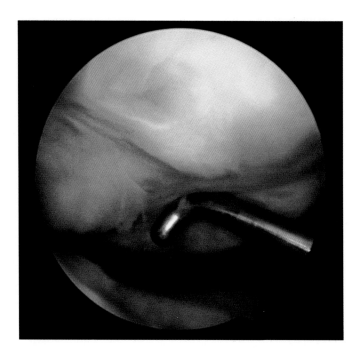
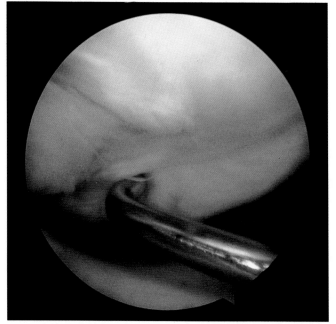

Figure 7

'Second-look' arthroscopy performed at 8 months following the initial curettage and debridement of the unstable osteochondritis dissecans lesion. A good quality of reparative fibrocartilaginous resurfacing was noted.

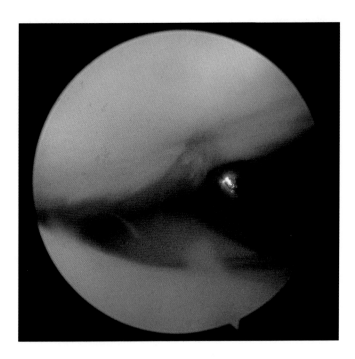

Figure 8

'Second-look' arthroscopic appearance of a healed osteochondritis dissecans lesion, 12 months following excision of the unstable osteochondritis dissecans lesion. The fibrocartilaginous surface was found soft on probing. This patient had an excellent clinical result.

primary gonarthrosis. Symptoms of degenerative arthritis began approximately 20 years after the diagnosis of OCD.

Management

The choice of surgical treatment depends on the site, size and the stability of the fragment. The lesion in situ will probably heal in the majority of cases, particularly in the young child. If it does not heal, then the movement of the fragment in the crater produces a feeling of repeated giving way. The fragment may hinge or become detached to form a loose body. While the fragment is loosening or hinging, the crater fills up with a fibrocartilaginous tissue and, later on, when the loose body has been separated for many years, it may be extremely difficult to identify the crater from which the fragment came.

Crawfurd et al. reviewed 28 patients (31 knees) with arthroscopically confirmed OCD of the femoral condyle and concluded that spontaneous healing is less likely to occur in the classical position on the medial femoral condyle.[96] There was no correlation between healing and the size of the lesion or the age of onset of OCD.

The patient should be assessed clinically and radiologically at regular intervals in order to monitor the healing response. It would be reasonable to restrict sporting activities but in a young athlete this may not be practical. If the symptoms persist despite conservative measures, then arthroscopy should be undertaken to assess the stability of the lesion.

If the fragment is stable on probing, it is left alone and conservative treatment is continued. Drilling of such a lesion through the articular surface has been suggested by Guhl.[73] The use of an image intensifier may accurately locate the site for drilling. The drilling can be performed either by the antegrade ('inside out') route or in a retrograde manner ('outside in'). The advantage of antegrade drilling is that the holes can be placed accurately and a second incision is avoided.[77] Internal fixation is usually not required for stable fragments.

The management of unstable or hinging lesions is controversial. Small, unstable fragments from non-weight-bearing surfaces of the femoral condyle may be excised if they become symptomatic. Larger lesions in such an area merit internal fixation. On the other hand, fragments from the weight-bearing area require careful consideration. Some authors[7,85] recommend excision of the fragment whilst others advocate internal fixation with or without bone grafting.

Smillie used small pins and screws for internal fixation of a detached osteochondral fragment resulting from OCD.[14] Scott and Stevenson used autogenous bone pegs and fine threaded Kirschner wires.[29] Guhl advocates curettage and debridement of the crater down to bleeding subchondral bone, and then fixation with Kirschner wires.[73] Occasionally, cancellous bone grafting to fill the base of the defect may be required.

Anderson et al. reported on the results of antegrade curettage, bone grafting and pinning of OCD in the skeletally mature knee.[24] Seventeen patients (average age at operation 17 years) were reviewed. The follow-up ranged from 5 to 7 years. Results were good or excellent for 65% of the patients, using the rating scale of Hughston et al.[72]

Recently, the absorbable bone pins and Herbert screw have become popular.[28,87] Meticulous preparation of the base of the crater is essential prior to the fixation.

The prognosis for knee function is relatively poor when there is a large defect involving the weight-bearing area.[72] Therefore, every effort should be made to reattach the large fragment that has separated from the weight-bearing surface of the femoral condyle. The articular surface should be restored, whenever possible, in large lesions of the weight-bearing area.[72,75,85] Excision of the fragment should be avoided except as a last resort.

Garrett reviewed 24 patients with osteochondral defects of the femoral condyle treated by fresh osteochondral allografts.[97] The transplantation was performed within 12 hours of harvesting. The follow-up ranged from 2 to 4 years in 10 cases and 1 to 2 years in the remaining 14. All patients improved in terms of pain, swelling, buckling and knee function, and none had lost more than 10° of knee movement. 'Second-look' arthroscopy was undertaken in 11 patients and the graft appeared viable in all 11 cases.

Thus, there are far too many treatment options and we agree with Hughston et al.[72] in that we are currently unable to treat OCD with consistently satisfactory results. We need to perform prospective randomized studies comparing different modalities of treatment. Moreover, a valid comparison between the various reported series is not possible, as the patient age group, size and location of the lesion, the type of treatment and the method of evaluation differ.[24] A universal documentation system is required for evaluation and comparison of the results, though the task is daunting.

Long-term outcome of OCD

Whether OCD of the knee will lead to degenerative changes in future depends upon various factors such as the age of the patient at the time of diagnosis, the size and site of the lesion and the method of treatment.

Lindén reviewed 67 knees with OCD after an average follow-up of 33 years and found that the incidence of osteoarthritis was higher in patients who had been diagnosed and treated after skeletal maturity.[27]

Hughston et al. examined 83 patients (95 knees) with OCD who were followed for 2 to 31 years.[72] In their series, 77% of the knees in the surgical group and 82% of those in the conservatively treated group had excellent or good results. Better results were obtained in knees in which the osteochondritic defect was small and was treated prior to epiphyseal closure, and in knees in which the fragment healed as compared with the ones from which the fragment was excised. The knees that were treated successfully by either conservative or surgical means showed little evidence of progressive long-term degeneration after follow-up of as long as 31 years.

Recently, Twyman et al. conducted a long-term follow-up study of 22 knees with OCD diagnosed before skeletal maturity.[98] The unstable lesion was excised in 13 knees. There was radiological evidence of grade II or III Ahlbäck (1968) degenerative changes in 32% of the knees at an average follow-up of 33.6 years (range 26–54 years) (Figure 9). About 50% of the knees had good or excellent functional result using the rating criteria of Hughston et al.[72] Their study suggested that in knees with a large area of denuded bone in a weight-bearing position the long-term prognosis is poor.

Osteochondritis dissecans patellae

This uncommon condition has been well reviewed by Edwards and Bentley.[99] The lesion may be associated with patellar subluxation. The fragment usually

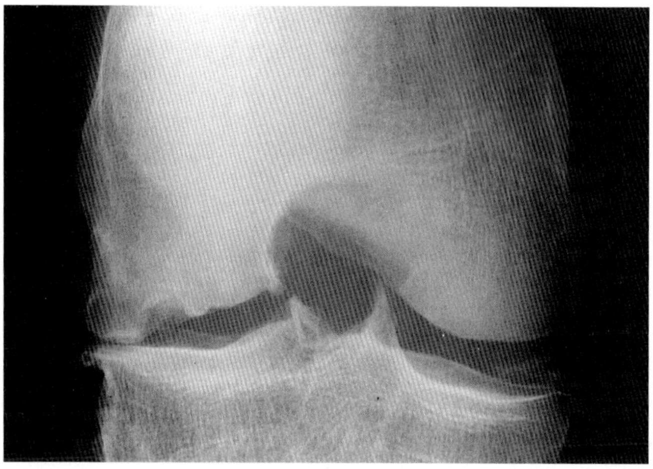

Figure 9

Plain radiograph showing a 32-year follow-up of osteochondritis dissecans involving the medial femoral condyle in a 10-year-old male child. Note the degenerative changes in the medial compartment of the knee.

remains in situ, producing retropatellar crepitus and pain, although a loose body may develop sometimes. The indication for surgery closely resembles that seen in osteochondritis dissecans of the femoral condyles. A loose fragment or a fragment partially detached from the articular surface of the patella is treated by excision of the affected area with drilling of the underlying bone.

Osteochondritis dissecans of the knee—a plan of management

(1) The lesion in situ in a young child will heal in most cases. Excessive activities are to be prevented and the child should be reviewed clinically and radiologically, and if necessary by radioisotope bone scan or MRI.

(2) If the fragment in the child remains symptomatic and in situ, then arthroscopy should be undertaken to assess the stability of the fragment. If the lesion is perfectly stable, drilling should be considered. However, if the fragment is found to be unstable, then internal fixation is advocated.

(3) In skeletally mature patients with OCD fragment in situ, early arthroscopic assessment is recommended as spontaneous healing is much less likely. If the fragment is found stable, drilling should be considered. In patients with unstable OCD lesion, internal fixation in situ should be undertaken.

(4) Every attempt should be made to reattach the large, unstable fragment from the weight-bearing surface of the femoral condyle. This may be achieved by arthroscopic or open internal fixation using a compression screw. Cancellous bone grafts are used in selective cases to restore surface congruity.

(5) In patients with severely fragmented unstable lesion, internal fixation may not be possible and the surgeon is left with no other choice than removal of the fragment. The resultant crater should be prepared with curette, powered instruments and burr so that bleeding subchondral bone is exposed.

(6) If the loose body has detached recently, as indicated by haemorrhage or a scanty fibrous tissue within the crater, and if congruous replacement is feasible, then internal fixation should be undertaken.

(7) Internal fixation is not recommended for long-standing loose bodies as accurate bone apposition is not possible. The established loose body with symptoms must be removed arthroscopically or via arthrotomy in difficult cases, and the crater should be inspected and if necessary curetted and debrided down to bleeding subchondral bone.

(8) The crater left after fragment excision should be reinspected arthroscopically at 6–9 months to assess the quality of fibrocartilaginous repair and to make sure that no further trimming of the edges is required.

(9) In patients with large defects on the weight-bearing surface, allografts should be considered.

Conclusions

(1) The precise aetiology of osteochondritis dissecans is still elusive.

(2) A high index of suspicion is required for the clinical diagnosis.

(3) Radioisotope bone scan and MRI are useful for the early detection of the lesion. Moreover, they also can be used to monitor the healing response and to determine the need for operative intervention.

(4) Arthroscopic assessment is vital to ascertain the stability of the fragment.

(5) The management of osteochondritis dissecans of the knee is controversial. Various modalities of treatment have been suggested but none of the methods has been able to produce consistently satisfactory results.

(6) Best results are obtained in children whose lesions heal before skeletal maturity.

(7) The fate of a massive defect on a long-term basis is not known.

(8) Prospective, randomized studies comparing the different treatment methods are required.

(9) Uniform documentation system is desperately needed to enable valid comparison amongst the various series.

References

1. **König F**, Ueber freie Körper in den Gelenken, *Deutsche Zeitschr Chir, Leipz* (1887–1888) **27**: 90–109.
2. **Barrie HJ**, Osteochondritis dissecans 1887–1987: a centennial look at König's memorable phrase, *J Bone Joint Surg (Br)* (1987) **69**: 693–695.
3. **Resnick D, Niwayama G**, In *Diagnosis of bone and joint disorders*, 2nd edn, ed Resnick D, Niwayama G (Philadelphia: WB Saunders, 1988).
4. **Nagura S**, The so-called osteochondritis dissecans of König, *Clin Orthop* (1960) **18**: 100–122.
5. **Paré A**, *The case reports and autopsy records of Ambroise Paré*, ed WB Hamby (Springfield, Ill.: Charles C Thomas, 1960).
6. **Paget J**, On the production of some of the loose bodies in joints, *St. Bartholomew's Hosp Reports* (1870) **6**: 1–4.
7. **Aichroth PM**, Osteochondritis dissecans of the knee: a clinical survey, *J Bone Joint Surg (Br)* (1971) **53**: 440–447.
8. **Fairbank HAT**, Osteochondritis dissecans, *Br J Surg* (1933) **21**: 67–82.
9. **Green JP**, Osteochondritis dissecans of the knee, *J Bone Joint Surg (Br)* (1966) **48**: 82–91.
10. **Hellström J**, Beitrag zur Kenntnis ders. g. Osteochondritis dissecans im Kniegelenk, *Acta Chir Scand* (1923) **55**: 190–221.
11. **Mouchet A, Bruas M**, Sur un cas d'ostéochondrite disséquante, *Lyon Chir* (1925) **22**: 510–512.
12. **Smillie IS**, *Diseases of the knee joint* (Edinburgh: Churchill Livingstone, 1974).
13. **Sommer R**, Osteochondritis dissecans (König). Eine klinische und pathologisch-anatomische Studie, *Bruns' Beit Klin Chir* (1923) **129**: 1–60.
14. **Smillie IS**, *Osteochondritis dissecans: loose bodies in joints: aetiology, pathology, treatment* (Edinburgh: E & S Livingstone, 1960).
15. **Rosenberg NJ**, Osteochondral fractures of the lateral femoral condyle, *J Bone Joint Surg (Am)* (1964) **46**: 1013–1026.
16. **Aichroth PM**, Osteochondral fractures and their relationship to osteochondritis dissecans of the knee: an experimental study in animals, *J Bone Joint Surg (Br)* (1971) **53**: 448–454.
17. **Langenskiöld A**, Can osteochondritis dissecans arise as a sequel of cartilage fracture in early childhood? An experimental study, *Acta Chir Scand* (1955) **109**: 206–209.
18. **Rehbein F**, Die Entstehung der Osteochondritis dissecans, *Arch Klin Chir* (1950) **265**: 69.
19. **Tallqvist G**, The reaction to mechanical trauma in growing articular cartilage, *Acta Orthop Scand* (1962) Suppl **53**: 1–112.
20. **Milgram JW**, Radiological and pathological manifestations of osteochondritis dissecans of the distal femur: a study of 50 cases, *Radiology* (1978) **126**: 305–311.
21. **Axhausen G**, Die Eetiologie der köhlerschen Erkrankung der Metatarsalköpfchen, *Beitr Z Klin Chir* (1922) **126**: 451.
22. **Green WT, Banks HH**, Osteochondritis dissecans in children, *J Bone Joint Surg (Am)* (1953) **35**: 26–47.
23. **Chiroff RT, Cooke CP III**, Osteochondritis dissecans: a histologic and microradiographic analysis of surgically excised lesions, *J Trauma* (1975) **15**: 689–696.
24. **Anderson AF, Lipscomb AB, Coulam C**, Antegrade curettement, bone grafting and pinning of osteochondritis dissecans in the skeletally mature knee, *Am J Sports Med* (1990) **18**(3): 254–261.
25. **Cahill BR, Phillips MR, Navarro R**, The results of conservative management of juvenile osteochondritis dissecans using joint scintigraphy: a prospective study, *Am J Sports Med* (1989) **17**(5): 601–606.
26. **Johnson LL, Uitvlugt G, Austin MD et al.**, Osteochondritis dissecans of the knee: Arthroscopic compression screw fixation, *Arthroscopy* (1990) **6**(3): 179–189.
27. **Lindén B**, Osteochondritis dissecans of the femoral condyles: a long-term follow-up study, *J Bone Joint Surg (Am)* (1977) **59**: 769–776.

28. **Lindholm S, Pylkkänen P**, Internal fixation of the fragment of osteochondritis dissecans in the knee by means of bone pins: a preliminary report on several cases, *Acta Chir Scand* (1974) **140**: 626–629.

29. **Scott DJ Jr, Stevenson CA**, Osteochondritis dissecans of the knee in adults, *Clin Orthop* (1971) **76**: 82–86.

30. **Zeman SC, Nielsen MW**, Osteochondritis dissecans of the knee, *Orthop Rev* (1978) **9**: 101.

31. **Carroll NC, Mubarak SJ**, Juvenile osteochondritis dissecans of the knee, *J Bone Joint Surg (Br)* (1977) **59**: 506.

32. **Koch W**, Ueber embolische Knochennekrosen, *Arch Klin Chir* (1879) **23**: 315.

33. **Rieger H**, Zur Pathogenese von Gelenkmausen, *Munch Med Wochenschr* (1920) **67**: 719.

34. **Watson-Jones R**, *Fractures and joint injuries*, 4th edn vol 1 (London: E & S Livingstone, 1952) 97.

35. **Enneking WF**, *Clinical musculoskeletal pathology*, (Gainesville, Fla: Storter Printing Co., 1977) 147.

36. **Rogers WM, Gladstone H**, Vascular foramina and arterial supply of the distal end of the femur, *J Bone Joint Surg (Am)* (1950) **32**: 867–874.

37. **Ficat P, Arlet J, Mazières B**, Osteochondritis dissecans and osteonecrosis of the lower end of the femur: value of functional investigation of the bone marrow, *Sem Hosp Paris* (1975) **51**: 1907–1916.

38. **Caffey J, Madell SH, Royer C et al.**, Ossification of the distal femoral epiphysis, *J Bone Joint Surg (Am)* (1958) **40**: 647–654.

39. **Langer F, Percy EC**, Osteochondritis dissecans and anomalous centres of ossification: a review of 80 lesions in 61 patients, *Can J Surg* (1971) **14**: 208–215.

40. **Phillips HO IV, Grubb SA**, Familial multiple osteochondritis dissecans: report of a kindred, *J Bone Joint Surg (Am)* (1985) **67**: 155–156.

41. **Ribbing S**, The hereditary multiple epiphyseal disturbance and its consequences for the aetiogenesis of local malacias – particularly the osteochondritis dissecans, *Acta Orthop Scand* (1955) **24**: 286–299.

42. **Smith AD**, Osteochondritis of the knee joint: a report of three cases in one family and a discussion of the etiology and treatment, *J Bone Joint Surg (Am)* (1960) **42**: 289–294.

43. **Bernstein MA**, Osteochondritis dissecans, *J Bone Joint Surg* (1925) **7**: 319–329.

44. **Fraser WNC**, Familial osteochondritis dissecans, *J Bone Joint Surg (Br)* (1966) **48**: 598.

45. **Gardiner TB**, Osteochondritis dissecans in three members of one family, *J Bone Joint Surg (Br)* (1955) **37**: 139–141.

46. **Hanley WB, McKusick VA, Barranco FT**, Osteochondritis dissecans with associated malformations in two brothers: a review of familial aspects, *J Bone Joint Surg (Am)* (1967) **49**: 925–937.

47. **Pick MP**, Familial osteochondritis dissecans, *J Bone Joint Surg (Br)* (1955) **37**: 142–145.

48. **Stougaard J**, The hereditary factor in osteochondritis dissecans, *J Bone Joint Surg (Br)* (1961) **43**: 256–258.

49. **Tobin WJ**, Familial osteochondritis dissecans with associated tibia vara, *J Bone Joint Surg (Am)* (1957) **39**: 1091–1105.

50. **Petrie PWR**, Aetiology of osteochondritis dissecans: failure to establish a familial background, *J Bone Joint Surg (Br)* (1977) **59**: 366–367.

51. **Clanton TO, DeLee JC**, Osteochondritis dissecans: history, pathophysiology and current treatment concepts, *Clin Orthop* (1982) **167**: 50–64.

52. **White J**, Osteochondritis dissecans in association with dwarfism, *J Bone Joint Surg (Br)* (1957) **39**: 261–267.

53. **Wiberg G**, Spontaneous healing of osteochondritis dissecans in the knee joint, *Acta Orthop Scand* (1943) **14**: 270–277.

54. **Woodward AH, Decker JS**, Osteochondritis dissecans following Legg–Perthes' disease, *South Med J* (1976) **69**: 943–944, 948.

55. **Lindén B**, The incidence of osteochondritis dissecans in the condyles of the femur, *Acta Orthop Scand* (1976) **47**: 664–667.

56. **Federico DJ, Lynch JK, Jokl P**, Osteochondritis dissecans of the knee: a historical review of etiology and treatment, *Arthroscopy* (1990) **6**(3): 190–197.

57. **Smith JB**, Osteochondritis dissecans of the trochlea of the femur, *Arthroscopy* (1990) **6**(1): 11–17.

58. **Wilson JN**, A diagnostic sign in osteochondritis dissecans of the knee, *J Bone Joint Surg (Am)* (1967) **49**: 477–480.

59. **Cahill BR**, Treatment of juvenile osteochondritis dissecans and osteochondritis dissecans of the knee, *Clin Sports Med* (1985) **4**: 367–384.

60. **Cahill BR, Berg BC**, 99m-Technetium phosphate compound joint scintigraphy in the management of juvenile osteochondritis dissecans of the femoral condyles, *Am J Sports Med* (1983) **11**: 329–335.

61. **McCullough RW, Gandsman EJ, Litchman HE et al.**, Dynamic bone scintigraphy in osteochondritis dissecans, *Int Orthop (SICOT)* (1988) **12**: 317–322.

62. **Mesgarzadeh M, Sapega AA, Bonakdarpour A et al.**, Osteochondritis dissecans: Analysis of mechanical stability with radiography, scintigraphy, and MR imaging, *Radiology* (1987) **165**: 775–780.

63. **Bradley J, Dandy DJ**, Osteochondritis dissecans and other lesions of the femoral condyles, *J Bone Joint Surg (Br)* (1989) **71**: 518–522.

64. **Matthewson MH, Dandy DJ**, Osteochondral fractures of the lateral femoral condyle: A result of indirect violence to the knee, *J Bone Joint Surg (Br)* (1978) **60**: 199–202.

65. **Milgram JE**, Tangential osteochondral fracture of the patella, *J Bone Joint Surg* (1943) **25**: 271–280.

66. **Kennedy JC, Grainger RW, McGraw RW**, Osteochondral fractures of the femoral condyles, *J Bone Joint Surg (Br)* (1966) **48**: 436–440.

67. **Landells JW**, The reactions of injured human articular cartilage, *J Bone Joint Surg (Br)* (1957) **39**: 548–562.

68. **O'Donoghue DH**, Chondral and osteochondral fractures, *J Trauma* (1966) **6**: 469–481.

69. **Edelstein JM**, Osteochondritis dissecans with spontaneous resolution, *J Bone Joint Surg (Br)* (1954) **36**: 343.

70. **Löfgren L**, Spontaneous healing of osteochondritis dissecans in children and adolescents: a case of multiple ossification centres in the distal epiphysis of the humerus and a rare "os epicondylitis medialis humeri", *Acta Chir Scand* (1954) **106**: 460–478.

71. **Van Demark RE**, Osteochondritis dissecans with spontaneous healing, *J Bone Joint Surg (Am)* (1952) **34**: 143–148.

72. **Hughston JC, Hergenroeder PT, Courtenay BG**, Osteochondritis dissecans of the femoral condyles, *J Bone Joint Surg (Am)* (1984) **66**: 1340–1348.

73. **Guhl JF**, Arthroscopic treatment of osteochondritis dissecans, *Clin Orthop* (1982) **167**: 65–74.

74. **Pappas AM**, Osteochondritis dissecans, *Clin Orthop* (1981) **158**: 59–69.

75. **Smillie IS**, Treatment of osteochondritis dissecans, *J Bone Joint Surg (Br)* (1957) **39**: 248–260.

76. **Salter RB, Field P**, The effects of continuous compression on living articular cartilage: an experimental investigation, *J Bone Joint Surg (Am)* (1960) **42**: 31–49.

77. **Bradley J, Dandy DJ**, Results of drilling osteochondritis dissecans before skeletal maturity, *J Bone Joint Surg (Br)* (1989) **71**: 642–644.

78. **Gepstein R, Conforty B, Weiss RE et al.**, Surgery for early stage osteochondritis dissecans of the knee in young adults: a preliminary report, *Orthopaedics* (1986) **9**: 1087–1089.

79. **Rae PJ, Noble J**, Arthroscopic drilling of osteochondral lesions of the knee, *J Bone Joint Surg (Br)* (1989) **71**: 534.

80. **Bandi W, Allgöwer M**, Zur Therapie der Osteochondritis dissecans, *Helv Chir Acta* (1959) **26**: 552.

81. **Bigelow DR**, Juvenile osteochondritis dissecans, *J Bone Joint Surg (Br)* (1975) **57**: 530.

82. **Gillespie HS, Day B**, Bone peg fixation in the treatment of osteochondritis dissecans of the knee joint, *Clin Orthop* (1979) **143:** 125–130.

83. **Johnson EW, McLeod TL**, Osteochondral fragments of the distal end of the femur fixed with bone pegs: report of two cases, *J Bone Joint Surg (Am)* (1977) **59:** 677–679.

84. **Lindholm S, Pylkkänen P, Österman K**, Fixation of osteochondral fragments in the knee joint: a clinical survey, *Clin Orthop* (1977) **126:** 256–260.

85. **Lipscomb PR Jr, Lipscomb PR Sr, Bryan RS**, Osteochondritis dissecans of the knee with loose fragments: treatment by replacement and fixation with readily removed pins, *J Bone Joint Surg (Am)* (1978) **60:** 235–240.

86. **Mackie IG, Pemberton DJ, Maheson M**, Arthroscopic use of the Herbert screw in osteochondritis dissecans, *J Bone Joint Surg (Br)* (1990) **72:** 1076.

87. **Thomson NL**, Osteochondritis dissecans and osteochondral fragments managed by Herbert Compression screw fixation, *Clin Orthop* (1987) **224:** 71–78.

88. **Bots RA, Slooff TJ**, Arthroscopy in the evaluation of operative treatment of osteochondritis dissecans, *Orthop Clin North Am* (1979) **10:** 685–696.

89. **Guhl JF**, Arthroscopic treatment of osteochondritis dissecans: a preliminary report, *Orthop Clin North Am* (1979) **10:** 671–683.

90. **Denoncourt PM, Patel D, Dimakopoulos P**, Arthroscopy Update: 1. Treatment of osteochondritis dissecans of the knee by arthroscopic curettage: follow-up study, *Orthop Rev* (1986) **XV:** 652–657.

91. **Ewing JW, Voto SJ**, Arthroscopic surgical management of osteochondritis dissecans of the knee, *Arthroscopy* (1988) **4:** 37–40.

92. **Convery FR, Akeson WH, Keown GH**, The repair of large osteochondral defects: an experimental study in horses, *Clin Orthop* (1972) **82:** 253–262.

93. **Homminga GN, Bulstra SK, Bouwmeester PSM et al.**, Perichondral grafting for cartilage lesions of the knee, *J Bone Joint Surg (Br)* (1990) **72:** 1003–1007.

94. **Bentley G**, Transplantation of isolated chondrocytes into joint surfaces, *J Bone Joint Surg (Br)* (1973) **55:** 209–210.

95. **Gross A, Langer, F**, Allotransplantation of partial joints in the treatment of osteoarthritis of the knee, *J Bone Joint Surg (Am)* (1974) **56:** 1540.

96. **Crawfurd EJP, Emery RJH, Aichroth PM**, Stable osteochondritis dissecans – Does the lesion unite?, *J Bone Joint Surg (Br)* (1990) **72:** 320.

97. **Garrett JC**, Treatment of osteochondral defects of the distal femur with fresh osteochondral allografts: a preliminary report, *Arthroscopy* (1986) **2(4):** 222–226.

98. **Twyman RS, Desai K, Aichroth PM**, Osteochondritis dissecans of the knee: a long-term study, *J Bone Joint Surg (Br)* (1991) **73:** 461–464.

99. **Edwards DH, Bentley G**, Osteochondritis dissecans patellae, *J Bone Joint Surg (Br)* (1977) **59:** 58–63.

9.2 Osteochondritis dissecans

James W. Stone and James F. Guhl

Introduction

Osteochondritis dissecans is a focal abnormality of articular cartilage and underlying subchondral bone that occurs in diarthrodial joints. It may result in the separation of the osteochondral fragment, nonunion, and subsequent development of a loose body. The term 'osteochondritis' is a misnomer, since it implies an infectious or inflammatory etiology for the disorder. Instead, the characteristic histologic appearance is more consistent with ischemic necrosis of the subchondral bone. The lesion would be more accurately termed an 'osteochondrosis' in that there is degeneration or necrosis of bone, cartilage or both followed by reossification and healing.[1,2]

The disorder can occur at the epiphysis of any joint, but is common in the knee, ankle, elbow, and hip. If the necrotic bone does not heal to the underlying healthy bone, then the fragment may become loose in the joint. This will predispose the patient to the development of early degenerative arthritis. The prognosis is particularly poor in the weight-bearing joints. The goal of therapy, therefore, is to encourage healing of the osteochondral fragment to the underlying healthy bone and to prevent articular incongruity and degeneration.

Discussions of the etiology of osteochondritis dissecans of the knee joint provoke much controversy. Early descriptions suggested that trauma plays an important role. It was proposed that direct abutment of the tibial spine against the femoral condyle causes osteochondral separation, but the importance of this mechanism has been difficult to prove.[1,3-5] Direct trauma to the patella with the knee in a position of approximately 135° of flexion also could result in damage to the medial femoral condyle. This is the most commonly noted location of osteochondritis dissecans.[6-8] Other categories of trauma, such as patellar dislocation or abnormal joint kinetics associated with ligament injuries, are related to the disorder. Of patients with osteochondritis dissecans, 40–50% report a history of trauma to the knee joint. It is, however, difficult to know whether a lesion was caused by a particular traumatic event or whether the finding was incidental to the event.

Enneking has proposed that the cause of this disorder is a primary ischemic event that results in the death of a wedge-shaped segment of subchondral bone.[9] His studies suggest that an area of potentially impaired circulation exists at the end-artery arcades located in the epiphysis. After osseous necrosis occurs, granulation tissue advances into the area between the necrotic fragment and the healthy bone. Healing may occur by creeping substitution, or nonunion may ensue. The only remaining support for the necrotic bone is the articular cartilage, and the fragment frequently detaches and floats into the joint.

Other proposed etiologies for osteochondritis dissecans include irregular ossification patterns in skeletally immature patients, endocrine imbalance, and genetic influences.

Osteochondritis dissecans of the knee is more common in males than females in an approximate ratio of 2:1 or 3:1. It presents most commonly in the second decade. It rarely presents before age 10 years or after age 50 years. There is medial femoral condyle involvement in 75% of cases, with the majority involving the intercondylar aspect. In a study of 95 cases of osteochondritis dissecans, Hughston et al. found that 82% were in the medial femoral condyle and 18% were lateral.[10] Of the medial lesions, 55% were in the intercondylar non-meniscal region (i.e., the classical position of knee-joint osteochondritis dissecans); another 25% were in the non-meniscal region (i.e., more centrally located on the medial femoral condyle).

A significant number of patients present with bilateral osteochondritis lesions. In the study of Hughston et al. 14% of the lesions were bilateral.[10] Guhl treated 50 patients with osteochondritis dissecans of the knee, and 24% of the cases were bilateral.[11]

The lesions themselves can be divided into groups based on the integrity of the overlying articular cartilage and the condition of the underlying subchondral bone. Although radiographic studies can help to predict the type of lesion, arthroscopic examination provides the most accurate means of staging these lesions. *Intact* lesions may have no breaks in the articular cartilage, although the hyaline cartilage may be discolored or softened. Careful palpation reveals that the underlying bone is not mobile. In a *separated* lesion, the bone moves under the articular surface, but there is no flaking or detachment of the articular cartilage. A *detached* lesion presents a portion of the surface articular cartilage flaking into the joint. The final category is the completely detached lesion —a *loose body*.

Cahill points out that 'juvenile osteochondritis dissecans' and 'osteochondritis dissecans' are not equivalent lesions.[12] The disease process in juvenile osteochondritis dissecans initiates prior to closure of the physis, whereas osteochondritis dissecans begins after physeal closure. The distinction between the two disorders is important because the degree of skeletal maturity influences the choice of treatment. Pappas further divides patients into three groups based on chronologic and skeletal age.[1] Category-I includes children through early adolescence up to skeletal age 11 years for females and 13 years for males. He feels that these patients have a high likelihood of healing the lesions with conservative treatment. Category-II includes males from skeletal age 14 years and females from skeletal age 12 years up to age 20 years approximately. These patients are in the final phase of growth and have less healing potential than the younger group. Some patients in this age group can be treated conservatively. Nevertheless, there may be indications for drilling the lesion in patients with intact lesions or for bone grafting in those with separated or detached lesions. Category-III includes patients older than 20 years. These patients have the least healing potential, and a more aggressive form of treatment is necessary to try to save the osteochondral fragment.

History and physical examination

Osteochondritis dissecans of the knee joint may be discovered as an incidental finding on radiographs obtained after trauma. Pain may be the sole presenting complaint. However, fragment separation or detachment usually causes symptoms of internal derangement with pain, swelling, catching, locking, or giving way. Unfortunately, symptoms may be minimal until detachment occurs. The physical examination may reveal a joint effusion, at times with limitation of range of motion and associated quadriceps atrophy. Tenderness may be medial or lateral, depending upon the location of the lesion. It may not be distinguishable from other types of internal derangement such as a torn meniscus.

Radiographic evaluation

Plain radiographic examination is usually diagnostic. The anteroposterior film usually reveals a lucency or incongruity of the intercondylar aspect of the medial femoral condyle, less commonly of the lateral condyle. In more advanced cases, the classic appearance of a well-circumscribed fragment of subchondral bone separated from the underlying condyle is present. The lesion may be better seen on the tunnel or intercondylar notch view. In the lateral projection, the lesion most frequently appears between a line extending along the posterior cortex of the femoral shaft and a line extending along the top of the intercondylar notch. The high incidence of bilateral osteochondritis dissecans lesions mandates the obtaining of plain radiographs of both knees, even if the contralateral knee is asymptomatic.

Anteroposterior and lateral conventional tomograms can further delineate the lesion and will frequently reveal more than one bone fragment. These studies are not useful in predicting whether the lesion is intact, separated, or detached, or whether the articular cartilage covering the lesion is intact. Arthrography rarely adds any useful information to the evaluation.

Bone scans will frequently reveal increased radiotracer uptake in active osteochondritis dissecans lesions. In addition, in an individual with other potential sites of osteochondritis dissecans, this study provides a screening procedure for all joints with minimal exposure to ionizing radiation. Cahill has demonstrated the usefulness of serial bone scans in monitoring treatment of juvenile osteochondritis dissecans.[13] He performed bone scans on 76 patients with osteochondritis dissecans in 92 knees at 8-week intervals. Technetium joint scintigraphy is a sensitive mechanism for monitoring healing of the lesion. There is an association between decreased activity and radiographic healing. Unfortunately, the bone scan at initial examination was not predictive of ultimate success or failure of conservative treatment.

Computed tomography (CT) can delineate osteochondritis dissecans in joints other than the knee, and can be useful in assessing healing. Unfortunately, axial sections of the knee yield little useful information. Sagittal or coronal reconstructions made from multiple axial views provide insufficient resolution to assist in evaluating lesion healing or the status of the articular cartilage.

Magnetic resonance imaging (MRI) holds promise in the evaluation of osteochondritis dissecans since it has the potential to visualize articular cartilage. The MRI can be formated in both the coronal plane and the sagittal plane for complete evaluation of the lesion. To date, however, we have not found it to be reliable in predicting the condition of the articular cartilage covering the bony lesion. In addition, it is unable to assess bone fragment healing.

Arthroscopy

Arthroscopy has developed into a significant tool both for the diagnostic work-up of osteochondritis dissecans and in treating the lesion. Despite the obtaining of any number of radiographic studies, arthroscopic examination gives the most accurate appraisal of the articular cartilage integrity, and the condition of the underlying bone fragment. It is not uncommon for the arthroscopic examination to alter significantly the preoperative radiographic assessment of the lesion.

In arthroscopy of the knee with osteochondritis dissecans, a complete evaluation of the joint should be performed prior to addressing the lesion itself. This complete evaluation should assess the entire joint for any associated abnormalities. Only then is the lesion itself assessed. If the lesion is intact and difficult to appreciate, light-dimming techniques and viewing with the 70° oblique arthroscope can assist in visualizing its extent. Methylene blue dye introduced into the joint and then washed out with saline will bring out the topography of the lesion in greater detail. The lesion should be gently probed to determine whether there is underlying separation. The articular cartilage should be evaluated for texture, thinning, friability, fibrillation, discoloration, softness, prominence, or depression. Fibrous tissue emanating from the surface margins of the lesion suggests the presence of separation beneath the articular surface. If the lesion is detached, the thickness and quality of any attached subchondral bone must be assessed. If little or no underlying bone is present on the undersurface of a detached lesion, there is no hope of healing. Attempts to replace and fix the lesion mechanically are futile.

Treatment alternatives

Nonoperative treatment

Particularly in young patients, there are frequent indications for a trial of nonoperative treatment of osteochondritis dissecans. In the minimally symptomatic patient without symptoms of effusion, locking, or giving way, activity limitation with avoidance of high-stress activities may be sufficient to relieve symptoms. At times, a period of restriction of weight bearing with crutches may be used to reduce acute symptoms. A hinged knee brace, either locked in a position of knee flexion or adjusted to limit the range of knee motion, may be useful. Use of knee immobilization with a cast is rare.

Arthroscopic drilling of osteochondritis dissecans

Drilling through the articular cartilage and bone fragment into the underlying condylar trabecular bone encourages revascularization of the lesion by vessels that traverse the predrilled holes. This method

of treatment is most applicable in a skeletally immature patient with an intact lesion that does not move below the articular surface when arthroscopically probed. The technique also may be used to supplement internal fixation with screws or autogenous bone pegs in the skeletally mature patient. Place the arthroscope in the anterolateral portal to obtain optimal visualization of common medial femoral condyle lesions. A lesion can usually be localized by noting subtle changes in the color, texture, and resiliency of the articular cartilage using careful probing techniques. If the lesion is difficult to locate, then methylene blue dye may be introduced into the joint, or image intensification may be used intraoperatively.

Use 0.062-inch Kirschner wire to place multiple drill holes through the lesion into healthy underlying trabecular bone. A smooth wire will cause less damage to the articular cartilage than a threaded wire or drillpoint. The use of a cannula from the small-joint arthroscopy set makes pin breakage less likely and guides precise placement of the wire through the soft tissue. Set the Kirschner wire so that approximately 1 inch protrudes from the end of the cannula. This prevents inadvertent deep penetration through the femoral condyle and ensures adequate penetration into healthy trabecular bone. Place approximately 6–8 holes in a lesion of 2 cm diameter. If a tourniquet is used during drilling, deflate it prior to completion of the procedure. Blood should emanate from the multiple drillholes. By using an arthroscopic pump without the tourniquet, a similar demonstration of blood oozing from the drillholes can be obtained by decreasing the pump pressure setting.

For medial femoral condyle lesions, introduce the cannula and Kirschner wire through a separate small portal located near the distal lateral border of the patellar tendon, or in a transpatellar tendon position. Ideal portal placement allows the cannula to be positioned perpendicular to the articular surface. Lesions of the lateral femoral condyle are frequently located more posteriorly and may be more difficult to reach. The cannula may need to be placed anteromedially or anterolaterally. The ideal position may be approximated using a 18-gauge spinal needle for localization.

Arthroscopic internal fixation using Kirschner wires

Internal fixation of osteochondritis dissecans lesions with threaded Kirschner wires and bone pegs was reported by Scott and Stevenson.[14] Fixation using smooth Kirschner wires was subsequently reported by Lipscomb.[15] The technique using smooth wires is preferred because the pins can be removed more easily, frequently in the office. The smooth wires

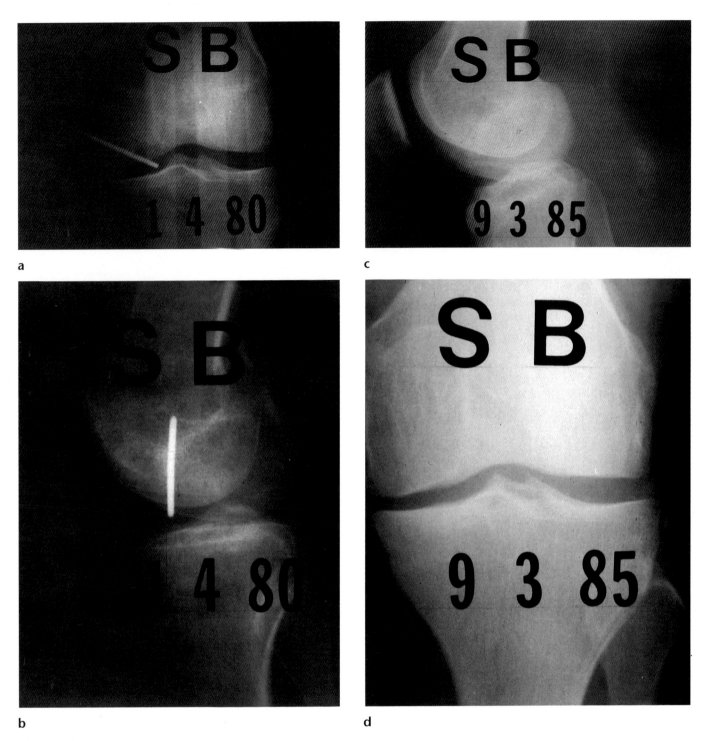

Figure 1

(a) Anteroposterior and (b) lateral radiographs demonstrate Kirschner wires placed from distal to proximal under arthroscopic guidance for treatment of osteochondritis dissecans of the medial femoral condyle. (c,d) Follow-up radiographs document healing of the lesion.

cause less injury to the articular cartilage. A pin partially threaded in the distal 3 inches is commercially available and is less likely to migrate than smooth wires. These partially threaded pins, however, are more difficult to remove and may be more likely to break at the junction of the threaded and nonthreaded portions.

The procedure can be readily performed arthroscopically with significantly less morbidity than with an arthrotomy. Its best application is for separated lesions in skeletally immature patients, or in lesions with thin bone fragments that are likely to splinter with screw fixation. Introduce the pins through a small cannula, to allow accurate placement without

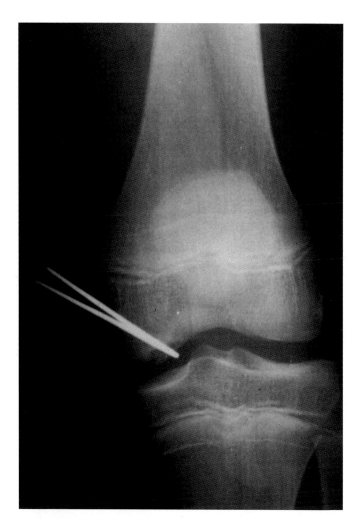

Figure 2

This radiograph demonstrates the technique of pinning for osteochondritis dissecans in the skeletally immature patient. The pins are placed from distal to proximal and carefully angled so as to exit the epiphysis, thus avoiding injury to the physeal plate.

bending, under direct arthroscopic visualization (Figure 1). In the skeletally immature patient, direct the pins to exit medially from the epiphysis instead of crossing the physis and exiting from the metaphysis (Figure 2). This careful positioning prevents injury to the physis. Image intensification may be useful to guide the pin placement. Once the pin exits the bone medially, make a small incision. While viewing arthroscopically, pull the pin back in a retrograde fashion until the tip just disappears below the articular cartilage surface. Alternately, an anterior cruciate ligament (ACL) reconstruction guide can be used to place a pin from proximal to distal directly into the lesion under arthroscopic control. Place the tip of the guide over the lesion, and place the extra-articular end of the guide accurately over the femoral

condyle. If using a partially threaded wire, advance it through the articular cartilage and withdraw it under direct visualization to 'cinch down' the lesion. With any of these methods, use multiple Kirschner wires to fix the lesions as solidly as possible.

Immobilize the knee until it is time for pin removal, usually 6–8 weeks postoperatively. After hardware removal, continue weight restriction until there is clinical and radiographic evidence of healing.

Arthroscopic internal fixation using cancellous screws

Use cancellous screws when desiring more rigid internal fixation than can be obtained with multiple Kirschner wires. This method is particularly applicable in patients nearing or past skeletal maturity, when healing of the osteochondritis dissecans fragment is more difficult to obtain. Compression across the bone fragment may enhance healing to the underlying trabecular bone. Although any cancellous screw may be used, a cannulated screw makes arthroscopic placement easier (Figure 3).

Disadvantages of cannulated screw fixation include potential guide-pin breakage by the drill or screw if either is misdirected over the guide-pin. In addition, screw fixation necessarily disrupts a larger surface area of the articular cartilage to accommodate the screwhead. Although a washer may provide more secure fixation by distributing the compression force over a greater area, its use also causes more articular cartilage destruction. Another disadvantage of screw fixation is the need for a second surgical procedure to remove the hardware. The second procedure, however, provides an opportunity to evaluate healing. In addition, the tracts left by the screws provide another channel for vascular ingrowth and healing of bone.

Approach the lesion under arthroscopic control. If the lesion is separated but not detached, advance the guide wire from an accessory portal so that it approaches the surface of the lesion perpendicularly. Over-drill the wire with a cannulated drill. Use the countersink, advance the appropriate length screw, and tighten it gently over the guide wire. If the lesion is raised or partially detached, elevate it gently while attempting to keep one corner as a hinge to prevent complete loosening of the fragment. When finding a completely detached or loose lesion, a decision must be made to remove it or to replace and internally fix it. The decision to replace and fix the lesion depends upon the size of the fragment, its location relative to the weight-bearing surface, and the length of time that the lesion has been loose. Consider an aggressive approach for large lesions comprising a significant portion of the weight-bearing surface. After several weeks a detached lesion will usually not fit into the

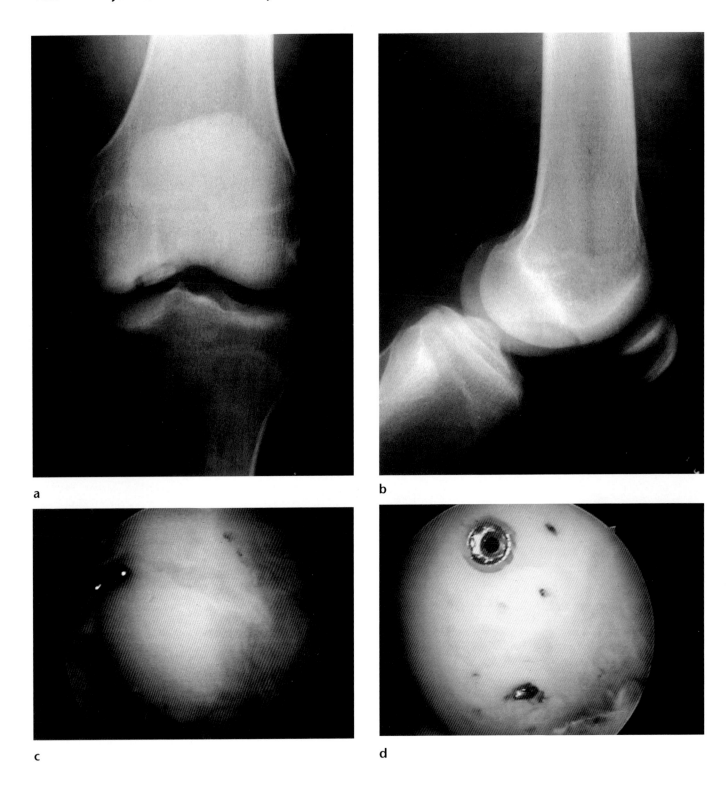

a

b

c

d

crater owing to distortion and remodeling of the fragment. Gently curette the base of the crater and the undersurface of the fragment and replace the lesion. If a large crater is present, supplemental bone graft may be placed into the defect prior to replacing the lesion. Perform screw fixation.

In any of these cases, internal fixation may be supplemented by drilling along the periphery of the lesion. In addition, supplemental bone grafting may be performed.

Immobilize the knee postoperatively, in a hinged knee brace locked in a moderate flexion for approximately 6 weeks. Gentle range of motion exercises can then commence if the screws have been countersunk below the articular surface. Leave the screws in place for approximately 12 weeks.

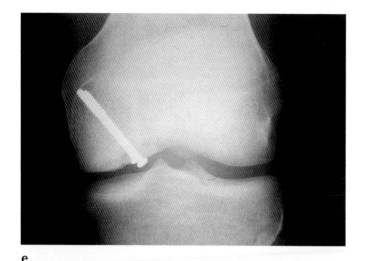

e

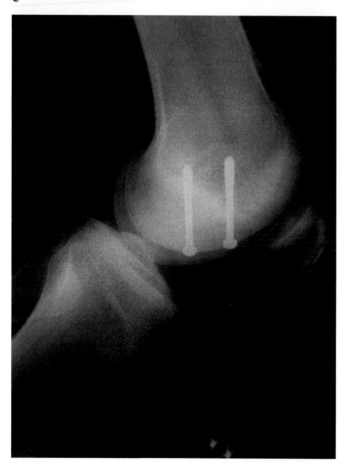

f

Figure 3

(a) Anteroposterior and (b) lateral radiographs of a 20-year-old male with symptomatic osteochondritis dissecans of the medial femoral condyle. (c) Arthroscopic examination revealed that the lesion was intact with only slight elevation of the fragment. (d) Internal fixation was performed with two cannulated 3.5-mm cancellous screws placed with the screwheads countersunk below the articular surface. (e) Postoperative anteroposterior and (f) lateral radiographs demonstrate the screws positioned in the two major bone fragments. The screws were removed 12 weeks postoperatively, and the patient has resumed full activities.

ing osteochondritis dissecans. Thomson reported its use in 18 patients with osteochondritis dissecans.[16] Although the follow-up was only 4–28 months, union was obtained in 16 patients. He recommended screw removal 6–8 weeks after the internal fixation procedure.

The indications for Herbert screw fixation are the same as those for fixation using cancellous screws. The method is similar. The screws are available in a cannulated form that allows guide-pin placement followed by drilling over the pin. As the trailing threads are engaged, compression of the fragment can be appreciated under direct arthroscopic visualization (Figure 4).

We recommend a period of non-weight bearing of approximately 8–12 weeks, depending upon the age of the patient and evidence of radiographic healing. Remove any fibrocartilage that covers the screw heads prior to screw removal. Replacement of the guide pin into the screw makes removal less complicated.

Removal of detached or loose fragments

Consider removing any loose multiple fragments that were displaced from the crater for more than a few weeks. The presence of only a thin layer of subchondral bone on a fragment of articular cartilage makes healing unlikely. Attempts at internal fixation will frequently result in the splintering of the bone fragment, inadequate fixation, and nonunion. If the fragment is removed, the crater should be debrided. The peripheral articular cartilage should be debrided to stable margins with a perpendicular edge. Place multiple drill holes into the underlying condylar bone, and begin early postoperative motion (Figure 5). Protected weight-bearing is recommended for several weeks to optimize formation of fibrocartilage over the surface of the lesion.

Arthroscopic internal fixation using Herbert screws

The Herbert screw provides compression across bone fragments based on the differential pitch of the leading and trailing threads. This property, along with the ability to bury the screw head completely below the articular surface, makes it useful in treat-

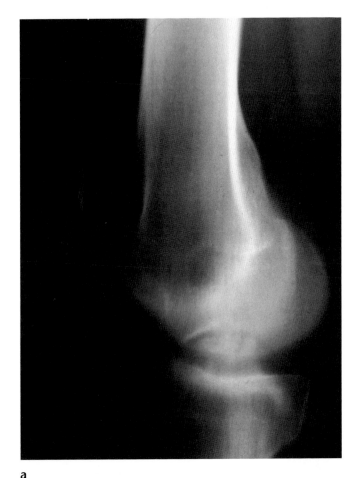

a

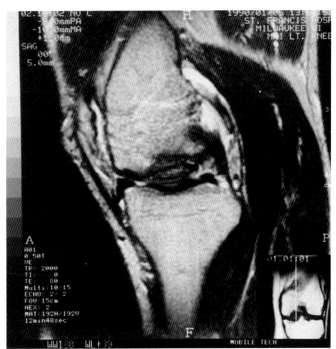

c

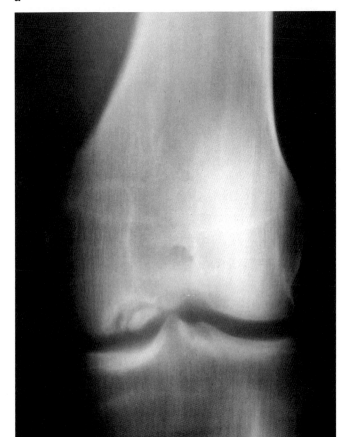

b

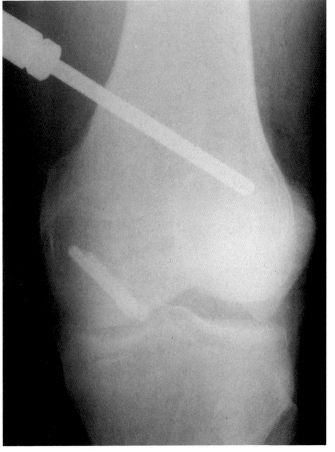

d

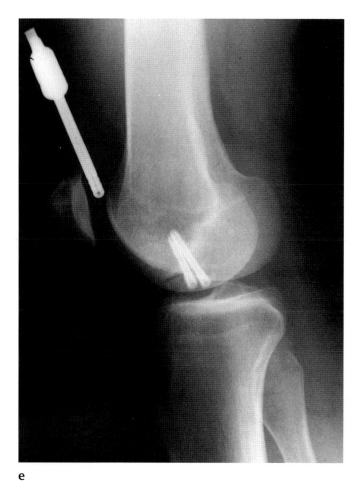

e

Figure 4

(a) Anteroposterior and (b) lateral tomograms demonstrate a large osteochondritis dissecans lesion of the medial femoral condyle in this 32-year-old male. (c) Magnetic resonance imaging study demonstrated the extent of the lesion. (d,e) At arthroscopic examination, the lesion was noted to be separated but not detached. The articular cartilage surface was elevated slightly. The lesion was fixed with two Herbert screws and multiple drillholes were placed with a 0.062-inch Kirschner wire. The Herbert screws were removed 12 weeks postoperatively.

Bone grafting of osteochondritis dissecans

Bone grafting of osteochondritis dissecans using corticocancellous bone pegs or cancellous graft has been used since the 1950s.[14,17–21] The procedure can be used in combination with internal fixation using screws or with concomitant drilling of the lesion. Grafting is particularly applicable in patients who are skeletally mature with separated or detached lesions.

Recently our trend has been to use internal fixation with screws for medial condyle lesions instead of bone grafting. Corticocancellous matchstick grafts can be placed arthroscopically or by arthrotomy (Figure 6). The arthroscopic technique is demanding and should be attempted only by experienced arthroscopic surgeons. A detached or loose fragment must be elevated and debrided prior to replacement in the defect. It may be held in place by a Kirschner wire, or a screw if supplemental fixation is desired. Harvest thin matchsticks of corticocancellous bone from the proximal tibia and taper one end to a sharp point. Place the grafts into predrilled holes using an arthroscopic cannula. Tamp them into position beneath the articular surface.

Cancellous bone grafting also may be accomplished in an antegrade fashion, inserting the bone into a tunnel from proximal to distal in the femoral condyle (Figure 7). This procedure can be performed arthroscopically, and is simplified by using an ACL reconstruction guide. After preparing the osteochondritis dissecans fragment, center the ACL guide tip on the lesion. Position the extra-articular portion of the guide over the femoral condyle. Advance a guide pin in a proximal to distal direction. Perform this under careful arthroscopic visualization so that the pin comes to lie just beneath the articular surface. Penetration, however, by the pin alone should cause no problem. If the patient is not skeletally mature, use image intensification to confirm that the appropriate angle of approach is achieved to avoid injury to the growth plate. Advance a 4–5-mm cannulated reamer over the guide-pin to create a tunnel into the osteochondritis dissecans lesion. Great care must be exercised to ensure that the large cannulated drill does not breach the articular surface. Insert autogenous cancellous bone graft into the tunnel and advance it to the subchondral position.

Although a similar method of grafting using distal-to-proximal insertion of the graft has been described, the technique requires the creation of a large defect in the articular surface. We do not recommend this procedure and prefer bone peg fixation or proximal-to-distal insertion of the graft to minimize articular cartilage damage.

If cancellous bone grafting is done without the use of screws, pins, or matchstick grafts, immobilize the knee for approximately 6 weeks postoperatively. Non-weight bearing is suggested. At the end of 6 weeks, allow gentle mobilization of the knee. Continue protected weight bearing until healing is achieved. Healing of osteochondritis dissecans is judged clinically by the absence of effusion, clicking, locking, giving way of the knee joint, and pain to palpation over the condyle. Plain radiographs and tomography may be useful to evaluate healing of the lesion. Examination by MRI may also aid in determining whether a lesion has healed.

It must be appreciated that lesions of the lateral femoral condyle are frequently located more posteri-

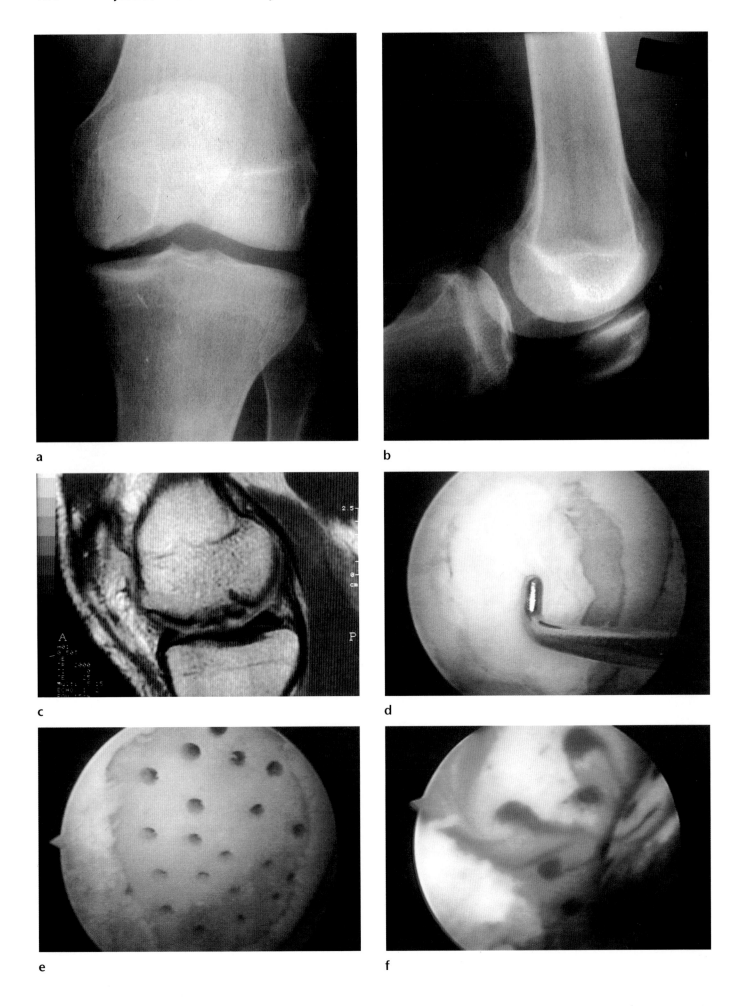

a

b

c

d

e

f

Figure 5

(a) Anteroposterior and (b) lateral radiographs of a 29-year-old male with medial pain, effusion, and locking of the knee. Osteochondritis dissecans of the medial femoral condyle with no significant subchondral bone fragment is seen. (c) Lateral magnetic resonance image outlines the osteochondritis dissecans lesion and suggests mainly a chondral lesion with little underlying bone. (d) Arthroscopic view demonstrates that the 2.5–3.0-cm lesion is comprised almost exclusively of articular cartilage with only a fine layer of subchondral bone. This lesion would not heal if internal fixation were attempted. (e) The lesion was debrided to a stable rim of articular cartilage and multiple drillholes were placed into the subchondral bone using a 0.062-inch Kirschner wire. (f) Deflation of the tourniquet demonstrates bleeding from the drillholes.

only than the typical medial femoral condyle lesion. The posterior location makes arthroscopic treatment with debridement, drilling, internal fixation, or bone grafting more difficult. Even an experienced arthroscopic surgeon may find that the procedure is more efficiently performed by open means. Often there is less damage to the intact articular surfaces and less chance of neurovascular complications. In addition, we recommend bone grafting laterally rather than internal fixation with screws, because of the difficulties of screw removal and possible articular cartilage damage.

Treatment recommendations

In formulating a plan of treatment for osteochondritis dissecans, the surgeon must assess the location of the lesion, the extent of weight-bearing surface involved, the degree of separation of the bone fragment, and the skeletal maturity of the patient. The size of the lesion and the degree of fragment separation are best assessed by arthroscopic examination. Since lesions in children tend to heal with fewer invasive approaches, they are usually treated conservatively. In contrast, patients nearing or past skeletal maturity are less likely to heal with conservative treatment. Therefore, an aggressive approach is appropriate.

It is useful to separate patients first by their degree of skeletal maturity. Patients who present for evalua-

tion prior to physeal closure have a better chance of healing the lesion with either conservative or surgical treatment. For the truly asymptomatic patient whose lesion is found incidentally on radiographic examination, a period of activity limitation and close clinical follow-up is indicated. The use of technetium bone scanning as advocated by Cahill may help assess the activity of the lesion and may be useful in following the healing process. Generally, there are no indications for operative intervention. If the patient later becomes symptomatic, an aggressive investigation with MRI scanning or direct arthroscopic assessment is indicated. The actual surgical procedure to be performed is based upon the arthroscopic appearance of the lesion. We recommend arthroscopic drilling of intact lesion in patients prior to skeletal maturity. Postoperatively, the patient is immobilized for 6 weeks, after which controlled motion is allowed. Generally, protected weight bearing should be enforced for approximately 12 weeks. It is helpful if radiographic evidence of healing is present during this interval, but this is often difficult to assess on plain radiographs. The use of an MRI scan can be helpful in this assessment, but clinical progress is most important in assessing healing. A 'second-look' arthroscopic procedure can be performed if there is any question regarding healing.

A partially separated or detached lesion should be fixed securely. In the skeletally immature patient, take care to avoid injury to the physis. Internal fixation with pins is generally successful and usually does not require a secondary surgical procedure for removal. Hardware is removed after 6–8 weeks. Again, protect the knee from weight bearing for approximately 12 weeks. We recommend internal fixation with a compression screw, especially for lesions of larger diameter and particularly for those with thicker bone fragments. We generally combine rigid internal fixation with drilling around the periphery of the lesion. We are satisfied with the cannulated Herbert screw for this purpose. It is easy to place it arthroscopically in medial lesions. Compression of the fragment can usually be seen arthroscopically as the screw is tightened. The use of this procedure necessitates later arthroscopic screw removal. This secondary procedure is helpful in assessment of healing and is useful in planning rehabilitation.

An attempt to internally fix a loose body with adequate attached bone should be performed in skeletally immature patients, particularly if the lesion occupies a significant portion of the weight-bearing surface. This procedure can be performed arthroscopically by an experienced surgeon. Nevertheless, if necessary, one should not hesitate to perform an arthrotomy, to obtain a perfect reduction and fixation. If the fragment has little attached bone, the surgeon has no choice but to remove the fragment and debride and drill the base.

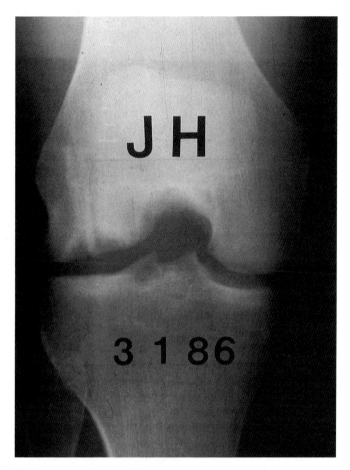

a

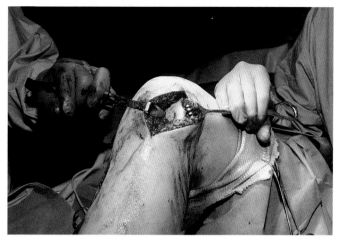

c

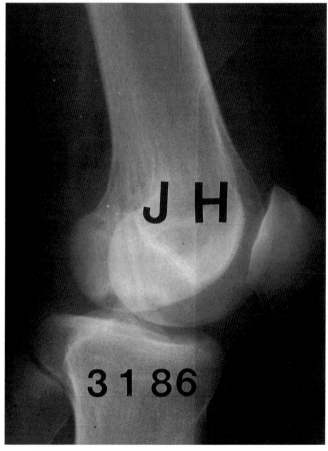

b

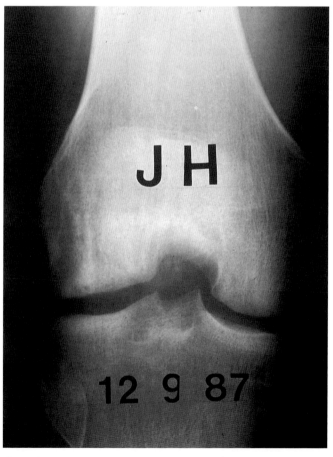

d

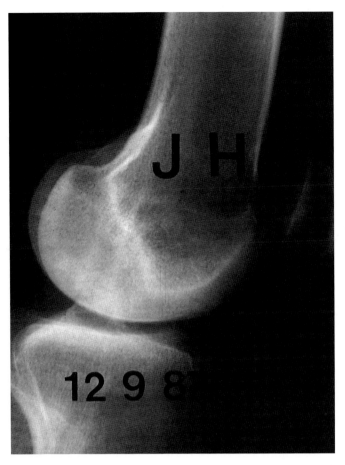

e

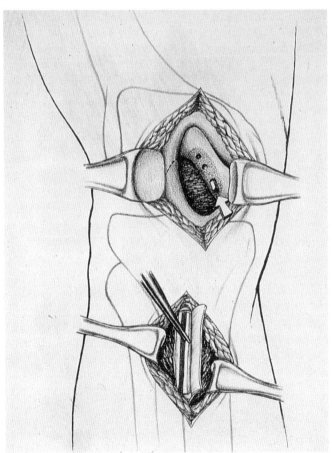

f

Figure 6

A 19-year-old male presented for treatment of osteochondritis dissecans of the lateral femoral condyle. He had undergone arthroscopic drilling of the lesion on two occasions at age 16 and 18 years. Arthroscopic examination revealed a 2- × 3-cm intact lesion of the lateral femoral condyle. Corticocancellous matchstick grafts were placed from distal to proximal through a lateral arthrotomy. (a) Anteroposterior and (b) lateral radiographs demonstrate the bone grafts in the lateral lesion. (c) Intraoperative photograph shows the arthrotomy incision and the lesion of the posterior aspect of the lateral femoral condyle. (d,e) A follow-up arthroscopic examination was performed 1 year later, and the lesion was noted to be healed with minimal chondromalacia of the lateral femoral condyle. Radiographs demonstrate the healed lesion. (f) Artist's sketch demonstrates the technique for open bone grafting.

The treatment recommendations for lesions of the medial femoral condyle apply as well to lesions of the lateral femoral condyle. Drilling of a lesion in the lateral femoral condyle can generally be performed arthroscopically. More complex procedures, such as bone grafting with pegs or cancellous graft and internal fixation with screws or wires, usually require arthrotomy. Separated or detached lesions should be internally fixed with multiple corticocancellous bone pegs. Loose bodies with adequate bone should be replaced and rigidly fixed.

Because the healing potential for osteochondritis dissecans in patients past skeletal maturity is less than for young patients, we take an aggressive posture in treating these patients. Preoperative radiographic studies are important in assessment of the lesion. Nevertheless, we do not recommend obtaining multiple costly studies that expose the patient to excessive radiation. Instead, obtain plain radiographs and either tomography or an MRI study. No doubt, as experience is gained using MRI in osteochondritis dissecans, there will be improved assessment of articular cartilage integrity.

After the basic radiographic assessment, arthroscopy is indicated both for diagnostic and therapeutic purposes. Arthroscopy gives the most accurate assessment of the integrity of the articular cartilage and the mobility of the underlying bone fragment. Therefore, it should be performed in all patients with

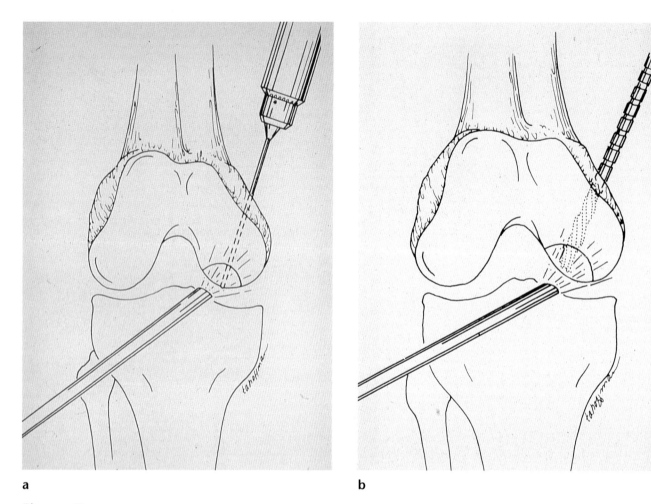

a

b

Figure 7

(a) Artist's sketch demonstrates the technique for 'proximal-to-distal' bone grafting of osteochondritis dissecans lesion. Under arthroscopic guidance, a guide-pin is introduced from the femoral metaphysis into the lesion. Placement of the pin is facilitated by the use of an anterior cruciate ligament guide, and may be confirmed using intraoperative image intensification or radiographs. (b) The guide-pin is carefully overdrilled with a 6–8-mm cannulated reamer, being careful not to breach the articular surface. Cancellous bone graft is then harvested from the iliac crest or proximal tibia and packed down the drillhole.

osteochondritis dissecans presenting after skeletal maturity. A treatment plan based upon accurate information can be formulated.

If arthroscopic examination reveals an intact lesion in the skeletally mature patient, we recommend bone grafting or internal fixation with compression screws and drilling of the lesion. Non-weight-bearing for at least 3 months is advised, and the internal fixation devices are usually removed then. Progression in weight-bearing depends upon radiographic appearance of the lesion and clinical examination.

A separated or detached lesion is internally fixed with compression screws or fixed with bone pegs. Earlier in our experience, bone grafting was preferred, but recently we have had good results with screw fixation. We use cannulated 3.5-mm cancellous screws or cannulated Herbert screws for this purpose.

Lesions of the lateral condyle in skeletally mature patients are treated aggressively, generally with an arthrotomy. Intact lesions are fixed with bone pegs, as are separated or detached lesions. Loose bodies are not usually amenable to reattachment and must be removed. The base is debrided and drilled.

Complications

The experience of the senior author (J.F.G) has included operative treatment of over 120 cases of osteochondritis dissecans and conservative treatment of an additional 20 over a 16-year period. We also have benefited from multiple consultations from other treating physicians nationwide. Many complications can occur in treating osteochondritis dissecans. Some relate specifically to the disease entity itself, and some relate to general complications of surgery. The latter include anesthetic complications, cardiovascular or pulmonary postoperative complications, deep vein thrombosis, etc. We will address only those complications specifically related to osteochondritis dissecans.

Failure to recognize osteochondritis dissecans on radiographs poses the risk of disease progression from an early, treatable form to one destined to progress to a loose body with crater formation. Patients with the earliest stage of the disorder may have minimal radiographic changes. These are easily overlooked by an orthopedist who is not cognizant of the potential diagnosis. Follow-up physical examination and radiographic studies are mandatory, especially in young patients with unexplained knee pain. The bone scan is a good screening study that should be obtained to rule out this possibility.

Even conservative treatment can result in complications. Usually, however, young patients can tolerate long periods of immobilization without adverse effects. Excessively long periods of immobilization can result in knee stiffness, quadriceps atrophy, quadriceps weakness, and flexion contracture.

Arthroscopic treatment must also be performed with meticulous attention to detail to avoid complications. Simple arthroscopic drilling can cause damage to articular cartilage or result in pin breakage. These complications can be avoided by directing the Kirschner wire with a small cannula to avoid bending on the wire. Take care not to penetrate the condyle too deeply and so run the risk of injury to critical neurovascular structures. This complication also can be avoided by use of the cannula. Set the Kirschner wire so that approximately 1–1.5 cm protrudes from the cannula tip.

Attempts to pin a detached or loose fragment can result in splintering of the small bone fragment or inadequate fixation. In addition, no less than anatomic positioning of the fragment can be tolerated. Fixation in a nonanatomic position is likely to result in treatment failure. In one case referred to the senior author for consultation, a large juxta-articular cyst developed at the site of pin insertion.

The cannulated compression screws and the cannulated Herbert screws use pins of small diameter to guide screw position. Take care when drilling over these wires to maintain accurate alignment so as not to sever the intraosseous portion of the wire. Washers placed under the screw head increase the area over which compressive forces distribute, but may cause significantly greater articular cartilage damage. The washers also can become loose within the joint. We do not recommend use of washers.

Cannulated screws can be removed easily by reinserting a guide-pin. Removal of noncannulated screws however, must be performed with great care to avoid a loose screw in the joint. Screws remaining in the joint after the initiation of motion require a careful follow-up radiographic examination. If there is any evidence that the screw has backed out, it must be removed. Otherwise, severe articular cartilage erosion can result.

Bone pegs inserted from distal to proximal can cause similar articular cartilage injury if not countersunk appropriately. Take care not to cross the physeal plate with bone pegs or screws. Similarly, insertion of bone graft from proximal to distal can cause damage to the epiphyseal plate if the tract crosses from the metaphysis into the epiphysis.

Separation of a fragment thought to be healed after surgical intervention is possible. A patient treated by the senior author experienced fragment separation 11 years after internal fixation with Smillie pins.

References

1. **Pappas AM**, Osteochondrosis dissecans, *Clin Orthop* (1981) **158**: 59–69.
2. *Dorland's illustrated medical dictionary*, 27th edn (Philadelphia: WB Saunders, 1988), sv 'Osteochondritis'.
3. **Smillie IS**, Treatment of osteochondritis dissecans, *J Bone Joint Surg (Br)* (1957) **39**: 248–260.
4. **Milgram JW**, The development of loose bodies in human joints, *Clin Orthop* (1977) **124**: 292–303.
5. **Phemister DB**, The causes of and changes in loose bodies arising from the articular surface of the joint, *J Bone Joint Surg* (1924) **6**: 278.
6. **Aichroth P**, Osteochondral fractures and their relationship to osteochondritis dissecans of the knee: an experimental study in animals, *J Bone Joint Surg (Br)* (1971) **53**: 448–454.
7. **Aichroth P**, Osteochondritis dissecans of the knee: a clinical survey, *J Bone Joint Surg (Br)* (1971) **53**: 440–447.
8. **Clanton TO, DeLee JC**, Osteochondritis dissecans: history, pathophysiology and current treatment concepts, *Clin Orthop* (1982) **167**: 50–64.
9. **Enneking WF (ed)**, *Clinical musculoskeletal pathology* (Gainesville, Fla: Storter Printing Company, 1977).
10. **Hughston JC, Hergenroeder PT, Courtenay BG**, Osteochondritis dissecans of the femoral condyles, *J Bone Joint Surg (Am)* (1984) **66**: 1340–1348.
11. **Guhl JF**, Arthroscopic treatment of osteochondritis dissecans. *Clin Orthop* (1982) **167**: 65–74.
12. **Cahill BR, Berg BC**, 99m-Technetium phosphate compound joint scintigraphy in the management of juvenile osteochondritis dissecans of the femoral condyles. *Am J Sports Med* (1983) **11**(5): 329–335.
13. **Cahill BR, Phillips MR, Navarro R**, The results of conservative management of juvenile osteochondritis dissecans using joint scintigraphy, *Am J Sports Med* (1989) **17**(5): 601–606.
14. **Scott DJ Jr, Stevenson CA**, Osteochondritis dissecans of the knee in adults, *Clin Orthop* (1971) **76**: 82–86.
15. **Lipscomb PR Jr, Lipscomb PR Sr, Bryan RS**, Osteochondritis dissecans of the knee with loose fragments: treatment by replacement and fixation with readily removed pins, *J Bone Joint Surg (Am)* (1978) **60**: 235–240.
16. **Thomson NL**, Osteochondritis dissecans and osteochondral fragments managed by Herbert compression screw fixation, *Clin Orthop* (1987) **224**: 71–78.

17. **Greville NR,** Osteochondritis dissecans: treatment by bone grafting, *South Med J* (1964) **57:** 886.
18. **Lindholm S, Pylkkänen P,** Internal fixation of the fragment of osteochondritis dissecans in the knee by means of bone pins, *Acta Chir Scand* (1974) **140:** 626–629.
19. **Bigelow DR,** Juvenile osteochondritis dissecans, *J Bone Joint Surg (Br)* (1975) **57:** 530.

20. **Johnson EW, McLeod TL,** Osteochondral fragments of the distal end of the femur fixed with bone pegs, *J Bone Joint Surg (Am)* (1977) **59:** 677–679.
21. **Gillespie HS, Day B,** Bone peg fixation in the treatment of osteochondritis dissecans of the knee joint, *Clin Orthop* (1979) **143:** 125–130.

9.3 Chondral and osteochondral lesions of the femoral condyles

David J. Dandy

Many clearly distinct chondral and osteochondral lesions are found in the knee. Terminology has been very loosely used in the past and this has led to needless controversy concerning the cause, diagnosis and management of the different disorders. In particular, 'osteochondritis dissecans' has sometimes been used as a generic term for any lesion involving the femoral condyles and 'chondromalacia' has been misused when describing pain arising from the patellofemoral joint.

There is a pressing need for agreement on the exact nature of the individual lesions and their characteristics. The definitions that follow are based on a review of the lesions seen on the femoral condyles in 5000 consecutive arthroscopies[1] with additional comments on lesions of the patella.

The incidence, age and sex distribution of different lesions of the femoral condyle were determined in a group of 5000 consecutive arthroscopic examinations during an 11-year period. Most of the examinations were elective procedures on patients admitted from the waiting list. The indications for arthroscopy were persistent mechanical symptoms, unexplained effusion, the absence of a diagnosis, or difficulty in deciding management. Arthroscopy was not performed for the investigation of asymptomatic radiological abnormalities or if the investigation was unlikely to have any immediate benefit for the patient. Many patients were managed without arthroscopy and the figures do not represent the total number of patients with lesions of the femoral condyles seen during the study period.

Figure 1 shows the types of lesion of the femoral condyle, and Figure 2 and Table 1 show statistics relating to the age of the patients with the different conditions. Table 2 shows the incidence and sex distribution of such conditions, with the incidence of haemarthrosis and intact cartilage.

Acute osteochondral fractures

Acute osteochondral fractures are caused by acute trauma, either direct or indirect. The fragments have one flat surface of fresh cancellous bone and a convex surface covered with articular cartilage (Figure 1A). Such fragments are almost always visible radiologically.[2]

Patients with acute osteochondral fractures have a haemarthrosis and a definite history of recent injury. All patients with a haemarthrosis in the study had acute osteochondral fractures. The average age of patients with acute osteochondral fractures in the 5000 knees reported is shown in Table 1.

Acute osteochondral fractures can be treated by removal of the fragment if it is small or by re-attachment if it is large and has a good mass of bone to take a pin or screw. Sometimes the bony part of the fragment is so flimsy that it cannot be firmly secured and curls up at the edges as soon as pins are inserted. In these circumstances it may be wiser to remove the fragment and allow the bed of the lesion to heal with fibrocartilage.

Although it is possible to secure these fragments under arthroscopic control without a formal arthrotomy, accurate repositioning is easier for many surgeons through a small arthrotomy.

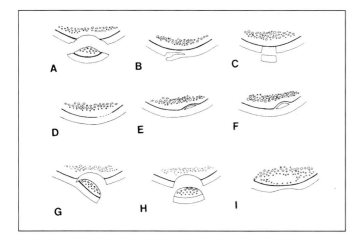

Figure 1

Types of lesion of a femoral condyle: (A) osteochondral fracture; (B) chondral flap; (C) chondral separation; (D),(E),(F) developing osteochondritis dissecans; (G) separating osteochondritis dissecans; (H) loose body from osteochondritis dissecans; (I) spontaneous osteonecrosis.

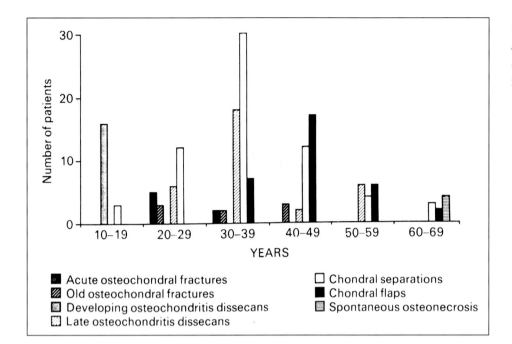

Figure 2

The age distribution of patients with osteochondral lesions of the femoral condyle.

Old osteochondral fractures

Patients were considered to have old osteochondral fractures if there was a loose body with one flat surface and one convex surface similar in shape to the fragment of a recent osteochondral fracture and a site of origin identifiable as a flattened area.

No difficulty was encountered in distinguishing between old osteochondral fractures and late osteochondritis dissecans using these criteria. The age distribution of the lesions is seen in Table 1.

Old osteochondral fractures seldom require any treatment apart from removal of the loose body. When the fragment is removed, the bed of the lesion is often so smooth and well-healed that there is great difficulty in identifying the site of origin of the loose body.

Chondral separations

Patients with normal radiographs and a full-thickness separation of normal articular cartilage with vertical margins (Figure 1C) surrounding exposed subchondral bone were considered to have chondral separations.[3-5] These lesions correspond with the type IV lesions of Bauer and Jackson.[6] Both longitudinal and circular separations were included in the study but old injuries and patients with extensive degenerative change were not included. Lesions less than 5 mm wide in any direction were disregarded.

Only recent lesions with clean, sharp margins in otherwise normal condyles were included to avoid difficulty in distinguishing between old chondral separations, chondral flaps and the lesions of degenerative osteoarthritis. Fragments of articular cartilage from chondral separations not visible radiologically were sometimes identified arthroscopically and removed. In others, the chondral fragment had become fragmented and remained as particulate debris within the joint.

Chondral flaps

Patients with isolated lesions involving only part of the thickness of the articular cartilage (Figure 1B) were considered to have chondral flaps.[3-5] These lesions correspond with the type III lesions of Bauer and Jackson.[6] Lesions less than 5 mm across were disregarded and knees with degenerative change on the affected condyle were not included.

These lesions may be treated by trimming the loose margins and leaving the bone untouched,[7] drilling of the subchondral bone, abrasion of the subchondral bone or excision of the cortex down to cancellous bone. There is no agreement on the best policy, but it is logical to convert lesions less than 1 cm across into what is, in effect, an osteochondral fracture by drilling, abrasion or excision. Excision of larger lesions may destabilize the weight-bearing area. It is the author's practice to remove all loose articular margins and remove the subchondral bone from lesions less than 1 cm in diameter. Larger lesions are drilled to leave cortical bridges.

Osteochondritis dissecans

Nowhere has the sloppy use of precise terminology led to more controversy than in the discussion of osteochondritis dissecans, and this probably explains

Table 1 Statistics relating to the age of the patients.

Condition	No.	Mean (years) [range]	Standard deviation	Standard error of mean	95% 't' confidence intervals
Acute osteochondral fracture	7	19.1 [16–22]	1.95	0.738	17.33–20.95
Old osteochondral fracture	8	34.9 [26–49]	8.7	3.09	27.57–42.18
Developing osteochondritis dissecans	16	13.6 [11–18]	1.9	0.47	12.55–14.57
Late osteochondritis dissecans	42	28.1 [18–44]	8.2	1.27	25.56–30.68
Chondral separation	64	32.3 [16–67]	10.9	1.37	33.12–38.6
Chondral flaps	32	45.6 [34–67]	8.32	1.47	41.62–47.63
Spontaneous osteonecrosis	5	67 [63–75]	4.64	2.07	61.24–72.76

Table 2 Details of patients.

Condition	No. of knees	Male (no.)	Female (no.)	Haemarthrosis No.	Haemarthrosis (%)	Intact articular cartilage (no.)
Acute osteochondral fracture	7	4	3	7	100	0
Old osteochondral fracture	8	8	0	0	0	0
Developing osteochondritis dissecans	16	13	3	0	0	16
Late osteochondritis dissecans	42	37	5	0	0	2
Chondral separation	64	52	12	0	0	0
Chondral flaps	32	21	11	0	0	0
Spontaneous osteonecrosis	5	4	1	0	0	0

why the subject remains controversial in spite of the many papers written on the subject.

Clanton and DeLee[8] identified two groups of osteochondritis dissecans, one occurring in children under the age of 15 and one in adults up to the age of 50 years. Smillie[9] described four lesions of articular cartilage, including an adult form of osteochondritis dissecans appearing after epiphyseal closure, but Green and Banks[10] reported the condition only in children.

Many different causes have been suggested, including trauma,[11,12] contact with the tibial spine,[13,14] abnormal ossification of the epiphyseal cartilage,[15,16] hereditary influences and generalised disorders such as multiple epiphyseal dysplasia and Fröhlich's syndrome.[9,17–19]

The role of trauma is particularly controversial. Both Paget[20] in the first description of the condition, and König,[21] who first used the term 'osteochondritis dissecans' in a report of eight patients with a definite history of minor injury, believed that trauma could not have been the sole cause, while Aichroth[11] found a history of significant trauma in 46% of his patients.

The explanation for these differences may be nothing more than a liberal interpretation of the term 'osteochondritis dissecans' to describe any condition in which there is separation of bone or articular cartilage from the underlying femoral condyle. Smillie,[14] for example, considered the condition now recognized as spontaneous osteonecrosis to be 'osteochondritis dissecans of the elderly' and Aichroth[11] described 100 patients with 'osteochondritis dissecans', including seven with osteochondral fractures, a few with radiological abnormalities of ossification and some which, in retrospect, were probably the result of osteochondral fractures caused by patellar dislocation.

As Barrie[22] has pointed out so eloquently, König had an ear for a euphonious title, and the harmony of the words has led to misuse.

Two patterns of osteochondritis dissecans can be recognized. *Developing osteochondritis dissecans* is characterized by lesions of the epiphysis in which a single area of ossification develops separately from the main body of an otherwise normal epiphysis (Figure 1D,E,F). Early radiographs show only an irregularity in the ossifying margin of the epiphysis (Type II[15]), but later radiographs show a separate concentric flake of bone (Type III[15]) which grows at the same rate as the epiphysis but remains separated from it by a transradiant line. Neither the fragment nor the defect is corticated.

Patients with irregular or patchy calcification of the epiphysis (Type I[15]) consistent with epiphyseal dysplasia were not included in this group. The lesions of developing osteochondritis dissecans were found only during the second decade of life. The articular cartilage was intact in all patients under the age of 18 years. All patients presented with pain and none had a haemarthrosis. The site of the radiological lesion could be identified at arthroscopy with a blunt probe in all knees. One patient had lesions in both knees.

Late osteochondritis dissecans is characterized by loose bodies arising from a concave defect on the femoral condyle with steeply sloping edges (Figure 1G,H). The shape of these defects distinguishes them from the flat sites of origin of osteochondral fractures. Both the fragment and the base of the condylar lesion are corticated with no exposed cancellous bone. Some patients whose radiographs showed a corticated fragment lying in situ within a condylar defect were found at arthroscopy to have intact articular cartilage over the lesion. These knees were also considered to have late osteochondritis dissecans.

The lesions of developing and late osteochondritis dissecans were found only at the 'classical' site on the medial femoral condyle. Careful search was made for these lesions at other sites on the condyles but none was found.

The lesions of late osteochondritis dissecans were not seen in patients under the age of 18 years. In some patients, the fragment had separated from its bed but remained attached on part of its circumference by a bridge of articular cartilage. Four patients had lesions in both knees and the articular cartilage over the lesion was intact in two patients over the age of 18 years.

Many lesions of osteochondritis dissecans before skeletal maturity can heal without any treatment,[23,24] but if there is no improvement within 6 months of diagnosis some form of surgical intervention is indicated. It is the author's practice to drill through the articular surface and the fragment into healthy bone and the results of this procedure are good.[25] In older patients in whom the fragment has begun to separate, it may be reattached with pin or screw. A cannulated screw with the same dimensions as the scaphoid screw of the ASIF system is available and allows the fragment to be drilled and screwed precisely under arthroscopic control.

Older knees in which the fragment has separated and the surfaces of the resulting loose body and the crater have become corticated may be treated in a variety of ways. The loose body can be removed and discarded or reattached, with or without grafting. If grafting is chosen it may be conducted either by an open procedure from inside the knee or by a closed procedure from the medial surface of the medial femoral condyle. Good results are reported for both procedures but there is no doubt that the immediate results of removing the loose body are better than those of grafting and fixation. No comparison of the late results is yet available.

Idiopathic osteonecrosis

Patients in whom the subchondral bone had disappeared to leave a cavity roofed by a plate of cortical bone (Figure 1I) were considered to have idiopathic osteonecrosis.[26,27] This is the same condition as Smillie's[14] 'osteochondritis dissecans of the elderly', but there is only a superficial similarity between the radiological or arthroscopic appearances. At arthroscopy, the cortical plate is unstable and the cavity contains soft amorphous tissue blending with the underlying bone without a corticated base, while patients with osteochondritis dissecans have a solid fragment with a corticated base. Idiopathic osteonecrosis is easily distinguished from the other conditions by the subchondral bone loss and absence of cortication visible either radiologically or arthroscopically.

The lesions of idiopathic osteonecrosis do not respond to any form of drilling or attempted vascularization. The patient is left with a crater in the medial femoral condyle which results in osteoarthritis. The loose tissue can be debrided to reduce the mechanical symptoms and an osteotomy is sometimes recommended to take weight off the effective medial side. Unicompartmental replacement is attractive but the soft necrotic bone provides a poor bed for the prosthesis and cement, and loosening has been reported.

Steroid osteonecrosis

The lesions of steroid osteonecrosis differ from those of osteochondritis dissecans and osteochondral fractures in the shape and size of the fragment, as well as the history of steroid administration. The fragments are large, corticated, irregular and involve large segments of the femoral condyle. The condition may be caused by massive dosage of steroids, as often seen in the early days of transplantation, and may also involve the femoral head. When the lesions are mature and the steroid dosage is reduced, replacement or fixation may be considered, but the underlying pathology in these patients may preclude definitive surgery.

Epiphyseal dysplasia

The appearances of epiphyseal dysplasia have been well described by Caffey et al.[15] but it must be remembered that they reported the appearances seen in routine examinations of the knee and the only patient in their series who developed symptoms was later found to have osteochondritis dissecans. The presence of these radiological abnormalities in the epiphysis does not indicate that pathology is present or that treatment is required.

In the study of Bradley and Dandy,[1] only those patients who had an effusion or mechanical symptoms of locking or catching underwent arthroscopy. Two knees meeting these criteria were examined arthroscopically during the study period.

Epiphyseal changes are seen in association with a discoid meniscus,[28] but I have not seen a patient with both a discoid meniscus and osteochondritis dissecans.

Lateral femoral condyle

A destructive lesion of the lateral femoral condyle is sometimes seen and two such knees were encountered in the 5000 knees reported. The lesion is flatter and shallower than that of osteochondritis dissecans of the medial condyle and the fragment is often decalcified. This pattern of lesion is not seen on the medial femoral condyle. The author has seen one example of this lesion in a lateral compartment which had a complete discoid lateral meniscus.

The radiological appearance of this lesion is more similar to an avascular pattern of osteochondritis such as Perthes' or Kienböck's disease than to the dissecting process seen on the medial condyle.

Treatment is difficult. The fragments seldom unite and the condition has a poor prognosis.

Articular surfaces

The articular surfaces were disrupted in all knees except the 16 with developing osteochondritis dissecans and two of the 42 (5%) with late osteochondritis dissecans.

Age of the patient

The ages of the patients with acute osteochondral fractures were significantly different (χ^2 test, $P<0.001$) from those with developing osteochondritis dissecans and the ages of those with chondral separations were significantly different (χ^2, $P<0.001$) from those with chondral flaps.

Patellar lesions

The paper by Bradley and Dandy[1] did not deal with the patella, but the following lesions were found.

Chondromalacia patellae

The word 'chondromalacia' means 'softening of cartilage' as 'osteomalacia' means softening of bone. It does not mean fissuring or splitting of the articular cartilage and still less does it mean a disorder or 'malaise' of cartilage as sometimes thought in North America.

The articular surface of the patella becomes progressively harder with age and most adolescent patellae are distinctly soft to the probing hook at arthroscopy. No satisfactory criterion has yet been decided for distinguishing normal and abnormal softening of the patella.

From a practical point of view, many teenage patients are seen with anterior knee pain, patellar tenderness, and even crepitus, whose patellae are found at arthroscopy to be intact but as soft as marshmallow. Shaving or drilling of these patellae is not likely to help and they are probably best left untouched provided that the patient and parents are given a very cautious prognosis. Many of these patellae later develop fissuring and splitting in the patients' early twenties.

Osteochondritis dissecans of the patella

A dissecting disorder of the patella is sometimes seen and was first described by Edwards and Bentley,[29] who reported six cases. Four such patellae were found in the 5000 knees described in this article. Patients with this condition can be managed as for osteochondritis dissecans of the medial femoral condyle, with drilling of the intact surfaces and debridement of late loose lesions. Some lesions heal but some separate and debridement of the underlying defect is then required. If the fragments are large and the symptoms severe, a later patellectomy may be required.

Osteochondral fractures of the patella

Osteochondral fractures of the patella are often found in patients with recurrent dislocation of the patella because the medial edge of the patella may fracture as it moves over the edge of the lateral condyle.

It is important to distinguish these lesions from areas of isolated calcification in the extra-articular structures on the medial side of the patella which result from ectopic ossification in the haematoma that follows capsular tears at the time of dislocation.

Longitudinal fissuring of the patella ('Sydney Opera House sign')

Longitudinal fissuring is sometimes seen on the medial half of unstable patellae. The fissures are oblique, so that the articular surface strips overlie each other. If the arthroscopic camera is turned through 180°, the lesion bears a slight resemblance to the interlocking shells of the Sydney Opera House.

This sign is of practical importance because it is only seen in patients who have subluxed or dislocated their patella and this diagnosis may escape even the most careful history and clinical examination. There is nothing to be done about these lesions except to treat the underlying instability.

Discussion

The main purpose of this study was to define osteochondritis dissecans and separate it from other conditions. Differentiation between osteochondritis dissecans and acute osteochondral fractures was straightforward. All patients with acute osteochondral fractures during the study period had a haemarthrosis, but a haemarthrosis was not found in any other condition. The appearances of the lesions were also different. Old osteochondral fractures were recognized by their characteristic shape, with one flat and one convex surface. The flat sites of origin were consistent with a tangential injury and differed markedly from the defects of osteochondritis dissecans.

The ages of the patients with developing or late osteochondritis dissecans were significantly different from those of the patients with osteochondral fractures in this study, and differed from those described by Matthewson and Dandy.[2] These differences in age distribution support the proposition that osteochondral fractures and osteochondritis dissecans are separate entities.

It is suggested that the diagnostic criterion for developing osteochondritis dissecans is an expanding lesion in an otherwise normal epiphysis. The only lesions meeting this criterion were found on the medial femoral condyle, at the classical site of osteochondritis dissecans, during the second decade of life. No such lesions were encountered at other sites on the condyles during the 11-year 5000-patient series, although four were seen on the patella. Similarly, the characteristic steep-sided defects of late osteochondritis dissecans were found only after skeletal maturity, at the 'classical' site on the medial femoral condyle. It is concluded from this that the lesions here called developing osteochondritis dissecans later become those of late osteochondritis dissecans, and that the mobile fragments attached at their periphery by articular cartilage represent the separation of an osteochondritic fragment from its bed.

The findings suggest strongly that osteochondral fractures are the result of acute trauma and not a 'dissecting' pathological process. This view agrees with that of Paget,[20] who believed that osteochondritis dissecans was a separate condition from osteochondral fracture and commented 'but how can such pieces of articular cartilage be detached from bone? They cannot be chipped off; no force can do this'.

The patients meeting the criteria for osteochondritis dissecans correspond closely with those described by Paget,[20] the category 3 patients of König,[21] and those of Green and Banks.[10] The recent use of 'osteochondritis dissecans' as a generic term for any disorder in which fragments separate from the femoral condyles either radiologically or mechanically has made discussion of osteochondritis dissecans needlessly complicated and should be discontinued.

Chondral separations, chondral flaps, steroid osteonecrosis and idiopathic osteonecrosis were easily distinguished from osteochondritis dissecans. The arthroscopic appearances and age distributions of each condition were different, and it is considered that these lesions are separate both from each other and from osteochondritis dissecans.

Caffey and his colleagues[15] studied the radiological appearances of the growing epiphysis in a group of asymptomatic knees, but only one of their patients met our criteria for osteochondritis dissecans. It is relevant that this patient was the only one in their study who later developed symptoms in the knee. This fact, and the difficulty in placing osteochondritis dissecans consistently into any one of the groups of Caffey and his colleagues,[15] suggests that their classification is not applicable to osteochondritis dissecans.

When local conditions affecting the articular surfaces within the knee are properly defined, many of the controversies vanish and a sensible discussion can be held on topics such as the relative advantages of screwing or grafting late osteochondritis and the wisdom of drilling chondral separations.

Provided that the above, or similar, guidelines are followed and the pathology is properly defined by arthroscopy and radiology before operation, considerable advances of the management of these lesions can be anticipated.

Summary

(1) The age and sex distribution of patients with lesions of the femoral condyles was studied in 5000 knees examined arthroscopically.

(2) The characteristics of developing and late osteochondritis dissecans, acute and old osteochondral fractures, chondral separations, chondral flaps and idiopathic osteonecrosis suggest that these are all separate conditions.

(3) Haemarthrosis was found only in the presence of acute osteochondral fractures.

(4) The characteristic feature of osteochondritis dissecans was an expanding concentric lesion at the 'classical' site on the medial femoral condyle, appear-

ing during the second decade of life and progressing to a concave steep-sided defect in the mature skeleton.

(5) The classification of Caffey and his colleagues (1958)[15] for epiphyseal dysplasia could not be applied to osteochondritis dissecans.

(6) Osteochondritis dissecans has a gradual onset without acute trauma.

(7) Much of the controversy surrounding osteochondral lesions is the result of imprecise nomenclature.

References

1. **Bradley J, Dandy DJ**, Osteochondritis dissecans and other lesions of the femoral condyles, *J Bone Joint Surg (Br)* (1989) **71**: 518–522.
2. **Matthewson MH, Dandy DJ**, Osteochondral fractures of the lateral femoral condyle: a result of indirect violence to the knee, *J Bone Joint Surg (Br)* (1978) **60**: 199–202.
3. **Dzioba RB**, The classification and treatment of acute articular cartilage lesions, *Arthroscopy* (1988) **4**(2): 72–80.
4. **Johnson-Nurse C, Dandy DJ**, Fracture-separation of articular cartilage in the adult knee, *J Bone Joint Surg (Br)* (1985) **67**: 42–43.
5. **Terry GC, Flandry F, Van Manen JW et al.**, Isolated chondral fractures of the knee, *Clin Orthop* (1988) **234**: 170–177.
6. **Bauer M, Jackson RW**, Chondral lesions of the femoral condyles: a system of arthroscopic classification, *Arthroscopy* (1988) **4**(2): 97–102.
7. **Hubbard MJS**, Arthroscopic surgery for chondral flaps in the knee, *J Bone Joint Surg (Br)* (1987) **69**: 794–796.
8. **Clanton TO, DeLee JC**, Osteochondritis dissecans: history, pathophysiology and current treatment concepts, *Clin Orthop* (1982) **167**: 50–64.
9. **Smillie IS**, *Osteochondritis dissecans: loose bodies in joints: aetiology, pathology, treatment* (Edinburgh: E & S Livingstone, 1960).
10. **Green WT, Banks HH**, Osteochondritis dissecans in children, *J Bone Joint Surg (Am)* (1953) **35**: 26–47.
11. **Aichroth PM**, Osteochondritis dissecans of the knee: a clinical survey, *J Bone Joint Surg (Br)* (1971) **53**: 440–447.
12. **Aichroth PM**, Osteochondral fracture and osteochondritis dissecans in sportsmen's knee injuries, *J Bone Joint Surg (Br)* (1977) **59**: 108.
13. **Fairbank HAT**, Osteochondritis dissecans, *Br J Surg* (1933) **21**: 67–82.
14. **Smillie IS**, *Diseases of the knee joint* (London: Churchill Livingstone, 1980).
15. **Caffey J, Madell SH, Royer C et al.**, Ossification of the distal femoral epiphysis, *J Bone Joint Surg (Am)* (1958) **40**: 647–654.
16. **Langer F, Percy EC**, Osteochondritis dissecans and anomalous centres of ossification: a review of 80 lesions in 61 patients, *Can J Surg* (1971) **14**: 208–215.
17. **Phillips HO IV, Grubb SA**, Familial multiple osteochondritis dissecans: report of a kindred, *J Bone Joint Surg (Am)* (1985) **67**: 155–156.
18. **Ribbing S**, The hereditary multiple epiphyseal disturbance and its consequences for the aetiogenesis of local malacias – particularly the osteochondritis dissecans, *Acta Orthop Scand* (1955) **24**: 286–299.
19. **Smith AD**, Osteochondritis of the knee joint: a report of three cases in one family and a discussion of the etiology and treatment, *J Bone Joint Surg (Am)* (1960) **42**: 289–294.
20. **Paget J**, On the production of some of the loose bodies in joints, *St Bartholomew's Hosp Rep* (1870) **6**: 1–4.
21. **König F**, Ueber freie Körper in den Gelenken, *Deutsche Z Chir, Leipz* (1887–1888) **27**: 90–109.
22. **Barrie HJ**, Osteochondritis dissecans 1887–1987: a centennial look at König's memorable phrase, *J Bone Joint Surg (Br)* (1987) **69**: 693–695.
23. **Edelstein JM**, Osteochondritis dissecans with spontaneous resolution, *J Bone Joint Surg (Br)* (1954) **36**: 343.
24. **Löfgren L**, Spontaneous healing of osteochondritis dissecans in children and adolescents: a case of multiple ossification centres in the distal epiphysis of the humerus and a rare "os epicondylitis medialis humeri", *Acta Chir Scand* (1954) **106**: 460–478.
25. **Bradley J, Dandy DJ**, Results of drilling osteochondritis dissecans before skeletal maturity, *J Bone Joint Surg (Br)* (1989) **71**: 642–644.
26. **Bauer GCH**, Osteonecrosis of the knee, *Clin Orthop* (1978) **130**: 210–217.
27. **Miller GK, Maylahn DJ, Drennan DB**, The treatment of idiopathic osteonecrosis of the medial femoral condyle with arthroscopic debridement, *Arthroscopy* (1986) **2**(1): 21–29.
28. **Glasgow MMS, Aichroth PM, Baird PRE**, The discoid lateral meniscus: a clinical review, *J Bone Joint Surg (Br)* (1982) **64**: 245.
29. **Edwards DH, Bentley G**, Osteochondritis dissecans patellae, *J Bone Joint Surg (Br)* (1977) **59**: 58–63.

9.4 Osteonecrosis of the knee: an overview

Dipak V. Patel and Paul M. Aichroth

The spontaneous osteonecrosis of the knee was first described as a distinct clinicopathological entity by Ahlbäck et al.[1] in 1968. Since then, numerous reports have appeared in the literature.[2-14] This entity is believed to be an important but underestimated cause of osteoarthritis of the knee.[1,4,10,13-16]

The condition commonly involves the medial femoral condyle but may also occur in the lateral femoral condyle[12] and medial tibial plateau.[5,9,17,18] Osteonecrosis of the knee can arise spontaneously without any predisposing factor or may be associated with various medical problems such as steroid therapy, renal transplantation, alcoholism, haemoglobino-pathies, Gaucher's disease, Caisson decompression sickness and systemic lupus erythematosus (SLE).

Mahood et al.[19] undertook a continuing prospective study which included 507 patients with SLE in 1986. Of 54 patients (10.6%) with osteonecrosis of any bone, 13 (2.6%) had symptomatic osteonecrosis of the knee. All patients had received systemic corticosteroid treatment for SLE. Two patients had been lost to follow-up, and of the remaining 17 knees (11 patients), the lateral femoral condyle was involved in 8 (47%). The authors mentioned that osteonecrosis of the knee in SLE may be a different process from that with spontaneous onset as the site of involvement is often different. They suggested that osteonecrosis of the lateral femoral condyle should be included in the differential diagnosis of knee pain in a patient with a history of SLE and systemic administration of corticosteroid.

The precise aetiology of the lesion is still unknown. The clinical course and the prognosis of the disease depend on the radiographic size of the lesion[2,8,13,14,16] and also on the pattern of the scintimetric uptake.[13,20]

The natural history of osteonecrosis of the knee

The clinical course and radiographic changes of the osteonecrosis of the femoral condyle in patients under conservative treatment have been assessed by Motohashi et al.[21] They observed 15 knees in 14 patients, averaging 62.8 years in age (range 23–79 years). The average follow-up was 4.9 years (range 1–12 years). Spontaneous osteonecrosis was found in 11 patients and steroid-induced osteonecrosis in 3.

The size of the osteonecrotic lesion was measured on plain radiographs as suggested by Ahlbäck et al.[1] A lesion of less than 10 mm width was regarded as small. Cases of small osteonecrotic lesions showed no remarkable changes with respect to staging of the lesion and limb alignment. The average size of the steroid-induced osteonecrotic lesion was significantly larger than that of the spontaneous type. At the follow-up examination, the size of the necrotic lesion increased by more than 18% of the initial size in 8 of the 12 knees.

Al-Rowaih et al. studied 40 patients with clinically suspected osteonecrosis of the knee using repeated plain radiography and scintimetry.[15] The mean age of the patients at the onset of osteonecrosis was 67 years (range 41–85 years) and the patients were followed for 1–7 years. In their series, 29 knees developed osteoarthrosis of at least Ahlbäck stage I. Of these 29 cases, 5 underwent unicompartmental arthroplasty, 3 had a total knee arthroplasty and 4 had an osteotomy.

Clinical features

The lesion typically occurs after the age of 60 years and is three times more common in females than in males.[10] It is characterized by a sudden onset of severe pain on the medial side of the knee. The pain may be worse on weight bearing, on ascending and descending stairs or at night. Many patients complain of pain at rest. The pain is initially very severe but gradually decreases during the first few months after onset. The clinical findings include a well-localized tenderness over the affected femoral condyle, and a mild synovitis with an effusion.

Differential diagnosis

Osteonecrosis of the knee should be distinguished from osteochondritis dissecans, osteoarthritis, menis-cal tears, stress fracture or pes anserinus bursitis.

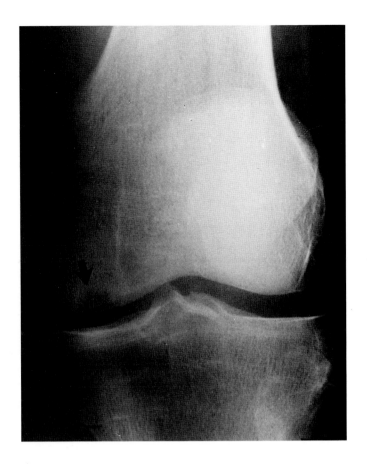

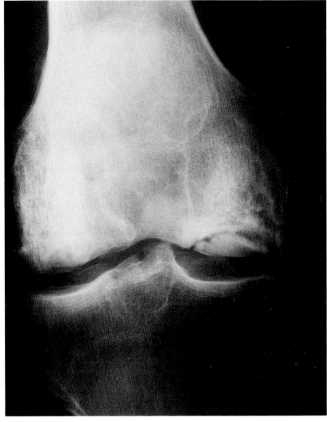

Figure 1

Plain radiograph of a 67-year-old woman with spontaneous osteonecrosis of the knee, affecting the medial femoral condyle. The lesion consists of a subchondral radiolucent area (arrow).

Figure 2

Plain radiograph of a 62-year-old man showing a large osteonecrotic lesion in the medial femoral condyle.

Radiological features

The plain radiographs are usually normal in the earlier course of the disease. Later, they may show a subchondral radiolucent area (Figure 1), usually surrounded by a sclerotic halo in the weight-bearing portion of the femoral condyle. As the disease process continues, a large area of osteonecrosis may be seen affecting a considerable portion of the femoral condyle (Figure 2). In the late stages, severe destruction with collapse of the femoral condyle occurs, leading to secondary osteoarthritis with axial malalignment (Figure 3).

The necrotic lesion can be graded according to Aglietti et al.[2] as modified by Koshino et al.[7]: Stage 1 = normal; Stage 2 = flattening of the affected weight-bearing portion of the femoral condyle; Stage 3 = typical lesion consisting of an area of radiolucency of variable size and depth, and surrounded proximally and distally by some sclerosis; Stage 4 = the radiolucent area is surrounded by a sclerotic halo and the subchondral bone has collapsed, and is visible as a calcified plate; Stage 5 = secondary degenerative changes with subchondral sclerosis of both femur and tibia, associated with some erosion.

However, it should be noted that the plain radiographs may be normal for a considerable period of time and sometimes normal throughout the entire course of the disease.[6,11,14,15] In contrast, radioisotope bone scans are positive in the early stage of the lesion, and are characterized by a high, localized uptake.

Pollack et al.[22] emphasized the value of magnetic resonance imaging (MRI) in the evaluation of suspected osteonecrosis of the knee, and Björkengren et al.[23] reported the usefulness of MRI in determining the prognosis. The advent of MRI has provided unparalleled ability to visualize bone marrow and to distinguish necrotic tissue from

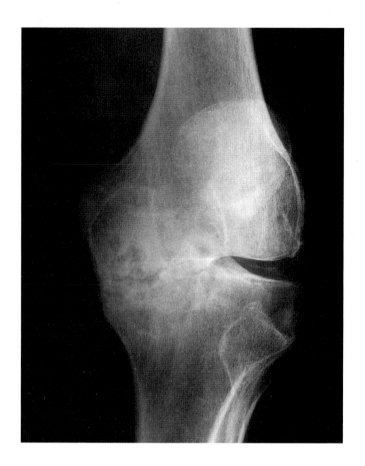

Figure 3

Radiograph showing extensive osteonecrosis with secondary osteoarthritic changes in the medial compartment, associated with varus deformity at the knee.

a

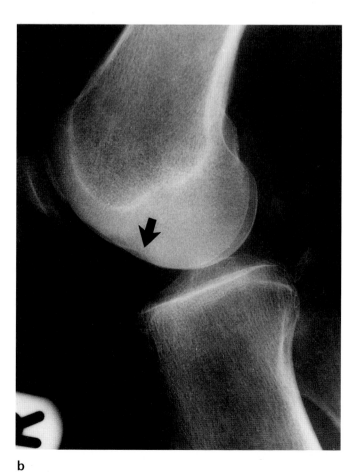

b

Figure 4

A 59-year-old woman with osteonecrosis involving the medial femoral condyle. The plain radiographs ((a) anteroposterior and (b) lateral views) taken 4 months after the onset of symptoms show an area of subchondral radiolucency (arrows).

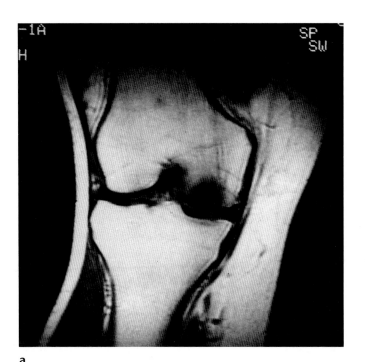

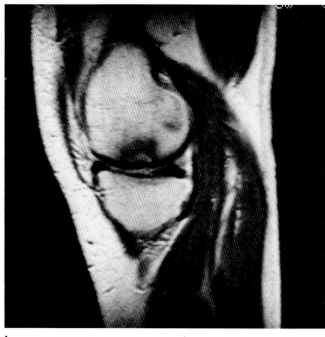

a   b

Figure 5

Magnetic resonance imaging of the same patient (shown in Figure 4) demonstrates the extent of the necrotic lesion.

viable segments with an extremely high level of sensitivity and specificity. Moreover, the extent of the osteonecrotic lesion as seen on MRI is often greater than that visualized on plain radiographs (Figures 4 and 5).

Prognosis

The prognosis of osteonecrosis has been described by Muheim and Bohne.[13] They noted development of osteoarthrosis in 18 out of 20 knees with osteonecrotic lesions followed for more than 2 years. They recommended conservative treatment for patients with small necrotic lesions less than 3.5 cm² in area, and tibial osteotomy with arthrotomy for those with larger osteonecrotic lesions exceeding 5 cm².

Rozing et al.[14] mentioned that the prognosis may depend on the size of the lesion and that osteoarthrosis is likely to develop in knees with lesions larger than 2.3 cm². They recommended surgery for cases in which conservative treatment failed to relieve symptoms or for cases with a large collapsed lesion associated with varus deformity and instability of the knee.

Aglietti et al. reported that the prognosis is unfavourable if the lesion is larger than 5 cm² and if its width is more than 40% of that of the condyle.[2]

Recently, Motohashi et al. mentioned two important criteria concerning the surgical indication: one is the change in the size of the necrotic lesion and the other is the significance of limb malalignment.[21] They suggested that high tibial osteotomy should be undertaken for a knee with painful osteonecrosis of the medial femoral condyle and varus deformity even if the lesion is smaller in size, as the necrotic lesions may not heal spontaneously under excessive weight-bearing pressure in the medial compartment and its stage may progress.

Lotke and Ecker reported that patients who never have a radiologically apparent lesion or who have a small lesion (less than 45% of the condylar width, or less than 3.5 cm²) have a favourable prognosis.[10] On the other hand, patients with a larger lesion (more than 50% of the width of the femoral condyle, or larger than 5 cm²) usually become disabled, with increasing pain, deformity and secondary osteoarthritis of the joint.

Treatment

Early recognition of this condition is vital. The conservative measures include physiotherapy, protected weight bearing, analgesics and anti-inflammatory drugs. Patients with more advanced stages of osteonecrosis may require surgical intervention. The various surgical procedures include arthroscopic debridement,[7,24] core decompression,[25] high tibial osteotomy,[2,6,14,16,26] drilling with or without bone grafting,[26] unicompartmental arthroplasty, total knee replacement,[2,6,14,16] or osteochondral allografts.[27–29]

Miller et al. reviewed five patients with idiopathic osteonecrosis treated by arthroscopic debridement.[24] The mean postoperative follow-up was 31 months (range 25–40 months). Using the Hospital for Special Surgery Rating System, four of the five patients were rated good postoperatively (average rating: preoperative 52 points, postoperative 82 points). Biopsies of two patients at repeat arthroscopy showed that fibrocartilage fills in the defects created by the debridement.

Jacobs et al. performed 28 core decompressions of the distal femur for pathologically confirmed avascular necrosis of the knee.[25] At a mean follow-up of 54 months (range 20–140 months) and using the Ficat staging, all 7 cases in stage I and stage II had good results. Of the 21 cases in stage III, 11 cases had good results, 4 had poor results and 6 required total knee replacement. The authors concluded that core decompression is a simple procedure with a low complication rate and offers an excellent chance of pain relief in patients with stage I and II disease and a 50% chance of pain relief in patients with stage III disease.

Koshino[26] performed a high tibial osteotomy in 37 knees with spontaneous osteonecrosis of the femoral condyle (35 medial and 2 lateral). Drilling or bone-grafting of the necrotic lesion was done concomitantly with the osteotomy in 23 knees. The mean postoperative follow-up was 61 months (range 24–102 months). Preoperative pain was relieved and walking ability was improved in 35 knees. The author concluded that bone-grafting or drilling into the necrotic lesion are effective in promoting healing of osteonecrosis, and that surgery should be undertaken in the early stages, prior to the onset of degenerative changes, in order to obtain maximum clinical and radiological improvement.

Aglietti et al.[2] reviewed 101 knees followed for an average of 5 years (range 2–16 years). Of the 22 knees that were treated conservatively, 80% were satisfactory (excellent or good). Of the 11 knees treated by arthrotomy (drilling alone or curettage and drilling of the base of the crater after removal of the fragment), 55% were satisfactory. Thirty-one knees were treated by tibial osteotomy (21 in conjunction with arthrotomy) and 27 of them (87%) had satisfactory results. Arthrotomy did not significantly improve the results of osteotomies. Thirty-seven knees underwent total knee replacement and 95% of these had satisfactory results.

We agree with Aglietti et al.,[2] Insall et al.[16] and Lotke and Ecker[10] in that the decision whether to perform a high tibial osteotomy or replacement arthroplasty should be made using the same criteria that would be used for a patient who has osteoarthritis. Younger, more active patients should be treated by proximal tibial osteotomy with or without bone grafting, whereas elderly patients with a lower level of activity and a greater deformity should be considered for prosthetic replacement. The choice between a total knee replacement and unicompartmental arthroplasty is still a subject of major debate.

Bayne et al. recommended fresh osteochondral allografts for traumatic osteonecrosis of the knee in young patients.[27] They suggested high tibial osteotomy in combination with allograft replacement in patients with associated malalignment. They noticed that patients with steroid-induced osteonecrosis did well initially after allograft replacement (for 6–18 months), especially in experiencing pain relief. However, because of the continuous use of high doses of steroids, revascularization of the allografts was poor, resulting in graft subsidence. Therefore, they do not recommend osteochondral allografts for steroid-induced osteonecrosis of the knee.

Steroid-related osteonecrosis of the knee

An association between prolonged corticosteroid administration and osteonecrosis of the knee has been reported previously.[3,30–33] The two most common disorders associated with steroid therapy are renal transplantation and systemic lupus erythematosus. In steroid-induced disease, 50% of the cases are bilateral, 60% affect the lateral femoral condyle, and in 90% there are multiple sites in other joints but symptoms are often minor as compared to those of lesions which involve an entire condyle.[2] The predilection for involvement of the femoral condyles, more specifically the lateral femoral condyle, is not fully understood.

Ahuja and Bullough reported a series of 11 patients (14 knees) with rheumatoid arthritis who had biopsy-proven osteonecrosis of the femoral condyles.[3] Ten of the 11 patients were on long-term corticosteroid therapy. In their series, lateral femoral condyle was involved in 11 of the 14 knees. The single largest reported series of steroid-related osteonecrosis of the femoral condyles is that of Sasaki et al.[32] They described 10 patients (18 knees) with a variety of underlying conditions. In their study, 80% of the cases were bilateral and the lateral femoral condyle was predominantly involved. The duration between the onset of steroid use and the development of symptoms ranged from 1.5 to 14.1 years (average 6.6 years) and the average cumulative dose was 29 g.

A high index of suspicion is required for the diagnosis of this condition. The clinical presentation in the knee begins with symptoms of pain and swelling. Later, symptoms of internal derangement appear, characterized by sensations of locking, catching and popping.[34]

The treatment of the steroid-induced osteonecrosis of the knee depends primarily on the stage of the disease process. In the very early stages, conservative measures are indicated, which include physiotherapy, protected weight bearing and activity modification. Later, when symptoms of internal derangement interfere with joint function, exploration and debridement (open or arthroscopic) may be indicated.

Wiedel reported his experience with the arthroscopic evaluation and treatment of 10 knees involved with steroid-induced osteonecrosis.[34] He suggested that arthroscopic debridement provides reasonable symptomatic relief of the impingement symptoms, allowing the patients to return to activities of daily living.

Disappointing results have been reported following the use of osteochondral allografts for steroid-induced osteonecrosis of the knee.[28] Total knee replacement should be considered in knees with severe destruction and deformity accompanied by marked degenerative changes.

References

1. Ahlbäck S, Bauer GCH, Bohne WH, Spontaneous osteonecrosis of the knee, Arthritis Rheum (1968) 11: 705–733.
2. Aglietti P, Insall JN, Buzzi R et al., Idiopathic osteonecrosis of the knee: aetiology, prognosis and treatment, J Bone Joint Surg (Br) (1983) 65: 588–597.
3. Ahuja SC, Bullough PG, Osteonecrosis of the knee: a clinico-pathological study in twenty-eight patients, J Bone Joint Surg (Am) (1978) 60: 191–197.
4. Bauer GCH, Osteonecrosis of the knee, Clin Orthop (1978) 130: 210–217.
5. Houpt JB, Alpert B, Lotem M et al., Spontaneous osteonecrosis of the medial tibial plateau, J Rheumatol (1982) 9: 81–90.
6. Houpt JB, Pritzker KPH, Alpert B et al., Natural history of spontaneous osteonecrosis of the knee (SONK): a review, Semin Arthritis Rheum (1983) 13: 212–227.
7. Koshino T, Okamoto R, Takamura K et al., Arthroscopy in spontaneous osteonecrosis of the knee, Orthop Clin North Am (1979) 10: 609–618.
8. Lotke PA, Abend JA, Ecker ML, The treatment of osteonecrosis of the medial femoral condyle, Clin Orthop (1982) 171: 109–116.
9. Lotke PA, Ecker ML, Osteonecrosis-like syndrome of the medial tibial plateau, Clin Orthop (1983) 176: 148–153.
10. Lotke PA, Ecker ML, Current concepts review: osteonecrosis of the knee, J Bone Joint Surg (Am) (1988) 70: 470–473.
11. Lotke PA, Ecker ML, Alavi A, Painful knees in older patients: radionuclide diagnosis of possible osteonecrosis with spontaneous resolution, J Bone Joint Surg (Am) (1977) 59: 617–621.
12. Marmor L, Osteonecrosis of the knee: Medial and lateral involvement, Clin Orthop (1984) 185: 195–196.
13. Muheim G, Bohne WH, Prognosis in spontaneous osteonecrosis of the knee: investigation by radionuclide scintimetry and radiography, J Bone Joint Surg (Br) (1970) 52: 605–612.
14. Rozing PM, Insall J, Bohne WH, Spontaneous osteonecrosis of the knee, J Bone Joint Surg (Am) (1980) 62: 2–7.
15 Al-Rowaih A, Lindstrand A, Björkengren A et al., Osteonecrosis of the knee: diagnosis and outcome in 40 patients, Acta Orthop Scand (1991) 62: 19–23.
16. Insall JN, Aglietti P, Bullough PG, Osteonecrosis, Surgery of the knee, ed Insall JN (New York: Churchill Livingstone, 1984) 527–549.
17. D'Anglejan G, Ryckewaert A, Glimet S, Ostéonécrose du plateau tibial intern, Extr Rheumat (1976) 8: 253–255.
18. Marmor L, Fracture as a complication of osteonecrosis of the tibial plateau: a case report, J Bone Joint Surg (Am) (1988) 70: 454–457.
19. Mahood J, Bogoch E, Urowitz M et al., Osteonecrosis of the knee in systemic lupus erythematosus, J Bone Joint Surg (Br) (1990) 72: 541.
20. Greyson ND, Lotem MM, Gross AE et al., Radionuclide evaluation of spontaneous femoral osteonecrosis. Radiology (1982) 142: 729–735.
21. Motohashi M, Morii T, Koshino T, Clinical course and roentgenographic changes of osteonecrosis in the femoral condyle under conservative treatment, Clin Orthop (1991) 266: 156–161.
22. Pollack MS, Dalinka MK, Kressel HY et al., Magnetic resonance imaging in the evaluation of suspected osteonecrosis of the knee, Skeletal Radiology (1987) 16: 121–127.
23. Björkengren AG, Al-Rowaih A, Lindstrand A et al., Spontaneous osteonecrosis of the knee: value of MR imaging in determining prognosis, Am J Roentgenol (1990) 154: 331–336.
24. Miller GK, Maylahn DJ, Drennan DB, The treatment of idiopathic osteonecrosis of the medial femoral condyle with arthroscopic debridement, Arthroscopy (1986) 2: 21–29.
25. Jacobs MA, Loeb PE, Hungerford DS, Core decompression of the distal femur for avascular necrosis of the knee, J Bone Joint Surg (Br) (1989) 71: 583–587.
26. Koshino T, The treatment of spontaneous osteonecrosis of the knee by high tibial osteotomy with and without bone-grafting or drilling of the lesion, J Bone Joint Surg (Am) (1982) 64: 47–58.
27. Bayne O, Langer F, Pritzker KPH et al., Osteochondral allografts in the treatment of osteonecrosis of the knee, Orthop Clin North Am (1985) 16: 727–740.
28. Ganel A, Israeli A, Horoszowski H et al., Osteochondral graft in the treatment of osteonecrosis of the femoral condyle, J Am Geriatric Soc (1981) 29: 186–188.
29. Gross AE, McKee NH, Pritzker KPH et al., Reconstruction of skeletal deficits at the knee: a comprehensive osteochondral transplant program, Clin Orthop (1983) 174: 96–106.
30. Havel PE, Ebraheim NA, Jackson WT, Steroid-induced bilateral avascular necrosis of the lateral femoral condyles: a case report, Clin Orthop (1989) 243: 166–168.
31. Kelman GJ, Williams GW, Colwell CW Jr et al., Steroid-related osteonecrosis of the knee: two case reports and a literature review, Clin Orthop (1990) 257: 171–176.
32. Sasaki T, Yagi T, Monji J et al., Steroid-induced osteonecrosis of the femoral condyle: a clinical study of eighteen knees in ten patients, J Jpn Orthop Assoc (1986) 60: 361–372.
33. Wiedel JD, Arthroscopy in steroid-induced osteonecrosis of the knee, Arthroscopy (1985) 1: 68–72.

9.5   Osteonecrosis of the knee

Kurt J. Kitziger and Paul A. Lotke

Osteonecrosis of the knee is a well-described but poorly understood pathological process. The disease itself is more precisely termed osteonecrosis of the femoral condyle or osteonecrosis of the tibial plateau. Indeed, one may question the use of the word 'osteonecrosis', since few authors have documented the presence of necrotic bone as the primary event in this perplexing lesion. Ahlbäck et al. first reported osteonecrosis of the medial femoral condyle as a painful radiolucent lesion associated with a focally active bone scan.[1] Most of their patients were not found to have any of the known associated risk factors for osteonecrosis of the hip. In the decades following their report little has been added to the description of the clinical syndrome, as most authors have addressed treatment issues. Osteonecrosis of the tibial plateau has been described, but in general this entity appears to occur less often and is not as well understood as the femoral process.

Osteonecrosis of the knee can be classified as follows:

I. Osteonecrosis of the femoral condyle
II. Osteonecrosis of the tibial plateau
III. Osteonecrosis of the knee associated with known risk factors

We do not believe it proper to ascribe the terms primary and secondary to the diagnosis of osteonecrosis because the pathogenesis of the disorder has not been clearly elucidated. The majority of this discussion will concern spontaneous, or idiopathic, osteonecrosis of the femoral condyle and tibial plateau. Osteonecrosis associated with diseases such as systemic lupus erythematosus (SLE) or with the use of steroids has a different clinical presentation and will be briefly discussed at the end of this contribution.

Osteonecrosis of the femoral condyle

Clinical presentation

Most patients with osteonecrosis of the knee are in the seventh decade of life, and females outnumber males in the ratio 3:1. The pain usually begins with an abrupt onset and is classically confined to the medial aspect of the knee. The pain is typically present at night, and most often no trauma can be related by the patient. More than 95% of cases have involved the medial side of the joint. Physical examination may reveal a minimal effusion, but the most common finding is focal tenderness over the affected condyle. This is to be distinguished from the joint-line tenderness that is commonly seen in meniscal lesions, an often-confused diagnostic issue. The range of motion is usually normal but may be limited by pain. Ligamentous examination is normal.

Imaging

Radiography

Koshino has developed a radiographic classification that has been modified by Insall.[2,3]

Stage I: radiographs are entirely normal. It is possible for the disease never to progress beyond this radiographic stage.
Stage II: slight flattening of the femoral condyle usually on the weight-bearing aspect of the convexity.
Stage III: focal area of radiolucency in the femoral condyle with a radiodensity distal to the lesion.
Stage IV: calcified plate with a radiolucency surrounded by a definite sclerotic halo.
Stage V: narrowing of the joint space with subchondral sclerosis and osteophyte formation on both sides of the joint.

The propensity toward progression of radiographic disease has been debated in the literature.[1,4–11] The discrepancy is due to different authors' criteria for admission into the Stage I or preradiographic phase of the disease. Aglietti and Buzzi have estimated that 50% of patients will develop radiographic changes of osteoarthritis by 1 year.[4] This will be discussed further under Natural History.

The radiographic extent of the disease can be measured in two ways. The first method requires measurement of the lesion on both the coronal and sagittal radiograph.[5,9] The topographic size of the lesion is then determined by multiplying the above

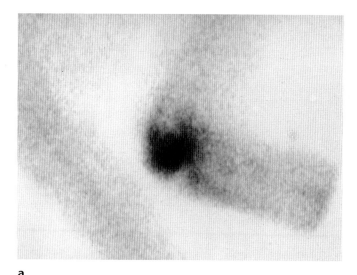

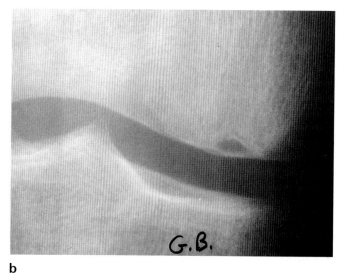

a

b

Figure 1

(a) The sagittal image on the bone scan clearly demonstrates increased uptake in the distal femur. (b) The radiograph demonstrates the typical appearance of a small osteonecrotic lesion in the medial femoral condyle. The lesion is Stage IV.

calculations. The problem with this method is that it is often difficult to measure the sagittal diameter owing to superimposition of the femoral condyles. In the second technique, the lesion is measured on the coronal view, and its size is expressed as a percentage of the total condylar width, which obviates the need for a lateral measurement.[8]

Scintigraphy

The hallmark of osteonecrosis is the scintigraphic finding of an intense increase in tracer uptake in one of the femoral condyles. Coronal and sagittal images assist in localization of the lesion (Figure 1). Many authors have felt that the scintigraphic findings are essential to the diagnosis of osteonecrosis.[1,12] These findings are to be distinguished from those seen in the knee with osteoarthritis, which tend to show a more diffuse pattern of tracer uptake.[9,13] The paradoxical finding of an active bone scan in the presence of osteonecrosis has been felt to represent bone remodeling around the necrotic lesion. In his initial description of the disease, Ahlbäck noted that the bone scan could be positive before the findings of osteonecrosis manifested themselves on plain radiographs. Numerous authors have identified a subgroup of patients with osteonecrosis of the knee who never develop radiographic changes consistent with osteonecrosis.[7,10,14] These patients present with a clinical history typical for osteonecrosis and have positive scinti-

graphic studies in the absence of any radiographic findings of osteonecrosis.

When the bone scan is repeated after the symptoms begin to abate, the study demonstrates less uptake and the radiographs remain unchanged. This has been called the 'self-resolving' bone scan.[5]

Magnetic resonance imaging (MRI)

This technique may eventually replace the technetium bone scan as the most valuable tool in diagnosing preradiographic osteonecrosis. Positive MRI findings consist of a discrete, well-marginated low signal area in the subchondral bone of the femoral condyle best seen on T_1-weighted images[3,7] (Figure 2). The dimensions of the lesion on MRI may be calculated and often appear larger than seen on radiographs.[15] In addition, an assessment of the articular cartilage can usually be made. One of the first signs of articular pathology is the buckling of the articular cartilage into the area of bone collapse.[15]

The problem with MRI in the diagnosis of osteonecrosis is that few authors have made pathologic correlation between the MRI findings and those seen at surgery. It is tempting to compare osteonecrosis of the knee to that of the femoral head, for which several studies have demonstrated good pathologic correlation between the images and the histopathologic findings.[16,17] The extrapolation of MRI data on the hip to the study of the knee should not obviate the need

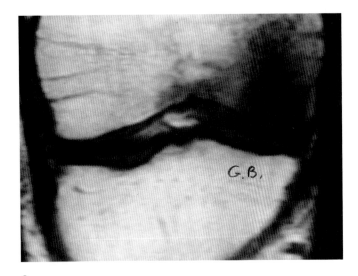

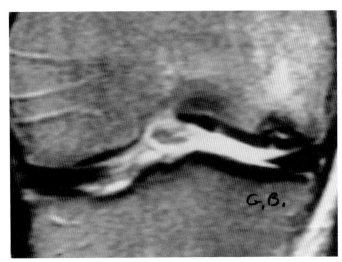

a   b

Figure 2

(a) The T_1-weighted magnetic resonance image of the same patient in Figure 1 shows a large area of decreased signal. (b) The T_2-weighted image highlights the necrotic area. Both magnetic resonance images suggest a greater area of involvement than that appreciated on the radiograph in Figure 1.

for tissue confirmation of MRI abnormalities in the knee. At any rate MRI appears to be of value in demonstrating the extent of involvement in the condyle, bone marrow changes in the absence of radiographic findings and the condition of the articular cartilage.

Pathology

Osteonecrosis is defined as the presence of dead bone in the subchondral weight-bearing region of the femoral condyle. Ahlbäck first noted that it is difficult to demonstrate the presence of necrotic bone in many lesions called osteonecrosis. Most often, patterns of revascularization are demonstrated on the pathologic studies.

Several studies have described quite well the histopathologic findings in osteonecrosis.[5,6,18,19] Gross examination of the femoral condyle in the earliest stage of the disease does not reveal any abnormalities. Through arthroscopic examination, Koshino delineated the sequence of articular changes.[3] The initial gross findings are slight flattening and discoloration of the articular cartilage. As the subchondral bone later begins to collapse, a flap tear of the articular cartilage can be noted. This flap tear eventually detaches, leaving an oval-shaped area of denuded necrotic bone with its long diameter based sagittally. Degenerative changes may eventually develop in the joint, and the lesion may fill with fibrous tissue or fibrocartilage. As mentioned above, microscopic examination of early

lesions reveals a predominance of revascularization.[4,6] Later in the course of the disease, empty lacunae will be found along with the invasion of abundant granulation tissue. The end stage of osteonecrosis consists of articular collapse and accelerated degenerative changes as documented in a histologic study of specimens resected for total knee arthroplasty.[18]

The difficulty in confirming the presence of necrotic bone in the early stages of this disease can be attributed to three reasons. The first is that most of the lesions are small and difficult to locate on biopsy, which leads to sampling error. The second potential reason is a delay in biopsy, during which revascularization and repair become the predominant histologic findings, obscuring the area of necrosis. The third reason is that many of the lesions will resolve spontaneously and surgery in these patients is not warranted. As a result of these difficulties, many authors have relied on clinical presentation and imaging studies to make the diagnosis of osteonecrosis. Limited pathologic confirmation of many of these early lesions has cast doubt on the validity of the term osteonecrosis. Indeed, a conceivable reason for the difficulty in demonstrating necrotic bone is that the cause for some patients' symptoms is a diagnosis other than osteonecrosis.

Pathogenesis

The etiology of osteonecrosis is unknown. The difficulty in postulating a cause for this disorder is made

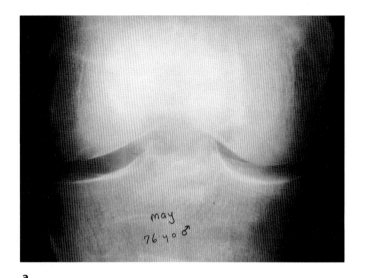
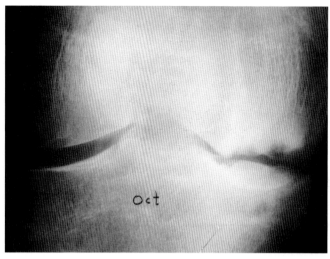

a

b

Figure 3

(a) This radiograph obtained at the onset of symptoms is normal. Bone scan and magnetic resonance imaging demonstrated a large lesion in the medial femoral condyle. (b) The radiograph after 5 months of continued pain shows extensive collapse of the condyle.

worse by the fact that the pathologic lesion has so rarely been identified in the early course of the disease. The two main etiologic theories are borrowed from the literature on femoral head necrosis. According to the vascular theory, the microcirculation of the femoral condyle is somehow interrupted, which leads to the formation of edema within the closed confines of condylar bone.[14,20-24] The resulting increase in pressure further interrupts the vascular supply to the subchondral bone, which then undergoes ischemic necrosis. During the period of revascularization, one of two events can occur. The first possibility is that the ingrowth of new blood vessels weakens the remaining bone, leading to subchondral collapse and progressive articular destruction. The second is that revascularization of the necrotic lesion succeeds before collapse can occur. The lesion thus heals, and a normal radiographic appearance is maintained.

According to the traumatic theory, the initiating event is a microfracture through osteoporotic subchondral bone.[25,26] Synovial fluid then leaks through the articular cartilage into the region of fracture, leading to an increased intraosseous pressure. The sequence of events is then similar to that outlined for the vascular etiology. Along these lines the actual finding of osteonecrosis would be considered a secondary event. Indeed, in some cases one could hypothesize the presence of microfractures followed by a phase of repair without any intervening stage consisting of osteonecrosis. This would help

to explain the difficulty in demonstrating the presence of osteonecrosis in such early lesions.

Natural history

The intense pain associated with the lesion persists for 2–3 months before it begins to resolve. The pain has usually dissipated by 12–15 months after onset. Persistence of symptoms is dictated by the presence of osteoarthritic changes following the insult. A significant percentage of elderly patients will have baseline osteoarthritis before the onset of acute symptoms.[27] Stage I patients, or those who have preradiographic lesions, progress to higher radiographic stages in only 50% or less of cases (Figure 3). This is markedly different from osteonecrosis of the femoral head, in which a much higher percentage of cases progress toward radiographic collapse.[28] The size of the lesion, rather than radiographic stage, appears to be a more important predictor of disease course.[7,9,10] Large lesions are those comprising greater than 50% of the condyle or measuring at least 5 cm². Several studies have shown that large lesions progress to radiographic collapse in a majority of cases. Those lesions which measure less than 50% of the individual condyle, or which measure less than 3.5 cm² in area are considered small and have a much more favorable prognosis. Small lesions usually resolve with minimal radiographic changes.

Differential diagnosis includes osteoarthritis, osteochondritis dissecans, pes anserinus bursitis, stress fracture, infection, neuropathy, and occult tumor.

Treatment

The initial form of treatment in most cases is conservative. The intense pain associated with the onset of this disease usually leads patients to present to the physician before radiographic changes of osteonecrosis are evident. As discussed previously, in many cases radiographic changes will never develop. Therefore, the most important consideration in the treatment of this disease is the recognition of it. By distinguishing osteonecrosis from other processes, unnecessary surgical procedures such as arthroscopic meniscectomy can be avoided. Bone scan and MRI may be needed to make the diagnosis in early stages. In the presence of a large radiographic lesion or in the case of symptomatic and radiologic progression, surgical treatment may be necessary.

Numerous surgical procedures have been described for femoral osteonecrosis, including arthroscopic debridement, high tibial osteotomy, drilling of the lesion with or without bone grafting, prosthetic replacement, and allograft replacement. The results of arthroscopic abrasion have been favorable in patients with small lesions; however, it is now felt that these lesions may indeed regress spontaneously.[29] Mechanical symptoms from a flap tear of articular cartilage may be relieved by debridement.

Jacobs et al. reported a small group of patients who underwent core decompression in a manner similar to that used in the femoral head.[14] Only two of the patients had spontaneous osteonecrosis and best results were seen in early radiographic stages. The authors felt that the risk of progression increased with higher radiographic stage at presentation. Size of the lesions was not specifically denoted. Most studies have focused on the options of high tibial osteotomy and prosthetic replacement. The indication for these procedures has been stated to be the same as for patients without osteonecrosis.[2,5,30] Many authors have recommended a high tibial osteotomy and have shown satisfactory results in those cases where minimal osteoarthritic changes are present, but investigators have disagreed on the amount of postoperative correction needed for a good result.[2,3]

The results of total knee arthroplasty have been excellent in patients with advanced osteoarthritic changes. Aglietti et al. reviewed 105 patients admitted with the diagnosis of femoral osteonecrosis at an average of 5 years of follow-up.[5] Results were satisfactory in 80% of the patients treated conservatively, but the authors noted that the success rate would probably have been higher if outpatients had been included. Satisfactory results following high tibial osteotomy and total knee arthroplasty were 87% and 95% respec-

tively. Lotke et al. reviewed 87 knees with osteonecrosis at an average of 3.5 years.[7] The authors used unicompartmental arthroplasty in approximately one-third of those patients with osteonecrosis who underwent prosthetic replacement. Because most patients are elderly, unicompartmental arthroplasty is favored over both total knee arthroplasty and high tibial osteotomy when involvement is limited to one compartment.

Allograft replacement has not been successful in most centers.[31,32] Bayne and associates reported six cases of allograft condylar replacement for osteonecrosis of which five failed.[31] Inability to comply with prolonged protected weight bearing was felt to be the main cause of failure.

Osteonecrosis of the tibial plateau

This entity is less well understood than osteonecrosis of the femoral condyle. The clinical syndrome has been termed osteonecrosis of the tibial plateau because it is quite similar to the process described in the femoral condyle. The studies describing this clinical entity, however, have offered little pathologic correlation between tissue findings and clinical findings.[33,34]

Clinical findings

The typical patient is in the sixth decade and has a sudden onset of pain along the medial aspect of the knee. Physical examination reveals tenderness confined to the joint-line and medial tibial plateau. The remainder of the knee examination is unremarkable.

Imaging studies

Plain radiographs usually do not show any lesions. Radiographic change, when present, consists of a collapsing lesion in the subchondral zone with an area of radiolucency surrounding a plate-like area of collapse in the subchondral bone. Concomitant osteoarthritic changes can be present. The most consistent imaging finding is that of a focally intense area of increased uptake with scintigraphy. Houpt and associates studied 21 knees and found most often that involvement was localized to the peripheral corner of the medial plateau.[33] Both coronal and sagittal views are used to identify the area in the tibial plateau. The findings of MRI are similar to those in femoral osteonecrosis (Figure 4).

Natural history

The period of intense pain usually lasts 6–9 months and then slowly begins to resolve. It appears that in

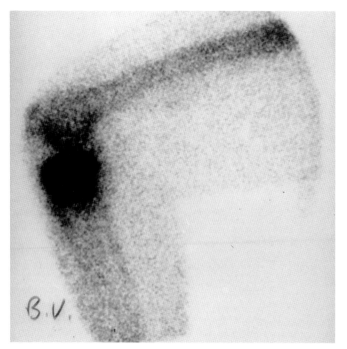

a

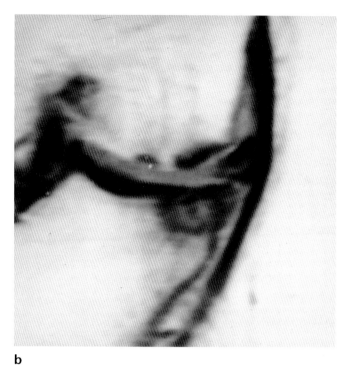

b

Figure 4

(a) The sagittal image on the bone scan clearly demonstrates increased uptake in the proximal tibia. (b) The corresponding T_1-weighted magnetic resonance image demonstrates a focal lesion of the medial tibial plateau that closely resembles osteonecrosis typically seen in the femoral condyle.

many cases no radiographic change whatsoever will occur. If radiographic collapse does occur, the patient will remain symptomatic and will eventually require surgical treatment. As with osteonecrosis of the femoral condyle, the etiology of this disorder is unknown.

Differential diagnosis

Differential diagnosis includes pes anserinus bursitis and meniscal tear. The importance of recognizing osteonecrosis is in the avoidance of unnecessary arthroscopic meniscal surgery.[30,35] The differential diagnosis also includes stress fracture of the tibia, which has been well described in the elderly population. A radiodense line becomes apparent sooner and the symptoms usually resolve more quickly.[36–38] Transient osteoporosis is a recently described clinical syndrome that appears to be quite similar to osteonecrosis of the tibial plateau.[39] Pathologic studies have not been useful in distinguishing these two syndromes.

Treatment

It appears that in most cases the syndrome will resolve during the course of symptomatic treatment. If a radiographic lesion does develop and progresses towards osteoarthritis, surgical treatment may be necessary. Again the indications for prosthetic replacement are similar to those in routine cases.

Osteonecrosis associated with risk factors

Osteonecrosis associated with corticosteroids, alcoholism, hemoglobinopathies, hyperbarism, and SLE has been well described.[20,40–46] Osteonecrosis may occur in either femoral condyle, tibial plateau, or in the patella. The lesion usually occurs in the metaphyseal bone and the femoral condyles, especially the lateral femoral condyle. The clinical presentation is quite similar to that of spontaneous osteonecrosis of the knee with the exception that one of the above risk factors can be elucidated. Although few authors have focused on this distinct entity, it is felt that these patients are more likely to progress to more advanced stages of disease and subsequent collapse. The treatment recommendations, however, are similar.

Controversies in the area of osteonecrosis of the knee should be worked out in the future. Prospective studies involving the correlation between MRI and pathologic findings are essential in the quest to determine the exact etiology of the disorder and to improve diagnostic accuracy. Treatment issues will focus on refining the indications for both unicompartmental and total knee arthroplasty. Allograft replacement is an exciting concept with an uncertain future.

References

1. Ahlbäck S, Bauer GCH, Bohne WH, Spontaneous osteonecrosis of the knee, *Arthritis Rheum* (1968) **11**: 705–733.
2. Insall JN, Joseph DM, Msika C, High tibial osteotomy for varus gonarthrosis: a long-term follow-up study, *J Bone Joint Surg (Am)* (1984) **66**: 1040–1048.
3. Koshino T, The treatment of spontaneous osteonecrosis of the knee by high tibial osteotomy with and without bone grafting or drilling of the lesion, *J Bone Joint Surg (Am)* (1982) **64**: 47–58.
4. Aglietti P, Buzzi R, Idiopathic osteonecrosis of the knee, *Italian J Orthop and Traumat* (1984) **10**: 217–226.
5. Aglietti P, Insall JN, Buzzi R, et al., Idiopathic osteonecrosis of the knee: aetiology, prognosis and treatment, *J Bone Joint Surg (Br)* (1983) **65**: 588–597.
6. Houpt JB, Pritzker KPH, Alpert B et al., Natural history of spontaneous osteonecrosis of the knee (SONK): A review, *Semin Arthritis Rheum* (1983) **13**: 212–227.
7. Lotke PA, Abend JA, Ecker ML, The treatment of osteonecrosis of the medial femoral condyle, *Clin Orthop* (1982) **171**: 109–116.
8. Lotke PA, Ecker ML, Osteonecrosis of the knee, *Orthop Clin North Am* (1985) **16**: 797–808.
9. Muheim G, Bohne WH, Prognosis in spontaneous osteonecrosis of the knee: investigation by radionuclide scintimetry and radiography, *J Bone Joint Surg (Br)* (1970) **52**: 605–612.
10. Rozing PM, Insall JN, Bohne WH, Spontaneous osteonecrosis of the knee, *J Bone Joint Surg (Am)* (1980) **62**: 2–7.
11. Williams JL, Cliff MM, Bonakdarpour A, Spontaneous osteonecrosis of the knee, *Radiology* (1973) **107**: 15–19.
12. Bauer GCH, Osteonecrosis of the knee, *Clin Orthop* (1978) **130**: 210–217.
13. Bauer GCH, Smith EM, ^{85}Sr scintimetry in osteoarthritis of the knee, *J Nucl Med* (1969) **10**: 109–116.
14. Jacobs MA, Loeb PE, Hungerford DS, Core decompression of the distal femur for avascular necrosis of the knee, *J Bone Joint Surg (Br)* (1989) **71**: 583–587.
15. Björkengren AG, Al Rowaih A, Lindstrand A et al., Spontaneous osteonecrosis of the knee: Value of MR Imaging in determining prognosis, *Am J Roentgenol* (1990) **154**: 331–336.
16. Robinson HJ Jr, Hartleben PD, Lund G et al., Evaluation of magnetic resonance imaging in the diagnosis of osteonecrosis of the femoral head, *J Bone Joint Surg (Am)* (1989) **71**: 650–663.
17. Seiler JG III, Christie MJ, Homra L, Correlation of the findings of magnetic resonance imaging with those of bone biopsy in patients who have stage-I or II ischaemic necrosis of the femoral head, *J Bone Joint Surg (Am)* (1989) **71**: 28–32.
18. Ahuja SC, Bullough PG, Osteonecrosis of the knee: A clini-copathological study in twenty-eight patients, *J Bone Joint Surg (Am)* (1978) **60**: 191–197.
19. Koshino T, Okamoto R, Takamura K et al., Arthroscopy in spontaneous osteonecrosis of the knee, *Orthop Clin North Am* (1979) **10**: 609–618.
20. Cruess RL, Osteonecrosis of bone: Current concepts as to etiology and pathogenesis, *Clin Orthop* (1986) **208**: 30–39.
21. Ficat RP, Idiopathic bone necrosis of the femoral head: Early diagnosis and treatment, *J Bone Joint Surg (Br)* (1985) **67**: 3–9.
22. Glimcher MJ, Kenzora JE, The biology of osteonecrosis of the human femoral head and its clinical implications. Part III: Discussion of the etiology and genesis of the pathological sequelae; comments on treatment, *Clin Orthop* (1979) **140**: 273–312.
23. Insall JN, Aglietti P, Bullough PG, Osteonecrosis, *Surgery of the knee*, ed Insall JN (New York: Churchill Livingstone, 1984) 527–549.
24. Zizic TM, Lewis CG, Marcoux C et al., The predictive value of haemodynamic studies in preclinical ischaemic necrosis of bone, *J Rheum* (1989) **16**: 1559–1564.
25. Arnoldi CC, Lemperg RK, Linderholm H, Intraosseous hypertension and pain in the knee, *J Bone Joint Surg (Br)* (1975) **57**: 360–363.
26. Lotke PA, Ecker ML, Alavi A, Painful knees in older patients: Radionuclide diagnosis of possible osteonecrosis with spontaneous resolution, *J Bone Joint Surg (Am)* (1977) **59**: 617–621.
27. Felson DT, Naimark A, Anderson J et al., The prevalence of knee osteoarthritis in the elderly: The Framingham osteoarthritis study, *Arthritis Rheum* (1987) **30**: 914–918.
28. Steinberg ME, Brighton CT, Corces A et al., Osteonecrosis of the femoral head: Results of core decompression and grafting with and without electrical stimulation, *Clin Orthop* (1989) **249**: 199–208.
29. Miller GK, Maylahn DJ, Drennan DB, The treatment of idiopathic osteonecrosis of the medial femoral condyle with arthroscopic debridement, *Arthroscopy* (1986) **2**: 21–29.
30. Kitziger KJ, DeLee JC, Failed partial meniscectomy, *Clin Sports Med* (1990) **9**: 641–660.
31. Bayne O, Langer F, Pritzker KPH et al., Osteochondral allografts in the treatment of osteonecrosis of the knee, *Orthop Clin North Am* (1985) **16**: 727–740.
32. Ganel A, Israeli A, Horoszowski H et al., Osteochondral graft in the treatment of osteonecrosis of the femoral condyle, *J Am Geriatr Soc* (1981) **29**: 186–188.
33. Houpt JB, Alpert B, Lotem M et al., Spontaneous osteonecrosis of the medial tibial plateau, *J Rheumatol* (1982) **9**: 81–90.
34. Lotke PA, Ecker ML, Osteonecrosis-like syndrome of the medial tibial plateau, *Clin Orthop* (1983) **176**: 148–153.
35. Lotke PA, Ecker ML, Current concepts review: osteonecrosis of the knee, *J Bone Joint Surg (Am)* (1988) **70**: 470–473.
36. Bauer G, Gustafsson M, Mortensson W et al., Insufficiency fractures in the tibial condyles in elderly individuals, *Acta Radiol Diagn* (1981) **22**: 619–622.
37. Engber WD, Stress fractures of the medial tibial plateau, *J Bone Joint Surg (Am)* (1977) **59**: 767–769.
38. Prather JL, Nusynowitz ML, Snowdy HA et al., Scintigraphic findings in stress fractures, *J Bone Joint Surg (Am)* (1977) **59**: 869–874.
39. Schneider R, Goldman A, Pellicci P et al., Transient regional osteoporosis of the knee. Presented at the 57th Annual Meeting of the American Academy of Orthopaedic Surgeons, New Orleans, Louisiana, USA (1990).
40. Havel PE, Ebraheim NA, Jackson WT, Steroid-induced bilateral avascular necrosis of the lateral femoral condyles, *Clin Orthop* (1989) **243**: 166–168.
41. Isono SS, Woolson ST, Schurman DJ, Total joint arthroplasty for steroid-induced osteonecrosis in cardiac transplant patients, *Clin Orthop* (1987) **217**: 201–208.
42. Kelman GJ, William GW, Colwell CW Jr et al., Steroid-related osteonecrosis of the knee: two case reports and a literature review, *Clin Orthop* (1990) **257**: 171–176.

43. **Marmor L,** Osteonecrosis of the knee: Medial and lateral involvement, *Clin Orthop* (1984) **185:** 195–196.

44. **Siemsen JK, Brook J, Meister L,** Lupus erythematosus and avascular bone necrosis: A clinical study of three cases and review of the literature, *Arthritis Rheum* (1962) **5:** 492–501.

45. **Susan LP, Braun WE, Banowski LH et al.,** Avascular necrosis following renal transplantation: Experience with 449 allografts with and without high-dose steroid therapy, *Urology* (1978) **11:** 225–229.

46. **Yamaguchi H, Masuda T, Sasaki T et al.,** Steroid-induced osteonecrosis of the patella, *Clin Orthop* (1988) **229:** 201–204.

9.6   Fresh small-fragment osteochondral allografts in the knee joint

Richard J. Beaver and Allan E. Gross

The restoration of articular congruity and absent bone stock about the knee in the young, relatively active patient remains one of the more difficult problems facing the orthopaedic surgeon. Realistically, only three options are possible; firstly, prosthetic replacement may be used; secondly, the joint may be arthrodesed; or, thirdly, the defect may be reconstructed using cadaveric osteochondral allograft. The last of these options will be discussed in this contribution.

A programme was instituted in 1972 by the senior author (A.E.G.) as part of the University of Toronto Orthopaedic Transplant Programme whereby fresh small-fragment osteochondral allografts were to be used for replacement of osteoarticular defects within the knee.[1-8] Because of the deleterious effects of freezing or lyophilization of bone even in the presence of cryo-preservatives, fresh non-frozen allograft offers the most hope of chondrocyte survival and continued function.[9]

Between January 1972 and November 1990 a total of 169 fresh osteochondral allografts have been performed and the patients have been followed prospectively. Previous papers have been published on this group of patients.[8,10,11] In addition, failed and retrieved osteochondral grafts in the knee have been analysed clinically, radiologically and histologically.[12,13] It was demonstrated that:

1. Although an immune response is mounted against the graft, rejection of the graft did not occur.
2. Chondrocyte viability was observed in most cases up to 92 months after transplantation.[12]
3. Failure of the graft was related to technical error, underlying disease or malalignment.

The technical errors related to graft failure were:

1. Use of a graft with a bony thickness less than 1 cm.
2. Inadequate fixation of the allograft to host bone.
3. Adjusting allograft thickness to correct knee malalignment.

Indications

A review of the first 100 cases was conducted in 1985 and it was recognized that the most favourable results were obtained in the correction of post-traumatic osteoarticular defects. Osteochondritis dissecans was felt to be a relative indication. Osteoarthritis and osteonecrosis are felt to be relative contraindications to the use of this technique.[10]

Harvesting of allograft

Fresh osteochondral allografts are procured according to the procedures established by the American Association of Tissue Banks.[14] It is recommended in addition, however, that the donor be less than 30 years of age in order to maximize cartilage quality.

The graft is procured as follows: Under strict aseptic precautions, within 24 (preferably 12) hours of donor death, the entire donor joint is excised, carefully preserving the joint ligamentous and capsular structures. After taking cultures for bacteria, fungi and mycobacteria, the joint is immersed in sterile Ringer's solution containing 1 g/l cefazolin and 50 000 units/l bacitracin and sealed within a container in a sterile fashion using adhesive plastic. This container is then triple-wrapped in towels and sterile plastic bags and stored at a temperature of 4°C (39°F) until it is ready to be used. Although an immune response is mounted by the host against allograft bone, this does not greatly affect the incorporation of the graft and, as shown by Langer and Gross in 1974,[15] chondrocytes appear to be relatively protected from immune assault by their surrounding matrix. Therefore, histocompatibility testing is not performed, nor is immunosuppression justifiable in these cases. The appropriate recipient is selected only on the basis of sex and sizing of the donor allograft. We believe that by not freezing the cartilage we are maximizing chondrocyte viability and consequently do not use stored or cryopreserved cartilage.[12]

Those patients who are judged to be suitable candidates for fresh osteochondral allografts are asked to be available at all hours either by telephone or pager. Once patients are notified they must make immediate arrangements for hospital admission. We are generally able to perform the surgery within 12–24 hours of graft procurement, with patients being brought in from all over North America and occasionally from overseas.

Pre-operative planning

(1) It is essential to correct joint malalignment prior to or simultaneously with the implantation of the allograft.

(2) It has been shown that attempts to correct malalignment using the height of the allograft leads to a high incidence of graft failure.[8,10,11]

(3) Correct varus deformities by high tibial valgus osteotomy (HTVO).

(4) Correct valgus deformities by distal femoral varus osteotomy (DFVO).

(5) When the allograft is to be implanted on the opposite side of the joint to the realignment procedure (e.g. DFVO plus allograft lateral tibial plateau or HTVO plus allograft medial femoral condyle), it is permissible to perform both procedures during the same operating session. However, when the two procedures are performed on the same side of the joint (e.g. HTVO plus allograft of the medial tibial plateau), it is recommended that the two procedures be staged several months apart. This prevents interference with the vascular bed of the allograft and obviates the technical difficulties of performing the two procedures together. On rare occasions, it has been necessary to perform proximal tibial *varus* osteotomy at the same time as allograft replacement of the lateral tibial plateau in order to maintain the plane of the knee joint horizontal.

Operative techniques

The most common scenario encountered is that of a valgus deformity with loss of the articular cartilage and subchondral bone of the lateral tibial plateau. The second most common scenario is that of a varus deformity with destruction of the medial femoral condyle.

Problem 1 – A valgus deformity with destruction of the lateral tibial condyle

The solution for this problem is a distal femoral varus osteotomy with allograft reconstruction of the lateral tibial plateau (Figure 1). A simplified version of the AO technique[16] for supracondylar varus osteotomy as performed at this institution has been described in previous publications and these should be consulted since it is vital for the success of the graft that alignment be corrected exactly.[17]

Preparation and implantation of allograft

Usually two operating teams are employed, one to prepare the allograft and the other to perform any realignment procedure and prepare the recipient bed.

After arthrotomy has been performed, the meniscus is inspected. Every attempt is made to preserve the patient's own meniscus but, in the case of an irreparable lateral meniscus, a meniscectomy is performed and a donor meniscus is implanted with the tibial allograft. In this case the meniscus is left attached to the donor plateau and sutured to the synovium and capsule of the recipient.

The damaged articular surface is resected and 'squared off' down to healthy, bleeding cancellous bone.

The corresponding segment of the donor joint is resected and trimmed to closely match the defect in the recipient. A tight fit is desirable.

If a meniscus is to be implanted as well, three or four absorbable mattress sutures are placed in the periphery of the meniscus and affixed to the capsule of the host. These sutures are not tied until after the graft is fitted.

The allograft is rigidly fixed to the tibia with AO 4.0 mm spongiosa screws. Because we wish to avoid making any breaches of the articular cartilage that may expose the graft to the immune response, it is important to place the screws well away from the articular

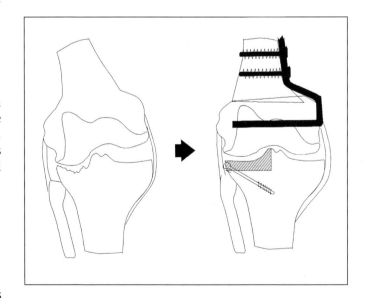

Figure 1

An osteoarticular defect in the weight-bearing portion of the lateral tibial plateau producing genu valgum deformity corrected by fresh osteochondral allograft of the tibial plateau. The allograft has been unloaded by a distal femoral varus osteotomy.

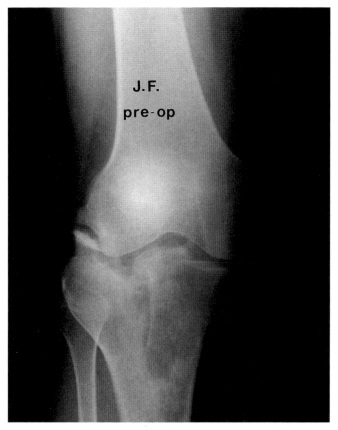

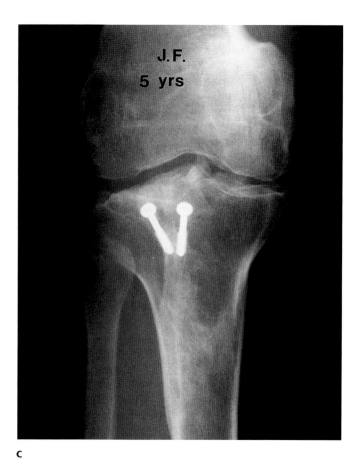

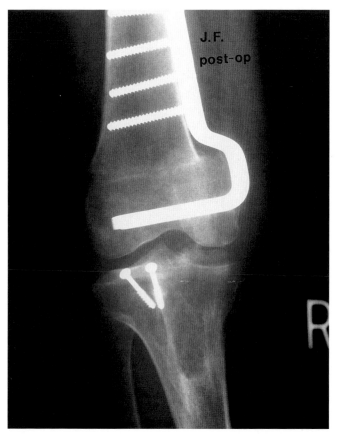

Figure 2

(a) Anteroposterior radiograph of the right knee of a 26-year-old female demonstrating a malunited lateral tibial plateau fracture with substantial loss of bone stock. (b) Following replacement of the deficient lateral tibial plateau with fresh osteochondral allograft. Distal femoral varus osteotomy has been performed to unload the allograft. (c) Five years following transplantation the allograft has completely united to the host with minimal subsidence. Hardware has been removed from the femur. The joint space is well preserved. Early degenerative changes are present.

cartilage and in a site not likely to cause impingement problems. This is usually immediately adjacent to the cartilage and through strong cortical bone.

Closure is performed over suction drains.

Postoperative management

During the learning curve portion of this programme the grafts were not rigidly fixed and it was found that, not uncommonly, manipulation of the knee was necessary to regain knee range of motion. However, since the introduction of rigid fixation and immediate postoperative continuous passive motion, this complication is no longer seen and most patients regain excellent range of motion. Continuous passive motion (CPM) on the operated knee is instituted immediately in the recovery room. It is felt that this will prevent the formation of intra-articular adhesions and optimize cartilage nutrition. We ensure that the CPM machine has been adjusted to allow maintenance of varus or valgus position throughout the whole joint range.

Patients are mobilized with partial weight bearing as soon as suction drains are removed. Partial weight bearing is maintained for at least a year by the application of an ischial-bearing long-leg orthosis. Union is usually radiologically evident between 3 and 6 months after transplantation.

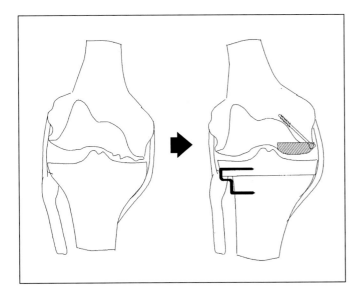

Figure 3

An osteoarticular defect in the weight-bearing portion of the medial femoral condyle producing genu varum deformity corrected by fresh allograft to the femoral condyle. The allograft is unloaded by proximal tibial valgus osteotomy.

An illustrative case is shown in Figure 2.

Problem 2 – A varus deformity with destruction of the medial femoral condyle

The solution to this problem is a proximal tibial valgus osteotomy with osteochondral allograft replacement of the medial femoral condyle (Figure 3).

Operative technique

The operative technique is similar to that outlined above. The specific techniques for proximal tibial valgus osteotomy have been well described by Coventry, Maquet and others[18–22] and will not be reproduced here. It has been the practice at this institution to perform a closing-wedge osteotomy 2 cm distal to the knee joint with a concomitant elevation of the tibial tubercle (Maquet procedure).[22]

With regard to exposure of the joint, it is often possible to obtain sufficient exposure of the medial femoral condyle by a medial parapatellar approach and subluxating the patella without completely dislocating it. As with the tibial plateau graft, considerable care should be given to obtaining an accurate press-fit of the allograft and rigidly fixing the graft using AO techniques. The postoperative use of continuous passive motion creates considerable shear stresses at the graft–host junction that would have deleterious effects on the union of a poorly fixed graft.

A case of fresh medial femoral condyle osteochondral allograft is shown in Figure 4. The allograft has been unloaded by proximal tibial valgus osteotomy.

Clinical results

A survivorship study of the clinical results of fresh osteochondral allografts in the knee has been performed. A total of 127 fresh, small-fragment allografts in 124 patients were able to be followed. The breakdown of these patients according to diagnosis is shown in Table 1. Where possible, each patient was brought back for review and a knee score was calculated using a modified Hospital for Special Surgery knee rating system (Table 2). If this was not possible because of distance or incapacity, the patient was contacted by telephone and a questionnaire was completed, thereby enabling assessment of the clinical success of the operation. This review process was purely clinical and no attempt was made to incorporate the radiological appearances in the knee rating. Failure was defined as an increment in the postoperative knee score of less than 10 points, any need for revision operations apart from removal of hardware,

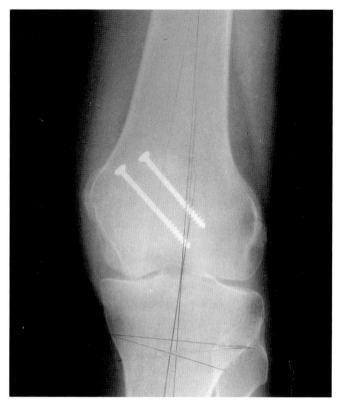
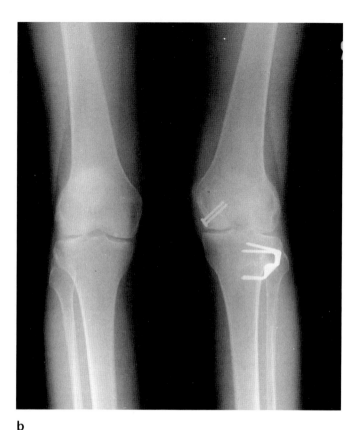

a

b

Figure 4

(a) Anteroposterior radiograph of the knee of a 33-year-old woman with a defect in the medial femoral condyle as a result of a motor vehicle accident 3 years previously. The patella has been internally fixed. (b) Four years after fresh osteochondral allograft replacement of the medial femoral condyle and proximal tibial valgus osteotomy. Note the preservation of joint space and lack of graft subsidence.

or a statement by the patient that the knee was worse than before the allograft procedure.

Life-table analysis according to the technique of Kaplan and Meier[23] was performed on the group of patients who received fresh osteochondral allografts for post-traumatic defects in the knee joint. There were a total of 92 grafts performed in 91 patients with an average follow-up of 68 months (range 4–174 months). There were 51 males and 40 females with an average age of 41.9 years (median age 46 years, range 17–75 years). The distribution of the grafts within the knee is shown in Table 3. Thirteen patients are known to have undergone revision surgery to their knee and a breakdown of these patients is shown in Table 4. A list of postoperative complications is shown in Table 5.

Survivorship analysis revealed that, at 5 years post-transplantation, 75% of cases were still rated clinical successes. The percentage of successes at 10 years and at 14 years was 64% (Figure 5). Log-rank analysis was used to compare the survival rates of unipolar grafts to bipolar grafts and a statistical trend towards improved

success rate was seen in the unipolar grafts (2-tailed P = 0.09 by linear interpolation) as seen in Figure 6. The unipolar grafts performed for trauma had a survival rate of 67% at 14 years. There was no statistical difference in the clinical performance of male patients as compared to female patients. Similarly, there was no statistical difference between the clinical success rate of those grafts performed in the tibia as compared to those performed in the femur, nor of those grafts performed on the medial side of the joint as compared to the lateral side of the joint. A comparison was made between the success rate of fresh grafts performed in those patients aged 60 years or more with those aged less than 60 years. A statistical trend was found towards improved success rate in the younger group of patients (2-tailed P = 0.08), but it is worth noting that the number of bipolar grafts was greater in the older group (6/12) than in the younger group (13/67) indicating more advanced degenerative changes in the older group. When those patients whose allograft was performed for post-traumatic defects were compared with those performed for all other diagnoses (with the

Table 1 A list of those diagnoses for which fresh osteochondral allografts have been performed in the knee joint. Those cases performed for reconstruction of defects following resection of tumours are not included in this review.

Diagnosis	Number of cases	Exclusions
Trauma	92	7
Osteoarthritis	18	1
Osteonecrosis	7	
Osteochondritis dissecans	10	
Total	127	8

Table 2 Modified Hospital for Special Surgery knee rating score.

Subjective (60 points)	
Pain	35
Instability	10
Walking Aids	5
Walking Distance	10
Objective (40 points)	
Extension	10
Flexion	20
Effusion	10
Total (normal knee)	100

Table 3 The distribution of unipolar grafts within the knee joint in this series. A unipolar graft is one that replaces only one side, tibial or femoral of a single compartment. There were 19 bipolar grafts of which 9 were lateral and 10 medial.

Lateral femoral condyle	12
Lateral tibial plateau	42
Medial femoral condyle	11
Medial tibial plateau	8

Table 4 Revision procedures known to have been performed on patients with fresh osteochondral allografts for post-traumatic defects in the knee.

Procedure	No.
Total knee arthroplasty	6
Arthrodesis	3
Retransplant	3
Curettage and drilling	1
Total	13

Table 5 Complications.

Stiffness requiring manipulation	3
Reflex sympathetic dystrophy	1
Wound haematoma	1
Rupture of the patellar tendon	1
Respiratory	2
Total	8

exception of tumours), the post-traumatic grafts were seen to have a significantly superior success rate as seen in Figure 7 (2-tailed $P = 0.002$). At 5 years post-transplantation, the post-traumatic group had a 72% survival rate as compared to 29% in the other diagnoses taken as a group.

Zukor et al. in 1989 published a clinical and radiographic review of the fresh osteochondral allografts performed for post-traumatic defects of the knee joint at Mount Sinai up to that time.[8,24] Only those patients with adequate radiographs and at least 2 years' follow-up were analysed. There were 55 transplants in 51 patients in this study group. The average age was 37.8 years and 33 patients were male and 18 female. Of these cases 76% were rated successes and 24% were failures.

Radiographic results

Establishment of graft–host union was obtained in all cases by 6–9 months following transplantation. The

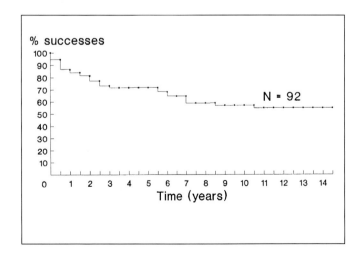

Figure 5

Kaplan–Meier survivorship analysis of those fresh osteochondral allografts performed for post-traumatic defects in the knee joint.

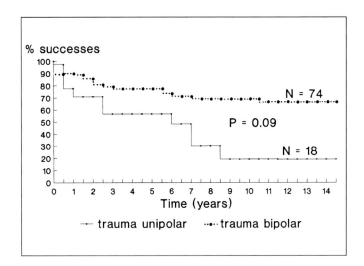

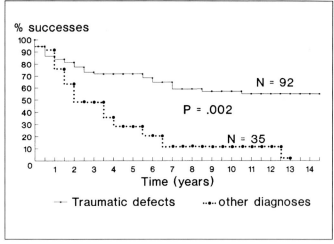

Figure 6

A comparison of the survivorship of unipolar (dotted line) and bipolar (solid line) grafts in the post-traumatic group. All *P* values are 2-tailed.

Figure 7

A comparison of the survivorship of the post-traumatic group (solid line) and that of all other diagnoses (dotted line) combined (osteoarthritis, osteochondritis dissecans and osteonecrosis).

average time required for establishment of normal bone density within the allograft was between 2 and 4 years.

There was evidence of subsidence of the grafts in most cases (70%) of from 1 to 3 mm, but most underwent no further collapse; 27.7% of the grafts subsided 4–5 mm and to date only one graft (1.9%) has collapsed completely.

Preservation of the joint space has been noted in 55% of the cases, mild to moderate decrease in 19% and complete loss or gross arthritis in 26%.

A small proportion (11%) of allografts underwent some degree of fragmentation close to their surface but there were no graft fractures. The significance of this is not clear but presumably represents evidence of degeneration of the allograft surface.

The long-term survival and function of meniscal allografts has not as yet been convincingly demonstrated in humans but very promising arthroscopic appearances have been seen in the menisci transplanted in association with fresh osteochondral allografts at this institution. Successful survival and apparent function have been observed as much as 8.5 years after transplantation.[25] Long-term analysis of retrieved menisci will be invaluable in determining their place in this type of surgery. The role of the menisci in cartilage nutrition and redistribution of joint contact forces is well accepted and it would seem prudent to preserve or replace them as required.[25]

A clinical and radiological analysis of failed fresh grafts at this institution has been performed by Oakeshott et al.[26] All bipolar allografts (simultaneous replacement of both sides of the joint) were failures. The majority of failed grafts occurred in patients whose limb alignment had not been corrected or in whom graft thickness had been used to correct malalignment, thereby overloading the graft. A high rate of failure was seen in those cases where rigid internal fixation was not achieved. Anatomical size mismatching between the host and the graft was seen in 50% of the failed grafts.

Chondrocyte viability

In 1990 Czitrom reported chondrocyte viability in biopsies of fresh osteochondral allografts obtained from patients between 1 and 6 years after transplantation.[12] He found that, when assessed by $^{35}SO_4$ and ^{3}H[cytidine] autoradiography, the percentage of viable chondrocytes ranged from 69% to 99% in three osteochondral allografts that were studied at 12, 24 and 41 months after transplantation and were producing proteoglycan. In a graft that had been implanted 6 years previously, 37% of chondrocytes were alive and actively producing proteoglycan. This was the first direct observation of the viability of articular cartilage in humans after allotransplantation. A previous study by Oakeshott et al. in 1988 of 18 failed fresh osteochondral grafts assessed chondrocyte viability indirectly by histological and electron-microscopic means.[26] They found that, even in failed grafts, 66% of the grafts had viable chondrocytes.

Complications

Complications related to the above procedures are relatively infrequent and are listed in Table 5. In addition, the case of reflex sympathetic dystrophy was also one of these patients. The single case of intraoperative rupture of the patellar tendon underwent immediate repair with good result. There were no superficial or deep infections.

Conclusions

(1) Fresh osteochondral allografts are preferable to stored allografts in the replacement of large post-traumatic articular defects in the knee.

(2) The best results for these grafts occur in relatively young patients with traumatically induced defects of the articular surface of the knee joint.

(3) Immunological rejection of the allograft does not appear to occur.

(4) It is essential to correct alignment of the limb prior to or simultaneous with implantation of the allograft.

(5) Rigid internal fixation of the allograft is vital.

(6) Bipolar and bicompartmental allografts perform poorly.

(7) Continuous passive motion in the immediate postoperative period, while not essential to the success of the procedure, appears to diminish the incidence and severity of postoperative knee stiffness. It is not clear, however, whether it improves chondrocyte survival in the short or long-term.

(8) Implantation of meniscal allograft appears to be associated with excellent functional results and biomechanically is to be recommended when the host meniscus is unsalvageable.

(9) Chondrocyte survival and continued function has been directly observed after fresh osteochondral transplantation.

Acknowledgments

While a Clinical Fellow at Mt Sinai Hospital, Dr Beaver was supported by grants from the University of Western Australia and the National Health and Medical Research Council of Australia.

References

1. Czitrom AA, Langer F, McKee N et al., Bone and cartilage allotransplantation: a review of 14 years of research and clinical studies, *Clin Orthop* (1986) **208**: 141–145.

2. Gross AE, Silverstein EA, Falk J et al., The allotransplantation of partial joints in the treatment of osteoarthritis of the knee, *Clin Orthop* (1975) **108**: 7–14.

3. Gross AE, Langer F, Osteochondral joint allografts in the management of osteoarthritis of the knee, *Transplant Proc* (1976) **VIII(2)**: 129–132, suppl 1.

4. Gross AE, McKee NH, Pritzker KPH et al., Reconstruction of skeletal deficits at the knee: a comprehensive osteochondral transplant programme, *Clin Orthop* (1983) **174**: 96–106.

5. Gross AE, Langer F, McKee N et al., A comprehensive orthopaedic transplant unit, *Transplantation Today* (1985) **2**: 38–44.

6. Gross AE, Langer F, McKee N et al., A comprehensive orthopaedic transplant unit, *Greffes de l'Appareil Locomoteur* (Paris: Masson, 1987) 127–131.

7. Gross AE, Farine I, Transplantation ostéocartilagineuse, *Les Publications de Biomat Cartilage '85*, ed Harmerut MF, Duccason D (1987) 287–293.

8. Zukor DJ, Gross AE, Osteochondral allograft reconstruction of the knee, part 1: A review, *Am J Knee Surg* (1989) **2(3)**: 139–149.

9. Jimenez SA, Brighton CT, Storage and preservation of viable articular cartilage. *Osteochondral allografts, biology, banking and clinical applications*, ed Friedlaender GE, Mankin HJ, Sell KW (Boston: Little, Brown, 1983) 73–79.

10. McDermott AGP, Langer F, Pritzker KPH et al., Fresh small-fragment osteochondral allografts: long-term follow-up study on first 100 cases, *Clin Orthop* (1985) **197**: 96–102.

11. Zukor DJ, Paitich B, Oakeshott RD et al., Reconstruction of post-traumatic articular surface defects using fresh small-fragment osteochondral allografts, *Bone transplantation*, ed Aebi M, Regazzoni P (Berlin: Springer-Verlag, 1989) 293–305.

12. Czitrom AA, Keating S, Gross AE, The viability of articular cartilage in fresh osteochondral allografts after clinical transplantation, *J Bone Joint Surg (Am)* (1990) **72**: 574–581.

13. Kandel RA, Gross AE, Ganel A et al., Histopathology of failed osteoarticular shell allografts, *Clin Orthop* (1985) **197**: 103–110.

14. Friedlander GE, Mankin HJ, Guidelines for the banking of musculoskeletal tissues, *Am Assoc Tissue Banks Newsletter* (1979) **3**: 2.

15. Langer F, Gross AE, Immunogenicity of allograft articular cartilage, *J Bone Joint Surg (Am)* (1974) **56**: 297–304.

16. Müller ME, Allgöwer M, Schneider R et al., *Manual of internal fixation*, 2nd edn (Berlin: Springer-Verlag, 1979) 376.

17. McDermott AGP, Finklestein JA, Farine I et al., Supracondylar varus osteotomy for valgus deformity of the knee, *J Bone Joint Surg (Am)* (1988) **70**: 110–116.

18. Bouillet R, Van Gaver P, L'arthrose du genou: étude pathogénique et traitement, *Acta Orthop Belg* (1961) **27**: 5–187.

19. Coventry MB, Osteotomy about the knee for degenerative and rheumatoid arthritis: Indications, operative technique and results, *J Bone Joint Surg (Am)* (1973) **55**: 23–48.

20. Jackson JP, Waugh W, Green JP, High tibial osteotomy for osteoarthritis of the knee, *J Bone Joint Surg (Br)* (1969) **51**: 88–94.

21. Maquet PGJ, *Biomechanics of the knee* (New York: Springer-Verlag, 1976).

22. Putnam MD, Mears DC, Fu FH, Combined Maquet and proximal tibial valgus osteotomy, *Clin Orthop* (1985) **197**: 217–223.

23. Kaplan EL, Meier P, Nonparametric estimation from incomplete observations, *Am Statist Assoc J* (1958) June: 457–481.

24. Zukor DJ, Oakeshott RD, Gross AE, Osteochondral allograft reconstruction of the knee, part 2: Experience with successful and failed fresh osteochondral allograft, *Am J Knee Surg* (1989) **2(4)**: 182–191.

25. Zukor DJ, Cameron JC, Brooks PJ et al., The fate of human meniscal allografts, *Articular cartilage and knee joint function*, ed Ewing JW (New York: Raven Press, 1990) 147–152.

26. Oakeshott RD, Farine I, Pritzker KPH et al., A clinical and histological analysis of failed fresh osteochondral allografts, *Clin Orthop* (1988) **233**: 283–294.

10

Synovial disorders

10.1 Synovial disorders: The role of arthroscopy

Dinesh Patel

The natural course of chronic joint inflammation or proliferating synovitis[1] from various disease processes is well known. Chronic synovitis or acute or chronic swelling in the knee or other joint damages architectural integrity of articular cartilage and soft tissue. Chronicity of this or failed medical treatment of such disorders invariably destroys the joint, causing chronic swelling, pain, loss of motion, deformity, and functional disability. In addition to the human sufferings, the cost to individuals, society, and government is known to be in the millions or billions of dollars.

Early removal of synovium, the offending target, has been shown to arrest or slow down the path of progressive destruction of joints. Surgical removal of the offending synovium—synovectomy—was first described in 1877 by Volkmann for tubercular arthritis.[2] The problems encountered by patients following open synovectomy[3,4] have included stiffness, loss of motion, muscle atrophy, prolonged rehabilitation, longer hospitalization, wound problems, neurovascular problems such as phlebitis, and ugly scars. Some of the problems have been minimized by early mobilization, selection of proper incision, early manipulation under anaesthesia, antibiotics, and anticoagulation. Despite all of these measures, there still remains significant morbidity[4-7] following open synovectomy.

The advent of arthroscopic technique with video TV monitoring and the use of hand and motorized instruments has revolutionized the diagnosis and treatment of disorders of many joints. Shibata,[8] Klein,[4] Dorfmann,[9] Rosenberg,[10] Patel,[11] and many others have written about arthroscopic synovectomy[10] and its value. One of the major benefits of arthroscopic surgery[12] has been our ability to diagnose and categorize different conditions which cause synovitis.

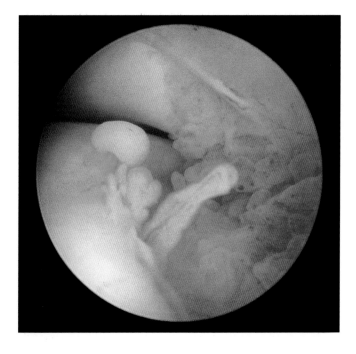

Figure 1

Rheumatoid arthritis.

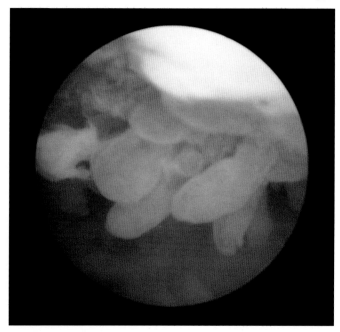

Figure 2

Rheumatoid arthritis.

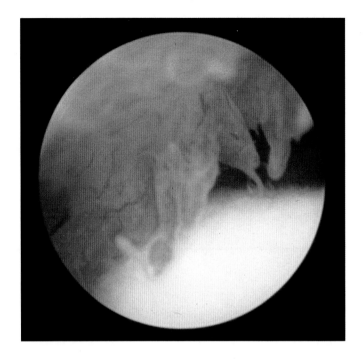

Figure 3

Synovial pannus in rheumatoid arthritis.

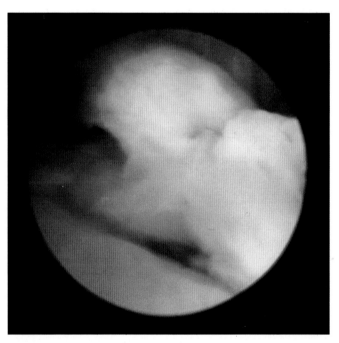

Figure 4

Microscopic view of rheumatoid arthritis.

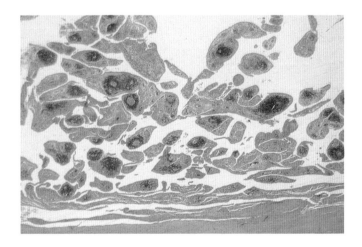

Figure 5

Microscopic view of rheumatoid arthritis.

Figure 6

Nodular pigmented villonodular synovitis.

The gross characteristics of synovium[12] in different synovial disease are now well understood. Apart from torn menisci, cruciate ligament injury, chondral and osteochondral injury, and degenerative arthritis, the following conditions cause synovitis:

1. Rheumatoid arthritis (see Figures 1–5)
2. Synovitis caused by or in association with psoriasis, systemic lupus erythematosus, Marie–Strümpell disease, inflammatory bowel disease, or crystal-induced synovitis (gout, pseudogout)

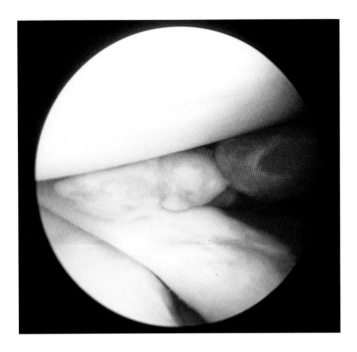

Figure 7

Multinodular pigmented villonodular synovitis.

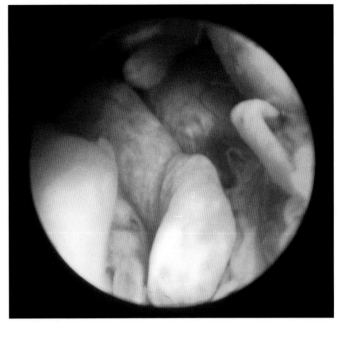

Figure 8

Diffuse nodular pigmented villonodular synovitis.

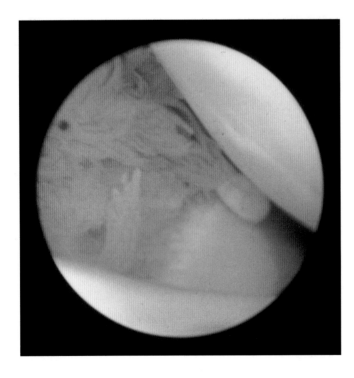

Figure 9

Diffuse nodular pigmented villonodular synovitis.

3. Pigmented villonodular synovitis—nodular and diffuse (Figures 6–12)
4. Synovial chondromatoses—osteochondromatoses (Figures 13–15)
5. Synovial hemangioma
6. Synovial fibroid tumor (Figure 16)
7. Plicae (Figures 17–19)
8. Intra-articular adhesion—scar tissue (Figure 20)
9. Sepsis, synovitis, adhesions
10. Hemophilic synovitis

The goals to be achieved in chronic synovial disorders are:

1. Reduction of synovial mass in all compartments
2. Removal of associated mechanical impediments
3. Preservation of all possible tissues—especially meniscus, cruciate ligaments, and articular cartilage
4. Least trauma to soft tissues

By fulfilling these goals, early mobilization and faster rehabilitation has been made possible. The advantages of arthroscopic synovectomy include short hospital stay, decreased postoperative morbidity and cost reduction. Most importantly, perhaps, further destruction of joint has been avoided, leading to possible long-term benefits.

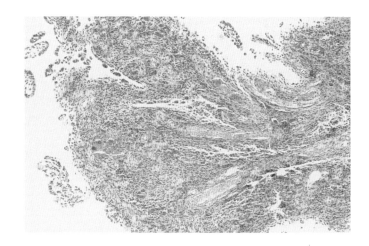

Figure 10

Photomicrograph of pigmented villonodular synovitis.

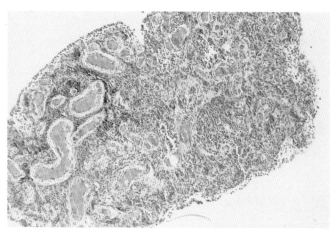

Figure 11

Photomicrograph of pigmented villonodular synovitis.

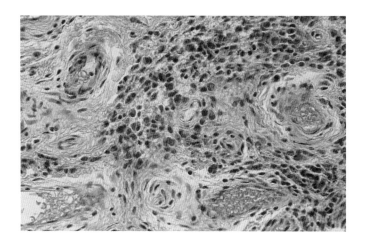

Figure 12

Photomicrograph of pigmented villonodular synovitis.

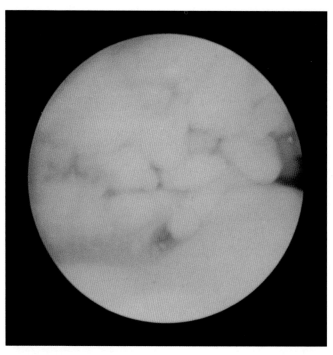

Figure 13

Synovial chondromatosis.

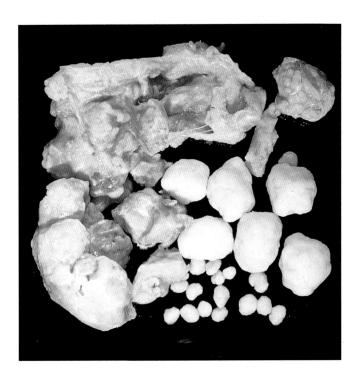

Figure 14

Gross loose bodies in synovial chondromatosis.

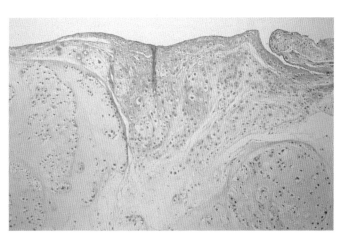

Figure 15

Microscopic view of synovial chondromatosis.

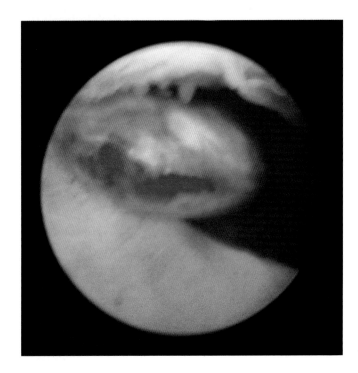

Figure 16

Fibroid tumor.

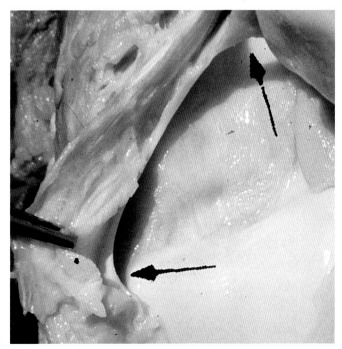

Figure 17

Plica—gross anatomy.

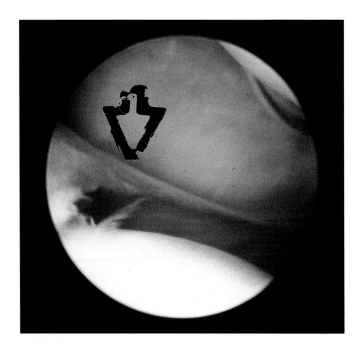

Figure 18

Arthroscopic view of medial plica.

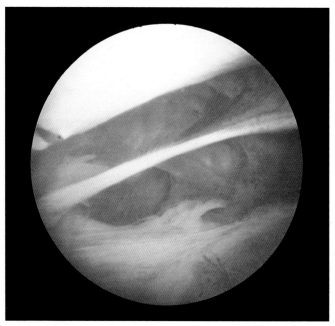

Figure 19

Arthroscopic view of medial plica.

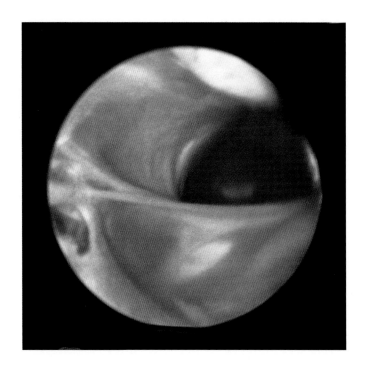

Figure 20

Intra-articular adhesions.

Environment—team approach

In order to achieve these goals, an arthroscopic 'high-tech' environment is absolutely necessary, with a fully equipped operating room giving ability to do such surgery using specialized hand and motorized instruments and a monitoring system.

1. Basic instruments, used for meniscectomies
2. Additional specific instruments, motorized instruments:

   (a) 3.5-mm to 5.5-mm synovial or full-radius resectors
   (b) Infusion pump; an adequate pump that maintains enough inflow when motorized instruments are used

3. Large-bore 5.5-mm to 6.0-mm inflow cannula
4. Ringer's lactate (3000 ml) with large bore Y tubing
5. Tourniquet, leg holder, and a good surgical assistant are essential.
6. Television monitor system:

   (a) 5-mm, 30° and 70° oblique telescopes
   (b) High-intensity light source
   (c) Small CCD camera

Additional small instruments such as basket punches or small-radius synovial resectors for removing synovium under the meniscus or gutters or posterior compartments are also essential.

Arthroscopic technique, knowledge of anatomy, different portals for arthroscopes and instruments, and a systematic approach are mandatory. I use the midpatellar approach with a 5-mm, 30° oblique telescope and use an inferomedial approach for synovectomies. A thorough systematic diagnosis is made initially and a plan is developed for synovectomy as follows.

1. Suprapatellar pouch
2. Patellofemoral joint
3. Plicae
4. Medial gutter
5. Medial compartment: (a) medial meniscus, (b) medial tibia, (c) medial femur
6. Ligamentum mucosum with fat pad
7. Anterior and posterior cruciate ligaments
8. Lateral compartment: (a) lateral meniscus, (b) lateral tibia, (c) lateral femur
9. Popliteus hiatus: (a) popliteus tendon, (b) fascicles
10. Lateral gutter

Investigate the same structures using probes and alternating portals.

Posteromedial portal

1. Posterior meniscosynovial area
2. Posterior cruciate ligament
3. Articular cartilages of the femur and tibia

The posterolateral portal has not been found to be necessary.

If the large bore 5.5–6.0-mm cannula is used, I use the superomedial portal for inflow using Y tube with 2000–3000 ml Ringer's lactate solution.

Technique of synovectomy

A systematic approach to resection of synovium and other mechanical offending tissues can be done in any manner, starting either from the suprapatellar pouch or from the medial or lateral compartments. I prefer the same approach as used for diagnosis. One of the problems encountered in synovectomies, specifically for other than pigmented villonodular synovitis (and perhaps also for that[13–15]), is how much to resect.

The synovium and fat pad or tissue underneath occasionally appear under the tourniquet the same yellowish white color, so in order to remove just the synovium and preserve other vital soft tissue, I have been using 6 ml of methylene blue in the knee joint before beginning the synovectomy. The methylene blue is kept in the knee for 2 minutes or so. The methylene blue stains the synovium or inner lining, including degenerative menisci and articular cartilage. The lesions in the menisci and damage to articular cartilage are well defined. Systematic removal of only the blue lining is the goal of synovectomy. Surgery is precise and technically less difficult, and vital tissues are not unnecessarily removed. Use of methylene blue as an adjunctive tool has additionally reduced the surgical time.

The following are particular points to be looked for in surgery.

(1) Neurovascular bundles in the posterior compartment. Keep the knee flexed at 90° and maintain the distension. Use 3.5-mm or full-radius blades. Remove large synovial blobs with pituitary rongeur. One may require two posteromedial punctures, one for the arthroscope and the other for hand or mechanized instruments. Occasionally, a 70° arthroscope introduced from the anterolateral or anteromedial portal and mechanized instruments from posterior compartment may work as well. A 5.5-mm plastic cannula placed permanently in the posteromedial compartment would be beneficial, as instruments can be exchanged easily using the same portal.

It is preferable to leave some proliferative synovium than to risk damaging vital structures in the posterior compartment.

(2) The popliteus hiatus gutter. The anterolateral portal is placed not too close to the patellar tendon — keeping the arthroscope at mid-patellar level will help remove the synovium. Similarly, keeping the arthroscope in the anterolateral compartment and using a midpatellar or higher approach for powered instruments will facilitate surgery in the lateral gutter, popliteus tunnel, and of course the entire suprapatellar pouch.

Because of chronicity, occasionally the suprapatellar plica[11,16,17] becomes thick, obliterating the communication between the suprapatellar bursa[18] and the main knee joint. One must remove the entire suprapatellar plica, as proliferative synovium, debris, or loose bodies may be hidden in the suprapatellar bursa.

(3) The undersurface of the menisci can be tackled by using small basket punches or powered instruments.

(4) There is considerable synovial tissue in the intercondylar notch and specifically around the cruciate ligaments.

I have occasionally done notchplasty, especially where the notch is stenotic in chronic synovitis, in order to remove the synovium in and around that area with ease.

The medial and lateral peripatellar synovium and inferior pole of the patella also need special attention because of the thickness of the retinaculum and patellar tendon.

Reinspection of all aspects of the knee is mandatory to make sure that the synovium is removed and that there is no damage to vital tissues. The surgical time is no more than 1½ hours. The tourniquet is released. The incisions are kept open and a bulky dressing is applied.

Postoperative regimen

After a few hours stay in surgical day care, the patient goes home with or without crutches and with or without a knee immobilizer. The determining factor has been the patient. All patients have been instructed in early mobilization of the knee and full weight bearing the same day or when they feel comfortable.

Structured physical therapy is not used for the first 7–10 days, but a program of exercises to prevent atrophy and stiffness is given. Patients are encouraged to use a stationary bicycle (high speed, low tension) as early as possible. The soft compression dressing is removed after 2 days. The patient is seen for follow-up in 7–10 days.

Patients are warned that the whole leg from the buttocks to the ankle may become black and blue or may swell. This happens very commonly because of extravasation of blood and fluid in the soft tissues. TED stockings are advised and early pumping exercises for the foot and ankle are encouraged. Because of the methylene blue that was injected in the knee, patients are also warned that the dressing and incision may appear black or blue and may be soaked with blood, which they should not worry about.

Amazingly, the narcotic requirements for pain control in patients with chronic synovitis has been much less than expected. By the time patients come back for follow-up, they have already achieved more than 90–100° of flexion. An appropriate regimen of structured physical therapy rehabilitation is used for 2–3 weeks or as necessary. Most patients suffering from rheumatoid arthritis have already been to physiotherapy for problems in other joints, so this is continued.

Complex technique and aggressive rehabilitation are certainly not necessary for excision of plica,[11,16,17,19,20] single nodules, or synovial osteochondromatoses.[9] Arthroscopic surgery has also been used selectively for septic knee[21-23] and hemophilic synovitis[24] with good results.

Complications

Infection, hematoma, neurovascular injury, phlebitis, inadequate surgery, cartilage damage or injury to other structures essentially do not differ from those in arthroscopic surgery. Patients who have been on steroids may have skin necrosis around the incision, so special precautions are taken to excise the skin edges before the dressing is applied. Since the technique demands a team approach with a good leader, complication perhaps may have some relationship to expertise, like anything else in surgery. The swelling in the knee remains for a considerable time, perhaps 3–4 months in some patients.

Conclusion

The availability of better optics, a videocamera monitor system, hand and mechanized instruments, and knowledge of the intricate anatomy of the knee has made it possible to diagnose different synovial disorders, and perhaps to study gross morphology and classify them.

Arthroscopic technique has certainly helped our understanding of the various knee pathologies in considerable detail. At the present time, most of the centers where there is a proper environment use arthroscopic synovectomy rather than open arthrotomy. Since there is less trauma to the skin and capsule, and as the quadriceps mechanism is spared, rehabilitation has been made easier and faster.

As complete removal of the synovium is possible with much less morbidity to the patient with cost containment, early referral and early arthroscopic synovectomy can be recommended in a patient who has obtained maximum benefit from medical management but is still symptomatic. The long-term benefit is certainly better than that of open surgery, but it is open to debate whether synovectomy will completely stop the disease process without any recurrence. Perhaps repeat of arthroscopic synovectomy or staged arthroscopic synovectomy is preferable, considering the known morbidity from open synovectomy.[8]

I have described various conditions of synovial disorders and explained the technique and salient features of synovectomy specifically for rheumatoid arthritis.[3,5,6,25-27]

In the future, perhaps electric surgery and laser surgery will make synovectomy easier.

References

1. **Sim FH**, Synovial proliferative disorders: Role of synovectomy, *Arthroscopy* (1985) **3**: 198–204.
2. **Volkmann R von** (1877), quoted in Mignon MA, Synovectomy of the knee, *Clin Orthop* (1964) **36**: 7.
3. **Laurin CA, Desmarchais J, Daziano L** et al., Long-term results of synovectomy of the knee in rheumatoid patients, *J Bone Joint Surg (Am)* (1974) **56**: 521–531.

4. **Klein W, Jensen K-U**, Arthroscopic synovectomy of the knee joint: indication, technique, and follow-up results, *Arthroscopy* (1988) **4**: 63–71.

5. **Barnes CG, Mason RM**, Synovectomy of the knee joint in rheumatoid arthritis, *Ann Phys Med* (1967) **9**: 83.

6. **Henderson MS**, Synovectomy for destructive arthritis of the knee joint, *Surg Clin North Am* (1924) **4**: 565.

7. **Marmor L**, Synovectomy of the knee joint, *Orthop Clin North Am* (1979) **10**: 211–222.

8. **Shibata T, Shiraoka K, Takubo N**, Comparison between arthroscopic and open synovectomy for the knee in rheumatoid arthritis, *Arch Orthop Trauma Surg* (1986) **105**: 257–262.

9. **Dorfmann H, De Bie B, Bonvarlet JP** et al., Arthroscopic treatment of synovial chondromatosis of the knee, *Arthroscopy* (1989) **5**(1): 48–51.

10. **Rosenberg TD**, Arthroscopic synovectomy—preliminary results and surgical technique (1982) (unpublished).

11. **Patel D**, Synovial lesions: plicae, *Operative arthroscopy*, ed McGinty JB (New York: Raven Press, 1991) 361–372.

12. **Watanabe M, Takeda S, Ikeuchi H**, *Atlas of arthroscopy* (Tokyo, New York: Springer-Verlag, 1979) 30–48, 131–133.

13. **Beguin J, Locker B, Vielpeau C** et al., Pigmented villonodular synovitis of the knee: results from 13 cases, *Arthroscopy* (1989) **5**(1): 62–64.

14. **Granowitz SP, Mankin HJ**, Localized pigmented villonodular synovitis of the knee: report of 5 cases, *J Bone Joint Surg (Am)* (1967) **49**: 122–128.

15. **Lopez-Vazquez E, Lopez-Peris JL, Vila-Donat E** et al., Localized pigmented villonodular synovitis of the knee: diagnosis and arthroscopic resection, *Arthroscopy* (1988) **4**(2): 121–123.

16. **Patel D**, Arthroscopy of the plica—synovial folds and their significance, *Am J Sports Med* (1978) **6**: 217–225.

17. **Dandy DJ**, Anatomy of the medial suprapatellar plica and medial synovial shelf, *Arthroscopy* (1990) **6**: 79–85.

18. **Pipkin G**, Knee injuries: the role of the suprapatellar plica and suprapatellar bursa in simulating internal derangements, *Clin Orthop* (1971) **74**: 161–176.

19. **Hardaker WT, Whipple TL, Bassett FH**, Diagnosis and treatment of the plica syndrome of the knee, *J Bone Joint Surg (Am)* (1980) **62**: 221–225.

20. **Jackson RW, Marshall DJ, Fujisawa Y**, The pathologic medial shelf, *Orthop Clin North Am* (1982) **13**: 307–312.

21. **Thiery JA**, Arthroscopic drainage in septic arthritides of the knee: a multicenter study, *Arthroscopy* (1989) **5**(1): 65–69.

22. **Jackson RW**, The septic knee: arthroscopic treatment, *Arthroscopy* (1985) **1**: 194–197.

23. **Smith MJ**, Arthroscopic treatment of the septic knee, *Arthroscopy* (1986) **2**: 30–34.

24. **Casscells CD**, Commentary: the argument for early arthroscopic synovectomy in patients with severe hemophilia, *Arthroscopy* (1987) **3**(2): 78–79.

25. **Ishikawa H, Ohno O, Hirohata K**, Long-term results of synovectomy in rheumatoid patients, *J Bone Joint Surg (Am)* (1986) **68**: 198–205.

26. **Mori M, Ogawa R**, Anterior capsulectomy in the treatment of rheumatoid arthritis of the knee joint, *Arthritis Rheum* (1963) **6**: 130–137.

27. **Geens S**, Synovectomy and debridement of the knee in rheumatoid arthritis, *J Bone Joint Surg (Am)* (1969) **51**: 617–625.

10.2   Arthroscopic synovectomy of the knee

Zaid Al-Duri, Paul M. Aichroth and Dipak V. Patel

Synovectomy (excision of the synovium) of the knee was first described by Volkman in 1877 for the treatment of tuberculosis.[1-3] Later investigations confirmed the good results of synovectomy for tuberculous arthritis.[3] Reports in non-tuberculous synovitis were traced back to 1887.[1] An inflamed synovium may have a deleterious effect on cartilage and bone and hence the necessity of performing a synovectomy before the damage is too advanced.[4]

Arthroscopy of the knee is not a new technique, as it has been in use for more than half a century. Lesions of the synovium are particularly amenable to inspection and biopsy by arthroscopic techniques.[5] The arthroscope may be of help as well in identifying the synovial lesions that may present as a mechanical knee disturbance. De la Caffinière[6] presented 30 cases in which problems related to internal derangement of the knee were found to be due to abnormalities of the synovium. Over a period of 3 years, 14% of the patients presenting with symptoms thought to be due to chondromalacia patellae or damage to the medial meniscus had synovial abnormalities of the knee. It was therefore, only natural that the arthroscope was put to use in attempting to remove the synovium.

Indications for synovectomy

Synovectomy is indicated generally in chronic synovitis. The indications remain the same whether the synovectomy is performed arthroscopically or by open surgery.[7] Ideally, synovectomy should be performed when the disease is limited to the synovium before the involvement of articular cartilage and bone, and when there has been a failure of a trial of adequate conservative treatment for at least 6 months.[2,8] Synovectomy is of least value when the arthritis is polyarticular. It is advisable that there should be no joint space narrowing.[2] To assess articular cartilage damage in the knee joint, the most sensitive technique is a weight-bearing radiograph with the knee in 45° posteroanterior flexion.[2] Some advise the performance of synovectomy after the subsidence of the acute stage.[8]

The most common indication for synovectomy today is rheumatoid arthritis.[2,8] However, there are other conditions in which synovectomy may be useful, such as:

1. Synovial chondromatosis and osteochondromatosis[2,8-10]
2. Pigmented villonodular synovitis[2,5,8,9,11 13]
3. Synovial haemangioma[8,9,14]
4. Crystalline synovitis[2,15]
5. Seronegative arthropathy such as psoriatic arthropathy, Marie–Strümpell disease, inflammatory bowel disease[2,3,15]
6. Non-specific synovitis[2,5]
7. Thorn synovitis[16,17]
8. Haemophilic synovitis[18-20]
9. Persistent synovitis following infection[2,3,8]
10. Synovial lipoma[8]
11. Pathological synovial plicae: their treatment when indicated is in many ways a form of partial synovectomy

Advantages of arthroscopic synovectomy

The great advantage of arthroscopic synovectomy is the reduction in the incidence of morbidity and stiffness. There is less pain and swelling in the knee joint and an improvement in the range of motion and knee function.[2,5] Arthroscopic synovectomy allows a more complete synovial excision and the menisci are spared.

Smiley and Wasilewski[21] presented a study evaluating the efficacy of knee synovectomy with arthroscopic technique. Nineteen patients (25 knees) were evaluated. There were 14 females and 5 males, with the median age being 42 years (range 16–66 years). Twenty-two knees were diagnosed as having rheumatoid arthritis or a variant, two as having psoriatic arthritis, and one as having pigmented villonodular synovitis. All 25 knees had a 6-month follow-up, 21 knees had a 2-year follow-up, and 14 knees were evaluated at least 4 years postoperatively. The results were: postoperative period 6 months, 96% good results; 2 years, 90% good; 4 years, 57% good.

Preoperative as well as postoperative follow-up weight-bearing radiographs were studied: at 2 years, 81% showed no progressive radiographic changes; at 4 years, 61.5% showed no radiographic deterioration.

The clinical results correlated well with the radiographic results. The conclusion was that arthroscopic synovectomy produced results similar to those previously reported with open synovectomy, with less operative and postoperative morbidity. The study supported the initial benefits of arthroscopic synovectomy for short-term relief.

Disadvantages of open synovectomy

The disadvantages of open synovectomy include the following:

1. Failure of the procedure to achieve thorough excision of the diseased synovium in the posterior compartment.[22]
2. Loss of motion leading to a disabling stiffness.[18,19,22] Thus a manipulation is frequently required after open synovectomy.[5]
3. Wound dehiscence, infection and cutaneous nerve injury.[2]
4. It is more expensive in terms of the hospital stay and care of the patient than arthroscopic synovectomy.

Possible disadvantages of arthroscopic synovectomy

Arthroscopic synovectomy should be performed by a proficient knee surgeon in an operating theatre well equipped with arthroscopic knee instruments. Special instruments are required and the surgeon needs to be skilled in the arthroscopic techniques[2] and use of all arthroscopic portals.

Technique of arthroscopic synovectomy

No technique for synovectomy allows for the total removal of the synovium.[9] However, synovectomy can be performed fairly completely using multiple portal techniques (Figures 1 and 2). While the technique of the individual operation depends on the pathology and its anatomical site within the knee joint, the discussion here will refer to total arthroscopic synovectomy.

Visualization can be difficult, especially if there is extensive proliferative villous formation of the synovium. Thus adequate distension of the knee joint cavity is essential for proper inspection.[5] A high-flow technique makes the procedure easier.[9] Wide-bore tubes and adequately large motorized resectors and shavers are essential.

The arthroscopist sets out to achieve complete resection of the synovium in all knee compartments. The main difficulty is in visualization and resection of the synovium in the posteromedial and posterolateral knee joint corners. Rosenberg et al.[22] described the 'six-portal arthroscopic synovectomy' of the knee joint as follows. The arthroscope (30°) is inserted through the anterolateral portal immediately adjacent to the infrapatellar tendon 1 cm above the joint-line. A similar method is used anteromedially. Both these portals are used to inspect the joint thoroughly and to take a synovial biopsy. A 70° scope is passed through the anterolateral portal into the posteromedial compartment. With the fluid inflow and subsequent distension, visualization is very good with the knee flexed to 90°. The posteromedial corner of the knee joint is next palpated externally to seek a point that is approximately 1 cm posterior to the femoral condyle and 1 cm above the joint-line. This portal is employed to remove the posteromedial synovium using a motorized suction-cutting resector under direct vision. Then pass the arthroscope from the anteromedial portal into the posterolateral compartment in a similar fashion, and repeat the steps. A 30° arthroscope is then inserted anterolaterally into the suprapatellar pouch. The suprapatellar synovium is approached by insertion of the motorized resector into the suprapatellar portal laterally or medially, alternating in portals with the scope. This system is clearly designed to cover all the knee regions under direct vision and to allow for a thorough resection.

Whilst the majority of surgeons recommend motorized shavers, O'Connor et al.[10] described their experience with arthroscopic synovectomy. The instruments they used before the advent of motorized cutting devices were a rongeur and a basket forceps. As the motorized devices became available, arthroscopic synovectomy became easier. However, it was felt that the motorized instruments had limited cutting tolerance and became clogged frequently. These authors reverted back to the old instruments. Posterior synovectomy of the knee joint was accomplished by viewing through the notch with an offset arthroscope and sweeping the synovium with motorized or hand-held instruments introduced through the posteromedial or posterolateral portals.

Postoperative management

It is advisable to apply compressive dressing after an arthroscopic synovectomy.[2,9] The patient is given crutches for partial weight bearing on the second

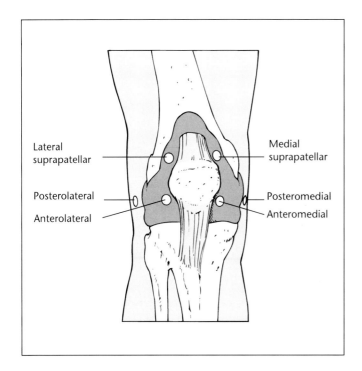

Figure 1

Arthroscopic portals.

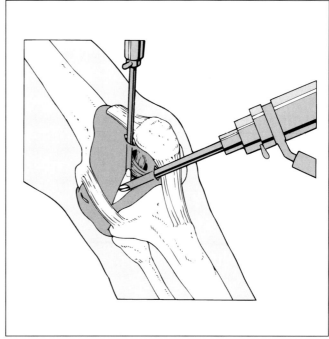

Figure 2

Triangulation technique. The arthroscope is in the suprapatellar portal.

postoperative day. The patient is allowed full weight bearing when it is possible to demonstrate full range of knee movement and good quadriceps strength.[9] The preoperative range of movement should be equalled or exceeded by the end of the fourth week.[2] Rosenberg et al.[2] advise physiotherapy only for those patients who continue to have difficulty in regaining motion. The continuous passive motion machine is useful.

Individual disease and the application of arthroscopic synovectomy

Juvenile chronic arthritis

Juvenile chronic arthritis (JCA) involving the knee joint in a child leads to a form of chronic synovitis that stimulates the adjacent growth plate, resulting in limb lengthening.[8,23] There is general agreement that in the children with the mild form of the disease, such as those with monoarticular or pauciarticular involvement, the results following synovectomy are good.[8,23] Poor results are encountered with synovec-

tomy of the knee joint in those children with systemic disease, those with the polyarticular form, and in those children under the age of 7 years, owing to their poor cooperation in the postoperative programme.[8] Ovregard et al.[4] performed a study aimed at evaluating the results of open synovectomies in various joints, including the knee joint in children with juvenile arthritis. They concluded that it was necessary to wait at least 3 years to evaluate the long-term effect of synovectomies, as good results tend to decrease with time.

Rheumatoid arthritis

The extent to which synovectomy impedes progression of damage to articular cartilage in adult rheumatoid arthritis is controversial, and the prophylactic effect is very difficult to assess.[24] Synovectomy is a palliative rather than a curative procedure in adult rheumatoid arthritis.[8] The knee joint is the most commonly involved joint in patients with rheumatoid arthritis. The indications for synovectomy in rheumatoid arthritis include failure of medical control of synovitis after 6 months of adequate conservative treatment, with resulting chronic effusion and a thickened synovium; minimal loss of joint space as confirmed by weight-bearing and stress films of the knee; a good range of knee movement with less than 20° flexion contracture; and no valgus deformity. Ideally the patient should be able to mobilize on crutches and participate in a physiotherapy programme.[9]

Shibata et al.[25] reported a comparison between arthroscopic and open synovectomy of the knee in rheumatoid arthritis. Ten surgical anterior capsulosynovectomies in 9 rheumatoid patients and 14 arthroscopic synovectomies in 11 patients were performed. In 3 patients with bilateral involvement at nearly the same stage (III), they operated on the knees simultaneously, using open capsulosynovectomy on one side and arthroscopic synovectomy on the other side. They assessed the postoperative course, the subjective evaluation of the patients, and the follow-up results. They remarked that surgical intervention is milder in the arthroscopic operation, and that postoperative knee pain during motion exercise is markedly less in the arthroscopic synovectomized knee. They concluded that, although the postoperative management was more complex for open capsulosynovectomized knees, the results obtained at 1–2 months after synovectomy showed no significant difference between the two procedures.

Cohen and Jones[27] evaluated the efficacy of arthroscopic synovectomy of the knee in rheumatoid arthritis. They reviewed 10 knees (9 patients) with chronic synovitis unresponsive to medical treatment. Postarthroscopically, patients were ambulatory and exhibited 90° of knee flexion on the day after surgery and were discharged at 24–48 hours. The joint tenderness and swelling improved postoperatively and was maintained for 1 year, and so did the range of movement of the knee in all the patients (a mean of 21°). Nine knees were followed up for at least 24 months and 4 required repeated surgery. The conclusion was that arthroscopic synovectomy was comparable to open synovectomy in short-term reduction of pain and swelling and that the chief benefit of arthroscopic synovectomy is a reduction in morbidity, hospital stay and postoperative rehabilitation.

Matsui et al.[37] reviewed the results of arthroscopic synovectomy (in 41 knees) in comparison with those of open synovectomy (in 26 knees) in patients with rheumatoid arthritis, with an average follow-up of 10 years. The clinical outcome was the same in both groups, but there was gradual deterioration after 8 years. Radiographic changes were worse in knees treated by open synovectomy compared to those treated by arthroscopic synovectomy. The conclusion was that arthroscopic synovectomy has many advantages and is better than open synovectomy for patients with rheumatoid arthritis.

Ogilvie-Harris and Babinski[28] reported on the results of arthroscopic synovectomy for rheumatoid arthritis performed in 96 knees. The follow-up period was 2–4 years. There was a statistically significant decrease in pain and synovitis while the range of movement was maintained. They concluded that arthroscopic synovectomy was at least a valuable palliative procedure for uncontrolled synovitis of the knee.

Mack and Clayton[9] state that the results of synovectomy in rheumatoid arthritis of the knee show good pain relief with suppression of the clinical activity. Recurrences approach 50% after several years, although function is still improved. The results and incidence of recurrence are time-dependent and proportional to the general activity of the disease as well as to the extent of joint damage present at the time of surgery. The long-term expectations of the procedure have not changed by doing the procedure arthroscopically as opposed to by open synovectomy. However, arthroscopic synovectomy has decreased the postoperative morbidity and recovery time and shortened hospital stay.

Radiological deterioration of an inflamed knee joint is delayed for approximately 3 years in rheumatoid arthritis patients who do not respond to conservative treatment within a period of 5 months and who undergo synovectomy.

Pigmented villonodular synovitis

Pigmented villonodular synovitis (PVNS) is a rare condition. The incidence of PVNS is estimated at 1.8 cases per million persons. The knee joint is most commonly affected, with an incidence varying from 28% to 76%;[12,29] others estimate the incidence of the knee joint involvement to be 90%.[9] Although histologically similar, the localized and diffuse forms of the pigmented villonodular synovitis are sufficiently different both clinically and in their response to treatment to be considered as different clinical entities.

Locker et al.[12] described 12 cases of PVNS. There were 9 females and 3 men, with an average age of 29 years (17–44 years). The average time between the first symptom and the first consultation was 2.5 years (range 3 months to 7 years). The diagnosis was made or confirmed by means of a percutaneous biopsy in one instance and by arthroscopy in 11 patients. They classified PVNS into the following types: (A) local lesions (1–7 cm), 7 patients; (B) diffuse lesion, 1 patient; (C) mixed lesions (localized and diffuse), 4 patients. The method of treatment undertaken included arthroscopic excision for the localized lesion in 2 patients and open synovectomy in 9 patients. The average follow-up in their series was 3.2 years (6 months to 9 years). The follow-up period was 1.7 years for the localized forms and 5.4 years for the others. Eight patients were totally asymptomatic (including 2 patients who had double meniscectomy (9 years follow-up). Four patients experienced some pain (after exhaustion or at the end of the day).

They fully acknowledge the value of arthroscopy in the elimination of the localized types of moderate or even larger lesions with the appropriate instrumentation. In the diffuse type, they state that synovectomy can be arthroscopic but is classically open. Finally, these authors stress the value of arthroscopy in monitoring the progress of the lesion by allowing an inspection of the results of treatment and determination of the re-activation of the lesion.

Ogilvie-Harris et al.[13] reviewed 22 patients with a histologically proven pigmented villonodular synovitis of the knee who were treated arthroscopically. The localized type of the lesion was present in 4 knees while 18 knees had the diffuse type of pigmented villonodular synovitis. The follow-up was 3.8 years. The patients in the diffuse group underwent a complete arthroscopic synovectomy (10 patients) using six portals, or a partial synovectomy (8 patients) removing just the area of pathological synovium. The patients who had the complete arthroscopic synovectomy showed a significant decrease in pain, increase in range of movement, and less synovitis. The recurrence rate was 9% following complete arthroscopic synovectomy and 43% following partial synovectomy. The time of recurrence was 1.8 years in the partial group and 3.5 years in the complete group. They concluded that for the localized PVNS, localized resection of the lesion is recommended. For the diffuse PVNS, complete arthroscopic synovectomy should be undertaken as it was statistically significantly better for all parameters than partial synovectomy.

Mack and Clayton[9] state that the treatment of choice for PVNS is arthroscopic synovectomy. The more complete the synovectomy, the better the result. The recurrence rate should be low as this is a localized disease. However, with recurrence, repeat arthroscopic synovectomy is indicated.

Synovial chondromatosis

Mack and Clayton[9] stated that the patient presents with internal derangement of the knee joint, with persistent effusion, pain and catching. Radiographs are often negative, although loose bodies may be seen. The treatment of choice is synovectomy. This can be accomplished arthroscopically using a wide-bore shaver. However, this may be impossible because of frequent clogging of the equipment with tiny loose bodies. The surgeon may revert to open classic synovectomy in this case. Medial and lateral parapatellar incisions are usually best for open synovectomy.

Coolican and Dandy[30] described three arthroscopic patterns of macroscopic appearances representing three different disease stages in 18 knees they reviewed. Such patterns included large lesions covered by normal synovium (22%), small cartilage fragments lying in or on synovium (56%) and free cartilage fragments in the joint cavity (22%). They reported the results of arthroscopic synovectomy and loose-body removal in 18 knees with primary chondromatosis after a mean follow-up of 3½ years (range 1–10 years): 14 were symptom-free or had only minor symptoms; 3 improved but were not cured; 1 knee was a failure. They concluded that their results were better than published results of open operation for this condition.

Dorfmann et al.[31] reviewed 39 patients with synovial chondromatosis; 29 of these patients (32 knees) were followed for an average of 3.5 years. Only one patient required synovectomy; the rest of the patients (31 knees) required removal of loose bodies only. They concluded that the simple arthroscopic removal of cartilaginous bodies without synovectomy is the treatment of choice for synovial chondromatosis of the knee. The essential prognostic factor for a good functional result is the condition of the tibiofemoral cartilage.

O'Connor et al.[10] advised removal of the loose bodies and synovectomy where appropriate.

Haemophilic synovitis

Kay et al.[32] reported the results of open synovectomies for the treatment of recurrent haemarthroses in 11 knees followed up for 29–76 months. The average number of bleeds was reduced postoperatively from 19 to 3 bleeds over a period of 12 months. Over the same period of follow-up, the same knee joints were found to have lost an average of 42° of mobility. Postoperatively 54% of the patients suffered from haemorrhages despite satisfactory levels of factor VIII. They concluded that synovectomy of the knee is to be avoided when other means of reducing the bleeding episodes are available.

Post et al.[33] reviewed the results of surgical synovectomy in 12 knees for an average of 59.6 months after the synovectomy. Their indication for surgery was a frequent or persistent haemorrhage in a joint with subacute or early chronic synovitis that did not respond to vigorous conservative management, including frequent factor-concentrate replacement. Additional indications included rapid deterioration of joint function, and chronic pain in the early chronic arthropathy. They stated that, while the incidence of bleeding is significantly decreased after surgical synovectomy, it was not necessarily associated with a cessation of the progression of the joint pathology. However, the reduced incidence of bleeds following surgical synovectomy may serve to delay reconstructive operations until a later period in life. They concluded that early surgical synovectomy for intractable chronic synovitis is recommended as a useful measure in the management of haemophilic arthropathy.

Klein et al.[18] reported on 7 patients who underwent arthroscopic synovectomy for haemophilic synovitis. All had frequent recurrent haemarthroses despite medical management. All had signs of degenerative arthritis preoperatively. The follow-up was 4 years on average. Regarding bleeding: 6 patients had reduced bleeding, with an average of 0.22 haemarthroses per week; 1 patient required significantly less factor VIII to control bleeding. Regarding motion: no patient lost more than 10° of motion; 3 patients had increased range of movement; 2 patients were unchanged as far as motion was concerned. Regarding radiographic changes: 5 patients had radiographic progression of the degenerative changes; 2 patients were unchanged. They recommend early arthroscopic synovectomy in the treatment of recurrent haemarthrosis in haemophilic patients.

Limbird and Dennis[19] reviewed 5 male patients with chronic and/or recurrent haemarthrosis due to haemophilia. The age range was 10–35 years. They underwent arthroscopic synovectomy of the knee followed by continuous passive motion (CPM). The CPM was begun in the recovery room and was continued for 5–7 days. The use of CPM and physiotherapy improved both the passive and active range of knee motion rapidly and by 3–6 months all patients (except one) achieved a better active range of movement than their preoperative range. All patients showed significant reduction of their documented bleeding episodes. They concluded that the combination of arthroscopic synovectomy and CPM in the treatment of haemophilic synovitis had been successful in maximizing the benefits and minimising the complications of synovectomy.

DeGnore and Wilson[20] performed open synovectomy on 16 knees of patients with haemophilic synovitis. The average follow-up was 4.8 years (range 7 months to 12 years). Postoperatively and during the first week, the knee was kept on a CPM device. As rehabilitation progressed, the time on the machine was gradually reduced to 12–18 hours per day. Two patients could not tolerate the CPM in the second postoperative week and required manipulation under anaesthesia. All patients gained on an average 2° of extension and lost 11° of flexion. Only one knee had no postoperative bleeding episode after an average follow-up of 4.2 years. On the whole, there is a decline in the number of bleeding episodes after surgery. The authors believe that there is no conclusive evidence that synovectomy significantly slows the progression of haemophilic arthropathy despite the reduction in destructive enzyme levels.

Wiedel[34] reported on a retrospective evaluation of 5–10 years of arthroscopic synovectomy of the knee in 8 patients (8 knees) with haemophilia. Seven patients had haemophilia A (age range 8–18 years) and one patient had haemophilia B (age 36 years). All patients experienced improvement in function. Two patients complained of pain on activity. Only one patient developed recurrent haemarthrosis. This occurred after a knee injury that occurred 18 months following the initial synovectomy. The author performed a repeat arthroscopic synovectomy 2½ years later and the patient has had no recurrent haemarthrosis to date. Regarding range of movement, the results were (A) *Flexion*: unchanged, 3 knees; improved, 3 knees; lost, 2 knees. (B) *Extension*: unchanged, 3 knees; improved, 2 knees; loss of extension, 2 knees.

The author expressed concern about the possibility of postoperative bleeding that occurred in one of the patients and resulted in loss of motion, despite the relatively less traumatic procedure of arthroscopic synovectomy. The conclusion was that arthroscopic synovectomy did offer some advantage in the immediate postoperative period but did not influence the ultimate outcome.

Synovial haemangioma

Haemangiomas seem to involve males and females equally. Synovial haemangiomas are a rare cause of recurrent knee effusions. The problem usually presents in childhood, but the diagnosis is often not made for many years. Seventy-five per cent of the patients will have symptoms before the age of 16 years. No cases of bilateral involvement have been reported.[9] Arthroscopy should be considered early to make the diagnosis and biopsy the tumour so that further treatment can be carried out.[35] In cases of spontaneous bleeding tendency, synovial haemangioma should be among the causes considered.[36] There are essentially two types of synovial haemangiomas: the localized sessile type and the infiltrated diffuse type. The localized type of the lesion is more amenable to total excision and offers a better prognosis. Where a total excision cannot be performed, recurrence is very common. Total synovectomy is indicated only in the case of the infiltrative type. Radiotherapy is another treatment modality.[9]

Meislin and Parisien[14] reported on a synovial haemangioma of the knee in a 33-year-old woman that was diagnosed and removed arthroscopically. Preoperatively this rare, benign soft-tissue lesion had caused recurrent swelling of the knee along with persistent pain and occasional buckling. Two years after surgery, the patient had a painless range of motion with no evidence of recurrence.

Juhl and Krebs[26] reporting on two cases of synovial haemangioma, concluded that synovial haemangioma will be discovered earlier and more frequently by arthroscopy and can be operated upon at once.

Thorn synovitis

Ramanathan and Luiz[16] reviewed 6 patients who had synovitis of the knee secondary to a prick by date-palm thorns. All the patients gave a definite history of palm-thorn injuries. The interval between the injury and the first hospital visit ranged from 3 days to 5 months. All had pain and effusion with restricted movement, and they all had routine blood test to help exclude septic arthritis. Despite the fact that four knees were treated satisfactorily by irrigation, two knees continued to show signs of synovitis and required arthrotomy and synovectomy. The results were satisfactory, as all knees became pain-free and regained full movement in a duration ranging from 4 to 13 months.

Doig and Cole[17] reported their experience with five children with chronic thorn synovitis. They advised the removal of the free thorn fragments and all macroscopically abnormal synovium in order that complete cure is achieved. Four of the children required total synovectomy for diffuse proliferative synovitis and one needed a partial synovectomy in the area where the thorn had penetrated the synovium. Partial synovectomy was not successful in children with diffuse synovitis.

Crystalline synovitis

Kalenak et al.[15] stated that the management of crystalline arthropathies (i.e. gout and pseudogout) is mainly medical. The authors suggest that arthroscopy might be useful in situations in which sepsis must be ruled out. Large deposits of crystalline material may require the use of a synovial resector to remove the bulk of the lesion.

Seronegative arthropathies

Reiter's syndrome and psoriatic arthritis rarely have indications for arthroscopic procedures. These conditions have to be differentiated from septic arthritis. In Reiter's syndrome there is no proliferative villous formation; however, a rich exudate may form abundantly. Therefore, lavage and debridement may become necessary. In psoriatic arthropathy, there is synovial hypertrophy and hyperaemia 'rabbit ear appearance'. Partial synovectomy and joint lavage may have a useful but limited role in this condition.[15]

Synovial plicae

Very rarely, a plica may become symptomatic, usually following a traumatic episode or with repetitive activity.[5,22] About 35% of persons will demonstrate a medial synovial plica, only a small percentage of whom are symptomatic. They will present with medial pain, snapping and occasionally buckling. The plica can be palpated under the medial retinaculum.[5] A pathological medial plica is inferred from observation of fibrotic thickening, inflamed synovium, and

evidence of impingement at the medial femoral condyle.[22]

Klein[38] reviewed 180 knees with medial patellar synovial plicae. Shelf fibrosis was present in 15.5% of them. Forty-three patients were treated by arthroscopic surgery. Plica excision was carried out in 17 knees. In 26 other patients, excision of the patellar plica was combined with other additional procedures such as intra-articular patellar shaving, lateral release, meniscectomy or local synovectomy. The best results were obtained in those patients with a medial shelf as the only abnormality in the knee joint. Knees with multiple lesions in addition to a medial patellar plica showed a relatively high amount of unsatisfactory results, the reason being the overlap of the other lesions by the plica.

Hansen and Boe[39] reported on a 43-month follow-up of 46 patients treated by arthroscopic resection of a medial synovial plica. Preoperatively, 40% of these patients had anterior knee pain on exertion, and 60% had mechanical symptoms. The symptoms were preceded by knee trauma in 50% of these patients. The results of this study were satisfying, with 80% excellent or good results according to the Lysholm score, and 59% of the patients were completely symptom free. It is interesting to note that the presence of chondromalacia of the patella or the femoral condyles or malalignment of the patella did not make the results worse. They therefore concluded that arthroscopic resection of a pathological medial synovial plica generally gives good results even if other pathology of the knee joint is present.

In a retrospective study of 89 patients undergoing 98 arthroscopies of the knee in which a medial synovial plica was noted, O'Dwyer and Peace[40] concluded that arthroscopic resection of a pathological plica is a worthwhile procedure.

Zanoli and Piazzai,[41] describing the synovial plica syndrome, emphasized that in certain circumstances (usually of mechanical origin) a normally innocuous synovial plica can undergo inflammatory changes resulting in fibrosis. If the diagnosis is made early, the results of the treatment are excellent.

Synovitis and infections

Arthroscopic synovectomy has been mentioned as an indication for the treatment of infection in joints.[2,8,42] However, the general reference is to irrigation and debridement of joints rather than actual synovectomy. Few reports on open synovectomy are mentioned here.

Torholm et al.[3] reviewed 20 patients with bacterial arthritis of the hip and knee joints who had either a delay in the diagnosis or no response to treatment. This figure presented a third of all the patients treated for bacterial arthritis during the study period. None of the patients treated with aspiration and antibiotics alone was included in this study. Fourteen of the patients had septic arthritis of the knee joint. The patients' ages ranged between 3 years and 79 years (4 patients under the age of 10 years). They were followed up for an average of 51 months (range 22–107 months). The criteria of infection in these patients included one of the following: positive culture taken by sterile aspiration, positive culture of the biopsy of the synovium, fistula formation from the joint, and radiographic evidence of osteomyelitis. The infective organisms were *Staphylococcus aureus* in 8 knees; *Staphylococcus aureus* and *Klebsiella* in 1 knee; *Mycobacterium tuberculosis* in 1 knee; *Proponibacterium acnes* in 1 knee; and no organism isolated in 3 knees.

The duration of the infection before synovectomy was 4–28 days with an average duration of 13 days, with only one knee undergoing a synovectomy after 6 months. The results were graded as good (a patient back to normal in terms of range of motion, activity of daily living, and normal radiographic appearance), fair (slight pain on weight bearing, slight limitation of mobility and a radiographic narrowing of the joint space of grade 2 Ahlbäck), and poor (the remaining patients). Twelve patients had good results and 2 had fair results. They concluded that synovectomy, even when performed after 5 days and up to 4 weeks later, could prevent knee joint destruction.

Tscherne et al.[42] stated that the treatment of pyogenic infection of the knee joint leads to unsatisfactory results. They recommended early synovectomy of the knee joint to 'excise' the focus of infection before the occurrence of articular cartilage damage. They reported on the excellent results after 26 knee-joint infections treated by thorough early synovectomy before cartilage damage and osteoarthritis occurred.

Antituberculous drugs, debridement and open synovectomy can be considered in the treatment of tuberculous synovitis of the knee if the synovium is extensively involved and studded with tubercles. Early bone involvement is no contraindication. Synovectomy can be undertaken in combination with other surgical procedures in the more advanced knee joint involvement with tuberculosis.[43]

All group studies

Calvisi et al.[44] reviewed 800 arthroscopic patients, among whom 7.6% (61 patients) had anterior knee pain due to synovial pathology. Of these there were 35 patients with symptomatic synovial plicae; 20 patients with specific hypertrophic synovitis; 12 patients with pigmented villonodular synovitis; and 5 patients with synovial ganglia of the cruciate ligaments. None of these patients had any form of systemic articular disease.

The arthroscopic treatment consisted mainly of partial or total synovectomy, removal of the plicae, decompression and removal of the synovial ganglia. At a follow-up of 1–4 years (using the Tegner activity score) the results were satisfactory in 83% of those patients with focal lesions; however, in those patients with widespread lesions that required total synovectomy, the results were satisfactory in only 69% of the patients. The best results were achieved in the treatment of synovial plicae, pigmented villonodular synovitis and synovial ganglia, with the satisfactory rate being 96% among these groups.

Rosenberg et al.[2] reviewed a series of 16 patients treated by arthroscopic synovectomy for the following synovial lesions: diffuse pigmented villonodular synovitis, 5 patients; rheumatoid arthritis, 5 patients; synovial chondromatosis, 3 patients; nonspecific monoarticular synovitis, 2 patients; not specified, 1 patient. The patients were evaluated at 2–4 years postoperatively. Subjectively, reported limitation of activity had improved in 14 patients. Based on clinical evaluation of the postoperative results, 87% of the patients obtained excellent to good ratings, which confirmed minimal or no swelling and a range of motion over 125°. Two arthroscopic synovectomies (for class III and IV rheumatoid arthritis) were failures. The authors also reported on a series reviewed by Ogilvie-Harris (personal communication, 1989) and included 33 patients who were operated on by arthroscopic synovectomy and followed up for 4 years. The results showed substantial improvement of pain, synovitis and functional impairment in the majority of the patients.

References

1. **Lloyd Jones JK**, Inflammatory arthritis, *Surgery of the knee joint*, ed Jackson JP, Waugh W (London: Chapman and Hall Medical, 1984) 338.
2. **Rosenberg TD, Tearse DS, Kolowich PA**, Synovectomy of the knee, *Operative arthroscopy*, ed McGinty JB (New York: Raven Press, 1991) 373–380.
3. **Torholm C, Hedstrom SA, Sunden G** et al., Synovectomy in bacterial arthritis, *Acta Orthop Scand* (1983) **54**: 748–753.
4. **Ovregard T, Hoyeraal HM, Pahle JA** et al., A three-year retrospective study of synovectomies in children, *Clin Orthop* (1990) **259**: 76–82.
5. **McGinty JB**, Arthroscopy of the knee, *Surgery of the knee*, ed Insall JN (New York: Churchill Livingstone, 1984) 125–126.
6. **de la Caffinière JY**, Les troubles engendrés par les anomalies synoviales du genou, *Int Orthop* (1982) **6**(2): 207–216.
7. **Sim FH**, Synovial proliferative disorders: role of synovectomy, *Arthroscopy* (1985) **1**(3): 198–204.
8. **Greer Richardson E**, Miscellaneous nontraumatic disorders, *Campbell's operative orthopaedics*, 7th edn, ed Crenshaw AH (St Louis: CV Mosby, 1987) 1007–1013.
9. **Mack RP, Clayton MC**, Synovial and bursal lesions about the knee, *Surgery of the musculoskeletal system*, 2nd edn, ed McCollister Evarts C (New York: Churchill Livingstone, 1990) 3539–3542.
10. **O'Connor RL, Salisbury RB, Shahriaree H**, Synovial disease, *O'Connor's textbook of arthroscopic surgery*, ed Shahriaree H (Philadelphia: JB Lippincott, 1984) 277–288.

11. **Flandry F, Hughston JC**, Current concepts review. Pigmented villonodular synovitis, *J Bone Joint Surg (Am)* (1987) **69**(6): 942–949.
12. **Locker B, Beguin J, Vielpeau C** et al., Pigmented villonodular synovitis of the knee: advantages of arthroscopy, *Surgery and arthroscopy of the knee*, ed Müller W, Hackenbruch W (Berlin: Springer-Verlag, 1988) 661–665.
13. **Ogilvie-Harris DJ, Zarnett R, McLean J**, Complete versus partial arthroscopic synovectomy for pigmented villonodular synovitis of the knee, *Abstracts of the Combined Congress of the International Arthroscopy Association and the International Society of the Knee. Toronto, Ontario, Canada*, 13–17 May 1991, paper No. 13.
14. **Meislin RJ, Parisien JS**, Arthroscopic excision of synovial hemangioma of the knee, *Arthroscopy* (1990) **6**(1): 64–67.
15. **Kalenak A, Hanks GA, Sebastianelli WJ**, Arthroscopy of the knee, *Surgery of the musculoskeletal system*, 2nd edn, ed McCollister Evarts C (New York: Churchill Livingstone, 1990) vol 4, 3386–3392.
16. **Ramanathan EBS, Luiz CP**, Date palm thorn synovitis, *J Bone Joint Surg (Br)* (1990) **72**(3): 512–513.
17. **Doig SG, Cole WG**, Plant thorn synovitis. Resolution following total synovectomy, *J Bone Joint Surg (Br)* (1990) **72**(3): 514–515.
18. **Klein KS, Aland CM, Kim HC** et al., Long-term follow-up of arthroscopic synovectomy for chronic hemophilic synovitis, *Arthroscopy* (1987) **3**(4): 231–236.
19. **Limbird TJ, Dennis SC**, Synovectomy and continuous passive motion (CPM) in haemophilic patients, *Arthroscopy* (1987) **3**(2): 74–79.
20. **DeGnore LT, Wilson F**, Surgical management of hemophilic arthropathy, *Instructional Course Lectures*, ed Barr JS (1989) vol. XXXVIII, 385–388.
21. **Smiley P, Wasilewski SA**, Arthroscopic synovectomy, *Arthroscopy* (1990) **6**(1): 18–23.
22. **Rosenberg TD, Paulos LE, Parker RD** et al., Arthroscopic surgery of the knee, *Operative orthopaedics*, ed Chapman MW (Philadelphia: JB Lippincott, 1988) vol 3, 1588–1590.
23. **Swann M**, The surgery of juvenile chronic arthritis: an overview, *Clin Orthop* (1990) **259**: 70–75.
24. **Insall JN**, Miscellaneous items: arthrodesis, the stiff knee, synovectomy, and popliteal cysts, *Surgery of the knee*, ed Insall JN (New York: Churchill Livingstone, 1984) 737–739.
25. **Shibata T, Shiraoka K, Takubo N**, Comparison between arthroscopic and open synovectomy for the knee in rheumatoid arthritis, *Arch Orthop Trauma Surg* (1986) **105**(5): 257–262.
26. **Juhl M, Krebs B**, Arthroscopy and synovial hemangioma or giant cell tumour of the knee, *Arch Orthop Trauma Surg* (1989) **108**(4): 250–252.
27. **Cohen S, Jones R**, An evaluation of the efficacy of the arthroscopic synovectomy of the knee in rheumatoid arthritis: 12–24 month results, *J Rheumatol* (1987) **14**(3): 452–455.
28. **Ogilvie-Harris DJ, Babinski A**, Arthroscopic synovectomy of the knee for rheumatoid arthritis, *Arthroscopy* (1991) **7**(1): 91–97.
29. **Flandry F, McCann SB, Hughston JC** et al., Roentgenographic findings in pigmented villonodular synovitis of the knee, *Clin Orthop* (1989) **247**: 208–219.
30. **Coolican MR, Dandy DJ**, Arthroscopic management of synovial chondromatosis of the knee. Findings and results in 18 cases, *J Bone Joint Surg (Br)* (1989) **71**(3): 498–500.
31. **Dorfmann H, De Bie B, Bonvarlet JP** et al., Arthroscopic treatment of synovial chondromatosis of the knee, *Arthroscopy* (1989) **5**(1): 48–51.
32. **Kay L, Stainsby D, Buzzard B** et al., The role of synovectomy in the management of recurrent haemarthroses in haemophilia, *Br J Haematol* (1981) **49**(1): 53–60.
33. **Post M, Watts G, Telfer M**, Synovectomy in hemophilic arthropathy: A retrospective review of 17 cases, *Clin Orthop* (1986) **202**: 139–146.
34. **Wiedel JD**, Arthroscopic synovectomy of the knee in hemophilia, *Abstracts of the Combined Congress of the International Arthroscopy Association and the International Society of the Knee. Toronto, Ontario, Canada*, 13–17 May 1991, paper 11.
35. **Paley D, Jackson RW**, Synovial haemangioma of the knee joint: diagnosis by arthroscopy, *Arthroscopy* (1986) **2**(3): 174–177.
36. **Boe S**, Synovial hemangioma of the knee joint — a case report, *Arthroscopy* (1986) **2**(3): 178–180.
37. **Matsui N, Taneda Y, Ohta H** et al., Arthroscopic versus open synovectomy in the rheumatoid knee, *Int Orthop* (1989) **13**(1): 17–20.
38. **Klein W**, The medial shelf of the knee. A follow-up study, *Arch Orthop Trauma Surg* (1983) **102**(2): 67–72.
39. **Hansen H, Boe S**, The pathological plica in the knee. Results of arthroscopic resection, *Arch Orthop Trauma Surg* (1989) **108**(5): 282–284.
40. **O'Dwyer KJ, Peace PK**, The plica syndrome, *Injury* (1988) **19**(5): 350–352.
41. **Zanoli S, Piazzai E**, The synovial plica syndrome of the knee. Pathology, differential diagnosis and treatment, *Ital J Orthop Traumatol* (1983) **9**(2): 241–250.
42. **Tscherne H, Giebel G, Muhr G** et al., Synovectomy as treatment for purulent joint infection, *Arch Orthop Trauma Surg* (1984) **103**(3): 162–164.
43. **Marks KE, McHenry MC**, Nonspinal tuberculosis, *Surgery of the musculoskeletal system*, 2nd edn, ed McCollister Evarts C (New York: Churchill Livingstone, 1990) vol 5, 4566–4567.
44. **Calvisi V, Collodel M, Are A** et al., Synovial pathology: a cause of anterior knee pain, *Abstract book of the Fourth Congress of the European Society of Knee Surgery and Arthroscopy* (1990) 150.

11

Children's knee derangements

11.1   Disorders of the knee in children

Paul M. Aichroth

The first sign of the limb bud in embryo is at the end of the 4th week. The mesenchyme then condenses axially and is converted initially into the cartilaginous skeleton and later into bone. The joint cavity forms at the 3rd month as a mass of undifferentiated mesenchyme which becomes looser and then forms a cavity, the cellular lining of which becomes synovium. Mesenchyme may persist in this cavitated area to form the articular menisci.

Ossification around the knee

The femur ossifies at the centre of the future shaft at the end of the 2nd month of intrauterine life. The ossific centre of the femoral condyles is usually present at birth. It appears in boys between the 8th month and birth, but in girls may appear as early as the 7th month of intrauterine life. The lower femoral epiphysis remains unfused until the age of 17 years in girls and until 18 or even 19 years in boys, when the epiphyseal line ossifies. The tibia is similarly ossified from centres in the shaft, the upper growing end and the lower epiphysis. The upper tibial epiphysis develops an ossific centre at the 8th month of intrauterine life in the female and just before or just after birth in the male. This proximal epiphysis may fuse as late as 19 or even 20 years in the male and 2–3 years earlier in the female. The upper tibial epiphysis includes the upper half of the tibial tubercle and there is usually an additional ossific centre here, appearing at the age of 12 or 13 years (Figure 1).

Patellar development

The patella is preformed in cartilage and is usually seen by the 3rd month of intrauterine life. It is cartilaginous at birth and a bony centre appears at the 3rd year in girls and the 4th or even 5th year in boys. Sometimes the ossific centre may be bipartite or multipartite and may be confused with a fractured patella by the unwary. Ossification is completed about the age of puberty.

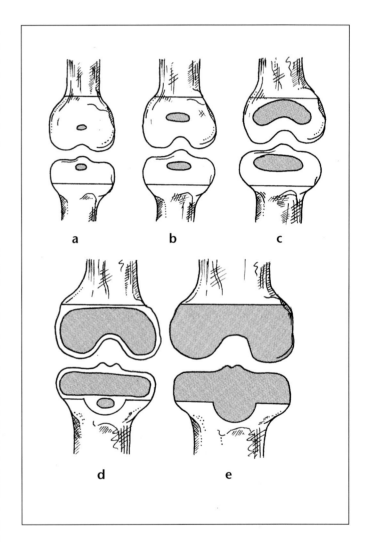

Figure 1

Ossification centres around the knee: (a) at birth; (b) end of 1st year; (c) 4th year; (d) 12th year; (e) fuses to shaft 17–20 years.

Irregularity of ossification of the femoral condylar epiphysis

Throughout childhood the edge of the ossific nucleus of the lower femur is irregular. At the distal epiphysis boundary the advancing front of ossification may

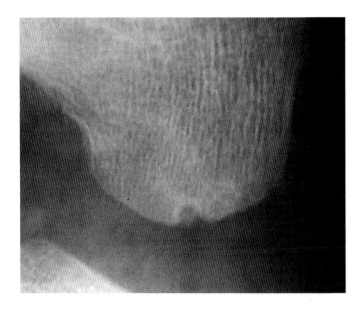

Figure 2

Ossification defect in the medial femoral condyle.

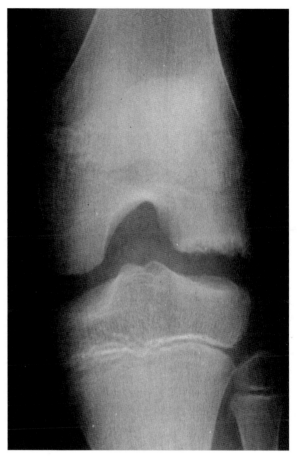

Figure 3

Osteochondritis dissecans of lateral femoral condyle.

produce multiple areas which resemble small loose bodies. This has given rise to confusion with osteochondritis dissecans and has been implicated in the aetiology of this condition. Smillie[1] feels that some cases of osteochondritis dissecans in the juvenile are actually ossification abnormalities. There is, however, a very definite difference in the radiological appearance of the two conditions. In the ossification irregularity producing an ossicle effect, the proximal edge of the fragment does not fit into a crater (Figure 2). In the child with osteochondritis dissecans the bony fragment fits exactly the crater in the epiphyseal bone (Figure 3). The articular cartilage in this latter situation is fractured and can be readily observed arthroscopically. Several patients with knee symptoms and ossification irregularity, as seen in Figure 4, have been examined arthroscopically by the author and no lesion has been seen. A definite 'fragment in crater' must therefore be identified radiologically before osteochondritis dissecans is suspected in a child of this age.

Special features of the immature knee

The child's knee is lax and especially so in the young girl. Although this state predisposes to easier patellar subluxation or dislocation, it does protect against significant ligament tears. Certainly major knee

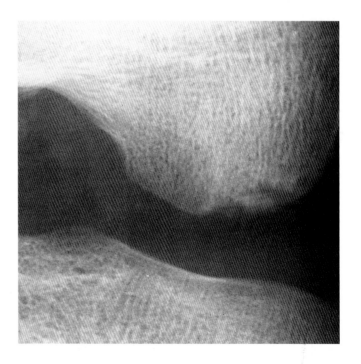

Figure 4

Ossification defect in the femoral condyle.

disruptions do occur in the child's knee, but fractures of the femur above, or the tibia below, are more common in the child whose teenage or adult counterpart would sustain a major ligament injury. Laxity of the ligaments allows a greater range of physiological varus, valgus and recurvatum at the knee and this must be borne in mind when examining the joint stability. Comparison with the other side is always necessary.

Ligament laxity certainly has its advantages in the child, for ligament and capsular strains are much less common. General joint laxity allows easy observation of the synovial cavity through the arthroscope in the child, for the bones may be readily separated by traction and by valgus and varus forces. In the child with congenital and sometimes familial joint laxity, recurrent dislocation of the patella may be present as well as congenital dislocation of the hip.

The details of physiological varus and valgus of the knee during development together with malalignment syndromes are well described by Andrew Jackson in this chapter.

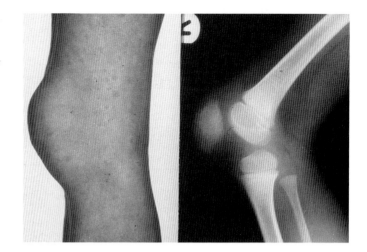

Figure 5

Patella magna.

Congenital abnormalities

Congenital abnormalities of this joint are rare. The discoid meniscus is the most commonly seen and is described in Chapter 12.

Congenital dislocation of the knee joint is reviewed by Barry Ferris later in this chapter.

Congenital short quadriceps muscle

This is another rare condition with progressive fibrosis of one or more components of the quadriceps musculature.[2] It may be seen with congenital heart defects, in which case the contracture may be acquired due to ischaemia of the quadriceps muscle following cardiac catheterization, for it has been seen in the same leg as the femoral arterial introduction of a catheter. Operative correction appears to be necessary with elongation of the quadriceps muscle.

Congenital dislocation of the patella

Congenital lateral dislocation of the patella is rare and is difficult to diagnose in the small baby. It is the cause of a fixed flexion contracture of the knee at birth and secondary deformities may develop in untreated cases.[3] The knee should be treated by operation when the infant is large enough to make patellar reposition possible. Quadriceps lengthening is usually necessary in a similar fashion to that described previously if it proves impossible to reposition the patella without full flexion of the joint.

Patellar ossification abnormalities

Bipartite or multipartite patellae are seen very regularly. The junior doctor may decide that such an abnormal radiological appearance indicates a patellar fracture but may be baffled by the minor nature of the injury which preceded the consultation. The vast majority of patellae with ossification defects of this type are normal in shape, size and articulation and are asymptomatic. There are some teenagers, however, whose patella is expanded and irregular, particularly on the lateral side, and in whom pain develops. The pain may be intermittent during activity and is due to abnormal articulation between the lateral expansion of the patella and the lateral femoral condyle. Eventually degenerative changes localized to this site may develop. Continued symptoms from this abnormal patellar lump and articulation may necessitate the removal of the separate ossicle through the epiphyseal–cartilage junction.

Other patellar abnormalities are rare and usually cause no symptoms. The child whose knee is illustrated in Figure 5 had a patella magna with a large knee cap malarticulating with the femur, producing pain and gross patellar crepitus.

Septic arthritis

Septic arthritis of the knee is now rarely seen in the West, for this is a joint which seems fairly resistant to infection. Nevertheless, an ill child may present with a high fever and an immobile lower limb, with a swollen, tender and slightly flexed knee joint. Any movement of the limb in general is painful and any attempt even to approach the knee is resisted by the child, who is greatly apprehensive of any local attention to this area.

The usual method of infection is by haematogenous spread, although direct inoculation of organisms into the synovial cavity may occur when the child kneels on a nail or spike. *Staphylococcus aureus* is still the most common organism, but *Haemophilus influenzae* and the pneumococci and meningococci have been detected with more recent frequency. *Escherichia coli*, salmonellae and brucella organisms are found rarely. Clinical diagnosis is usually relatively easy with the features described above. Investigations include a high white cell count and polymorphonuclear leucocytosis, a high ESR and a positive blood culture in some cases. The radiograph usually shows an effusion and at a much later stage erosions and joint destruction will become obvious.

The major differential diagnosis is between a primary septic arthritis and lower femoral osteomyelitis, where the most distal part of the metaphysis is within the synovial area of the suprapatellar pouch. The septic arthritis is characterized by more swelling with a tight effusion and even a minimal amount of joint movement produces acute agony. The effusion which accompanies a lower femoral osteomyelitis is smaller and the tenderness is localized to the lower femur, with the joint being a little more mobile. The radiograph will give no help in the early stage but an isotope bone scan will usually localize the increased blood flow to the metaphyseal region of the femur in osteomyelitis and to a much more diffuse region of the whole knee area in a septic arthritis.

Treatment

Antibiotics are administered, preferably intravenously, as soon as the blood culture sample has been taken. A combination is necessary and this should be a synthetic penicillin of a cloxacillin type (e.g. flucloxacillin) or alternatively fusidic acid (fucidin) to take care of the penicillin-resistant staphylococci. Ampicillin, a cephalosporin or some other antibiotic which is active against *Haemophilus influenzae* and the other Gram-negative organisms should be given. The antibiotic must be reviewed as soon as the first cultures are obtained from either the blood or synovial sample.

Aspiration of the joint must be undertaken under a general anaesthetic as soon as the child can be prepared. Decompression at the earliest stage is vital to preserve the articular cartilage from enzymatic attack due to bacterial infection within the synovial cavity. The synovial sample will reveal either frank pus or a very cloudy synovial fluid which should be

Gram stained as well as cultured and sent for sensitivities. Once bacterial infection is confirmed, the joint must be fully decompressed and irrigated, either by open operation or preferably by arthroscopic irrigation. The latter technique is ideal, allowing synovial crevasses, recesses and pockets to be washed out. Once this technique has been used the operator will realize how much more efficient this method is compared to even wide open inspection. Redivac drains must then be inserted and this is again very easy to perform through the arthroscope. Irrigation and drainage may then be undertaken using two Redivac tubes, and an antibiotic or a Noxyflex-type irrigation fluid is used. The joint should be splinted until it is more comfortable and all signs of infection have resolved. Slow return to weight bearing then occurs and the antibiotics should be administered for several weeks, certainly well beyond the time when the ESR returns to normal.

It is only by early and vigorous treatment along these lines that a destructive arthropathy is avoided. Chronic granulomatosis infection with tuberculosis is seen rarely and the diagnosis and treatment follow the same principles. The destructive effect is decreased by synovectomy and in some cases prolonged splintage and non-weight bearing are important. If the joint surface destruction is very severe a knee fusion will be necessary when the child is large enough and calliper control may be necessary in the interim period.

The irritable knee

The swollen, painful knee may be due to a major infection as described above or, more commonly, to a traumatic or transient synovitis. Traumatic synovitis occurs with a direct blow to the knee and is common in the normal active child. Direct injury causes an outpouring of synovial fluid from the traumatized synovial epithelium. In severe direct injuries haemarthroses may occur from synovial damage, but osteochondral fractures, cruciate ligament or capsular tears must be suspected if frank blood is aspirated from a very swollen, painful joint.

There are many other causes of a transient synovitis similar to those seen more commonly in the hip joint. The child may have an infection, such as rubella or mumps, producing a synovitis which develops before the overt stage of the disease. A monarticular synovitis may again develop without obvious cause, but frequently a history of recent infection of the upper respiratory tract or the gastrointestinal tract is given. In some children the monarticular synovitis may be the first sign of a specific arthropathy (juvenile chronic arthritis). In others there may be a mechanical internal derangement or patellar abnormality. The effusion may persist and the child will tend to limp and the quadriceps musculature will waste.

Full investigation to exclude all the specific diagnoses outlined above must be undertaken vigorously and appropriate treatment instituted. However, there still remains a group of children in whom a definite diagnosis cannot be made, and although some of these will turn out to be a pauciarticular type of rheumatoid arthritis, many continue with a persistent, slowly resolving synovitis or even recurrent synovitis. It is presumed that these are due to a viral infection, although this is never proved. Arthroscopy and synovial biopsy through the arthroscope are indicated whenever the synovitis persists. The discoid meniscus is frequently missed clinically but detected arthroscopically, and with the use of this instrument other pathologies may become evident.

It is important to rest the child's knee in the acute irritable stage, but when a chronic non-specific synovitis persists, normal activities and even quadriceps building exercises from a physiotherapist may be necessary to prevent muscle wasting. Further immobility may actually lead to more synovial effusion. There is a group of children, particularly young teenage girls, in whom traumatic or simple synovitis persists by producing an immobilization syndrome, sometimes voluntarily. Those children with emotional problems may then become 'knee cripples' and their treatment depends upon a combination of sympathetic but firm physiotherapy and psychotherapy.

Mechanical derangements

Table 1 lists the various abnormalities seen in 130 consecutive patients with a painful swollen knee who were reviewed at the 'problem knee clinics' set up at the Westminster Children's Hospital and the Hospital for Sick Children, Great Ormond Street, London. The most common derangements were found to be the unstable patella and osteochondritis dissecans.

Table 1 Abnormalities seen in the knees of 130 children (up to age 14).

Dislocating patella	50
Osteochondritis dissecans	38
Irritable knee	16
Meniscus	
Tears	3
Discoid	9
Cysts	3
Proven chondromalacia patellae	4
Others	7

The other internal derangements included the meniscus abnormalities, but of these the discoid lateral meniscus abnormality was the most common.

Symptoms

Although knee pain in the child is certainly a feature of knee pathology it may be caused by abnormalities in other areas, for example hip abnormalities, especially transient hip synovitis. Perthes' disease and slipped capital femoral epiphysis often produce pain which the child describes as being in the knee region. Thigh pain is rare in knee pathology but the knee symptoms may radiate inferiorly, particularly when the lateral compartment is involved. Swelling in the knee is obvious and especially so when the muscles are wasted above. A feeling of 'giving way' is usually described in the child who has instability due to patellar subluxation or due to movement of a loose body. A child complaining of locking must be carefully interrogated because surgical locking where there is a mechanical block to extension, is always indicative of a true internal derangement with a meniscal tear or loose body. A feeling of 'catching' as felt in osteochondritis dissecans or chondromalacia patellae is sometimes interpreted as locking. Stiffness of the joint may also be a parental synonym for locking. A loose body may be recognized by a child, and may be the source of some classroom amusement, as it acts like a 'joint mouse' popping in and out of various parts of the joint. Clicking of the joint may be described accurately and the classic loud snap of the discoid meniscus may be demonstrated by the child to the surgeon or to the amused party audience, for it is frequently painless and often very loud.

Examination

This is performed along the same lines as for the adult. However, a greater deal of ligament and joint laxity must be allowed for in the normal paediatric knee. The patella and its instability must be carefully assessed because this derangement is so common. The popliteal fossa must be carefully examined as a Baker's cyst may be found in this site.

Special investigations

Radiographic examination is as for the adult.

Arthrography

This has a place in the diagnosis of internal derangements and is also important in assessing the synovial cavity and its various abnormalities. A discoid meniscus and a torn meniscus may be diagnosed by arthrography, but as a general anaesthetic usually has to be given for this investigation in the young child, it is often thought preferable to view the joint through an arthroscope. The accuracy of arthrography in general radiological departments is in the region of 70%, and this figure may rise in very specialized units to 95%.[4]

Magnetic resonance imaging (MRI)

Magnetic resonance imaging is now playing an important role in the diagnosis of various internal derangements. It is important in the assessment of menisci and ligaments and, being totally non-invasive, it is taking over the diagnostic role which arthrography used to play. The accuracy is now very high but the same problems of diagnosis in the child's knee are present in MRI scanning as in arthrography since the child must remain very still for a relatively long time. As these scanning machines progress, they will be of increasing importance in the diagnosis of knee disorders.

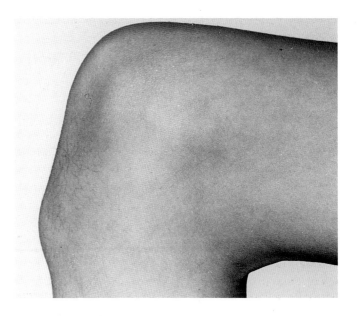

Figure 6

The tibial tubercle swelling in Osgood–Schlatter's disease.

Arthroscopy

This is now the most important and definitive of the diagnostic tools used in the child's knee. Before the introduction of the arthroscope the clinical accuracy of diagnosis of internal derangements, even in the easier adult, remained in the region of 70% and in the child very much lower.[5,6] The improved diagnostic accuracy when using the arthroscope is remarkable and in experienced hands approaches 100%.[7] The technique in children is exactly as for the adult. The child's lax joint makes inspection even easier than in most adult knees and derangements of the menisci and femoral condyles may be seen without problem.

Discoid lateral meniscus is fully reviewed in Chapter 12.

Osgood–Schlatter's disease

Avulsion of a minor flake from the bone at the tibial tubercle occurs in this condition, which particularly affects the vigorous young teenager. The male is more commonly affected but the athletic schoolgirl does not escape. The child complains of pain, tenderness and swelling at the insertion of the patellar tendon into the tibial tubercle. Exercise, especially kicking and jumping, aggravates the symptoms, which are most marked during and after activity. A direct blow or fall onto the swollen tubercle produces excessive pain. On clinical examination, the joint itself is normal but the tubercle is prominent and selectively tender. There may be a bursa at the tendon insertion

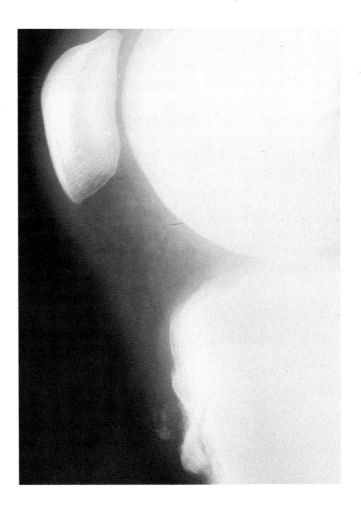

Figure 7

The avulsion flake in Osgood–Schlatter's disease.

and this produces a fluctuant mass which adds to the prominence of the tubercle (Figure 6).

The radiological appearance is that of an avulsion flake from the tibial tubercle, combined with reparative callus at this site (Figure 7). As the disease continues, the bony mass may enlarge and become quite ugly. There has been much discussion over the years of the aetiology of this condition, with an osteochondrosis being commonly implicated. There seems little doubt, however, that the problem is one of an avulsion flake fracture.

Treatment

In most children the symptoms settle spontaneously. For a period of time during the acute symptoms the avoidance of the heaviest sports activities should be recommended, but it seems excessive to immobilize the knee joint further. If the symptoms do persist for more than 18 months to 2 years, exploration may be advocated.

Removal of the avulsed fragment from within the tendon, removal of the associated bursa and drilling of the bone–tendon junction have all been advocated. The same results might have occurred if the child, the parents and the surgeons had waited for natural resolution of the pain. The prominence of the tibial tubercle, however, usually persists.

Larsen–Johansson syndrome

A similar avulsion flake with associated pain and tenderness may occur at the superior insertion of the patellar tendon to the lower pole of the patella. The symptoms are rather similar to those of Osgood–Schlatter's disease, with pain during and after exercise, and the disease particularly affects high-jumpers. There is selective tenderness at this site. The radiographic appearance is shown in Figure 8. Rest and controlled physical activity are all that are required in most cases but, in some children with chronic local pain, exploration and curettage of the bone fragments appear to be curative.

Osteochondritis dissecans is fully reviewed in Chapter 9.

Dislocation of the patella is described in Chapter 8.

Bursae around the knee

Every tendon at and around the knee has a potential bursa in relationship (Figure 9). The commoner cystic swellings in this region are described below.

Baker's cyst

Morrant Baker in the last century described a cystic mass in the popliteal fossa of children. The cyst is the constantly swollen bursa in relationship to the semimembranosus tendon and, although it arises from this medial hamstring, it usually presents as a central popliteal fossa mass. It is fluctuant and trans-illuminant, and it can reach moderately large proportions but rarely produces symptoms apart from the presence of a lump noted by the parent when the child's knee is fully extended. The majority of Baker's cysts appear spontaneously, often persisting for 1 or 2 years before resolution. Exploration and excision are advisable if the cyst rapidly increases in size or if there is any doubt whatsoever concerning the diagnosis. The differential diagnoses include enlarged popliteal lymph nodes, tumours attached to the popliteal nerve, soft-tissue sarcomas and a popliteal aneurysm. A cyst however, which is definitely fluctuant and trans-illuminant, is most likely to be this semimembranosus bursa of Baker and should be left alone.

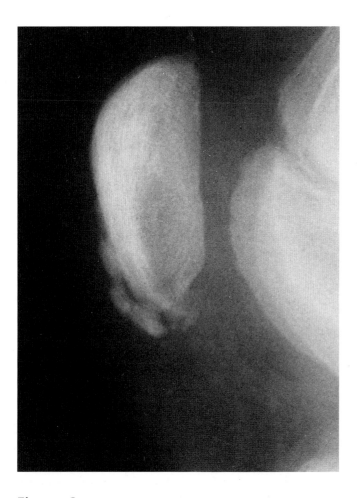

Figure 8

Larsen–Johansson syndrome.

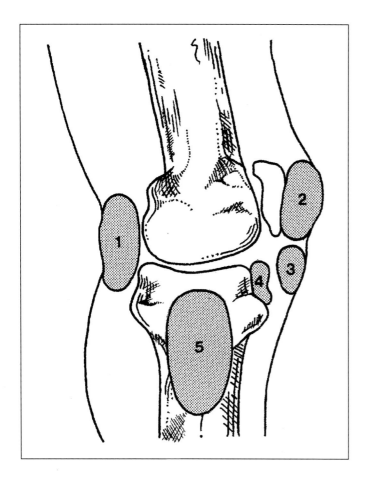

Figure 9

Bursae around the knee: (1) semimembranosus bursa; (2) prepatellar bursa; (3) infrapatellar bursa; (4) subpatellar tendon bursa; (5) subsartorial bursa.

The adult's knee sometimes presents with a similar semimembranosus bursa, but more commonly there is a mass of synovium or a knee joint synovial pouch which swells in the popliteal fossa owing to an associated knee effusion, synovitis or other pathology affecting the joint as a whole. This posterior synovial pouch may become large and may interfere with venous return from the leg. The posterior synovial cyst may also burst and leak synovial fluid into the popliteal fossa and into the calf musculature, producing a synovial 'pseudocyst'. Pain and swelling of the lesion may be mistaken for a sudden deep-vein thrombosis and many patients have been hospitalized and anticoagulated with this mistaken diagnosis.

Prepatellar bursa (housemaid's knee)

The normal bursal sac separating the anterior patella from skin and scanty subcutaneous tissue may become swollen owing to the constant irritation of kneeling or to a direct blow on the prominence of the patella. A fluctuant mass develops over the patella which may rapidly become inflamed and frequently secondarily infected. The portal of entry of bacteria may be a graze or laceration near the knee, infected eczema or athlete's foot more distally. Treatment of the inflamed bursa depends upon the prevention of further mechanical irritation, rest and anti-inflammatory medication. In the cellulitic infective stage antibiotics will be effective but pus rapidly forms and the large abscess which results will require incision and drainage.

Infrapatellar bursa (vicar's knee)

The bursal sac which is present superficial to the patellar tendon may be also inflamed by prolonged 'kneeling in prayer' position. The 'high-jumper's' lesion is a strain of the upper attachment of the patellar tendon to the bone of the inferior pole of the patella and this patellar tendonitis may be associated with an infrapatellar bursa. The treatment follows that outlined above.

Tibial tubercle bursa

The bursal sac becomes inflamed in association with Osgood–Schlatter's disease deep to the inferior attachment of the patellar tendon at the tibial tubercle. If Osgood–Schlatter's disease is treated surgically, it is important to look for this bursa and to remove it.

Subsartorial bursa (pes anserinus bursa)

This occurs over the medial upper tibia, well below the joint-line where it should not be confused with a meniscal cyst. The lump may become large and painful and may interfere with joint function. It is a swelling of the normal bursal sac in relationship to the insertion of sartorius, gracilis and semitendinosus tendons into the upper medial tibia. Its excision is usually necessary since it does produce increasing symptoms.

Biceps femoris bursa

A less common bursa may be found in relationship to the biceps tendon insertion into the fibular head. It may also be related to the tendon at a higher point in the lateral popliteal fossa. The bursa may be confused with a ganglion arising from the superior tibiofibular joint and both abnormalities usually require excision.

References

1. **Smillie IS**, *Osteochondritis dissecans* (Edinburgh: E & S Livingstone, 1960).
2. **Hnêkovský O**, Progressive fibrosis of the vastus intermedius muscle in children: a cause of limited knee flexion and elevation of the patella, *J Bone Joint Surg (Br)* (1961) **43**: 318–325.
3. **Green JP, Waugh W**, Congenital lateral dislocation of the patella, *J Bone Joint Surg (Br)* (1968) **50**: 285–289.
4. **Freiberger RH, Kaye JJ**, *Arthrography* (New York: Appleton-Century-Crofts, 1979).
5. **Zaman M, Leonard MA**, Meniscectomy in children, *J Bone Joint Surg (Br)* (1978) **60**: 436.
6. **Bedford A, Aichroth PM, Hutton P**, Arthroscopy – the first hundred are the worst, *J R Soc Med* (1979) **72**: 6.
7. **Jackson RW, Dandy DJ**, *Arthroscopy of the knee* (New York: Grune and Stratton, 1976).

11.2 Knock knee and bow leg in children

Andrew M. Jackson

Normal development

The normal child is bow-legged at birth and during infancy. Alignment corrects to neutral at the age of about 2 years before swinging to an exaggerated valgus angle at the beginning of the fourth year. Morley[1] noted that at this age 22% of the population have an intermalleolar interval in excess of 5 cm but by the age of 7 years less than 2% have a knock knee of this magnitude. Spontaneous correction is the rule (Figure 1).

To quantify these changes, Salenius and Vankka[2] in a radiological study found a mean value of 16° varus for the tibiofemoral angle in the newborn. By the age of 3 years this had shifted a remarkable 27° to a value of 11° valgus and by the age of 9 years the normal adult alignment had been realized. Whilst most bow legs correct, a few of the more severe examples will progress to true Blount's disease. Measurement of the upper tibial metaphysis/diaphysis angle of Levine and Drennan[3] defines the magnitude of the upper tibial deformity and its contribution to the total bowing as a whole. This measurement may help to predict the outcome, but in practice all children with obvious bowing require follow-up. The behaviour of the deformity becomes obvious with time. Measurement of the bow-leg interval, radiographs and clinical photographs are the parameters required to make good clinical records.

Clinical assessment of knee deformity

The bow-leg interval is defined as the distance between the medial femoral condyles when the medial malleoli are in contact and the knees are extended. The measurement is made with the patient lying supine, as is the intermalleolar interval of knock knee. The radiographs should be taken standing when possible and with the patellae pointing directly

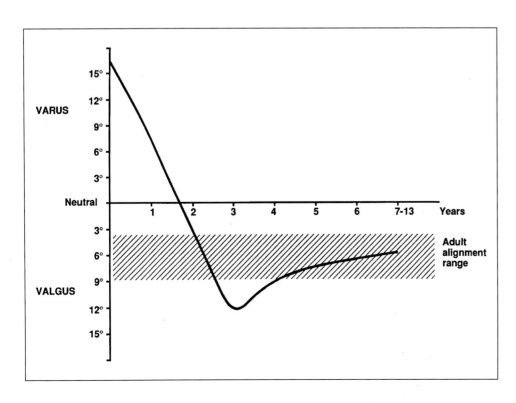

Figure 1

Graph constructed from the data of Salenius and Vankka,[2] to show the mean tibiofemoral angle in childhood in relation to age.

forwards. Medial beaking of the femoral and tibial metaphysis, tapering ossific nuclei and thickening of the medial tibial cortex are the usual radiological findings in physiological bow leg.

Physiological or pathological?

The predominance of anxious parents and physiological knee deformities in the clinic should not lull the surgeon into a false sense of security. In every case, the following five questions must be answered in order to exclude pathological deformity:

1. Is the child short or disproportioned? (Think of a bone dysplasia or endocrine disturbance.)

2. Is the deformity asymmetrical or unilateral? (Think of growth plate damage due to either trauma or infection.)

3. Is there a family history of severe knock knee or other bony abnormality? (Think of bone dysplasias, syndromes, or inherited varieties of renal rickets.)

4. Has a physiological deformity progressed to such a degree that it can no longer be regarded as a normal variant? (Blount's disease. Also a knock knee with an intermalleolar gap greater than 9 cm in the younger child or greater than 10 cm in the older child is cause for suspicion.)

5. Is the deformity opposite to that which is the usual physiological deformity at that age? (For example, a newborn with a knock knee deformity is abnormal.)

Blount's disease (tibia vara)

Blount described a growth disturbance of the medial aspect of the upper end of the tibia associated with a sharp angular varus deformity at this site combined with internal tibial torsion (Figure 2).[4]

The condition is rare, having an estimated incidence of 0.05 per 1000 live births, though this may vary a little from population to population.[5] The condition has been subdivided into two separate clinical entities by the age of onset, though in practice the distinction may not always be so clear-cut.

Infantile Blount's disease

It is often impossible to make the distinction between a severe physiological bow leg and Blount's disease when the child is first seen. If the deformity fails to improve by 2 or 3 years or increases, then Blount's disease must be suspected.

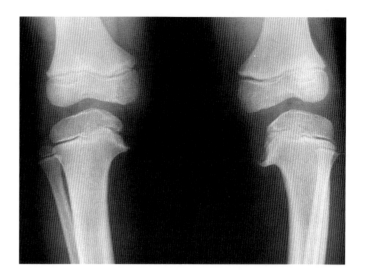

Figure 2

Blount's disease.

The cause is unknown, but there is evidence to suggest that early walking and excessive weight in a patient with physiological bow leg cause increased stress on the inner side of the upper tibia.[6] The normal resolution is prevented and a physiological deformity progresses to become a pathological condition. The first sign that this has occurred is the radiological appearance of fragmentation of the medial metaphyseal beak. This irregularity may appear at any time between the age of 18 months and 4 years and until it is seen the diagnosis of Blount's disease should not be made.

Once Blount's disease is established the prognosis is poor if it is left untreated. By the time adolescence is reached, pain on weight bearing, progressive deformity, and superimposed ligamentous instability can make walking unaided an impossibility, especially when the knee deformity is accompanied by extreme obesity. To some extent the medial femoral condyle may enlarge in order to compensate for the varus deformity and hypertrophy of the medial meniscus has also been described.

Treatment

The treatment of Blount's disease is difficult and unpredictable at any age and it is wise to warn the parents of the risk of recurrence and possible further surgical procedures. A sensible management policy depends on a number of factors; the age of the patient, the amount of growth remaining, the severity of the deformity and the presence of ligamentous laxity. Once a bone bridge is present, a simple corrective osteotomy stands no chance of achieving a lasting correction. Epiphysiodesis may be more acceptable in bilateral disease than in the unilateral case. The following guidelines may prove useful.

(a) The management of pre-Blount's disease is to watch and wait. Most of these deformities will resolve spontaneously. The role of splintage is unproven.

(b) Definite Blount's disease under the age of 8 years if left untreated is very likely to progress. To delay in treatment is a mistake. Langenskiöld has shown that an osteotomy of the tibia and fibula correcting the rotation as well as the varus into the normal physiological valgus will usually effect a cure.[7] If the varus deformity recurs, it is likely to be due to a missed medial bony bar. If such a bar is suspected on the plain radiographs, and perhaps in all children over 6 years old, biplanar tomography or CT scans of the growth plate should be performed.

(c) When there is a unilateral deformity with a bony bar and the child is under the age of 10 years, consider resection of the bone bridge combined with a corrective osteotomy. The bone bridge resection may be quite large. A dental burr may prove useful for the excavation. Various interposition materials including fat, silastic, bone cement and cranioplast have been used and each substance has its advocates. Fat is not haemostatic and may float away from the surface of the resection, leaving a space in which haematoma may organize and in which new bone may form. Fat also gives no support and a more solid material may be necessary if the excavation has been large. If this sort of method is attempted, the periosteum must be excised in order to lower the risk of recurrent bar formation.

(d) After the age of 9 or 10 years when there is a bone bridge and especially in bilateral cases, consider corrective osteotomy combined with epiphysiodesis in order to prevent further growth on the lateral aspect of the tibia and at the head of the fibula. Avoid epiphysiodesis in an already short extremity.

(e) In the late neglected case at or near skeletal maturity where considerable deformity may be complicated by collateral ligament instability, consider corrective osteotomy combined with elevation of the medial tibial plateau.[8] Lateral epiphysiodesis may also be necessary if there is still growth to come.

Adolescent Blount's disease

This condition is first noticed between the ages of 6 and 13 years and is due to a medial growth plate arrest of uncertain aetiology. Perhaps trauma or low-grade infection may be incriminated. The deformity is usually unilateral and less severe than infantile Blount's disease and patients may present with pain in the knee before the progressive varus is noticed. The radiological changes are less pronounced and there is no medial metaphyseal beak. Internal tibial torsion is unusual and shortening of about 2 cm may become apparent as growth proceeds towards maturity. Once diagnosed, the deformity progresses. Corrective osteotomy is probably the most reliable method of treatment.

Other forms of growth plate disturbance

The lower femoral growth plate is more susceptible to injury than that of the upper tibia. Whilst the Salter/Harris classification of epiphyseal injuries is in general a useful guide in forecasting any future growth disturbance, the lower femur is an unpredictable place.[9,10] Here it seems that growth disturbance may follow virtually any epiphyseal injury. The distal femoral growth plate has a large surface area and injury to it requires considerable force. The germinal layer may be damaged by crushing on the compression side of the injury, and this may not be obvious on the early radiographs. Furthermore, Ogden has pointed out that the undulating nature of the epiphysis may result in the line of shear passing through the germinal layer in certain places.[10] An osseous bridge and consequent deformity is therefore a common sequel to such injuries.

Infection is seen in its most severe form in the neonate when extensive damage to the growth plate occurs, followed by a disturbance of ossification of the epiphysis. Indeed, the early appearances may suggest extreme destruction of the epiphysis usually on the lateral side. However, the knee remains stable and an arthrogram will show the cartilaginous anlage intact and ultimately the whole epiphysis will ossify. Since 70% of the longitudinal growth of the femur occurs at its lower end, a growth arrest at this site will result in considerable shortening as well as deformity. It has been our practice to manage this situation with two or three corrective osteotomies performed over the years in order to keep up with growth. The final osteotomy may be combined with an epiphysiodesis on the growing side of the growth plate and femoral lengthening then being undertaken. In the future, application of the Ilizarov principle, which enables correction of deformity and lengthening to be undertaken at the same time, is likely to become more popular.

Bone dysplasias and syndromes

Knock-knee and bow-leg deformities in patients with bone dysplasias often need correction. Joint laxity may be severe and in the very wobbly knee the aim of surgery may be simply to make the knee 'brace-able', which is always a difficult problem in patients with short stocky legs. The valgus knee is difficult to control in a brace, whilst the problem with bracing a bow leg is that pressure is exerted over the head of the fibula.

As a rule the slight varus seen in the achondroplast does not seem to progress or to produce significant osteoarthritis in later life and it is therefore usually accepted. However, many other deformities are progressive, partly because the collateral ligaments stretch and partly because abnormal joint loading increases the bony deformity, especially at the later end of growth when the child is getting heavier. The decision to operate should be based on serial observations. If progressive deformity is corrected by early surgery, the parents should be warned that further osteotomies may be necessary as growth proceeds. We have observed the rapid return of deformity after surgery in Morquio's disease and the Ellis–Van Creveld syndrome, whilst in epiphyseal and metaphyseal dysplasias the correction may be well maintained. If one attempt at early correction fails, it is probably best to put off the final correction until near the time of skeletal maturity or as long as the deformity can be tolerated.

In bone dysplasias it is not uncommon for valgus deformity to be associated with patellar subluxation and even dislocation (Figure 3). The bony incongruity of the patellar and trochlear groove means that the bony anatomy contributes little to stability and the problem is compounded by joint laxity. These knees may require prolonged bracing postoperatively if a lasting improvement is to be achieved.

It is traditional to correct angular deformity in dwarfs by osteotomy, taking special care not to further shorten the leg. However, in some patients an impressive growth spurt can be induced by growth hormone, and against this background stapling may become a possible alternative. In syndromes such as diaphyseal aclasis or Beckwith's syndrome, where the patient is nearer normal height and the growth plates look normal, staples have proved a very effective means of achieving correction, providing they are correctly placed and substantial enough to do the job.

Dysplasia epiphysealis hemimelica is a rare condition which is worthy of mention (Figure 4). It was probably originally described by Mouchet and Belot in 1926, but in the United Kingdom it is known as 'Trevor's disease'. In children this disease can present at the knee as asymmetrical cartilaginous overgrowth of the epiphysis affecting either the medial or lateral side of the joint. The histology is indistinguishable from an osteocartilaginous exostosis and at maturity the appearance may be similar to an exostosis or the epiphysis may be simply enlarged and irregular. Malignant change has not been reported. The ankle and tarsal bones of the same limb should be scrutinized because they may also be involved. Boys are affected three times as commonly as girls.[11]

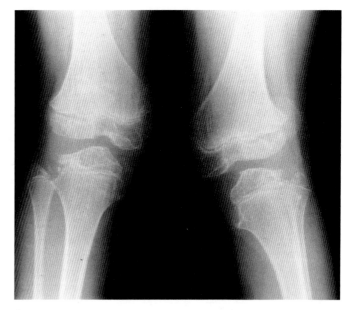

a

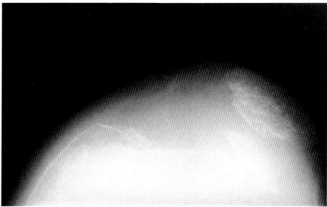

b

Figure 3

(a and b) Knock knee in multiple epiphyseal dysplasia complicated by lateral dislocation of the patella. A low femoral osteotomy to correct valgus and flexion deformity, together with quadriceps realignment, was required.

Swelling and deformity are the usual presenting features and there may be slight overgrowth or undergrowth of the affected limb. Deformity tends to progress with age and large lesions of the tibial epiphysis have been known to involve the meniscus.

The asymmetrical overgrowth of one side of the joint causes swelling and deformity. Bony prominences and exostoses can be excised, but not to such a degree as to render the joint unstable. Residual deformity may need to be corrected by osteotomy. It is wise to leave the surgery as long as possible because of the huge growth potential at the lower end of the

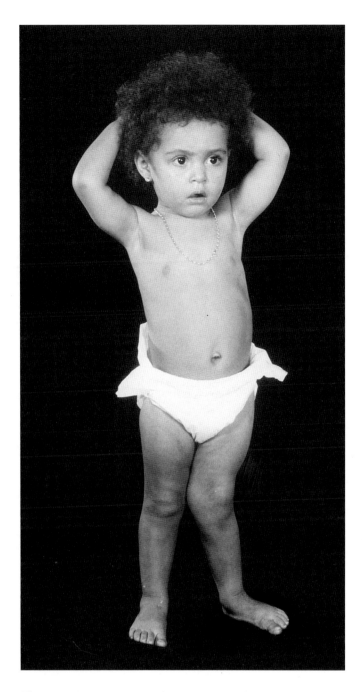

Figure 4

Dysplasia epiphysealis hemimelica. Note the unilateral deformity with swelling on the inner side of the knee.

Rickets

Rickets of any type typically presents as a bow leg rather than a knock knee and, appreciating this fact, many physicians tend to perform biochemical screening in all children with bow leg. Such screening is really only necessary if there are other clinical or radiological features of the disease; for example, if the diet is poor, if there is a family history of rickets or if the child is small and failing to thrive. The well-known clinical features are wrist and ankle swelling, the rib rosary and cranial bossing, whilst radiologically the epiphyses are widened and irregular and the metaphyses are 'cupped'. The lower limb deformity is not usually confined to the level of the knee joint, there being complex three-dimensional midshaft deformities often associated with Looser's zones and stress fractures (Figure 5). Anterior bowing of the tibia at the junction of the middle and lower thirds is very common. Metaphyseal dysplasia may have a similar radiological appearance to rickets but the biochemistry is normal.

No matter whether the cause of rickets be a dietary deficiency, malabsorption, or renal disease, the radiological appearances are the same. If the cause is nutritional, correction of the diet with supplements of vitamin D, calcium and phosphate will invariably be followed by correction of the deformity. In resistant rickets, delay in diagnosis and non-compliance of patients with therapy may lead to persistent deformity which will require surgical correction. Hypophosphataemic rickets is now the commonest type of the disease to present in our clinics. This condition is transmitted by autosomal dominant inheritance and is caused by a life-long leak of phosphate through the kidneys. Patients who require large doses of vitamin D may become seriously hypercalcaemic if suddenly immobilized. It is therefore, sensible to stop the vitamin D treatment a week or two before the proposed date for surgery.

Whilst there are always pressures to correct deformities on cosmetic grounds, the following guidelines for undertaking orthopaedic surgery in metabolic rickets have proved useful.[12]

1. The life expectancy should be good.
2. The deformity should be amenable to simple correction.
3. Some means of controlling the disease metabolically should be available.
4. The patient's intelligence should be normal and motivation good.
5. The deformity should be symptomatic.

In our experience, delay in union has not been a problem.

As well as knee deformity, some of these patients develop chondral separations from the articular surface of the femoral condyles and present with the

femur and the risk of superimposing an iatrogenic growth disturbance on an already difficult condition.

Sadly, severe knee deformities are occasionally encountered in children with conditions such as glycogen storage disease and hypophosphatasia, where the overall prognosis is poor. Surgery in these cases is of course contraindicated.

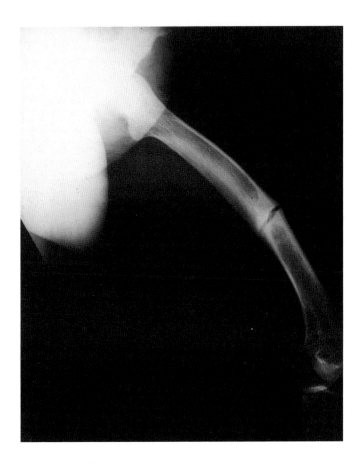

Figure 5

Looser's zone in the mid-femoral shaft of a young adult with hypophosphataemic rickets. This appearance may persist for months without proceeding to fracture.

symptoms of loose bodies within the joint, though these cannot be seen radiologically.

Trauma

There is one particular fracture of the knee that requires special mention in the context of knee deformity and that is the incomplete fracture of the proximal tibial metaphyses which is usually seen in the younger child. The fracture line is incomplete, extending laterally from the medial aspect of the upper tibia. The injury results from a valgus force and the fibula escapes intact.

Clearly, the aim of treatment is to correct the deformity and hold the position in a cast for 6 weeks until union is assured. There may, however, be difficulty in maintaining the reduction because the distal fragment has a tendency to spring back to valgus deformity. This is in part due to the greenstick component at the lateral cortex, but sometimes the periosteum becomes interned at the fracture site.

Whether the greenstick is completed or whether interned periosteum is cleared from the fracture site, the surgeon must employ a 'no-hands' technique after the manipulation to ensure that the tibia does not spring back into deformity.

Once an adequate reduction is ensured, a further problem may lie in store. The valgus deformity sometimes recurs once union is complete owing to accelerated growth at the medial side of the physis. This delayed-action deformity phenomenon may perhaps be triggered off by the release of periosteal tension or by the asymmetry of the fracture and its vascular response. The tethering effect of an intact fibula and the iliotibial band have also been incriminated. The recurrence of deformity occurs within a matter of weeks from removal of the cast and then tends to stabilize. A period of observation is advised since this deformity may correct slowly over the following 2 or 3 years (Figure 6). If it does not, a corrective osteotomy will be needed. When faced with this fracture the parents are best forewarned of what might transpire.

Miscellaneous deformities

Significant knock-knee deformity requiring treatment is sometimes seen in heavy patients with paralytic conditions such as meningomyelocoele, juvenile rheumatoid arthritis and endocrine diseases. In patients with polio who walk with the leg in external rotation for stability, the valgus deformity noted clinically and on standing radiographs may be due in part to laxity of the medial ligament. Although this looks impressive, it is seldom painful and does not progress once skeletal maturity has been achieved.

In the rare condition of neuropathic osteonecrosis of the lateral femoral condyle, collapse of the condyle will result in valgus deformity and osteotomy may help to place more load on the intact medial compartment.[13] However, with the passage of time these knees may become so disorganized that they require arthrodesis.

Congenital short femur is frequently associated with retroversion of the hip and a valgus deformity at the knee. The patella may be small and subluxing laterally, in which case it is safest to correct the valgus knee deformity before embarking on any leg lengthening procedure. In patients with congenital short tibia, knee deformity is less common but there is often evidence of ligamentous laxity, especially in the anteroposterior plane.[14]

Recently attention has been drawn to the condition of focal fibrocartilaginous dysplasia.[15,16] At first sight, the deformity looks similar to Blount's disease but the radiograph is quite distinct. The lesion is on the medial aspect of the upper tibia and produces a kinked appearance. The histology shows fibrocarti-

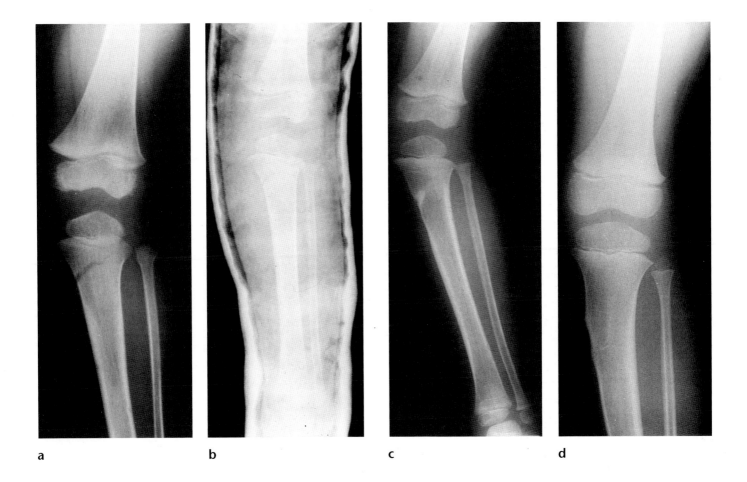

a   b   c   d

Figure 6

(a) Metaphyseal fracture of childhood. (b) Straightened and held in a cast. (c) Delayed-action valgus deformity at 9 months. (d) Correcting with no treatment after 2½ years.

laginous tissue with dense fibrous tissue at the margins. Conservative treatment is recommended in the first instance since the deformity tends to correct on its own accord.

The choice of osteotomy and possible complications

Choosing the level of osteotomy

Logic would dictate that a corrective osteotomy should be performed at the site of the deformity, but there are other considerations. The gross clinical appearance obviously reflects the underlying bony deformity but on occasion it belies the complexity of the situation. When two or more deformities are present, if similar they may combine with one another, whilst opposite deformities will tend to compensate or cancel each other out. Also, it is important to understand the effect of the knee deformity on the hip and ankle and to predict the effect of corrective osteotomy at these levels. Bear in mind that if the ankle is tipped into varus by a knee osteotomy, this will be poorly tolerated. For these reasons full-length scanograms are essential and standing or stress films will ensure that any ligamentous laxity is also taken into account.

The choice between proximal tibial or supracondylar osteotomy depends very much on which operations will make the knee joint horizontal. Again, the scanogram will help. In the younger patient and when ossification is not sufficiently advanced, an arthrogram or MRI scan can be most helpful in defining the joint-line. Clinical examination of the hip and ankle is also important; for example, in severe bow leg, the patient stands with the hips abducted; before correcting the knee deformity it is as well to make sure the hips will adduct to neutral or the patient will be walking on a very broad-based gait.

Soft-tissue release of the hips may be required as a supplement to correction of the knee.

Remember that the proximity of the tibial tubercle is a 'no-go' area for osteotomy in the immature skeleton. Physeal damage will result in tibia recurvatum. Care must also be exercised when doing a high fibular osteotomy, and perhaps the risks to the common peroneal nerve do not justify this level as the routine site for fibular division.

Choosing the type of osteotomy

If a bent bone is straightened, its length will be increased, as will the length of the limb as a whole. The amount of increase in the length of the extremity depends on the site and magnitude of the deformity corrected, the distance at which the osteotomy is performed from the site of maximum deformity and the femoral neck offset effect. In severe bow leg, the apparent femoral length is increased if its vertical alignment is corrected by a tibial osteotomy. It is probably easier and more accurate to predict the change in limb length from tracings rather than calculations should this be considered necessary.

In addition, the type of osteotomy can also influence the outcome. Canale and Harper showed that the absolute amount of length gained by a closing or opening wedge osteotomy is estimated at one-half the base of the osteotomy wedge.[17] The closing wedge is well tried and has inherent stability, especially if one cortex is left intact. Whilst one may wish to gain a little length with an opening wedge, stability is lost and early satisfaction with the postoperative radiograph can fade into disappointment as the graft site collapses down and deformity recurs. If an opening wedge is to be attempted then a small length of fibula placed on its side is probably the strongest and most convenient graft to keep the osteotomy open.

The dome osteotomy fashioned by making multiple drill holes and joining them with a small osteotome is stable and does not of itself significantly alter the limb length. A modified Hohman's osteotomy applied to the tibia is stable and allows some side-to-side displacement of the proximal on distal fragments.

More recently, the proponents of external fixation have described various methods of correcting angular deformity. The frame can simply be used as a fixation device following osteotomy and this is most suited to tibial osteotomy in the growing child.

In an alternative technique, a gradual and asymmetrical distraction force can be applied once callus has started to form. This technique is similar to that employed in leg lengthening and indeed makes an appropriate entrée to a leg lengthening if angular deformity is combined with a leg length discrepancy. The great advantage of the external fixator is that it allows the limb to be observed throughout the healing period and the position can be fine-tuned by minor adjustments to the apparatus. An all-round frame gives greater stability than a unilateral bar fixator.

Complex bony deformities affecting both the femur and the tibia are encountered most frequently in osteogenesis imperfecta and hypophosphataemic rickets. Shaft deformities are best treated by multiple osteotomy and intramedullary nailing using a kebab technique. Not only does the intramedullary rod hold the position while the osteotomy joins but subsequently it reinforces the bone, which is inherently weak. Penetration of the epiphyseal plate by relatively small-diameter rods does not seem to disturb growth and the commonest problem has proved to be the bone growing off the nail, with subsequent recurrence of deformity. Re-nailing may perhaps be required three or four times during growth in patients with severe osteogenesis imperfecta. The advent of the telescopic intramedullary rod has dramatically reduced the frequency of re-rodding procedures, but these rods are more difficult to insert and are not without their own special problems (Figure 7).

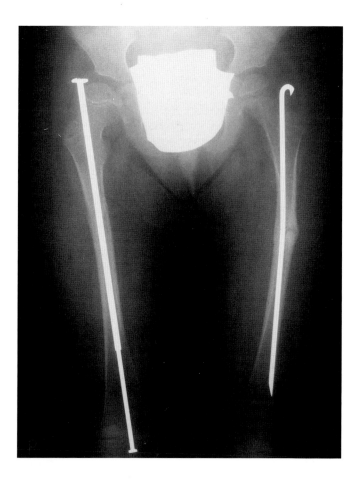

Figure 7

Osteogenesis imperfecta, showing the advantage of the telescoping nail reducing the number of 'nailings' required during growth. Initially the rod in the left femur did not prevent a minor fracture.

Complications of osteotomy

(1) Malunion occurs because of failure to hold the corrected position until union is secure or because a spurious correction was accepted postoperatively in the plaster cast. Percutaneous pins in the tibia on either side of the osteotomy have the advantage of added stability when incorporated in a cast, and they also ensure that bone is corrected on bone and that a false correction has not been achieved in the presence of collateral ligament laxity at the knee. It is a short step from percutaneous pins incorporated in the cast, which was common practice some years ago, to the adoption of a more solid external fixator in the controlling of childhood osteotomies, and this is often the method of choice. Remember that smaller bones demand smaller-diameter pins if fractures through the pin holes are to be avoided.

(2) Recurrence of deformity after union is achieved may occur because an osseous bone bridge had not been recognized on the preoperative films. Deformity may also recur in uncontrolled rickets and osteogenesis imperfecta.

(3) Non-union is very rare but should be anticipated, for example, when growth plate damage and deformity are the result of high-dose radiotherapy, and osteotomy is required through poorly vascularized bone.

(4) Two types of vascular complications have been recorded following tibial osteotomy. First, there is the anterior compartment syndrome and an awareness of this should lead to its early detection when it occurs postoperatively. The diagnosis has been made easier now that there are simple techniques for measuring intracompartmental pressure at the bedside. Better still, a prophylactic fasciotomy adds little to the procedure especially if an incision has already been made over the anterior compartment. Gibson has shown the importance of a vacuum drain in lowering the intracompartmental pressure postoperatively.[18] Backslabs are safer than a complete plaster and dorsiflexing the foot further reduces the risk of raised intracompartmental pressure. The use of an external fixator rather than plaster allows closer observation. Current enthusiasm by anaesthetists for regional and caudal blocks in the relief of postoperative pain risks removing some of the important signs and symptoms of impending disaster. If these techniques are used, we must be especially vigilant.

Second, there is acute vascular occlusion which should very rapidly become obvious once the tourniquet is released. This potential disaster may simply be due to kinking of a major vessel as a result of angular rotational correction at the osteotomy site. Should this complication occur, the limb should be returned to the pre-osteotomy position immediately. If the peripheral circulation is not rapidly restored after this manoeuvre, an arteriogram will be necessary. With this sort of complication in mind, it is obviously unwise to use any kind of cumbersome internal fixation and the adjustability of the external fixator may prove a very positive advantage. The circulation should always be checked upon release of the tourniquet.

(5) Mention has already been made of the risk to the common peroneal nerve when high fibular osteotomy is performed. Less well recognized is the risk of stretching the same nerve when employing a supracondylar osteotomy to correct a severe valgus deformity at the knee, and especially if the knee is maintained in extension in the postoperative period. Rarely, a tardy common peroneal nerve palsy may come on 2 or 3 days after tibial osteotomy. The exact cause of this is obscure and recovery is the rule.

(6) If the length of a bone is increased when it is straightened, it follows that the soft tissues will be relatively shortened and a soft tissue 'contracture' may be created. For example, the posterior compartment muscles of the tibia are often found to be tight when multiple osteotomies are used to correct a predominantly anterior bowing deformity in rickets or osteogenesis imperfecta. Either a segment of bone must be excised at one of the osteotomy sites, or the toe flexors and even the heel cord may need to be lengthened.

Acknowledgment

Parts of this chapter, including Figure 1, are reproduced from Jackson AM, 'Knock knee and bow leg', *Current Orthop* (1990) 4: 47–58 by kind permission of the Editor.

References

1. **Morley M**, Knock knee in children, *Br Med J* (1957) **2**: 976.
2. **Salenius P, Vankka E**, The development of the tibio-femoral angle in children, *J Bone Joint Surg (Am)* (1975) **57**: 259–261.
3. **Levine AM, Drennan JC**, Physiological bowing and tibia vara: The metaphyseal–diaphyseal angle in the measurement of bowleg deformities, *J Bone Joint Surg (Am)* (1982) **64**: 1158–1163.
4. **Blount WP**, Tibia vara: Osteochondrosis deformans tibiae, *J Bone Joint Surg* (1937) **19**: 1–29.
5. **Zayer M**, *Natural history of osteochondrosis tibiae*, ed Louis CWK (Gleerup, 1973) 25.
6. **Bateson EM**, The relationship between Blount's disease and bow legs, *Br J Radiol* (1968) **41**: 107–114.
7. **Langenskiöld A**, Tibia vara: Osteochondrosis deformans tibiae, *Clin Orthop* (1981) **158**: 77–82.
8. **Siffert RS**, Intraepiphyseal osteotomy for progressive tibia vara: case report and rationale of management, *J Paediatr Orthop* (1982) **2**: 81–85.
9. **Salter RB, Harris WR**, Injuries involving the epiphyseal plate, *J Bone Joint Surg (Am)* (1963) **45**: 587–622.
10. **Ogden JA**, *Skeletal injury in the child* (Philadelphia: Lea and Febiger, 1982).
11. **Kettelkamp DB, Campbell CJ, Bonfiglio M**, Dysplasia epiphysealis hemimelica: a report of fifteen cases and a review of the literature, *J Bone Joint Surg (Am)* (1966) **48**: 746–766.

12. **Cattell HS, Levin S, Kopits S et al.**, Reconstructive surgery in children with azotemic osteodystrophy, *J Bone Joint Surg (Am)* (1971) **53**: 216–228.

13. **Citron ND, Paterson FWN, Jackson AM**, Neuropathic osteonecrosis of the lateral femoral condyle in childhood, *J Bone Joint Surg (Br)* (1986) **68**: 96–99.

14. **Thomas NP, Jackson AM, Aichroth PM**, Congenital absence of the anterior cruciate ligament: a common component of knee dysplasia, *J Bone Joint Surg (Br)* (1985) **67**: 572–575.

15. **Bell SN, Campbell PE, Cole WG et al.**, Tibia vara caused by focal fibrocartilagenous dysplasia, *J Bone Joint Surg (Br)* (1985) **67**: 780–784.

16. **Bradish CF, Davies SJM, Malone M**, Tibia vara due to focal fibrocartilaginous dysplasia: the natural history, *J Bone Joint Surg (Br)* (1988) **70**: 106–108.

17. **Canale ST, Harper MC**, Biotrigonometric analysis as practical applications of osteotomies of tibia in children, *Instructional course lectures, AAOS* (St Louis: CV Mosby, 1981) **30**: 85–101.

18. **Gibson MJ, Barnes MR, Allen MJ et al.**, Weakness of foot dorsiflexion and changes in compartment pressures after tibial osteotomy, *J Bone Joint Surg (Br)* (1986) **68**: 471–475.

11.3   Congenital dislocation of the knee

Barry D. Ferris

Incidence

Congenital dislocation of the knee is said by Shattock to have been first described by Chatelaine in 1822.[1] It is a rare condition; the incidence is variously reported as 0.017 per 1000 live births[2] or about 1 per 100 000 live births.[3] It is said to be between 40 times[4,5] and 84 times[5] rarer than congenital hip dislocations. Thus, although there have been many publications, most have been case reports and there are only a small number of series.

Heredity, race and sex

Most cases are sporadic. There are a number of reviews that have detected a familial tendency. Provenzano[6] found seven families with a positive history in his review of 200 cases. McFarlane[7] reported a family in which a mother and her three children were all affected; however, each child had a different father! There have been case reports of the condition occurring in twins[8] but most series do not report a family history.[9–12] Curtis and Fisher[13] described a very rare form of congenital knee dislocation in five patients with anterior subluxation of the tibia on the femur in extension (see below) that occurred in families. They suggested that this was inherited and coined the term heritable congenital tibiofemoral subluxation. Ferris and Jackson[14] reported a further four patients with this condition in which no family history was evident. Although rare in Caucasians, congenital dislocation of the knee is said to occur more commonly in African communities,[15] but hyperextension of the knee is so common that it is not worth reporting.[16]

The condition seems to be more prevalent in girls. Provenzano[6] found a male-to-female ratio of 1:1 and Katz et al.[17] found a ratio of 1:8, but most reviewers have found a ratio of about 1:3.5.[4,9,10,12,16]

Classification

Congenital dislocation of the knee encompasses a spectrum of pathology ranging from simple genu recurvatum to full-blown dislocation of the tibiofemoral joint. Finder[18] identified five different types; however, Laurence[16] modified this to three types and this seems to be the most widely accepted classification. He distinguished congenital recurvatum, subluxation and dislocation (Figure 1). In the first, the knee merely hyperextends with no disruption of the joint (Figure 2). Subluxation and dislocation are self-explanatory in that hyperextension of the knee is associated with anterior subluxation or dislocation of the tibia on the femur (Figure 3). This is often associated with increasing difficulty in flexing the knee. Nogi and MacEwen[12] have observed that it may be difficult to distinguish congenital dislocation of the knee from that of subluxation. Bell et al.[11] suggested that, although widely used, this classification did not give any indication of the likely response of the condition to treatment – an observation that is similar to the author's experience.[9]

There does, however, exist a very rare form of congenital knee dislocation in which hyperextension of the knee is not a feature. In this condition, the tibia subluxes anteriorly on the femur in extension and reduces with a 'clunk' at roughly 30° flexion (Figure 4). Sixteen knees in nine patients have been described by two centres[13,14] and the term habitual anterior subluxation of the tibia in extension has been suggested.[14] The feature of this is that, although initially it is possible to reduce the subluxation passively, as time progresses the subluxation becomes fixed.

The diagnosis of congenital dislocation of the knee is usually obvious at birth as hyperextension is the main feature, although it may be overshadowed by other more pressing associated anomalies (see below). Indeed, there has been a report of a prenatal diagnosis made on an abdominal radiograph taken for other reasons.[19]

Associated conditions

Carlson and O'Connor[20] identified three different types of patients: those with an isolated dislocation,

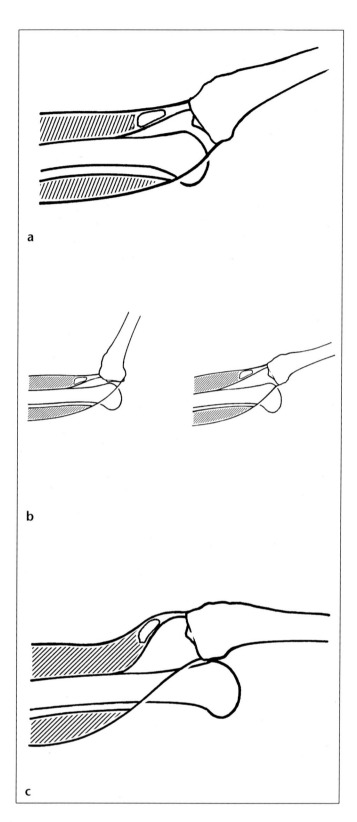

Figure 1

Classification of congenital dislocation of the knee as described by Laurence.[16] (a) Hyperextension – knee hyperextends more than 15° but fully flexes; (b) subluxation – knee hyperextends more than 15°. There is some restriction of flexion or the knee feels unstable; (c) dislocation – the knee is unstable and extension/flexion are variable. Reproduced by permission of the author and the British Editorial Society of Bone and Joint Surgery.

multiple dislocations, and syndromes. The latter two, they felt, were more resistant to conservative treatment. This was certainly the author's experience.

Conditions that are commonly associated with congenital knee dislocation include congenital hip dislocation,[9–11,17] club foot,[1,9,10,17] arthrogryposis[10,11] and Larsen's syndrome.[9] Rarer associated conditions include dislocated elbows[10,15,17] and coxa valga,[15] dislocated radial heads,[21] digital anomalies,[9,10] achondroplasia,[9] Streeter's syndrome,[10] dislocated ulnae,[10] vertical talus[10] and Down's syndrome.[11]

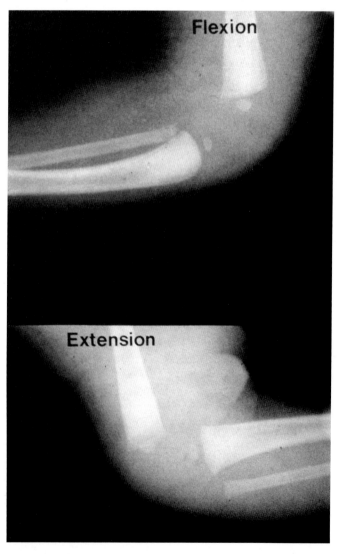

Figure 2

Radiograph of congenital hyperextension of the knee demonstrating the range of movement possible.

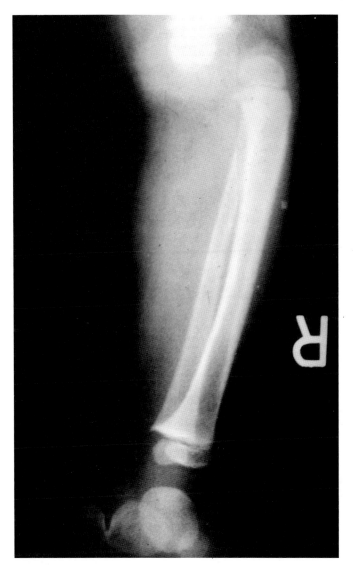

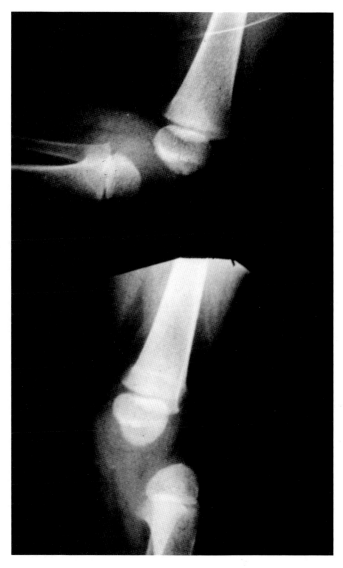

Figure 3

Radiograph of congenital dislocation of the knee demonstrating the tibia anterior to the femur. The knee is fully flexed and required surgery.

Figure 4

Radiographs of habitual anterior subluxation of the tibia in extension. The tibia is subluxed anteriorly on the femur in the extended position but reduced in flexion.

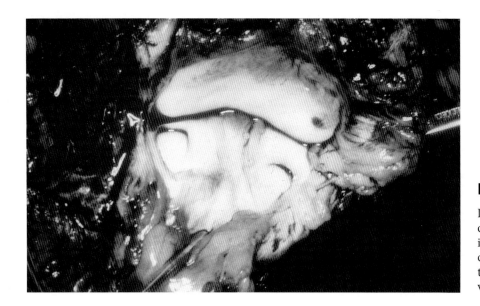

Figure 5

Peroperative photograph of a congenital knee dislocation. The femur is superior, the quadriceps has been divided and turned down. The broad, thick anterior cruciate ligament is visible.

Pathology

Birth trauma was suggested by Mauclaire as a cause of congenital knee dislocation; however, this has never been seriously considered as it has been shown that in the fetus, displacement of the distal femoral epiphysis will occur before the knee is disrupted.[17] Fetal moulding due to oligohydramnios or extended breech position was suggested by Shattock[1] and supported by Niebauer and King.[5] Certainly Johnson et al.[10] found a 41% incidence of breech presentation in their series, but although a contributory factor this could not account for most of the dislocations.

Abnormality of the anterior cruciate ligament was suggested by Katz et al.[17] as the cause of congenital knee dislocation. This was based on their findings at operation of an attenuated hypoplastic anterior cruciate ligament. However, Laurence[16] demonstrated that no single ligamentous abnormality could give rise to the condition. Curtis and Fisher[4] and most other authors believe the cruciate ligament abnormality to be a secondary feature. Middleton[22] emphasized the fibrosis seen in the quadriceps muscle and considered a quadriceps contracture to be the cause of congenital knee dislocation. Certainly most authors agree with this, because, at operation, fibrosis of the quadriceps is usually seen particularly in its distal part.[4,9–11,15,16,21,23,24]

Although this could explain the surgical findings on the basis of mechanics, the aetiology of the quadriceps fibrosis remains obscure. A suggestion has been made that it could be due to intrauterine ischaemia (analogous to the process found in the sternomastoid) but there is no evidence for this.[9]

Anatomically there is shortening of quadriceps with fibrosis. The tibia is subluxed or dislocated anteriorly on the femur, and the anterior cruciate ligament is usually broadened and flattened (Figure 5). These are the constant findings. Depending on the degree of subluxation or dislocation, the hamstrings and the iliotibial band may be subluxed anteriorly, which may then act as extensors of the knee thus perpetuating the deformity.

A variable finding is obliteration of the suprapatellar pouch, which may indicate a more resistant deformity.[16]

Treatment

Congenital hyperextension of the knee does not require treatment. There is no doubt that untreated congenital dislocations and subluxations result in poorly functioning stiff painful knees.[9,10] As long ago as 1913, Mayer[23] recognized that if conservative treatment was started early, good results may be obtained. For a good result from conservative management, treatment should have commenced before 3 months of age.[9,21,23] However, if it is started as late as 6 months the chances of a good result fall to 33%.[21] Laurence[16] recommended an arthrogram by 2 months of age if conservative treatment had not succeeded in increasing the range of flexion or reducing the dislocation. If no suprapatellar pouch could be demonstrated, he considered that the prognosis was poor and that surgery should be undertaken. Some series have reported using arthrography occasionally,[10] but other authors have not found arthrography to be particularly useful.[4,9]

Conservative management

Classical conservative management of congenital dislocation of the knee consists of a combination of traction, manipulation and serial (weekly) splintage[9,16,21,23] in order to flex the knee with the dislocation or subluxation reduced. Curtis and Fisher[4] found that all patients who required surgery were unable to flex their knees beyond 35° despite conservative management.

There have been a number of recent reports of the successful use of the Pavlik harness in managing congenital knee dislocation.[12,25] The advantage of this is that the commonly associated ipsilateral congenital hip dislocation may be treated at the same time.

Surgical management

Patients who require surgery have usually presented at later than 6 months or may have a syndrome of which congenital dislocation is a part and thus fall into the 'recalcitrant' group described by Laurence.[16] There may be restriction of flexion[4] or obliteration of the suprapatellar pouch.[10,16] Surgery may give good results if undertaken as late as 2 years of age.[4,9,21,23] Surgery is usually through a midline incision. A fibrotic quadriceps is usually found, but the suprapatellar pouch may or may not be obliterated. An abnormality of the anterior cruciate ligament is common, which is usually broad and thick (Figure 5). The medial hamstrings may be dislocated, as may be the iliotibial band. The essential abnormality is the quadriceps fibrosis with a contracture, thus requiring the quadriceps to be lengthened. This may be done as an inverted V–Y-plasty in the distal part as recommended by Curtis and Fisher[4] or by a Z-plasty of the quadriceps. The former operation is usually performed. Additional length may be achieved by proximal division of the rectus femoris and mobilization of the quadriceps off the femur prior to the V–Y-plasty.[11]

In order to achieve reduction, the iliotibial band may have to be divided and reconstituted with or without lengthening, as may the medial hamstrings. Occasionally the anterior cruciate ligament may require advancement.[10,17] Certainly it should not be divided, as this will result in early degenerative change in the knee.[9] The knee is splinted in flexion prior to mobilization.

The conservative treatment of habitual anterior subluxation of the knee in extension is unsuccessful. Surgery partially relieved the phenomenon using an extra-articular tenodesis from the iliotibial band as in the MacIntosh procedure for anterolateral rotatory instability.[14] Division of the biceps femoris tendon has been reported as being successful in controlling this condition.[13]

References

1. **Shattock SG**, Genu recurvatum in a foetus at term, *Trans Pathol Soc Lond* (1891) **42**: 280–292.
2. **Jacobsen K, Vopalecky F**, Congenital dislocation of the knee, *Acta Orthop Scand* (1985) **56**: 1–7.
3. **Kopits E**, Beiträge zur Pathologie und Therapie den angeborenen Kniegelenkssubluxationen, *Arch Orthop Unfall Chir* (1925) **23**: 593–609.
4. **Curtis BH, Fisher RL**, Congenital hyperextension with anterior subluxation of the knee: surgical treatment and long-term observations, *J Bone Joint Surg (Am)* (1969) **51**: 255–269.
5. **Niebauer JJ, King DE**, Congenital dislocation of the knee, *J Bone Joint Surg (Am)* (1960) **42**: 207–225.
6. **Provenzano RW**, Congenital dislocation of the knee. Report of a case, *N Engl J Med* (1947) **236**: 360–362.
7. **McFarlane AL**, A report on four cases of congenital genu recurvatum occurring in one family, *Br J Surg* (1947) **34**: 388–391.
8. **Dungy CI, Leuppe M**, Congenital hyperextension of the knees in twins, *Clin Pediatr (Phila)* (1984) **23**(3): 169–172.
9. **Ferris B, Aichroth P**, The treatment of congenital knee dislocation: a review of nineteen knees, *Clin Orthop* (1987) **216**: 135–140.
10. **Johnson E, Audell R, Oppenheim WL**, Congenital dislocation of the knee, *J Paediatr Orthop* (1987) **7**(2): 194–200.
11. **Bell MJ, Atkins RM, Sharrard WJW**, Irreducible congenital dislocation of the knee: aetiology and management, *J Bone Joint Surg (Br)* (1987) **69**: 403–406.
12. **Nogi J, MacEwen GD**, Congenital dislocation of the knee, *J Paediatr Orthop* (1982) **2**: 509–513.
13. **Curtis BH, Fisher RL**, Heritable congenital tibiofemoral subluxation: clinical features and surgical treatment, *J Bone Joint Surg (Am)* (1970) **52**: 1104–1114.
14. **Ferris BD, Jackson AM**, Congenital snapping knee. Habitual anterior subluxation of the tibia in extension, *J Bone Joint Surg (Br)* (1990) **72**: 453–456.
15. **Ahmadi B, Shahriaree H, Silver CM**, Severe congenital genu recurvatum, *J Bone Joint Surg (Am)* (1979) **61**: 622–624.
16. **Laurence M**, Genu recurvatum congenitum, *J Bone Joint Surg (Br)* (1967) **49**: 121–134.
17. **Katz MP, Grogono BJS, Soper KC**, The etiology and treatment of congenital dislocation of the knee, *J Bone Joint Surg (Br)* (1967) **49**: 112–120.
18. **Finder JG**, Congenital hyperextension of the knee, *J Bone Joint Surg (Br)* (1964) **46**: 783.
19. **Lage J de A, Guarniero R, de Barros TEP et al.**, Intrauterine diagnosis of congenital dislocation of the knee, *J Paediatr Orthop* (1986) **6**(1): 110–111.
20. **Carlson DH, O'Connor J**, Congenital dislocation of the knee, *Am J Roentgenol* (1976) **127**: 465–468.
21. **Stern MB**, Congenital dislocation of the knee, *Clin Orthop Rel Res* (1968) **61**: 261–268.
22. **Middleton DS**, The pathology of congenital genu recurvatum, *Br J Surg* (1935) **22**: 696–702.
23. **Mayer L**, Congenital anterior subluxation of the knee: description of a new specimen, summary of the pathology of the deformity and discussion of its treatment, *Am J Orthop Surg* (1913) **10**: 411–437.
24. **Gilbert RJ, Larsen LJ, Ashley K et al.**, Open reduction with patellar tendon elongation for congenital dislocation of the knee, *J Bone Joint Surg (Am)* (1975) **57**: 133.
25. **Iwaya T, Sakaguchi R, Tsuyama N**, The treatment of congenital dislocation of the knee with the Pavlik harness, *Int Orthop* (1983) **7**: 25–30.

Congenital discoid lateral meniscus in children

12.1 Congenital discoid lateral meniscus in children: An overview and current clinical perspectives

Paul M. Aichroth and Dipak V. Patel

The intermittent and vague symptoms caused by the presence of a discoid meniscus may produce difficulty and delay in the clinical diagnosis. Young,[1] in 1889, first described a discoid lateral meniscus in a cadaver specimen, but the term 'snapping-knee syndrome' was attributed to this anomaly by Kroiss (1910).[2] Since then, there have been numerous reports on the discoid lateral meniscus and its associated clinical syndrome.[3–26]

Incidence

Various authors[5,17,27–30] have reported the incidence of the lesion to be between 1.4% and 15.5%, with Ikeuchi[13] reporting a 16.6% incidence in the Japanese population. However, it should be noted that Ikeuchi studied a preselected group of patients having knee symptoms. Studies based on evaluation of a large group of cadaver knees are more accurate and have shown the incidence to be 5%.[31]

Smillie[21] reported on 29 discoid menisci in 1300 meniscectomies, an incidence of 2.2%. Later, in 1970, he reported a 4.7% incidence of discoid menisci in a group of approximately 10 000 meniscectomy patients.[30] A study of meniscectomies at the Hospital for Joint Disease (New York) from 1957 to 1967 revealed 30 discoid menisci in 1219 surgical specimens, an incidence of 2.5%.[18] Noble[32] in a postmortem series reported an incidence of 7%, but followed this in 1980 with a clinical study giving an incidence of 0.5%.[33] Dickason et al., in a retrospective study, examined 14 731 menisci; of the 8040 medial menisci 10 (0.12%) were discoid; and of the 6691 lateral menisci 102 (1.5%) were discoid.[34]

Familial incidence of discoid lateral meniscus has been reported by Dashefsky,[35] whereas bilateral discoid lateral meniscus in identical twins has been reported by Gebhardt and Rosenthal.[10]

Aetiopathology of the discoid meniscus

Ellis in 1932 mentioned that the lizard is the only possessor of a discoid meniscus.[36] On critical review of the literature, however, it appears that no one has claimed to have actually observed a discoid meniscus in any animal.[14] Numerous hypotheses have been proposed concerning the aetiopathology of congenital discoid meniscus.[14,21,29,37–39] Smillie attributed this anomaly to an atavistic phenomenon and failure of the normal meniscus to undergo gradual absorption in the central area during the course of development.[21] He classified discoid menisci into three types: primitive, intermediate, and infantile.

Kaplan refuted Smillie's theory by studying menisci in all the stages of fetal development and discovered that at no stage in the development of the human fetus was the meniscus discoid in nature.[37] Clark and Ogden, on the basis of 109 fetal dissections, demonstrated that the menisci assumed their characteristic semilunar shape early in prenatal development.[40]

The intermediate zone between the femur and the tibia which appears very early in the embryological development of the knee is known as the intermediate disc. This disc develops into two semilunar menisci, so that even in the first few days of development the general shape of the meniscus is similar to that in the adult. Kaplan dissected the knees of a young gorilla, three chimpanzees, one orangoutang, one gibbon, two rhesus monkeys, one lemur, one bear, one pig, one sheep, one bullfrog, one iguana, one lion, one alligator, several birds, and numerous cats and dogs.[14] In his series, not a single animal was found with a meniscus, either medial or lateral, which resembled a disc, although some of them did have circular menisci. Dissections in animals showed that the posterior horn was not attached to the tibial plateau, but instead was found attached to the lateral aspect of the medial femoral condyle by a meniscofemoral ligament, popularly known as the ligament of Wrisberg.

On the basis of the embryological and anatomical studies, Kaplan established that neither in human fetuses nor in the animals examined (representing mammals, birds, amphibians and reptiles) is there a meniscus which has the form of a disc.[14]

Kaplan[14] noticed that the Wrisberg ligament did not permit the lateral meniscus to move completely forward during full extension, but dislocated the meniscus into the intercondylar space. At each flexion, the lateral meniscus, being released from the pull of the meniscofemoral ligament, was pulled laterally by the coronary ligament and the popliteus tendon. It was this abnormal mediolateral movement which Kaplan thought frequently produced an audible 'clunk'. He also proposed that this increased abnormal movement led to a hypertrophied meniscus, which has been described as discoid. He concluded that patients with discoid lateral menisci were born with menisci normal in shape but abnormal in attachments to the tibia and femur. In these individuals, as in all animals but man, the meniscofemoral ligament is attached to the medial femoral condyle.

Pathology

The discoid meniscus is a solid mass of fibrocartilage, oval or roughly circular in shape and varying in thickness from 5 mm to 13 mm. The lateral tibial plateau is usually entirely covered by the discoid meniscus, which at its inner margin is attached throughout its length along the intercondylar space and the cruciate ligaments. Occasionally, the anterior horn and the body of the discoid form a solid mass, whereas the posterior horn is normal. Cystic degeneration can occur within the discoid meniscus leading to formation of central cavities (Figure 1). Histological examination usually shows some degree of mucoid degeneration in all specimens.

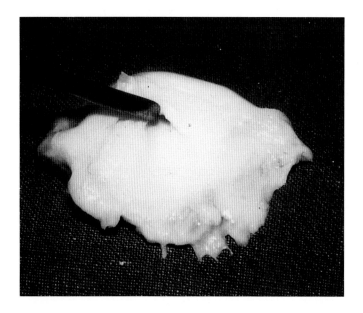

Figure 1

Specimen of a lateral discoid meniscus showing central cavity.

Clinical features

The condition is often asymptomatic in infancy and early childhood. The youngest known case of a 'popping knee' associated with a discoid lateral meniscus was reported by Barnes et al.[3] They described the management of discoid lateral meniscus in a 6-month-old child who initially presented with an audible and palpable 'pop' on movement of the knee.

The lateral meniscus is commonly affected, though occasionally the condition may occur in the medial meniscus.[18,21,27,34,39,41–47] The condition is often bilateral. There is no sex predilection.

The symptoms of a discoid lateral meniscus usually do not develop until adolescence. The complete or incomplete type of the discoid meniscus in a child's knee may remain asymptomatic and hence may not be diagnosed until the discoid lesion tears or the child undergoes arthroscopic examination for an unrelated cause. On the other hand, children with Wrisberg-ligament type of the discoid may present early with lateral pain with or without audible or palpable clunk.

The clinical symptoms of a discoid meniscus include pain, swelling, limping, giving way, locking, clicking or snapping, and reduced sporting activities. The clinical signs include quadriceps wasting, effusion, joint-line tenderness and block to extension. The McMurray's test may not be positive for pain and clunk in all cases of discoid menisci.

Smillie (1948) described snapping in only four of 29 patients studied.[21] Nathan and Cole studied 26 patients with discoid menisci and found that 20 patients (77%) presented with clicking.[18] Hayashi et al. reviewed 46 children (53 knees) with discoid lateral meniscus and found that the McMurray's test and the Watson–Jones test were positive in about one-half to two-thirds of the knees.[11] Recently, Aichroth et al.[48] reviewed 52 children (62 knees) with discoid lateral menisci and noted that the classical clunk was present in only 39% of the knees.

In the differential diagnosis of a discoid meniscus, the following conditions which cause 'snapping knee' in infancy and childhood should be considered: subluxation or dislocation of the patellofemoral joint, meniscal cyst, snapping of the tendons around the knee, congenital subluxation of the tibiofemoral joint or subluxation/dislocation of the proximal tibiofemoral joint.

Radiological investigations

Numerous authors have reported on the plain radiographic findings indicative of a discoid lateral meniscus.[42,49,50] These include widening of the lateral joint space, squaring-off of the lateral femoral condyle, cupping of the lateral aspect of the tibial plateau, oblique alignment of the articular surface of the lateral tibial condyle, high fibular head, minimal hypoplasia of the lateral intercondylar tibial spine and questionable dysmorphia of the femoral condyles.

However, Dickhaut and DeLee noticed that these radiological findings are often absent in a child with discoid meniscus.[5] They reviewed 18 patients with arthroscopically proven discoid lateral meniscus and found that only three had widening of the lateral joint space. Cupping of the lateral aspect of the tibial plateau was present in two of these three patients.

Aichroth et al.[48] in a series of 52 children (62 discoid menisci) found plain radiographs to be of limited value. In their study, widening of the lateral joint space was seen in five knees (Figure 2) and a sclerotic lateral tibial plateau was noted in two. Cupping of the lateral tibial plateau was present in three knees. None of the radiographs showed squaring-off of the lateral femoral condyle. The most remarkable feature of this series was an associated osteochondritis dissecans affecting the lateral femoral condyle in seven knees and ossification defects involving the lateral femoral condyle in four.

Contrast arthrographic studies have been used for diagnosing discoid menisci and, according to Hall,[51] the hall mark of the arthrographic diagnosis is the demonstration of an abnormally large and elongated meniscus. He developed a classification system of discoid meniscus based on size and shape as seen arthrographically, and described six types: slab type, biconcave type, wedge type, asymmetric anterior type, forme fruste, and grossly torn type. However, Hall did not indicate specifically which types of discoid lateral meniscus were prone to be symptomatic. Haveson and Rein stressed the significance of viewing the posteroanterior projection and suggested that the diagnosis of discoid lateral meniscus should be made only when the meniscus can be demonstrated extending up to the intercondylar notch.[49]

Computed tomographic scanning and magnetic resonance imaging (MRI) may be helpful in diagnosing the discoid meniscus, which appears as a hypertrophied mass of tissue. We do not recommend routine use of MRI in the diagnosis of discoid lateral meniscus. We believe that, with better resolution techniques, MRI may provide better definition of the Wrisberg ligament, which is usually difficult to visualize at arthroscopy.

Diagnosis

The clinical diagnosis of a discoid meniscus in a child's knee is often difficult, as the presenting symptoms are usually intermittent and vague and the

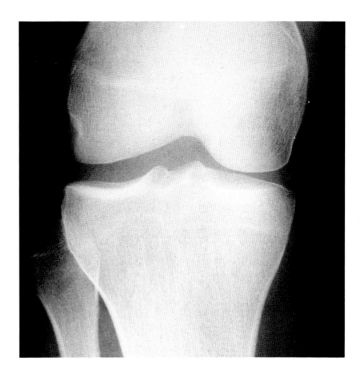

Figure 2

Plain radiograph showing widening of the lateral joint space in a 16-year-old girl with lateral discoid meniscus.

clinical signs often uncertain and not conclusive. The plain radiographs usually provide inadequate information. Arthrography has been recommended by some authors,[49,51,52] but we believe that in a small child this is not practical as general anaesthesia is usually necessary for a good arthrogram. If a general anaesthetic is to be administered, then arthroscopic assessment is preferable.

We believe that the diagnosis of a discoid meniscus should be confirmed by arthroscopy (Figures 3 and 4). Arthroscopy permits more precise diagnosis of the lesion.[12,13,26,53] Arthroscopic examination confirms the clinical diagnosis of discoid meniscus, facilitates its morphological description and can identify an associated tear.[4]

At arthroscopy, it may sometimes be difficult to enter the lateral compartment if a discoid meniscus is present. In such instances it is advisable to use the medial portal first. Several portals may be required for adequate visualization and probing of the discoid meniscus, especially for a Wrisberg-ligament type of the discoid (Figure 5). It has been said that visualization of the Wrisberg ligament is difficult. However, with the skilful use of an arthroscopic hook, it may be possible to see the meniscofemoral ligament of Wrisberg which extends from the posterior aspect of the discoid to the lateral aspect of the medial femoral condyle (Figure 6). The peripheral

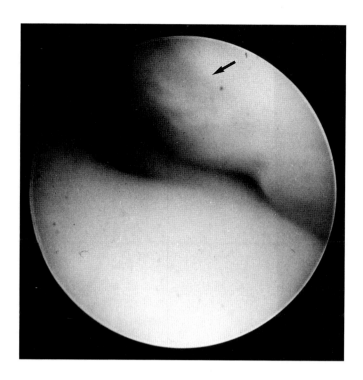

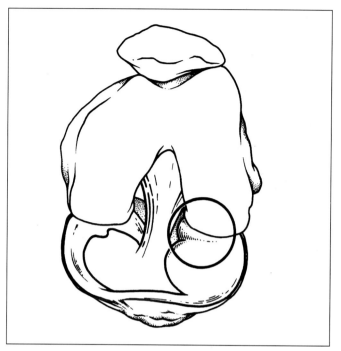

Figure 3

Arthroscopic view of complete discoid lateral meniscus. Note the associated osteochondritis dissecans involving the lateral femoral condyle (arrow).

Figure 4

Diagram of the area seen in Figure 3.

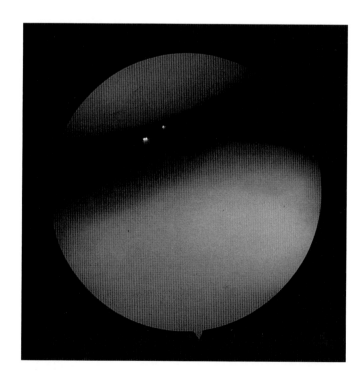

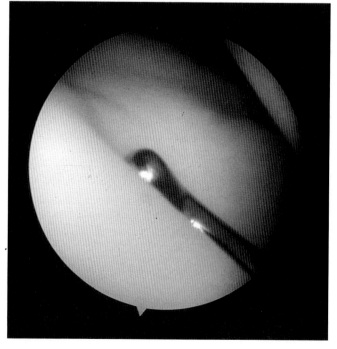

Figure 5

Arthroscopic view of the Wrisberg-ligament type of the lateral discoid meniscus. In this photograph, the area of Wrisberg ligament attachment is not seen.

Figure 6

A probe is used to show the area of attachment to the meniscofemoral ligament of Wrisberg. The posterior instability of the discoid must be assessed using the probe.

attachment of the meniscus, its stability, and whether it is torn or not should be determined using an arthroscopic probe.

The thickness of a discoid meniscus, its poor vascularization[54,55] and a flimsy attachment of the posterior area of the discoid to the capsule make it more susceptible to mechanical stress.[11] The tears of the discoid meniscus can be of various types including longitudinal, horizontal, bucket-handle, radial and complex tears. Hayashi et al. made an important point that excising the meniscus in one piece is the only way to confirm the shape and the extent of the tear postoperatively.[53] The most common site of the tear is at the posterior segment and inside the middle segment.[11] The recognition of the tear on arthrography may be difficult or impossible especially when there is a horizontal tear in the mid-substance or a transverse cleavage in the middle segment.[51]

O'Connor mentioned that the normal lateral meniscus covers 20% of the tibial plateau and that a discoid lateral meniscus should be described by the percentage of the tibial plateau covered.[56] On the other hand, Watanabe et al. classified discoid menisci (as seen arthroscopically) into three categories; the Complete, Incomplete or the Wrisberg-ligament type.[26] However, it must be pointed out that the distinction between the Complete and Incomplete types is based purely on the size of the discoid alone, and thus arthroscopic differentiation is entirely subjective[5] and left to the discretion of the surgeon who performs arthroscopic assessment.

Management of the discoid meniscus

In the pre-arthroscopy era, total excision of the meniscus was the only surgical treatment available. With the advent of arthroscopy, it became possible to differentiate between the various types of discoid menisci and treat them accordingly.

The currently accepted method of classification for the discoid lateral meniscus is that of Watanabe et al., who described three types: Complete, Incomplete or the Wrisberg-ligament type, based on the degree of coverage of the lateral tibial plateau and the presence or absence of normal posterior meniscotibial attachment.[26]

The management of the discoid meniscus is based on this system of classification. *Torn* discoid menisci—Complete or Incomplete type—should be partially resected to a stable peripheral rim.[5,9,11,13,16,20,23] Even though Ikeuchi recommends partial meniscectomy, his study concluded that patients who underwent total meniscectomy did better than those who had partial meniscectomy.[13] Kurosaka et al. reported long-term results of total meniscectomy (20–26 years of follow-up) and found that 71% of the knees had

excellent or good results on clinical examination. Over 85% of the patients younger than 20 years at the time of the operation showed excellent or good results. Radiologically, moderate to severe degenerative changes were seen in 75% of the knees.[15]

Total meniscectomy is recommended for the Wrisberg-ligament type of the discoid.[5,14,20,24,57]

Most authors agree that the intact discoid lateral meniscus of the Complete or Incomplete type should be left unresected.[5,16,23,57]

Prior to 1979, the differentiation between Complete, Incomplete and the Wrisberg-ligament type of discoid meniscus was not possible owing to lack of awareness and the absence of preceding arthroscopy. Since then, our management protocol has evolved gradually. Currently, we follow the classification system suggested by Watanabe et al.[26] We became aware that the majority of the children treated in the past decade had the Wrisberg-ligament type of discoid meniscus with posterior instability. This is in contrast to other series where no Wrisberg-ligament type of discoid lesions were reported.[4,11,25]

We certainly do not advocate total lateral meniscectomy for all knees with discoid lateral meniscus. Various authors have recommended arthroscopic partial or total meniscectomy for discoid lateral menisci.[4–6,9,11,13,19,25] This is undoubtedly a good technique, but certainly demands considerable skill and experience.

The arthroscopic surgery of the discoid meniscus is more difficult than lesions of the normal meniscus, principally owing to the increased size and thickness of the discoid, which considerably narrows the joint space required to manoeuvre the arthroscopic instruments.[13] Moreover, there may be reactive synovial hypertrophy which obscures good visualization of the discoid meniscus.[19] The difficulty of arthroscopic total meniscectomy for a lateral discoid meniscus often resides in the resection of the anterior horn.[4] In fact, the earlier techniques described by Fujikawa et al. and Ikeuchi were semiarthroscopic meniscectomies.[9,13]

Fujikawa et al. reviewed seven children who underwent partial meniscectomy for symptomatic discoid lateral meniscus.[9] This procedure, modifying the discoid meniscus to the normal semilunar shape, was indicated only when the discoid showed slight degeneration or a minimal tear; when it was not abnormally thickened nor of Wrisberg type; when it was not hypermobile; and when the capsular attachment was intact. They stressed that these conditions should be accurately confirmed prior to operation by double-contrast arthrography and arthroscopy. The results on a short-term basis were excellent clinically, radiologically and arthroscopically. The rehabilitation period was shortened to half that required for total meniscectomy and the residual meniscus functioned entirely normally.

However, there are some doubts concerning the long-term results of partial meniscectomy in children with discoid meniscus. The arrangement of collagen fibres of the discoid meniscus is different from that of a normal meniscus[58] and it is likely that further tearing or degeneration of the residual rim of the meniscus could occur after this procedure.

Ikeuchi reported on 45 patients (49 knees) who had torn Complete or Incomplete discoid lateral menisci.[13] Of these 45 patients, 22 patients (24 knees) underwent a follow-up evaluation. The mean follow-up was 4.3 years (range 1.4–7.7 years). Overall, 78% of the knees had excellent or good results and 22% had fair results. There were no poor results. It was noteworthy that the results in the group treated by total meniscectomy were better than those in the group treated with partial meniscectomy.

Hayashi et al. reviewed 53 knees with symptomatic discoid lateral menisci treated by arthroscopic partial, subtotal or total meniscectomy, at an average follow-up of 31.2 months.[11] They noticed that the extent of meniscectomy depended on the site and shape of the tear, as did the symptoms and signs. They also tried to establish the width of partial meniscectomy of a discoid that would prevent new tears. They suggested that a rim of 6 mm should be left for Complete type of the discoid and a rim of 8 mm should be left for Incomplete type of the discoid meniscus. The authors stated that a further study with a long-term follow-up is in progress to evaluate the results of preserving the meniscal rim and to determine whether the proposed width is ideal.

We suggest arthroscopic partial lateral meniscectomy for *torn*—Complete or Incomplete type of the discoid menisci—with stable posterior tibial attachment. However, in children with Wrisberg-ligament type or hypermobile discoid lateral meniscus, we believe that partial meniscectomy would be inappropriate as it would merely leave an unstable rim of the meniscus, which becomes symptomatic in the future.[5,13–15,20,24,26] Therefore, a total meniscectomy is recommended in such circumstances.

Rosenberg et al. described a case report of arthroscopic peripheral attachment after central partial meniscectomy of a Wrisberg-ligament type of lateral discoid meniscus in a 19-year-old male athlete.[59] They also documented healing at 'second-look' arthroscopy, 12 months following the surgery. This is certainly an attractive concept which demands considerable technical skill and experience. Reports such as this, using a larger number of patients with a long-term follow-up, are needed before definitive conclusions can be drawn. It may well be the technique of choice in future for the management of Wrisberg-ligament type of the discoid meniscus.

Discussion

The clinical symptoms and signs of the discoid lateral meniscus are often vague and intermittent, causing considerable delay in presentation and clinical diagnosis. It is possible that the toleration of the meniscal abnormalities by the children may have contributed to this delay.

We believe that pain is the more common presenting symptom rather than the conventionally taught click or clunk. The pain is most likely to be due to the abnormal movement of the meniscus as a result of the instability and its lack of posterior capsular attachment. On clinical examination, the classical clunk may not be present in all cases.

Contrary to Picard,[50] we do not feel that radiographs play a significant role in diagnosis of the discoid meniscus. The plain radiographs usually provide inadequate information. Double-contrast arthrography has been suggested by some authors, but we feel that because of the frequent necessity to administer a general anaesthetic in order to perform an arthrogram in a young child, and the often equivocal results, the child should be spared this investigation.

Recently, Vandermeer and Cunningham in a series of 25 discoid lateral menisci found arthrography of limited value, with only one-fourth yielding the correct preoperative diagnosis.[25] We believe that the diagnosis and assessment of the discoid meniscus should be undertaken arthroscopically.

Following a total lateral meniscectomy, an adequate 'pseudomeniscus' develops[48] (Figures 7 and 8). However, we are aware that some authors believe that regeneration of the discoid meniscus after total excision is unlikely to occur as the absence of the blood supply at the area of the popliteal tendon precludes the development of the meniscal tissue.[54,55]

One must note that these studies were performed using cadaveric knees of adult and elderly patients. Arnoczky and Warren[54] studied 20 cadaveric knees of patients between 53 and 94 years of age, whereas Danzig et al.[55] investigated 25 lower limb, fresh cadaveric specimens of patients ranging in age from 40 to 80 years. We believe that the child's knee behaves differently.

Total meniscectomy of a lateral non-discoid meniscus often leads to osteoarthritis.[60–63] This remains true for discoid menisci in adults as well. However, our experience suggests that in children the results are different. A similar observation has been reported by others.[64–67] It has been said that the prognosis after total meniscectomy is better in children than in adults.[65] Recently, Hayashi et al. reported that the axial alignment of the extensor mechanism and the pliability of the tissue may be forgiving in children, leading to reasonable adaptation of the knee joint to the stresses of activity.[64]

Hayashi et al. reviewed 46 children (53 knees) with symptomatic discoid lateral menisci treated by arthroscopic partial or total meniscectomy, and found no degenerative changes at an average follow-up of 31.2 months (range 20–53 months).[11]

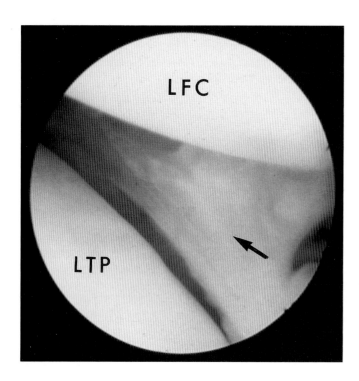

Figure 7

Arthroscopic appearance of the 'pseudomeniscus' (black arrow), 24 months following total lateral meniscectomy. LFC = lateral femoral condyle; LTP = lateral tibial plateau.

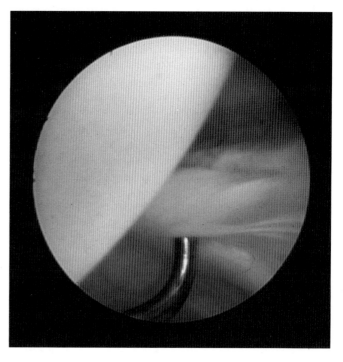

Figure 8

'Second-look' arthroscopy, performed 18 months after a total lateral meniscectomy in a 12-year-old child. A substantial 'pseudomeniscus' is seen.

Zaman and Leonard emphasized the hazards of total meniscectomy in children.[63] They reported the results of meniscectomy carried out in 49 children (59 knees), at an average follow-up of 7.5 years (range 1.5–16 years). It should be noted that only 11 children in their series had discoid lateral menisci and one-third of all the excised menisci were found normal at operation. The average age of the children at the time of meniscectomy was 13 years. There was a statistically significant correlation ($P<0.01$) between the clinical results and the meniscal lesions; poorer results were seen in children where a normal meniscus had been removed. Early degenerative changes were seen in 11 knees (19%) on radiological examination. They concluded that meniscectomy is not a benign procedure in children and that preoperative assessment should include arthroscopy and possibly arthrography.

Long-term results of total meniscectomy in children

Kurosaka et al. reported 20–26 years of follow-up of total meniscectomy for discoid lateral meniscus.[15] In their series, good subjective results were achieved in over 85% of the cases, although moderate to severe degenerative changes were seen in 75% of the cases on radiological examination.

Aichroth et al.[48] reviewed 52 children with 62 discoid lateral menisci. Forty-eight knees with symptomatic, *torn* discoid menisci underwent total lateral meniscectomy, six knees had arthroscopic partial meniscectomy and eight knees with minimal symptoms but arthroscopically proven intact discoid menisci were left alone. The mean postoperative follow-up was 5.5 years (range 2–18 years). On radiological examination, early degenerative changes (positive Fairbank sign, Figure 9) were noted in only three cases at the time of latest review (Figure 10).

Recently, Abdon et al. reviewed 89 children who underwent total meniscectomy.[68] It should be pointed out that in this series only 12 children had discoid menisci (10 lateral and two medial) and the remaining children had undergone meniscectomy for various post-traumatic meniscal lesions. The mean postoperative follow-up was 16.8 years (range 10–28 years).

Overall, 74% of the patients were pleased with the outcome of surgery. Forty-six patients (52%) had an excellent or satisfactory result as classified by the scoring system of Tapper and Hoover[69] and 52

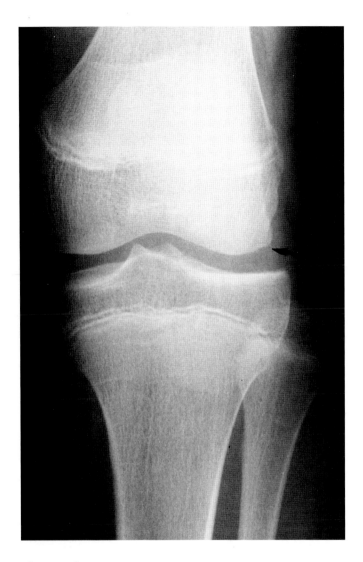

Figure 9

Early degenerative changes (positive Fairbank sign, arrow) in the lateral compartment following a total lateral meniscectomy in a 7-year-old child. The postoperative follow-up was 11.5 years.

patients (58%) had excellent or satisfactory results according to the scoring system of Johnson et al.[70] They noted significantly poorer results with lateral meniscectomy. Minor instabilities were recorded in 45% of the patients and major instabilities in 15%. Radiologically, grade I gonarthrosis was seen in 39% of the surgically treated knees and grade II or III gonarthrosis in 9%.

Conclusions

Children with congenital discoid lateral menisci often present with vague and intermittent symptoms leading to considerable delay in the clinical diagnosis. Pain is the major presenting symptom rather than

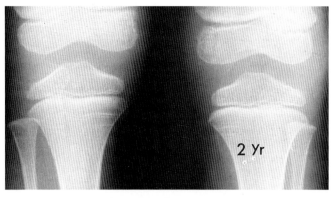

a

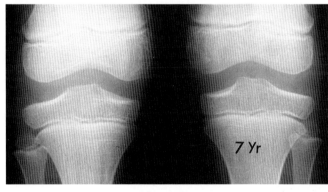

b

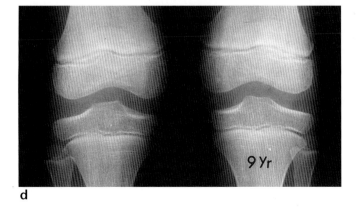

c

d

Figure 10

Series of plain radiographs showing postoperative follow-up of bilateral total lateral meniscectomy undertaken in a 5-year-old child with extremely shredded, torn discoid menisci.

the traditionally taught classical clunk. Search should be made for an associated osteochondritis dissecans involving the lateral femoral condyle.

We recommend arthroscopic examination at an earlier stage in a child presenting with recurrent symptoms of pain, clunk, swelling, locking or giving way suggestive of a meniscal abnormality. Arthroscopic partial meniscectomy is indicated only when the posterior attachment of the discoid meniscus is found to be stable. In children with Wrisberg-ligament type of the discoid, a total meniscectomy is recommended.

Acknowledgments

We are grateful to Dina Stanford for her assistance. The authors would like to thank the Medical Photography Department at Westminster Hospital for their help with the illustrations.

References

1. **Young RB**, The external semilunar cartilage as a complete disc, In *Memoirs and memoranda in anatomy*, ed Cleland J, Mackay JY, Young RB (London: Williams and Norgate, 1889) 1: 179.
2. **Kroiss F**, Die Verletzungen der Kniegelenkszwischenknorpel und ihrer Verbindungen, *Beitr Klin Chir* (1910) 66: 598–801.
3. **Barnes CL, McCarthy RE, VanderSchilden JL** et al., Discoid lateral meniscus in a young child: case report and review of the literature, *J Paediatr Ortho* (1988) 8: 707–709.
4. **Bellier G, Dupont Jean-Yves, Larrain M** et al., Lateral discoid menisci in children, *Arthroscopy* (1989) 5(1): 52–56
5. **Dickhaut SC, DeLee JC**, The discoid lateral-meniscus syndrome, *J Bone Joint Surg (Am)* (1982) 64: 1068–1073.
6. **Dimakopoulos P, Patel D**, Partial excision of discoid meniscus: arthroscopic operation of 10 patients, *Acta Orthop Scand* (1989) 60(6): 40–41.
7. **Engber WD, Mickelson MR**, Cupping of the lateral tibial plateau associated with a discoid meniscus, *Orthopaedics* (1981) 4: 904–906.
8. **Fairbank HAT**, Internal derangement of the knee in children and adolescents, *Proc R Soc Med* (1937) 30(Part I): 427–432.
9. **Fujikawa K, Iseki F, Mikura Y**, Partial resection of the discoid meniscus in the child's knee, *J Bone Joint Surg (Br)* (1981) 63: 391–395.
10. **Gebhardt MC, Rosenthal RK**, Bilateral lateral discoid meniscus in identical twins, *J Bone Joint Surg (Am)* (1979) 61: 1110–1111.
11. **Hayashi LK, Yamaga H, Ida K** et al., Arthroscopic meniscectomy for discoid lateral meniscus in children, *J Bone Joint Surg (Am)* (1988) 70: 1495–1500.
12. **Hayashi LK, Yamaga H, Mori R** et al., Clinical and arthroscopic study of discoid lateral meniscus in infants, *Central Jpn J Orthop Traumat Surg* (1987) 30: 639–645.
13. **Ikeuchi H**, Arthroscopic treatment of the discoid lateral meniscus: technique and long-term results, *Clin Orthop* (1982) 167: 19–28.
14. **Kaplan EB**, Discoid lateral meniscus of the knee joint: nature, mechanism and operative treatment, *J Bone Joint Surg (Am)* (1957) 39: 77–87.
15. **Kurosaka M, Yoshiya S, Ohno O** et al., Lateral discoid meniscectomy: a 20-year follow-up, presented at the American Academy of Orthopedic Surgery Meeting, San Francisco, January 1987.
16. **Metcalf RW**, Operative arthroscopy of the knee, *Instructional course lectures*, The American Academy of Orthopedic Surgeons (St Louis: CV Mosby, 1981) 30: 357–396.
17. **Middleton DS**, Congenital disc-shaped lateral meniscus with snapping knee, *Br J Surg* (1936) 24: 246–255.
18. **Nathan PA, Cole SC**, Discoid meniscus: a clinical and pathologic study, *Clin Orthop* (1969) 64: 107–113.
19. **Pellacci F, Stilli S, Pignatti G**, Arthroscopic surgical technique in the treatment of lesions of the discoid meniscus, *Ital J Orthop Traumatol* (1988) XIV (3): 357–362.
20. **Sisk TD**, *Campbell's operative orthopaedics*, 7th edn, ed Crenshaw AH (St Louis: CV Mosby, 1987) 2323–2324.
21. **Smillie IS**, The congenital discoid meniscus, *J Bone Joint Surg (Br)* (1948) 30: 671–682.
22. **Smillie IS**, *Injuries of the knee joint*, 5th edn (London: Churchill Livingstone, 1978).
23. **Stone RG, Miller G**, Discoid lateral meniscus: diagnosis and treatment, *Arthroscopy* (1986) 2(2): 113.
24. **Tachdjian MO**, *Paediatric orthopaedics* (Philadelphia: WB Saunders, 1990) 1539–1551.
25. **Vandermeer RD, Cunningham FK**, Arthroscopic treatment of the discoid lateral meniscus: results of long-term follow-up, *Arthroscopy* (1989) 5(2): 101–109.
26. **Watanabe M, Takeda S, Ikeuchi H**, *Atlas of arthroscopy*, 3rd edn (Berlin: Springer-Verlag, 1979).
27. **Cave EF, Staples OS**, Congenital discoid meniscus: a cause of internal derangement of the knee, *Am J Surg* (1941) 54: 371–376.
28. **Jeannopoulos CL**, Observations on discoid menisci, *J Bone Joint Surg (Am)* (1950) 32: 649–652.
29. **Nemoto HN**, Study on discoid meniscus of the knee, *Nigata Med J* (1950) 64: 404–410.
30. **Smillie IS**, *Injuries of the knee joint*, 4th edn (Edinburgh: Churchill Livingstone, 1970).
31. **Casscells SW**, Gross pathological changes in the knee joint of the aged individual: a study of 300 cases, *Clin Orthop* (1978) 132: 225–232.
32. **Noble J**, Lesions of the menisci: autopsy incidence in adults less than fifty-five years old, *J Bone Joint Surg (Am)* (1977) 59: 480–483.
33. **Noble J, Erat K**, In defence of the meniscus: a prospective study of 200 meniscectomy patients, *J Bone Joint Surg (Br)* (1980) 62: 7–11.
34. **Dickason JM, Del Pizzo W, Blazina ME** et al., A series of ten discoid medial menisci, *Clin Orthop* (1982) 168: 75–79.
35. **Dashefsky JH**, Discoid lateral meniscus in three members of a family: case reports, *J Bone Joint Surg (Am)* (1971) 53: 1208–1210.
36. **Ellis VH**, Congenital abnormality of the external semilunar cartilage, *Lancet* (1932) 1: 1359.
37. **Kaplan EB**, The embryology of the menisci of the knee joint, *Bull Hosp Joint Dis* (1955) 16: 111–124.
38. **Paolou EC, Lopez UCL, Mateu JMD**, Menisco discoideo, estudio embriogenico, *Revista de Ortopedia y Traumatologia* (1983) 27-IB: 63–74.
39. **Ross JA, Tough ICK, English TA**, Congenital discoid cartilage: report of a case of discoid medial cartilage, with an embryological note, *J Bone Joint Surg (Br)* (1958) 40: 262–267.
40. **Clark CR, Ogden JA**, Development of the menisci of the human knee joint: morphological changes and their potential role in childhood meniscal injury, *J Bone Joint Surg (Am)* (1983) 65: 538–547.
41. **Basmajian JV**, A ring-shaped medial semilunar cartilage, *J Bone Joint Surg (Br)* (1952) 34: 638–639.
42. **Berson BL, Hermann G**, Torn discoid menisci of the knee in adults: four case reports, *J Bone Joint Surg (Am)* (1979) 61: 303–304.
43. **Dwyer FC, Taylor C**, Congenital discoid internal cartilage, *Br Med J* (1945) 2: 287.

44. **Murdoch G**, Congenital discoid medial semilunar cartilage, *J Bone Joint Surg (Br)* (1956) **38**: 564–566.

45. **Riachi E, Phares A**, An unusual deformity of the medial semilunar cartilage, *J Bone Joint Surg (Br)* (1963) **45**: 146–147.

46. **Richmond DA**, Two cases of discoid medial cartilage, *J Bone Joint Surg (Br)* (1958) **40**: 268–269.

47. **Weiner B, Rosenberg N**, Discoid medial meniscus: association with bone changes in the tibia: a case report, *J Bone Joint Surg (Am)* (1974) **56**: 171–173.

48. **Aichroth PM, Patel DV, Marx CL**, Congenital discoid lateral meniscus in children: a follow-up study and evolution of management, *J Bone Joint Surg (Br)* (1991) **73**: 932–936.

49. **Haveson SB, Rein BI**, Lateral discoid meniscus of the knee: arthrographic diagnosis. *Am J Roentgenol Radium Ther Nucl Med* (1970) **109**: 581–585.

50. **Picard JJ**, Radiological aspects of the discoid menisci, *J Radiol Elect* (1964) **45**: 839–841.

51. **Hall FM**, Arthrography of the discoid lateral meniscus, *Am J Roentgenol* (1977) **128**: 993–1002.

52. **Fujikawa K, Tomatsu T, Matsu K** et al., Morphological analysis of meniscus and articular cartilage in the knee joint by means of arthrogram, *J Jpn Orthop Assoc* (1978) **52**: 203–215.

53. **Hayashi LK, Yamaga H, Hattori T** et al., Arthroscopic study on the lateral discoid meniscus tears, Paper read at the Sixty-ninth Meeting of the Central Japanese Orthopaedic Association, Matsue, Japan, October 1987.

54. **Arnoczky SP, Warren RF**, Microvasculature of the human meniscus, *Am J Sports Med* (1982) **10**: 90–95.

55. **Danzig L, Resnick D, Gonsalves M** et al., Blood supply to the normal and abnormal menisci of the human knee, *Clin Orthop* (1983) **172**: 271–276.

56. **O'Connor RL**, *Arthroscopic surgery* (Philadelphia: JB Lippincott, 1984) 158–162.

57. **Griffin PP**, The lower limb, *Paediatric orthopaedics*, ed Lovell WW, Winter RB (Philadelphia: JB Lippincott, 1986) 887.

58. **Amako T**, On the injuries of the menisci in the knee joint of Japanese, *J Jpn Orthop Assoc* (1960) **33**: 1289–1322.

59. **Rosenberg TD, Paulos LE, Parker RD** et al., Discoid lateral meniscus: Case report of arthroscopic attachment of a symptomatic Wrisberg-ligament type, *Arthroscopy* (1987) **3**(4): 277–282.

60. **Fairbank TJ**, Knee joint changes after meniscectomy, *J Bone Joint Surg (Br)* (1948) **30**: 664–670.

61. **Kurozawa H, Koide K, Nakajima H**, Results of meniscectomy, *Orthop Surg* (1976) **27**: 825–832.

62. **Manzione M, Pizzutillo PD, Peoples AB** et al., Meniscectomy in children: a long-term follow-up study, *Am J Sports Med* (1983) **11**: 111–115.

63. **Zaman M, Leonard MA**, Meniscectomy in children: results in 59 knees, *Injury* (1981) **12**: 425–428.

64. **Hayashi LK, Yamaga H, Ida K** et al., Long-term results of total meniscectomy of the lateral discoid meniscus in young patients: osteoarthritis and axial alignment, Paper read at the Seventieth Meeting of the Central Japanese Orthopaedic Association, Nagoya, Japan, May 1988.

65. **Kobayashi A, Uezaki N, Mitsuyasu M**, Discoid meniscus of the knee joint, *Clin Orthop Surg Jpn* (1975) **10**: 10–24.

66. **Yoshida N, Koshino T, Yasutake S** et al., The knee problem in children: meniscus problems in the infants and results of meniscectomy, *Kanto Soc Orthop Traumatol* (1983) **14**: 377–380.

67. **Yoshiya S, Okada Y, Ono S**, Late results after meniscectomy in children and adolescents, *Orthop Surg* (1984) **27**: 2037–2038.

68. **Abdon P, Turner MS, Pettersson H** et al., A long-term follow-up study of total meniscectomy in children, *Clin Orthop* (1990) **257**: 166–170.

69. **Tapper EM, Hoover NW**, Late results after meniscectomy, *J Bone Joint Surg (Am)* (1969) **51**: 517–526.

70. **Johnson RJ, Kettelkamp DB, Clark W** et al., Factors affecting late results after meniscectomy, *J Bone Joint Surg (Am)* (1974) **56**: 719–729.

12.2 Discoid meniscus in children

Kyosuke Fujikawa

Discoid meniscus in the child's knee joint has recently been of increasing interest as its clinical pathology has been elucidated by means of double-contrast arthrography and arthroscopy. However, because of the ambiguity of the patients' complaints, uncertainty of the clinical signs and the inadequate information provided by plain radiography, numerous patients are inadequately treated owing to misdiagnosis.

The majority of meniscus problems in children are due to lateral discoid meniscus and not associated with injury to ligaments such as the anterior cruciate and posterior cruciate which, in this context, represents the main difference between children and adults.

Development of the menisci

According to our studies on the development of the meniscus using 203 embryos and fetuses, at the 6th week, the knee joint consists of three layers: the femoral and tibial chondrogenous layers and the intermediate layer inbetween, which develops into menisci later.

At the 7th week, a space appears between the femoral chondrogenous layer and the intermediate layer, and the intermediate layer begins to show the ultimate figure of the meniscus.

At the 8th week, a space also appears between the tibial chondrogenous layer and the intermediate layer so that the figure of the meniscus becomes more well defined (Figure 1). At this stage, as the lateral condyle of the femur declines more than the medial condyle against the tibial plateau, the space between the lateral femoral condyle and the tibial plateau is much wider than that between the medial femoral condyle and the tibial plateau, particularly at the intercondylar side. Accordingly, the lateral intermediate layer is much thicker than the medial.

The difference in the shape and angle between the lateral and the medial femoral condyle becomes the cause of the abnormal generation of the discoid meniscus in the lateral compartment of the knee joint which is described later.

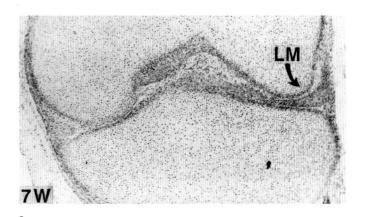

a

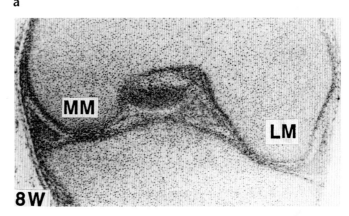

b

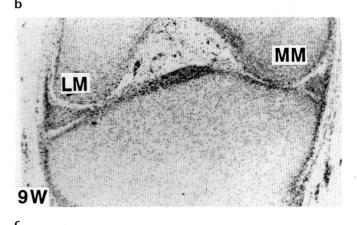

c

Figure 1

Development of menisci: (a) 7th; (b) 8th; (c) 9th week of fetal life. LM, lateral meniscus; MM, medial meniscus.

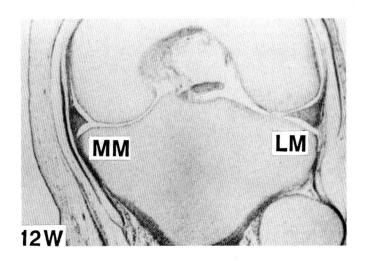

Figure 2

Development of menisci (12th week of fetal life).

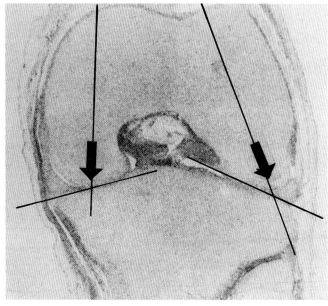

a

As the development of the knee joint progresses, the intercondylar side of the intermediate layer disc starts to be resorbed from the posterior segment towards the anterior in the medial compartment so that the medial intermediate layer becomes semilunar in shape.

At the 9th and 10th weeks, the lateral intermediate layer disc becomes semilunar in shape from its posterior part, as in the medial, as the angle of the lateral femoral condyle against the tibial plateau decreases.

At the 12th week, the medial and lateral intermediate layers become semilunar in shape, as those in the adult knee joint. However, the medial meniscus develops faster than the lateral (Figure 2).

Origin of lateral discoid meniscus

Ishidoh, Yamauchi, Nemoto and Gotoh reported that the lateral discoid meniscus was congenital in origin on the basis of their studies using fetuses over 5–6 months old. On the other hand, Amako observing fetuses over 5 months old could find no discoid meniscus and concluded that the medial and lateral menisci were all semilunar in shape.[1] According to Smillie, the meniscus was all discoid cartilagenous mass at the initial stage of fetal life, and would develop into a semilunar cartilage as time passed; a normal meniscus was the result of a gradual resorption of the central part of an original complete plate during fetal life.[2] Thus, when a discoid meniscus appears in the mature joint this would simply be the

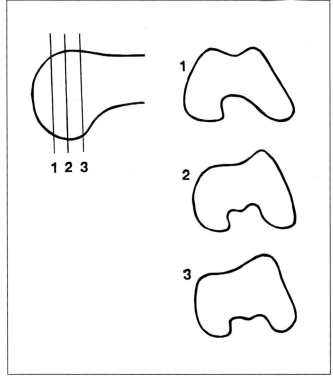

b

Figure 3

Cause of discoid meniscus appearance in the lateral femorotibial compartment. When reduction of the lateral femoral condylar angle which is more declined than that of the medial femoral condyle is delayed in fetal development, the lateral meniscus remains discoid in shape.

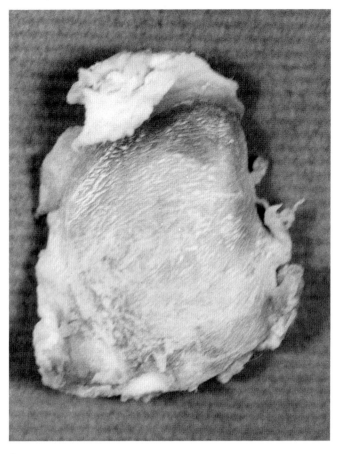

a

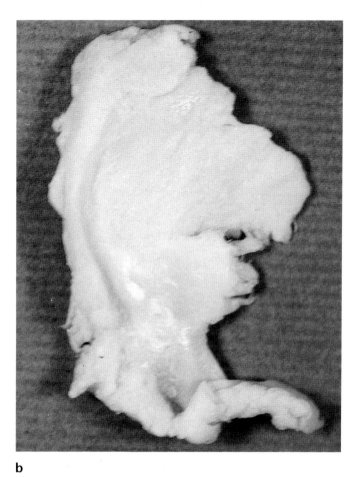

b

Figure 4

Classification of discoid meniscus. (a) Complete type; (b) incomplete type; (c) anterior megahorn type.

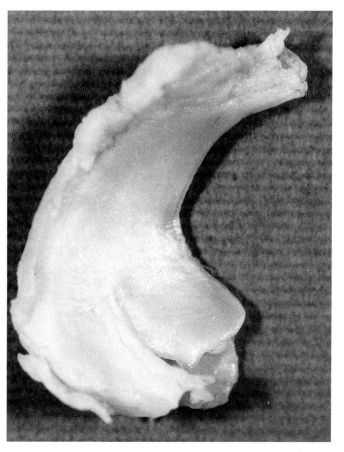

c

result of interruption of the resorption process. Kaplan reported in certain rare cases that the lateral meniscus had a circular form at birth and was unattached to the posterior aspect of the tibial plateau, as in the knee joint of other anthropoids, and was held in place by the meniscofemoral (Wrisberg) ligament, which was too short to adapt the meniscus to the normal movement of the knee.[3] Its constant mediolateral motion in growing children produced secondary thickening, transforming this initially normal meniscus into a discoid, thick fibro-cartilaginous mass assuming a solid irregular form. However, as growth of the meniscus occurs as early as 6–10 weeks in the fetus, development of discoid meniscus cannot be investigated by observing it in the later stage of the fetal life or after birth.

According to our study of the development of the meniscus, discoid meniscus is a congenital deformity normally observed on the lateral side because the angle of the lateral femoral condyle against the tibial condyle is more declined than that of the medial, so that in the medial compartment the intermediate layer can develop easily and early into the semilunar form (Figure 3). On the other hand, in the lateral compartment as the declining angle of the lateral femoral condyle decreases, the intermediate layer develops gradually into the semilunar shape from the posterior section. When reduction of the angle of the lateral femoral condyle is delayed, the lateral meniscus remains discoid in shape (Figure 4). Further, an anterior megahorn discoid can appear when the posterior part of the intermediate layer is only resorbed and its anterior part remains intact. Hence, the discoid meniscus is usually observed in the lateral compartment and very rarely in the medial.

Clinical cases

During the past 15 years, meniscectomy was performed in 134 joints of children under 15 years of age, of which 109 were lateral discoid menisci, 10 for damage to a normal semilunar lateral meniscus and 15 for damage to normal semilunar medial meniscus (Figure 5). Accordingly, it can be said that the majority of meniscal disturbances in the child's knee joint are caused by lateral discoid meniscus.

The youngest patient was a 3-year-old boy. Generally, the number of patients increased in direct proportion to age, although the age distribution of the patients showed a peak around 9 years, when children become more active in their daily life and sports. All patients except two under the age of 12 years had lateral discoid menisci, and over 13 years of age lateral and medial semilunar meniscus damage were included, the pattern of meniscal tear being very similar to that of adults.

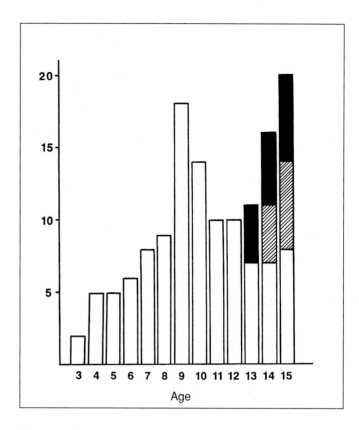

Figure 5

Operated cases: lateral discoid (open columns); semilunar lateral (shaded); semilunar medial (solid).

The lateral menisci of both knee joints were discoid in shape in all but two cases. In these patients with symptoms secondary to discoid menisci, the operation was performed on one side in 95 children and on both knees in 7 children.

This confirms our previously reported observation on arthrographic and arthroscopic study that the menisci are almost always of the same shape in right and left joints.[4] This was so in 98.7% of patients on the lateral side and 99.3% of patients on the medial side. The present series confirms that there are many clinically silent discoid menisci in children. There are little or no degenerative changes or damage, not only in the meniscus itself but also in the articular cartilages in the knee joint with a silent discoid meniscus.

On the other hand, the symptomatic discoid meniscus is often associated with considerable damage or degeneration, the cause of which is not a single trauma but repeated minor trauma and shearing stress in the activities of daily living.

The degenerative changes of the discoid meniscus are usually observed in the central part of the tibial side, and the femoral surface is smooth without any pathological changes macroscopically. In the case

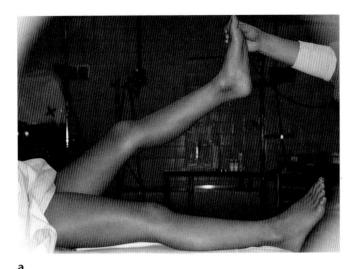

a

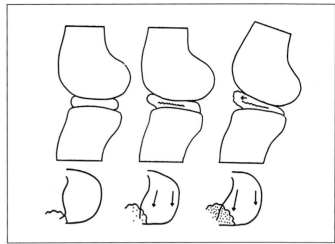

b

Figure 6

(a) Extension block of the knee joint with discoid meniscus under anaesthesia, and (b) its cause.

with persistent extension block of the knee joint, erosive changes, ulcerations or defects of the articular cartilage of the femoral condyle are often observed.

It is generally accepted that the discoid meniscus seldom appears on the medial side, the reason for which is as previously described.

Clinical symptoms

Subjective symptoms of discoid meniscus disturbance in children are ambiguous, so that their parents or schoolteachers are often conscious of abnormal behaviour appearing first as lameness, followed by lack of full extension of the knee joint (extension block), spare-built thigh, and so on, such symptoms leading parents to present the children for clinical examination.

Pain is not a major complaint in children as it is in adults, which again is a significant difference between children and adults.

The major objective signs are quadriceps atrophy, positive manual rotating friction test (pain or/and snap or click under rotation flexion stress), extension block of the knee, pain on activities, tenderness over the affected joint-space, locking and joint effusion. The first three signs are most often observed.

Extension block, which is often mistaken for locking, is a disturbance of full extension of the knee and it occurs because the femoral surface of the horizontally torn discoid meniscus moves more anteriorly than the tibial surface at knee extension and forms a mass with the proliferated infrapatellar fat pad thus blocking full extension of the knee (Figure 6).

The snap or click in the manual test or even in active knee motion occurs as a result of sudden change in the relationship between the meniscus and the femoral and tibial condyle when the femoral condyle flips the torn flap, thick margin or degenerated bent part of the discoid meniscus.

Diagnosis

Fifty-five children in this series were treated inadequately elsewhere with the diagnosis of joint sprain, contusion, developmental pain, simple monarthritis, and so on, before they visited our clinic.

Although as described earlier the subjective complaints are variable and not distinct at the initial stage, it is not difficult to diagnose correctly by careful observation. Plain radiographs can rarely provide any information on discoid meniscus in children.

The diagnosis is easily made by double-contrast arthrography and arthroscopy. Synovial pleat syndrome (plica syndrome), tangential osteochondral fracture of the patella, osteochondritis dissecans, solitary pigmented villonodular synovitis and so-called chondropathia patellae should be differentially diagnosed.

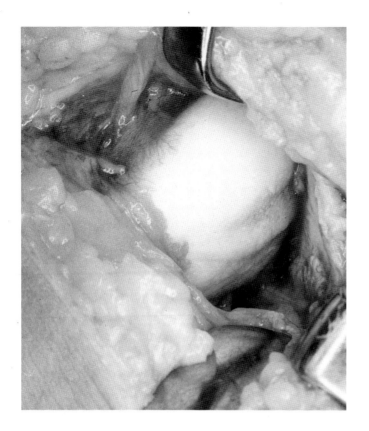

Figure 7

Degenerative change on the lateral femoral condyle due to persistent extension block of the knee joint.

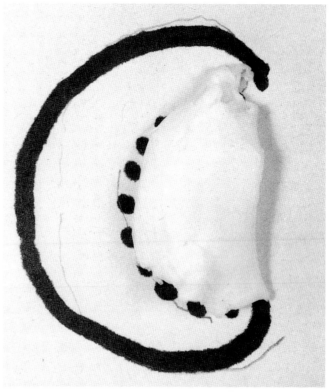

Figure 8

Partial resection of discoid meniscus moderating to the semilunar shape.

Treatment

Total or subtotal resection has been the recommended treatment for symptomatic discoid meniscus only after failure of conservative methods of treatment such as local rest, short-term immobilization in brace or plaster and quadriceps drill. Surgical treatment has been restricted to those patients with repeated or persistent locking, a block to extension or severe pain. In these cases, double-contrast arthrography or arthroscopy may show rapid secondary degenerative changes of the articular cartilage and bone demonstrating the adverse effects of the symptomatic discoid meniscus on the joint (Figure 7).

In general, excellent clinical results have been obtained in over 90% of our patients who have undergone total or partial resection, but some degenerative changes of the joints are unavoidable postoperatively.

For the past 10 years partial resection of the free edge of the discoid meniscus has been undertaken in 26 cases at Keio University Hospital, modifying it to the normal semilunar shape in order to minimize the effect of meniscectomy.

Partial resection of discoid meniscus

Indications

This procedure is indicated when the discoid meniscus shows only slight degeneration or a minimal tear; when it is not extraordinarily thickened or of the Wrisberg type; when it is not hypermobile; and when the capsular attachment is intact.[5]

These conditions should be conclusively confirmed before operation by double-contrast arthrography and/or arthroscopy.

Operative procedure

Initially the operation was carried out via a 3 cm anterolateral incision under a pneumatic tourniquet with the knee flexed to 90° over the end of the table. Subsequently, the procedure has been performed with arthroscopic assistance.

No abnormality is usually apparent on the femoral surface of the discoid meniscus, but slight degeneration or a minimal tear may be seen on its tibial

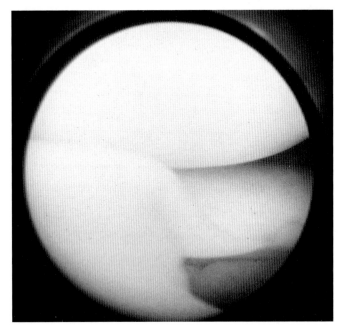

a

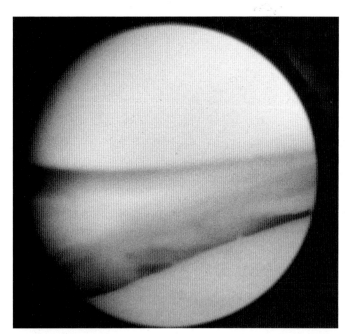

b

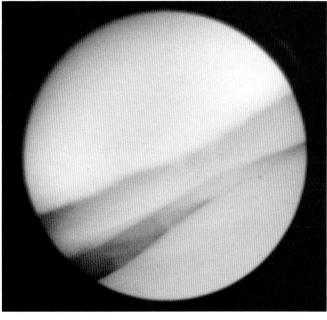

c

Figure 9

Arthroscopic findings of partial resection of the discoid meniscus. (a) Before resection (incomplete type); (b) just after partial resection; (c) 2 years after partial resection.

surface or within its structure. Palpation of the femoral surface with a probe, moving from the capsular side to the free edge, may locate a slight sagittal irregularity (Figure 8). The meniscus is incised along the line of this irregularity using a small knife and scissors in as clean a manner as possible. The anterior insertion of the meniscus is left untouched, and by pulling the free edge of the anterior part towards the intercondylar fossa it is possible to complete partial resection of the central and posterior parts of the meniscus. The posterior insertion of the meniscus is left intact. The resected portion of the meniscus is almost circular in shape (see Figure 9).

In some cases, the discoid meniscus was resected piece-by-piece under arthroscopy.

It is then necessary to confirm that the residual rim of the meniscus is free from any degeneration or tears. If degeneration or tears are observed, total or subtotal resection of the meniscus should be performed.

Postoperative care

One day after operation quadriceps drill and exercise for knee motion on the continuous passive motion device are commenced. A full range of movement

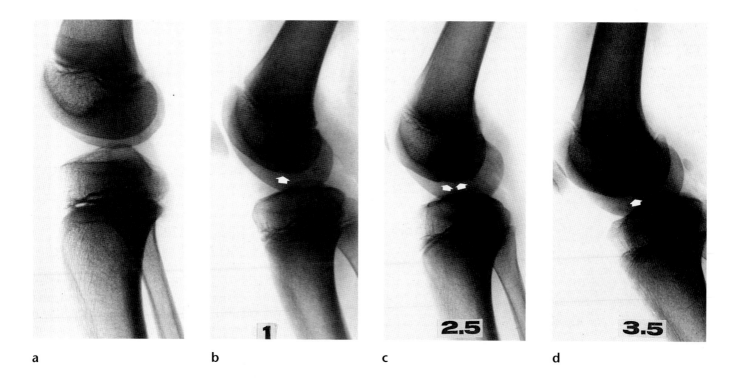

a   b   c   d

Figure 10

Osteochondritis dissecans-like lesion. (a) Before meniscectomy; (b) 1 year after operation; (c) 2.5 years after operation; (d) 3.5 years after operation when the lesion had been improved by conservative treatment.

should be achieved within a week or so, but if extension has been blocked for a considerable time before operation it will take longer to regain full extension, and intermittent traction may be required in combination with the other exercises. The period of rehabilitation is less than half that required for total meniscectomy.

Results and complications

The prognosis of discoid meniscectomy in children is generally excellent, not only for activities of daily living but also for sports activities, although varying degrees of secondary osteoarthritic changes on radiographs are unavoidable. However, in six cases in this series, osteochondritis dissecans-like change on radiographs was observed after lateral discoid meniscus resection (Figure 10). One case showed this change bilaterally after bilateral discoid meniscal resection.

The lesion was localized to the lateral part of the lateral femoral condyle in four cases, at the centre in one case, and was located broadly from the lateral part to the medial part of the lateral femoral condyle in one case.

Four cases improved with conservative treatment, such as non-weight-bearing with crutches and muscle drilling, although it took much longer than in cases with ordinary osteochondritis dissecans. One case in which the lesion spread broadly required drilling under arthroscopy. In one case, after continued sports activities, the osteochondral fragment dropped into the joint cavity, becoming a loose body.

Discussion

In the past, abnormalities of the meniscus in children posed difficulties in diagnosis. However, recently precise diagnosis has become possible by arthroscopy. The majority of the meniscal problems in children are due to lateral discoid meniscus without any ligamentous lesion, which is the main difference between children and adults.

The initial management of these problems in children should be conservative, with operation reserved for those patients who do not improve, and the results are generally satisfactory for a long period, although considerable secondary osteoarthritic changes on the radiographs are unavoidable.

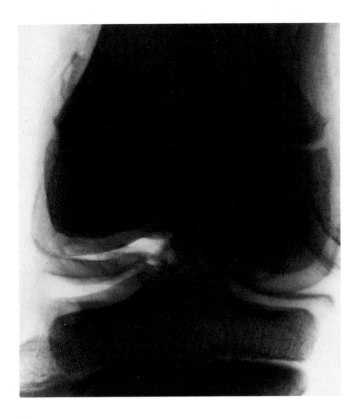

Figure 11

Clinically silent discoid (double-contrast arthrography).
No tear in the discoid meniscus or degeneration of the
articular cartilage was seen.

However, these secondary degenerative changes are
usually not related to the clinical symptoms.

When conservative treatment fails, total or partial
resection of the discoid meniscus is generally
indicated in children, but recent biomechanical
studies of knee function have revealed the importance of the menisci in load transmission—even if it
is discoid in shape as there are not only a number of
complete-type discoids which are clinically silent
without any tear or degeneration (Figure 11) but also
functional menisci which have been found acciden-
tally in older people. Therefore, partial resection of
the symptomatic discoid meniscus is being done for
the torn semilunar meniscus in adults and has been
reported with excellent results.

Adaptation of the residual rim of the discoid meniscus in partial resection could often be seen in this
series. Should the long-term results in partial resection of the discoid meniscus be as good as those of
total resection, this technique would be recommended for the treatment of symptomatic discoid
meniscus in children under the strict indications
described earlier.

However, when this procedure is performed for the
complete-type, extraordinarily thick discoid meniscus, there are some doubts concerning the long-term
results of this procedure as the arrangement of collagen fibres is different in the semilunar and complete-
type discoid meniscus[1] and it is possible that further
tearing or degeneration of the residual meniscus
could occur after surgery.

Resection of a thick and broad discoid meniscus
can cause a sudden change of articulation between
the lateral femoral condyle and the tibial plateau, and
after operation this change can cause repeated minor
trauma to the immature subchondral area of the
lateral femoral condyle of children in activities of
daily living and sports activities, which may become
the cause of this osteochondritis dissecans-like lesion.
However, as this lesion was observed in only a few
cases in a series of about 150, there could be other
intrinsic factors operating simultaneously. Long-term
follow-up is thus necessary for resection of discoid
meniscus in children.

References

1. **Amako T**, On the injuries of the menisci in the knee joint of
   Japanese, *J Jpn Orthop Assoc* (1960) **33**: 1289–1322.
2. **Smillie IS**, The congenital discoid meniscus, *J Bone Joint Surg*
   (1948) **30**: 671–682.
3. **Kaplan EB**, Discoid lateral meniscus of the knee joint: nature,
   mechanism and operative treatment, *J Bone Joint Surg (Am)*
   (1957) **39**: 77–87.
4. **Fujikawa K, Tomatsu T, Matsu K** et al., Morphological analysis of meniscus and articular cartilage in the knee joint by
   means of arthrogram, *J Jpn Orthop Assoc* (1978) **52**: 203–215.
5. **Fujikawa K, Iseki F, Mikura Y**, Partial resection of the discoid
   meniscus in the child's knee, *J Bone Joint Surg (Br)* (1981) **63**:
   391–395.

Bibliography

1. **Aarstrand T**, Treatment of meniscal rupture of the knee joint:
   a follow-up examination of material where only the ruptured
   part of the meniscus has been removed, *Acta Chir Scand* (1954)
   107: 146–157.
2. **Cargill AOR, Jackson JP**, Bucket-handle tear of the medial
   meniscus: a case for conservative surgery, *J Bone Joint Surg (Am)*
   (1976) **58**: 248–251.
3. **Cox JS, Nye CE, Schaefer WW** et al., The degenerative effects
   of partial and total resection of the medial meniscus in dogs'
   knees, *Clin Orthop* (1975) **109**: 178–183.
4. **Fairbank TJ**, Knee joint changes after meniscectomy, *J Bone
   Joint Surg (Br)* (1948) **30**: 664–670.
5. **Gray DJ, Gardner E**, Prenatal development of the human knee
   and superior tibio-fibular joint, *Am J Anat* (1950) **86**: 235–
   287.
6. **Ikeuchi H**, Total meniscectomy of the complete discoid meniscus under arthroscopic control. A case report, *J Jpn Orthop Ass*
   (1970) **44**: 374.
7. **Ikeuchi H**, Supplementary study of arthroscopic anatomy of
   the knee joint. Part 2: menisci, *J Jpn Orthop Ass* (1978) **52**:
   11–24.

8. Jackson JP, Degenerative changes in the knee after meniscectomy, *Br Med J* (1968) **2**: 525–527.

9. Kettelkamp DB, Jacobs AW, Tibiofemoral contact area-determination and implications, *J Bone Joint Surg (Am)* (1972) **54**: 349–356.

10. Kobayashi A, Discoid meniscus of the knee joint, *Clin Orthop Surg Jpn* (1975) **10**: 10–24.

11. McGinty JB, Geuss LF, Marvin RA, Partial or total meniscectomy: a comparative analysis, *J Bone Joint Surg (Am)* (1977) **59**: 763–766.

12. Mikura Y, Fujikawa K, Takeda T et al., Development of the human knee: special reference on the meniscal development, *J Joint Surg Jpn* (1985) **4**: 603–611.

13. Ritchie D, Meniscectomy in children, *J Bone Joint Surg (Br)* (1965) **47**: 596–597.

14. Seedhom BB, Hargreaves DJ, Transmission of the load in the knee joint with special reference to the role of the menisci. Part II. Experimental results, discussion and conclusion, *Eng Med* (1979) **8**: 220–228.

15. Takao T, An experimental study on the development of osteoarthritis of the knee joint with special reference to the degree of resection of the meniscus, *J Jpn Orthop Assoc* (1971) **45**: 731–742.

16. Yamauchi Y, Static research on the semilunar cartilage and ligament of the knee joint, *J Anat* (1933) **6**: 188–216.

12.3 Congenital discoid lateral meniscus in children: A long-term follow-up study and evolution of management

Paul M. Aichroth, Dipak V. Patel and Clare L. Marx

Young (1889) was the first to describe a discoid lateral meniscus in a cadaver specimen and the term 'snapping-knee syndrome' was attributed to this anomaly by Kroiss (1910).[1] The vague and intermittent symptoms caused by the presence of a discoid meniscus may produce difficulty and delay in the clinical diagnosis. Recently, arthroscopy has permitted more precise diagnosis of the lesion.[2-6] Arthroscopic examination confirms the clinical diagnosis of discoid meniscus, facilitates its morphological description and can identify an associated tear.[7]

On review of the literature, we found that this is the largest series of congenital discoid lateral menisci described, with a maximum follow-up of 18 years. The purpose of the present study was to report our experience with the arthroscopic assessment and overall strategy of management of the discoid lateral meniscus, and to determine the long-term clinical, functional and radiological results of operative treatment.

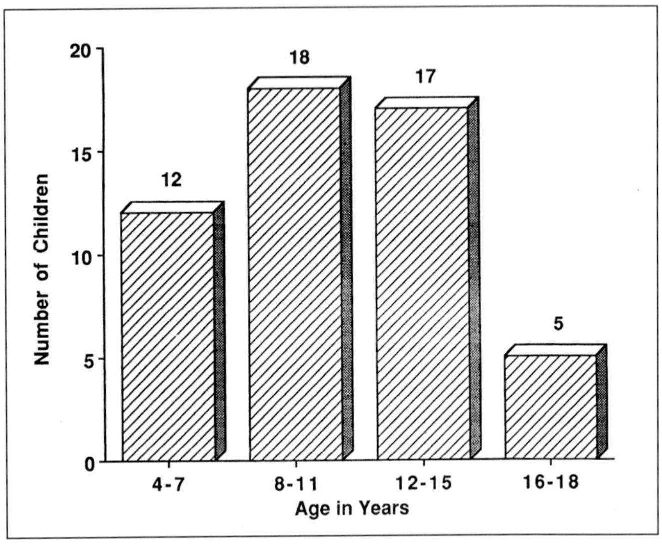

Material and methods

In the past 25 years, 52 children with 62 discoid lateral menisci were treated at the Hospital for Sick Children, Great Ormond Street, London, and at Westminster Children's Hospital, London. Their average age at the time of operation was 10.5 years (range 4–18 years). The age distribution of the children at the time of surgery is shown in Figure 1. The mean follow-up was 5.5 years (range 2–18 years). There were 28 boys and 24 girls. The right knee was involved in 27 cases and the left in 35. Ten children had bilateral discoid menisci. The duration between the onset of symptoms and the clinical diagnosis varied from 3 months to 96 months, the average being 24 months (Figure 2). This delay could possibly be attributed to the presence of intermittent symptoms or to the tolerance of meniscal anomalies by the children.

Figure 1

Age distribution of the children at operation.

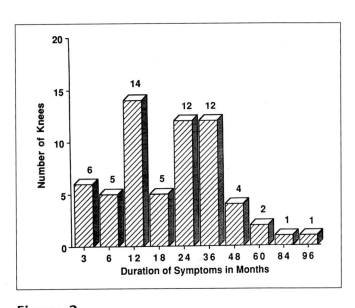

Figure 2

Duration of preoperative symptoms.

Preoperative clinical and radiological features

The details of the preoperative clinical symptoms are given in Table 1. Pain was the predominant symptom in the majority of the cases. Thirty children (36 knees) complained of click or clunk in the knee. However, on examination, the traditionally taught clunk so characteristic of the discoid meniscus was elicited in only 24 knees. Only 7 of the 17 knees which presented with the symptom of locking were actually found to be locked. Of these, 4 were persistent and 3 were intermittent. The details of the preoperative physical signs are shown in Table 2.

Routine anteroposterior, lateral and intercondylar ('tunnel') views were taken. Widening of the lateral joint space was seen in 5 knees and a sclerotic lateral tibial plateau was noted in 2. None of the radiographs showed squaring-off of the lateral femoral condyle. Cupping of the lateral tibial plateau was present in 3 knees. The most remarkable feature of this series was an associated osteochondritis dissecans affecting the lateral femoral condyle in 7 knees (Figure 3) and ossification defects involving the lateral femoral condyle in 4. The diagnosis of osteochondritis dissecans was confirmed at arthrotomy or arthroscopy in all 7 cases. The unstable fragment of osteochondritis dissecans was excised in 3 knees.

The diagnosis of the discoid meniscus was confirmed at arthrotomy in 18 children (treated before 1974) or by arthroscopy in the remaining 34 (treated after 1974). Arthrography was performed in some cases but in a small child this was not practical as a general anaesthesia was usually necessary for a good arthrogram. If a general anaesthetic is to be administered, then arthroscopic assessment is preferable. Magnetic resonance imaging was not performed in any of the children in our series.

At arthroscopy, the first indication of a discoid meniscus was the difficulty in entering the lateral compartment. Five children in our series were arthroscoped at other hospitals. In each case the operative records showed that the lateral compartment had been difficult to enter and the diagnosis of the discoid lateral meniscus had not been initially made. In such instances, it is advisable to use the medial portal first.

Several portals may be required for adequate visualization and probing of the discoid meniscus, especially for a Wrisberg-ligament type of the discoid (Figures 4 and 5). The skilful use of the probe is required to confirm the Wrisberg ligament attachment. The stability of the discoid and whether it is torn or not should be determined using a hook.

Arthrotomy/arthroscopy findings

There were 26 untorn and 36 torn discoid menisci. The untorn menisci had in many cases an attachment

Table 1 Preoperative clinical symptoms

Symptom	No. of knees
Pain	55
Click or clunk	36
Swelling	30
Locking	17
Giving way	12
Preceding injury	5

Table 2 Preoperative clinical signs

Physical sign	No. of knees
Locked knee	7
Joint-line tenderness	22
Effusion	12
Clunk	24
Patellar signs	4
No signs	12

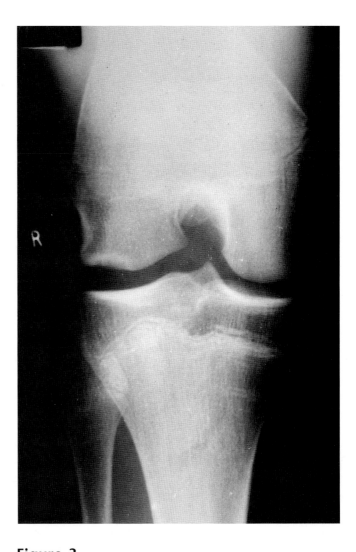

Figure 3

Osteochondritis dissecans of the lateral femoral condyle in a child with discoid lateral meniscus.

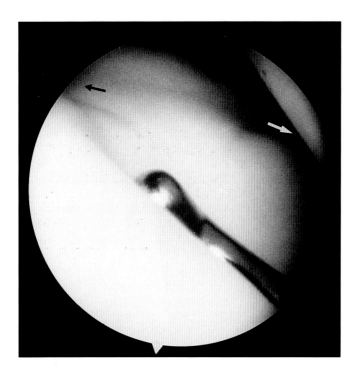

Figure 4

Wrisberg-ligament type of discoid. Black arrow shows attachment to the ligament of Wrisberg; white arrow indicates site of posterior instability.

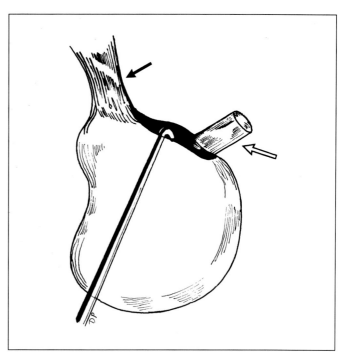

Figure 5

Diagram of the area seen in Figure 6. Black arrow shows attachment to the ligament of Wrisberg; open arrow indicates popliteus tendon.

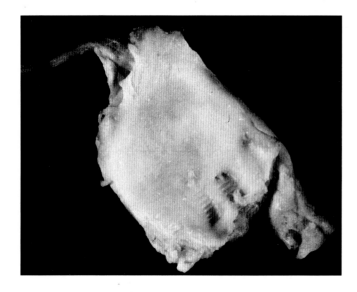

Figure 6

Pathological specimen of a discoid lateral meniscus with unusual attachment to the popliteus tendon.

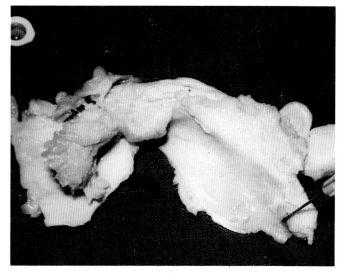

Figure 7

Specimen of a discoid lateral meniscus showing gross shredding and multiple tears.

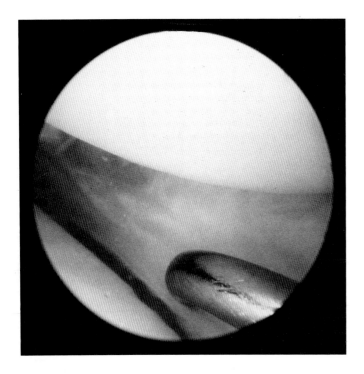

Figure 8

Arthroscopic appearance of the 'pseudomeniscus' following total lateral meniscectomy.

Table 3 The knee rating system (after Ikeuchi[5], Vandermeer and Cunningham[9])

Grade	Description
Excellent	No mechanical symptoms (click, locking), no pain, full range of movement
Good	No mechanical symptoms, occasional mild pain on motion, full range of movement
Fair	Mechanical symptoms, mild to moderate pain on motion, full range of movement
Poor	Mechanical symptoms, moderate to severe pain on motion or pain at rest, limitation of movement

Overall, 40 children (48 knees) in this study were treated by open total excision of the discoid and 6 had arthroscopic partial lateral meniscectomy. Six children (8 knees) with minimal clinical symptoms but arthroscopically proven untorn discoid meniscus were left alone.

Repeat arthroscopy

'Second-look' arthroscopies were performed in 4 knees, at an average of 18 months postoperatively (range 10–22 months). An adequate peripheral fibrous rim ('pseudomeniscus') was seen in 3 knees (Figure 8) and the popliteal tendon was found covered. No degenerative changes were noted in the lateral compartment.

Results

Clinical assessment

The results were analysed using Ikeuchi's grading system.[5,9] (Details in Table 3.) Results were excellent for 37% of the knees, good for 47% and fair for 16%. None of the knees had a poor result.

Of the 46 children treated by open total or arthroscopic partial lateral meniscectomy, 7 complained of mild to moderate pain and 5 complained of swelling on exertion. None of them presented with recurrent episodes of locking or giving way. On examination, none of the knees had persistent effusion or joint-line tenderness. They all had a full range of knee movement.

to the Wrisberg ligament as described by Watanabe et al.[6] and Dickhaut and DeLee;[8] however, these menisci had no posterior meniscotibial attachment and therefore were extremely unstable posteriorly, and the whole meniscus could be brought forwards on probing. An abnormal attachment to the popliteus tendon was noted in two cases (Figure 6).

Of the 36 torn discoid menisci, 7 were cystic and the tears were of various types including bucket-handle tears, longitudinal and horizontal tears. In 13 cases, the menisci were extremely shredded (Figure 7), producing gross symptoms and signs.

Treatment

In the pre-arthroscopy era, total excision of the meniscus was the only surgical treatment available. With the advent of arthroscopy, it became possible to differentiate between the various types of discoid menisci and deal with them accordingly.

In one child the pain was severe enough to warrant an arthroscopic assessment where no further abnormality was noted but an excellent 'pseudomeniscus' was seen. One child with bilateral discoid menisci and bilateral osteochondritis dissecans presented with a persistent, painless clunk in both knees.

Of the 6 children with intact discoid menisci who were left untreated, 2 had mild pain and 1 had a persistent clunk, at the time of latest review. One of them had a stable osteochondritis dissecans involving the lateral femoral condyle at arthroscopy.

Radiological assessment

Early degenerative changes (grade 1 Fairbank)[10] were seen in the lateral compartment in only 3 knees. These were older children (>16 years of age) with 11, 13 and 18 years of follow-up, respectively, after total meniscectomy. None of the radiographs showed narrowing of the joint space postoperatively. The osteochondritis dissecans lesion had healed spontaneously in 4 cases where the stable fragment was left in situ.

Discussion

The present series revealed several points of interest. Pain was the most common preoperative symptom rather than the conventionally taught clunk. The pain is most likely to be due to the abnormal movement of the meniscus as a result of the instability and its lack of posterior capsular attachment. On clinical examination, the classical clunk was present in only 39% of the knees.

We also noted that the clinical symptoms and signs of the discoid lateral meniscus are often vague and intermittent, causing considerable delay in presentation and accurate diagnosis. It is possible that the tolerance of the meniscal abnormalities by the children may have contributed to the delay.

Contrary to Picard,[11] we do not feel that radiographs play a significant role in diagnosis. In our series, only 5 knees had the classical lateral joint space widening which has been described in previous reviews.[7,8] It was noteworthy on plain radiographs that 7 children had osteochondritis dissecans of the lateral femoral condyle and a further 4 had ossification defects involving the lateral femoral condyle. The presence of such changes on the radiographs might well serve to alert the clinician to the possibility of a concurrent lateral meniscal abnormality.

We feel that because of the frequent necessity to administer a general anaesthetic in order to perform an arthrogram in a young child, and the often equivocal results, the child should be spared this investigation. Recently, Vandermeer and Cunningham

reviewed 22 patients (25 knees) with discoid lateral menisci.[9] In their series, the average age of the patients at the time of surgery was 31.9 years (range 2–61 years). They found arthrography to be of limited value, with only one-fourth yielding the correct preoperative diagnosis. We believe that the diagnosis and assessment of the discoid meniscus should be undertaken arthroscopically.

In the earlier part of our series (before 1979), the differentiation between Complete, Incomplete and the Wrisberg-ligament type of discoid meniscus was not possible owing to lack of awareness and the absence of preceding arthroscopy. Since then, our management protocol has evolved gradually. Currently, we follow the classification system suggested by Watanabe et al.[6] We became aware that the majority of the children treated in the past decade had Wrisberg-ligament type of discoid meniscus with posterior instability. This is in contrast to other series where no Wrisberg-ligament type of discoid lesions were reported.[9,12]

In the current series, 40 children (48 knees) with symptomatic torn discoid menisci underwent open total lateral meniscectomy. We certainly do not advocate open total lateral meniscectomy for all knees with discoid lateral meniscus. Various authors have recommended arthroscopic partial or total meniscectomy for discoid lateral menisci.[5,7–9,12,13] This is undoubtedly a good technique, but certainly demands considerable skill and experience. The difficulty of arthroscopic total meniscectomy for a lateral discoid meniscus resides in the resection of the anterior horn.[7] In fact, the earlier techniques described by Fujikawa et al. and Ikeuchi were semiarthroscopic meniscectomies.[5,13]

We suggest arthroscopic partial lateral meniscectomy for *torn*, Complete or Incomplete type of discoid menisci with stable posterior meniscotibial attachment. However, in children with Wrisberg-ligament type of lateral discoid, we believe that partial meniscectomy would be inappropriate as it would merely leave an unstable rim of the meniscus, which becomes symptomatic in the future. Therefore, a total meniscectomy is recommended in such circumstances.

Rosenberg et al. described a case report of arthroscopic peripheral attachment after central partial meniscectomy of a Wrisberg-ligament type of lateral discoid meniscus in a 19-year-old male athlete, with documentation of healing at 'second-look' arthroscopy 12 months following the surgery.[14] This is certainly an attractive concept which demands considerable technical expertise.

We noticed that after total lateral meniscectomy, an adequate 'pseudomeniscus' was seen arthroscopically in three knees. We are aware that some authors believe that regeneration of the discoid meniscus after total excision is unlikely to occur as the absence of the blood supply at the area of the popliteal tendon precludes the development of the meniscal tissue.[15,16] However, these studies were performed in cadaveric knee specimens of adult and elderly patients, and we believe that the child's knee behaves differently.

Total meniscectomy of a lateral non-discoid meniscus often leads to osteoarthritis.[10,17–19] This remains true for discoid menisci in adults as well. Our experience suggests that in children the results are different. Recently, Hayashi et al. reported that the axial alignment of the extensor mechanism and the pliability of the tissue may be forgiving in children, leading to reasonable adaptation of the knee to the stresses of activity.[12]

Hayashi et al. reviewed 53 discoid menisci treated by arthroscopic partial or total lateral meniscectomy, and found no degenerative changes at an average follow-up of 31.2 months.[12] Zaman and Leonard emphasized the hazards of total meniscectomy in children.[19] They reported the results of meniscectomy carried out on 59 knees, at an average follow-up of 7.5 years. In their series, early degenerative changes were seen in 19% of the knees on radiological examination. In our series, only 3 knees were noted to have early degenerative changes (grade I Fairbank) on radiological assessment at the time of latest review. As only 4 out of 62 knees had 'second-look' arthroscopy, we are unable to comment on the arthroscopic evidence of degenerative changes in the articular surfaces. Whether osteoarthritis will develop in any of these knees in future is a matter for conjecture.

Conclusions

Children with congenital discoid lateral menisci often present with vague and intermittent symptoms leading to considerable delay in the clinical diagnosis. In our series, pain was the major presenting symptom, but on examination the classic clunk was elicited in only 39% of the knees. Seven children had an associated osteochondritis dissecans involving the lateral femoral condyle.

We recommend arthroscopic examination at an earlier stage in a child presenting with recurrent symptoms of pain, click or clunk, swelling, locking or giving way suggestive of a meniscal abnormality. Arthroscopic partial lateral meniscectomy is indicated in children with symptomatic, *torn* discoid meniscus—Complete or Incomplete type—only when the posterior meniscotibial attachment of the discoid is found stable. In children with Wrisberg-ligament type of the discoid, a total meniscectomy is indicated.

Acknowledgments

Many of the early children described in this series were under the care of the late G.C. Lloyd-Roberts. We are grateful to Dina Stanford for her assistance. The authors would like to thank the Medical Photography Department at Westminster Hospital for their help with the illustrations.

References

1. **Kroiss F**, Die Verletzungen der Kniegelenkszwischenknorpel und ihrer Verbindungen, *Beitr Klin Chir* (1910) **66**: 598–801.
2. **Hayashi LK, Ida K, Oishi Y** et al., Arthroscopic management of discoid lateral meniscus in children, Paper read at the First Knee Section of the Western Pacific Orthopaedic Association Meeting, Penang, Malaysia, November 1987.
3. **Hayashi LK, Yamaga H, Hattori T** et al., Arthroscopic study on the lateral discoid meniscus tears, Paper read at the Sixtyninth Meeting of the Central Japanese Orthopaedic Association, Matsue, Japan, October 1987.
4. **Hayashi LK, Yamaga H, Mori R** et al., Clinical and arthroscopic study of discoid lateral meniscus in infants, *Central Jpn J Orthop Traumat Surg* (1987) **30**: 639–645.
5. **Ikeuchi H**, Arthroscopic treatment of the discoid lateral meniscus: technique and long-term results, *Clin Orthop* (1982) **167**: 19–28.
6. **Watanabe M, Takeda S, Ikeuchi H**, *Atlas of arthroscopy*, 3rd edn (Berlin: Springer-Verlag, 1979).
7. **Bellier G, Dupont Jean-Yves, Larrain M** et al., Lateral discoid menisci in children, *Arthroscopy* (1989) **5**(1): 52–56.
8. **Dickhaut SC, DeLee JC**, The discoid lateral-meniscus syndrome, *J Bone Joint Surg (Am)* (1982) **64**: 1068–1073.
9. **Vandermeer RD, Cunningham FK**, Arthroscopic treatment of the discoid lateral meniscus: results of long-term follow-up, *Arthroscopy* (1989) **5**(2): 101–109.
10. **Fairbank TJ**, Knee joint changes after meniscectomy, *J Bone Joint Surg (Br)* (1948) **30**: 664–670.
11. **Picard JJ**, Radiological aspects of the discoid menisci, *J Radiol Elect* (1964) **45**: 839–841.
12. **Hayashi LK, Yamaga H, Ida K** et al., Arthroscopic meniscectomy for discoid lateral meniscus in children, *J Bone Joint Surg (Am)* (1988) **70**: 1495–1500.
13. **Fujikawa K, Iseki F, Mikura Y**, Partial resection of the discoid meniscus in the child's knee, *J Bone Joint Surg (Br)* (1981) **63**: 391–395.
14. **Rosenberg TD, Paulos LE, Parker RD** et al., Discoid lateral meniscus: case report of arthroscopic attachment of a symptomatic Wrisberg-ligament type, *Arthroscopy* (1987) **3**(4): 277–282.
15. **Arnoczky SP, Warren RF**, Microvasculature of the human meniscus, *Am J Sports Med* (1982) **10**: 90–95.
16. **Danzig L, Resnick D, Gonsalves M** et al., Blood supply to the normal and abnormal menisci of the human knee, *Clin Orthop* (1983) **172**: 271–276.
17. **Kurozawa H, Koide K, Nakajima H**, Results of meniscectomy, *Orthop Surg* (1976) **27**: 825–832.
18. **Manzione M, Pizzutillo PD, Peoples AB** et al., Meniscectomy in children: a long-term follow-up study, *Am J Sports Med* (1983) **11**: 111–115.
19. **Zaman M, Leonard MA**, Meniscectomy in children: results in 59 knees, *Injury* (1981) **12**: 425–428.

Fractures around the knee

13.1 Fractures around the knee: An overview

Mason Hohl

In this chapter the background and management of supracondylar fractures of the femur and tibial plateau fracture are covered, emphasizing the problems that through the years have frustrated surgeons in closed and open treatment of these fractures. Although rigid internal fracture fixation is favored, the difficulties of applying modern fixation techniques in the elderly osteoporotic patient are recognized. Other means of managing fractures must be in the armamentarium of fracture surgeons.

The succinct review of repair of articular cartilage after fracture damage should be known by all who treat joint fractures. I give much credit to Haldeman who, in 1939, studied defects of articular cartilage in dogs, and noted repair by fibrocartilage only when the subchondral bone was fractured. Dr Vernon Luck and I noted in a primate study of articular cartilage defects in subchondral bone, simulating fracture, that these healed by pannus emanating from the bone and synovial tissues. If the knee was immobilized in a cast for 2 months, scar tissue encompassed much of the affected compartment. On the other hand, if the monkey was permitted cage ambulation with active knee movement, scar tissue was not a feature and the articular defect healed by a hyaline cartilage-like tissue. This observation established in our mind the necessity of promoting movement in fractured joints. In the 1950s the only way to accomplish this was treatment in traction. Developments in internal fixation materials and techniques have made possible the rigid fixation of many fractures about the knee joint, allowing early joint mobilization. Many other investigators have contributed to this science, among them Salter, whose concept of continuous passive motion is being used clinically.

The important principles in the treatment of fractures about the knee are accurate articular reconstruction, restoration of joint stability and early knee movement.

Supracondylar fractures

The AO classification of supracondylar fractures is comprehensive and should be used today in preference to others that have been popular in the past. It lends itself well to the principles and techniques of open reduction and aids communication between clinicians.

Socioeconomic factors now dictate operative treatment whenever possible, to decrease hospital expense. The argument against open techniques is discussed in detail, leaving readers to make their own conclusions. One of these arguments concerns the difficulties of internal fixation in the elderly osteoporotic patient.

Preoperative planning is emphasized as the secret of consistently good reduction and rigid fixation with a condylar screw device. The importance of accurate reduction of the intercondylar fracture is obvious and can be obtained as a rule with the femoral distractor condylar screw fixation. The best way of dealing with the comminuted distal femoral metaphysis, whether by anatomic reduction and grafting or by collapsing the fragments into the most stable position and fixing shaft to the condyles, is an interesting debate. I believe that closing dead space with living bone, especially in older individuals, is preferable to anatomic reduction and bone grafting.

Postoperative management is the key to obtaining a good functional result when it is considered that operative reduction adds much soft-tissue dissection to the fracture damage and this combination evokes a great healing reaction that tends to cause permanent loss of knee movement. Certainly, continuous passive motion or at least early active movement is the key to a good functional result after supracondylar fracture.

Tibial plateau fractures

The important background subjects in relation to mechanism of production of plateau fractures and associated soft tissue injuries are covered. Among the important points with which I agree is that meniscal injuries are likely to be found in larger numbers of plateau fractures with the advent of magnetic resonance imaging and arthroscopy. Some injury to the menisci will probably be found in more than 50% of patients. I fully endorse preserving the meniscus unless it has been irreparably damaged.

Ligament injuries, on the other hand, have been well documented to occur in nearly 25% of plateau fractures. Diagnosis of ligament injury should be made early and I believe that collateral ligament injuries should be repaired along with the bony injury to stabilize the knee.

There is little doubt that within the next decade a universally acceptable method of classifying fractures will be adopted. The AO group has made a promising start in this direction and with some modification it shows promise of allowing clinical researchers to communicate about results with greater specificity. Meanwhile I favor a classification that is simple and names fracture types logically.

Concerning examination of the knee, I believe that there is much to be learned by knowing whether there is tenderness at ligament attachments and whether the knee is clinically unstable. Of course, instability is usually due to bony instability or depression, and if the knee is unstable a stress radiograph will essentially demonstrate whether there is ligament incompetence. Tomograms are certainly very satisfactory for local compression or split compression fractures but are very difficult to interpret in bicondylar fractures. Computed tomography scans are especially useful for seeing articular displacement in axial projections.

Treatment considerations must include the restoration of stability to the knee. Therefore, it is important to know whether there is instability before a decision about treatment is made. One must not forget the Rasmussen contribution, that if surgery is performed only on unstable plateau fractures with the objective of restoring stability the results will be very satisfactory. Surgical indications include 8–10 mm of depression of the joint surface, widening of the tibial condyles or meniscal interposition. I add the indication of restoring joint stability when stress testing reveals instability.

The difficulties of reconstructing bicondylar fractures is emphasized, and two plates should not be used unless absolutely necessary. The main problem, aside from accurate reduction, is wound healing.

Experienced surgeons obtain better results with fewer problems than inexperienced surgeons, as noted in several articles. Also, medial plateau fractures had fewer good results.

Among the newer approaches to treating plateau fractures is the arthroscope, which can allow direct visualization of the articular damage and associated soft tissue injuries. A tourniquet may be advisable if the procedure is done within a few hours of injury, or if cleaning out of clots and debris causes much bleeding. Percutaneous cancellous screw fixation is described for split fractures. For depressed fractures the use of iliac bone grafts is suggested. The trend in the United States has been to use sterile bank bone to fill defects and to add mechanical stability.

Schatzker's series had 27% complications after operative treatment. It was noted that instability led to a high incidence of post-traumatic arthritic change.

The treatment of tibial plateau fractures emphasizes reconstruction of joint surfaces, restoration of knee alignment and repair of soft tissue injuries. Whatever treatment method is used, it should permit early movement of the knee joint.

13.2   Fractures around the knee

Timothy D. Bunker

Despite recent advances in classification, planning, approach, fixation and assessment, the distal femoral fracture remains a severe challenge to the fracture surgeon, particularly when the patient is old and frail and the bone weak and slow healing. This contribution will look at the recent developments in the management of distal femoral fractures from basic science to clinical results.

Tibial plateau fractures have always been a source of controversy to the fracture surgeon. In particular, the debate about conservative versus operative management is bound to engender a heated exchange whenever two orthopaedic surgeons meet. Recent advances have been in the field of preoperative assessment, tomography, computed tomography (CT) scanning and in particular three-dimensional CT scanning; minimally invasive and percutaneous arthroscopically controlled reduction and fixation; and finally postoperative assessment.

The ideal of management of fractures around the knee should strive to preserve motion, alignment and the soft tissues while preventing complications, particularly infection and neurovascular impairment.

Fracture healing in the knee

The knee is anatomically the most complex of the major weight-bearing joints. The knee differs from the hip and ankle in that it lacks bony congruity, particularly in the saddle-shaped lateral compartment. Because of this, knee function depends on the shape of the menisci, a complex system of ligaments, and the coordination of ten musculotendinous units which cross the joint. An injury severe enough to fracture the bone around the knee may damage menisci, ligaments and muscle, adding to the complexity of reconstruction. Thus the fracture surgeon must also be a knee surgeon, understanding the complexity of the anatomy and function of the soft tissues of the knee, and not base treatment solely on the radiographic appearance of the knee.

This contribution will discuss in most detail intra-articular fractures of the knee, for these are the most difficult to manage. In 1850, Sir James Paget wrote

'There are no instances . . . in which a wounded piece of cartilage has been repaired with new and well formed cartilage in the human subject.' However, recent experimental evidence has shown that perfect healing with hyaline (Type II) cartilage can occur in both mature and immature small mammals after accurate fixation and joint movement. Salter et al.[1] used the model of the intra-articular fracture in the rabbit knee, which was then rigidly fixed with a lag screw. The rabbits were split into three groups. Those treated in plaster had grossly limited motion and easily visible fracture lines at 4 weeks; those caged had a normal range of motion but visible fracture; those on continuous motion had a full range of movement and in 80% the fracture line had disappeared.

Mitchell and Shepard[2] studied intra-articular fracture healing in mature rabbits. Three groups were studied: incomplete reduction, adequate but non-rigid fixation, and finally accurate rigid fixation with compression. The results were studied at 7 weeks to 1 year with transmission and scanning electron microscopy. The first two groups healed with fibrocartilage but the rigidly fixed group healed with tissue which by electron microscopy appeared to be Type II hyaline cartilage. These animal studies suggest that the surgeon should attempt to accurately reconstruct the joint surface and rigidly fix the fracture with interfragmentary compression in order to allow early joint excursion in man.

The knee, however, is a privileged site. It has been shown that the thickness of articular cartilage is directly proportional to the incongruity of the joint. Thus the knee has the thickest cartilage of the major weight-bearing joints, and by implication the greatest reserve. The knee is also privileged in having intra-articular menisci that appear to protect the hyaline cartilage beneath them, which also means that the joint normally functions as a hyaline cartilage-to-fibrocartilage articulation as well as a hyaline-to-hyaline cartilage articulation. This may have implications in articular surface repair, particularly under the lateral meniscus in lateral plateau fractures, where Hohl and Luck[3] showed macroscopically and microscopically that defects in the tibial plateau in rhesus monkeys filled in with fibrocartilage. Similar observations have been made in humans with arthrography[4] and arthrotomy.[5] This may be the basis on which radiological results are not always directly proportional to functional results following fractures in the knee. Burri et al.[6] showed that in the hands of an inexperienced surgeon radiological results were good, yet clinically 22% of patients needed a stick to walk, mainly as a result of excision of the lateral meniscus in order to visualize the fracture of the tibial plateau.

The argument that the knee may be forgiving is not an excuse for neglecting fractures around the knee, or for treating them with any lack of precision, but is stated mainly as a plea to preserve the soft tissues of the knee at the same time as treating the fracture, so that early movement of the knee can be instituted to prevent stiffness while the fracture management protects against malunion and malalignment.

Classification of supracondylar fractures

Many different systems of classification have been used for supracondylar fractures. In the literature the most commonly used is that of Neer et al.,[7] in which there are three groups. The first group is that of minimal displacement; the second is with displacements of the condyles, either medially (2a) or laterally (2b); the third group is a conjoined supracondylar and shaft fracture. The problem with this classification is that it is rather simplistic and does not address the unicondylar fractures or the extra-articular supracondylar fractures.

Giles et al.[8] have used Seinsheimer's classification of fractures, which divides the fracture into four groups. The first group is an undisplaced supracondylar fracture; the second is a displaced supracondylar fracture with no intra-articular element; the third is an intra-articular fracture of either one condyle or both condyles; and the fourth group is comminuted intra-articular fracture but also includes fractures of the edges of the condyles which come through the articular surface rather than through the intercondylar notch.

Perhaps the best method of classification of these fractures is now the AO classification.[9] The reason for this is that it is comprehensive, it is understandable, and the prognosis and outcome varies from good to poor as the classification increases. Thus the prognosis for A1 extra-articular, supracondylar, minimally displaced, simple fracture is good, whereas the prognosis for a C3 multifragmentary, intra-articular and shaft fracture is poor.

The AO classification divides fractures of the supracondylar femur into three clear sections. The first or A series is an extra-articular fracture, varying from A1, simple, to A2, metaphyseal wedge, to A3 metaphyseal complex.

The B series is a partial articular fracture: B1, lateral condyle sagittal; B2, medial condyle sagittal; B3, condyle fracture in the frontal plane.

The C group of the AO classification is a complete articular fracture. C1 is articular simple, metaphyseal simple; C2 is articular simple, metaphyseal multifragmentary; C3 is multifragmentary.

However, all classifications fall down in that they only describe the radiographic appearance of the fracture and do not describe the patient. This is relevant in particular to supracondylar fractures, where there is a great difference in the prognosis for the fit, healthy motorcyclist compared to the porotic 90-year-old lady.

Most surgeons would now have no hesitation in recommending open reduction and internal fixation followed by early joint movement in a fit, young motorcyclist with good quality bone. However, decision making is far more difficult in the elderly lady who has a minimally displaced fracture with grossly porotic bone. The problem here is not the fracture but the quality of the bone, as there is a very high incidence of failure to hold the fracture with internal fixation in poor-quality bone in a patient who no longer has the coordination or the will to touch weight bear. Unfortunately, the alternative treatment of traction in such an elderly patient is not without problems of its own in terms of systemic complications and pressure sores.

Investigation

In the majority of patients, following a careful clinical examination of peripheral perfusion, sensibility and motor power, the only investigation required is a good-quality anteroposterior and lateral radiograph of the knee and the distal femur. The interpretation of these radiographs is not quite as straightforward as it would seem and Neer et al.[7] have shown in cadaver studies how a small amount of displacement can be interpreted as an anterior tilt of the distal femur due to the pull of gastrocnemius when in fact it is a rotational projection of the X-ray beam. In the severely comminuted fracture, a radiograph of the normal side is required for fracture-planning purposes.

Injury to the femoral or popliteal artery is a well-known complication of this particular fracture. However, Stewart et al.,[10] in a review of 442 patients, state that major nerve or vascular injury is uncommon in this fracture and they had seven patients requiring amputation, two with severe mangling injuries and vascular injuries, one caused by a shotgun blast into the popliteal fossa and one with a comminuted ipsilateral tibial fracture with vascular insufficiency. In Neer's series of 100 patients, one patient had a severed popliteal artery as the fracture exited under the arch of adductor magnus, where the artery is bound to the shaft. In patients in whom vascular insufficiency is considered clinically, an arteriogram or digital subtraction angiography should be immediately performed.

Treatment

There has been a great debate in the orthopaedic literature upon whether supracondylar fractures should be treated by closed methods or by surgical methods. This debate is clearly naive, for, as has already been stated, the choice of management depends not only upon the fracture but also upon the patient, the patient's age, motivation and bone quality. Not all of these factors can be assessed from radiographs, and this is where the clinical skills of the experienced fracture surgeon take over.

Advances in the management of fractures take a surprisingly long time to filter through into quality publications. For this reason papers which are now only of historical interest may often hold sway in fracture decision making. In particular, the paper of Stewart from the Campbell Clinic has biased the management of supracondylar fractures of the femur for over a generation and, as Colton puts it, 'the ghost of Stewart's paper still haunts orthopaedic mythology'.[11] Stewart's paper recommending non-operative treatment for supracondylar fractures needs to be seen in context. Firstly, a glance at the illustrations from the paper will show that the methods of internal fixation were appropriate at the time in the 1940s and 1950s, the period upon which the paper is based, but today would be regarded as entirely historical. None of the fixations was of a rigid nature as championed by the AO group. The second reason for regarding this paper as historical is that the results were graded as good if the patient had only occasional pain, a slight limp or slight arthritis, and fair if the patient had less than 90° of flexion. Today's patient would in no way consider such an outcome fair or good.

The three reasons quoted against open reduction and internal fixation of supracondylar fractures are inadequate fixation, infection, and a high incidence of non-union. Inadequate fixation remains the greatest problem in osteoporotic patients, those in the elderly group. The most adequate form of fixation is the AO dynamic condylar screw or Richards supracondylar screw device, both of which have the security of interfragmentary compression of intercondylar fractures as well as a strong plate to join the condylar section to the shaft. However, these depend on the hold of the screws in the cortical bone.

Methods attempted to give a stronger fix in porotic bone have been the use of an AO nut on the end of the screw, but this involves dissection of the medial side of the bone and further stripping of muscle, and injection of methyl methacrylate cement down the screw tracks prior to screw insertion in the condyles and the diaphysis (keeping the fracture clear of cement as this tends to delay union). Finally, the use of a plastic Gallanaugh plate on the medial side, into which the screws may be passed, does add to fracture stability but once more requires further stripping of quadriceps from the distal shaft and medial side of the femur.

Deliberate non-rigid fixation can be used in extra-articular fractures, such as Rush nails, Ender's nails or the Zikel supracondylar device. Use of the Zikel device has been published by Wilde et al.,[12] who treated 21 cases over a 3-year period. Six of their patients were young, 13 were elderly patients with minor trauma and 2 had metastatic malignant fractures. The functional results were considered excellent in 10, good in 6 and poor in 5. There were two cases of superficial wound infections. All cases united after 3–6 months. The best functional results were in those patients below 60 years of age or with a pathological fracture.

In the majority of series, the infection rate for open reduction and internal fixation of supracondylar fractures varies from 0 to 5.8%. The highest incidence is in the paper of Olerud,[13] who reported on the extended approach using what has been termed 'the inverted Mercedes Benz incision' for severe type C supracondylar fractures. Obviously, in a limited series of markedly severe fractures treated by an extended open approach, the incidence will be higher than in series which include minimally displaced simple fractures that can be treated through a short incision with short surgical times. In 16 patients, one developed osteomyelitis, one was termed a metallosis, though the authors felt that this might have been a low-grade infection, there was one septic arthritis and there was one tibial infection.

The last reported reason against open reduction and internal fixation has been a high incidence of non-union. However, this high incidence has drifted downwards from the historical papers of Stewart and Neer, who both quote a 14% incidence of non-union with historical methods of non-rigid internal fixation. This has become a non-union rate of zero in recent papers on AO fixation such as those of Giles et al.[8] and Olerud.[13] With modern forms of internal fixation the non-union rate is now lower following internal fixation than following non-operative management.

Non-operative treatment

Two forms of traction have been championed. The first form is the double pin technique as reported by Stewart, Sisk and Wallace[10] and the second, and easier, form of traction is the tibial pin traction as reported by Neer, Grantham and Shelton.[7]

Stewart et al. state that there are four large muscle groups which influence the fracture position during traction and treatment.[10] The quadriceps and hamstrings produce longitudinal tension, which tends to shorten the fracture; more importantly gastrocnemius may cause angulation of the distal femur owing to the strong force it imparts through its origin in the popliteal fossa to this distal fragment. Finally, the adductors may cause a valgus deformity by pulling the proximal fragment in a varus direction, whereas they do not influence the distal fragment, causing a valgus malunion at the fracture site.

Stewart et al. suggested that treatment should be by a tibial pin with the pull of 67 N (15 lb) in the line of the femur. There is indication for a second wire placed transversely through the femoral condyles at the level of the superior pole of the patella if the periosteum and soft tissues on the posterior side of the femur are disrupted, producing the tendency towards posterior angulation or rotation of the distal fragment. Provided that the skin is clean and strict sterile technique is used, the authors do not hesitate to pass the wire through a comminuted or even an open fracture.

Neer suggested that treatment by a simple tibial pin was effective in the majority of cases. Moreover, he suggested that traction with the knee fully flexed was not often required, as uncontrolled flexion of the distal fragment caused by the pull of gastrocnemius was not seen in his study except when the impact of injury or the overriding femoral shaft had tilted the distal segment. Neer elegantly showed how a false radiographic appearance of flexion of the distal fragment could be produced by rotation of the fragment, and this is shown by radiograph studies of cadaver osteotomies in his paper. In contradistinction to Stewart's paper, Neer found that the commonest deformity encountered was inward rotation and varus of the distal segment. Neer concluded that uncontrollable flexion of the distal segment is an exaggerated concept, inviting unnecessarily complicated treatment.

Surgical management of supracondylar fractures

The rationale of open reduction and internal fixation of supracondylar fractures lies in the fact that rigid internal fixation circumvents the problems of malunion and allows early movement of the joint and early mobilization of patients and their return to the community (Figure 1).

Fracture planning

Prior to embarking on open reduction and internal fixation, the procedure should be planned by drawing the fragments separately on pieces of tracing paper and reassembling the fracture on paper (Figure 2). This may be aided either by using a reversed outline of the uninjured femur or by using the AO templates of the normal anatomical axis of the knee. It is important when planning the fixation of this fracture that correct alignment of the leg is achieved. Templates of the fixation device, usually the AO dynamic condylar screw, are then placed under the assembled fracture and copied into place. From this the various screw positions can be worked out and it can be determined which should be lag screws and which will act as neutralization screws. Areas needing grafting can be assessed so that the patient is prepared with access to the iliac crest or not as required. It is far better when embarking on what can be quite technically difficult fracture fixations to have gone through the process preoperatively on paper so that any problems may be anticipated both by the surgeon and by the scrub team.

Prophylactic intravenous wide-spectrum antibiotics are used in high dose at induction and for two doses postoperatively.

Incision

The incision runs along the lateral border of the distal thigh, starting to pass obliquely at some 5 cm above the knee, to run along the lateral retinaculum of the patella and then down along the lateral border of the patellar tendon and lateral to the tibial tuberosity.

The old 'inverted Mercedes Benz' approach is no longer used for fixation of this fracture as it led to too high a complication rate, with skin necrosis in the centre of the Y.

The fascia lata and lateral patellar retinaculum is divided in the line of the skin incision. The superior lateral genicular vessels are ligated and divided, and the quadriceps is taken forward, exposing the distal femur. If the fracture has an intra-articular component, the synovium of the knee joint is opened and the knee is exposed. The exposure can be extended either by performing an osteotomy of the tibial tubercle and lifting a plug of bone with the patellar tendon after it has been predrilled and tapped, or by performing the Olerud oblique extra-articular patellar osteotomy. Using either of these techniques, the whole of the distal femur can be fully exposed.

Operative method

Fracture reduction may be assisted by placing the AO femoral distractor from the shaft of the femur above the fracture to the tibial metaphysis. This allows gentle traction upon the fracture and also has the advantage of holding the fracture in a relatively stable configuration while the initial lag screws are

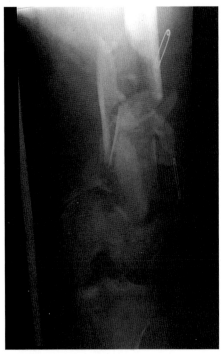

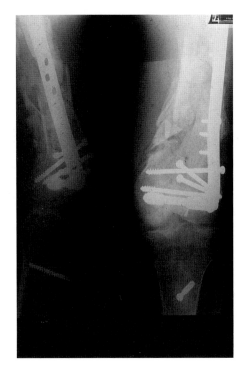

a   b

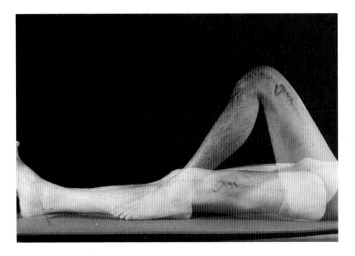

c

Figure 1

(a) A severe distal femoral fracture. (b) Treated by extended approach with tibial tubercle osteotomy and biological fixation with bone grafting. (c) Following early movement.

inserted. There is now a move towards the Jeff Mast technique of biological fixation. This involves careful exposure and reconstruction of the intra-articular fragments with lag screws and the cross-screw of the dynamic condylar screw, followed by the use of the blade of the dynamic condylar screw to attach the reassembled condylar fragments to the undamaged diaphysis of the femur above the fracture in the correct rotation and alignment but without any attempt at anatomical reduction of the comminuted metaphyseal portion of the supracondylar fracture (Figure 3). In so doing, this comminuted section is not stripped of its blood supply from the periosteum and quadriceps but is grafted and allowed to heal

naturally. The dynamic condylar screw acts to maintain length and alignment and allows knee joint movement while nature heals the comminuted portion of the fracture.

Postoperative management

Following open reduction and internal fixation, the limb is rested in the 90°/90° position on three pillows or is placed on a continuous passive motion machine. Early supervised active and passive mobilization of the knee joint is instituted as soon as is possible according to the patient's postoperative pain and

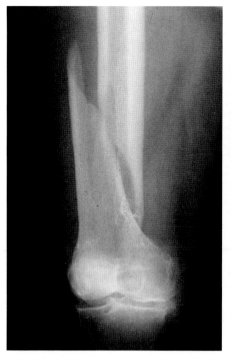

a

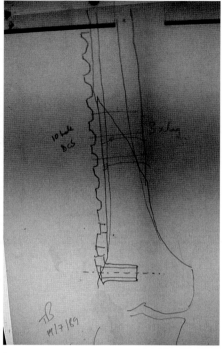

b

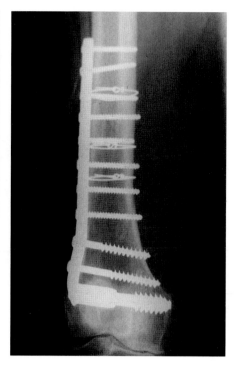

c

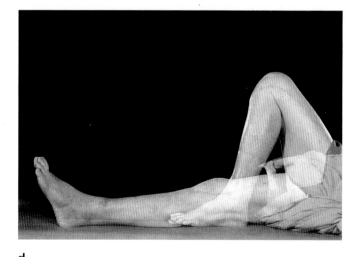

d

Figure 2

(a) Simple supracondylar fracture in an elderly lady. (b) Plan devised to fix the fracture. (c) Plan turned in reality. (d) A good range of movement is obtained.

tolerance. Depending on the classification of the fracture and the rigidity of the internal fixation, the patient is then allowed up, touch weight bearing with crutches, for a period of 6 weeks and then partial weight bearing for 3 months. Radiographic control is instituted postoperatively and at 6 weeks and 3 months, and beyond that as needed (Figure 4).

Results of treatment

Methods of treatment have evolved and improved so much that there is now no point in comparing opera-

tive with non-operative treatment. Therefore, it is best to look at the 'gold standard' papers in the literature in an historical context and to report on these results in the context of the fractures treated not as a comparison of one method of treatment against another.

Stewart, Sisk and Wallace[10]

The review consisted of 422 fractures of the distal third of the femur seen at the Campbell clinic over a 20-year period. Of these, 213 were followed for 1 year or longer and 144 of these were by closed methods.

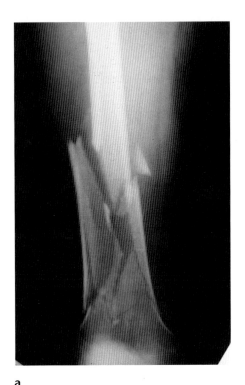
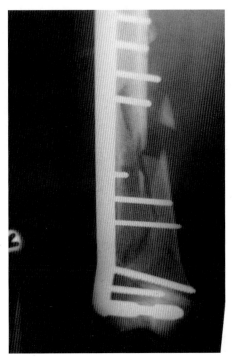

a   b

Figure 3

(a) Comminuted supracondylar fracture. (b) Fracture treated with biological
fixation.

Results were excellent or good for 67% and rated as
fair or poor for 33%. One-third of the patients in the
closed group were treated by plaster immobilization
only and two-thirds by skeletal traction. The results
were the same with both methods.

Those patients treated with skeletal traction stayed
an average of 62 days in hospital and clinical stability was usually achieved in 5–8 weeks.

Neer, Grantham and Shelton[7]

These authors studied 110 cases treated between 1942
to 1966 in New York. Of these patients 71 were
treated by traction or plaster and the patients were
assessed on a 100-point chart, function being given
70 units and anatomy 30 units. An excellent result
was above 85 units, satisfactory was above 70 units
and failure was below 55 units. These authors
concluded that closed treatment yielded satisfactory
results in 90% of the patients evaluated and in 84%
of those with displaced supracondylar fractures.
However, it should be noted that Neer states that
most patients were satisfied so long as they had
strong extensor power and could flex the knee to 70°,

which enabled them to walk on stairs normally,
while a lesser range of flexion forced them to climb
the stairs sideways. It is unlikely that patients now
would consider knee flexion of only 70° satisfactory.
Average hospital stay was 60 days. The most common
deformity was one of varus and internal rotation.

The authors conclude that the prognosis regarding
range of motion and development of arthritic change
in the knee joint could be estimated with considerable accuracy at the end of 1 year. Whilst the range
of motion improved beyond expectation during the
initial 9 months, it did not increase more than 20°
between the ends of the first and second years after
injury. Arthritic changes were evident on radiographs
at 1 or 2 years.

Mize, Bucholz and Grogan[14]

Thirty supracondylar fractures were stabilized using a
95° condylar plate according to the standard AO
recommendations. Evaluation was based on the criteria of Schatzker and Lambert. Excellent rating
required loss of flexion of less than 10°, full extension, no varus, valgus or rotatory deformity, no pain

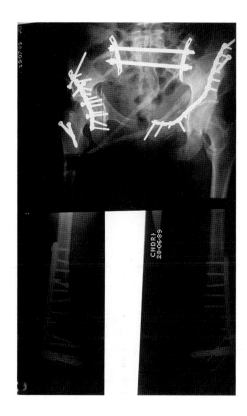

Figure 4

A complex fracture fixation allowing early postfracture mobilization.

and perfect joint congruency. Good meant not more than one of the following: loss of flexion of more than 20°; loss of extension of more than 10°; varus or valgus deformity of more than 10°; or minimum pain. Fair meant any two of the criteria listed in the good category. Failure meant any of the following: flexion to 90° or less; varus or valgus deformity exceeding 15°; joint incongruency; or disabling pain no matter how perfect the radiographic appearance.

In this series 14 had an excellent result, 10 had a good result, 5 had a fair result and there was one failure. Fracture union occurred in all limbs. One patient had a deep infection and union was delayed. Time to full weight bearing averaged 4 months. There were two malunions, both being valgus deformities, one of 5° and one of 10°; both of these patients were elderly women with advanced osteoporosis.

Giles, DeLee, Heckman and Keever[8]

These authors reported on 26 patients using the AO supracondylar blade plate. All the fractures united. The average hospital stay was 7 days. Time to full weight bearing without protection averaged 3.7 months. The average range of postoperative knee motion was 120°. Three patients failed to achieve full extension of the knee and only three patients had less than 100° of knee flexion, one of whom had had a previous patellectomy with a stiff knee prior to fracture. In only one patient was reduction lost due to severely osteopenic bone. In no patient was traumatic arthritis evident clinically or radiologically.

Tibial plateau fractures

Classification

The usual form of injury to the tibial plateau is a combination of axial loading and valgus with the knee straight, causing the lateral femoral condyle to crush or split the lateral tibial plateau.[15] Fractures thus occur usually to the lateral plateau; the split or compressive elements may occur alone or in the more severe fracture they may occur together. The incidence of associated meniscal injury varies from 17% to 85%. Schatzker[16] found 16 meniscal tears in 70 patients: 14 of these tears were peripheral and could be repaired. Sometimes the meniscus may prolapse within the split component of the fracture and this interposition prevents closed reduction of the fracture. All authors agree that the meniscus must be preserved if at all possible.

Associated ligament damage is surprisingly uncommon. This is because the forces which cause the fracture are compressive rather than distractive. This was confirmed experimentally on cadavers by Kennedy and Bailey.[17] The incidence of ligament damage varies from 4% to 25%. Generally, joint instability following plateau fracture is caused by residual joint surface depression rather than ligament rupture.

Rasmussen and Sørensen[18] stated that collateral and cruciate tears were of minor importance compared to bony deformity. They also felt that the soft-tissue fibrosis occurring around the knee during fracture healing often led to ligamentous stability.

Roberts[15] found in 5 of 9 patients in whom the medial collateral ligament was diagnosed but not repaired a degree of instability of the knee at follow-up. Schatzker et al.[16] state that repair of ruptured collateral ligaments is essential for stability. However, Porter[19] detected anterior cruciate laxity in 6 out of 137 patients under review; none had been noted primarily and only one was significant.

Various classifications have been used for tibial plateau fractures. The commonest is that of Hohl and Luck.[3] In their study, 24% had an undisplaced fracture; 26% a local compression fracture; 26% a combination of split and compression; and the others fell into three groups—total condylar depression, split and comminuted. Roberts,[15] Porter,[19] Rasmussen and Sørensen[18] and Schatzker et al.[16] have all described their own methods of classification, but the fracture patterns are similar.

The AO group have classified fractures of the proximal tibia in a very understandable way. The A series of fractures of the tibia are extra-articular, and these will not be discussed here. The B series are the three simple forms of tibial plateau fractures, B1 being a pure split, B2 a pure depression and B3 the combination of split and depression. This accounts for over 75% of all tibial fractures. Group C are complete articular fractures, C1 being a simple articular fracture and simple metaphyseal fracture, C2 the articular simple but the metaphyseal multifragmentary, and C3 multifragmentary or comminuted.

The healing of tibial plateau fractures

There is controversy whether joint surface depression seen on radiographs corresponds to actual joint surface cartilagenous depression following healing. Hohl and Luck[3] created a depressed tibial fracture in rhesus monkeys and showed both microscopically and macroscopically that the defect filled in with a fibrocartilage. Similar observations have been made in humans, using arthrography[4] and arthrotomy.[5] Drennan et al.[20] and Porter[19] speculated that this infilling may account for good functional results in the face of radiographic depression. However, Schatzker et al.[16] stated that there was no evidence that articular defects could fill in.

There is a direct correlation between the depth of radiographic depression and prognosis. Porter[19] found that results in patients with minimal depression were good, those with less than 10 mm of depression were nearly all acceptable (28 out of 29); those with between 10 and 14 mm of depression were acceptable in two-thirds (15 out of 21); but those with more than 14 mm of joint depression were unacceptable in one-third of the cases (8 unacceptable out of 28).

Hohl and Luck[3] found that patients with under 1 cm of depression had 77% excellent results whereas those with over 1 cm had only 61% acceptable results. This has to be taken in the light of the grading which was used in 1956, where a 90° total range of motion was considered good, whereas this may not be considered good in modern fracture practice.

The knee is an exceptional joint in that it has meniscal cartilages. In particular, the lateral meniscus of the knee is very broad and local joint depression fractures of the lateral tibial plateau may indeed be hidden under the broad anterior horn of the lateral meniscus. This being the case, the femoral articular surface may be protected by the lateral meniscus from the step in the tibial articular surface. This is borne out by the results following excision of the meniscus in tibial plateau fractures. Excision of the meniscus leads to very poor results.

Investigation of tibial plateau fractures

Following a careful clinical examination of the patient, the knee, the distal perfusion, sensibility and motor power, plain anteroposterior and lateral radiographs of the knee should be taken. Sometimes the degree of joint depression can be difficult to gauge from these plain radiographs as a depressed but comminuted joint surface may appear as only faint lines sunk within the metaphysis of the tibia. For this reason, many surgeons recommend tomography of the knee in order to assess the degree of joint depression better. Computed tomography (CT) may be used in the investigation of plateau fractures, but thin transverse slices must be used for if the joint depression is 8 mm it may show on only one cut when 4-mm slices are used. For this reason, plain tomography may be more helpful than CT, although the movement and the need for removal of splints for plain tomography are avoided by CT scanning.[21,22]

More information may be gleaned with three-dimensional CT reconstruction where the femur can be subtracted and the image viewed from any position.

Without the use of contrast, plain radiographs, tomograms and CT cannot show the status of the lateral meniscus, and for this reason some investigators have used arthroscopy in the investigation and treatment of tibial plateau fractures. Good views can be obtained of the articular surface at arthroscopy as long as this is performed relatively early before a clot cast forms in the knee joint. Patience must be used in clearing blood from the joint and at all costs the temptation to inflate the joint with gas must be avoided, as there have been two reported deaths from air embolism following arthroscopic investigation of lateral tibial plateau fractures using room air which entered the circulation and led to the patients' death when the tourniquet was removed.

The management of tibial plateau fractures

Every conceivable form of orthopaedic management has been used to treat tibial plateau fractures, from plaster to cast brace, to traction and surgery. In undisplaced fractures it is quite acceptable to treat the patient conservatively in a plaster. Drennan et al.[20] reported on the use of conservative treatment with plaster in 53 patients at an average of 4 years. Results were excellent or good for 85%. Of the eight unsatisfactory results, all were stated to have unlimited walking distance, only two had slight pain and two had a fixed flexion deformity. Both Schatzker[16] and Hohl and Luck[3] reported 100% excellent or good results following undisplaced fractures treated in plaster. Hohl and Luck's excellent and good results dropped to 90% if the knee was immobilized for more than 1 month. For this reason most surgeons would change to a cast brace at between 2 and 4 weeks.

For patients in whom there is minimal joint depression, treatment with skeletal traction through a tibial pin on a split bed gives excellent results. Apley[23] studied 60 patients evaluated at both 1 and 10 years by his functional method. Excellent or good knees were rated in 83%. Apley's assessment of results was that excellent meant that the knee was normal, did not interfere with the patient's work or play, did not ache or swell, and had a full painless range of movement. Good meant that the knee was barometric, that is aching in damp weather, or had slight limitation of full flexion but was otherwise normal and did not interfere with work or play. Fair meant that the knee hampered the patient slightly, ached after exercise, swelled sometimes and had a limitation of movement. Poor was any knee worse than fair. Interestingly, Apley found that the radiographs were of no help as a guide to either treatment or prognosis; indeed, he states that radiographs are probably irrelevant. His paper, although written some 35 years ago, is still worth reading for its wonderful use of English alone.

The method of treatment by tibial skeletal traction is to insert a Steinman pin, with the patient anaesthetized, 1–2 inches below the fracture. An attempt is made at reduction and the patient returned to bed with the knee and calf resting on a pillow and 45 N (10 lb) traction. Knee straightening and leg raising exercises are begun the following day and knee bending exercises are begun as soon as the patient can maintain a straight leg raise. Apley's treatment consisted of skeletal traction up to 6 weeks followed by crutch walking with partial weight bearing for a further 6 weeks. Many authors would now reduce the hospital time by reducing the traction to about 3 weeks when most patients can achieve 100° of flexion and then mobilizing the patient partially weight bearing with crutches in a cast brace to 8 weeks.

Surgical treatment of tibial plateau fractures

The indications for surgical management of tibial plateau fracture are significant joint depression (8–10 mm), widening of the tibial condyles or meniscal interposition.

The incision has to be carefully planned. Tibial plateau fractures used to be termed 'bumper fractures' or 'fender fractures', however, only a small proportion of tibial plateau fractures are actually caused by a pedestrian being struck on the tibia by the bumper or fender of a car. In Apley's series, only 5 of 60 patients were injured in this manner; in Roberts' series, 13% were hit by cars and in Bachalim's series

25% were hit by cars. In this admittedly small proportion of patients, great care must be taken, for the skin and soft tissues over the tibia may have been severely damaged but often do not declare their death until about 3 days following the fracture. There is hardly anything more galling than the skin over the tibia turning black 2 days after one has operated on a tibial plateau fracture. The consequences of infection in this area are severe since the soft tissue covering of the bone is so thin and osteomyelitis, once present, is very difficult to irradicate. However, in those patients who have not been struck directly with great force over the skin (and these account for the majority of patients with tibial plateau fractures) the wound usually heals without difficulty.

An oblique incision is made from the lateral femoral condyle, passing obliquely across the patellar retinaculum and then down the side of the tibial tendon and the tibial tuberosity.

Gerdy's tubercle is then elevated with an osteotome and the iliotibial tract is displaced laterally. A fasciotomy is performed of the anterior tibial compartment and the muscles are stripped from the lateral border of the tibia in order to expose the fracture.

It is essential that the meniscus is preserved at all costs and a surgical approach has been described whereby the lateral meniscus is divided at the origin of the anterior horn from the intercondylar area and swung out on the split part of the fracture as though opening a book. At the end of the procedure, the meniscus is re-sutured. Some authors in the past have recommended the removal of the meniscus to permit a good view, but further understanding of the fracture has demonstrated that it is absolutely essential that the meniscus is preserved. Once the split element of the fracture has been opened like a book, the depressed fragments are elevated and iliac crest bone graft is packed below them to hold them up. Choice in the use of internal fixation depends upon the severity of the fracture. A simple split fracture may be treated by cancellous lag screws, with washers alone, but if the fracture is more severe then an AO 'L' plate or the new AO hockey plate may be used. This plate is used in buttress mode.

Bicondylar fractures are more difficult to fix but often one plateau is minimally displaced, and if this is the case it is best to avoid the soft-tissue stripping involved in putting plates on both sides and to use a plate on the most depressed side with lag screws into the second condyle. Bicondylar fractures are often caused by extreme energy and it is in these fractures that the likelihood of skin breakdown is the highest.

Burri et al.[6] reviewed 278 patients who had been treated surgically at an average of almost 3 years following their fracture. Although the anatomical results were good, the price was poor function. The results were shown to depend upon the surgeon; surgeons were classified as being experienced if they had performed more than seven procedures. Inexperienced surgeons had only 66% excellent or good results and a 15% infection rate; only 19% of these patients could walk over 10 km and 22% needed a stick to walk. Radiological arthritis was shown to be present in 53–82% but the definition of radiological arthritis was very strict. The experienced surgeons had the better results: 97% of cases were good or acceptable, yet only 43% could walk over 10 km. In this group, the infection rate was 0.7%.

Schatzker et al.[16] looked at the Toronto experience of 70 patients evaluated at over 2 years. Only 50% were treated by operation. Split compression B3 fractures had 66% excellent or good results. Joint surface depression of greater than 5 mm led to valgus malalignment and poor results. Medial plateau fractures had the worst results. They tended to occur in an older population with soft bone. The complication rate here was high at 27%. The most common complication was peroneal nerve palsy; all recovered. There were two infections at the graft donor site and one infection of the knee wound.

Arthroscopic reduction and internal fixation of tibial plateau fractures

Patients in whom there is an intra-articular fracture without a metaphyseal element may be treated by arthroscopic reduction and percutaneous internal fixation. With the patient under a general anaesthetic, the knee joint is assessed arthroscopically. A tourniquet is used to prevent further bleeding during the procedure and the knee joint is first washed out. If a clot cast has formed within the knee joint, then an attempt may be made to remove this with an arthroscopic shaver system, but if this is not rapidly feasible the operation should be abandoned and open reduction and internal fixation carried out. The knee is copiously irrigated until all the blood within the knee has been removed and the field of view is cleared.

The difficulty posed by blood within the joint has persuaded some surgeons to attempt to inflate the joint with air, which has led to two reported deaths in the literature from air embolism from the air pumped into the fracture surfaces on release of the tourniquet. Obviously, this should never be attempted. If a clear field of view cannot be gained, then the arthroscopic procedure should be abandoned and the knee joint opened.

With a clear field of view the fracture is identified and inspected. If there is a simple split fracture, then the split may be closed by a percutaneous reduction and then by the lag screw effect of percutaneously introduced AO 6.5 mm cancellous lag screws. If there is comminution with joint depression, then a small incision is made some 4 cm below the comminuted

surface. A cortical window is made and a punch is inserted to elevate the depressed segment under arthroscopic control. Percutaneous lag screws are then inserted to close the split element and to act as reinforced steel girders below the elevated segment. Graft may be harvested from the iliac crest and punched in underneath this surface, but this has been found not to be necessary. At the end of the procedure, the portals are steristripped, the short incisions for the lag screws and the cortical window are closed and radiographic controls are taken. The patient is then put into a cast brace with partial weight bearing for a period of 6 weeks.

This minimally invasive technique allows rapid return to early joint movement but is still in the developmental phase.

Complications of lateral plateau fractures

Rasmussen and Sørensen[18] looked at the question of incidence of osteoarthritis following tibial plateau fractures in great detail. They showed that there was a lack of correlation between the functional and anatomical end results. Thus, although 89% of patients with poor functional results had radiographic arthritis, there were some patients with a poor functional result who had an excellent anatomical end result, and conversely some patients with an excellent functional end result had a poor anatomical end result. They noted that many other studies confirmed these findings.

These authors defined osteoarthritis radiographically as narrowing of the joint space with or without subchondral sclerosis. Of their patients 26% were found to have these changes at follow-up.

There was a statistically significant difference in the incidence of arthritis according to the severity of the fracture. Lateral fractures only had 16%, medial fractures 21% and the severe bicondylar fractures 42%. The incidence of osteoarthritis was also statistically correlated with knee alignment. Normally aligned knees had a 13% chance of developing arthritis, valgus knees 31% chance and varus knees 79% chance.

Instability was also correlated with the development of osteoarthritis. Knees which were stable in extension had a 14% chance and knees unstable in extension a 46% chance of developing arthritis.

Surprisingly, Rasmussen and Sørensen[18] found no correlation between joint depression and radiological joint space narrowing or subchondral sclerosis. However, there was a link between condylar widening and osteoarthritis.

Iatrogenic complications can occur following surgery for tibial plateau fractures. Surgical repair of tibial plateau fractures requires great experience.

Schatzker et al.[16] stated that it should be emphasized again and again that the results of poor open reduction are far worse than the results of poor non-operative treatment. In Schatzker's series, the complication rate was 27% for those treated surgically. The most common complication was peroneal nerve palsy. It was not possible to say how many were iatrogenic and all recovered. There were two infections at the graft donor site and one infection of the knee wound (7.3%).

Burri et al.[6] showed a great difference in the complication rate for surgeons who had operated on fewer than seven plateau fractures (14% haematomas and 15% infection) compared with experienced surgeons (6% haematomas and 0.7% infection).

The key to the management of the tibial plateau fracture is to preserve motion by careful attention to reconstruction of the joint surface, the soft tissues and the ligaments. The second important point is to preserve the normal alignment of the knee joint and to treat the patient by a method that allows early controlled movement of the knee joint.

References

1. **Salter RB, Simmonds DF, Malcolm BW** et al., The biological effect of continuous passive motion on the healing of full-thickness defects in articular cartilage, *J Bone Joint Surg (Am)* (1980) 62: 1232–1251.

2. **Mitchell N, Shepard N,** Healing of articular cartilage in intra-articular fractures in rabbits, *J Bone Joint Surg (Am)* (1980) 62: 628–634.

3. **Hohl M, Luck JV,** Fractures of the tibial condyle. A clinical and experimental study, *J Bone Joint Surg (Am)* (1956) 38: 1001–1018.

4. **Dovey H, Heerfordt J,** Tibial condyle fractures, *Acta Chir Scand* (1971) 137: 521–531.

5. **Reitel DB, Wade PA,** Fractures of the tibial plateau, *J Trauma* (1962) 2: 337–352.

6. **Burri C, Bartzke G, Coldewey J, Muggler E,** Fractures of the tibial plateau, *Clin Orthop* (1979) 138: 84–93.

7. **Neer CS, Grantham SA, Shelton ML,** Supracondylar fracture of the adult femur: a study of 110 cases, *J Bone Joint Surg (Am)* (1967) 49: 591–613.

8. **Giles JB, DeLee JC, Heckman JD** et al. Supracondylar–intercondylar fractures of the femur treated with a supracondylar plate and lag screw, *J Bone Joint Surg (Am)* (1982) 64: 864–870.

9. **Müller ME, Nayaria S, Kach P,** *The AO classification of fractures* (Berlin: Springer-Verlag, 1988).

10. **Stewart MJ, Sisk TD, Wallace SL Jr,** Fractures of the distal third of the femur, *J Bone Joint Surg (Am)* (1966) 48: 784–807.

11. **Colton CL,** AO fixation, *Injury* (1990) 21: 287–289.

12. **Wilde P, Griffiths J, Dooley B** et al., Management of supracondylar fractures of the femur with Zickel supracondylar nails, *Aust NZ J Surg* (1989) 59(3): 243–248.

13. **Olerud S,** Operative treatment of supracondylar–condylar fractures of the femur, *J Bone Joint Surg (Am)* (1972) 54: 1015–1032.

14. **Mize RD, Bucholz RW, Grogan DP,** Surgical treatment of displaced, comminuted fractures of the distal end of the femur, *J Bone Joint Surg (Am)* (1982) 64: 871–879.

15. **Roberts JM,** Fractures of the condyles of the tibia, *J Bone Joint Surg (Am)* (1968) 50: 1505–1521.

16. **Schatzker J, McBroom R, Bruce D,** The tibial plateau fracture, *Clin Orthop* (1979) 138: 94–104.

17. **Kennedy JC, Bailey WH,** Experimental tibial-plateau fractures, *J Bone Joint Surg (Am)* (1968) 50: 1522–1534.

18. **Rasmussen PS, Sørensen SE,** Tibial condylar fractures, *Injury* (1973) 4: 265.

19. **Porter BB,** Crush fractures of the lateral tibial table, *J Bone Joint Surg (Br)* (1970) 52: 676–687.

20. **Drennan DB, Locher FG, Maylahn DJ,** Fractures of the tibial plateau, *J Bone Joint Surg (Am)* (1979) 61: 989–995.

21. **Rafi M, Lamont JG, Firooznia H,** Tibial plateau fractures: CT evaluation and classification, *CRC Crit Rev Diagn Imaging* (1987) 27(2): 91–112.

22. **Dias JJ, Stirling AJ, Finlay DB** et al., Computerized axial tomography for tibial plateau fractures, *J Bone Joint Surg (Br)* (1987) 69(1): 84–88.

23. **Apley AG,** Fractures of the lateral tibial condyle treated by skeletal traction and early mobilization, *J Bone Joint Surg (Br)* (1956) 38: 699–708.

14

Osteoarthritis: Conservative surgery

14.1 Arthroscopic debridement for degenerative arthritis of the knee: An overview

Dipak V. Patel and Paul M. Aichroth

Degenerative changes in the knee joint are seen with increasing frequency in patients past the third decade of life. The management of degenerative arthritis (following previous meniscectomy, fracture or instability) in younger patients remains a difficult therapeutic dilemma. Arthroscopic debridement seems to be a reasonable alternative in those patients who present with persistent symptoms despite adequate conservative treatment.

Magnuson[1] advocated open debridement or the 'house-cleaning' procedure for degenerative arthritis of the knee. Pridie[2] introduced the concept of drilling of the bare subchondral bone to encourage fibrocartilaginous repair. His procedure was later reviewed by Insall.[3,4]

However, there are well-known disadvantages of open debridement, including prolonged hospitalization, lengthy rehabilitation period and increased morbidity. In the past decade, various authors have reported on arthroscopic surgery for osteoarthritis of the knee (details in Table 1). Advantages of arthroscopic surgery include low incidence of complications, shorter rehabilitation period and decreased hospital stay.

Indications for surgery

Casscells[20] pointed out that patients for arthroscopic debridement must be selected carefully. Patients with osteoarthritis who present with persistent pain, swelling, joint irritability, mechanical locking and limitation of activities of daily living despite adequate conservative measures, are selected for arthroscopic debridement. Those with ligamentous instability or significant malalignment (>15°) should be excluded.

The natural history of untreated osteoarthritis of the knee

Hernborg and Nilsson[21] reviewed 71 patients (94 knees) with osteoarthritis of the knee at 10–18 years' follow-up. The course of the disease could not be evaluated in 7 knees owing to other major disability. Of the remaining 87 knees, only 17% of the knees improved; 27% remained unchanged and 56% became worse.

Recently, Odenbring et al.[22] reported a 16-year follow-up study of 189 knees with medial compartment osteoarthritis. After 14 years, tibial osteotomy was performed in 85 knees and arthroplasty in 33 knees. No major surgery was undertaken in 71 knees; of these 71 knees, 31 patients (40 knees) had died. Of the remaining 23 patients (31 knees) the majority had an unsatisfactory result. This study strongly supports the unfavourable prognosis of medial compartment gonarthrosis and confirms that the majority of the patients with this condition will eventually require a major knee surgery.

Discussion

In recent years there has been renewed interest in debriding and irrigating the arthritic knee endoscopically. Arthroscopic debridement is now an increasingly accepted technique for the treatment of a painful, degenerative knee.

Several factors—such as patient's age; severity, nature and duration of symptoms; physical findings (degree of axial malalignment); extent of radiological changes; and patient compliance with rehabilitation—should be considered before undertaking arthroscopic surgery. In degenerative arthritis of the knee a 'cure' in its true sense is not possible, for there cannot be restoration of the articular surface to normal by any known treatment method. Our aim, therefore, is to treat patients' symptoms with the hope of improving joint function.

In the early stage of osteoarthritis, plain radiographs are often normal, but the chondral degenerative changes are readily seen at arthroscopic examination. However, when advanced radiological changes are present, little new information is gained by arthroscopy. In future, magnetic resonance imaging (MRI) may allow non-invasive evaluation of

Table 1 Previous reviews on arthroscopic surgery for osteoarthritis of the knee

Author and year	No. of patients (no. of knees)	Type of surgery	Mean follow-up in months (range)	Results
Del Pizzo et al. (1980)[5]	51 (54)	Arthroscopic debridement	–	67% good
Sprague (1981)[6]	63 (69)	Arthroscopic debridement	13.6 (6–21)	74% good
Shahriaree et al. (1982) [7]	275	Arthroscopic debridement	26 (13–84)	76% good
Jackson and Rouse (1982)[8]	47 (51)	Arthroscopic partial meniscectomy	30 (6–67)	82% good or excellent
Richards and Lonergan (1984)[9]	22	Arthroscopic drilling of chondral or osteochondral defect	25.1 (12–39)	80% good
	21	Arthroscopic partial meniscectomy	40.6 (16–62)	81% good
Friedman et al. (1984)[10]	41	Abrasion arthroplasty and debridement—medial compartment	12 (6–18)	53% improved
	37	Arthroscopic debridement of medial compartment	12 (6–18)	32% improved
McBride et al. (1984)[11]	17	Arthroscopic partial meniscectomy	35 (24–55)	65% satisfactory
Salisbury et al. (1985)[12]	41 (48)	Arthroscopic debridement	27.5	53% good
Rand (1985)[13]	84 (87)	Arthroscopic partial meniscectomy	24	84% improved
Johnson (1986)[14]	95 (99)	Abrasion arthroplasty	Minimum 24	75% improved
Jackson et al. (1987)[15]	166 (202)	Arthroscopic debridement	39.6 (24–112)	68% improved
Bert and Maschka (1989)[16]	67	Arthroscopic debridement	60	66% good or excellent
	59	Abrasion arthroplasty and arthroscopic debridement	60	51% good or excellent
Chan (1989)[17]	250	Arthroscopic debridement	55 (24–87)	72% excellent or good
Baumgaertner et al. (1990)[18]	44 (49)	Arthroscopic debridement for severe arthritis		At the time of maximum improvement, 52% had good or excellent results. The maximum improvement was maintained for an average of 15.4 months (range 3–52 months). At the time of final follow-up, 40% had good or excellent results. The final follow-up examination averaged 33 months (range 17–69 months).
Hedtmann et al. (1990)[19]	1125	Arthroscopic debridement	23	75% of patients had subjective improvement

the articular surfaces with considerable accuracy. It is worth mentioning here that the interpretation of the MRI scans requires experience and one must be aware of the false positives.

There are numerous intra-articular pathological problems that could be dealt with arthroscopically, including degenerative meniscal tears, fibrillated articular cartilage, loose bodies, impinging osteophytes and hypertrophic synovitis.

The degenerative meniscal tears are usually confined to the posterior segment of the meniscus. The excision of degenerative flap or tag tear leads to significant pain relief. Large, impinging osteophytes, particularly in the intercondylar area of the femur, should be excised. Loose, desquamated chondral fronds should be excised to provide a smooth articular surface. At the end of the procedure, the joint

must be thoroughly lavaged. We recommend a localized abrasion for lesions less than 10–15 mm in diameter. The depth of the abrasion should be no more than 1 mm. The completed abrasion creates furrows that are usually 1 mm in depth on the bony surface.[23] Later in this chapter (contribution 14.3) Lanny Johnson describes the current status of arthroscopic abrasion arthroplasty with magnificent histological illustrations.

The role of arthroscopic debridement in older patients (>50 years of age) has been evaluated by Baumgaertner et al.[18] They performed arthroscopic debridement in 49 knees in 44 patients. Two-thirds of the patients had radiographic evidence of severe arthritis. In their series, surgery offered no benefit for 39% of the patients. Good or excellent results were obtained in 52% of the patients and were maintained through the final follow-up examination in 40% of the patients. Of these, two-thirds had no visible deterioration within a 33-month average follow-up period. Symptoms of longer duration, arthritic severity as seen on radiographs, and malalignment predicted poor results. Conversely, shorter duration of symptoms, mechanical symptoms, mild to moderate arthritis, and crystal deposition correlated with improved results.

Conclusions

(1) Arthroscopic debridement is a valuable therapeutic alternative in the management of degenerative arthritis of the knee. This procedure is recommended for well-motivated, carefully selected patients who have symptomatic osteoarthritis of the knee, despite adequate conservative measures. Patients with ligamentous instability or significant malalignment (>15°) are not suitable candidates for this procedure.

(2) The procedure can be repeated, if needed, and does not complicate future realignment osteotomy or replacement arthroplasty. It delays or postpones major open knee surgery for a substantial period. Patients with grade I or II degenerative changes have better results than those with grade III or IV changes.

(3) Arthroscopic surgery demands considerable technical skill and expertise. This technique *must not* be misused.

(4) The assessment of pain relief following this operation is difficult, as pain is a subjective symptom and therefore difficult to quantify. Visual Analogue Scale (VAS) may be one way of dealing with this problem. A uniform evaluation and documentation system is required to enable a valid comparison between the various reported series.

(5) There is an increasing need to improve upon the Outerbridge classification system[24] for grading of the degenerative changes in the articular surfaces.

(6) Further studies with a longer-term follow-up are necessary to determine the duration of symptomatic benefit, and the incidence of subsequent surgical intervention.

(7) We still do not have enough knowledge concerning the biomechanical strength of the fibrocartilage that forms following arthroscopic abrasion.

References

1. **Magnuson PB**, Joint debridement: Surgical treatment of degenerative arthritis, *Surg Gynaecol Obstet* (1941) **73**: 1–9.
2. **Pridie KH**, A method of resurfacing osteoarthritic knee joints, *J Bone Joint Surg (Br)* (1959) **41**: 618–619.
3. **Insall JN**, Intra-articular surgery for degenerative arthritis of the knee: a report of the work of the late KH Pridie, *J Bone Joint Surg (Br)* (1967) **49**: 211–228.
4. **Insall JN**, The Pridie debridement operation for osteoarthritis of the knee, *Clin Orthop* (1974) **101**: 61–67.
5. **Del Pizzo W, Fox JM, Blazina ME et al.**, Operative arthroscopy for the treatment of problems of the medial compartment of the knee, *Orthopaedics* (1980) **3**: 984–986.
6. **Sprague NF**, Arthroscopic debridement for degenerative knee joint disease, *Clin Orthop* (1981) **160**: 118–123.
7. **Shahriaree H, O'Connor RL, Nottage WM**, Seven years' follow-up on arthroscopic debridement of the degenerative knee, *Field of View* (1982) **1**: 1–7.
8. **Jackson RW, Rouse DW**, The results of partial arthroscopic meniscectomy in patients over 40 years of age, *J Bone Joint Surg (Br)* (1982) **64**: 481–485.
9. **Richards RN, Lonergan RP**, Arthroscopic surgery for relief of pain in the osteoarthritic knee, *Orthopaedics* (1984) **7**: 1705–1707.
10. **Friedman MJ, Berasi CC, Fox JM et al.**, Preliminary results with abrasion arthroplasty in the osteoarthritic knee, *Clin Orthop* (1984) **182**: 200–205.
11. **McBride GG, Constine RM, Hofmann AA et al.**, Arthroscopic partial medial meniscectomy in the older patient, *J Bone Joint Surg (Am)* (1984) **66**: 547–551.
12. **Salisbury RB, Nottage WM, Gardner V**, The effect of alignment on results in arthroscopic debridement of the degenerative knee, *Clin Orthop* (1985) **198**: 268–272.
13. **Rand JA**, Arthroscopic management of degenerative meniscus tears in patients with degenerative arthritis, *Arthroscopy* (1985) **1**: 253–258.
14. **Johnson LL**, Arthroscopic abrasion arthroplasty – historical and pathological perspective: present status, *Arthroscopy* (1986) **2**: 54–69.
15. **Jackson RW, Marans HJ, Silver RS**, The arthroscopic treatment of degenerative arthritis of the knee, Presented at the Eighth Combined Meeting of the Orthopaedic Associations of the English-speaking World, Washington DC, 1987.
16. **Bert JM, Maschka K**, The arthroscopic treatment of unicompartmental gonarthrosis: a five-year follow-up study of abrasion arthroplasty plus arthroscopic debridement and arthroscopic debridement alone, *Arthroscopy* (1989) **5**: 25–32.
17. **Chan KM**, Arthroscopic debridement and lavage for osteoarthrosis of the knee: a prospective study of 250 patients with a minimum follow-up of 2 years, *Abstracts of the 6th Congress of the International Society of the Knee*, Rome, 8–12 May, 1989.
18. **Baumgaertner MR, Cannon WD Jr, Vittori JM et al.**, Arthroscopic debridement of the arthritic knee, *Clin Orthop* (1990) **253**: 197–202.
19. **Hedtmann A, Rosenthal A, Moraldo M et al.**, Results of arthroscopic surgery in osteoarthrosis of the knee, *Abstracts of the XVIII World Congress of SICOT*, Montreal, 9–14 September, 1990.
20. **Casscells SW**, What, if any, are the indications for the arthroscopic debridement of the osteoarthritic knee? (Editorial), *Arthroscopy* (1990) **6**: 169–170.
21. **Hernborg JS, Nilsson BE**, The natural course of untreated osteoarthritis of the knee, *Clin Orthop* (1977) **123**: 130–137.
22. **Odenbring S, Lindstrand A, Egund N et al.**, Prognosis for patients with medial gonarthrosis: a 16-year follow-up study of 189 knees, *Clin Orthop* (1991) **266**: 152–155.
23. **Schonholtz GJ**, Arthroscopic debridement of the knee joint, *Orthop Clin North Am* (1989) **20**: 257–263.
24. **Outerbridge RE**, The etiology of chondromalacia patellae, *J Bone Joint Surg (Br)* (1961) **43**: 752–757.

14.2 Arthroscopic debridement for degenerative joint disease of the knee: A prospective review of 276 knees

Dipak V. Patel, Paul M. Aichroth and Simon T. Moyes

Many patients with degenerative gonarthrosis of the knee can be managed successfully by conservative measures, whilst others require corrective osteotomy or replacement arthroplasty. However, there remains a third group of patients who, because of age, level of symptoms or inclination are not suitable candidates for major open knee surgery and yet are dissatisfied with the results of conservative treatment.[1]

Magnuson[2,3] and Haggart[4,5] recommended open debridement for degenerative arthritis of the knee. With recent advances in both arthroscopic technique and instrumentation, many procedures previously performed through arthrotomy incisions are now being executed percutaneously under arthroscopic visualization.[1,6-17]

The aim of this prospective study was to evaluate the symptomatic improvement (extent and duration), to assess the clinical results and to determine any predictive indicators of the likely success of this procedure.

Materials and methods

Between 1977 and 1988, 280 patients underwent arthroscopic debridement and irrigation for degenerative joint disease (DJD) of the knee at Westminster Hospital. All operations were either performed or supervised by the senior author (P.M.A.). Twenty-six patients were lost to follow-up, leaving 254 available for clinical and radiological assessment.

All patients were personally interviewed by one author (D.V.P.) and were asked to give their opinion on the degree and duration of the symptomatic improvement and whether they had undergone any additional knee surgery. The same author also performed detailed clinical examination of all the knees.

Two-hundred and seventy-six knees (146 right and 130 left) in 254 patients (184 males and 70 females) were assessed at an average follow-up of 44 months (range 24–140 months). Thirty per cent of the patients had more than 5 years of follow-up and 15% had more than 7 years of follow-up. Their mean age at the time of operation was 49 years (range 28–82 years). Forty-nine per cent of the patients were <50 years of age and 51% were >50 years of age.

Indication for surgery

Patients with DJD who had persistent pain, recurrent swelling, joint irritability, mechanical locking and restriction of daily functional activities despite adequate conservative measures were selected for arthroscopic debridement. Patients with ligamentous instability or significant malalignment (>15°) were excluded.

Previous surgery

Fifty patients (20%) had had previous operations on their knees (Table 1).

Table 1 Previous operations in 50 patients.

Operation	Number
Open medial meniscectomy	22
Open lateral meniscectomy	7
Arthroscopic medial meniscectomy	11
Arthroscopic lateral meniscectomy	4
Open synovectomy	1
Arthrotomy and removal of loose bodies	2
Arthroscopic removal of loose bodies	2
Patellectomy	1
High tibial osteotomy	1
Exploration of popliteal fossa and excision of massive pseudocyst from calf	1

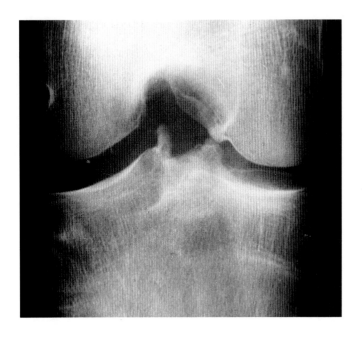

Figure 1

Radiograph ('tunnel' view) showing impinging osteophytes in the intercondylar notch of the femur in a 48-year-old male with degenerative gonarthrosis.

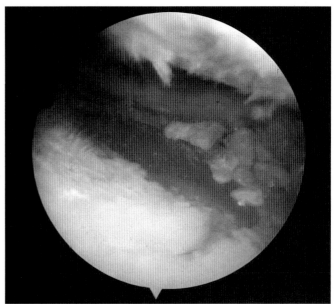

Figure 2

Arthroscopic appearance of the eburnated tibial plateau (grade IV Outerbridge changes) and degenerative medial femoral condyle in a 55-year-old man with medial compartment osteoarthritis.

Preoperative assessment

Clinical assessment

Preoperatively, 83% of the knees had moderate pain and 17% had severe pain. Night pain was recorded in 15% of the knees. There was mild to moderate swelling in 76% of the knees. A feeling of instability or giving-way was noted by 54% of the patients. This was probably due to the degenerative meniscal lesion, as the joint was stable on clinical examination. Thirty-six per cent of the patients complained of locking.

Joint-line tenderness was noted in 87% of the knees and 68% had demonstrable effusion. The McMurray's test was positive for pain in 62% of the knees. The mean preoperative flexion was 120° (range 90–140°). None of the knees had major collateral or cruciate ligament instability; 30% of the knees had a 5–10° flexion contracture. Prior to the onset of disabling symptoms 60% of the patients had participated in recreational sports.

Radiological assessment

Routine weight-bearing anteroposterior, lateral, intercondylar ('tunnel') and skyline views were taken. The 'tunnel' view was particularly useful for demonstrating impinging osteophytes (Figure 1).

Preoperative degenerative changes were graded according to Ahlbäck[18] (Table 2). Radiographs were normal for 33% of the knees. However, these knees were noted to have early degenerative changes on arthroscopic examination. Thirty-nine per cent of the knees showed grade I Ahlbäck changes, 18% showed grade II changes, 8% had grade III changes and 2% had grade IV changes. The medial compartment was involved in 80% of the knees, the lateral in 14% and both in 6%.

Operative technique

The patient was placed in a supine position under general anaesthesia. Examination under anaesthetic was performed and the findings were carefully recorded. A tourniquet was applied to the thigh after exsanguination. The joint was aspirated and the

Table 2 Ahlbäck radiological grading system (1968).

Grade I	Joint-space narrowing
Grade II	Joint-space obliteration
Grade III	Minor bone attrition
Grade IV	Moderate bone attrition
Grade V	Severe bone attrition
Grade VI	Severe bone attrition with subluxation

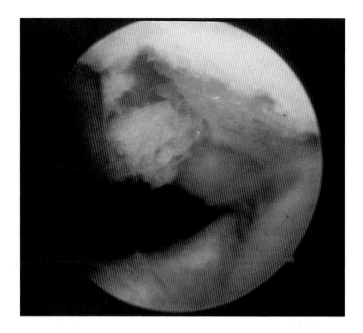

Figure 3

Large osteophyte is excised from the intercondylar notch of the femur using a small osteotome.

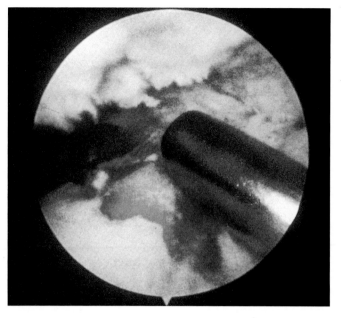

Figure 4

The ensheathed powered burr abrading the eburnated tibial plateau.

synovial fluid was sent for crystal studies. The joint was then distended with approximately 100 ml of normal saline.

Standard anteromedial and anterolateral arthroscopy portals were used. A 30° wide-angle arthroscope was generally employed. A television monitoring system and video circuit were routinely used. Visualization of the posteromedial and posterolateral compartments was accomplished by slipping the arthroscope through the intercondylar notch from one of the anterior portals, or by making a separate posteromedial or posterolateral portal in selective cases. A variety of arthroscopic instruments, including punches, rongeurs, knives, scissors and powered meniscotome were used for meniscal or chondral debridement.

The degenerative meniscal tears were excised and trimmed down to a stable peripheral rim. Frayed, degenerative articular surfaces (Figure 2) were shaved and debrided, and the loose bodies were removed. Large, impinging osteophytes, particularly in the intercondylar area of the femur, were excised using a small osteotome (Figure 3) and then removed with a rongeur, taking care to avoid creating a loose body.

In patients with severe, generalized hypertrophic synovitis, a limited synovectomy was performed using powered instruments. The eburnated tibial plateau (<1–1.5 cm in diameter) was abraded using a powered burr until bleeding subchondral bone was exposed (Figures 4 and 5). The femoral condylar surfaces were similarly abraded if eburnated bone was seen.

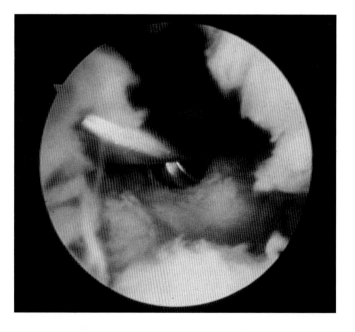

Figure 5

The powered burr is used to expose the bleeding subchondral bone.

Table 3 Outerbridge grading system (1961).

Grade I	Soft, discoloured superficial fibrillation
Grade II	Fragmentation <1.3 cm^2
Grade III	Fragmentation >1.3 cm^2
Grade IV	Erosion down to subchondral bone (eburnation)

Table 4 Non-meniscal pathology.

Pathology	Number of knees	Percentage
Articular cartilage degeneration		
Mild to moderate	204	74
Severe (subchondral bone exposed)	72	26
Loose bodies	50	18
Chondrocalcinosis	42	15
Intra-articular adhesions	10	4

Table 5 Meniscal pathology.

Pathology	Number of knees	Percentage
Previous meniscectomy		
Medial	32	11.6
Lateral	10	4.0
Both	1	0.4
Total	43	16.0
Meniscal tears		
Medial	179	65
Lateral	34	12
Both	11	4
Total	224	81

The stability of the remaining meniscus was ascertained using a probe. At the completion of the procedure, the tourniquet was released and the joint was thoroughly irrigated with normal saline to remove small meniscal or chondral fragments and joint debris. The arthroscopy portals were closed using a single nylon stitch and a bulky compression dressing was applied. The mean operative time was 50 minutes.

Postoperative management

The compression bandage was reduced to a tubigrip the next morning and active straight leg raising and range of motion knee exercises were commenced to mobilize and strengthen the quadriceps to the maximum. The patients were encouraged to bear weight when comfortable. The average hospital stay was 48 hours.

Operative findings

Eighteen per cent of the knees in this review had grade I Outerbridge[19] (Table 3) degenerative changes, 36% had grade II changes, 20% had grade III changes and 26% had grade IV changes in the articular surfaces. Details of non-meniscal pathology are listed in Table 4.

Forty-three knees (16%) had had previous open or arthroscopic meniscectomy. There were 235 meniscal tears (190 medial and 45 lateral) in 224 knees. Eleven knees had both menisci involved. The remaining 52 knees had degenerative menisci without any obvious tears or had stable peripheral rim following previous meniscectomy. Details of meniscal pathology are shown in Table 5.

The most frequent lesion was a degenerative flap or a tag tear involving the posterior segment of the medial meniscus, seen in 65% of the knees. The observed patterns of meniscal tears are given in Table 6 and the location of the tears is shown in Table 7. Twenty-seven tears involved both the midportion and the posterior segment of the medial meniscus, and 7 tears involved middle and posterior one-third of the lateral meniscus. Forty-three knees (16%) had impinging osteophytes around the intercondylar notch and these were excised using a small osteotome.

Postoperative assessment

A simple and practical grading system was used to evaluate the result of the knee (Table 8), with emphasis on pain, swelling, range of movement and daily activities. The routine preoperative radiographs were repeated. The data were analysed using the chi-squared test and Student's t-test.

Results

Subjective assessment

At the time of review, 22% of the knees had no pain, 60% had occasional ache or discomfort and 18% had moderate pain. Fifty-seven per cent of the knees had no swelling, 25% had mild swelling on strenuous exertion and 18% had moderate swelling. Eighty per cent of the patients were back to work at an average of 10.4 days following arthroscopic surgery, and 20% had retired.

Seventeen per cent of the patients were able to return to their previous sports and 25% were participating in various recreational sports such as tennis, squash, golf, badminton, etc. The mean time for return to sports was 76 days.

Table 6 Pattern of meniscal tears (224 knees).

	Radial	Horizontal cleavage	Parrot-beak	Flap or tag	Bucket-handle	Complex tear	Tear in discoid meniscus
Medial	4	10	0	145	22	9	0
Lateral	3	6	10	20	3	1	2

Table 7 Location of meniscal tears (224 knees).

	Anterior third	Middle third	Posterior third	Combined middle and posterior third	Total
Medial	4	6	153	27	190
Lateral	3	10	25	7	45

Table 8 Criteria for grading of results.

Result	Grade	Description
Satisfactory	Excellent	No pain or swelling Full range of knee movement Normal daily activities Return to previous sports (if applicable)
	Good	Occasional discomfort not interfering with daily activities No swelling or minor swelling after strenuous exertion Knee movement—full range or 10° restriction of flexion Improved daily activities Return to recreational sports (if applicable)
Unsatisfactory	Fair	Moderate pain reducing daily activities Analgesics required Moderate swelling Knee movement—more than 10° restriction of flexion Daily activities unchanged Reduced sporting activities
	Poor	Pain and swelling are either unchanged or worse Daily activities reduced No sports possible or Patient underwent major open knee surgery

Clinical examination

Thirty-two per cent of the knees were noted to have minimal varus deformity and 8% had minor valgus deformity at the time of follow-up. Twelve per cent of the knees had mild to moderate joint-line tenderness. Eleven per cent of the knees had minimal effusion and 18% had moderate effusion. Forty-two per cent of the knees had a full range of movement (0–140°), 37% had a 10° restriction of terminal flexion and 21% had >10° limitation of flexion.

Radiological assessment

Twenty-eight per cent of the knees demonstrated progression of degenerative changes by Ahlbäck grade I.

Grading of results

Seventy-five per cent of the knees had satisfactory results and 25% had unsatisfactory results (Table 9).

Table 9 Post-operative results.

Grade	Number of knees	Percentage		
Excellent ⎤ Satisfactory	50	18 ⎤ 75		
Good ⎦	156	57 ⎦		
Fair ⎤ Unsatisfactory	42	15 ⎤ 25		
Poor ⎦	28	10 ⎦		

Table 10 Subsequent operations.

Operation	Number of knees
Repeat arthroscopy	20
High tibial osteotomy	6
Distal femoral osteotomy	1
Unicompartmental arthroplasty	7
Total knee replacement	4

There was a statistically significant correlation ($P < 0.005$) between the result and the length of follow-up. The results deteriorated with passage of time (Figure 6). Thirty-six patients (14%) had a subsequent operation following arthroscopic debridement (Table 10) at an average of 46 months (range 14–78 months).

We found that age significantly affected the outcome. Those less than 60 years of age had 78% satisfactory results compared to 55% satisfactory results in the over 60 years of age group ($P < 0.008$).

We noticed that the outcome from surgery correlated significantly ($P < 0.001$) with preoperative radiological Ahlbäck grading (Figure 7). Similarly, there was a significant correlation ($P < 0.001$) between Outerbridge grading and the result (Figure 8). Patients with more advanced arthrosis had less satisfactory results.

No significant correlation was seen between the type or location of the meniscal tear and the result. The presence or absence of previous surgery did not influence the outcome significantly.

Complications

There was a superficial stitch infection in one patient that responded to local wound care. There were no deep infections. Two patients with large haemarthrosis were treated by aspiration and compression bandage.

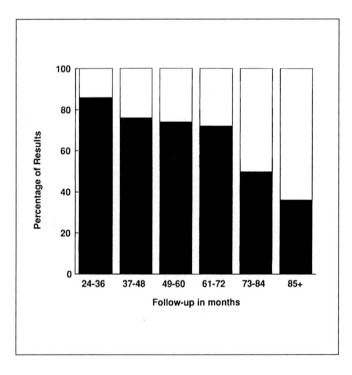

Figure 6

The percentage of satisfactory results (solid columns) deteriorated with passage of time.

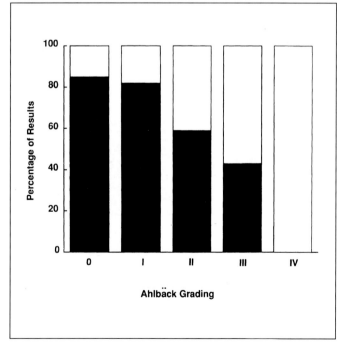

Figure 7

The relationship between Ahlbäck radiological grading and the result. Solid columns represent satisfactory results.

Patient satisfaction

Of the patients, 67% were pleased and 18% were satisfied with the result; 11% were dissatisfied and 4% expressed reservation about the outcome of the procedure.

Discussion

For many years, open debridement or the 'house-cleaning' operation was the only possible surgical procedure for moderate degenerative arthritis of the knee.[2-5,20] Both Magnuson and Haggart described methods of wide joint exposure, shaving of fibrillated cartilage, removal of torn menisci and loose bodies, trimming of osteophytes, patellectomy if needed, and rarely synovectomy. Pridie (1959) used a less extensive procedure and introduced drilling of the bare subchondral bone to encourage fibrocartilaginous repair.[21] His procedure was later reviewed by Insall.[22,23]

In our study, 142 knees (51%) were treated by a combined meniscal and chondral debridement, and this was associated with 68% excellent or good results. Those with less severe degenerative changes and treated by meniscal debridement alone (104 knees), had 86% excellent or good results. Chondral debridement either alone or in combination with meniscal debridement was performed in 62% of the knees and a localized abrasion arthroplasty was undertaken in 28%.

The results of arthroscopic partial meniscectomy in the older patient with osteoarthritis are encouraging.[13,24,25] In our series, 65% of the knees had a flap or tag tear involving the posterior segment of the medial meniscus that is typical of a degenerative tear.[13,24]

Following initial report by Burman,[26] various authors have noticed a marked reduction in joint discomfort following arthroscopic lavage.[7,17,27] This is particularly noticeable in patients with chondrocalcinosis (Figure 9). Possible explanations for the beneficial effect include mechanical removal of the debris, alteration of enzymes within the joint or stretching and distension of the joint capsule. In our series, all patients underwent thorough arthroscopic lavage postoperatively.

Abrasion arthroplasty has been used with varying success in the management of osteoarthritis of the knee.[10,12] Recently, Bert and Maschka[6] reported 51% excellent or good results in 59 patients treated by a combined abrasion arthroplasty and arthroscopic debridement for unicompartmental osteoarthritis.

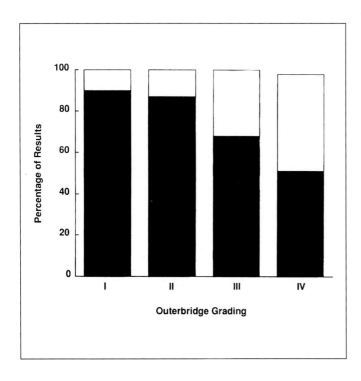

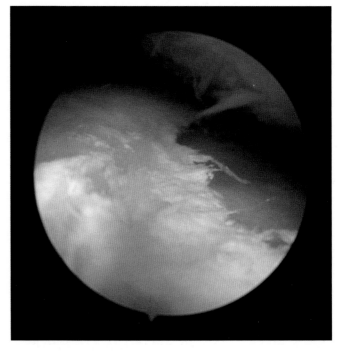

Figure 8

The relationship between Outerbridge grading and the result. Solid columns represent satisfactory results.

Figure 9

Arthroscopic view showing chondrocalcinosis in a 60-year-old male patient with degenerative arthritis of the medial compartment of the knee.

They concluded that the results of this combined procedure were totally unpredictable.

In our series, the eburnated tibial plateaux were perforated using a powered burr, but no major abrasion arthroplasty was undertaken. We agree with Dandy[7] in that drilling or abrading small areas of exposed bone (usually less than 1 cm in diameter) produces satisfactory results and there is no evidence that it is harmful.

The relationship between the severity of osteoarthritis and results after arthroscopic debridement has been variable. Shahriaree et al.[16] and Richards and Lonergan[14] reported less favourable results with advanced osteoarthritis, whereas Sprague[1] found no significant correlation. In our study, patients with more advanced degenerative changes had a less satisfactory outcome.

The relation between the patient's age at operation and the final result is reported to be unclear. Sprague[1] and Jackson and Rouse[24] observed no significant correlation between the two, but Shahriaree et al.[16] noted poor results with advanced age. In our series, statistically significant correlation ($P < 0.008$) was noticed between age at operation and the result.

In the present series, 75% of the knees had excellent or good results. A direct comparison between our study and the various reported series would be inappropriate as the patient age group, location, severity and extent of the degenerative changes, and the methods of evaluation differ. None the less, our results compare with the series of Ewing,[9] who reported 79% good results in patients with unicompartmental arthritis treated by arthroscopic surgery.

The high percentage of satisfactory results obtained in our series could be attributed to various factors. Firstly, the patients were in relatively younger age group (49% were less than 50 years of age). Secondly, the majority of them had less-severe degenerative changes (54% of the knees had grade I or II Outerbridge changes) involving single compartment. Thirdly, our follow-up was relatively short (average 44 months).

The natural history of untreated degenerative arthritis of the knee has been studied by Hernborg and Nilsson.[28] They reported on 71 patients (94 knees) who had osteoarthritis for 10–18 years. In their series, only 17% of the knees improved, 27% remained unchanged and 56% became worse. A much longer-term follow-up is needed to determine whether arthroscopic debridement alters the natural history of osteoarthritis of the knee.

It is likely that the results following arthroscopic debridement will deteriorate with time. However, a useful period is gained during which the level of symptoms is reduced and major open knee surgery is postponed. We agree with Sprague[1] that the knowledge gained during the arthroscopy may be helpful in planning the future reconstructive procedure that may subsequently be needed.

Arthroscopic debridement and irrigation is recommended in well-motivated, carefully selected patients with early, symptomatic, degenerative joint disease of the knee. This procedure burns no bridges and, if it is unsuccessful, there is still recourse to corrective osteotomy or replacement arthroplasty.

Acknowledgments

The authors thank Miss Dina Stanford for the computer analysis of the data. Our thanks are also due to the Medical Photography Department at Westminster Hospital for their help with the illustrations. We are grateful to Miss Linda Terrett for typing this manuscript.

References

1. Sprague NF, Arthroscopic debridement for degenerative knee joint disease, *Clin Orthop* (1981) **160**: 118–123.
2. Magnuson PB, Joint debridement: Surgical treatment of degenerative arthritis, *Surg Gynaecol Obstet* (1941) **73**: 1–9.
3. Magnuson PB, Technique of debridement of the knee joint for arthritis, *Surg Clin North Am* (1946) **26**: 249–266.
4. Haggart GE, Surgical treatment of degenerative arthritis of the knee joint, *New Engl J Med* (1947) **236**: 971–973.
5. Haggart GE, The surgical treatment of degenerative arthritis of the knee joint, *J Bone Joint Surg* (1940) **22**: 717–729.
6. Bert JM, Maschka K, The arthroscopic treatment of unicompartmental gonarthrosis: a five-year follow-up study of abrasion arthroplasty plus arthroscopic debridement and arthroscopic debridement alone, *Arthroscopy* (1989) **5**(1): 25–32.
7. Dandy DJ, Abrasion chondroplasty, *Arthroscopy* (1986) **2**(1): 51–53.
8. Del Pizzo W, Fox JM, Blazina ME et al., Operative arthroscopy for the treatment of problems of the medial compartment of the knee, *Orthopaedics* (1980) **3**(10): 984–986.
9. Ewing JW, Unicompartmental gonarthritis of the knee managed by arthroscopic surgical techniques, *Eighth International Seminar on operative arthroscopy*, Maui, Hawaii, 18–25 October, 1986.
10. Friedman MJ, Berasi CC, Fox JM et al., Preliminary results with abrasion arthroplasty in the osteoarthritic knee, *Clin Orthop* (1984) **182**: 200–205.
11. Jackson RW, Marans HJ, Silver RS, The arthroscopic treatment of degenerative arthritis of the knee, Presented at the Eighth Combined Meeting of the Orthopaedic Associations of the English-speaking World, Washington DC, 1987.
12. Johnson LL, Arthroscopic abrasion arthroplasty – Historical and pathological perspective: present status, *Arthroscopy* (1986) **2**(1): 54–69.
13. Rand JA, Arthroscopic management of degenerative meniscus tears in patients with degenerative arthritis, *Arthroscopy* (1985) **1**(4): 253–258.
14. Richards RN, Lonergan RP, Arthroscopic surgery for relief of pain in the osteoarthritic knee, *Orthopaedics* (1984) **7**(11): 1705–1707.
15. Salisbury RB, Nottage WM, Gardner V, The effect of alignment on results in arthroscopic debridement of the degenerative knee, *Clin Orthop* (1985) **198**: 268–272.
16. Shahriaree H, O'Connor RL, Nottage WM, Seven years'

follow-up on arthroscopic debridement of the degenerative knee, *Field of View* (1982) **1**(1): 1–7.

17. Watanabe M, Takeda S, Ikeuchi H, *Atlas of arthroscopy*, 3rd edn (Berlin: Springer-Verlag, 1979).

18. Ahlbäck S, Osteoarthritis of the knee: a radiographic investigation, *Acta Radiol (Stockh)* (1968) (Suppl) **277**: 7–72.

19. Outerbridge RE, The etiology of chondromalacia patellae, *J Bone Joint Surg (Br)* (1961) **43**: 752–757.

20. Isserlin B, Joint debridement for osteoarthritis of the knee, *J Bone Joint Surg (Br)* (1950) **32**: 302–306.

21. Pridie KH, A method of resurfacing osteoarthritic knee joints, *J Bone Joint Surg (Br)* (1959) **41**: 618–619.

22. Insall JN, Intra-articular surgery for degenerative arthritis of the knee: a report of the work of the late KH Pridie, *J Bone Joint Surg (Br)* (1967) **49**: 211–228.

23. Insall JN, The Pridie debridement operation for osteoarthritis of the knee, *Clin Orthop* (1974) **101**: 61–67.

24. Jackson RW, Rouse DW, The results of partial arthroscopic meniscectomy in patients over 40 years of age, *J Bone Joint Surg (Br)* (1982) **64**: 481–485.

25. McBride GG, Constine RM, Hofmann AA et al., Arthroscopic partial medial meniscectomy in the older patient, *J Bone Joint Surg (Am)* (1984) **66**: 547–551.

26. Burman MS, Finkelstein H, Mayer L, Arthroscopy of the knee joint, *J Bone Joint Surg* (1934) **16**: 255–268.

27. Jackson RW, Abe I, The role of arthroscopy in the management of disorders of the knee, *J Bone Joint Surg (Br)* (1972) **54**: 310–322.

28. Hernborg JS, Nilsson BE, The natural course of untreated osteoarthritis of the knee, *Clin Orthop* (1977) **123**: 130–137.

14.3 Arthroscopic abrasion arthroplasty: What is known and what is unknown?

Lanny L. Johnson

Arthroscopic abrasion arthroplasty remains a controversial topic. Many misunderstandings still prevail concerning the procedure. Some of the misconceptions are that debridement was advocated of intact degenerative cartilage to promote secondary repair; that the abrasion includes removal of the subchondral bone cortex, exposing the cancellous bone; that postoperative joint protection was unnecessary; that I have said that the regenerated tissue was normal hyaline cartilage; that only noncartilaginous fibrous tissue regenerated; that the regenerated tissue always disappeared with time; that the regenerated tissue did not histochemically stain positive for glycopolysaccharides; that no type II collagen would exist in the regenerated fibrocartilage; and last, but not least, that the patients did not derive any benefit from the procedure.

The purpose of this contribution is to clarify these misconceptions. Information will be provided on what is known about arthroscopic abrasion arthroplasty. In addition, those issues which are undocumented or not known at this time will be presented.

Historical review of articular cartilage repair

The attempts at surgical repair by conventional open treatment of full-thickness articular cartilage lesions was restricted to drilling or resection of cortical bone. Magnuson first described the open debridement 'house-cleaning' procedure. The Pridie procedure popularized by Insall was the prevailing surgical approach to the localized area of full-thickness articular cartilage injury.

Animal experiments in injury and repair of articular cartilage indicated that partial thickness lacera-

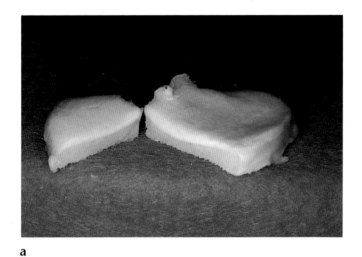
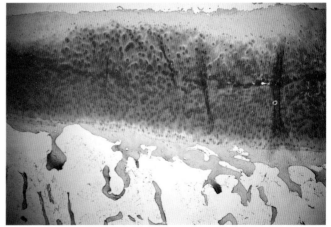

a
b

Figure 1

Normal hyaline cartilage. (a) Gross anatomy of normal tibial plateau from autopsy. Hemisection is made through the specimen. (b) Low-power photomicrograph of normal hyaline cartilage. Safranin-O, ×105.

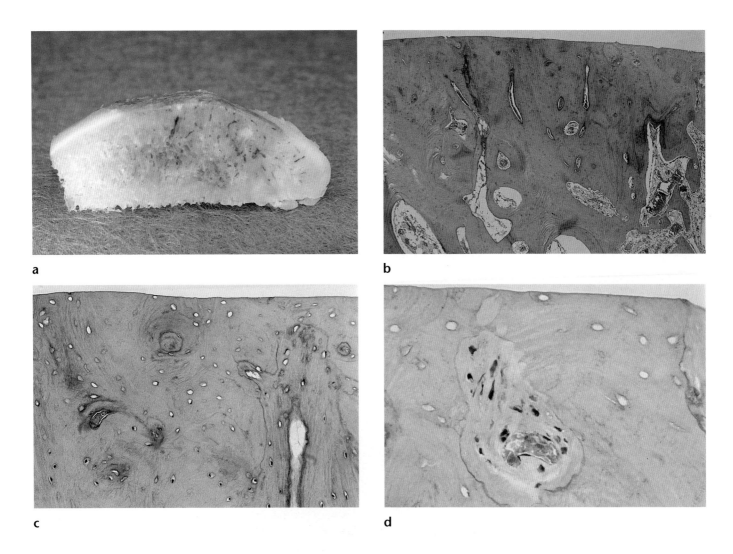

a **b** **c** **d**

Figure 2

Pathology of the sclerotic lesion. (a) Photograph of gross specimen of sclerotic lesion of femoral condyle. The specimen was removed during total knee replacement surgery and subjected to formic acid decalcification. Notice the hypervascularity (dark lines) in the dense bone beneath the sclerotic lesion. (b) Photomicrograph of same specimen showing sclerotic lesion, dense bone, hypervascularity, and empty osteons at the surface. Hematoxylin and eosin, ×8122. (c) Photomicrograph showing surface of the sclerotic lesion with sclerosis and lacunae empty of cells. Hematoxylin and eosin, ×8384. (d) Photomicrograph shows small blood vessels at the surface. Hematoxylin and eosin, ×1048.

tions did not heal.[1] Drilling into subchondral bone was necessary for bleeding to occur in the partial thickness lesion. This drilling was followed by an inflammatory response. A full-thickness lesion created in normal articular cartilage of a rabbit would repair in small lesions (2 mm diameter drillholes).[2] Salter proposed that drilling into the subchondral bone released a pleuripotential cell for the articular repair. Full-thickness lesions of a large diameter did not repair and led to degenerative arthritis.[3] It was agreed that if the subchondral cancellous bone was exposed, the bleeding followed by an inflammatory response resulted in a fibrous tissue repair.[1,4,5] This fibrous tissue would not form cartilage or histo-

chemically stain positive for mucopolysaccharides. In addition, the fibrous repair would always fail and disappear with time.

Other conventional surgical procedures recommended for severe degenerative arthritis are osteotomy and total knee replacement.[6-16]

Normal hyaline cartilage

Inspection of normal hyaline cartilage surfaces gives a basis for comparison with the sclerotic lesion of degenerative arthritis.[17] The gross specimen of

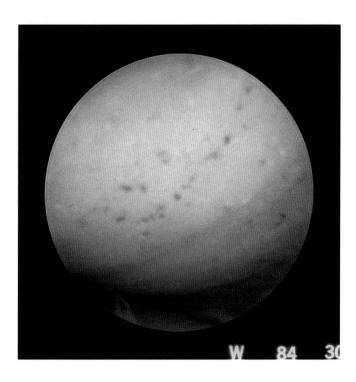

Figure 3

The sclerotic lesion. Arthroscopic view of the sclerotic lesion on the femoral condyles of medial compartment. The lesion is yellow in color and has 'dots' on the surface that represent the small vessels at the surface.

hyaline cartilage shows the bone surface covered with white, glossy hyaline cartilage (Figure 1a). Hyaline cartilage tissue is thick and the surface is smooth. The cells are arranged in orderly vertical rows (Figure 1b). There is an abundance of pericellular material that stains positive for glucoaminoglycans. The tidemark is evident. The normal subchondral bone has a layer of cortex above cancellous bone with thin trabeculae. Osseous vascularity is minimal.

Pathology of the sclerotic lesion

The sclerotic lesion (Grade IV) occurs after the loss of articular cartilage in progressive degenerative arthritis of the knee (Figure 2a–d).[18] Although little attention is given to the sclerotic lesion in the literature,[19,20] these lesions are easily recognized during diagnostic arthroscopy of the knee joint (Figure 3). The sclerotic lesion has a surface with dead osteons interspersed with patches of fibrocartilage repair (Figure 2b). The bone beneath the sclerotic lesion is very dense. There is hypervascularity within the sclerotic lesion (Figure

2b). In fact, on occasion spontaneous hemorrhage and subsequent clot formation have been observed on the surface of a sclerotic lesion during diagnostic arthroscopy (Figure 4). Gross pathological inspection of the sclerotic lesion shows yellow areas of exposed bone surrounded by adjacent yellow-white fragmented degenerative hyaline cartilage[21] (Figure 5). The sclerotic lesion has scattered, small white patches. The patches are well secured both biologically and mechanically to the surface (Figure 5b). There are also scattered pin-point dark dots seen by arthroscopy (Figure 3). The dots represent blood vessels. The presence of the white fibrocartilage patches and dark vessels gives a 'salt-and-pepper' appearance to the sclerotic surface. The cortical bone beneath the lesion is dense with hypervascularity (Figure 2).

Histologically, the sclerotic surface is covered with dead osteons interrupted with islands of cartilage tissue (Figure 2). These islands of cartilage stain positive on Safranin-O for glycosaminoglycans (Figure 5b).[22] This naturally occurring regenerative fibrocartilage is localized to the cortical level and does not penetrate into the cancellous area. The dark dots seen on gross inspection are blood vessels when viewed microscopically (Figure 2b,c,d). The cortical bone is increased in density with thickened trabeculae (Figure 2a). The vascularity in the sclerotic bone is increased over that of adjacent cortical bone under intact articular cartilage. The vessels penetrate through the cortex to the surface. In some cases, focal areas of hemorrhage are seen on the surface by arthroscopy (Figure 4).

Reconstruction of the natural history of the sclerotic lesion

The histological picture, coupled with arthroscopic findings, gives clues to the natural history of the sclerotic lesion. When articular cartilage tissue becomes degenerative, blood vessels penetrate the tide mark (Figure 2b,c). Following complete loss of the hyaline cartilage, the subchondral bone thickens with absence of the articular cartilage cushion (Figure 2a). The surface of the exposed bone becomes necrotic. The reactive bone is hypervascular. Small vessels penetrate to the surface. With weight bearing and friction, the surface vessels rupture and a blood clot is formed[23,24] (Figure 4). The focal area of the blood clot undergoes an inflammatory response, and organization results in fibrous tissue. The fibrocartilage island develops as the spread of the repair is limited by the surrounding surface of dead osteons (Figure 5). This process results in a sclerotic lesion with patches of repair fibrocartilage and small surface blood vessels with an occasional hemorrhage on the surface.

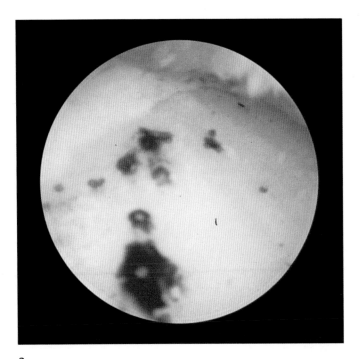
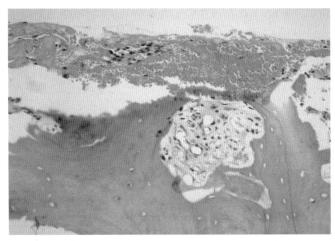

a   b

Figure 4

Natural pathological history of sclerotic lesion with surface bleeding. (a) Arthroscopic view during diagnostic arthroscopy and prior to surgery shows naturally occurring hemorrhage on the surface of the sclerotic lesion. (b) Photomicrograph of biopsy of the same lesion shows hemorrhage and blood clot attached to the surface of the sclerotic lesion. Hematoxylin and eosin,×262.

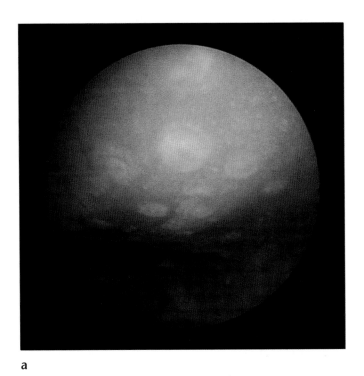
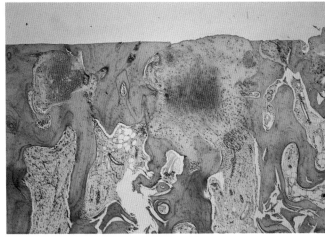

a   b

Figure 5

Natural history of the pathological attempt to resurface the sclerotic lesion. (a) Arthroscopic view of the medial compartment shows the sclerotic lesion on the femoral surface. Notice the small patches of fibrocartilage on the sclerotic lesion. (b) Photomicrograph of a similar sclerotic lesion showing patches of fibrocartilage in dense bone surface with hypervascularity below. Safranin-O, ×104.8.

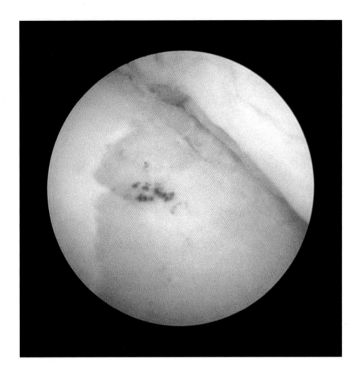

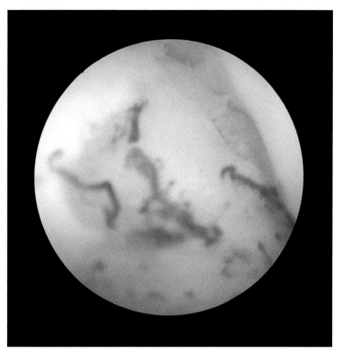

Figure 6

Arthroscopic determination of vascularity. Arthroscopic view of abraded sclerotic lesion with a deeper defect (dimple) into the cortex. The dimple shows red blood vessel on wall within cortical bone.

Figure 7

Arthroscopic determination of vascularity in dense bone of sclerotic lesion. Arthroscopic view following abrasion of femoral condyle with joint decompression. Notice the streaming of blood from the small superficial vessels exposed by the abrasion.

Observations of postosteotomy joint space widening and articular tissue growth

Reports of fibrocartilage growth following osteotomy are probably the result of an improved local environment (decreased pressure) for spontaneous tissue regeneration.[3,9,25] Radiographic evidence of joint-space widening was observed, although no intraarticular surgery was performed. The 'second-look' arthroscopic inspections showing tissue growth had no previous videotape record for control comparison at the site in question.[25]

My early arthroscopic debridement procedures

From 1975 to 1979, arthroscopic debridement procedures were performed in my practice for degenerative arthritis of the knee joint, but no abrasion was performed on areas of the sclerotic lesion. The postoperative management of these patients included one month of non-weight-bearing crutch ambulation. Although most of these patients with degenerative changes had a reduction in their symptoms of pain and swelling, those with sclerotic lesions (Grade IV) were no better. They often came to a second arthroscopic procedure. When a comparison was made between the 'second-look' and the previous arthroscopic videotapes, there was no change observed on the surface of the sclerotic lesion, although repair was seen in other tissues. In addition, patients with unabraded sclerotic lesions showed no widening of the joint spaces on postoperative radiographs which might reflect growth of tissue.

Potential for repair of sclerotic lesion by arthroscopic surgery

In 1979, the question was raised as to what could be done by arthroscopy to stimulate repair in the area of the sclerotic lesion. Open surgical drilling procedures were advocated in the literature to

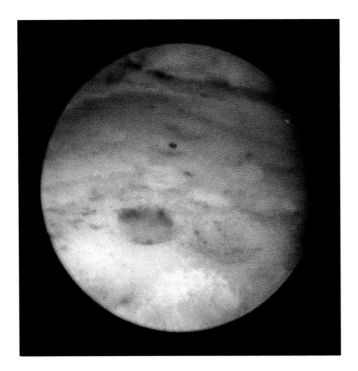

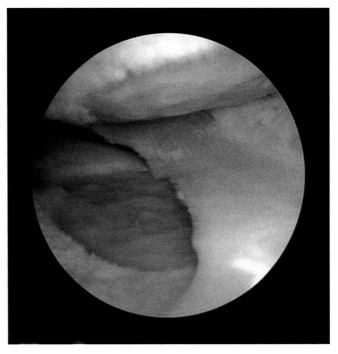

Figure 8

Healing of multiple dimples on sclerotic lesion. 'Second-look' arthroscopic view at 5 weeks after surgical creation of multiple dimples on the tibial surface. There is no coalescence of regrown tissue. The gross appearance of the patches is red, showing residual of blood clot at 5 weeks.

Figure 9

Immediate postoperative arthroscopic view of abrasion arthroplasty. Notice the yellow abraded area on opposing surfaces of both femur and tibia. The meniscus was intact in this patient.

stimulate fibrocartilaginous growth.[26–31] Therefore, multiple drillholes were attempted by arthroscopy through the surface of the sclerotic lesion. It was not technically possible to drill a hole in the posterior areas of the condyles. The arthroscopic surgical exposure did not facilitate a proper angle for drilling a hole. The question arose of how this area, inaccessible to the drill bit, could be exposed to the vascularity. In other words, how deep is the blood supply in the sclerotic lesion of degenerative arthritis? I was not aware, at the time, of the pathological nature of the sclerotic lesion. A defect was made in the sclerotic surface by hand using a curette (Figure 6). This showed that the intracortical vessels were within 1–2 mm of the surface. The confirmation of the superficial position of the vessels was facilitated by decompression of the joint with suction on the arthroscope. The blood streamed out of the small vessels (Figure 7). Isolated small defects were created with a curette in the sclerotic lesion. 'Second-look' arthroscopy performed for academic purposes showed islands of repair tissue at the site of the superficial defects (Figure 8).

In subsequent cases, multiple superficial dimples were created with a motorized burr rather than drillholes on the sclerotic lesion. 'Second-look' arthroscopy showed healing of each dimple but, again, no coalescence of repair tissue between the sparsely placed defects (Figure 9). These were in effect superficial drillholes. There was minimal clinical improvement.

In an attempt to achieve complete reparative covering of the sclerotic defect, an abrasion was performed on the entire sclerotic lesion with a motor-driven burr. These patients reported reduction of symptoms, especially if they had preoperative rest or night pain. Initially, the surgery was limited to one joint surface even if the opposite surface was involved, because of concern for transcondylar fibrous adhesion and resultant ankylosis.

The next step was to create the surface debridement on sclerotic lesions of opposing surfaces. Intermittent active motion was utilized during the postoperative period to reduce the chance of intra-articular adhesion. 'Second-look' arthroscopy between 5 weeks and 2½ years of these single surface repairs showed complete coalescence on the abraded side and no adhesions to the opposing surface.

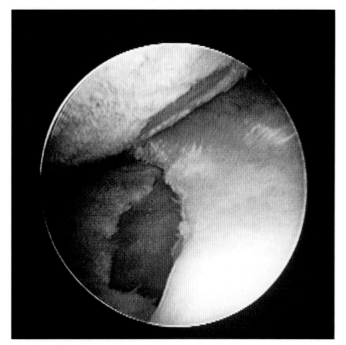

a

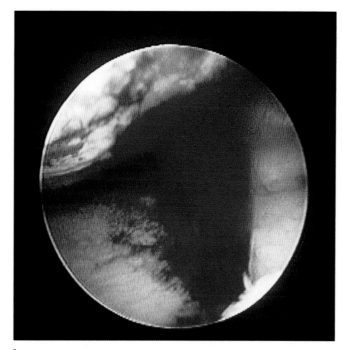

b

Figure 10

Immediate postoperative bleeding and blood clot formation. (a) This arthroscopic view was taken immediately following the abrasion on femur and tibia. There was an inner margin meniscectomy. (b) This arthroscopic view is of same patient 7 minutes later. The tourniquet was released. Bleeding occurred from the arthroscopic portals. Blood clot formed within 7 minutes. The joint was cleansed of blood and unattached blood clot. Notice immediate blood clot attachment to the areas incised and resected during the arthroscopy.

Source of postoperative blood clot

Although I knew it was not necessary to expose cancellous bone area to create bleeding, I originally thought that the arthroscopic abrasion of the sclerotic area must expose vascularity. The vascularity was demonstrated by joint decompression. The surgeon watched for blood to stream out of the debrided cortical bone (Figure 7). Subsequently, I observed that the major volume of blood that would cover the surgical abrasion site came from other sources. The immediate postoperative bleeding came from the intracortical abraded bone, and from the arthroscopic portals and synovial incisions (Figure 10).[32] Redistension and washing after 5–7 minutes show blood clots attached to the abraded sclerotic lesion (Figure 10a). In addition, blood clots form on all areas of surgical incision or debridement: meniscal tissue, hyaline cartilage, and synovium.

Sources of cellular healing

What are the sources of cellular repair of the abraded sclerotic lesion? Salter has proposed a pleuripotential

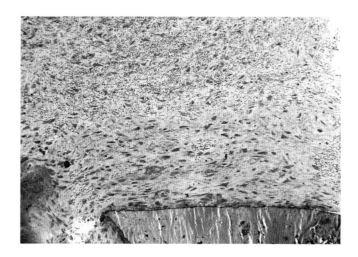

Figure 11

Early healing process shows spindle cell fibrous tissue. Photomicrograph of regrown tissue at 8 weeks following abrasion of sclerotic lesion in patient who protected the joint from weight bearing. Notice the bone below and the avascular spindle cells attached to the surface. Hematoxylin and eosin, ×1048.

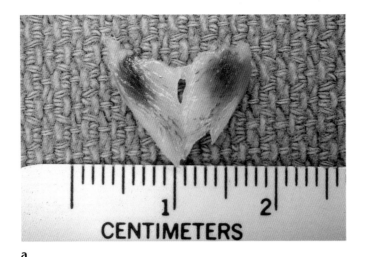

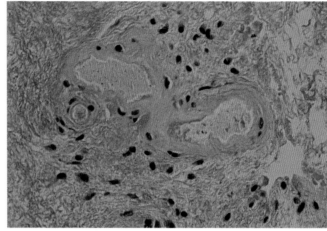

a   b

Figure 12

Deleterious effects of failure to protect joint after abrasion. (a) Photograph of gross specimen taken 1 year after abrasion arthroplasty in a bilateral case in which it was impossible for patient to comply with postoperative non-weight-bearing protocol. Note the vascularity in the specimen. (b) Photomicrograph of fibrous and vascular tissue reaction to immediate ambulation, showing no signs of cartilage cells at 1 year post-operation. Hematoxylin and eosin, ×1048.

cell from the cancellous bone area as a source of articular cartilage repair following drillholes through intact hyaline cartilage in rabbits. This should not directly apply to abrasion arthroplasty, since the debridement does not penetrate into cancellous bone and is not performed in normal joints.

The parent tissue contributes to healing in synovium and bone, but is not a contributor in articular cartilage.[4,5] Unfortunately, hyaline cartilage adjacent to a laceration or a partial-thickness lesion demonstrates no healing contribution to the lesion.[33] There is adjacent cellular mitosis in the early stages of degenerative arthritis, but there is no cellular contribution demonstrated.[1,4,5,33] Little evidence has been reported of local cellular contribution to articular cartilage healing. In a study of loose bodies, Barrie suggested that local cartilage cells proliferate, causing fibrous tissue sealing of surface defects.[34] Carlson reported 'atypical chondrones' adjacent to articular lesions.[35] Aspiration of human knee joint effusion in the presence of a torn meniscus shows monocytes, lymphocytes, and synovial cells. Potenza showed that free cells in the synovium contribute to cellularization and fibrous tissue formation of acellular 14.5-year-old freeze-dried tendon grafts placed free within the animal knee joint.[36] There was cellular covering of the surface and filling of open spaces within the freeze-dried graft. This nonangioblastic, avascular source of cells may contribute to the sealing of the edge of the meniscus and the healing of loose bodies, articular cartilage partial-thickness lesions, and other disrupted intraarticular tissues that are often seen at 'second-look' arthroscopy.

Blood has many components that contribute to tissue repair. Arnoczky reported the importance of the fibrin clot in dog knee joint meniscal healing.[37,38] The nonangioblastic cellular contribution was demonstrated in vitro with human meniscus specimens.[39] Growth factors, such as platelet-derived growth factor (PDGF) and monocyte-macrophage derived growth factor (MDGF) have been identified.[40,41] In-vivo experiments using diffusion-chamber barriers in the subcutaneous tissue of animals showed the differentiation of monocytes into fibroblasts.[23] Allgower and Volkman reported supporting evidence for monocyte transformation into fibroblasts.[42,43] The blood clot contained the cells for the initial inflammatory response.[23]

Necessity of joint protection during early postoperative course

The postoperative events of bleeding, blood clot formation and organization, followed by fibrous tissue replacement take 8 weeks. During this time the clot and the tissue are soft and loosely attached to the abraded tissue. The mechanical force of weight bearing would disrupt or remove the tissue. For both pathological and clinical reasons, the routine of 2 months with non-weight-bearing crutches was instituted early in the series. The patients who protected the joint with non-weight-bearing showed coalescence of avascular spindle cells (Figure 11). These clinical and pathological observations demonstrated the advantages of postoperative joint protection and limited subsequent patient selection for this procedure to those who could and would protect the joint. Patients who walked immediately on their surgically treated extremity had pain and swelling. In addition, 'second-looks' showed that the tissue response was different in the patients who walked on the knee from that in those who protected the joint (Figure 12). Biopsies taken during 'second-look' arthroscopies at 2 months in unprotected knees showed hypervascular granulation tissue. By 4–6 months, the tissue has differentiated into fibrocartilage characterized by round cells surrounded by lacunae (see Figure 17b). At 9 months, there is adherence to the subchondral bone and adjacent articular cartilage (see Figure 16).

Clinical presentation

The patient with a sclerotic lesion accompanying degenerative arthritis presents with a pain complaint greater than anticipated by the physical examination or radiographic changes. The pain occurs even at rest, especially at night. The pain symptom is similar to that experienced by a patient with localized condylar osteonecrosis. The patient also has swelling and joint crepitus. The physical examination confirms the joint degeneration, but is nonspecific for the presence of the sclerotic lesion.[44]

Surgical indications and patient selection

The indications for arthroscopic debridement procedure in degenerative joint disease of the knee include pain, effusion, joint warmth, and loss of function. The indication for the abrasion aspect is dependent upon observing exposed bone at the time of diagnostic arthroscopy. The patient selection has evolved to include a low-activity patient with pain at rest and a minimal alignment problem. In addition, patients must be willing and able to comply with 2 months' postoperative non-weight-bearing ambulation. They also must recognize that there is no expectation for an increased activity level (see Results).

Occasionally, the presence of a sclerotic lesion may not be suspected clinically and is first recognized at surgery. The abrasion aspect of the debridement procedure is usually deferred because the patient has not been prepared for the prolonged postoperative convalescence. Therefore, in all patients with degenerative arthritis undergoing arthroscopic debridement procedures, the possibility of a sclerotic lesion should be considered and the consequences of abrasion discussed prior to surgery. The postoperative extremity protection period may require scheduling to accommodate the patient's calendar.

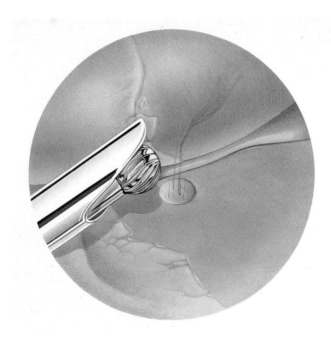

Figure 13

Surgical method of determining depth of blood vessels. Graphic illustration of dimple created by motorized instrumentation in an attempt to assess depth of the intracortical vessels.

Preoperative radiographic evaluation

The radiographic evaluation should include a standing anteroposterior view with the knee at both the extended and 45° flexion positions to determine anterior and posterior joint space.[45] A bilateral Merchant view at 45° flexion provides additional patellofemoral assessment.[46] The loss of joint space is indicative of loss of articular cartilage and a sclerotic lesion.

Pathological criteria

The general pathological indication is restricted to degenerative arthritis. Patients with inflammatory arthritis have little benefit from this procedure. The specific pathological indication for the addition of the abrasion is the presence of exposed bone. Only sclerotic lesions are abraded. Existing articular cartilage surfaces, even though significantly degenerative should be preserved. The debridement on intact degenerative cartilage surfaces should be superficial, preserving existing tissue.

Figure 14

Cutting too deeply is not abrasion. (a) Arthroscopic view of the medial compartment of left knee after complete removal of the cortical bone. The knee was painful. The biopsy site shows thin layer of fibrous tissue even 1 year later. These findings are very different from those if abrasion had been performed and cortex remained intact. (b) Photomicrograph shows thin fibrous layer on osteoporotic bone. There is no cortical bone remaining. Hematoxylin and eosin, ×262. (c) Histological sections of same patient showed thin layer of hypervascular fibrous tissue over cancellous bone. Hematoxylin and eosin, ×1048.

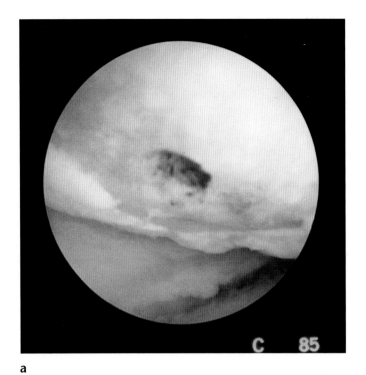

a

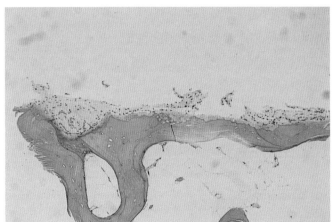

b

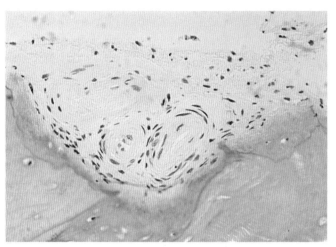

c

Rationale of arthroscopic surgical abrasion

The rationale for the abrasion of the sclerotic lesions is based upon changing the local environment to one which would promote fibrocartilaginous regeneration. Removal of the dead osteons provides a suitable environment for attachment of new tissue (Eugene Mindell, personal communication). The superficial abrasion preserves the supporting cortical bone. Exposure of the superficial vessels is one measure of adequate surgical depth, and provides one source of blood (Figure 7). Blood also accumulates on the debrided area from other surgically disrupted sites (Figure 10).[32] This concept should not be so foreign, in that the natural history of a sclerotic lesion shows aborted attempts at repair (Figure 5).

Surgical technique

The procedure is arthroscopic. The term abrasion indicates that the debridement is superficial, similar to dermabrasion performed in plastic surgery. The name arthroplasty describes an operation including a number of procedures that accompany and usually precede the actual abrasion: synovectomy, meniscectomy, chondroplasty, loose-body removal, lateral patellar release, plus the abrasion to the sclerotic surface. The actual abrasion is performed with motorized instrumentation (Figure 13). A rotation burr is coupled with a suction device, providing clarity of visualization. The abrasion is restricted to areas of exposed sclerotic bone (Grade IV lesions). The abrasion is performed systematically over the lesion. The depth of the cut is restricted to the cortical bone,

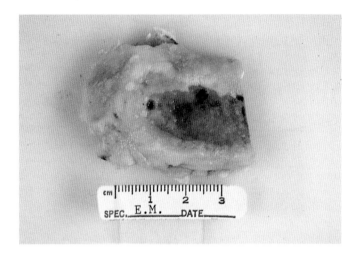

Figure 15

48 hours after abrasion arthroplasty. Photograph of gross specimen shows abraded area with blood clot (dark) attached to abraded area. This early postoperative specimen provides rare opportunity for pathological study. I am indebted to a senior surgeon at another institution who performed an elective total knee arthroplasty 48 hours after a junior surgeon performed abrasion arthroplasty. The senior partner was reportedly dismayed with the surgical judgment and procedure performed by the junior arthroscopic surgeon and performed the total knee arthroplasty as a salvage procedure at this early moment.

usually 1–2 mm. The objective of the debridement is to remove the dead surface osteons and provide a recessed crater for blood attachment (Figures 2, 10b). The proper depth of debridement should not be judged by evidence of vascularity, even though joint decompression and suction applied to the arthroscope will cause bleeding to come from an otherwise apparently avascular cortical surface (Figure 7). If 2 mm of cortical bone have been removed and a depression has been created, there is no reason to resect deeper (Figure 14). In fact, a deep exposure into cancellous bone is counterproductive. Abrasion arthroplasty is not the same procedure reported by Pridie and Insall or created in animals by Salter.[2,10,11,31] The configuration of the Pridie lesion is in reality, an avulsion fracture of the joint surface. This type of lesion results in increased postoperative morbidity and fibrous tissue type healing that lacks longevity (Figure 14).[47] The lesion created by Salter was a full-thickness drillhole into cortical bone. Recently, Salter has published an experiment on abrasion plus continuous passive motion.[54]

The immediate postoperative bleeding from the arthroscopic portals or synovial incision will produce ample blood clot to attach to the abraded surface (Figure 10).[32] Within 6 minutes, a blood clot has formed over the abraded area. The clot is there at 48 hours (Figure 15). The abraded cortical bone is hypervascular (Figure 14b,c).

The configuration produced by the arthroscopic surgical abrasion creates a depression in the bone. There are often a series of grooves produced by the spherical shape of the burr. The irregularity of the surface is thought to facilitate the mechanical attachment of future fibrocartilage. The concave surface will provide a secure housing for the subsequent blood clot[32] (Figure 10b). If the abrasion is too deep, including removal of the cortical bone, then the fibrous tissue that regenerates is thin, vascular, and without cartilaginous nature[47] (Figure 14b). The width of the abrasion continues a few millimeters beyond the exposed bone, so there is a clean smooth junction with the adjacent existing articular cartilage to facilitate biological adhesion to the surrounding cartilage. If this is not performed during the abrasion, the resulting fibrous tissue patch will not coalesce with the adjacent tissue and will appear as an island surrounded by exposed bone.

Observation of the reparative process

The technique of arthroscopy provides means of careful inspection of the pathological lesion, the surgical site, and the immediate postoperative events, and an opportunity for a 'second-look' and biopsy of the operative site with minimal patient risk or morbidity. In addition, the original procedure was recorded on videotape for subsequent comparison. Correlation of the pathological process seen by arthroscopy can be made from biopsy and surgical specimens following an occasional subsequent total knee replacement (Figure 16).

In those patients who came to subsequent high tibial osteotomy, there were small areas of regenerated fibrocartilage. These cases provided an opportunity for biopsies for histological and collagen type studies.

Nature of the regenerated articular cartilage

The regenerated tissue is *not* hyaline cartilage. Normal hyaline cartilage is characterized by its glassy gross appearance. The normal color is white and it is firm to palpation. The color becomes yellow and the surface becomes soft with degeneration. Histologically, normal hyaline cartilage has a sparse round cellular pattern in the normal matrix (Figure 17a). The cells have surrounding lacunae. Normal hyaline cartilage stains positive for glycosaminoglycans with Safranin-O, especially around the cells.[2,31,40,48] Hyaline cartilage is uniquely characterized by the presence of type II collagen.[49]

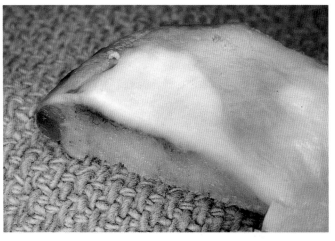

a

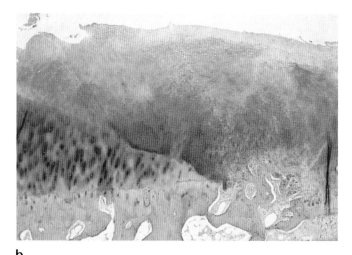

b

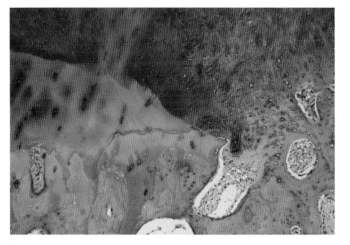

c

Figure 16

Regenerated fibrocartilage at 9 months after abrasion. This specimen was obtained at the time of total knee arthroplasty in a patient who had gross instability of the knee and in whom the arthroscopic procedure would not now be performed. (a) Photograph of gross specimen of femoral condyle shows the regenerated fibrocartilage higher in profile than the adjacent tissue. (b) Photomicrograph of the same specimen shows regenerated fibrocartilage to the right and existing hyaline cartilage in left lower corner. Notice the biological adherence to the bone beneath and the adjacent hyaline cartilage. Safranin-O, ×104.8. (c) Photomicrograph at higher magnification shows tidemark, hypervascularity beneath regenerated fibrocartilage. Safranin-O, ×262.

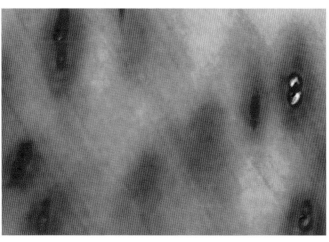

a

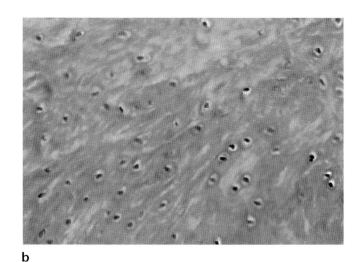

b

Figure 17

Comparison of cellularity of hyaline and regenerative fibrocartilage at 9 months. (a) Photomicrograph of hyaline cartilage. Notice the cellular pattern in clumps with pericellular increased density of histochemical stain for mucopolysaccharide. Safranin-O, ×1048. (b) Photomicrograph of regenerative fibrocartilage. This pattern is more cellular. The pattern is irregular. The cells are smaller, although having lacunae. The histochemical staining is diffuse. The matrix is fibrous in nature. Safranin-O, ×1048.

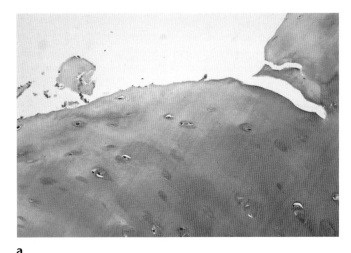

a

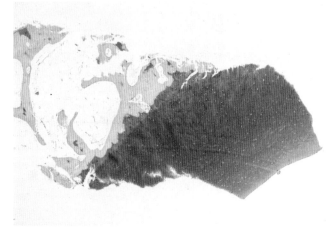

a

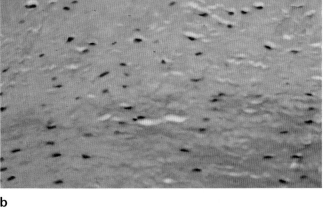

b

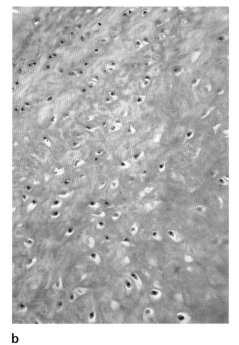

b

Figure 18 (above)

Comparison of surface of degenerative and regenerative articular cartilage at 9 months after abrasion. (a) Photomicrograph of surface of degenerative hyaline cartilage. Notice the fissure. Safranin-O, ×1048. (b) Photomicrograph of surface of regenerated fibrocartilage. Notice the flattened cellular layer similar to normal lamina splendins. Safranin-O, ×1048.

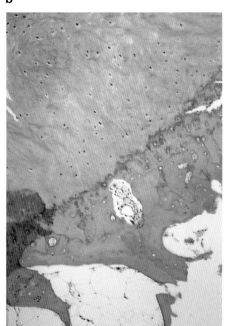

c

The regenerated fibrocartilage following abrasion arthroplasty does not have the physical properties of hyaline cartilage. It is not glassy in appearance (Figure 16). It is biomechanically different, being easily compressible to palpation. The reparative fibrocartilage differs histologically from adjacent degenerative hyaline cartilage (Figure 17b). The cells are smaller and more numerous. The matrix staining with Safranin-O shows a diffuse concentration of proteoglycans rather than closely surrounding the cells as in the normal tissue. The tidemark does not exist under the repair at this time (Figure 16b). This area is very vascular compared to the adjacent degenerative area, which has only an occasional vascular penetration of the tidemark. The surface of the reparative fibrocartilage is smooth compared to the adjacent fragmented degenerative cartilage (Figure 18). This fibrocartilage develops type II collagen, but not in the same quantities as normal hyaline cartilage.

Restoration of the tidemark

'Second-look' arthroscopies and biopsies have been performed up to 5 years following abrasion of a sclerotic lesion. This opportunity occurs with subsequent injury to or surgery on the opposite knee. The tidemark was not seen at 2 years, but was observed in specimens at 4, 5 and 9 years (Figure 19c).

Development of type II collagen in regenerated fibrocartilage

The histological nature of the reparative tissue is fibrocartilaginous. The presence of type II collagen would liken the regrown tissue to hyaline cartilage.[12,50] Collagen typing was performed in Keely's laboratory at Toronto Children's Hospital in Canada on 14 patients when opportunity presented. These were performed between 1 year and 9½ years following the original surgery. The regenerated articular tissue from the area of the previously debrided sclerotic lesion was examined and biopsied. There was no type II collagen in two specimens taken at 1 year or at 9 years. Two specimens had 10% of the normal type II collagen at the 1-year interval. Two others had 20% at 2 years postoperatively. One had 75% at 5 years. Three specimens had 100% of the normal amount of type II collagen; one was only 1 year post-abrasion.

These preliminary data on a small number of patients demonstrated that the regenerative fibrocartilage has the potential to develop type II collagen. The amounts increase between 1 and 5 years, but not in concentrations of normal cartilage. The issue of maintenance of that type of collagen was questioned when the longest-surviving tissue specimen (over 9 years) in our series had no type II in their fibrocartilage.

Durability of the regenerated articular cartilage

The presence of the regenerated tissue following abrasion arthroplasty can be determined by two methods. The first would be circumstantial evidence from comparison of pre- and postoperative radiographs (Figure 20). The creation and maintenance of a wider joint space would suggest the presence of regenerative tissue. The second method would be by 'second-look' arthroscopy or inspection of open surgical specimens (Figure 16).

Comparison radiographs in the first series (1979–1980) of 105 patients showed 64 to have standing anteroposterior radiographs available for comparison studies 2 years following surgery. Half of them showed development and maintenance of a wider joint space. Fifteen of the 20 patients with bone on bone developed a wider joint space at 2 years postoperatively. Only 5 patients of the 64 developed a narrower joint space during the 2 years after surgery.

The regenerative fibrocartilage tissue has survived up to 9½ years following abrasion debridement (Figure 17). Arthroscopic 'second-looks' were possible with surgery on the other knee, injury to involved knee, or failure of first procedure. The covering, although complete, is usually fibrillated and soft.

Figure 19

'Second-look' arthroscopy at 5 years following abrasion arthroplasty provides biopsy specimen. (a) Photomicrograph of the core biopsy of healed area. Notice the surface to the right and the bone to the left. The fibrocartilage is richly stained histochemically for mucopolysaccharides. Safranin-O, ×104.8. (b) Photomicrograph of central area of cellular pattern typical of mature regenerated fibrocartilage. Safranin-O, ×8384. (c) Photomicrograph of regenerated tide mark at 5 years following abrasion arthroplasty. Safranin-O, ×262.

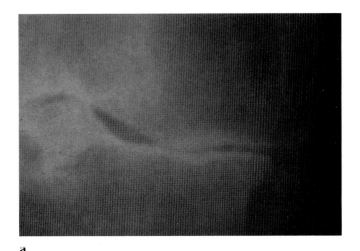

a

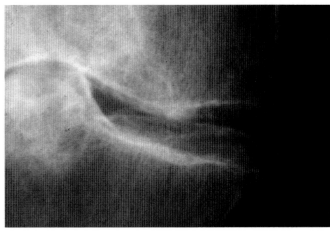

b

Figure 20

Comparison standing radiographs. (a) Preoperative standing anteroposterior plain radiographs show absence of medial joint space. (b) Radiographs at 2½ years following surgery show widened joint space, indicative of regenerated fibrocartilage.

Maintenance of regenerated articular cartilage has been reported in patients coming to total knee replacement between 9 months and 2 years, even though the clinical result was unsatisfactory (Figure 16).[51]

Clinical response

The preceding discussion of the pathology and tissue response is of importance only if the patient benefits from the procedure. My clinical results have been assessed on three occasions.

Original series; two-year follow-up

This was reported in 1982 at the AAOS annual meeting in Anaheim, California. The material was submitted, but not accepted for publication. The following is a summary of those data.

One-hundred-and-five patients underwent abrasion of a sclerotic lesion during an arthroscopic debridement procedure between 1979 and 1980. All patients had pain at rest, especially during the night. They had a joint effusion confirmed at surgery. There was radiographic evidence of degenerative arthritis. Forty-five patients had previous open surgical procedures on their knees at an average of 8.6 years before the present surgery. It should be noted that all 105 patients were considered candidates in those years for open surgery: arthrotomy, osteotomy, or total knee

replacement. There were 59 men and 46 women. The age range was 29–88 years with an average of 60 years. Preoperatively, 33 patients had agreed to a 'second-look' arthroscopy for research purposes between 5 weeks and 2½ years. This prior agreement provided information on the healing response.

The minimum follow-up was 2 years. Ninety-five patients responded to questionnaires. Forty-two patients (44 knees) returned for a follow-up examination.

The composite response to the questionnaire on the 99 knees (95 patients) showed 7 the same, 74 better, and 15 worse than before surgery. Three patients did not respond to that question. Further analysis did not find a significant relationship between the result and age, sex, previous surgery, the side involved, the site of the lesion, the size of the lesion, any combination of lesion sites, the combination of the debridement performed, the existence of mild varus or valgus, the presence of the meniscus, preoperative radiographic joint space, and, perhaps significantly, the widening of the postoperative radiographic joint space.

Of the 42 patients examined in the office, 5 knees were reported the same, 35 were better, 1 was worse, and 3 patients did not answer the question. Half of the 44 knees had no night or standing pain. Pain and symptoms were related to activity. No stiffness or swelling was reported by 52%; 25% said they had stiffness or swelling with activity. Seven of the 42 patients used a cane. Sixteen patients made a postoperative doctor's visit for treatment; six were given a cortisone shot.

Physical examination

Grating on physical examination was present in 55% of those knees examined. The range of motion showed minimal loss.

Subsequent surgery

Ten of the 105 patients had repeat surgery within the first 2 years. Five arthroscopic surgical procedures were performed, including two therapeutic lavages, a second abrasion over a wider area, and one repeat abrasion for a new lesion. An arthrotomy was performed by another surgeon for a loose body. Two patients had osteotomies. There were two total knee replacements, with one performed at 4 months postoperatively in another city. That patient subsequently returned for an abrasion of the other knee, because the total knee had ankylosis. The other total knee replacement was performed on a poorly selected case for abrasion, having marked preoperative ankylosis.

Radiographic evaluation

Radiographic comparisons were possible on 64 patients; 50% had a wider joint space (Figure 20).

Complications

There were no hemorrhages, thromboembolic phenomena, surgical deaths, or infections.

Five-year follow-up on original series

The 1979–1980 series was reviewed again at a minimum of 5 years following surgery. The results are summarized here.

Forty-six patients (50 knees) were examined a minimum of 5 years following the initial surgery. Another 27 patients (28 knees) responded by questionnaire.

The chance of another operation in this first series (1979–1980) was 22% at 5 years. Three had a subsequent arthroscopic procedure. Eighteen patients' knees (out of 105) had a subsequent open operation. There were 7 osteotomies, 7 total knee replacements, and 4 arthrotomies. There was little patient selection in this series. It included multiple compartment disease, ankylosis, morbid obesity, and instabilities. These are now recognized as contraindications. It is important to recall that in 1979–1980 the original choice of procedure would have been an open operation in all of these patients, but only 18 had open surgery in this unselected group even after 5 years.

Physical examination

Of the 50 examined knees, there was tenderness in 25. Forty-five knees had crepitus in the patellofemoral joint. There were two existing mild effusions at the time of the examination. The range of motion averaged 4.5° extension and 122° flexion. The range of motion observed is superior to those reported following total knee joint replacement.[6,7,10-16]

1988 Review of entire experience

In the fall of 1988, a review was initiated on the entire experience with abrasion arthroplasty.

1983–1986 series

There were 399 patients undergoing 423 arthroscopic debridement procedures that included an abrasion arthroplasty between 1983 and 1986. This gives a maximum follow-up of 5 years and a minimum of 2 years.

Fifty-three percent of the patients (217 patients/228 knees) responded to a questionnaire to evaluate their subjective result and the incidence of reoperation. The summary is as follows:

No complaint of any type: 12%
Pain: 66%
Use medication: 44%
Loss of motion: 24%
Limp: 36%
Use of cane/crutch: 12% at some time
Restriction of activity: 99%
Under a doctor's care: 25%
Had subsequent surgery: 14% (31 of 228 patients)
Type of subsequent surgery:
    Arthroscopic: 13
    Open: 15
    Osteotomy: 1
    Total knee replacement: 12
    Unicompartmental replacement: 2
    Unspecified knee surgery: 3

Reoperation incidence by the individual year

The incidence of reoperation in this recent series was 11% at 2 years, 16% at 3 years, 9% at 4 years, and 16% after 5 years.

The follow-up on 228 patients reporting by questionnaire in the 1983–1986 series was 31 knee reoperations. This is a 14% reoperation rate. Thirteen procedures were arthroscopic. There was one osteotomy. There were 12 total knee replacements and 2 unicompartmental surgeries. There were three unspecified knee surgeries.

The 5-year follow-up from 1983 showed a 16% incidence of reoperation. There were 5 arthroscopic procedures, 1 osteotomy, and 6 total knee replacements.

In 4 years of follow-up from 1984, there was a 9% incidence of reoperation. There were 4 total knee replacements, and 2 arthroscopic procedures.

In a 3-year follow-up from 1985, there was a 16% incidence. There were 6 arthroscopic procedures, 1 osteotomy, 1 total knee, and 1 unicompartmental replacement.

In a 2-year follow-up from 1986, there was an 11% incidence of reoperation. There were 2 arthroscopic procedures and 2 total knee replacements.

The incidence of reoperation 2–5 years after abrasion and osteotomy is 11%, or 2 out of 19.

Management of malalignment

Many patients with severe osteoarthritis have axial malalignment with joint space collapse. Although it seemed that both the surface and alignment problems should be corrected, it was not technically possible in 1980 for me to perform both the arthroscopic debridement and osteotomy in a reasonable operative time. Many patients were elderly or had medical problems that placed restraints on the duration of anesthesia. Also, the surgical equipment used at that time was not as perfected as the motorized instrumentation of today. In early 1980, primitive transcutaneous burrs without suction were being utilized and the arthroscopic debridement lasted 1½ hours. Therefore, the arthroscopic procedure was performed first and the angulation osteotomy was planned for 6–8 weeks later. Many patients experienced immediate relief of pain after the debridement procedure that included the abrasion of the sclerotic lesion and therefore, declined the osteotomy. They opted for testing the result of arthroscopic debridement procedure. The opportunity was seized to observe the results of the arthroscopic abrasion arthroplasty procedure. Subsequently, only 7 of the first 105 knees came to osteotomy within the next 5 years.

A retrospective review of the incidence of abrasion arthroplasty and accompanying osteotomy shows an increased incidence of the combined procedure in my practice. The decreased total numbers of this type of surgery during 1989 and 1990 reflected a reduction in my total surgical volume. I reduced my clinical practice to one surgery day per week to accommodate an increased research schedule (see Table 1).

Results of combined abrasion and osteotomy

In our first survey, 29 out of 83 cases of combined abrasion with osteotomy between 1983 and 1986

responded to the questionnaire. Nineteen had persistent pain. Thirteen took medication. Six experienced loss of motion. Thirteen walked with a limp. Three used a cane or crutch. Nineteen had restricted activity. Six were under a doctor's care for their knees. There were two reoperations. There was one total knee replacement and one unicompartmental procedure in minimum 2-year and maximum 5-year follow-up. A new study is presently underway.

Present status of combined procedure: abrasion and osteotomy

Presently, osteotomies are routinely performed in combination with knee abrasion arthroplasty, when varus deformity exceeds 5° or valgus exceeds 12°. In addition, an osteotomy is recommended in patients who walk with a lurch, are obese, or desire a higher activity level. The osteotomy is contraindicated if opposite compartment or patellofemoral joint has severe degeneration or there is mechanical instability with shift of the tibia on the femur. Recent results would indicate a better result than if abrasion had been the only procedure in patients with measured malalignment.

Summary of what is known about abrasion arthroplasty in 1991

Patient selection
Patient selection plays a major role in the outcome of this procedure. The ideal patient is one with low activity level, rest or night pain, satisfactory axial alignment, and no mechanical instability. The patient must be compliant with 2 months of non-weight-bearing protocol following surgery and wait a 6–12 month period for maximal benefit. The patient often selects this procedure as an alternative to total knee replacement when the lesion is confined to only one compartment.

Contraindications
The contraindications are morbid obesity, ankylosis, instability, severe angulatory deformity, multiple compartment exposed bone, inflammatory arthritis,

Table 1

Year	1980	1981	1982	1983	1984	1985	1986	1987	1988	1989	1990
AAA cases[a]	110	151	141	138	122	76	87	47	56	9	6
Osteotomies	4	0	6	7	12	30	34	13	29	25	20

[a]AAA = Arthroscopic abrasion arthroplasty.

and anticipated failure of compliance with the postoperative regimen of non-weight-bearing ambulation.

Pathologic basis for superficial abrasion

The pathologic observations show that the vascularity of a sclerotic lesion is abundant and at the surface. Therefore, only a superficial debridement is required to expose vessels. When an articular cartilage traumatic avulsion lesion occurs, subchondral cortical bone is exposed. No abrasion is required in acute traumatic cases, as the crater is created from the cartilage surface and the vessels have been traumatically exposed. Trimming of the hyaline cartilage margins may be all that is required.

Surgical technique

Most surgeons make too deep an abrasion. Cutting too deeply is a common technical error resulting in worsening of pain and prolonged recovery or failure to benefit. The surgical technique of abrasion requires only a 2-mm-deep crater to be created over the area of the sclerotic lesion. Deeper debridement is not only unnecessary, but results in increase patient morbidity and non-cartilaginous repair, perhaps even propagating further degenerative changes in the knee.

Role of the osteotomy

An angulation osteotomy is combined with the arthroscopic procedure in unicompartmental cases with significant axial malalignment.

Postoperative management

Two months of non-weight-bearing ambulation is necessary for proper healing and maturation of the regenerative tissue. A noncompliant patient will have a painful, swollen knee joint. The regenerated tissue will remain hypervascular (Figure 7). Continuous passive motion is used only in the osteotomy patients. It is limited to 3–4 days during their hospitalization.

Morbidity

There is minimal surgical discomfort from the abrasion procedure. There is no hospital admission for arthroscopic debridement and abrasion. The postoperative complications are nonexistent. The postoperative non-weight-bearing ambulation for 2 months is inconvenient, but necessary for success of this procedure.

The reparative process

The immediate postoperative bleeding from the joint and adjacent vessels form a blood clot on the surface. This clot is vulnerable to mechanical disruption. If protected the clot organizes and forms fibrous tissue by 8 weeks (Figure 11). A fibrocartilage will be seen by 4 months (Figure 17).

What happens to the regenerated tissue? The tissue will survive. It has been seen at 'second-look' arthroscopy on many occasions (Figure 20). The longest documented survival at this time is 9½ years in one patient. The entire surface was covered. The tissue was soft and fragmented. It stained positive for glycosaminoglycans, but had no type II collagen.

Unfortunately, the survival of the reparative fibrocartilage is not consistent. It has greater chance of survival in traumatic lesions. The survival incidence is less when generalized or progressive degenerative arthritis exists, and in the presence of axial malalignment or mechanical or ligamentous instability.

Is the growth of regenerated fibrocartilage a benefit? It is not known whether the existence of reparative fibrocartilage is correlated with a clinical benefit. In my 2-year analysis of the 1979–1980 series, a comparison was made of clinical benefit and the presence of a widened joint space at minimum 2 years. The absence of a wider joint space indicative of no tissue growth did not adversely affect the patient assessment of benefit. A report by Jack M. Bert showed that regeneration was associated with poor clinical result.[51]

Results of other surgeons

Friedman et al. had modest success even though their patients did not conform to the postoperative regimen.[52] Rand[53] has not had success in salvaging previous osteotomy or in reducing the incidence of subsequent total knee replacement. Rand reported reoperation in high percentage of his patients. A report by Bert showed no correlation between growth and maintenance of the tissue and a beneficial clinical result. In addition, Bert reported poorer clinical results in patients with an abrasion as compared to a similar group without abrasion even though tissue was produced and retained following abrasion during the debridement procedure.[51] Inspection of the illustrations of surgical technique suggests the debridement was deeper than an 'abrasion.'

My results

My results are better than those reported or what other surgeons personally communicate. I believe the main reason for poor results is lack of preoperative assessment of the patient's objectives and expectations. The procedure has to be understood as palliative, not curative. Patients have to be selected with this type of outcome in mind. Many surgeons cut too deeply, thereby creating an iatrogenic avulsion fracture which will result in immediate postoperative pain and a poor tissue repair. Another reason for poor results is the failure to insist on postoperative joint protection of the immature fibrous tissue with 2 months of non-weight-bearing ambulation. In the absence of the protection, the newly forming tissue is mechanically destroyed.

Seventy-five percent of my patients report that they are improved at 2 years compared to their memory of the preoperative condition. Eighty-eight percent of my patients (minimum 2-year follow-up) had some complaint; the most common was activity restriction; two-thirds complained of pain. Although they complained of decreased range of motion, the measured motions after abrasion arthroplasty were better than those reported after total knee replacement.[6,7,10,11,13–16] The reoperation rate in my patients is low.

At the time of their surgery, these patients would have been considered candidates for an open conventional surgery, arthrotomy, osteotomy, or total knee replacement. After minimum of 5 years following abrasion arthroplasty, only a small percentage submitted to such surgery (see above results). Arthroscopic abrasion arthroplasty remains a reasonable alternative to open surgical treatment.

References

1. **Mankin HJ**, Current concepts review: The response of articular cartilage to mechanical injury, *J Bone Joint Surg (Am)* (1982) **64**: 460–466.
2. **Salter RB, Simmonds DF, Malcolm BW et al.**, The biological effect of continuous passive motion on the healing of full-thickness defects in articular cartilage: an experimental investigation in the rabbit, *J Bone Joint Surg (Am)* (1980) **62**: 1232–1251.
3. **Coventry MB**, Osteotomy about the knee for degenerative and rheumatoid arthritis: indications, operative technique and results, *J Bone Joint Surg (Am)* (1973) **55**: 23–48.
4. **Mankin HJ**, The reaction of articular cartilage to injury and osteoarthritis. Part I, *N Engl J Med* (1974) **291**: 1285–1292.
5. **Mankin HJ**, The reaction of articular cartilage to injury and osteoarthritis. Part II, *N Engl J Med* (1974) **291**: 1335–1340.
6. **Aglietti P, Rinonapoli E**, Total condylar knee arthroplasty: A five-year follow-up study of 33 knees, *Clin Orthop* (1984) **186**: 104–111.
7. **Bae DK, Guhl JF, Keane SP**, Unicompartmental knee arthroplasty for single compartment disease: clinical experience with an average four-year follow-up study, *Clin Orthop* (1983) **176**: 233–238.
8. **Convery FR, Akeson WH, Keown GH**, The repair of large osteochondral defects: an experimental study in horses, *Clin Orthop* (1972) **82**: 253–262.
9. **Coventry MB**, Upper tibial osteotomy for gonarthrosis: the evolution of the operation in the last 18 years and long-term results, *Orthop Clin North Am* (1979) **10**: 191–210.
10. **Insall J, Walker P**, Unicondylar knee replacement, *Clin Orthop* (1976) **120**: 83–85.
11. **Insall JN, Hood RW, Flawn LB et al.**, The total condylar knee prosthesis in gonarthrosis: a five to nine-year follow-up of the first one hundred consecutive replacements, *J Bone Joint Surg (Am)* (1983) **65**: 619–628.
12. **Jackson RW, Burdick W**, Unicompartmental knee arthroplasty, *Clin Orthop* (1984) **190**: 182–185.
13. **Laskin RS**, Unicompartmental tibiofemoral resurfacing arthroplasty, *J Bone Joint Surg (Am)* (1978) **60**: 182–185.
14. **Mallory TH, Dolibois JM**, Unicompartment total knee replacement: a 2–4 year review, *Clin Orthop* (1978) **134**: 139–143.
15. **Scott RD, Volatile TB**, Twelve years' experience with posterior cruciate-retaining total knee arthroplasty, *Clin Orthop* (1986) **205**: 100–107.
16. **Windsor RE, Lotke PA, Ecker ML et al.**, Long-term results after total condylar knee replacement, *Orthop Trans* (1983) **7**: 415–416.
17. **Weiss C**, Normal and osteoarthritic articular cartilage, *Orthop Clin North Am* (1979) **10**: 175–189.
18. **Outerbridge RE**, The etiology of chondromalacia patellae, *J Bone Joint Surg (Br)* (1961) **43**: 752–757.
19. **Byers PD**, The effect of high femoral osteotomy on osteoarthritis of the hip: an anatomical study of six hip joints, *J Bone Joint Surg (Br)* (1974) **56**: 279–290.
20. **Jaffe HL**, *Metabolic, degenerative and inflammatory diseases of bones and joints* (Philadelphia: Lea & Febiger, 1972) 735.
21. **Johnson LL**, Arthroscopic abrasion arthroplasty historical and pathologic perspective: present status, *Arthroscopy* (1986) **2**: 54–69.
22. **Rosenberg L**, Chemical basis for the histological use of Safranin O in the study of articular cartilage, *J Bone Joint Surg (Am)* (1971) **53**: 69–82.
23. **Petrakis NL, Davis M, Lucia SP**, The in vivo differentiation of human leukocytes into histiocytes, fibroblasts, and fat cells in subcutaneous diffusion chambers, *Blood* (1961) **17**: 109–118.
24. **Ross R, Oldland G**, Human wound repair. II. Inflammatory cells, epithelial-mesenchymal interrelations, and fibrogenesis, *J Cell Biol* (1968) **39**: 152–168.
25. **Fujisawa Y, Masuhara K, Shiomi S**, The effect of high tibial osteotomy on osteoarthritis of the knee: an arthroscopic study of 54 knee joints, *Orthop Clin North Am* (1979) **10**: 585–608.
26. **Campbell CJ**, The healing of cartilage defects, *Clin Orthop* (1969) **64**: 45–63.
27. **Magnuson PB**, Technique of debridement of knee joint for arthritis, *Surg Clin North Am* (1946) **26**: 249–266.
28. **Meachim G, Roberts C**, Repair of the joint surface from subarticular tissue in the rabbit knee, *J Anat* (1971) **109**: 317–327.
29. **Meachim G, Osborn GV**, Repair of the femoral articular cartilage surface in osteoarthritis of the hip, *J Pathol* (1970) **102**: 1–8.
30. **Mitchell N, Shepard N**, The resurfacing of adult rabbit articular cartilage by multiple perforations through the subchondral bone, *J Bone Joint Surg (Am)* (1976) **58**: 230–233.
31. **Pridie KW**, A method of resurfacing osteoarthritic knee joints, *J Bone Joint Surg (Br)* (1959) **41**: 618–619.
32. **Johnson LL**, Characteristics of the immediate postarthroscopic blood clot formation in the knee joint, *Arthroscopy* (1991) **7**: 14–23.
33. **Ghadially FN**, *Fine structure of synovial joints* (London: Butterworths, 1983).
34. **Barrie HJ**, Intra-articular loose bodies regarded as organ cultures in vivo, *J Pathol* (1978) **125**: 163–169.
35. **Carlson H**, Reactions of rabbit patellar cartilage following operative defects, *Acta Orthop Scand* (1957) suppl. 28.
36. **Potenza AD, Herte MC**, The synovial cavity as a "tissue culture in situ" – science or nonsense? *J Hand Surg* (1982) **7**: 196.
37. **Arnoczky SP, Warren RF**, Microvasculature of the human meniscus, *Am J Sports Med* (1982) **10**: 90–95.
38. **Arnoczky SP, McDevitt CA, Warren RF et al.**, Meniscal repair using an exogenous fibrin clot: An experimental study in the dog, *Trans Orthop Res Soc* (1986) **11**: 452.
39. **Johnson LL, Bull R, Flo G et al.**, Meniscal healing: non-angioblastic cellular contribution, AANA Annual Meeting, San Francisco (1986).
40. **Deuel TF, Huang JS**, Platelet-derived growth factor: Structure, function, and roles in normal and transformed cells, *J Clin Invest* (1984) **74**: 669–676.
41. **Ross R, Raines E, Bowen-Pope D et al.**, *General concepts of growth factors: A progress report on platelet-derived growth factor* (Departments of Pathology and Biochemistry, University of Washington School of Medicine, Seattle, Wash.) 27–34.
42. **Allgower M, Hulliger L**, Origin of fibroblasts from mononuclear blood cells: a study on in vitro formation of the collagen precursor, hydroxyproline, in buffy coat cultures, *Surgery* (1960) **47**: 603–610.

43. **Volkman A,** The origin and fate of the monocyte, *Ser Haemat,* vol III (1970) **2:** 62–92.

44. **Johnson LL,** Arthroscopic surgery, principles and practice (St Louis: CV Mosby, 1986) 732–773.

45. **Rosenberg TD, Paulos LE, Parker RD et al.,** The forty-five-degree posteroanterior flexion weight-bearing radiograph of the knee, *J Bone Joint Surg (Am)* (1988) **70:** 1479–1483.

46. **Merchant AC, Mercer RL, Jacobsen RH et al.,** Roentgenographic analysis of patellofemoral congruence, *J Bone Joint Surg (Am)* (1974) **56:** 1391–1396.

47. **Richmond JC, Gambadella PG, Schelling S et al.,** A canine model of osteoarthritis with histologic study of repair tissue following abrasion arthroplasty, Presented at the Annual Meeting of the North American Arthroscopy Association, Boston, Mass. (1985).

48. **Sokaloff L,** *The joints and synovial fluid,* vols 1 and 2 (Orlando, Fla.: Academic Press, 1980).

49. **O'Driscoll SW, Salter RB, Keely FW,** A method of quantitative analysis of ratios of Type I and II collagen in small samples of articular cartilage, *Anal Chem* (1985) **145:** 277–285.

50. **Freeman MAR,** *Adult articular cartilage,* 2nd edn (Tunbridge Wells, Kent: Pitman Medical, 1979).

51. **Bert JM, Maschka K,** The arthroscopic treatment of unicompartmental gonarthrosis: a five-year follow-up study of abrasion arthroplasty plus arthroscopic debridement and arthroscopic debridement alone, *Arthroscopy* (1989) **5:** 25–32.

52. **Friedman MJ, Berasi CC, Fox JM et al.,** Preliminary results with abrasion arthroplasty in the osteoarthritic knee, *Clin Orthop* (1984) **182:** 200–205.

53. **Rand JA, Ritts GD,** Abrasion arthroplasty as a salvage for failed upper tibial osteotomy, *J Arthroplasty* (1989) **4**(suppl.) S45–S48.

54. **Kim HKW, Moran ME, Salter RB,** The potential for regeneration of articular cartilage in defects created by chondral shaving and subchondral abrasion: an experimental investigation in rabbits, *J Bone Joint Surg (Am)* (1991) **73:** 1301–1315.

15

Osteotomy in osteoarthritis

15.1   High tibial osteotomy for degenerative arthritis of the knee: An overview

Zaid Al-Duri, Dipak V. Patel and Paul M. Aichroth

Since the description of proximal tibial osteotomy by Jackson in 1958 and Wardle in 1962, it has become a standard and generally a successful surgical treatment for patients with primary degenerative medial unicompartmental arthritis of the knee associated with angular deformity. Yet the popularity of high tibial osteotomy has lately waxed and waned as the results of knee arthroplasty improved.[1,2] Many, though, believe that high tibial osteotomy is an operation that preserves the joint[2] and is even curative to a point.[3] They believe that despite the fact that there are those who think that current patterns of condylar replacement give such good results that the need for the osteotomy will be eliminated, such a position has not yet been reached.

The bottom line of the argument is in the perception of the effect of such an operation. Is it a procedure employed to 'buy-time' till the patient is old enough to have a knee arthroplasty, or is it a procedure in its own right that is employed to preserve a joint and even reverse the degenerative disease that has set in?

This contribution will examine these possibilities carefully.

Historical review

The operation was first reported by Jackson and Waugh.[4,5] Their original osteotomy was performed just below the tibial tubercle. Wardle[6] reported on the osteotomy at the junction of the upper and middle thirds of the tibia. The operative site was next moved proximal to the tibial tubercle.[7,8]

Biomechanics

We do not intend to give a detailed biomechanical account here. The purpose is to review some of the essential findings of relevance to high tibial osteotomy.

In the case of a varus knee, overpressure beyond tolerance of the tissues destroys the medial articular cartilage, which causes or aggravates the varus knee. The knee then enters a vicious circle of osteoarthritis; that is, once angular deformity and cartilage loss occur, the severity of the deformity and of arthritis tend to increase with time. The prerequisite for a biological healing of the joint is a significant reduction of the articular compressive forces.[9] When high tibial osteotomy is performed, there is ample evidence that regeneration of the articular cartilage occurs.[3,9–16]

Is the relief of pain afforded by high tibial osteotomy due to decompression of the hypertensive intramedullary vascular bed?[17] Is it due to mechanical causes or others? The majority of authorities tend to agree that the main effect of the high tibial osteotomy operation is mechanical.[9,16,18] Therefore, there is increase in joint space, i.e. reduction of the high pressure on the involved compartment with cartilage regeneration, correction of the deformity and therefore less stretching of the supporting tissue components of the joint. Maquet[9] stated that 'It appears that osteoarthritis of the knee is likely to regress. The regeneration of the joint is tantamount to healing.' Tjörnstrand et al.[16] reported that the increased load on the other compartment does not seem to harm the articular cartilage.

Principle of the osteotomy

The principle of high tibial osteotomy is best described by Coventry,[3] who wrote: 'The concept arose, at least in my mind, as a result of the success achieved by intertrochanteric osteotomy for the osteoarthritic hip.' Improvement in congruity of the joint surfaces, opening of the joint space, and lessening of sclerotic changes in the bone of both acetabulum and the femoral head were achieved by this operation. The reason for this was a lessening of loading force and an increase in surface contact of the femoral head and acetabulum.

It followed that a comparable biological improvement should occur if the overload on the involved compartment (medial or lateral) in unicompartmental osteoarthritis of the knee was relieved. In medial compartment osteoarthritis, a vicious cycle occurs in which cartilage and bone destruction lead to more varus which, in turn, causes more overload and more destruction. The cycle can be reversed by changing the tibiofemoral angle and placing load stresses on the relatively normal cartilage and bone of the lateral compartment. This is the principle behind the use of the upper tibial osteotomy for degenerative arthritis (i.e., 'osteoarthrosis' and 'osteoarthritis').

Maquet[9] stated that logical surgery of the osteoarthritis must aim at restoring an equilibrium between the mechanical stresses in the knee joint and the resistance of the tissues. The only practical way consists of reducing the stresses sufficiently to make them tolerable. That is possible by reducing the force transmission through the joint and distributing the force over larger articular surfaces.

Advantages of high tibial osteotomy

1. It is made near the deformity (i.e. knee).[3,19]
2. It is made through cancellous bone that heals rapidly.[3,18,19]
3. The compressive forces of the quadriceps mechanism act to advantage.[3]
4. The risk of delayed union and non-union is minimized when early weight bearing is allowed.[18]
5. It permits exploration of the knee through the same incision should that prove necessary.[19]
6. Owing to reasonably large surface area of cancellous bone, it permits fragments to be held firmly in position either by one or two staples[19] or by reliance on good opposition in a cast.[20]
7. Prolonged immobilization in a cast postoperatively is not necessary.[19]

Indications for high tibial osteotomy

These include the following:

1. Disabling pain caused by unicompartmental osteoarthritis of the knee.[3,18,19,21-24] The pain should be localized to the medial joint line or the medial tibial tubercle in a varus knee, or conversely to the lateral area in a valgus knee. The pain is associated with stress, especially weight bearing, and is usually relieved by rest.[3,24] Such pain interferes with employment and recreation.[19]
2. Evidence on weight-bearing radiographs of degenerative arthritis that is confined to one compartment with a corresponding varus or valgus deformity.[3,19,25]

3. The knee should have a range of flexion of 90–100° or more.[22,23]
4. It should be a stable knee.[20,21-23,25]
5. Good vascular status without serious arterial insufficiency or large varicosities.[19]
6. The ability of the patient to use crutches after the operation and the possession of sufficient strength and motivation to carry out a rehabilitation programme.[19]

There are areas of some disagreement among surgeons owing to the variety of the methods of treatment, experiences of the surgeons and patient requirements, as follows.

The degree of varus–valgus deformity has been addressed by many. Insall et al.[20] advised a high tibial osteotomy only in knees with no more than 10° of varus angulation. Jackson and Waugh[22] stated that the limit to the coronal tibiofemoral varus angle is 5° in the case of tibial osteotomy carried above the tibial tuberosity. If angulation is greater than 5° of varus, then a Maquet type osteotomy should be carried out. Maquet[9] extended his indications to severe joint deformities and even subluxed joints.

Age is another issue of marginal controversy. Coventry[3] mentioned that the patient's age is not an important factor in itself and that it is a matter of developing 'physiological' age and expected activity of the patient. The results in the older age group are as good as those in the younger group. Some agree with Coventry's view.[1,26,27] Others believe that the younger patient (50–60 years) is better suited to tibial osteotomy and that beyond that age arthroplasty might be a better choice.[22-24] Maquet et al., reporting on 881 osteotomies in patients from 15 to 90 years of age, had better and more durable results when the patient was younger.[54]

However, proximal tibial osteotomy is frequently indicated in less than ideal situations. Kettelkamp[23] concluded that, as a general rule, the younger the patient, the greater his or her weight, and the more strenuous the occupational requirements, the more likely would be the recommendation of osteotomy in less than ideal circumstances.

Contraindications to high tibial osteotomy

There are contraindications to high tibial osteotomy to which a consensus exists. They include:

1. Instability secondary to previous surgery or trauma.[19,22]
2. Bone loss with medial compartment depression of subchondral bone of more than a few millimeters.[19,22,23]

3. Valgus deformity greater than 12°[3,19,23] and a varus deformity more than 15°.[19]
4. Flexion contractures degree varies as follows: (a) Jackson and Waugh:[22] 10°; (b) Richardson:[19] >15°; (c) Kettelkamp:[23] >20°; (d) Insall et al.[20] and Vainionpää et al.:[18] >30°.
5. An arc of motion of: <75° (Insall et al.[20]); <60° (Vainionpää et al. [18]); <90° (Richardson[19]).
6. Bicompartmental arthritis of the knee.[19]
7. Serious arterial insufficiency in the affected limb.[19]

There are areas of conflict of opinion. One of these is obesity. Obesity had a negative effect on the outcome of surgery in many series.[24,28,29] Many would agree in view of the possible general postoperative complications of obesity as well as the problems of postoperative application of the cast and early mobilization. It is rational that if a patient is overweight, then the weight should be brought to near normal before surgery.[3]

Another area is patellofemoral arthritis associated with another compartmental arthritis of the knee. Kettelkamp[23] considers severe patellofemoral arthritis a relative contraindication. Most surgeons, however, believe that the presence of patellofemoral arthritis does not affect the results of high tibial osteotomy and therefore is not a contraindication.[3,7,20,30,31]

Examination

Adequate clinical assessment before and after operation and a standardized radiographic technique are essential.[2] It is important to examine the range of motion of the knee, the cruciate stability, collateral ligament status, and the integrity of the peroneal nerve. The circulatory status of the limb should be assessed and recorded.[18]

The patient should be observed during walking for thrust. A thrust is defined as a sideways movement of the knee in the coronal plane on walking.[32] If there is excessive lateral thrust (i.e. adduction moment), the prognosis for improvement after osteotomy may not be good.[3] A knee is considered unstable when it shows medial or lateral thrust as the patient walks, as such a thrust indicates collateral ligament laxity.[18,32] There is a close relation between deformity and instability according to Insall.[33] Knees with less than 10° of deformity when standing are nearly always stable, but when deformity exceeds 10°, instability is found more often. When the deformity is more than 15°, the instability attributable to a combination of loss of substance and soft-tissue stretching can be expected to prejudice the result of osteotomy.

All varus knees have degenerated medial menisci with varying degrees of tears. A similar situation occurs laterally in the valgus knee. Coventry[3] advises against removing such menisci, as long-term studies have shown that they cause no symptoms once they are unloaded by the osteotomy.

Arthroscopy has been used as an aid in the assessment of the condition of the knee. If used before and after the surgery it should confirm the extent of articular cartilage damage and show whether or not repair takes place if the optimal conditions of the high tibial osteotomy are achieved.[2] Others feel that there is little or no correlation between what one sees at arthroscopy and the clinical result from osteotomy.[27] They advise arthroscopy only if there are symptoms of internal derangement.[3,23]

Investigations

Radiographs are important not simply in measuring the degree of the deformity but also to document the amount of arthritis in the various knee compartments, and the degree of subluxation when present.

Radiographic examination should include anteroposterior (weight-bearing), lateral and intercondylar notch views. Weight-bearing views on a single leg at a time are preferred when feasible because this prevents knock knees from disguising the actual extent of the deformity.[32] Also, since the knee is maximally stressed during the one-legged period of the gait,[9] this is a further reason to check the actual amount of knee deformity in a one-legged stance. Kettelkamp[23] recommends Merchant's views for patellofemoral joint assessment.

The coronal tibiofemoral angle (anatomic axis) can be measured. The axial line of the femur passes from the centre of the diaphysis to the intercondylar notch; the line of the tibia passes from the centre of the diaphysis to a point on the proximal tibial metaphysis equidistant between the cortices, and this line projects close to, if not directly over the lateral tibial spine. Insall[33] is in agreement with Coventry that the normal tibiofemoral angle is 5–8°. Others agree with the figure but believe that there is no reliable scientific information about the normal coronal tibiofemoral angle in relation to age and sex.[2]

Many surgeons now prefer *the angle of deviation of the mechanical axis* because this helps avoid difficulties caused by curves in the shafts of the bones.[2] It is determined from weight-bearing radiographs. The weight-bearing axis normally passes from the centre of the hip through the centre of the knee to the centre of the ankle. Maquet[9] believed that only such a radiograph would permit a reliable measurement of the angle formed by the tibia and the femur. Insall[33] doubts the validity of this method for the following reasons:

1. Normal knee loading is predominantly medial.
2. There is a discrepancy between the mechanical axis in the static weight-bearing and the dynamic weight-bearing status. In the former, there is a vertical reaction from the floor passing through the centre of the knee with no horizontal forces. In the latter, there is an additional horizontal component to the floor reaction, causing the vector to be directed medially to the knee.

Gait analysis studies show that varus deformity was associated with a high medial plateau load (as much as 100% with the coronal tibiofemoral angle of 20° varus). At 7° valgus, the medial load is about 60%. However, even in severe valgus deformity (up to 30° valgus) the medial plateau load never fell below 30%.[2]

Vainionpää et al.[18] described how *subluxation* could be measured on anteroposterior weight-bearing views: One line was drawn tangential to the most lateral point on the lateral aspect of the lateral femoral condyle and another line was drawn parallel to the first line through the most lateral point on the lateral aspect of the lateral tibial condyle (ignoring changes caused by osteophytes). The distance (in millimetres) between these two lines was the measurement of the subluxation.

It was thought that *joint tilt* following tibial osteotomy was not of relevance. Harding[31] defined joint tilt as the tibial plateau/horizontal angle and not the tibial plateau/tibial angle. He stated that the actual magnitude of the tilt in valgus knees is of little importance directly in influencing the quality of the results, until a limit of about 15° is exceeded.

Stress radiography has been advised by Kettelkamp.[23] This would assess the ligament stability and demonstrate the presence of a joint space on the unaffected plateau.

Radioisotope scanning is useful in cases of suspicion of whether more than one compartment is involved.[3]

Arthrography as an aid to identification of the intra-articular pathology has been mentioned.[23]

Arthroscopy has been discussed under examination.

Preoperative planning

It is important to predetermine the size of the bone wedge to be removed preoperatively. In planning a valgus osteotomy for a varus knee, one should add 4° to the normal anatomical axis of 5° of valgus, and thus attain 9° of valgus in the tibiofemoral angle. Likewise, in a varus osteotomy for a valgus deformity, an overcorrection of 5° (bringing the knee to neutral axis) is necessary.[3] Maquet[9] believes as well that overcorrection is necessary in cases of varus and valgus knees.

A very popular method of wedge calculation is that described by Bauer et al.[21] It describes a wedge with a 1 cm base as giving a correction of 10°, as 1 mm equals 1° of correction. Insall et al.[20] believe that this method does not take into account the individual size of the tibia. They believe that it is a close enough approximation for women, but that in men the correction will be somewhat less. For the average man's tibia, a wedge with 1 cm base produces approximately 8° of correction.

Operative technique

The majority of the surgeons, including the authors, prefer *a closing wedge osteotomy*.[3,11,20,34,35] Maquet[15] described *a dome osteotomy* which provides correction of the deformity in the coronal plane and also allows *anterior displacement of the tibial tubercle*, thus decompressing the patellofemoral joint. The same principle has been applied by others in the form of *a close wedge osteotomy plus elevation of the tibial tubercle*.[36–38] Some centres employ an *open wedge osteotomy*. The disadvantage of such an osteotomy is the prolonged immobilization time required for the incorporation of the bone graft. Graft collapse with loss of correction is an added hazard.

It is important here to discuss the fibular part of the procedure. Unless the base of the tibial wedge is entirely above the fibular head, the fibula will exert a tethering effect and prevent closure of the osteotomy.[33] In order to achieve that effect, several methods have been designed:

1. Osteotomy of the fibular shaft:[22] this osteotomy in effect involves the removal of a small portion of bone by two parallel oblique cuts.
2. Removal of the fibular head together with the tibiofibular ligaments:[29,39] this permits direct visualization of the proximal tibia.
3. Division of the superior tibiofibular joint: this joint is subluxed either by carefully levering the fibula posteriorly or by sharp dissection. Removing the ligament between the fibula and the tibia allows the fibular head to slide cephalad, but impingement of the proximal fragment against the lateral tibial condyle may occur and prevent complete correction or contribute to the nonunion.[3]
4. Removing only the inferomedial portion of the fibular head and neck: thus the lateral collateral ligament and the biceps tendon need not be reattached to the fibular neck.[19] It also removes the part of the head that protrudes into the osteotomy, preventing the closure of the wedge.[2]

The authors agree with Insall[33] that the fibular shaft osteotomy is unnecessary.

Complications

High tibial osteotomy has generally proved to be a relatively simple and complication-free procedure even in the elderly. Yet serious complications can occur.[33] Complications may be general or local.

General complications

Deep venous thrombosis

Analysing the complications in 10 series totalling 804 operations, Insall[33] reported 29 cases of deep venous thrombosis. Vainionpää et al.[18] reviewed 103 operations with deep venous thrombosis in 5 patients.

Pulmonary embolism

The incidence is as follows: Insall:[33] 1.6%; Insall et al.:[20] 2.1%; Vainionpää et al.:[18] 1%.

Local complications

Intra-articular fractures

The reported incidence in series is: Bauer et al.:[21] 9.5%; Insall:[33] 1%; Vainionpää et al.:[18] 1%; Jackson and Waugh:[22] 13.4% (in 67 wedge osteotomies) and 18.7% (in 16 curved osteotomies carried out above the tuberosity).

Recognition of such a problem and the need for accurate cuts has prompted many to develop jigs to facilitate the osteotomy.[40]

Delayed union and non-union

This is of a rare occurrence. The incidence of non-union in the literature is variable: Myrnerts et al.:[40] 1.3%; Tjörnstrand et al.:[41] 3.6%; Jackson and Waugh:[22] 1.2%.

The incidence of delayed union reported by Vainionpää et al.[18] is as follows: 4% in osteotomies performed proximal to the tibial tubercle; 14% in osteotomies performed distal to the tibial tubercle.

According to Schatzker et al.[42] motion between the osteotomy fragments appears to be the cause of non-union in high tibial osteotomy. In treating the non-union, one needs to ensure that enough proximal bone stock is preserved, that the deformity is corrected, and that knee motion is achievable.[43]

Tjörnstrand et al.[41] believe that patients with non-union following high tibial osteotomy should undergo resection of the pseudoarthrosis and transfixation compression as the treatment of choice. Endoprosthetic replacement then can be used as a salvage procedure if it is needed. In a series of 280 high tibial osteotomies performed for osteoarthritis of the knee between 1969 and 1975, there were 10 cases of pseudoarthrosis, an incidence of 3.6%. These 10 knees (and an additional 2 referred cases) were re-operated on. In most cases the pseudoarthrosis was resected and stabilized with the Charnley transfixation–compression method. Other procedures involved resection without compression (one knee), compression blade-plate fixation, and arthroplasty with a hinge endoprosthesis. All osteotomies healed eventually with the knee in satisfactory position. In spite of the initial non-union and repeated operations, all 12 patients eventually had satisfactory correction of the pre-osteotomy deformity and none had a loss in walking ability.

Schatzker et al.[42] reported on 3 patients with non-unions following high tibial osteotomy for medial compartment osteoarthritis of the knee. They used the special AO/ASIF threaded external fixator with double clamps, which achieved excellent stability and rapid union while maintaining joint motion. They consider resection of the pseudoarthrosis as advocated by Tjörnstrand et al.[41] as unnecessary and harmful because it jeopardizes the integrity of the small proximal fragment, removes valuable fibrocartilage that has osteogenic potential, and renders the hypertrophic non-union unstable. Although theoretically cancellous bone grafting is not necessary, they used it. They criticized the continued immobilization of the knee in plaster employed by other authors.

Wolff et al.[43] argue against the use of external fixation in treatment of non-unions of proximal tibial osteotomy that has been reported by some authors.[41,42] While infections in most cases of external fixation devices are temporary and limited, the proximity of the site to the knee joint and the likelihood of a future desire to convert the high tibial osteotomy to a total knee replacement make external fixation less desirable. Internal fixation was used in six cases of high tibial osteotomy non-unions. Healing of the non-union was obtained in all six cases. Realignment of the angulatory deformity was achieved, in addition to creating an improved substrate for a later total knee replacement. The method of internal fixation depended on the available bone, but blade-plate fixations were the favourites.

Peroneal nerve palsy

Variable incidences have been reported in the literature:

Coventry:[7] 3.3% (in 30 osteotomies), weakness of dorsiflexors.

Jackson et al.:[44] 11.4% (in 70 osteotomies), weakness of dorsiflexors.

Jackson and Waugh:[45] 11.9% (in 229 osteotomies), in most cases recovery was complete.

Vainionpää et al.:[18] 2% (in 103 osteotomies), permanent peroneal nerve palsy.

In reviewing the complications in ten series totalling 804 operations, Insall[33] noted that some complications seem to be related to particular techniques and that 66% of cases of peroneal nerve palsies were related to the use of transfixing pins and external frames. Other possible causes include pressure on the nerve from a plaster cast or tight bandage,[11] or direct injury to the nerve, traction on the nerve, injury to the peroneal vessels and increased pressure in the anterior compartment. Despite the fact that the incidence in the Vainionpää et al.[18] series was equally divided between a distally divided fibula and division of the superior tibiofibular joint, we prefer to release the proximal tibiofibular joint or excise a portion of the fibular head rather than perform a fibular osteotomy. The majority of these patients usually recover completely, although a few may have residual weakness.

Possible vascular injuries

This is a rare complication but is one of the most severe complications of tibial osteotomy.[23] Jackson and Waugh[22] have appreciated the possibility of injury to the peroneal and anterior tibial vessels and believe that this might cause a compartment syndrome after operation. The peroneal veins and the anterior tibial vessels are close to the fibula in the upper half of its shaft. It may be that damage to these vessels could cause compartment syndrome.

It is essential to observe the foot carefully after operation; severe pain in the lower leg is a warning symptom which must not be ignored. The plaster cast should immediately be removed. If compartment syndrome is suspected, then a fasciotomy should be performed.

Perforation of the popliteal artery has been reported.[23]

Infections

When skin infection occurs, it is usually superficial and resolves with treatment. The use of transfixing pins and external frames can be associated with infection, and it accounted for 61.7% of the infected cases reported by Insall.[33]

The recurrence of varus deformity

Most studies have found less recurrence of the deformity in upper tibial osteotomy if overcorrection is made.[2,14,20,40,41,46,47] Postosteotomy loss of correction and particularly recurrent varus is implicated as a cause of deterioration of the clinical results.[11,18,20,27,48] It seems that the degree of valgus achieved at surgery is not, by itself, successful in preventing a recurrent varus deformity. This apparent unpredictability in the maintenance of the femorotibial alignment may be explained in part by the study of Prodromos et al.[48] They found that 100% of the patients with low adduction moments had good results, compared to 50% of the patients with high adduction moments. They also observed that patients with high adduction moments experienced recurrent varus angulation and that postoperative alignment did not change much in patients with low adduction moments.

These patients may be treated by a repeated osteotomy or a total knee arthroplasty depending upon the age of the patient, the severity, and the extent of osteoarthritis.

Stuart et al.[49] reviewed 113 knees (in 95 patients) with medial gonarthrosis that were treated by valgus-producing proximal tibial osteotomy and followed clinically and radiographically for a minimum of 5 years (mean 6.3 years). The tendency for varus recurrence greater than 5° and progression of medial or lateral compartment arthritis was evaluated. They found that varus recurred in 18%, lateral compartment arthritic progression in 60%, and medial compartment arthritic progression in 83% by 9 years after the surgery. They stated that the probability of arthritic progression is much higher than the probability of significant varus recurrence in long-term radiographic follow-up studies of patients with valgus-producing proximal tibial osteotomies. This study demonstrated a small average loss of correction with time (1.5°) with only an 18% probability of varus recurrence greater than 5° by 9 years after surgery. A substantial number of patients, however, experienced moderate to severe pain despite maintenance of a femorotibial angle within 5° of that achieved at surgery. Radiographic standing film analysis revealed medial and lateral compartment arthritic progression with time. These changes can occur irrespective of alterations in the postoperative limb alignment.

Unicompartmental osteoarthritis in association with patellofemoral arthritis

Debate continues regarding the effect of patellofemoral arthritis on high tibial osteotomy and vice versa. Does patellofemoral arthritis contraindicate high tibial osteotomy? Is high tibial osteotomy of any beneficial effect to patellofemoral arthritis pathology and therefore symptoms?

As far as surgical indications are concerned, many surgeons believe that the presence of patellofemoral arthritis does not affect the results of high tibial osteotomy.[3,7,20,25,30,31] Even radiographically severe patellofemoral osteoarthritis was not regarded as a contraindication to high tibial osteotomy.[20] Some believe that patellofemoral symptoms often improved after the operation, either for reasons that could not be explained[25] or owing to a subtle alteration in patellar tracking.[20] Others felt that should postoperative symptoms be thought to emerge from the patellofemoral joint, then observation is recommended. Should it later prove to be the cause, then tibial tubercle elevation or even patellectomy could be done.[22] However, they performed only one patellectomy in

229 operations. Kettelkamp[23] considers severe patello-femoral arthritis a relative contraindication to high tibial osteotomy.

Maquet,[14] Ferguson,[50] and Radin[51] have demonstrated the relief of patellofemoral joint symptoms with elevation osteotomy of the tibial tubercle. Some surgeons have felt that the operations of high tibial osteotomy plus the Maquet procedure form a theoretically attractive option. Hofmann et al.[36] reported on the combined Coventry–Maquet procedure for two-compartment degenerative arthritis. The procedure was investigated in a prospective study of 14 patients (13 with medial compartment and patellofemoral osteoarthritis and 1 with lateral compartment and patellofemoral osteoarthritis), with an average age of 56 years (range 36–65 years) and a follow-up duration of 23–30 months. There were no excellent results, one good result, and 13 poor results. They stated that the combined Coventry–Maquet procedure required too much dissection, had too high a complication rate, and yielded a minimal improvement in knee function and pain. *They thus advise alternative surgery such as total knee arthroplasty in cases of combined two compartment osteoarthritis.*

Putnam et al.[38] reported on the effect of combined Maquet and proximal upper tibial valgus osteotomy. They reviewed 34 knees (31 patients) with an average age of 59.6 years at the time of surgery and followed them up for 6–36 months (mean follow-up period 16 months). Sixty-eight per cent of the patients were graded as good to excellent, 20% as fair, and 12% had failed. They concluded that the applicability of this combined osteotomy remains rather unclear, partly because of the difficulty in assessing the patient's disease, goals and life span, and partly because of the increasing reliability of total knee arthroplasty. However, the morbidity of the combined osteotomy as they described it is much more favourable than comparable figures reported for total knee arthroplasty, the only other available salvage procedure for this group of patients. *Overall, this combined osteotomy is applicable in many situations currently being treated by total knee arthroplasty and should be seriously considered in the physiologically young individual capable of a vigorous rehabilitation programme.*

Nguyen et al.[37] reviewed the effect of adding the Maquet tibial tubercle elevating procedure to a valgus high tibial osteotomy in combined medial and patellofemoral disease and compared it to the procedure of high tibial osteotomy performed alone in dual compartment arthritis. A modified Hospital for Special Surgery assessment (maximum 100 points) was used with an optimum pain score of 30 points. All were followed radiographically with grading of the three knee compartments. In both groups, the total and pain scores improved significantly post-operatively. *Although high tibial osteotomy was a good procedure for pain relief for dual-compartment disease, the addition of Maquet procedure did not improve the results.*

Combined high tibial osteotomy and joint debridement

Joint debridement has been advocated as an adjunct to high tibial osteotomy by MacIntosh and Welsh.[52] They reviewed 105 patients who had the combined procedure of high tibial osteotomy and debridement and followed them up for an average period of 11 years. They consider it the treatment of choice for unicompartmental osteoarthritis of the knee whenever return to vigorous activity is contemplated. They also state that such a procedure should be considered strongly before any definitive arthroplastic technique is used, especially in patients who are neither decrepit nor elderly.

Such a claim has been doubted by some[20] or received cautiously by others who stress the importance of proper methods of evaluation of surgical results to determine whether procedures like debridement really influence the results.[2]

Varus osteotomy for a valgus deformity

Lateral compartment osteoarthritis is relatively uncommon, and most patients have fairly advanced changes in the joint when they are first seen. In such a situation osteotomy may not be suitable, but in a small number of patients who have pain and whose radiographs show only loss of articular cartilage, correction of the deformity can achieve satisfactory results.[2]

Correction of a valgus deformity of the knee produces an obliquity or tilting of the knee joint axis in the coronal plane.[33] Harding[31] defined joint tilt as the tibial plateau/horizontal angle. While some believed the joint tilt to be of no significance,[21] others felt that it was not compatible with good clinical results.[29,31,32] The actual magnitude of the tilt has little importance directly in influencing the quality of the results until a limit of about 15° is exceeded.[31] When the tilt exceeds 15°, the mechanical effect is to shift the loading of the joint from the lateral compartment only as far medially as the tibial spine and not as intended to the more normal medial compartment, which in due course causes the femur to sublux medially on the tibia, leading to a varus angulation.[33]

In these knees in which the joint is oblique to the horizontal, a supracondylar femoral osteotomy, rather than a tibial osteotomy is indicated.[2] Disadvantages of high tibial osteotomy for valgus deformity therefore include a possible conversion of a valgus deformity to a varus one (in cases of joint tilt exceeding 15°) and increased medial collateral laxity and therefore a predisposition to joint instability.[33]

Results

In the past two decades, various series have shown encouraging long-term results following upper tibial osteotomy.[10,18,20,25,34,46,47,53] Whilst the majority of the authorities agree that there is a gradual decline in the quality of the result with time, neither Harding[31] nor Coventry[3,10] have found predictable decreases in the quality of the results with similar length studies in similar populations.

Aglietti et al.[25] in a review of 139 knees that had high tibial osteotomy, noted excellent and good results in 64% of the knees after a follow-up period of at least 10 years. The average age was 62 years (range 40–77 years). The conclusion of the study was that a high tibial osteotomy is a reliable method for relieving pain in the varus osteoarthritic knee. However, a tendency for results to deteriorate with time was observed, but 64% of the knees with more than 10 years' follow-up evaluation, 87% of the knees with 2–5 years', and 70% of the knees with 6–10 years' had satisfactory results.

These authors consider high tibial osteotomy the procedure of choice in early medial compartment osteoarthritis. Relatively young, active patients with unilateral disease are those most likely to gain maximum benefit from the operation. Other conclusions included:

(a) In general the results in the knees that had more than 10° of varus angulation prior to operation were inferior to those in knees with less deformity.

(b) The best results were obtained with an alignment of 6–10° or 6–15° of valgus. They advise, therefore, a limited overcorrection of 5°.

(c) Age, sex, bilaterality, and level of osteotomy did not appear to influence the results to a significant degree.

(d) Some progression of degeneration was observed in 58% of the knees with unsatisfactory results but in only 7% of those with satisfactory results.

(e) The degree of patellofemoral osteoarthritis remained unchanged or tended to deteriorate slightly with time. The so-called patellar symptoms often improved after the operation, for reasons that cannot entirely be explained.

(f) The surgical technique is not a crucial determinant of clinical results, but the authors have found the lateral closed wedge osteotomy the safest, simplest and most precise technique.

Insall et al.[20] evaluated the results in 83 patients (95 knees) who had had a high tibial osteotomy for either unicompartmental osteoarthritis or osteonecrosis. The mean follow-up period was 8.9 years (range 5–15 years). The early results were promising: at 2 years 97% and at 5 years 85% of the knees had either an excellent or a good result. At a subsequent follow-up, however, only 60 knees (63%) had an excellent or

good result, and in the remainder recurrent pain developed. Twenty-three per cent of the knees had been revised to a total knee replacement. The passage of time was the most important factor in determining the result, as 37% of the knees that had been followed up for more than 9 years were pain-free. Thus, the results of high tibial osteotomy frequently deteriorated with time; in fact, the passage of time seemed to be by far the most important determinant of the result.

Healy and Riley[26] evaluated 25 patients for high tibial osteotomies performed for varus gonarthrosis. The age of the patients at the time of surgery ranged from 39 to 67 years (mean 60 years) and the follow-up period ranged from 2 years to 14 years (mean 5.5 years). Preoperative tibiofemoral angulation averaged 7° varus. Postoperative tibiofemoral angulation averaged 5° valgus. Eighty-eight per cent claimed postoperative improvement, 8% were unchanged, and one patient was worse. Ninety-two per cent had excellent or good results, according to Coventry's criteria and the HSS knee score. Eighty-eight per cent had no further surgery. Excellent/good results deteriorated from 92% at 2 years to 88% at 5 years, to 91% at 7 years, and to 80% at 9 years. This is a smaller rate of deterioration than noted in other series. Factors contributing to success included careful patient selection, correction of limb to mechanical axis, and precise surgical technique.

Vainionpää et al.[18] reviewed 103 knees (92 with a varus deformity and 11 with normal alignment) treated by tibial osteotomy and followed up for an average of 6.9 years. In 68 knees, the result was good or fair. In the 11 knees with normal preoperative alignment, the osteotomy was designed to shift the load to the compartment in which there was less osteoarthritic involvement. In 9 of these 11 knees there was an average change in angulation (varus or valgus) of 5.3° (range 3–9°) and the result was good or fair. All osteotomies united without re-operation. No internal fixation was used for the tibial osteotomies performed for varus knees above the tibial tubercle (71 knees); L-shaped blade-plate was used for osteotomies below the tibial tubercle. At an average of 3.4 years after the osteotomy, deterioration was demonstrable in 26 knees in which the initial result had been good. This is a higher incidence of deterioration than in previously published series. In 16 of the 103 knees, a total arthroplasty was subsequently performed because of a poor result, at an average of 7.6 years after the osteotomy.

Valenti et al.[53] reported on 100 high tibial valgus osteotomies with a mean follow-up of 11 years (range 8–16.3 years). In their series, patients with mild to moderate osteoarthritis had the best results.

Rudan and Simurda[35] prospectively reviewed 79 knees treated by a valgus closing wedge high tibial osteotomy at an average follow-up of 5.8 years (range 3–9 years). Eighty per cent of the patients had good or excellent results. They noted that correction to a tibiofemoral angle between 6 and 14° of femorotibial valgus was associated with an optimal clinical result. Undercorrection to less than 5° of the femorotibial valgus was associated with a 62.5% failure rate.

Ivarsson et al.[34] reported long-term clinical and radiographic results of high tibial osteotomy performed for medial compartment osteoarthritis of the knee. They reviewed 99 knees at 1–2 years, 81 knees at a mean of 5.7 years, and 65 knees at a mean of 11.9 years. At 1–2 years and at 5.7 years, over 50% were good and over 75% acceptable. At 11.9 years, 43% were good and 60% acceptable. The best results were seen in knees with preoperative grade I or grade II Ahlbäck osteoarthritis.

Conclusions

High tibial osteotomy has long been recognized as an effective procedure in the management of medial compartment osteoarthritis of the knee. The operation is best used for the young active patient with predominant unicompartmental osteoarthritis, particularly before the stage of bony collapse or subluxation. Long-term follow-up studies have shown that it provides reasonable pain relief and improves joint function.

Preoperative planning and a meticulous operative technique are vital for a successful clinical result. In the operative technique, an additional 3–5° of overcorrection is recommended to obtain approximately 10° of anatomical tibiofemoral valgus alignment.

Recently, unicompartmental resurfacing arthroplasty has gained increasing popularity and equally good or even better results have been obtained. A prospective, randomized, clinical study is needed to compare the effectiveness of tibial osteotomy against unicompartmental arthroplasty. Various factors, such as the age of the patient, degree of activity, and severity and extent of the arthritis, must be considered before contemplating either of the two procedures. It may be that with continuing advances in the prosthetic design, replacement arthroplasty may supersede the osteotomy in the future.

References

1. Cass JR, Bryan RS, High tibial osteotomy, *Clin Orthop* (1988) **230**: 196–199.
2. Waugh W, Tibial osteotomy in the management of osteoarthritis of the knee, *Clin Orthop* (1986) **210**: 55–61.
3. Coventry MB, Osteotomy about the knee: Principles of treatment, *Operative orthopaedics*, ed Chapman MW (Philadelphia: JB Lippincott, 1988) vol. 1, 705–710.
4. Jackson JP, Osteotomy for osteoarthritis of the knee, *J Bone Joint Surg (Br)* (1958) **40**: 826.
5. Jackson JP, Waugh W, Tibial osteotomy for osteoarthritis of the knee, *J Bone Joint Surg (Br)* (1961) **43**: 746–751.
6. Wardle EN, Osteotomy of the tibia and fibula, *Surg Gynecol Obstet* (1962) **115**: 61–64.
7. Coventry MB, Osteotomy of the upper portion of the tibia for degenerative arthritis of the knee: A preliminary report, *J Bone Joint Surg (Am)* (1965) **47**: 984–990.
8. Gariépy R, Correction du genou flechi dans l'arthrite, *Proc Int Soc Orthop Surg Traumatol* (1960) **8**: 884–886.
9. Maquet P, The biomechanics of the knee and surgical possibilities of healing osteoarthritic knee joints, *Clin Orthop* (1980) **146**: 102–110.
10. Coventry MB, Upper tibial osteotomy for gonarthrosis: The evolution of the operation in the last 18 years and long-term results, *Orthop Clin North Am* (1979) **10**: 191–210.
11. Coventry MB, Current concepts review: Upper tibial osteotomy for osteoarthritis, *J Bone Joint Surg (Am)* (1985) **67**: 1136–1140.
12. Fujisawa Y, Masuhara K, Shiomi S, The effect of high tibial osteotomy on osteoarthritis of the knee: an arthroscopic study of 54 knee joints, *Orthop Clin North Am* (1979) **10**: 585–608.
13. Insall JN, Shoji H, Mayer V, High tibial osteotomy: a five-year evaluation, *J Bone Joint Surg (Am)* (1974) **56**: 1397–1405.
14. Maquet P, Valgus osteotomy for osteoarthritis of the knee, *Clin Orthop* (1976) **120**: 143–148.
15. Maquet PGJ (ed), *Biomechanics of the knee: with application to the pathogenesis and the surgical treatment of osteoarthritis*, 2nd edn (Berlin: Springer-Verlag, 1984).
16. Tjörnstrand BAE, Egund N, Hagstedt, BV, High tibial osteotomy: A seven-year clinical and radiographic follow-up, *Clin Orthop* (1981) **160**: 124–136.
17. Brookes M, Helal B, Primary osteoarthritis: Venous engorgement and osteogenesis, *J Bone Joint Surg (Br)* (1968) **50**: 493–504.
18. Vainionpää S, Läike E, Kirves P et al., Tibial osteotomy for osteoarthritis of the knee: A five to ten-year follow-up study, *J Bone Joint Surg (Am)* (1981) **63**: 938–946.
19. Richardson EG, Miscellaneous nontraumatic disorders, *Campbell's operative orthopaedics*, 7th edn, ed Crenshaw AH (St Louis: CV Mosby, 1987) 1022–1026.
20. Insall JN, Joseph DM, Msika C, High tibial osteotomy for varus gonarthrosis, *J Bone Joint Surg (Am)* (1984) **66**: 1040–1048.
21. Bauer GCH, Insall J, Koshino T, Tibial osteotomy in gonarthrosis (osteo-arthritis of the knee), *J Bone Joint Surg (Am)* (1969) **51**: 1545–1563.
22. Jackson JP, Waugh W, Osteoarthritis of the knee, *Surgery of the knee joint*, ed Jackson JP, Waugh W (London: Chapman and Hall, 1984) 290–314.
23. Kettelkamp DB, Tibial osteotomy, *Surgery of the musculoskeletal system*, 2nd edn, ed Evarts CM (New York: Churchill Livingstone, 1990) vol. 4, 3551–3567.
24. Matthews LS, Goldstein SA, Malvitz TA et al., Proximal tibial osteotomy: Factors that influence the duration of satisfactory function, *Clin Orthop* (1988) **229**: 193–200.
25. Aglietti P, Rinonapoli E, Stringa G et al., Tibial osteotomy for the varus osteoarthritic knee, *Clin Orthop* (1983) **176**: 239–251.
26. Healy WL, Riley LH Jr, High tibial valgus osteotomy: A clinical review, *Clin Orthop* (1986) **209**: 227–233.
27. Keene JS, Monson DK, Roberts JM et al., Evaluation of patients for high tibial osteotomy, *Clin Orthop* (1989) **243**: 157–165.
28. Brueckmann FR, Kettelkamp DB, Proximal tibial osteotomy, *Orthop Clin North Am* (1982) **13**: 3–16.
29. Coventry MB, Osteotomy about the knee for degenerative and rheumatoid arthritis: Indications, operative technique, and results, *J Bone Joint Surg (Am)* (1973) **55**: 23–48.
30. Engel GM, Lippert FG, Valgus tibial osteotomy, *Clin Orthop* (1981) **160**: 137–143.

31. **Harding ML**, A fresh appraisal of tibial osteotomy for osteoarthritis of the knee, *Clin Orthop* (1976) **114**: 223–234.

32. **Shoji H, Insall J**, High tibial osteotomy for osteoarthritis of the knee with valgus deformity, *J Bone Joint Surg (Am)* (1973) **55**: 963–973.

33. **Insall JN**, *Surgery of the knee* (New York: Churchill Livingstone, 1984) 551–585.

34. **Ivarsson I, Myrnerts R, Gillquist J**, High tibial osteotomy for medial osteoarthritis of the knee: 5 to 7 and an 11 to 13 year follow-up, *J Bone Joint Surg (Br)* (1990) **72**: 238–244.

35. **Rudan JF, Simurda MA**, High tibial osteotomy: a prospective clinical and roentgenographic review, *Clin Orthop* (1990) **255**: 251–256.

36. **Hofmann AA, Wyatt RWB, Jones RE**, Combined Coventry–Maquet procedure for two-compartment degenerative arthritis, *Clin Orthop* (1984) **190**: 186–191.

37. **Nguyen C, Rudan J, Simurda MA et al.**, High tibial osteotomy compared with high tibial and Maquet procedures in medial and patellofemoral compartment osteoarthritis, *Clin Orthop* (1989) **245**: 179–187.

38. **Putnam MD, Mears DC, Fu FH**, Combined Maquet and proximal tibial valgus osteotomy, *Clin Orthop* (1985) **197**: 217–223.

39. **Gariépy R**, Genu varum treated by high tibial osteotomy, *J Bone Joint Surg (Br)* (1964) **46**: 783–784.

40. **Myrnerts R**, Clinical results with the SAAB jig in high tibial osteotomy for medial gonarthrosis, *Acta Orthop Scand* (1980) **51**: 565–567.

41. **Tjörnstrand B, Hagstedt B, Perrson BM**, Results of surgical treatment for non-union after high tibial osteotomy in osteoarthritis of the knee, *J Bone Joint Surg (Am)* (1978) **60**: 973–977.

42. **Schatzker J, Burgess RC, Glynn MK**, The management of nonunions following high tibial osteotomies, *Clin Orthop* (1985) **193**: 230–233.

43. **Wolff AM, Krackow KA**, The treatment of nonunion of proximal tibial osteotomy with internal fixation, *Clin Orthop* (1990) **250**: 207–215.

44. **Jackson JP, Waugh W, Green JP**, High tibial osteotomy for osteoarthritis of the knee, *J Bone Joint Surg (Br)* (1969) **51**: 88–94.

45. **Jackson JP, Waugh W**, The technique and complications of upper tibial osteotomy, *J Bone Joint Surg (Br)* (1974) **56**: 236–245.

46. **Coventry MB, Bowman PW**, Long-term results of upper tibial osteotomy for degenerative arthritis of the knee, *Acta Orthop Belg* (1982) **48**: 139–156.

47. **Kettelkamp DB, Wenger DR, Chao EYS et al.**, Results of proximal tibial osteotomy, *J Bone Joint Surg (Am)* (1976) **58**: 952–960.

48. **Prodromos CC, Andriacchi TP, Galante JO**, A relationship between gait and clinical changes following high tibial osteotomy, *J Bone Joint Surg (Am)* (1985) **67**: 1188–1194.

49. **Stuart MJ, Grace JN, Ilstrup DM et al.**, Late recurrence of varus deformity after proximal tibial osteotomy, *Clin Orthop* (1990) **260**: 61–65.

50. **Ferguson AB**, Elevation of the insertion of the patellar ligament for patellofemoral pain, *J Bone Joint Surg (Am)* (1982) **64**: 766–771.

51. **Radin EL**, Anterior tibial tubercle elevation in the young adult, *Orthop Clin North Am* (1986) **17**: 297–302.

52. **MacIntosh DL, Welsh RP**, Joint debridement: A complement to high tibial osteotomy in the treatment of degenerative arthritis of the knee, *J Bone Joint Surg (Am)* (1977) **59**: 1094–1097.

53. **Valenti JR, Calvo R, Lopez R et al.**, Long term evaluation of high tibial valgus osteotomy, *Int Orthop* (1990) **14**: 347–349.

54. **Maquet P, Watillon M, Burney F et al.**, Traitement chirurgical conservateur de l'arthrose du genou, *Acta Orthop Belg* (1982) **48**: 204.

15.2   Curvilinear osteotomy of the tibia

Jacques Wagner

Biomechanics

In a normal knee, when the patient stands on one foot, the resultant of the load and the muscular forces is exerted axially between the two tibial plateaus. If a medial or a lateral displacement of this resultant occurs, the medial or the lateral tibial compartment is overloaded; in these cases, a concentration of compressive stresses alters the cartilage and the subchondral bone. A secondary deformity of the knee joint can appear later.[1-14] From a mechanical point of view, at this stage, a conservative surgical treatment has to be considered: the axial recentering of the resultant of the forces. This goal can be obtained by the tibial curvilinear osteotomy.[15,16]

Indications

The tibial osteotomy is planned more often for the correction of the varus deformity of the knee than for a valgus deformity.[17-21] For the latter deformity, like Maquet and the others, we recommend performing a lower femoral osteotomy rather than a tibial one, because the obliquity of the joint in the valgus persists in creating a conflict between the external condyle and the tibial spines.[7]

Surgical procedure

Drawing

On radiographs (in the frontal plane) of the whole loaded lower limb we draw two lines from the center of the femoral head to the center of the knee and from this point to the center of the ankle. Normally, these two lines constitute the mechanical axis of the lower limb. In the case of a varus deformity, these lines determine an angle which will be essential to know for the correction obtained by the tibial osteotomy.[7,22,23]

Material

To perform a curvilinear osteotomy of the tibia we need an *osteotomy guide* that is curved and gives the possibility of drawing, on the bone and behind the patellar tendon, the exact line of osteotomy. The second piece, also created by Paul Maquet, consists of *an angular guide* for the insertion of two Steinman pins in the tibia. This guide presents a graduated scale for choosing the angular correction in degrees. Moreover, the distance between the two pins can be modified as the aiming device consists of two mobile parts. For the fixation of the two Steinman pins, we use the *external fixation* of Müller.

Procedure

The patient lies on his back, the leg being raised on a package of draw-sheets. A tourniquet is set around the thigh. At the level of the middle third or lower third of the fibula, a lateral small incision (3–4 cm) allows one to divide the muscular groups (peroneal and soleus) and to cut the bone obliquely with an electric saw. An incision, lateral to the anterior tuberosity of the tibia (10 cm) is performed. After the disinsertion of the tendon of 'the pes anserinus,' the osteotomy guide is set behind the patellar tendon close to its lower insertion. Small holes are made through the guide in the tibia in order to draw a mark.

The tibial osteotomy is started with special curved osteotomes; after having used prototypes from André Danis, we now recommend those made by Citieffe because these osteotomes can easily glide behind the patellar tendon (Figure 1). Under fluoroscopy, a Steinman pin is inserted through the upper part of the tibial epiphysis, over the osteotomy. The angle of correction, calculated on the radiographs, is fixed on the angular guide; the angle plus 3° of overcorrection. The guide, being slid on the first upper pin, gives the direction for the second Steinman pin. This second pin is introduced under fluoroscopic control up to the medial cortex of the tibial shaft.

With the knee bent (40°), the osteotomy is finalized after a retractor has been set behind the bone to protect the vessels (Figure 2). The calculated correction in valgus of the leg is then obtained by setting the Steinman pins in parallel. The lower pin can be pushed through the medial skin. An external fixator of Müller linking the two pins stabilizes the tibial curvilinear osteotomy.

A drainage is set and the tibial and fibular wounds are sutured. A cast is made for the first postoperative days to increase comfort.

Postoperative care

Fraxiparine is given to the patient up to the time of walking. The drainage is removed after 2–3 days and the cast after 6 days. Sutures are removed after 2 weeks. The Müller fixator is removed after 6 weeks, at the time of the bone healing (Figure 3).

Revalidation

The revalidation starts the day after the operation by mobilization of the patella and of the knee joint. After a week, the patient can sit in a chair and walks with a partial weight bearing on the operated leg. Complete weight-bearing is allowed after 3 weeks.

During a revalidation of three months, the development of lateral muscles reinforces the valgus correction.

Recommendations

In the sagittal plane, the osteotomy must be strictly perpendicular to the tibial axis in order to rid an anterior gliding of the upper part of the tibia.

The location for dividing at the mid-shaft of the fibula is less hazardous than in the upper part close to the external sciatic popliteal nerve.

The use of four Steinman pins (two upper, two lower) was abandoned because the fixation in this case was too rigid and would lead to delayed bone healing.

This procedure, allowing a correction in the frontal plane, can also be associated with an anterior displacement of the tibial shaft to obtain a decompression of the patellar cartilage (Maquet's procedure).[24]

Very often we add to the curvilinear osteotomy a cutting of the external patellar ligament and the capsule, obtaining a release of the patella.

References

1. **Blaimont P, Burnotte J, Baillon JM et al.**, Contribution biomécanique à l'étude des conditions d'équilibre dans le genou normal et pathologique, *Acta Orthop Belg* (1971) **37:** 573–591.

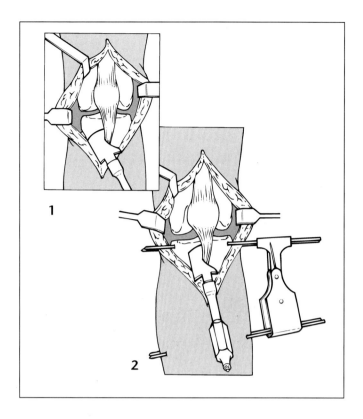

Figure 1

Tibial osteotomy using curved osteotomes.

Figure 2

The osteotomy is finalized; a retractor is placed behind the bone to protect the vessels.

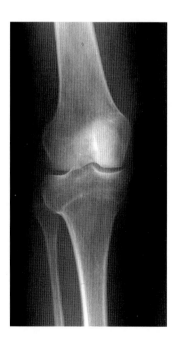

Figure 3

Radiograph showing bone healing.

2. **Frankel VH, Burstein AH,** *Orthopaedic biomechanics* (Philadelphia: Lea and Febiger, 1970).

3. **Kummer B,** Gait and posture under normal conditions with special reference to the lower limbs, *Clin Orthop* (1962) **25:** 32–41.

4. **Kummer B,** Biomechanischer Grundlage "beanspruchungsändernder" Osteotomiën im Bereich des Kniegelenks, *Z Orthop* (1977) **19:** 923–928.

5. **Maquet P,** Biomécanique des membres inférieurs, *Acta Orthop Belg* (1966) **32:** 705–728.

6. **Maquet P,** The biomechanics of the knee and surgical possibilities of healing osteoarthritic knee joints, *Clin Orthop* (1980) **146:** 102–110.

7. **Maquet P,** *Biomechanics of the knee,* 2nd edn (Berlin: Springer-Verlag, 1984).

8. **Paul JP,** Magnitude of forces transmitted at hip and knee joints, *Lubrication and wear in joints,* ed Wright V (London: Sector Publishing, 1969) 77–78.

9. **Pauwels F,** *Gesammelte Abhandlungen zur funktionellen Anatomie des Bewegungsapparates* (Berlin: Springer-Verlag, 1965).

10. **Pauwels F,** *Biomechanics of the locomotor apparatus* (Berlin: Springer-Verlag, 1980).

11. **Radin EL, Paul IL, Rose RM,** Role of mechanical factors in pathogenesis of primary osteoarthritis, *Lancet* (1972) 519–522.

12. **Wagner J, Bourgois R, Hermanne A,** Comportement mécanique du cadre tibio-péronier dans les genoux varum et valgum, *Acta Orthop Belg* (1982) **48:** 57–93.

13. **Walker PS, Erkman MJ,** The role of the menisci in force transmission across the knee, *Clin Orthop* (1975) **109:** 184–192.

14. **Wolff J,** *Das Gesetz der Transformation der Knochen* (Berlin: Hirschwald, 1892).

15. **Blaimont P,** L'ostéotomie curviplane dans le traitement de la gonarthrose, *Acta Orthop Belg* (1982) **48:** 97–109.

16. **Maquet P,** Osteotomy, *Arthritis of the knee,* ed Freeman MAR (Berlin: Springer-Verlag, 1980).

17. **Coventry MB,** Osteotomy of the upper portion of the tibia for degenerative arthritis of the knee: a preliminary report, *J Bone Joint Surg (Am)* (1965) **47:** 984–990.

18. **Coventry MB,** Osteotomy about the knee for degenerative and rheumatoid arthritis. Indications, operative technique and results, *J Bone Joint Surg (Am)* (1973) **55:** 23–48.

19. **Jackson JP, Waugh W,** Tibial osteotomy for osteoarthritis of the knee, *Acta Orthop Belg* (1982) **48:** 93–96.

20. **Shoji H, Insall J,** High tibial osteotomy for osteoarthritis of the knee with valgus deformity, *J Bone Joint Surg (Am)* (1973) **55:** 963–973.

21. **Weill D, Schneider M,** Les ostéotomies du genou dans le traitement de la gonarthrose. A propos d'une expérience de douze ans et de plus de 500 interventions, *Acta Orthop Belg* (1982) **48:** 131–138.

22. **Ramadier JO, Buard JE, Lortat-Jacob A et al.,** Mesure radiologique des déformations frontales du genou. Procédé du profil vrai radiologique, *Rev Chir Orthop* (1982) **68:** 75–78.

23. **Van de Berg A, Collard P, Quiriny M,** Gonarthrose et déviation angulaire du genou dans le plan frontal, *Acta Orthop Belg* (1982) **48:** 8–27.

24. **Wagner J, Cheval P, Nelis JJ,** Incidence du degré d'avancement du tendon rotulien sur les contraintes fémoro-patellaires, *Acta Orthop Belg* (1982) **48:** 639–650.

15.3 Technique of upper tibial osteotomy with wedge excision

Paul M. Aichroth

Figure 1

Osteotomy at the knee must be undertaken accurately to allow full correction of the malalignment and in many situations very slight overcorrection is beneficial. The malalignment at the knee must be assessed on weight bearing and this can only be calculated accurately from a long film, which includes the hip, knee and ankle.

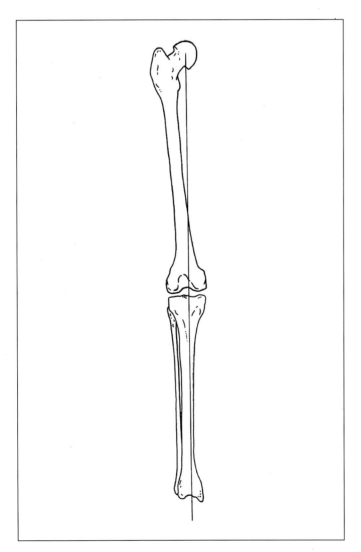

Figure 1

Figure 2

The degree of malalignment is the angle of variation from the mechanical axis and this is fully outlined in contribution 21.6. The exact angle must be measured and from this the correction is calculated. A metal foil template should be cut at this corrective angle.

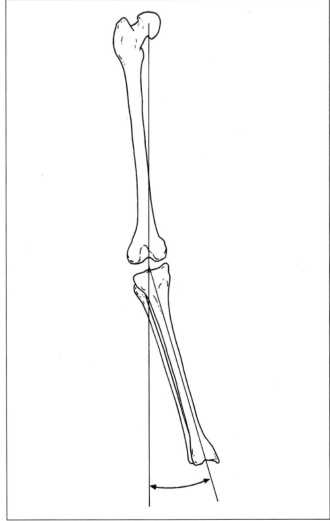

Figure 2

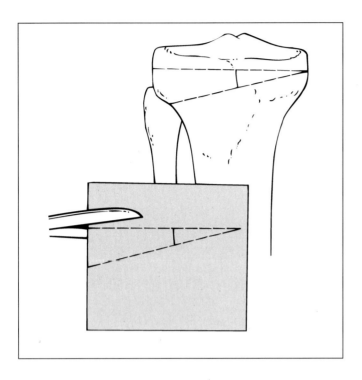

Figure 3

Figure 3

The incision is transverse – half-way between the joint-line and the tibial tubercle. The fat layer is undermined and the capsule, expansions and patellar tendon are revealed.

Figure 4a

The upper tibial bone surfaces are exposed by vertical incision of the expansions on each side of the patellar tendon. The joint-line is identified and conveniently marked by needles. A transverse incision of the expansion parallel to the joint-line but 1 cm inferior is made. The fascial flaps are developed subperiosteally and stripped distally.

Figure 4b

The fibular collateral ligament is exposed and the capsule is incised vertically along its anterior border. This ligamentous layer is removed from the fibular head by sharp dissection and this flap is then developed laterally and posteriorly. The fibular head is exposed fully and the upper 1.5 cm is removed with a saw or osteotome. The soft tissues are then progressively stripped from the lateral and posterolateral aspects of the tibia and their position is maintained with a bone spike.

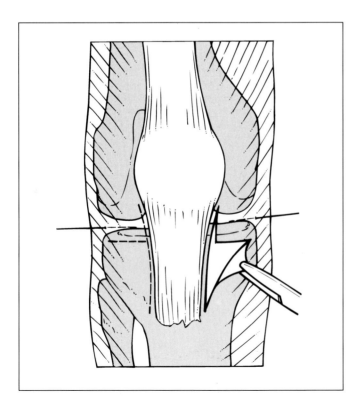

Figure 4a

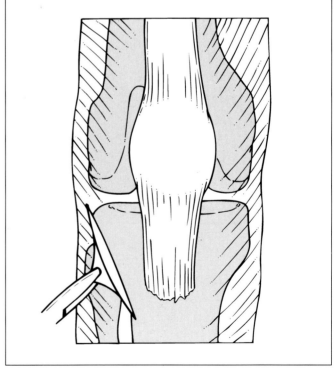

Figure 4b

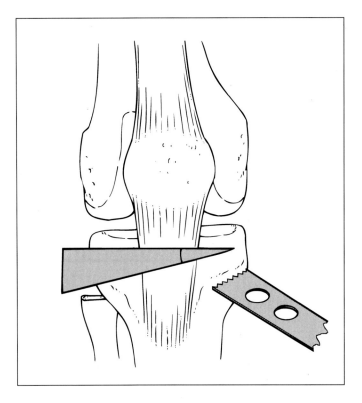

Figure 5

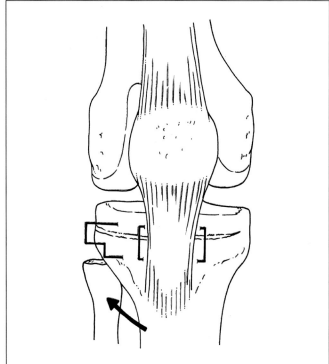

Figure 6

Figure 5

The tibial bone cut is then marked out with an osteotome, making sure that the angle is no more than that indicated by the metal foil template applied to the upper tibia. The periosteum is retracted posteromedially and posterolaterally. The bone cut is made accurately with an oscillating saw up to, but not including, the medial cortex for a corrective valgus osteotomy. The lateral cortex is preserved if the correction is varus.

Figure 6

The tibia is then bent at the osteotomy site and, if the correct amount of medial or lateral cortex is maintained, the bone surface will bend or infarct rather than fully fracture.

Internal fixation staples are positioned as shown and the lateral side will require an off-set shaped staple. Care must be taken not to fracture the proximal tibial fragment and the staple must not enter the joint. The wound is closed in layers with drainage. A split cylinder cast is applied for 3 weeks only.

Postoperative course

At 3 weeks the cast is removed and the knee is mobilized with the help of a physiotherapist. A constant passive motion machine is helpful during the first 48 hours. Minimal weight bearing is maintained until the 8th week and progressive full weight bearing thereafter.

Lower femoral osteotomy

If the knee is in marked valgus, a lower femoral osteotomy is preferable. Very minor degrees of valgus can be corrected at the upper tibial site.

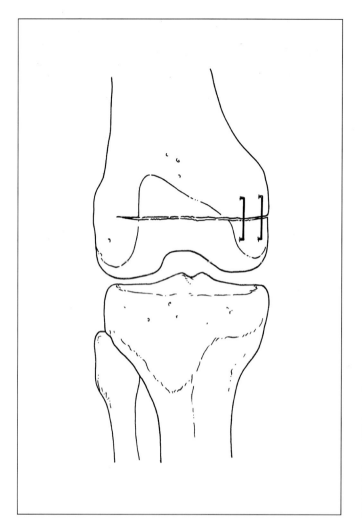

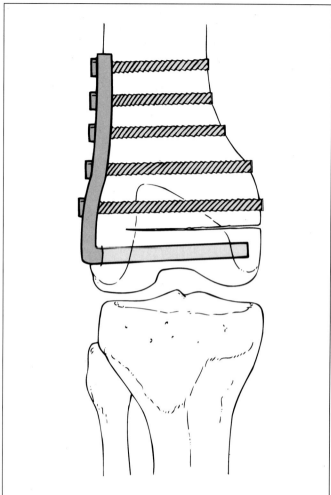

Figure 7

Figure 8

Figure 7

If the valgus correction is of a few degrees only, the osteotomy at the supracondylar site may be closed and stabilized with staples.

Figure 8

If the correction is 10–15° or more, then an appropriate blade-plate must be used to maintain position and to allow early and full knee mobility.

16

Unicompartmental replacement arthroplasty

16.1   Unicompartmental total knee arthroplasty

Richard D. Scott

Despite almost two decades of controversy, the status of unicompartmental knee replacement remains uncertain. In the early 1970s, several authors reported early discouraging results with unicondylar arthroplasty and questioned its role except perhaps in lateral compartmental disease.[1,2] During the next 10 years, more favorable results began to appear.[3-5] These were largely the result of refined surgical technique and the narrowing of patient selection to those candidates ideally suited for the procedure.

The concept of unicompartmental total knee replacement is attractive as an alternative to tibial osteotomy or tricompartmental replacement in the elderly osteoarthritic patient with unicompartmental disease confirmed at arthrotomy. Compared to osteotomy, unicompartmental arthroplasty has a higher initial success rate and fewer early complications.[4,6] Any internal derangement can be relieved at the time of the arthrotomy. Intra-articular debridement can lead to an improvement in range of motion. Patients with bilateral disease can have both knees operated on during the same anesthetic with full recovery within 3 months of surgery. Osteotomies in the same patient should probably be spaced from 3 to 6 months apart and as much as a year may be required to achieve full recovery from the time of the initial procedure.

Compared to tricompartmental arthroplasty, unicompartmental replacement has the advantage of preserving both cruciate ligaments, yielding a knee with nearly normal kinematics.[7,8] A study of 42 patients with a bi- or tricompartmental arthroplasty on one side and a unicompartmental replacement on the other showed that more patients preferred the unicompartmental side because it felt more like a normal knee and had better function.[9]

Another potential advantage over tricompartmental replacement is the preservation of bone stock in the patellofemoral joint and opposite compartments. Theoretically, this should make revision easier to perform should it become necessary. So far, however, this theoretical advantage has not been supported by two different studies of revision of unicompartmental replacements.[10,11] Results of revision were not superior to those seen after revision of bi- or tricompartmental replacement and bone stock deficiency in the femoral condyle or tibial plateau often had to be augmented with bone graft or special components. These deficiencies are often the result of poor surgical techniques or prostheses that invade the bone stock unnecessarily. More modern techniques using surface replacements on the femoral and tibial sides should make the procedure as conservative in practice as it is in theory.[12]

Survivorship analyses have been reported for tricompartmental replacement, indicating that survivorship with or without cruciate retention can be above 90% after 10 years of follow-up.[13-15] So far, 10-year survivorship studies generated from early unicompartmental series show that survivorship is not as good at 10 years, dropping into the 85% range.[16] This series was generated, however, at a time when patient selection was still evolving and surgical techniques were not yet perfected.

Patient selection

Osteotomy remains the procedure of choice in the young, heavy, active patient with unicompartmental osteoarthritis. Rest pain and poor range of motion are relative contraindications to osteotomy. Internal derangement is not a contraindication to osteotomy but should be relieved by an arthroscopic procedure prior or subsequent to the osteotomy. Subluxation and extreme angular deformity are a contraindication to both osteotomy and unicompartmental replacement. Metallic interpositional arthroplasty may occasionally be advisable when osteotomy is contraindicated and the patient is considered too young or too heavy to be a candidate for total knee replacement.[17,18]

Once an arthroplasty has been chosen over osteotomy, the final decision between unicompartmental replacement versus bi- or tricompartmental replacement is made at arthrotomy.[4,7,8] Although the patient may be an ideal candidate for unicompartmental arthroplasty from clinical examination and radiography, several contraindications to the procedure may be discovered at the time of arthrotomy. The author considers an absent anterior cruciate ligament a significant contraindication to unicompartmental replacement because this is usually accompanied by a degree of ligamentous laxity that can promote eventual lateral subluxation of the tibia on the femur and secondary opposite compartment disease. Inspection of the opposite compartment and patellofemoral joint may show significant degenerative changes that make unicompartmental arthroplasty inadvisable. Mild chondromalacia in the opposite compartment can be accepted, but areas of eburnated bone are definite contraindications. In a varus osteoarthritic knee with medial compartment arthritis, a secondary lesion appears on the medial aspect of the lateral femoral condyle with early lateral subluxation. This is usually accompanied by intercondylar osteophyte formation. If the subluxation is slight and the lesion is small, it can be debrided and corrected by unicompartmental arthroplasty. If the subluxation is great and the lesion large, bi- or tricompartmental arthroplasty is advisable.

Eburnated bone in the patellofemoral compartment is also a fairly significant contraindication to unicompartmental arthroplasty. There are some surgeons, however, who will accept patellofemoral degeneration including areas of eburnated bone and still proceed with unicompartmental arthroplasty. This author will accept significant chondromalacia in the patellofemoral joint, but not eburnated bone.

A third contraindication discovered at arthrotomy consists of a significant inflammatory component to the patient's disease. This may be in the form of a very dramatic synovial reaction or the discovery of diffuse crystal deposits from either gout or pseudo-gout. Inflammatory disease in any form substantially increases the risk of secondary degeneration of the opposite compartment in subsequent years.

Implant design

Over the past two decades, many lessons have been learned concerning the ideal design features of a unicompartmental arthroplasty. Many early femoral components were narrow in their medial–lateral dimension and suffered a high incidence of subsidence of the component into the condylar bone.[4,16] The ideal component should be wide enough to maximally cap the resurfaced condyle, widely distributing the weight-bearing forces and decreasing the chance of subsidence and loosening. For this reason, multiple sizes should be available to accommodate both small and large patients. Revision studies have shown the inadvisability of deeply invading the condyle with fixation methods.[10,11] Relatively small fixation lugs appear to be sufficient as long as there are two present to gain rotational

fixation to the bone or some sort of fin is provided for this purpose. The posterior metallic condyle should fully cap the posterior condyle of the patient to allow physiologic range of motion without impingement. The amount of bone resection required for insertion should be minimal. Preferably, the femoral component can be supported on top of the distal subchondral bone without any resection, but this requires sacrifice of more bone from the tibial side. The ideal compromise is perhaps to resect between 2 and 4 mm of distal condyle, still retaining part of the subchondral bone for adequate purchase, and 4–6 mm of distal femoral bone to allow easy conversion to a bicompartmental prosthesis. At the same time, this 2–4 mm of distal resection of the femur preserves an equivalent amount of proximal resection from the tibia.

The articulating topography must also consist of a compromise. A flat surface on the femoral component articulating with a flat surface on the tibial component may potentially improve metal-to-plastic contact but is too difficult technically to line up accurately and avoid edge contact. An articulating surface with a small radius of curvature articulating on the tibial side with a flat surface creates too much point contact. A femoral surface with a small radius of curvature matched to a similarly small radius on the tibial side can create too much constraint. The ideal surfaces, for both components therefore, are probably those with a relatively large radius of curvature that allow adequate metal-to-plastic contact without excessive constraint. The anterior-to-posterior topography of the articulating surface of the tibial component can be sloped in front and in back to help guide the femoral component into proper anterior–posterior positioning in the central 50% of the articulating surface so as to avoid abnormal anterior or posterior subluxation.

The shape of the tibial component as it sits on the tibial plateau should probably be anatomic. This will maximize contact between the prosthesis and the bone and widely distribute the weight-bearing forces to resist subsidence and loosening. This will necessitate an asymmetric shape with right and left components. As is necessary on the femoral side, multiple sizes will be required on the tibial side to accommodate both small and large patients.

Metal-backing of the tibial component is controversial. This was initiated in the early 1980s in order to more uniformly distribute the weight-bearing forces to the cut surface of the plateau. Early results with metal-backed components were superior to those with all-polyethylene components, but probably because of improved patient selection and operative technique rather than the use of the metal-backing.[12] When metal-backed components were followed for more than 5 years, failures were seen because of wear-through of the polyethylene to the metal-backing. This resulted when there were areas of polyethylene thickness of less than 4 mm and design flaws in the method of fixation of the polyethylene to the metal. These problems were similar to those seen with metal-backed patellar components.[19,20] Depending on the type of metal utilized (titanium vs chrome cobalt), the minimal composite thickness of the tibial component must be 8–10 mm. This necessity makes metal-backing less attractive than previously thought and there may be a trend back to all-polyethylene tibial components.

Operative technique

The surgical technique is critical to the success of the procedure.[4,8,21] A vertical incision centered over the medial one-third of the patella is recommended. It is usually about 12 cm long and begins proximally over the mid-shaft of the femur and ends distally just medial to the tibial tubercle. A medial parapatellar capsulotomy is performed to allow eversion of the patella and adequate exposure.

For medial compartmental replacement, the coronary ligament is incised at the anterior horn of the medial meniscus, and a periosteal sleeve is elevated from the anteromedial aspect of the tibia. To allow eversion of the patella, the lateral dissection is performed within the fat pad anterior to the coronary ligament, avoiding derangement of the anterior horn of lateral meniscus. For lateral compartmental replacement, the coronary ligament is left intact medially, avoiding derangement of the anterior horn of the medial meniscus. The ligament is incised lateral to the mid-line and a periosteal sleeve is elevated from the anterolateral aspect of the tibia as far as Gerdy's tubercle.

Alternatively, some surgeons recommend a lateral parapatellar incision for a valgus deformity and lateral compartment replacement.[22] This will provide excellent exposure of the lateral compartment but may make bicondylar replacement more difficult if that is deemed necessary and the surgeon is not familiar with the lateral approach.

After adequate exposure has been achieved, the three compartments of the knee are carefully inspected and a decision is made concerning the number of compartments that need replacement. Unicompartmental arthroplasty is contraindicated if there is an inflammatory synovitis or there are crystalline deposits of uric acid or calcium pyrophosphate. The anterior cruciate should be intact. The cartilage in the opposite compartment should appear to be healthy. Chondromalacia in the patellofemoral compartment is not a contraindication to unicompartmental arthroplasty but eburnated bone on the patella or trochlea is probably an indication for a tricompartmental replacement.

Intercondylar osteophytes

As osteoarthritis of the medial compartment progresses, there is usually a tendency for lateral subluxation of the tibia on the femur during weight bearing. As a result, the lateral tibial spine impinges on the medial aspect of the lateral femoral condyle, and 'kissing' osteophytes develop, accompanied by erosion of the medial aspect of the lateral femoral condyle. If these osteophytes are not removed, intercondylar impingement can persist after unicompartmental replacement, with pain on weight bearing. If the 'kissing' erosion lesion is large, bicompartmental or tricompartmental arthroplasty may be necessary.

As lateral compartment osteoarthritis progresses, lateral subluxation of the tibia on the femur usually does not occur until the deformity is so severe that unicompartmental replacement is not appropriate. The medial collateral ligament and medial capsule gradually elongate as the valgus deformity progresses. With significant medial laxity, the knee can no longer be stabilized by unicompartmental replacement and bicompartmental arthroplasty accompanied by lateral release is necessary to stabilize the knee.

Peripheral osteophytes

In an osteoarthritic knee with a varus deformity, peripheral osteophytes build up on the periphery of the medial femoral condyle and medial plateau of the tibia. The medial collateral ligament and capsule may be tented over these osteophytes, resulting in relative shortening of the structures and preventing passive correction of a varus deformity. When the osteophytes are removed there is relative lengthening of the medial collateral ligament and capsule, allowing passive correction of the varus deformity.

Femoral component

Placement

The femoral component should be placed in the center of the medial–lateral dimension of the femoral condyle, measured after removal of peripheral and intercondylar osteophytes. If, for example, in a medial compartmental arthroplasty, the femoral component is placed laterally, too close to the intercondylar notch, the procedure may fail for the following reasons. If the tibial component utilized provides no medial–lateral constraint, medial subluxation of the tibial component will occur and the femoral component will impinge on the medial tibial spine. If, however, the laterally placed femoral component is mated to a medial tibial component with intercondylar constraint, the tibia will move laterally on the femur when the components are seated and the lateral tibial spine will impinge on the lateral femoral condyle.

The femoral component should extend far enough anteriorly to cover the weight-bearing surface that comes in contact with the tibia in full extension. The anterior extent of the weight-bearing surface is usually well defined by the junction between the eburnated bone of the femoral condyle and the intact cartilage remaining in the trochlear groove. The leading edge of the femoral component must be countersunk into this junction to prevent patellar impingement during flexion of the knee. The same principles apply to placement of a femoral component onto the lateral femoral condyle.

Size

The femoral component used should be of a size that reproduces most accurately the anterior–posterior dimension of the femoral condyle. In borderline cases, the larger size should always be inserted first to conserve bone. The posterior condylar bone should be resected to at least the thickness of the metallic implant. It is better to resect slightly too much of the posterior condyle than too little, to avoid making the components too tight in flexion.

Tibial component

Placement

The tibial component should be positioned on the tibia so that, with the knee correctly aligned, this component is directly under the femoral component in the medial–lateral dimension and the articulating surfaces of the two components are congruent during weight bearing. The congruency of components should be determined with the knee in full extension. It should not be judged while the knee is flexed and the patella is everted, because in that position the displaced quadriceps mechanism artificially externally rotates and laterally subluxes the tibia on the femur. If there is a preoperative quadriceps contracture, the force of the displaced quadriceps is even greater. After placement of the tibial component, proper congruency in the frontal plane should be judged by observing the tracking of the components as the knee is flexed and extended with the patella located in the trochlear groove. Viewed from the front, the line of resection of the tibial plateau should be within 5° of a right-angle to the longitudinal axis of the tibia. Viewed from the side, the line of resection can vary from 0 to 10° depending on the individual case. Three to five degrees of posterior slope is usually appropriate.

Size

Ideally, the proper thickness of the tibial component is that which is necessary to restore the worn tibial plateau to its normal height after resection. In a varus knee, if the medial collateral ligament and capsule have been properly released by removal of medial osteophytes, correction of the deformity should be possible without resorting to thicker tibial components. If the articulated components are too tight, the tibia will subluxate toward the opposite compartment and produce excessive pressure there. After medial compartmental replacement, the medial compartment should open up 1–2 mm when valgus stress is applied with the knee in full extension. The same principles apply to replacement of the lateral compartment.

Postoperative rehabilitation

A postoperative regimen following unicompartmental arthroplasty will be similar to that following bi- or tricompartmental arthroplasty. It is often noted, however, that rehabilitation goals are met faster and the patients suffer from less postoperative pain, swelling, and blood loss.[9] Following closure of the capsule, a note is made of the patient's potential flexion against gravity, since it is unreasonable to expect improvement on this during the initial postoperative period. Our current postoperative protocol includes the use of low-dose Coumadin (started the night prior to surgery) combined with pulsatile compression stockings to minimize the chance of postoperative venous thrombosis.

Continuous passive motion (CPM) is begun immediately in the recovery room starting at 30–40° of flexion if a general anesthetic has been utilized or 70–90°, if a long-acting spinal or continuous epidural anesthetic has been administered. The motion machine is used during the day and a knee immobilizer is applied at night to minimize the chance of the development of a significant flexion contracture. The CPM machine is advanced 10–20° per day as tolerated until 90° is achieved and maintained. Quadriceps setting exercises and attempts at straight-leg raising are initiated on the second postoperative day, when the patient also begins bed–chair transfers. By the third day, the patient ambulates with a walker or crutches and 50% weight bearing. A knee immobilizer is used during ambulation until the patient has a secure ability to straight-leg raise. Most patients achieve adequate flexion and independence by the 7th to 9th day, when they are discharged home. They remain on protected weight bearing with full-time support until they are 6 weeks following surgery, when they graduate to a cane outdoors and no support for short distances. The cane is discontinued completely at 3 months post-surgery.

Cementless unicompartmental arthroplasty

The role of cementless unicompartmental arthroplasty is uncertain. In theory, it is appealing if it can be shown to be conservative compared to cemented unicompartmental arthroplasty. In practice, a cementless unicompartmental arthroplasty is actually more radical than a cemented procedure. For most cementless components, more bone resection is required on the femoral side. Failure rates are reported to be higher in terms of loosening on both the femoral and tibial sides.[23] Metal-backed components are most likely required on the tibial side. Cementless unicompartmental arthroplasty must therefore remain experimental until better methods and results are reported.

Summary

Despite two decades of experience, the role of unicompartmental arthroplasty remains controversial and uncertain. It would appear to offer an attractive alternative to osteotomy or tricompartmental replacement in elderly patients with unicompartmental osteoarthritis. Compared to osteotomy, there is a higher initial success rate and fewer early complications. Compared to tricompartmental replacement, there tends to be a better-quality result with a faster recovery and improved function. The procedure is conservative regarding preservation of both cruciate ligaments and bone stock in the opposite compartment and patellofemoral joint. Ten-year survivorship curves, however, have shown that bi- and tricompartmental replacements done in the 1970s have a longer survivorship than unicompartmental replacements from the same era. This appears to be explainable by errors made in patient selection and operative technique as well as prosthetic design. When the appropriate requirements in these areas have been met, unicompartmental knee replacement should assume its appropriate role in our armamentarium.

References

1. Insall JN, Walker PS, Unicondylar knee replacement, *Clin Orthop* (1976) 120: 83–85.
2. Laskin RS, Unicompartmental tibiofemoral resurfacing arthroplasty, *J Bone Joint Surg (Am)* (1978) 60: 182–185.
3. Marmor L, Unicompartmental knee arthroplasty: ten- to thirteen-year follow-up study, *Clin Orthop* (1988) 226: 14–20.
4. Scott RD, Santore RF, Unicondylar unicompartmental replacement for osteoarthritis of the knee, *J Bone Joint Surg (Am)* (1981) 63: 536–544.
5. Bae DK, Guhl JF, Keane SP, Unicompartmental knee arthroplasty for single compartment disease: clinical experience with an average four-year follow-up study, *Clin Orthop* (1983) 176: 233–238.
6. Broughton NS, Newman JH, Baily RAJ, Unicompartmental replacement and high tibial osteotomy for osteoarthritis of the knee: a comparative study after 5–10 years' follow-up, *J Bone Joint Surg (Br)* (1986) 68: 447–452.
7. Kozinn SC, Scott RD, Current concepts review: unicompartmental knee arthroplasty, *J Bone Joint Surg (Am)* (1989) 71: 145–150.
8. Thornhill TS, Scott RD, Unicompartmental total knee arthroplasty *Orthop Clin North Am* (1989) 20: 245–256.
9. Cobb AG, Kozinn SC, Scott RD, Unicondylar or total knee replacement: The patient's preference, *J Bone Joint Surg (Br)* (1990) 72: 166.
10. Barrett WP, Scott RD, Revision of failed unicondylar unicompartmental knee arthroplasty, *J Bone Joint Surg (Am)* (1987) 69: 1328–1335.
11. Padgett DE, Stern SH, Insall JN, Revision total knee arthroplasty for failed unicompartmental replacement, *J Bone Joint Surg (Am)* (1991) 73: 186–190.
12. Kozinn SC, Marx C, Scott RD, Unicompartmental knee arthroplasty: a 4.5 to 6-year follow-up study with a metal backed tibial component, *J Arthroplasty* (1989) 4(suppl.): S1–S10.
13. Ranawat CS, Oheneba BA, Survivorship analysis and results of total condylar knee arthroplasty: eight- to 11-year follow-up period. *Clin Orthop* (1988) 226: 6–13.
14. Scuderi GR, Insall JN, Windsor RE et al., Survivorship of cemented knee replacements, *J Bone Joint Surg (Br)* (1989) 71: 798–803.
15. Rand JA, Ilstrup DM, Survivorship analysis of total knee arthroplasty: Cumulative rates of survival of 9200 total knee arthroplasties, *J Bone Joint Surg (Am)* (1991) 73: 397–409.
16. Scott RD, Cobb AG, McQueary FG et al., Unicompartmental knee arthroplasty: eight to twelve-year follow-up with survivorship analysis, *Clin Orthop* (1991) 271: 96–100.
17. Emerson RH, Jr, Potter T, The use of the McKeever metallic hemiarthroplasty for unicompartmental arthritis, *J Bone Joint Surg (Am)* (1985) 67: 208–212.
18. Scott RD, Joyce MJ, Ewald FC et al., McKeever metallic hemiarthroplasty of the knee in unicompartmental degenerative arthritis: long-term clinical follow-up and current indications, *J Bone Joint Surg (Am)* (1985) 67: 203–207.
19. Bayley JC, Scott RD, Ewald FC et al., Failure of the metal-backed patellar component after total knee replacement, *J Bone Joint Surg (Am)* (1988) 70: 668–674.
20. Lombardi AV Jr, Engh GA, Volz RG et al., Fracture/dissociation of the polyethylene in metal-backed patellar components in total knee arthroplasty, *J Bone Joint Surg (Am)* (1988) 70: 675–679.
21. Scott RD, Robert Brigham unicondylar knee surgical techniques, *Techn Orthop* (1990) 5: 15–23.
22. Keblish PA, Valgus deformity in total knee replacement: The lateral retinacular approach, *Orthop Trans* (1985) 9: 28–29.
23. Bernasek TL, Rand JA, Bryan RS, Unicompartmental porous coated anatomic total knee arthroplasty, *Clin Orthop* (1988) 236: 52–59.

16.2   Unicompartmental replacement of the knee

John H. Newman

Osteoarthritis of the knee is a common condition in which involvement of one compartment frequently predominates. In the early stages symptoms can be improved by anti-inflammatory agents, intra-articular steroid injection or arthroscopic washout. However, once articular cartilage becomes significantly worn, pain tends to persist. Since much of the joint is relatively well-preserved, it is not surprising that surgeons try to help their patients by replacing merely the diseased part of the knee.

Early unicompartmental replacements

In the late 1970s and 1980s several reports of good results from unicompartmental replacement were published,[1-4] though others were less encouraging.[5] A particularly worrying report was that from Insall and Aglietti,[6] who presented a group of patients who initially had a satisfactory result but when followed up at 6 years had deteriorated badly so that only about a third were then regarded as good or excellent.

In the 1970s the most widely accepted surgical treatment for unicompartmental arthritis of the knee was an upper tibial osteotomy. This usually gave symptomatic improvement, though the published success rate following the procedure varied from 56%[7] to 97% at 2 years.[8] The latter authors, though, subsequently reported a deterioration of these results with time.

Comparison of tibial osteotomy and unicompartmental replacement[25]

In Bristol the early experience of unicompartmental replacement using the St Georg 'sledge' prosthesis had been encouraging,[9] but at that time the follow-up was short. Since the obvious alternative procedure was an upper tibial osteotomy, it was decided to carry out a retrospective study of patients who had undergone either an osteotomy or a unicompartmental replacement using the same assessment criteria for both groups. The objective was to try to determine whether one procedure was superior to the other in terms of either the quality or the longevity of result.

All patients treated surgically in Bristol for osteoarthritis of the knee by unicompartmental replacement or upper tibial osteotomy between 1974 and 1979 were studied, thus giving a follow-up period of between 5 and 10 years. Forty-nine osteotomies were available for study and these were compared with 42 unicompartmental replacements. All osteotomies had been performed by resecting a wedge of bone above the tibial tubercle in order to fully correct the coronal tibiofemoral angle. The fibula was released in a variety of ways. Postoperatively the knee was usually immobilized in plaster for 6 weeks.

The unicompartmental replacements were all of the St Georg 'sledge' type, cemented in place, with a deliberate effort being made to minimally undercorrect the deformity (Figure 1).

The selection of patients for the two procedures was determined purely by the pattern of referral from general practitioners. At that time the unicompartmental replacements were carried out by the late Mr R.A.J. Baily and the late Mr W.G.J. Hampson and their teams, while the tibial osteotomies were carried out by other Bristol surgeons. There was no evidence of cross-referral. The preoperative parameters of the two groups were broadly similar (Table 1) and it was therefore felt that retrospective comparison was justified.

All patients were assessed by history plus clinical and radiological examination between 5 and 10 years from operation. An objective assessment was made using the Baily knee score, which was adapted from that used by the Hospital for Special Surgery and has a maximum score of 50. Thirty-five or more is rated as good, 30–34 fair and less than 30 poor. The radiological features of arthritis were graded according to the system of Kellgren and Lawrence[10] and the coronal tibiofemoral angles were measured on long weight-bearing radiographs.

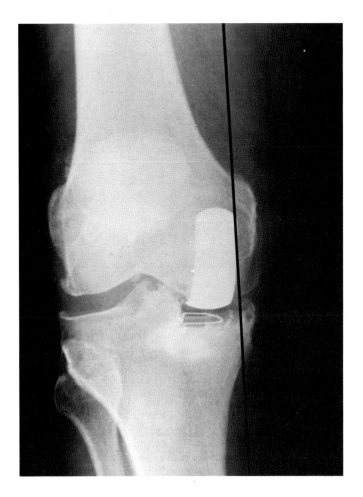

Figure 1

5 year follow-up radiograph of St Georg 'sledge' prosthesis. The load line shows deliberate under-correction of the original varus deformity.

Table 1 Comparison of the preoperative condition of the unicompartmental and osteotomy groups.

	Replacement	Osteotomy
Average age (years)	71	63
Sex F:M	31:11	38:11
Preoperative deformity:		
Varus	36°	33°
Valgus	6°	16°
Average deviation from coronal tibiofemoral angle of 7° valgus (degrees)	10.2	9.9
Average Kellgren–Lawrence score in		
Affected compartment	3.2	3.3
Unaffected compartment	1.9	2.0
Patellofemoral joint	2.0	2.4

Table 2 Comparison of overall results.

	Osteotomy	Replacement
Good	21	32
Fair	11	4
Poor	7	3
Failed	10	3

Statistical significance, $P<0.01$.

Results

Overall assessment

The unicompartmental replacements showed significantly better results than the osteotomies (Table 2). Seventy-six per cent of the unicompartmental group were classified as having a good result, whereas only 43% of the osteotomies were viewed in that light ($P<0.01$). Twenty per cent of the osteotomies had been revised to a knee replacement, whereas only 7% of the unicompartmental replacements had required further surgery.

Pain

Although pain represented 30% of the overall score, most patients regard this as the most important factor and it was therefore assessed separately. Of those patients who had not undergone further surgery, 67% of the unicompartmental group had no pain as compared with 26% in the osteotomy group.

Radiological changes

Not all cases had adequate radiographs to allow full assessment, but it can be seen from Table 3 that following tibial osteotomy the affected compartment rarely deteriorated but the loaded compartment usually did, and half the time the patellofemoral joint

Table 3 Incidence of radiological deterioration in compartments.

Compart-ment	Replacement		Osteotomy	
	Deterior-ation	No deterior-ation	Deterior-ation	No deterior-ation
Affected	–	–	2	15
Unaffected	2	18	12	5
Patello-femoral joint	3	16	8	8

became more worn. Following unicompartmental replacement with deliberate undercorrection of the deformity, radiological deterioration of either of the other two compartments was unusual.

Thus, on the criteria studied, the unicompartmental group appeared to do better when reviewed between 5 and 10 years. The study is open to criticism because it was retrospective and also because the average follow-up of the osteotomies was slightly longer. However, this did not appear to affect the results and in Bristol it seems that patients get a better quality of result and are less likely to need further surgery within 10 years following unicompartmental replacement than following upper tibial osteotomy. The differences were very apparent for the varus knee but were even more striking for the small number of valgus knees, which did particularly well with unicompartmental replacement.

A comparison of unicompartmental and total knee replacement

Because the early reports of unicompartmental replacement were variable, some surgeons thought that the procedure should not be performed and that patients with unicompartmental disease would be better treated by either osteotomy or total knee replacement. Such an approach denied many patients the undoubted benefits that can be derived from the relatively simple procedure of unicompartmental replacement, though, as the results of total knee replacement improve, the need for other procedures diminishes.

In Bristol the group of patients previously discussed who underwent unicompartmental replacement between 1974 and 1979 were compared retrospectively with patients who underwent total knee replacement at the same time. At an average follow-up of 7 years it was found that 76% of the unicompartmental group were still rated as having a good result, as compared with 50% of those undergoing total knee replacement. However, the prosthesis being used at that time was the Sheehan semiconstrained arthroplasty and the results of this group of patients would undoubtedly now be much improved by using a total condylar type of prosthesis.

A second retrospective comparison was therefore made between a group of patients undergoing unicompartmental replacement and those treated with a resurfacing Kinematic total knee replacement during 1982 and 1983. These two groups of patients were compared at the time of their 2-year follow-up using standard knee arthroplasty assessment forms with a maximum score of 100. The average score for

Table 4 Knee flexion at 3 weeks postoperatively (as found in a prospective study with 50 patients in each group).

| | Prosthesis | |
Regime	Sledge	Kinematic
Flexion	91°	84°
Extension	79°	70°
CPM	90°	80°
Preoperatively	96°	93°

the total knee replacement group rose from a preoperative figure of 44 to one of 80, while that for the unicompartmental group rose from 55 to 86. It therefore seems that in Bristol patients undergoing unicompartmental replacement fare slightly better at 2 years than those who have had a total knee replacement, but it is to be noted that they were a group who had slightly less severely damaged knees in the first place.

Further studies in Bristol of various postoperative regimens[11] demonstrated that knees treated by unicompartmental replacement remobilized more rapidly than those undergoing total knee replacement (Table 4) and it was found that this advantage was maintained at 6 months. The unicompartmental group had approximately 10° more flexion whether treated in the immediate postoperative period by a flexion or extension regime or by early continuous passive motion.[12]

The Swedish multicentre prospective knee replacement study[13] demonstrated that at 6 years there was a slightly smaller risk of a unicompartmental replacement failing than was seen with a bicompartmental or tricompartmental replacement. The same study also demonstrated a lower infection rate following unicompartmental replacement; a finding that was also demonstrated in Bristol where the infection rate after unicompartmental replacement was approximately half that seen after total resurfacing replacement.[14]

These various factors would tend to support the contention that there is a place for unicompartmental replacement, but most of the studies mentioned were retrospective and none had matched material. With the improving results of total knee replacement, the place of the various procedures will need more accurate definition. This can only be done by controlled, randomized, prospective study but as yet no such work has been published. Clearly, though, there will be limits beyond which unicompartmental replacement is ill-advised, and a recent review in Bristol has suggested that 10° or more of fixed flexion should be regarded as a contraindication, while rather greater varus or valgus angulation can usually be corrected (Newman, J.H., unpublished).

Recent results of unicompartmental replacement

In 1988 Mackinnon et al.[15] published the most recent review of the Bristol unicompartmental experience. They reported on 138 knees followed between 2 and 12 years and demonstrated good or excellent results in 86%, with an even higher rate of patient satisfaction. Many others have also reported satisfactory long-term results which seem comparable to those obtained by total knee replacement. Kozinn and Scott[16] report an 83% survivorship at 10 years and the Swedish multicentre study demonstrates a 90% survivorship at 6 years for medial compartment prostheses.[13] Marmor[17] presents 87% continued pain relief at between 10 and 13 years, while Goodfellow and O'Connor,[18] using a meniscal bearing unicompartmental replacement, report good results but caution that the anterior cruciate must be intact.

Patterns of failure of unicompartmental replacement

Now that unicompartmental replacements have been used for over 15 years, failures are inevitably being seen. The precise pattern of failure will probably depend on the individual prosthesis; for example, occasional femoral fractures occur with the St Georg 'sledge' prostheses (Figure 2) and a high rate of tibial loosening has been reported for the metal-backed tibial component of the PCA Uni when used uncemented.[19] Despite these individual problems, some patterns are beginning to emerge.

Failure will frequently occur if the disease is not truly unicompartmental and it is to be noted that in the series reported by Insall and Aglietti[6] in which early failure occurred, over 50% had already undergone a previous patellectomy, so that the disease was not truly unicompartmental. There is debate about

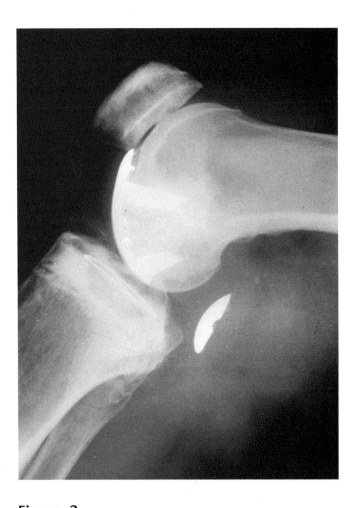

Figure 2

Fracture of the femoral component at 4 years.

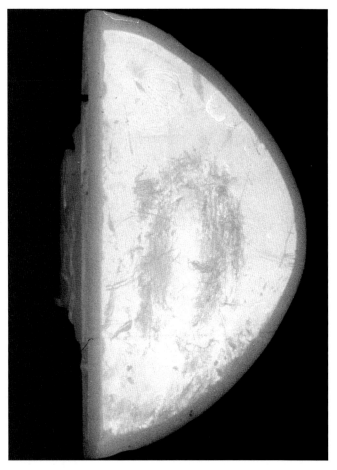

Figure 3

Tibial component removed at 4 years. The maximum depth of wear was 0.4 mm.

the importance of patellofemoral arthritis, with some authors regarding it as a contraindication while others feel it is largely irrelevant.[20] Significant damage to the articular cartilage of the opposite compartment is clearly an indication for total knee replacement despite the fact that most authors advise slight under-correction of the deformity so as to load the pros-thesis rather than the opposite articular cartilage, which will almost inevitably be substandard. If applied to total knee replacement, this policy of undercorrection would lead to failure, and it may well do so in the long-term. As yet, few series of unicompartmental replacement over 10 years have been published, but most results do not suggest rapid loosening or subsidence of the loaded component.

Møller et al.[21] have suggested from cadaveric studies that an intact anterior cruciate ligament is necessary for long-term survival of an unconstrained implant, and recently Goodfellow and O'Connor[18] have presented clinical data to support this theory. The need for an intact anterior cruciate suggests that the procedure is inappropriate for correction of gross collateral instability unless this is purely due to loss of bone.[22]

Most unicompartmental prostheses have a relatively flat tibial polyethylene surface and rely on ligamentous integrity for stability. A round femoral component articulating with a flat polyethylene tibia might be expected to wear badly, but the few speci-mens removed in Bristol have demonstrated a wear rate of about 0.1 mm per year (Figure 3), which is very comparable to that seen in Charnley hip replace-ment.[23]

Conclusions

Unicompartmental replacement has proved success-ful in many hands, with 10-year follow-ups showing over 80% survival.[16,17] Excellent 10-year results have also been reported from total knee replacement, though in a different patient population many of whom suffer from rheumatoid arthritis. Clearly, proper prospective studies are required before the definitive place of the two procedures is established.

Osteoarthritis of the knee progresses with time and the best procedure for the patient will depend upon the severity of the disease. In the younger patient with early unicompartmental disease, there is little doubt that osteotomy is the most appropriate form of surgery. Once the disease has progressed to involve other compartments and fixed flexion is developing, then total knee replacement is required. Between these two lies the unicompartmental replacement. In the United Kingdom patients tend to be referred late, so that in 1989 in Bristol many more total knee replacements were performed than unicompartmen-tal replacements. Only a small number of tibial

osteotomies was carried out during this period. However, in Sweden as long ago as 1980 patients tended to present earlier, thus allowing a more conservative surgical approach, so that approximately a third of the patients with gonarthrosis were treated with each of the three procedures.[24] It is hoped that this will eventually happen elsewhere, so that as much as possible of the patient's own joint can be preserved.

Acknowledgment

I would like to acknowledge the contributions to this paper made by the late Mr R.A.J. Baily, Mr P.H. Roberts and Mr C.E. Ackroyd. Most of the figures quoted from Bristol represent an accumulation of the results of cases operated on by our four teams, all of which are assessed pre- and postoperatively in a standard way.

Tables 1 and 3 are reproduced from the *Journal of Bone and Joint Surgery* with permission.

References

1. Inglis GS, Unicompartmental arthroplasty of the knee: a follow-up of 3 to 9 years, *J Bone Joint Surg (Br)* (1984) **66**: 682–684.
2. Marmor L, Marmor modular knee in unicompartmental disease, *J Bone Joint Surg (Am)* (1979) **61**: 347–353.
3. Scott RD, Santore RF, Unicondylar unicompartmental replace-ment for osteoarthritis of the knee, *J Bone Joint Surg (Am)* (1981) **63**: 536–544.
4. Thornhill TS, Unicompartmental knee arthroplasty, *Clin Orthop* (1986) **205**: 121–131.
5. Laskin RS, Unicompartmental tibiofemoral resurfacing arthroplasty, *J Bone Joint Surg (Am)* (1978) **60**: 182–185.
6. Insall J, Aglietti P, A five to seven-year follow-up of unicondy-lar arthroplasty, *J Bone Joint Surg (Am)* (1980) **62**: 1329–1337.
7. Harding ML, A fresh appraisal of tibial osteotomy for osteoarthritis of the knee, *Clin Orthop* (1976) **114**: 223–234.
8. Insall JN, Joseph DM, Msika C, High tibial osteotomy for varus gonarthrosis: a long-term follow-up study, *J Bone Joint Surg (Am)* (1984) **66**: 1040–1048.
9. Staniforth P, Baily RAJ, St Georg "Sledge" resurfacing of the tibiofemoral joint, *J Bone Joint Surg (Br)* (1982) **64**: 246–247.
10. Kellgren JH, Lawrence JS, Radiological assessment of osteoarthrosis, *Ann Rheum Dis* (1957) **16**: 494–502.
11. Newman JH, Ackroyd CE, Baily RAJ et al., A comparison of flexion and extension regimes after knee replacement, *J Bone Joint Surg (Br)* (1985) **67**: 488–489.
12. Ackroyd CE, Newman JH, Roberts PH et al., La rééducation après arthroplastie du genou, *Ann Orthop de l'Ouest* (1988) **20**: 51–83.
13. Knutson K, Lindstrand A, Lidgren L, Survival of knee arthro-plasties: a nation-wide multicentre investigation of 8000 cases, *J Bone Joint Surg (Br)* (1986) **68**: 795–803.
14. Johnson DP, Bannister GC, The outcome of infected arthro-plasty of the knee, *J Bone Joint Surg (Br)* (1986) **68**: 289–291.
15. Mackinnon J, Young S, Baily RAJ, The St Georg Sledge for unicompartmental replacement of the knee: a prospective study of 115 cases, *J Bone Joint Surg (Br)* (1988) **70**: 217–223.

16. Kozinn SC, Scott RD, Current concepts review: Unicondylar knee arthroplasty, *J Bone Joint Surg (Am)* (1989) **71**: 145–150.

17. Marmor L, Unicompartmental knee arthroplasty: Ten- to 13-year follow-up study, *Clin Orthop* (1988) **226**: 14–20.

18. Goodfellow JW, O'Connor JJ, Clinical results of the Oxford knee: surface arthroplasty of the tibiofemoral joint with a meniscal bearing prosthesis, *Clin Orthop* (1986) **205**: 21–42.

19. Bernasek TL, Rand JA, Bryan RS, Unicompartmental porous coated anatomic total knee arthroplasty, *Clin Orthop* (1988) **236**: 52–59.

20. Goodfellow JW, Tibrewal SB, Sherman KP et al., Unicompartmental Oxford meniscal knee arthroplasty, *J Arthroplasty* (1987) **2**: 1–9.

21. Møller JT, Weeth RE, Keller JØ et al., Unicompartmental arthroplasty of the knee: cadaver study of the importance of the anterior cruciate ligament, *Acta Orthop Scand* (1985) **56**: 120–123.

22. Cartier P, Cheaib S, Unicondylar knee arthroplasty, *J Arthroplasty* (1987) **2**: 157–162.

23. Wroblewski BM, Direction and rate of socket wear in Charnley low-friction arthroplasty, *J Bone Joint Surg (Br)* (1985) **67**: 757–761.

24. Bauer GCH, Treatment of gonarthrosis, *American Academy of Orthopaedic Surgeons, Instructional Course Lectures* (St. Louis: CV Mosby, 1982) **31**: 152–166.

25. Broughton NS, Newman JH, Baily RAJ, Unicompartmental replacement and high tibial osteotomy for osteoarthritis of the knee: a comparative study after 5–10 years' follow-up, *J Bone Joint Surg (Br)* (1986) **68**: 447–452.

16.3 Unicompartmental arthroplasty of the knee using the Robert Brigham prosthesis: A prospective study with a 3–7-year follow-up

Dipak V. Patel and Paul M. Aichroth

Unicondylar arthroplasty has been a somewhat controversial procedure in the management of unicompartmental osteoarthritis of the knee.[1] However, in the past decade, various authors have reported excellent clinical results using the different unicompartmental prostheses.[2–6] Encouraging results have also been reported using the Robert Brigham prosthesis.[7–10]

The purpose of this contribution is to report the clinical and radiological results of Robert Brigham unicompartmental arthroplasty of the knee.

Material and methods

This is a prospective study of 35 patients (36 knees) who underwent unicompartmental arthroplasty of the knee. There were 20 males and 15 females; the right knee was involved in 19 cases and the left in 17. One patient had bilateral unicompartmental replacement. The average age of the patients at the time of surgery was 64.5 years (range 52–82 years) and the mean follow-up was 4.8 years (range 3–7 years). The medial compartment was replaced in 34 cases and the lateral in 2.

All patients had single compartmental osteoarthritis of the knee with minimal or no changes in the contralateral compartment or the patellofemoral joint. The majority of the patients had an arthroscopic assessment prior to surgery.

All patients in this study had substantial pain which failed to respond to adequate conservative treatment in the form of quadriceps rehabilitation, analgesics and non-steroidal anti-inflammatory drugs.

Preoperatively, 64% of the knees presented with severe pain and 36% had moderate pain. All patients had an adequate trial of conservative treatment. The walking distance was 500–1000 m in 6% of the patients, 100–500 m in 51% and 50–100 m in 43%. Eighty per cent of the patients were using walking aids (usually a single stick) preoperatively. The average preoperative knee flexion was 121° (range 100° to 135°). Flexion contracture of an average of 8° (range 5–12°) was present in 22 knees (63%). The mean preoperative varus deformity was 9.5° (range 5–13°) and the average valgus deformity was 9° (range 7–11°).

The patients were evaluated using the BASK (British Association for Surgery of the Knee) scoring system. The average preoperative BASK score was 48.6 points (range 37–65 points). The results were graded as excellent, good, fair and poor; knees with a score between 91 and 100 were regarded as excellent; between 75 and 90 as good; between 60 and 74 as fair; and less than 60 as poor.

The standard weight-bearing short radiographs were obtained for the majority of the patients; long radiographs were available in 10 cases. The radiographs were evaluated for alignment, presence of radiolucent lines, component position and subsequent migration. The radiolucent lines were noted as complete or incomplete for each of three zones on the anteroposterior and lateral views for the tibial interfaces, and for four zones on the lateral view for the femoral interfaces.

Indications for unicompartmental arthroplasty

The operation is recommended for the elderly, less-active patients who have single compartment osteoarthritis of the knee with minimal or no changes in the opposite compartment or the patellofemoral joint. The patient's age, occupational and recreational demands, the preoperative range of knee movement, the extent of varus or valgus malalignment, the degree of flexion contracture and the intra-articular pathology must be considered.

Patients with a varus or valgus malalignment of less than 15° and a flexion contracture of less than 10° are suitable candidates for unicompartmental knee

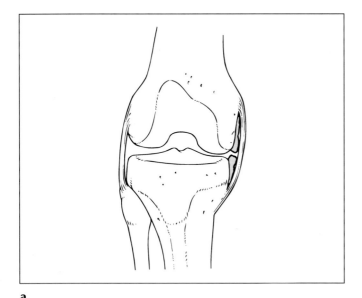

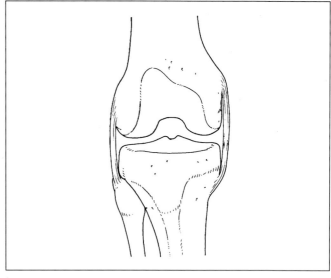

a   b

Figure 1

(a) Peripheral osteophytes on the femur and tibia. (b) The deformity can be passively corrected by removal of these osteophytes.

replacement. In some cases, the final decision to perform unicondylar replacement should be made after an arthroscopy or arthrotomy has been performed and the status of articular surfaces has been examined. It is worth emphasizing that both cruciate ligaments should be intact to ensure best clinical results after unicompartmental arthroplasty.

Patients with rheumatoid or other inflammatory arthritis are not suitable for this procedure owing to synovial involvement of the contralateral compartment.

Operative technique

A detailed description of the operative technique is reported by Scott.[11] A mid-line longitudinal skin incision that runs slightly medial to the centre of the patella is used. A standard medial parapatellar capsulotomy is performed and the patella is everted laterally as the knee is flexed. For medial compartment replacement, the coronary ligament is incised at the anterior horn of the medial meniscus and a periosteal sleeve is elevated from the anteromedial aspect of the tibia. The dissection is carried laterally as far as the infrapatellar bursa, but the coronary ligament is protected beyond this point to avoid derangement of the anterior horn of the lateral meniscus. For lateral compartment replacement, the coronary ligament is incised lateral to the mid-line and a periosteal sleeve is elevated from the antero-lateral aspect of the tibia as far as Gerdy's tubercle.

The hypertrophic peripheral (Figure 1) and intercondylar osteophytes (Figure 2) are removed using an osteotome or rongeur. This provides passive correction of the angular deformity and eliminates any intercondylar impingement with weight bearing. Soft-tissue release is usually not necessary after removal of the osteophytes.

The placement of the femoral component should be in the centre of the femoral condyle, measured after removal of the osteophytes. The femoral component must extend far enough anteriorly to cover the weight-bearing surface in contact with the tibia in extension. The junction between the eburnated bone in the arthritic compartment and the normal cartilage of the trochlea (Figure 3) should be marked by bringing the knee into full extension.

A burr is used to remove a small area of subchondral bone to allow the leading edge of the femoral component to be inset into the femur (Figure 4). The posterior condylar cutting jig is then used with its leading edge set into the recess created by the burr (Figure 5). The jig should be oriented vertically on the distal end of the femur (Figure 6). The thickness of the posterior condyle to be resected should be at least as great as that of the prosthesis chosen to replace it, to avoid making the components too tight in flexion.

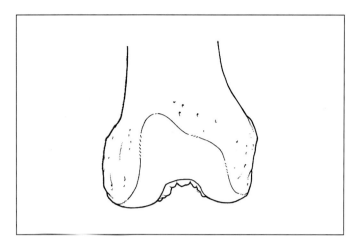

Figure 2

Osteophytes in the intercondylar notch of the femur should be removed to relieve impingement.

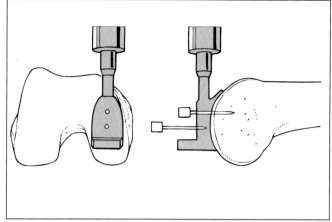

Figure 5

The posterior condylar cutting jig is pinned to the femur.

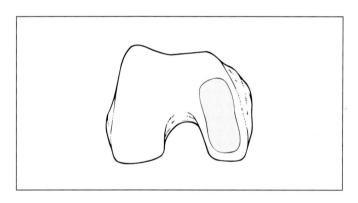

Figure 3

The junction between the eburnated bone and the intact trochlear articular cartilage is identified.

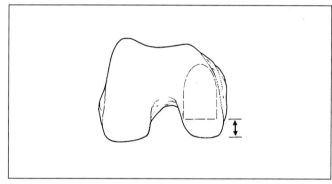

Figure 6

Excessive internal or external rotation of the femoral component should be avoided. Approximately 8–10 mm of the posterior condyle is resected. (As suggested by Richard Scott).[11]

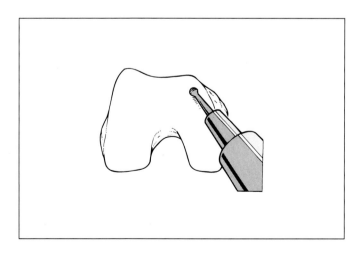

Figure 4

A burr is used to recess the leading edge of the femoral component.

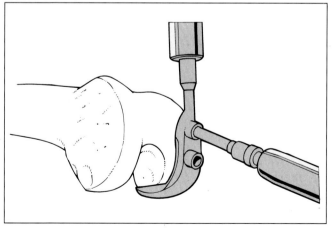

Figure 7

A drill enlarges the pinholes to receive the femoral fixation lugs.

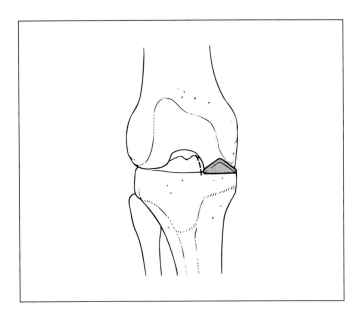

Figure 8

A mark is made along the tibial spine to establish the correct rotatory alignment of the tibial component.

A drill guide is used to orient the angulation of the fixation lugs of the femoral component (Figure 7). A femoral trial is then inserted and its fit is assessed.

With the femoral trial component in place, the knee is brought into full extension, and a mark is made along the tibial spine 2 mm from the edge of the femoral component to orient the rotational and mediolateral positioning of the tibial component in relation to the femoral component (Figure 8). The tibial alignment guide is then used. This guide consists of a femoral trial component with an extension that drops over the tibial plateau when the knee is extended (Figure 9a). A transverse line is drawn along the proximal tibia parallel to the guide (Figure 9b). This line should be within 10° of being oriented at a right-angle to the long axis of the tibia. A proximal tibial marker can be used to check this orientation (Figure 10).

A telescoping tibial alignment/cutting guide is used to determine the precise level and orientation of the proximal tibial resection. After applying this guide, the cutting platform is adjusted so that it is parallel with the line drawn on the tibia (Figure 11a). The cutting platform is then raised proximally to the level of minimal bone resection (Figure 11b). As viewed from the lateral side, this cut should be angled slightly posteriorly to allow rollback of the femur during flexion (Figure 11c).

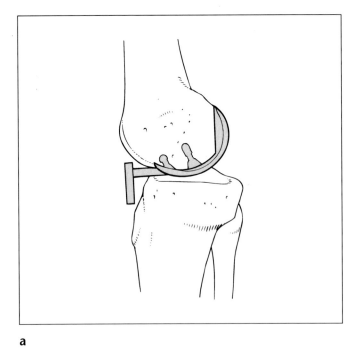

a

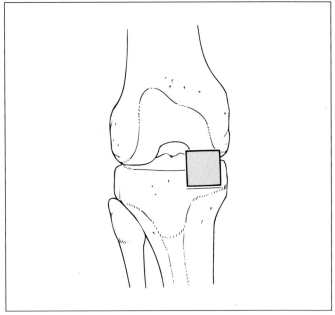

b

Figure 9

(a) The tibial alignment guide is inserted and the knee is extended. (b) A line is drawn on the tibia parallel to the guide.

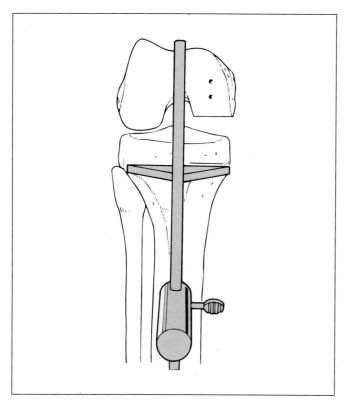

a

Figure 10

A proximal right-angle tibial marker is used to check the orientation of the tibial alignment.

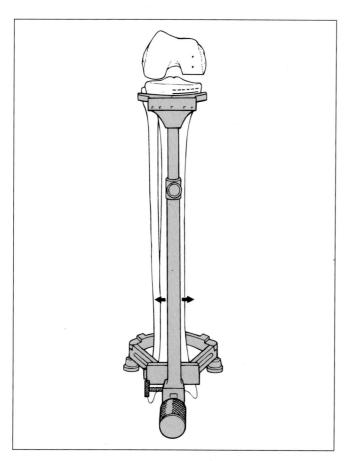

a

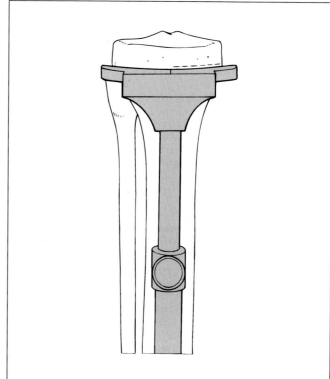

b

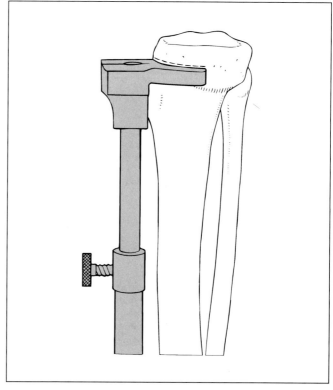

c

Figure 11

(a) A tibial guide is applied and adjusted so that the cutting platform is parallel with the established tibial component alignment. (b) The platform is raised proximally to the point of minimal resection. (c) The cut is angled posteriorly between 0° and 10°.[11]

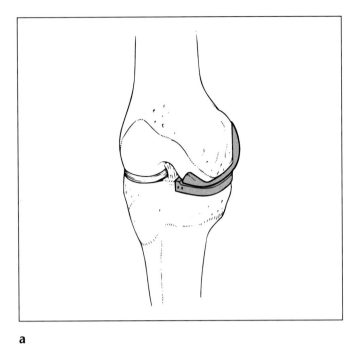

a

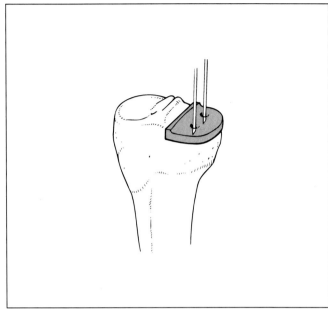

b

Figure 12

(a) The femoral and tibial trial components are inserted. (b) The holes for the fixation lugs of the tibial component are marked.

A tibial trial is now inserted, followed by the femoral trial, and the knee is brought into full extension (Figure 12a). Two sizes of tibial components are available (small and large) in three thicknesses (8, 10 and 12.5 mm). The stability and congruence should be tested using the different thicknesses. On application of valgus stress, the knee should open up at least 2 mm, otherwise the fit may be considered too tight. When the proper size, thickness and orientation of the tibial component have been determined, the positions of the fixation lugs are marked through the appropriate holes in the tibial trial (Figure 12b). The holes are eventually deepened to about 6 mm (Figure 13).

The tibial component is now inserted and should be flush with the resected surface of the tibial plateau. The femoral component is then inserted and it should also fit flush (Figure 14). There should be good mediolateral and rotational congruence of the components (Figure 15a). Their articulating surfaces should be parallel. The knee should be stable in extension, opening up 1–2 mm on valgus stress. If the components are too tight in flexion, more posterior femoral condyle might have to be resected, requiring a smaller femoral component or repositioning of the lug holes more anteriorly on the femur. The patella should track well without imping-ing on the leading edge of the femoral component (Figure 15b). The tibial component should not protrude beyond the peripheral bony cortex. If it does, then a small tibial component should be used, or the component should be moved closer to the tibial spine.

A pulsed lavage system is used to cleanse the bony surfaces prior to the fixation of the definitive prostheses with bone cement. The tibial component is cemented first. Care must be taken to remove the excess cement with a curette, especially from the posterior aspect of the tibial prosthesis. Then the femoral component is placed with cement packed in the posterior housing of the prosthesis to ensure good posterior condyle-to-bone contact.

Postoperative management

A compression dressing is applied for 24 hours. On the first or second postoperative day, a continuous passive mobilization machine is used, and muscle strengthening and mobilizing exercises are commenced. Assisted weight-bearing ambulation is started on the 3rd postoperative day, or as soon as the patient is comfortable.

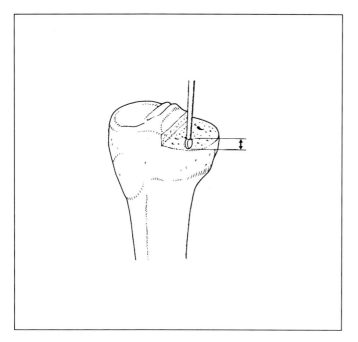

Figure 13

The lug holes are deepened to approximately 6 mm.

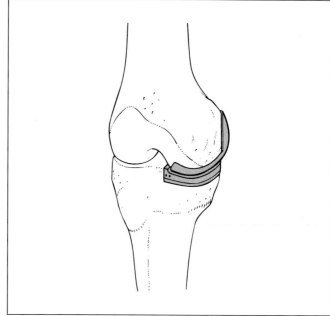

Figure 14

The definitive components are inserted without cement and tested.

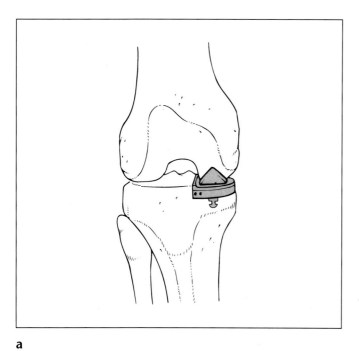

a

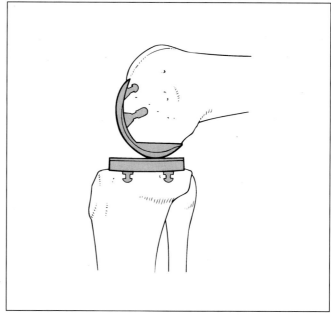

b

Figure 15

(a) In extension, the articulating surfaces of the components should be parallel and there should be good rotational and mediolateral congruency. (b) The leading edge of the femoral component should be recessed enough to avoid patellar impingement.

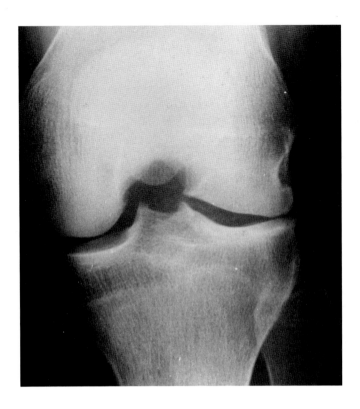

Figure 16

Preoperative radiograph of a 67-year-old man with lateral compartment osteoarthritis of the knee.

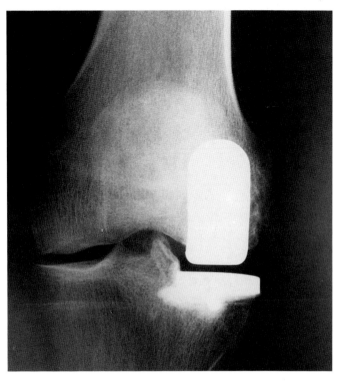

Figure 17

Postoperative radiograph of the patient in Figure 16, 5.5 years following the unicompartmental replacement. The patient had an excellent clinical result.

Results

Clinical results

Fifty-six per cent of the knees had an excellent result, 36% had a good result and 8% had a fair result. None of the patients had a poor result. The mean postoperative BASK score was 89.2 (range 70–99). At the time of latest follow-up, 89% of the knees had no pain and 11% had mild discomfort on strenuous exertion.

The walking distance had improved to greater than 1 km in 74% of the patients and to 0.5–1 km in 26%. Sixty-three per cent of the patients required no walking aids, whereas 37% used a walking stick for outdoor activities only. The average postoperative knee flexion was 118° (range 85–135°). Postoperatively, a residual flexion contracture of an average of 4.2° (range 3–7°) was seen in 8 knees.

Radiological results

The tibiofemoral alignment was measured on standard weight-bearing radiographs. The average postoperative alignment was 3.8° of valgus (range 2°

of varus to 8° of valgus). Thirty-six per cent of the knees had non-progressive, incomplete radiolucent line of less than 1 mm width under the metal-backed tibial component. No radiolucent lines were seen under the femoral component. No subsidence of the femoral or tibial components was seen on progressive radiographs. Figures 16 and 17 show preoperative and postoperative radiographs of a 67-year-old man who underwent unicompartmental resurfacing arthroplasty for lateral compartment osteoarthritis of the knee. This patient had an excellent clinical result.

Complications

There were no superficial or deep infections in this series. One 65-year-old woman presented with a history of locking in her right knee, 10 months after unicondylar replacement for medial compartment osteoarthritis. The radiographs showed a small fragment of cement in the posterolateral compartment of the knee (Figure 18). We feel that this fragment arose from the excess of cement at the posterior aspect of the tibial prosthesis. The patient subsequently had no further symptom of locking and we trust that the loose fragment is lying quietly

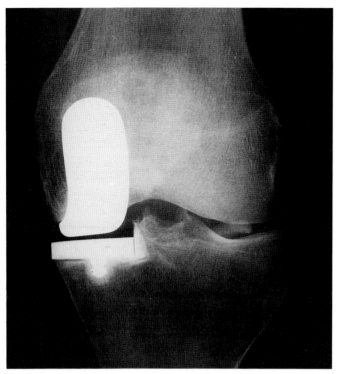
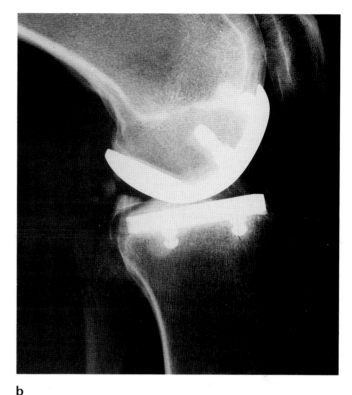

a   b

Figure 18

(a) Anteroposterior view showing a fragment of cement in the lateral compartment. (b) However, on the lateral view, the fragment was seen to lie in the posterior compartment.

in the posterior compartment of the knee. From this experience, we would emphasize that care should be taken to remove the excess of cement from the posterior aspect of the tibial and femoral components.

Five patients required manipulation under anaesthetic at an average of 14 days postoperatively in view of the limited range of knee movement. All five patients obtained more than 90° of knee flexion after manipulation, and all had maintained their knee movement at the time of latest review.

Patient satisfaction

Twenty-nine patients (83%) were very pleased and 6 (17%) were satisfied with the outcome of surgery.

Discussion

In patients with predominantly unicompartmental knee involvement, total knee replacement seems irrational, especially in patients who are in their fifth and early sixth decade. The high tibial osteotomy is suitable for younger patients who have early osteoarthritis with malalignment. However, the results of tibial osteotomy in patients with advanced arthritis are less encouraging. Unicondylar replacement offers a reasonable alternative to total knee replacement, which may be too radical, and to corrective osteotomy, which gives unpredictable results, particularly in elderly patients.[12]

Unicompartmental arthroplasty has many advantages when compared to a total knee replacement.[8,13] A minimum resection of the bone is required, and the meniscus and the articular cartilage of the uninvolved compartment are preserved. The anterior and the posterior cruciate ligaments are retained, as are the patellofemoral and the contralateral tibiofemoral compartments. The preoperative range of movement is maintained and may be improved upon. Moreover, the morbidity of the procedure is lower, with a shorter operating time, less blood loss, a lower sepsis rate, and a shorter period of hospitalization.

The potential advantages of unicondylar knee replacement over high tibial osteotomy include shorter time to full weight-bearing ambulation, higher initial long-term success rates, and fewer complications.[10,14–16]

The status of the patellofemoral joint, the affected compartment and the opposite compartment was carefully assessed at the time of preceding arthroscopy in the majority of the cases in our series. It is important here to point out that all patients in our series had an intact anterior cruciate ligament. In patients with osteoarthritis, it is difficult to determine with absolute certainty by clinical examination whether or not the anterior cruciate ligament is intact.[2] Preoperative examination under anaesthetic and arthroscopic examination is certainly helpful in noting the stability of the anterior cruciate ligament.

In some cases, the final decision whether to perform unicompartmental or total knee replacement should be made during the operation. It is important to note that both under- and overcorrection of the varus or the valgus deformity must be avoided. An overall alignment of 3–7° of valgus has been suggested.[10,17] We are aware that some surgeons prefer a slight undercorrection of the angular deformity in order to avoid deterioration of the opposite compartment from overloading.

On review of the orthopaedic literature, a mixed opinion concerning the unicompartmental knee arthroplasty has been reported.[18-20] However, more recently, encouraging intermediate and long-term clinical results following unicondylar knee replacement have been published, with results comparable to total knee replacement and better than those for corrective osteotomy.[3,4,6,10,21,22]

Marmor[6] reported 10–13-year follow-up results on 60 consecutive unicompartmental modular knee arthroplasties and found that 70% of the knees were satisfactory and 87% had continued relief of pain. Broughton et al.[12] compared the results of unicompartmental arthroplasty to those of high tibial osteotomy, with a 5–10-year follow-up period. The unicondylar arthroplasties had 76% good results as compared to 43% for osteotomy. The disadvantages of tibial osteotomy in the elderly patients include unsatisfactory pain relief and general difficulty in remaining partial weight bearing during the prolonged rehabilitation phase. Moreover, the initial good results deteriorate with passage of time.

Summary and conclusions

We prospectively reviewed 35 patients (36 knees) who underwent unicompartmental resurfacing arthroplasty of the knee with a Robert Brigham prosthesis. The average age of the patients at the time of operation was 64.5 years (range 52–82 years) and the mean postoperative follow-up was 4.8 years (range 3–7 years). All patients had unicompartmental osteoarthritis with minimal or no degenerative changes in the contralateral compartment or the patellofemoral joint.

The patients were evaluated using the BASK (British Association for Surgery of the Knee) scoring system. Fifty-six per cent of the knees had an excellent result, 36% had a good result, 8% had a fair result and none had a poor result. Eighty-three per cent of the patients were pleased and 17% were satisfied with the outcome of surgery.

Careful patient selection and meticulous surgical technique are vital for a successful result. We recommend unicompartmental arthroplasty as a therapeutic alternative to high tibial osteotomy in sedentary, less-active patients with single-compartment osteoarthritis of the knee. The intermediate-term results are encouraging and certainly justify the continued use of the Robert Brigham prosthesis on a long-term basis.

References

1. **Kozinn SC, Scott R,** Current concepts review: Unicondylar knee arthroplasty, *J Bone Joint Surg (Am)* (1989) **71:** 145–150.
2. **Goodfellow JW, Kershaw CJ, Benson MKD'A et al.,** The Oxford knee for unicompartmental osteoarthritis: the first 103 cases, *J Bone Joint Surg (Br)* (1988) **70:** 692–701.
3. **Goodfellow JW, Tibrewal SB, Sherman KP et al.,** Unicompartmental Oxford meniscal knee arthroplasty, *J Arthroplasty* (1987) **2:** 1–9.
4. **Knutson K, Lindstrand A, Lidgren L,** Survival of knee arthroplasties: a nation-wide multicentre investigation of 8000 cases, *J Bone Joint Surg (Br)* (1986) **68:** 795–803.
5. **Mackinnon J, Young S, Baily RAJ,** The St. Georg sledge for unicompartmental replacement of the knee: a prospective study of 115 cases, *J Bone Joint Surg (Br)* (1988) **70:** 217–223.
6. **Marmor L,** Unicompartmental knee arthroplasty: ten- to 13-year follow-up study, *Clin Orthop* (1988) **226:** 14–20.
7. **Cobb AG, Kozinn SC, Scott RD,** Unicondylar or total knee replacement: the patient's preference, *J Bone Joint Surg (Br)* (1990) **72:** 166.
8. **Kozinn SC, Marx C, Scott RD,** Unicompartmental knee arthroplasty: A 4.5 to 6-year follow-up study with a metal-backed tibial component, *J Arthroplasty* (1989) **4**(suppl.): S1–S10.
9. **Marx C, Scott RD, Kozinn S,** Unicompartmental knee arthroplasty, *J Bone Joint Surg (Br)* (1989) **71:** 336.
10. **Scott RD, Santore RF,** Unicondylar unicompartmental replacement for osteoarthritis of the knee, *J Bone Joint Surg (Am)* (1981) **63:** 536–544.
11. **Scott RD,** Robert Brigham unicondylar knee surgical technique, *Techn Orthop* (1990) **5:** 15–23.
12. **Broughton NS, Newman JH, Baily RAJ,** Unicompartmental replacement and high tibial osteotomy for osteoarthritis of the knee: a comparative study after 5–10 years' follow-up, *J Bone Joint Surg (Br)* (1986) **68:** 447–452.
13. **Magnussen PA, Bartlett RJ,** Cementless PCA unicompartmental joint arthroplasty for osteoarthritis of the knee, *J Arthroplasty* (1990) **5:** 151–158.
14. **Coventry MB,** Current concepts review: Upper tibial osteotomy for osteoarthritis, *J Bone Joint Surg (Am)* (1985) **67:** 1136–1140.
15. **Insall JN, Joseph DM, Msika C,** High tibial osteotomy for varus gonarthrosis: a long-term follow-up study, *J Bone Joint Surg (Am)* (1984) **66:** 1040–1048.
16. **Pachelli AF, Kaufman EE,** Long-term results of valgus tibial osteotomy, *Orthopaedics* (1987) **10:** 1415–1418.

17. **Kennedy WR, White RP**, Unicompartmental arthroplasty of the knee: postoperative alignment and its influence on overall results, *Clin Orthop* (1987) **221**: 278–285.

18. **Insall J, Aglietti P**, A five to seven-year follow-up of unicondylar arthroplasty, *J Bone Joint Surg (Am)* (1980) **62**: 1329–1337.

19. **Laskin RS**, Unicompartmental tibiofemoral resurfacing arthroplasty, *J Bone Joint Surg (Am)* (1978) **60**: 182–185.

20. **Mallory TH, Danyi J**, Unicompartmental total knee arthroplasty: a five- to nine-year follow-up study of 42 procedures, *Clin Orthop* (1983) **175**: 135–138.

21. **Larsson S-E, Ahlgren O**, Reconstruction with endoprosthesis in gonarthrosis: a report of 111 consecutive cases operated upon from 1973 through 1977, *Clin Orthop* (1979) **145**: 126–135.

22. **Shurley TH, O'Donoghue DH, Smith WD et al.**, Unicompartmental arthroplasty of the knee: a review of three to five-year follow-up, *Clin Orthop* (1982) **164**: 236–240.

17

Total knee replacement

17.1   Total knee replacement arthroplasty

Paul M. Aichroth

Total knee replacements are doing well! This chapter outlines the general development of condylar knee replacement and Michael Freeman's 21 years' experience of this progress is unique. The various versions of condylar replacement, their clinical progress, and their long-term survival are discussed. Knee replacement arthroplasty operations are now increasing at a fast rate throughout the world after initial scepticism. It is quite clear that in well-selected patients a condylar prosthetic replacement has a higher success rate than that achieved in total hip replacement arthroplasty. The survivorship at 10 years is now 97% for the posterior stabilized condylar replacement arthroplasty.

The geometry, mechanics, component fixation and function are described by Peter Walker in this chapter. He is now Professor of Biomedical Engineering at the Institute of Orthopaedics in London. His concepts of kinematics and design have influenced many condylar prostheses and his contribution is important.

The review of posterior stabilized total condylar knee (Insall–Burstein design) was undertaken in London in several centres by a range of surgeons (both Senior Registrar and Consultant). The overall results and problems in a 'general hospital situation', with a variety of surgeons operating, is described with 86% excellent and good results and 90% patient satisfaction. The general safety, reliability and versatility of this prosthetic replacement is clearly stated.

Most arthritic knees may now be replaced with a condylar type of resurfacing. The modular prosthesis described by George Dowd and Paul W. Allen shows the importance of a modular system and the PFC knee (press fit condylar) is most versatile in this respect. There is now no reason to use the hinge design unless major areas of bone are being replaced in tumour surgery.

The important features of operative technique are stressed by the contributors in this chapter, and Carroll Laurin and David Zukor demonstrate, by beautiful diagrams and text, the adjustments to be made during the insertion of a trial prosthesis to produce perfect alignment and stability in both flexion and extension.

The Insall–Burstein Mark II prosthesis is described at an early stage. The instrumentation for this prosthetic replacement is now superb and it was felt important therefore to report the early results of the IB-II condylar arthroplasty.

The long survivorship of knee condylar prostheses has been demonstrated by various authors.[1,2] Some, however, do fail with mechanical and rarely infection problems. The revision of such prosthetic complications is described by Norman Scott of New York and Kevin Hardinge of Wrightington, England, in Chapter 18. The practical details and good results of revision are well stated.

References

1. **Vince KG, Insall JN, Kelly MA**, The total condylar prosthesis. 10–12 year results of a cemented knee replacement, *J Bone Joint Surg (Br)* (1989) **71**: 793–797.
2. **Ranawat CS, Boachie-Adjei O**, Survivorship analysis and results of total condylar knee arthroplasty; 8–11 year follow-up period. *Clin Orthop* (1988) **226**: 6–13.

17.2 Total knee replacement at the Royal London Hospital: 21 years' experience

Michael A. R. Freeman

This contribution describes the evolution of a series of prostheses, each a modification of its predecessor. The first of these was entitled the Freeman–Swanson prosthesis; the second the ICLH (Imperial College/London Hospital) prosthesis, and the third the Freeman–Samuelson prosthesis. As this contribution is written, the third version of the prosthesis has been modified in certain respects and is known as the Freeman–Samuelson Modular prosthesis.

Work began on the design of this prosthesis in 1968 in the Biomechanics Unit at the Department of Mechanical Engineering at Imperial College, then directed by Professor S.A.V. Swanson and the present author. We sought a device which would resurface the whole of the tibiofemoral joint with a polythene component articulating with a metallic femoral component. Both components were to be attached to the bone with the aid of polymethylmethacrylate cement.

It was intended that this device should be used for the severely damaged knee. To realign such knees, it was anticipated that the cruciate ligaments would have to be resected. A further reason for resecting the cruciate ligaments was to abolish the roll-back/forward that was then believed to occur between the femur and tibia during flexion and extension. By abolishing this movement it was planned to provide an area of contact between femoral and tibial components by making both surfaces curved with the same radius. Only by doing this did it seem possible, by calculation, to provide acceptably low stresses on the polyethylene surface.

The resultant prosthesis (Figure 1) was first implanted at the London Hospital in 1969. So far as the author is aware, this represented the first implantation of a total knee replacement prosthesis of the condylar kind.

The tibial component was initially attached to the tibia with the aid of two staples, whose function was simply to steady the prosthesis while the cement set. This proved an unsatisfactory method of fixation. The femoral component did not replace the whole of the patellofemoral joint and was of only one size, so that in a large knee the short anterior flange was

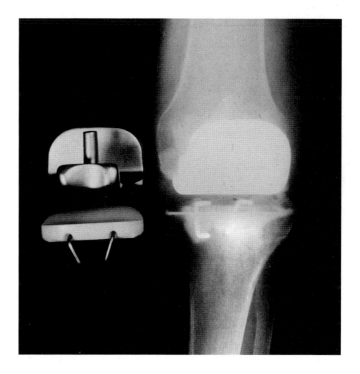

Figure 1

The Freeman–Swanson prosthesis inserted at the London Hospital in 1969.

buried within the femur. The result was to produce an irregular surface over which the patella travelled. This potential problem was addressed initially by carrying out a patellectomy. Wound healing following patellectomy proved difficult in the first 10 knees, and thereafter the patella was left in place. The posterior flange of the femoral component was not divided at the intercondylar notch, in order to increase the contact area with the polyethylene tibial component. As a consequence, it was difficult to extract cement from the posterior aspect of the knee.

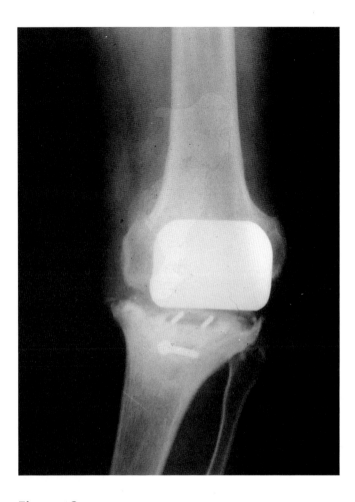

Figure 2

Tibial component loosening with downward medial migration: a common complication in the early series of prostheses.

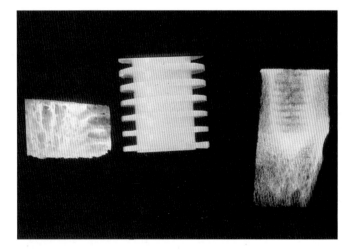

Figure 3

Macerated post-mortem specimen (left) and radiograph (right) to show interlock between a flanged polyethylene peg (centre) and the tibia.

Over the first 10 years of clinical experience at the London Hospital, a number of problems and complications were encountered which were enumerated in the *Journal of Bone and Joint Surgery* in 1978.[1] In that paper the authors concluded that the operation of condylar knee replacement was clearly possible and that the short-term results were encouraging. However, attention was drawn to four major problems: an unacceptably high incidence of tibial component migration and loosening; an unacceptable incidence of patellar pain; wear of the polyethylene component; and finally, an inability reliably to align and stabilize the knee in extension. In the following years these problems were addressed, and in doing so both the prosthesis and the operative technique were modified.

Tibial component loosening and migration

The initial tibial component was made in only one size and, therefore, was smaller than the top of the tibia in most knees. A radiograph illustrating a typical consequence is shown in Figure 2.

In 1978, Bargren et al.[2] proposed, on the basis of cadaver studies in the laboratory, that larger tibial components should be available which would cover the whole of the top of the transsected bone and that the tibia should be resected as proximally as possible since the bone was point-for-point stronger proximally than distally. Clinical studies with the modified device showed that the loosening rate was indeed reduced but that it was still not acceptable.

Because of wear produced by cement debris (a subject discussed below), the method of tibial fixation was then modified to permit fixation without cement. The resultant prosthesis was attached to the tibia by medial and lateral flanged pegs which could be expected to interlock with the cancellous bone of the tibia (Figure 3). Early experience with this device, fixed both with and without cement[3] showed an acceptable early loosening rate.

By the early 1970s, the need to develop a technique for revision arthroplasty had become evident. In many knees requiring this procedure the bone of the proximal tibia was significantly damaged. Accordingly, in 1978, an additional component was designed consisting of a horizontal metal element upon which the polyethylene tibial component was placed. The 'metal back' had a stem on its under surface. Because of the fear of infection following revision arthroplasty, it was decided not to cement the stem but instead to use cement simply to fill defects in the bone under the horizontal component. The early results of this revision technique were reported by Bertin et al.,[4] who drew attention to the fact that at a maximum follow-up of 5 years there had been no case of aseptic tibial loosening.

Thus, by 1983, four techniques of tibial fixation were available: the purely polyethylene component fixed with cement, the polyethylene component fixed without cement, and the polyethylene component placed on a metal-back and stem, the latter having cement under its horizontal surface or being entirely without cement. In the short-term it proved difficult to distinguish between the rival merits of these four possibilities, in particular because Blaha et al.[3] had demonstrated that conventional radiography was an insensitive method of measuring component migration (migration of less than 2 mm and of less than 3° could not be detected).

Fortunately, in the late 1980s, the technique of roentgen stereophotogrammetric analysis (RSA), introduced initially by Selvik, was reported in its application to the early measurement of tibial migration by Ryd.[5] We were fortunate at the Royal London Hospital in being able to work in co-operation with Ryd in Lund and in so doing were able to compare the quality of early fixation achieved by the alternatives then in clinical use. In 1990, Albrektsson et al.[6] reported that, without cement, the purely polyethylene component was statistically significantly less stable both at 1 and at 2 years than was the same component placed upon a metal-back and stem. These workers not only reported that the metal-back and stem was more stable but also that the reduction in migration concerned particularly the tendency of the component to tilt into varus/valgus and antero/ posteriorly. This finding was of particular interest because a short experience of an uncemented, metal-backed device without a stem had produced an obvious increase in early loosening as compared with the purely polyethylene device.[6] It thus appeared that rigidity made fixation worse but that this disadvantage could be more than offset by the addition of a stem.

In clinical practice, it was found that the use of the stem in primary arthroplasty carried with it a difficulty: if such a stem was too long, there was a danger that it might contact the inner cortex in short or unusually curved tibiae. If the tip of the stem contacts the inner cortex, it tends to displace the upper horizontal portion of the prosthesis and thus makes fixation worse. Clinical experience suggested that most tibiae could be accommodated by an 80-mm stem but that some tibiae required a 50-mm stem. Two investigations were therefore carried out. Firstly, the 80-mm stem fixed without cement was evaluated by RSA and compared with the same device having cement under the horizontal surface.[7] This study demonstrated that the 80-mm stem was on average slightly more stable than the earlier 110-mm stem used by Albrektsson et al., but not to a statistically significant degree. On the other hand, the addition of cement produced a statistically significant

Table 1 Tibial component fixation: early migration measured by RSA vs late revision rate.

Prosthesis and fixation	MTPM (mm) at 1 year	Revision rate
Polyethylene press fit	2.0	17% at 10 years
Metal-back 110 mm plus stem	1.5	10% at 8 years
Press fit 80 mm	1.3	
Metal-back plus stem proximal cement	0.5	0% at 10 years

improvement in early migration, mean total point motion (MTPM) now falling to 0.5 mm at the end of the first postoperative year. This figure represents the lowest value for early tibial MTPM so far recorded in the literature. Secondly, a modular version of the tibial component (the prosthesis being known as the Freeman–Samuelson modular prosthesis) was introduced to enable the surgeon to adjust the length of the stem to suit the particular tibia under operation.[6]

Although demonstrating that certain configurations were more stable in the first year or two postoperatively, RSA is open to the criticism that it may have no relevance to the long-term failure rate. It is interesting, therefore, to note that studies at the Royal London Hospital of the long-term failure rate of the various configurations studied by RSA produce a ranking order identical to that of their stability at 1 year (Table 1).[18]

In summary, it would appear that a tibial component placed as proximally as possible, covering the whole of the tibia and having a metal-back, a medial and lateral peg and a central stem 50–80 mm in length can be securely fixed to the proximal tibia with the aid of cement placed only under the horizontal surface. Cement used in this way produces no significant invasion of the bone and appears to have no obvious disadvantages. Having said that, the author is at present evaluating a cementless device having exactly the same configuration but with hydroxyapatite on the undersurface of the metal-back in the hope that this may provide even lower early migration rates.

Patellar pain and the evolution of the femoral component

Anterior pain was a major problem in the early years and was attributed to the fact that the unreplaced patella had to make its way across an uneven, bony and metallic surface. In 1973, the posterior surface of the patella was replaced and the anterior flange of the femoral component was lengthened. The latter step

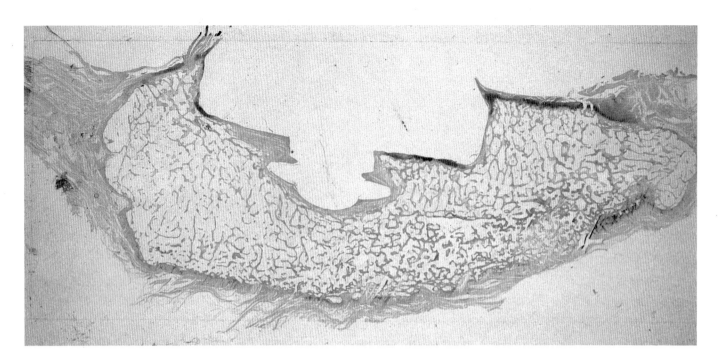

Figure 4

The histological appearances of the patella beneath a press-fit polyethylene component. Note the presence of chondroid metaplasia where the interface is loaded in compression.

necessitated the introduction of femoral components of varying anteroposterior size.

Initially it was feared that patellar component loosening might represent a major hazard and, therefore, an attempt was made to design a relatively unconstrained patellofemoral joint so as to reduce the shear stresses that might otherwise have been generated at the patellar bone–prosthesis interface. The resultant prosthesis had a flat anterior flange in the mediolateral direction and was known as the 'ICLH'. Unfortunately, lack of constraint at the patellofemoral joint, although it was indeed associated with a low incidence of component loosening, was also associated with an unacceptable incidence of lateral patellar subluxation.[8] However, in patellae in which tracking was satisfactory, anterior knee pain almost disappeared.[9]

In view of these findings, it was decided to provide the anterior part of the femoral surface with a deep groove having a single radius as viewed from the side. The patellar component was made of polyethylene and was saddle-shaped to provide, firstly, an area contact (and thus low stresses) when articulating with the femoral component and, secondly, a significant area laterally to resist lateral patellar dislocation. The design of this part of the prosthesis was particularly attri-

butable to the work of Dr K.N. Samuelson. The patellar component could be fixed with or without cement.

A review of the results of this mode of reconstruction was reported by Elias et al.[10] A summary of their findings is contained in Table 2, from which it can be seen that the incidence of patellofemoral complications has now fallen to an acceptable level. We have measured, in a small unpublished series, the rate of forward migration of the patellar component through the patella when fixed without cement over the course of 7 years. The average migration rate was found to be 0.1 mm per year.

Table 2 Patellar complications after patellar replacement: 122 uncemented and 18 cemented prostheses.[a]

Anterior pain requiring analgesia	1
Fracture	
Intra-operative	2
Postoperative	2
Subluxation	2
Dislocation	0
Aseptic loosening	0

[a]Inserted 1980–1987; average follow-up 5 years.

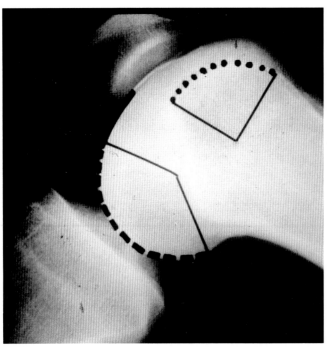

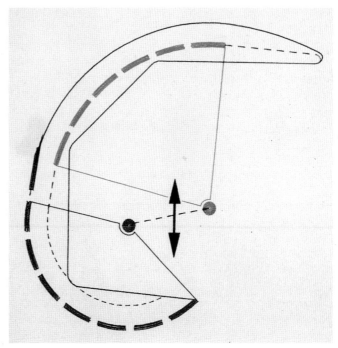

a   b

Figure 5

(a) A lateral radiograph of the knee and (b) a diagram of the prosthesis to show the circular patella and tibial surfaces of the femur.

Histological studies of well-functioning knees retrieved at postmortem have shown that the patellar component is contained in a fibrous tissue bed which undergoes chondroid metaplasia where it is loaded in compression (Figure 4). Since the patellar component is recessed into the patella, rather than being placed on its transsected surface, the peripheral portion of the original articular surface of the patella also carries load. This surface also becomes covered with soft tissue which, as in the bed of the prosthesis itself, undergoes chondroid metaplasia.

Certain features of the patellofemoral reconstruction are of importance. Firstly, it has been reported[11] that in the natural knee exhibiting recurrent patellar subluxation, the anatomical defect is in the proximal extremity of the lateral prominence of the femoral condyle so that patellar maltracking starts between 0° and 10°. In view of this, it seems appropriate to provide the femoral component with an anterior flange of sufficient height to engage the patella throughout its range of extension.

Secondly, the natural femoral surface around which the patella tracks is circular as viewed from the side (Figure 5). In a similar way the patellar articular surface of the femoral prosthesis should be circular to provide smooth tracking for the patella throughout

the range of flexion (Figure 5).[10] It is important that the patellar component should be adequately recessed into the bone and that the patellar articular surface of the femur should be anatomically placed anterodistally. If the femoral component is displaced forwards or the patella is made too thick by replacement, the extensor mechanism is rendered unduly tense as the knee flexes. This may contribute to 'pull-off' lateral patellar fractures, to limitation of flexion, and perhaps to anterior pain.

With regard to its tibial surface, the essential feature of the femoral component is that it has a single radius articulating with a tibial trough of the same radius. Two things follow from this geometry. Firstly, all the femoral components may be interchanged with all the tibial components and, secondly, the stresses on the polyethylene may be reduced to acceptable levels. Rostocker and Gallante[12] have argued on the basis of experimental data that polythene stresses should not rise appreciably above 1000 lb/in². For the medium size of Freeman/Samuelson prosthesis, this stress is produced by the application of three times the bodyweight using the existing conforming geometry. Thus, for relatively flat tibial components (having a larger radius of curvature than their matching femur), the operating stresses must be above the levels recommended by Rostocker and Gallante.

A consequence of a fully conforming tibiofemoral joint which is not at the same time meniscal is that anteroposterior translation of the femur on the tibia during flexion and extension cannot occur. Neither can axial tibial rotation. Space does not allow these topics to be entered into in detail here, but two observations may be made. Firstly, it is the author's view that the amount of obligatory posterior translation occurring during flexion of the femur (at least on the medial side) is negligible and can certainly be neglected if the anterior cruciate ligament (ACL) is divided. Translation does indeed occur in the lateral compartment but this is simply a manifestation of axial tibial rotation. This subject has been discussed in the context of posterior cruciate resection by the author elsewhere.[13] Secondly, it is not clear to the author that there is any particular disadvantage in providing some rotational constraint within the prosthesis as is done by a roller-in-trough geometry. Certainly, there does not appear to be a functional penalty: patients do not complain that their tibia will not rotate axially. Rotational component migration can be demonstrated by RSA[14] but actual rotational loosening has, so far as the author is aware, never been demonstrated for any prosthesis, although it has always been asserted that a rotationally constrained bearing would fail in this way. Paradoxically, the amount of rotational migration occurring in Ryd's studies of various prostheses was greater in unconstrained implants than in constrained ones.[5] This may perhaps be because in constrained devices rotation is actually prevented by soft-tissue adhesions, whereas in the unconstrained device rotation does occur but in so doing friction plus ploughing generates a significant torque on the tibial components.

When it is stated that the roller-in-trough geometry is relatively constrained, it is important to appreciate that the degree of constraint which it provides has been studied experimentally in the cadaver.[2] If the femoral roller is articulated with the tibial trough and rotated while an axial compressive load of three times the body weight is applied, the femur will eventually 'climb' out of the tibial trough, transmitting to the latter a certain torque which reaches a maximum (in much the same way as would that transmitted by a torque wrench) the magnitude of which is dependent on the depth of the trough. The rotational torque generated by the Freeman–Samuelson geometry can easily be resisted (in the cadaver) by a number of methods of tibial fixation.[2] Of course, in clinical practice the tendency of the femoral component to rotate and climb is resisted not simply by the tibiofemoral geometry but mainly by the tibiofemoral soft tissues, thus further reducing the torque which is actually transmitted to the tibial component interface.

Isolated femoral component loosening has not represented a major problem.[15] This is presumably because (i) the femoral component is of a shape which makes it intrinsically more stable on the lower femur than is the tibial component on the proximal tibia, and (ii) the bone of the femur is stronger point-for-point than that of the tibia. We have not demonstrated statistically that cement improves femoral fixation, although there has been a trend in this direction (a recent unpublished review showing an incidence of femoral loosening of 0 out of 225 in cemented devices as against 3 out of 180 uncemented pressfits).

Wear

The third problem identified in 1978[1] was that of wear of the tibial component produced by impacted fragments of polymethylmethacrylate. Initially, the posterior flange of the femoral component was not split centrally, so as to increase the tibiofemoral contact area. This made it difficult to extract excess cement from the back of the tibial and femoral components. Furthermore, it was not appreciated that the tibia could be fully subluxed forwards when the tibial component was implanted, a feature of modern techniques which makes the extraction of posterior cement more reliable. To facilitate the removal of posterior cement, we followed Insall and Walker in dividing the posterior flange of the femoral component so that the posterior compartment could be reached through the intercondylar notch, the posterior cruciate ligament having been removed. A disadvantage of this step was that it reduced the contact area and thus increased the contact stresses in the tibiofemoral joint. Two other features aimed at reducing wear have already been mentioned. Firstly, the component was fixed without the use of cement with the object of eliminating cement debris as an abrasive. Secondly, a conforming tibiofemoral articulation has been used from the outset to reduce the contact stresses on the polyethylene, a feature peculiar to this series of prostheses and to implants of the meniscal type.

A tibial component having been fixed without cement retrieved at post-mortem 11 years postoperatively is shown in Figure 6. In this figure, the machining marks on the original polythene surface can be seen and the imprint made by the femoral component is evident. This imprint is partly due to creep and partly due to wear. Were this the only pattern to be seen, the wear problem might be viewed with some equanimity. Unfortunately, some polyethylene components demonstrate subsurface fatigue leading to the separation of flakes of polyethylene from the articular surface (Figure 7). At the present time, it is not clear why there is this variation in the behaviour of an

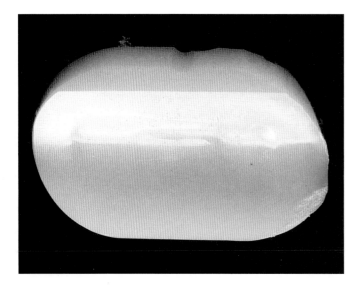

Figure 6

A tibial component retrieved at post-mortem examination 11 years postoperatively showing polishing but no other material wear.

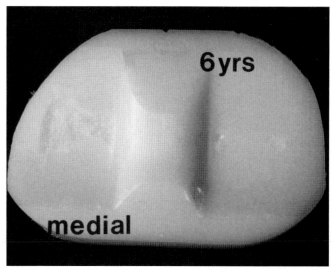

Figure 7

A second polyethylene tibial component removed 6 years after operation, at revision for infection showing significant wear in the medial compartment.

apparently similar articulation. It is, however, worth noting that similar variation, also unexplained, occurs with regard to wear at the acetabulum.

In the early 1980s, Tuke (confirmed by McKellop et al.[16]) showed that Delrin could be used as a bearing material against polyethylene. Polyethylene wear against Delrin was 62% less than against CoCr and the combined wear rates of the two materials was 10% less. In view of this, an experimental series of Freeman–Samuelson prostheses were implanted in 1981 and 1982 in which the femoral component was made of Delrin and not CoCr (Figure 8). To date, one post-mortem specimen has been retrieved at 8 years: no visible wear was present. These findings are clearly encouraging but await further study and publication.

One further aspect of wear should be considered: the problem of wear of a polyethylene surface when it is articulating against bone at the fixation surface. In practice wear of this kind is not a clinical problem unless (1) the component loosens, and (2) the interface is under a compressive load sufficient to crush the soft tissue which otherwise separates polyethylene from bone. This combination of loosening and direct polyethylene–bone contact certainly produces unacceptable polyethylene abrasion (and it was partly for this reason that a metal-back was placed on the undersurface of the tibial component). In contrast to the tibial component, this problem has never been seen at the patella (Figure 4) where fixation with an uncemented, purely polyethylene device has proved satisfactory (Table 2). (It is interesting to note that

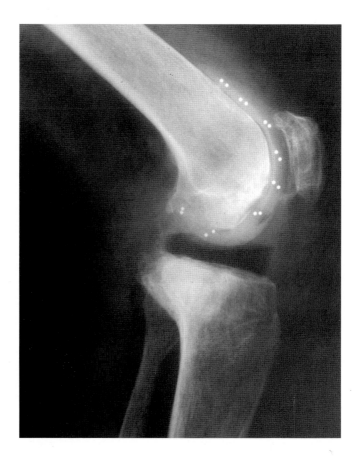

Figure 8

The postoperative radiograph of a knee in which the femoral component was made of Delrin.

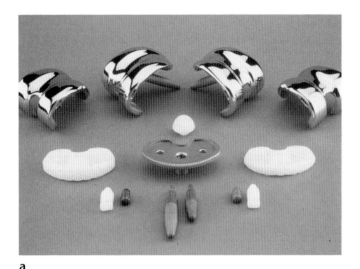

a

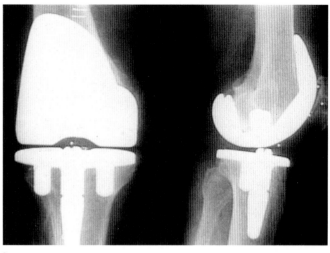

b

Figure 9

(a) The Freeman–Samuelson modular prosthesis showing the separated components and (b) a postoperative radiograph.

the purely polyethylene device appears to have functioned better than similar metal-backed devices: perhaps the adverse effect of rigidity noted at the tibia is equally applicable to the patella.)

The appearance of the prosthesis as it had evolved in the light of these findings by 1990 is shown in Figure 9.

The surgical technique

The discussion to this point has concerned itself with the evolution of the prosthesis. It should be emphasized, however, that the results of knee arthroplasty today do not depend on the remaining small differences between one condylar prosthesis and another. On the contrary, they do depend, critically, upon the quality of the surgical technique. This in its turn is dependent on the surgeon and upon the concepts and instruments being used. Unfortunately, space does not allow a detailed description of the evolution and present concepts underlying the surgical technique, which are fully dealt with elsewhere (manufacturer's literature). Certain points are, however, worth making in summary form.

Firstly, it is essential that the knee should be appropriately aligned and stabilized in extension: failure to do this reliably was an important cause of early failure.[1] The ideal alignment should result in a resultant load acting through the centre of the tibial component. This in turn means that the knee should be aligned in about 7° of valgus (i.e. 7±3° valgus) or, to put the same anatomical fact another way, with the centres of the hip, knee and ankle in straight alignment. To achieve this in a knee with preoperative fixed varus or valgus deformity, it is necessary to understand how to release the soft-tissue contractures which produce the deformity. At the start of the author's experience in 1969, the concept of medial and lateral soft-tissue release procedures was not understood and it has been a critical part of the evolution of knee arthroplasty in the ensuing 21 years that now the required techniques are fully appreciated.

Not only must the soft tissues be released to produce the requisite alignment, but at the same time they must be placed under balanced and appropriate tension in extension so as to result in a stable knee. In the early days of unlinked condylar arthroplasty, it was thought to be impossible to achieve this, and thus linkages of various kinds were proposed. It is now known that, by appropriately adjusting the relationship between the thickness of the prosthesis and the separation of the proximal tibial and distal femoral osteotomies, the knee can be satisfactorily stabilized. This concept was first introduced in the Freeman–Swanson arthroplasty in the early 1970s. The results were reported in 1978,[1] the first report so far as the author is aware of soft-tissue release applied to total knee arthroplasty (Figure 10).

Stability at 90° flexion has not been as widely discussed as stability in extension. However, the knee must be stabilized in this (and intermediate) positions

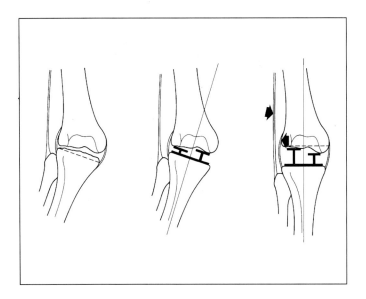

Figure 10

A semidiagrammatic representation of the concept of a soft-tissue release procedure (here shown for a valgus deformity) and the use of the 'tensor' (reproduced with the kind permission of the Editor of the *Journal of Bone and Joint Surgery (Br)* (1978) **60**: 3).

if it is to function satisfactorily, particularly in activities such as stairclimbing. It is of course possible to rely on both the cruciate ligaments to provide stability. However, if the tibial component has a stem, the ACL must be resected (and of course it is often absent). With the author's present prosthesis, the PCL can be left in place but no special advantage for this has as yet been demonstrated in the author's view.[13] If one or both of the cruciate ligaments are to be resected, anteroposterior stability depends upon the relationship between the height of the gap between the posterior femoral osteotomy and the proximal tibial osteotomy on the one hand and the thickness of the prosthesis on the other. If the prosthesis is thicker than the gap, the knee will not flex. If the prosthesis is thinner than the gap, the femoral roller can move over the anterior (or rarely the posterior) lip of the tibial component to produce an unstable knee. Thus, the requirement is to produce an appropriate relationship between the thickness of the prosthesis and the gap both in flexion and in extension and at the same time correctly to align the knee in extension.

As has been mentioned, in 1978 the author described an instrument, the tensor, with which these objectives could be achieved in extension.[1] The instrument has since been modified to enable the flexion objective to be met with the same device as follows. The posterior femur and proximal tibia are resected. The tensor is introduced into the gap in flexion and the femur is tensed away from the tibia. The instrument automatically measures the height of the gap.

The knee is now extended and the two compartments (medial and lateral) are tensed open separately (accompanied by whatever soft-tissue release is needed) until the knee is both stable and correctly aligned. The tensor now transfers the gap measured in flexion into the extended knee, referencing from the already cut tibia to indicate the correct level and valgus/varus attitude of distal femoral section. This technique can be used with both extramedullary or intramedullary alignment. The difference between these two is a matter of convenience provided that the hip is found radiologically if extramedullary alignment is used. If intramedullary alignment is to be accurate, the femoral shaft must be neither obstructed nor deformed.

Anteriorly, the femur must be resected so as to enable the anterior flange of the femoral component to be placed on the anterior femoral cortex. Posteriorly, the femur must be resected so that the resected femur will fit one of the available sizes of femoral component.

The proximal tibia should be resected perpendicular to the long axis of the tibia, and for this an extramedullary technique is the author's preference. Resection should be as high as practicable provided that an adequate thickness of polythene can be inserted.

In view of these considerations the sequence of bone resections preferred by the author is as follows.

1. The anterior femur is cut flush with the anterior cortex.
2. The posterior cortex is cut so as to provide an adequate posterior fixation surface to fit one of the three sizes of femur.
3. The proximal tibia is cut as high as possible and perpendicular to the long axis of the bone.
4. The tensor is used to determine what thickness of prosthesis will be appropriate, to control the alignment of the knee in extension, and to determine the valgus/varus attitude and proximal/distal position of the distal femoral cut.
5. The distal femur is then cut perpendicular to the anterior femoral osteotomy as viewed from the side.
6. Finally, a single chamfer cut is made anterodistally to fit the femoral component. It is important that this cut be sufficiently deep to enable the patella to track anatomically.
7. The patella is drilled, not transected, to receive a prosthesis. The femur and tibia are similarly drilled to receive fixation pegs and stems.

The results

The results of condylar arthroplasty in general are well known and are no different (so far as the author is aware) using the author's prosthesis and techniques from those achieved with other well-known devices. In round terms, 95% of replaced knees should not require analgesia postoperatively.[17] Two or three percent of patients will require analgesia for undetermined reasons. The average range of motion obtained is about 110° but this depends mainly upon the preoperative arc. The remainder will develop painful aseptic loosening in the first 10 years.

On average, knees starting with a preoperative arc of less than 90° will gain 30° with a maximum in the author's experience (operating on a knee preoperatively stiff) of 110°. (At operation the tibiofemoral joint will always flex fully: it is indeed impossible to implant the tibial component unless this is done. The postoperative arc thus depends upon the elasticity of the extensor mechanism and the patellofemoral reconstruction.)

Patients are able to walk essentially unlimited distances postoperatively, although it is the author's view that they should be encouraged to conserve their prosthesis mechanically because of the long-term danger of wear. Unless patients are over 70 years of age or have rheumatoid arthritis, virtually all can walk 30 minutes or more at any one time and can join in such activities as golf (although again it is probably wise to recommend the avoidance of this activity postoperatively). They should be able to rise from a chair without the use of their hands and ascend and descend stairs of ordinary steepness, again without using their hands and in a natural fashion.

Revision for aseptic loosening is now a routine procedure using techniques referred to briefly above. The early results using these techniques were reported by Bertin et al.[4] A recent review[18] of 99 consecutive revisions for aseptic loosening with a maximum follow-up of 9 years revealed no case of recurrent loosening and only one re-revision for infection.

Infection remains an important hazard. We have employed single-stage revision using gentamicin-impregnated Palacos cement as a fixative, for infected loose prostheses. Debridement and antibiotics may be tried initially for well-fixed implants.[19] On a recent study of 18 loose infected prostheses, 16 appear to have been cured.[20] Two other cases developed further infections but it was felt that these did not represent true recurrence (one was secondary to an infected leg ulcer and one occurred in an immunosuppressed patient who suffered multiple infections elsewhere).

Publications

During the past 21 years, knee replacement at the Royal London Hospital has been advanced by the work of many surgeons from the UK and overseas. Their publications are listed at the end of this contribution.

Conclusion

Knee replacement of the condylar variety started at the London Hospital 21 years ago and has since undergone a process of continuous evolution. The operation can now be said to have come of age. The essential features of the operative technique and (less importantly) of the prosthesis are clear. The operation appears to be as reliable as hip replacement and provides results of a similar symptomatic kind at a slightly lower functional level. Revision is possible in the event of aseptic loosening or in the event of sepsis. Today, therefore, it is possible to say that any knee can if necessary be replaced. Fortunately, most knees do not need it.

References

1. Freeman MAR, Todd RC, Bamert P et al., ICLH arthroplasty of the knee: 1968–1977, *J Bone Joint Surg (Br)* (1978) **60**: 339–344.
2. Bargren JH, Day WH, Freeman MAR et al., Mechanical tests on the tibial components of non-hinged knee prostheses, *J Bone Joint Surg (Br)* (1978) **60**: 256–261.
3. Blaha JD, Insler HP, Freeman MAR et al., The fixation of a proximal tibial polyethylene prosthesis without cement, *J Bone Joint Surg (Br)* (1982) **64**: 326–335.
4. Bertin KC, Freeman MAR, Samuelson KM et al., Stemmed revision arthroplasty for aseptic loosening of total knee replacement, *J Bone Joint Surg (Br)* (1985) **67**: 242–248.
5. Ryd L, Micromotion in knee arthroplasty. A Roentgen stereophotogrammetric analysis of tibial component fixation, *Acta Orthop Scand* (1986) suppl. 220: 857.
6. Albrektsson BEJ, Ryd L, Carlsson LV et al., The effect of a stem on the tibial component of knee arthroplasty: A Roentgen stereophotogrammetric study of uncemented tibial components in the Freeman–Samuelson knee arthroplasty, *J Bone Joint Surg (Br)* (1990) **72**: 252–258.
7. Albrektsson BEJ, Freeman MAR, Carlsson LV et al., Proximally cemented versus uncemented Freeman–Samuelson knee arthroplasty: A prospective randomised study, *J Bone Joint Surg (Br)* (1992) **74**: 233–238.
8. Levai J-P, Freeman MAR, Les complications patellaires de la prosthese du genou ICLH, *Rev de Chir Orthop* (1984) **70**: 41.
9. Levai J-P, McLeod HC, Freeman MAR, Why not resurface the patella? *J Bone Joint Surg (Br)* (1983) **65**: 448–451.
10. Elias SG, Freeman MAR, Gokcay EI, A correlative study of the geometry and anatomy of the distal femur, *Clin Orthop* (1990) **260**: 98–103.
11. Kujala UN, Osterman K, Kormano M et al., Patellofemoral relationships in recurrent patellar dislocation, *J Bone Joint Surg (Br)* (1989) **71**: 788–792.
12. Rostocker W, Gallante JO, Contact pressure dependence of wear rates of ultra high molecular weight polyethylene, *J Biomed Mater Res* (1979) **13**: 957–964.
13. Freeman MAR, Railton GT, The current status of total replacement of the knee with special reference to prostheses of the condylar variety, *Current trends in orthopaedic surgery*, ed Galasko CSB, Noble J (Manchester University Press, 1988) 221.
14. Freeman MAR, Samuelson KM, Elias SG et al., The patellofemoral joint in total knee prostheses: Design considerations, *J Arthroplasty* (1989) **4**(suppl.): S69–S74.
15. Colley J, Cameron HU, Freeman MAR et al., Loosening of the femoral component in surface replacement of the knee, *Arch Orthop Traum Surg* (1978) **92**: 31–34.

16. McKellop H, Hossenian A, Tuke M et al., Superior wear properties of an all-polymer hip prosthesis, *Trans Orthop Res Soc* (1985) **10**: 322.

17. Brach Del Prever EM, MacPherson IS, Freeman MAR et al., Esperienza clinica con la protesi di ginocchio Freeman–Samuelson (1980–1985) *G Ital Ortop Traumatol* (1988) **XIII**(4): 423.

18. Freeman MAR, Rimmer M, Grewat R, Early migration of prostheses related to long-term survivorship: Comparison of tibial components in knee replacement, *J Bone Joint Surg (Br)* (1992) **74**: 239–242.

19. Freeman MAR, Sudlow RA, Casewell MW et al., The management of infected total knee replacements, *J Bone Joint Surg (Br)* (1985) **67**: 764–768.

20. Freeman MAR, Goksan SB, One-stage reimplantation for infected total knee arthroplasty, *J Bone Joint Surg (Br)* (1992) **74**: 78–82.

Bibliography

Freeman MAR, Plastics in orthopaedics, *Br J Hosp Med* (1969) **2**(5): 1007.

Freeman MAR, Swanson SAV, Heath JC, The production characterization and biological significance of the wear particles produced in vitro from cobalt–chromium–molybdenum total joint replacement prostheses, *Br J Surg* (1969) **56**: 701.

Heath JC, Freeman MAR, Swanson SAV, Carcinogenic properties of wear particles from prostheses made in cobalt–chromium alloy, *Lancet* (1971) **7699**: 564–566.

Freeman MAR, Swanson SAV, Zahir A, Total replacement of knee using metal/polyethylene two-part prosthesis, *Proc R Soc Med* (1972) **65**: 374.

Swanson SAV, Freeman MAR, A new prosthesis for the total replacement of the knee, *Acta Orthop Belg* (1972) **38**(suppl 1): 55–62.

Freeman MAR, Swanson SAV, Total prosthetic replacement of the knee, *SICOT 12 Abstracta Part II* (1972): 574.

Freeman MAR, Swanson SAV, Total prosthetic replacement of the knee, *J Bone Joint Surg (Br)* (1972) **54**: 170.

Freeman MAR, Bio-engineering in joints with special reference to the hip and knee (summary), *Proc R Soc Med* (1972) **65**: 1120–1121.

Freeman MAR, Swanson SAV, Todd RC, Total replacement of the knee: Design considerations and early clinical results, *Acta Orthop Belg* (1973) **39**: 181–202.

Swanson SAV, Freeman MAR, Heath JC, Laboratory tests on total joint replacement prostheses, *J Bone Joint Surg (Br)* (1973) **55**: 759–773.

Freeman MAR, Swanson SAV, Todd RC, Total replacement of the knee using the Freeman–Swanson knee prosthesis, *Clin Orthop* (1973) **94**: 153–170.

Freeman MAR, Swanson SAV, Heath JC, Biological properties of the wear particles generated by all cobalt–chrome total joint replacement prostheses. *Arthroplasty of the hip*, ed Chapchal G (Stuttgart: George Thieme Verlag, 1973) 8.

Swanson SAV, Freeman MAR, A new approach to the total replacement of the knee joint, *Digest, 10th International Conference on Medical and Biological Engineering, Dresden* (1973) 125.

Freeman MAR, Todd RC, Swanson SAV, The results of 100 Freeman–Swanson arthroplasties, *International Congress on the Knee Joint, Rotterdam*, 15 September, 1973.

Swanson SAV, Freeman MAR, Heath JC, Some biological properties of the wear particles generated by all cobalt–chrome total joint replacement prostheses, *J Bone Joint Surg (Br)* (1973) **55**: 424.

Andersson GBJ, Jessop J, Freeman MAR et al., MacIntosh arthroplasty in rheumatoid arthritis, *Acta Orthop Scand* (1974) **45**: 245–259.

Freeman MAR, Total replacement of the knee, *Orthop Rev* (1974) **III**: 21.

Freeman MAR, The problems and hazards of replacement of the knee. *J Bone Joint Surg (Am)* (1974) **56**: 1308 (Summary of communication).

Evans EM, Freeman MAR, Miller AJ et al., Metal sensitivity as a cause of bone necrosis and loosening of the prosthesis in total joint replacement, *J Bone Joint Surg (Br)* (1974) **56**: 626–642.

Freeman MAR, General considerations in the design of prostheses for the total replacement of joints, *Recent advances in orthopaedics* No. 2, ed McKibbin B (Edinburgh: Churchill Livingstone, 1975) 93–114.

Freeman MAR, Swanson SAV, Todd RC, Replacement of the knee with the Freeman–Swanson prosthesis: Current developments and the results of a clinical trial with a standard prosthesis, *Proceedings of the Institution of Mechanical Engineers Conference on Total Knee Replacement, September 1974* (1975) p 102.

Vernon-Roberts B, Freeman MAR, Morphological and analytical studies of the tissues adjacent to joint prostheses: Investigations into the causes of loosening of prostheses, *Advances in artificial hip and knee joint technology*, ed Schaldach M, Hohmann D (Berlin: Springer-Verlag, 1976) 148–186.

Freeman MAR, Some disadvantages of cemented intramedullary stem fixation and their remedies, *Advances in artificial hip and knee joint technology*, ed Schaldach M, Hohmann D (Berlin: Springer-Verlag, 1976) 127–137.

Freeman MAR, Unlinked surface replacement, *Proc R Soc Lond* (1976) **B192**: 199.

Freeman MAR, Current state of total joint replacement, *Br Med J* (1976) **2**: 1301–1304.

Bargren JH, Freeman MAR, Swanson SAV et al., ICLH (Freeman/Swanson) arthroplasty in the treatment of arthritic knee: A 2 to 4-year review, *Clin Orthop* (1976) **120**: 65–75.

Sculco TP, Freeman MAR, Todd RC, I.C.L.H. total knee arthroplasty in severely damaged knees, *J Bone Joint Surg (Am)* (1976) **58**: 730.

Freeman MAR, Wear and tissue reaction in failed knee arthroplasty (Discussion), *J Bone Joint Surg (Br)* (1976) **58**: 366–367.

Freeman MAR, Sculco TP, Todd RC, Replacement of the severely damaged arthritic knee by the ICLH (Freeman–Swanson) arthroplasty, *J Bone Joint Surg (Br)* (1977) **59**: 64–71.

Freeman MAR, Bargren J, Miller I, A comparison of osteotomy and joint replacement in the surgical treatment of the arthritic knee, *Arch Orthop Unfall-Chir* (1977) **88**: 7–18.

Vernon-Roberts B, Freeman MAR, The tissue response to total joint replacement prostheses. *The scientific basis of joint replacement*, ed Swanson SAV, Freeman MAR (Tunbridge Wells: Pitman Medical, 1977) 86–129.

Freeman MAR, A three to five years' follow-up of the Freeman–Swanson replacement arthroplasty of the knee, *J Bone Joint Surg (Br)* (1977) **59**: 119.

Freeman MAR, Todd RC, Cundy AD, A technique for recording the results of knee surgery, *Clin Orthop* (1977) **128**: 216–221.

Freeman MAR, Todd RC, Cundy AD, The presentation of the results of knee surgery, *Clin Orthop* (1977) **128**: 222–227.

Freeman MAR, Insall JN, Besser W et al., Excision of the cruciate ligaments in total knee replacement, *Clin Orthop* (1977) **126**: 209–212.

Freeman MAR, Intramedullare Schaftverankerung, ihre Nachteile und deren Vermeidung (Some disadvantages of cemented intramedullary stem fixation and their remedies), *Orthopäde* (1978) **7**: 55.

Bargren JH, Day WH, Freeman MAR et al., Mechanical properties of four non-hinged knee prostheses, *Trans Orthop Res Soc* (1978) **3**: 155.

Revell PA, Weightman B, Freeman MAR et al., The production and biology of polyethylene wear debris, *Arch Orthop Traum Surg* (1978) **91**: 167–181.

Freeman MAR, Hammer A, Patellar fracture after replacement of the tibio-femoral joint with the ICLH prosthesis, *Arch Orthop Traum Surg* (1978) **92**: 63–67.

Aichroth P, Freeman MAR, Smillie IS et al., A knee function assessment chart, *J Bone Joint Surg (Br)* (1978) **60**: 308–309.

Moreland JR, Thomas RJ, Freeman MAR, ICLH replacement of the knee: 1977 and 1978, *Clin Orthop* (1979) **145:** 47–59.

Day WH, Brown GC, Revell PA et al., A method for obtaining immediate direct fixation of polyethylene to cancellous bone, *Proc Orthop Res Soc* (1979) **4:** 223.

Samuelson KM, Freeman MAR, Day WH, Salvage of failed total knee replacements: Is a hinge necessary? *Proc Orthop Res Soc* (1979) **4:** 232.

Freeman MAR (ed), *Arthritis of the knee* (Berlin: Springer-Verlag, 1980).

Freeman MAR, ICLH arthroplasty of the knee joint, *Total knee replacement*, ed Savastano AA (New York: Appleton-Century-Crofts, 1980).

Freeman MAR, Blaha JD, Insler HP, Replacement of the knee in rheumatoid arthritis using the ICLH prosthesis, *Med Orthop Tech* (1980) **100:** 124.

O'Riordan SM, Freeman MAR, Salvage of the failed ICLH knee replacement, Communication to the European Rheumatoid Arthritis Surgical Research Society, Vienna (1980).

Freeman MAR, The surgical anatomy and pathology of the arthritic knee, *Arthritis of the knee*, ed Freeman MAR (Berlin: Springer-Verlag, 1980) 31.

Todd RC, Freeman MAR, Gschwend N, Clinical assessment, *Arthritis of the knee*, ed Freeman MAR (Berlin: Springer-Verlag, 1980) 57–76.

Freeman MAR, Charnley J, Arthrodesis, *Arthritis of the knee*, ed Freeman MAR (Berlin: Springer-Verlag, 1980) 142–147.

Freeman MAR, Insall J, Tibio-femoral replacement using two unlinked components and cruciate resection (The ICLH and total condylar prostheses), *Arthritis of the knee*, ed Freeman MAR (Berlin: Springer-Verlag, 1980) 254.

Freeman MAR, Blaha JD, Insler HP, Replacement of the knee in rheumatoid arthritis using the Imperial College London Hospital (ICLH) prosthesis, *Reconstruct Surg Traumatol* (1981) **18:** 147.

Freeman MAR, Reconstructive surgery in arthritis, *Current surgical practice*, ed Hadfield J, Hobsley M (Maidenhead: Edward Arnold, 1981) **3:** 211.

Freeman MAR, Trends in arthroplasty of the knee, *Clinical trends in orthopaedics* (New York: Thieme-Stratton Inc, 1982) **30:** 262.

Freeman MAR, Blaha JD, Bradley GW et al., Cementless fixation of the ICLH tibial component, *Orthop Clin North Am* (1982) **13:** 141–154.

Freeman MAR, Bradley GW, Revell PA, Observations upon the interface between bone and polymethylmethacrylate cement, *J Bone Joint Surg (Br)* (1982) **64:** 489–493.

Freeman MAR, Bradley GW, Blaha JD et al., Cementless fixation of the tibial component for the ICLH knee, *J R Soc Med* (1982) **75:** 418–424.

Bargren JH, Blaha JD, Freeman MAR, Alignment in total knee arthroplasty: correlated biomechanical and clinical observations, *Clin Orthop* (1983) **173:** 178–183.

Freeman MAR, McLeod HC, Levai J-P, Cementless fixation of prosthetic components in total arthroplasty of the knee and hip, *Clin Orthop* (1983) **176:** 88–94.

Freeman MAR, Levai J-P, Replacement of the knee in rheumatoid arthritis using the Imperial College London Hospital (ICLH) prosthesis, 1977–1979, *Ann Acad Med Singapore* (1983) **12:** 213.

Freeman MAR, McLeod HC, Revell PA, Bone ingrowth and graft incorporation in polyethylene pegs in man, *Proc Orthop Res Soc* (1983) **8:** 133.

Levai J-P, Freeman MAR, La prothese du genou ICLH dans la polyarthrite rheumatoide: Résultats et complications, *Rev Chir Orthop* (1984) 70. SOFCOT, reunion annuelle, November 1983.

Levack B, De Alencar PGC, Freeman MAR, The Freeman–Samuelson knee: evolution and current results, *Acta Orthop Belg* (1985) **51:** 478–497.

Freeman MAR, Samuelson KM, Bertin KC, Freeman–Samuelson total arthroplasty of the knee, *Clin Orthop* (1985) **192:** 46–58.

Freeman MAR, Knee flexion: The cruciate ligaments and posterior stability in the flexed knee, *Total arthroplasty of the knee. Proceedings of the Knee Society 1985–1986*, ed Rand J, Dorr L (Gaithersburg: Aspen, 1986) 3–22.

Freeman MAR, Levack B, British contribution to knee arthroplasty, *Clin Orthop* (1986) **210:** 69–79.

Samuelson KM, Fixation in total knee arthroplasty: Interference fit, *Total arthroplasty of the knee. Proceedings of the Knee Society 1985–1986*, ed Rand J, Dorr L (Gaithersburg: Aspen, 1986) 249–256.

Bradley GW, Freeman MAR, Albrektsson BEJ, Total prosthetic replacement of ankylosed knees, *J Arthroplasty* (1987) **2:** 179–183.

Samuelson KM, Bone grafting and noncemented revision arthroplasty of the knee, *Clin Orthop* (1988) **226:** 93–101.

Freeman MAR, Railton GT, Should the posterior cruciate ligament be retained or resected in condylar nonmeniscal knee arthroplasty? The case for resection, *J Arthroplasty* (1988) **3**(suppl.): S3–S12.

Railton GT, Waterfield, A, Nunn D et al., The effect of a metal-back without a stem upon the fixation of a tibial prosthesis, *J Arthroplasty* (1990) **5**(suppl.): S67–S71.

Railton GT, Levack B, Freeman MAR, Unconstrained knee arthroplasty after patellectomy, *J Arthroplasty* (1990) **5:** 255–257.

17.3   Design of total knee replacement

Peter S. Walker

There are now several follow-up studies which show that the cemented condylar replacement type of knee prosthesis can provide satisfactory and trouble-free function in 95% of cases for up to 10 years, with no signs of impending deterioration at that time. A study of the many different designs that have been used provides evidence for the characteristics which are responsible for success and, conversely, the factors responsible for failure or inadequate performance. In general, successful results are achieved when the bearing surfaces are moderately conforming, pegs or posts of sufficient size and surface area are used for fixation, and the alignment is within a few degrees of ideal. Consistency of results depends upon instrumentation and a technique which ensures the alignment and enables correct ligament tensions to be obtained.

Geometry and mechanics

In the normal knee, the profiles of the femoral and tibial surfaces, together with the cruciate ligaments, control the major characteristics of the kinematics in the sagittal plane.[1] When the joint forces and moments are accounted for, the joint surfaces and ligaments define the boundaries of laxity and guide the motion within those boundaries.[2] The ligaments extend from their resting length by only 3–5 mm during motion[3] so that small deviations in the sagittal profiles of prosthetic components can be expected to change the joint kinematics significantly, leading to either reduced motion or excess laxity. This means that the femoral profile should be closely anatomical in shape, the component must be placed accurately at surgery, and there need to be sufficient sizes, probably at least five. The profile from anterior to distal is important to the patellar tracking, where geometrical deviations can overstretch patellar expansions, producing a tight region during the flexion range or, at the other extreme, reducing the quadriceps lever arm. The patellar groove needs to be anatomical, with a normal profile angle of 140°[4] in order to provide the optimum surface for tracking of a retained patella. Allowance is necessary for the

various laxities and motions of the patella relative to the femur which occur during normal function. The most important of these is 2–5 mm of lateral deviation of the patella in extension, central tracking after about 30° of flexion, and 5° of internal–external and varus–valgus rotations during the full range of flexion.[5,6] Given an anatomical patellar groove, the surface of an artificial patella must also resemble anatomical to be consistent with the groove shape and to allow normal motions. However, an axisymmetric shape has the practical advantage of ease of alignment at surgery, the important feature being the skyline profile.

The most normal knee kinematics is achieved for correctly positioned unicompartmental replacement, or for total replacements when both cruciates are preserved and the tibial surface is close to being flat[7,8] (Figure 1). This arrangement evidently results in normal contact point locations, allowing the muscles to function at their correct lever arms. If the anterior cruciate is absent or sacrificed, a flat tibial surface can again allow almost normal function, but excessively posterior contact points can occur as might be expected so that posterior upsweep of the tibial surface is ideally required to substitute for the anterior cruciate function. Such dishing provides restriction to anterior–posterior displacements under weight-bearing conditions by a potential-energy mechanism called the 'uphill principle'.[9] Excessive curvature, however, restricts the laxity to the extent that ligament tensions become restrictive and loss of motion results. In addition, high shear forces and torques are transmitted to the components, leading to interface failure. If both cruciates are sacrificed, both posterior and anterior tibial dishing are necessary for stability, but when posterior shear forces act on the tibia, the femoral–tibial contact points can be too anterior, reducing the quadriceps lever arm. This leads to a compensatory gait whereby the posture of the limbs and body reduce the flexing moment at the knee, avoiding the excess force which would otherwise be needed in the quadriceps for equilibrium.[10] This situation has an adverse effect on more demanding activities such as climbing up or down steep stairs. Possible solutions to this problem include the scheme of Freeman[11] whereby the tibial dishing is

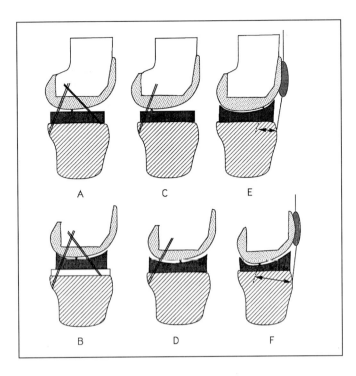

Figure 1

Geometrical schemes for condylar replacement. The small crosses show contact point locations. A, An ideal situation for normal kinematics. B, An ideal situation with reduced bearing stresses (sliding meniscus type). C, A flat tibial surface and absent ACL can result in posterior contact points. D, A posterior upsweep mechanically substitutes for the ACL. E, An absent ACL and PCL can allow anterior contact points, reducing the quadriceps lever arm. F, A posteriorly located cylindrical bearing restores the quadriceps lever arm.

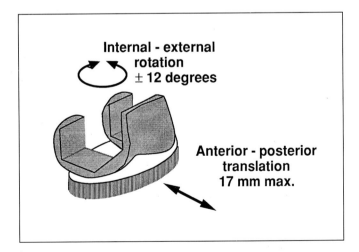

Figure 2

Rotation and translation in a condylar total knee in activities of everyday living (mean ± one SD).

posterior, or the stabilizer type of designs where intercondylar cams guide the contact points throughout flexion.

An important observation in knee joint motion is the variety of patterns between individuals. During activity, the motion of the knee can be described by six degrees of freedom – three translations and three rotations, the most important being flexion–extension, internal–external rotation, and anterior–posterior translation. Average or normative patterns of movement have been determined for normal knees.[12] For example, during the stance phase of walking, this pattern is flexion during early stance, extension during mid-stance, followed by rapid flexion during late stance, with a total range of 15°, accompanied by an internal–external rotation of 5°.

In cadaveric specimens, during a full range of flexion, internal–external rotation averaged 20°, and anterior–posterior translation 8 mm.[13] In groups of normals and total knee replacement patients, similar patterns were observed but with slightly reduced magnitude.[14] The two groups also gave similar mean results to each other. However, the standard deviations in both groups were considerable, being of the order of ±4° and ±4 mm in the mid-flexion range. This presents a problem of variable motion requirements in different individuals.

A reasonable guideline for the motions to allow in a prosthesis design is to specify the mean plus and minus one standard deviation (Figure 2). However, the translation as shown may be excessive, as will be explained later.

Component fixation

The relative positions of the femoral and tibial components, in combination with the forces and moments acting[15] will result in various stresses at the component–bone interfaces. These stresses can be considered in an overall sense, across the entire implant–bone interface, or at a local trabecular level. The stresses affect the response of the bone both biologically and mechanically. In general terms, if the stresses deviate substantially from normal or if the stress pattern changes substantially during activity cycles, interface bone resorption is likely to occur, leading to progressive sinkage, deformity and symptomatic loosening.

Undesirable stress patterns can originate in several ways. Where the overall alignment of the leg deviates from normal, the most common being inadequately corrected varus deformity, the forces on the medial side will be excessive, producing radiolucent zones at the interface[16] indicative of trabecular microfractures and bone resorption.[17] If the femoral–tibial contact points move along an anterior–posterior direction during activity, owing to ligamentous instability or to improper component placement at surgery, the stresses at the anterior and posterior aspect of the component will oscillate between being too high and too low, even to the point of applying tensile stresses.[18,19]

From the clinical experience so far, the most reliable interface has been cemented. The most likely reason for this is that the forces are transferred to the trabeculae over the entire surface such that individual trabeculae are not stressed beyond their limit. The efficiency of load transfer is optimized when there is a uniform cement penetration of 2–3 mm so as to encase horizontal trabecular struts as well as vertical ones.[20,21] Such uniform penetration is not easy to achieve, particularly at the peripheries of components where there is pressure loss when the components are applied at surgery. Localized cement application techniques using small nozzles or the drilling of small holes are methods for achieving peripheral cement penetration.[22]

At a trabecular level, intimate cement–bone contact is not achieved if fluid or debris are present at the time of cement and component application, leading to bone resorption from interface micromotion. The exact mechanism is not fully understood but is associated with non-physiological strains on bone cells. The stresses and micromotions at the interface affect the recruitment or differentiation of cells, leading to an osseointegrated, fibrocartilaginous or fibrous tissue interface. In the long term, migration of polyethylene and cement wear particles as a result of the pumping action due to interface micromotion can lead to the recruitment of macrophage and foreign-body giant cells. These cells, once activated, secrete the enzyme collagenase and factors such as prostaglandin and interleukin which lead to the differentiation and recruitment of osteoclasts.

Many cement–bone interfaces which appear to be well fixed radiographically are found to consist of intervening fibrous membranes between the cement and bone when examined at retrieval.[23] Evidence that this may be a more general situation is provided from the micromotion data using the Roentgen stereophotogrammetry (RSM) technique.[24] This technique is an important one in that it may provide indicators about the fixation viability of different component designs within a time as short as 2 years. A migration of less than 1 mm which has stabilized at 2 years may indicate stability, while progressive migration may indicate impending fixation failure.

The relative motions between components and the bone surface are shown in Figure 3. The distinction between relative rigid body motion and relative micromotion due to elastic deformations is shown.

The tibia and the component are defined as rigid bodies by the coordinates of three points in each body; B1, B2 and B3; and C1, C2 and C3. After a certain time, such as 1 year, radiographic measurement of the reference points typically shows that the

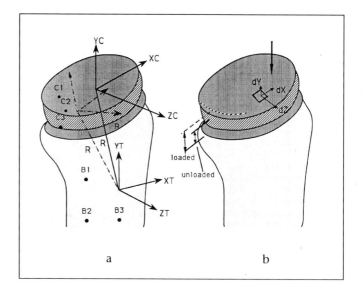

Figure 3

(a) Relative rigid body motion as detected by the RSM technique and (b) relative micromotion as detected by local displacement transducers. For terms, see text.

component axis system has moved relative to the tibial axis system. The movement is defined as three translations (defined as R–R) and three rotations. Individual elements such as vertical migration along YT, and frontal plane rotation about ZT can be calculated. Micromotion, on the other hand, is defined locally and results from relative rigid body motions as well as from local elastic deformations of the materials. For example, if a tibial component is loaded axially, the tibia expands radially outwards,[25] producing relative shear micromotions dX and dZ. Local separation is expressed as displacement dY.

Uncemented interfaces have received a great deal of attention in recent years, the impetus being the perceived need for an uncemented solution for the younger and more active patient. Direct metal-to-bone interfaces, so-called 'press-fit', have been shown to be durable in design configurations such as McKeever tibial plateaus and condylar replacements.[26] On surgical implantation, the metal–bone contacts are localized at small discrete areas, which predictably fail owing to microfractures, leading progressively to the formation of surface densification of bone from healed microfractures, resembling a new subchondral bone plate, with an intervening fibrous tissue layer adjacent to the metal.[27] Such an interface may be more sensitive to uneven or oscillating stresses than a cemented one, and is therefore more dependent on design, benefiting from enhanced stem or peg fixation.[28] The absence of potentially degradable and abrasive cement at the interface may prove to be a long-term advantage of press-fit interfaces.

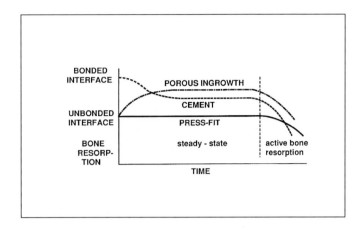

Figure 4

A theoretical model for the changing status of different interfaces with time.

Porous surfaces offer the possibility of bone interlock over the interfaces, but retrieval studies of specimens of different designs and types of porous surface have shown great variations in the extent of the bone ingrowth.[29] Typically, tibial components have shown bone ingrowth into localized regions, usually adjacent to fixation posts or screws, with the remaining area showing ingrowth of fibrous tissue only. There has often been bone densification just beneath the level of the porous surface, similar to that seen for press-fit metal interfaces. The reason for the incomplete bone ingrowth, particularly of tibial components, is the interface micromotion which occurs during weight-bearing activities. Even for symmetrical loading of a tibial component, the radial expansions of the elastically deformable upper tibia, relative to the rigid metallic component, lead to shear micromotions of up to about 100 μm.[25]

For asymmetric loading, micromotions of more than 500 μm have been measured.[30] Interface micromotion cannot be entirely eliminated owing to the elastic deformations of the materials. The bone in particular displays a wide range of elastic properties, as well as a range of distribution in the proximal region.[31] However, micromotion can be reduced by effective design of auxiliary fixation. Central posts reduce motion due to varus–valgus loading; posts or keels in the lateral and medial sides resist torques and shear forces;[32] while screws are most effective at minimizing initial motion.[33] In general, micromotion will be minimum in the vicinity of such fixations and will increase more or less linearly with the distance. In the long term, interface stability may be influenced by other factors such as the age of the patient, the concentration of metallic ions, the accumulation

of debris generated at the interface and the ingress of polyethylene wear particles. Polyethylene has been shown to be much more aggressive in resorption than cement and particularly more so than metal.[34] A model for comparing different types of interface is shown in Figure 4. This model suggests an initial 1–2 year phase, followed by a longer steady-state phase, and a final phase during which time deterioration takes place due to the long-term factors described above.

The use of materials

The most reliable performance to date has been achieved for a femoral component made from cast cobalt–chrome alloy with the tibial and patellar bearing components made from ultra-high-molecular-weight polyethylene (UHMWPE). The friction coefficient of around 0.1 seems to be acceptably low,[35] and the steady wearing of the plastic material reported for hip replacements has not been a general observation for the knee.[36,37]

In recent years, titanium alloy has been used for femoral components, giving an advantage in uncemented mode owing to its high degree of biocompatibility, and the reduced possibility of adverse bone remodelling as a result of the lower elastic modulus. However, considering it as a bearing material, if hard particles intervene between metal and plastic, damage to the metal surface can occur, with subsequent acceleration of both metal and plastic wear. Increasing the surface hardness of the metal, by nitriding or by nitrogen ion implantation, for example, improves the wear resistance,[38] but the protective layers are thin and can evidently break down with time.[39]

Metal-backing of the tibial component provides an advantage in a more uniform distribution of load to the interface and a reduction in the bending stresses on the cement.[40] On the other hand, all-plastic components result in transfer of the force at the interface in a localized region beneath the femoral contact point, and the plastic can warp or cold-flow over time. Metal-backing, however, does mean a reduction in plastic thickness for a given total thickness of the component. This becomes a concern when a small total component thickness is used on the grounds of minimizing the resection of strong trabecular bone from the upper tibia.[41]

The reduction in plastic thickness leads to an increase in the contact stresses at the femoral–tibial contact points with the risk of accelerated wear, complete penetration and even component splitting. Such failures lead to metal-on-metal contact, with the generation of large quantities of particulate metal debris. Empirically, a thickness of plastic below about 6 mm appears to be inadequate, although the femoral–tibial conformity will affect this value. A tenable position is that metal-backing is only necessary when the bone quality is inadequate, such that progressive trabecular failure would occur over time. However, for uncemented application, whether by porous coating or press-fit, metal-backing is needed, while uncemented all-plastic components are liable to plastic wear at the interface, a known cause of bone resorption.

The use of metal-backing in patellar components is difficult to defend owing to the small available component thicknesses at the sides of the component, which is where the highest forces are concentrated during activities where flexion angles exceed about 60°.[42] Furthermore, numerous failures of various designs of metal-backed patellar components have been well documented.[43] Nevertheless, metal-backing continues to be used in uncemented porous-coated components and in such designs the metal substrate needs to avoid subsurface stress concentrations to minimize the failure risk.

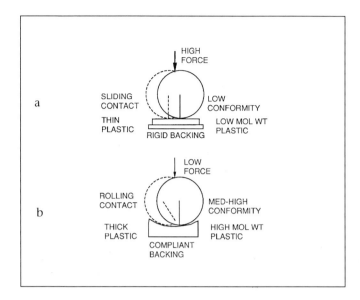

Figure 5

Factors in total knee design which can increase (a) or decrease (b) the wear and deformation of the plastic.

Wear and deformation of plastic

A potential limitation to condylar knees is the wear and deformation of the plastic, leading to excessive joint deformity from asymmetrical wear, complete wearing through to the metal-backing, or particulate debris ingressing along the interface eliciting a bone resorptive response. Retrieval studies have revealed striking anomalies in wear behaviour, some components showing severe wear and deformation, with others of similar design showing only polished areas with small indentations.[37] Flat plastic tibial components which would be expected to display the greatest wear, are often minimally affected. The deleterious effect of cement particles has been well documented.[37] These particles become entrapped between the bearing surfaces, producing local cutting of the plastic. They also increase the local friction, causing further cutting and surface shredding of the plastic. If the cement particles fragment, this leads to three-body wear. Highly dished tibial surfaces are most susceptible to this type of wear, evidently because of the difficulty of escape of the particles.

In the absence of abrasive particles, there are several factors which affect the wear of sliding surfaces (Figure 5). For bearings where the contact stresses are within the elastic limits of the materials, wear is found to be proportional to force (the force pressing the bearing surfaces together) times the sliding distance. On this basis alone, there will be a wide variation in the wear between the knees of different individuals. To obtain a comparison, for a particular activity such as level walking, the product of force times sliding distance can be obtained for each stance phase. Recalling the variations in motion patterns discussed earlier, one

individual may have a flexion–extension range of 15° with sliding taking place, giving an integrated force times distance of A newton-mm. In another knee the flexion–extension during stance may be small, together with low values of anterior–posterior translation. This represents a 'stiff-knee' gait pattern which is typical of many knee replacement patients. In this case, the summation of force times sliding distance will be, say, B newton-mm. It is obvious that B is much smaller than A, so that the wear would be expected to be proportionately smaller. A further mode of motion that would reduce sliding distance is rolling contact, so that, even if there was up to 15° of flexion–extension during stance, if rolling rather than sliding occurred the summation of force times sliding distance would be small.

Such variations in motion patterns between individuals can at least partially account for the anomalies in wear behaviour described earlier. It is noted that such variations in sliding behaviour are much less in the hip than in the knee. For the hip, the flexion–extension range does not have a wide variation between individuals and there is minimal possibility for linear translation or rolling, so that all of the rotations lead to sliding across the interfaces, the sliding distance being proportional to ball diameter. Despite this, a wide range of wear rates has been determined that has been ascribed to a combination of weight, activity level, cement debris and quality of the plastic material, factors which will also apply to the knee.

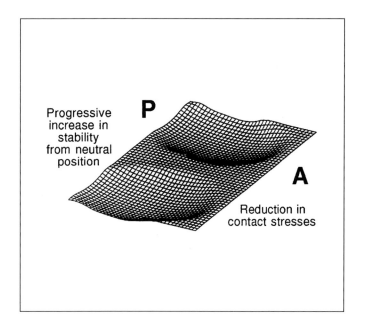

Figure 6

A moderately conforming surface providing a compromise between the ideal requirements for function and wear. P: posterior; A: anterior.

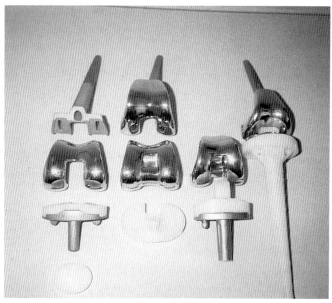

Figure 7

A typical condylar replacement showing some modular parts and an adjustable cutting jig using the intramedullary canal, the anterior cortex and the posterior condyles as reference.

Superimposed on the effect of sliding distance and type of motion, the geometry of the bearing surfaces will play an important role.[44] For high conformity, seen particularly in the sliding meniscus designs, the contact stresses are nominally low. For low conformity, often seen in unicondylar designs, the contact stresses are high. From studies of retrieved specimens, the wear mechanism in highly stressed contacts is in the form of surface and subsurface cracks, leading to the release of particles and the gradual break-up of the surface. Such a mechanism, which is termed delamination wear, seems to depend not only on high contact stresses but on repeated sliding across the surface. Cyclic loading at a fixed location, or rolling contact, evidently does not produce severe delamination wear, even for low-conformity surfaces.

In summary, the factors which minimize the wear of the UHMWPE are minimization of sliding, low contact stresses and the absence of abrasive particles. For the standard condylar replacement, a moderately conforming plastic surface reasonably satisfies the requirements of stability and contact stresses (Figure 6).

Total knee systems

The need for a range of prosthesis types from unicompartmental to fixed hinges has been recognized for many years. In recent years there has been a focus on the condylar replacement type as being the most generally applicable to a wide range of problems (Figure 7). Despite their clinical success, unicompartmentals are not extensively used, while improved instrumentation and technique have extended the use of condylar replacements to situations where hinges would have been used in the past. Most condylar systems have five or more sizes, with variable thicknesses of tibial components. Modular snap-in plastic inserts facilitate surgery and reduce inventory. For the filling of tibial defects, metal wedges are available,[45] while add-on stems are used for revision cases where extra fixation is required. Stabilizer components are used to substitute for the cruciate ligaments and are used routinely by many surgeons who prefer this approach. Superstabilizer designs with a tibial post housed in an intercondylar recess of the femoral component are used when varus–valgus stability is required. When linkage is necessary, rotating hinges are usually preferred over fixed hinges because of the reduced rotational shear stresses at the interfaces. For the most severe cases, particularly in revisions, customized designs are probably the most appropriate.

References

1. O'Connor JJ, Shercliff TL, Biden E et al., The geometry of the knee in the sagittal plane, *Proc Inst Mech Engrs* (1989) **203**(H4): 223.

2. Blankevoort L, Huiskes R, De Lange A, The envelope of passive knee joint motion, *J Biomechanics* (1988) **21**: 705–720.

3. Reuben JD, Rovick JS, Schrager RJ et al., Three-dimensional dynamic motion analysis of the anterior cruciate ligament deficient knee joint, *Am J Sports Med* (1989) **17**(4): 463–471.

4. Ficat P, *Pathologie femoro-patellaire* (Paris: Masson, 1970).

5. Kaltwasser P, Uematsu O, Walker PS, The patello-femoral joint in total knee replacement, *Trans Orthop Res Soc* (1987) **12**: 292.

6. Van Kampen A, Huiskes R, The three-dimensional tracking pattern of the human patella, *J Orthop Res* (1990) **8**: 372–382.

7. Weinstein JN, Andriacchi TP, Galante JO, Factors influencing walking and stairclimbing following unicompartmental knee arthroplasty, *J Arthroplasty* (1986) **1**: 109–115.

8. Whittle MW, Jefferson RJ, Functional biomechanical assessment of the Oxford meniscal knee, *J Arthroplasty* (1989) **4**: 231–243.

9. Walker PS, Wang CJ, Masse Y, Joint laxity as a criterion for the design of condylar knee prostheses, *Proceedings of the Conference on Total Knee Replacement*, Institution of Mechanical Engineers, London, September, 1974, 22–29.

10. Andriacchi TP, Stanwyck TS, Galante JO, Knee biomechanics and total knee replacement, *J Arthroplasty* (1986) **1**: 211–219.

11. Freeman MAR, Railton GT, Should the posterior cruciate ligament be retained or resected in condylar non-meniscal knee arthroplasty? The case for resection, *J Arthroplasty* (1988) (suppl.) **3**: S3–S12.

12. Chao EY, Laughman RK, Schneider E et al., Normative data of knee joint motion and ground reaction forces in adult level walking, *J Biomech* (1983) **16**: 219–233.

13. Kurosawa H, Walker PS, Abe S et al., Geometry and motion of the knee for implant and orthotic design, *J Biomech* (1985) **18**: 487–499.

14. El Nahass BE, Madson MM, Walker PS, Motion of the knee after condylar resurfacing, *Trans Orthop Res Soc* (1990) **15**: 476.

15. Morrison JB, Function of the knee joint in various activities, *Biomed Eng* (1969) **4**: 573–580.

16. Hsu HP, Garg A, Walker PS et al., Effect of knee component alignment on tibial load distribution with clinical correlation, *Clin Orthop* (1989) **248**: 135–144.

17. Miegel RE, Walker PS, Nelson PC et al., A compliant interface for total knee arthroplasty, *J Orthop Res* (1986) **4**: 486–493.

18. Walker PS, Ranawat CS, Insall JN, Fixation of the tibial components of condylar replacement knee prostheses, *J Biomech* (1976) **9**: 269–275.

19. Manley MT, Stulberg BN, Stern LS et al., Direct observation of micromotion at the implant–bone interface with cemented and non-cemented tibial components, *Trans Orthop Res Soc* (1987) **12**: 436.

20. Krause WR, Krug W, Miller J, Strength of the cement–bone interface, *Clin Orthop* (1982) **163**: 290–299.

21. Walker PS, Soudry M, Ewald FC et al., Control of cement penetration in total knee arthroplasty. *Clin Orthop* (1984) **185**: 155–164.

22. Wixson RL, *Lectures on total knee replacement* (personal communication, Northwestern University, Chicago, Ill., 1990).

23. Ryd L, Linder L, On the correlation between micromotion and histology of the bone–cement interface: report of three cases of knee arthroplasty followed by roentgen stereophotogrammetric analysis, *J Arthroplasty* (1989) **4**: 303–309.

24. Selvik G, *A roentgen stereophotogrammetric method for the study of the kinematics of the skeletal system* (Thesis, University of Lund, Sweden, 1974) [Reprinted in *Acta Orthop Scand* (1989) **60**(suppl. 232)].

25. Garg A, Walker PS, The effect of the interface on the bone stresses beneath tibial components, *J Biomech* (1986) **19**: 957–967.

26. Yamamoto S, Nakata S, Kondoh Y, A follow-up study of an uncemented knee replacement: the results of 312 knees using the Kodama–Yamamoto prosthesis, *J Bone Joint Surg (Br)* (1989) **71**: 505–508.

27. Walker PS, Rodger RF, Miegel RE et al., An investigation of a compliant interface for press-fit joint replacement, *J Orthop Res* (1990) **8**: 453–463.

28. Albrektsson BEJ, Ryd L, Carlsson LV et al., The effect of a stem on the tibial component of knee arthroplasty: a roentgen stereophotogrammetric study of uncemented tibial components in the Freeman–Samuelson knee arthroplasty, *J Bone Joint Surg (Br)* (1990) **72**: 252–258.

29. Turner TM, Urban RM, Sumner DR et al., Bone ingrowth into the tibial component of a canine total condylar knee replacement prosthesis, *J Orthop Res* (1989) **7**: 893–901.

30. Branson PJ, Steege JW, Wixson RL et al., Rigidity of initial fixation with uncemented tibial knee implants, *J Arthroplasty* (1989) **4**: 21–26.

31. Wixson RL, Elasky N, Lewis J, Cancellous bone material properties in osteoarthritic and rheumatoid total knee patients, *J Orthop Res* (1989) **7**: 885–892.

32. Walker PS, Hsu HP, Zimmerman RA, A comparative study of uncemented tibial components, *J Arthroplasty* (1990) **5**: 245–253.

33. Voltz RG, personal communication, Knee Society, 1990.

34. Mirra JM, Marder RA, Amstutz HC, The pathology of failed total joint arthroplasty, *Clin Orthop* (1982) **170**: 175–183.

35. Thatcher JC, Zhou XM, Walker PS, Inherent laxity in total knee prostheses, *J Arthroplasty* (1987) **2**: 199–207.

36. Hood RW, Wright TM, Burstein AH, Retrieval analysis of total knee prostheses: a method and its application to 48 total condylar prostheses, *J Biomed Mater Res* (1983) **17**: 829–842.

37. Landy MM, Walker PS, Wear of ultra-high-molecular-weight polyethylene components of 90 retrieved knee prostheses, *J Arthroplasty* (1988) suppl. **3**: S73–S85.

38. Crowninshield R, Lower JH, Gilbertson L et al., Simulating total knee replacement wear in vivo: comparison of Ti-6Al-4Va and nitrogen ion implanted Ti-6Al-4Va, *Trans Orthop Res Soc* (1990) **15**: 470.

39. Davidson JA, Kovacs P, Lanzer WL, Metal ion release during articulation of ion implanted Ti-6Al-4Va alloy against UHMWPE, *Trans Orthop Res Soc* (1990) **15**: 460.

40. Bartel DL, Burstein AH, Santavicca EA et al., Performance of the tibial component in total knee replacement: conventional and revision designs, *J Bone Joint Surg (Am)* (1982) **64**: 1026–1033.

41. Hvid I, Jensen J, Cancellous bone strength at the proximal human tibia, *Eng Med* (1984) **13**: 21–25.

42. Reilly DT, Martens M, Experimental analysis of the quadriceps muscle force and patello-femoral joint reaction force for various activities, *Acta Orthop Scand* (1972) **43**: 126–137.

43. Bayley JC, Scott RD, Ewald FC et al., Failure of the metal-backed patellar component after total knee replacement, *J Bone Joint Surg (Am)* (1988) **70**: 668–674.

44. Walker PS, Bearing surface design in total knee replacement, *Eng Med* (1988) **17**: 149–156.

45. Brooks PJ, Walker PS, Scott RD, Tibial component fixation in deficient tibial bone stock, *Clin Orthop* (1984) **184**: 302–308.

17.4 Posteriorly stabilized (Insall–Burstein) total condylar knee arthroplasty: A 2–7-year follow-up study of 157 knees

Dipak V. Patel, Paul M. Aichroth and Jonathan S. Wand

The posteriorly stabilized (Insall–Burstein) condylar prosthesis was introduced in 1978 as a modification of the Total Condylar I prosthesis. Since then, successful results have been reported by various authors.[1-7]

The purpose of this review was to assess the results, with special reference both to patellar complications, which are reported to be more frequent with this modification,[3] and to fixation of the tibial component, which may be put at risk by the cam and post mechanism which provides the posterior stability.[8] We have also analysed the incidence of mechanical loosening and the extent of radiolucent zones beneath the tibial plateau with respect to component positioning, overall knee alignment and the type of knee pathology.

Materials and methods

Between 1982 and 1987, 140 patients underwent posteriorly stabilized total condylar knee replacement arthroplasty at Westminster Hospital, London. Six patients had died due to unrelated causes and 16 patients (17 knees) were lost to follow-up, thus leaving 118 patients (157 knees) available for detailed clinical and radiological assessment.

There were 41 males and 77 females. The right knee was involved in 88 cases and the left in 69. Thirty-nine patients had bilateral knee arthroplasty. All patients were reviewed by one of us (D.V.P.). Their average age at the time of operation was 69 years (range 47–85 years) and the mean follow-up was 42 months (range 24–84 months).

The details of preoperative diagnosis are shown in Table 1. Forty-two patients had had previous operations on their knees (Table 2). Preoperatively, 104 knees (66%) had a varus deformity (Figures 1 and 2) and 53 knees (34%) had a valgus deformity (Figures 3 and 4). The mean preoperative varus deformity was 15° (range 5–30°) and the average preoperative valgus deformity was 14° (range 6–35°). Thirty knees (19%) had a flexion contracture of a mean of 13° (range 10–35°).

Table 1 Preoperative diagnosis in 118 patients (157 knees).

Diagnosis	No. of patients	No. of knees	Percentage of knees
Osteoarthritis	77	102	65
Rheumatoid arthritis	31	45	29
Osteonecrosis	5	5	
Posttraumatic arthritis	3	3	
Paget's disease + secondary osteoarthritis	1	1	6
Synovial osteochondromatosis + secondary osteoarthritis	1	1	

Table 2 Previous operations in 42 patients (51 knees).

Operation	No. of knees
Open medial meniscectomy	12
Open lateral meniscectomy	4
High tibial osteotomy	11
Synovectomy	7
Arthroscopic debridement (medial compartment)	7
Arthroscopic debridement (lateral compartment)	3
Supracondylar femoral osteotomy	2
Patellectomy	2
Osteotomy for femoral and tibial bowing (Paget's disease)	1
Open reduction and internal fixation for fracture of the lateral tibial plateau	1
Arthrotomy and removal of loose bodies	1

All patients had significant limitation of daily functional activities despite adequate conservative measures. The walking distance was markedly reduced in the majority of the patients. The mean preoperative BASK (British Association for Surgery of the Knee) score was 43 points (range 3–65 points).

Operative technique

The surgical technique employed was identical to that reported by Insall et al.[3] and Aglietti and Buzzi.[1]

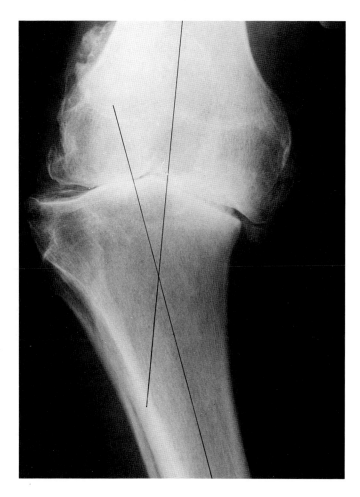

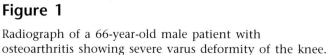

Figure 1

Radiograph of a 66-year-old male patient with
osteoarthritis showing severe varus deformity of the knee.

Routine soft-tissue release was undertaken in patients
with moderate to severe deformities to facilitate insertion of the prosthesis without excessive bone
removal.

An economical tibial resection at 90° to the long
axis of the tibia is essential. Dorr[9] mentioned that in
a varus knee not more than 5 mm of bone on the
medial and 10 mm on the lateral side should be
removed, so as to preserve the stronger subchondral
bone.[10] Flexion contractures of 20–25° were corrected
by an appropriate distal femoral resection.

Postoperative management

A well-padded compression bandage and side slabs
were applied. Continuous passive mobilization was
started after 48–72 hours when the patient was
comfortable. Weight-bearing mobilization using a
walker was encouraged on the third or fourth postop-

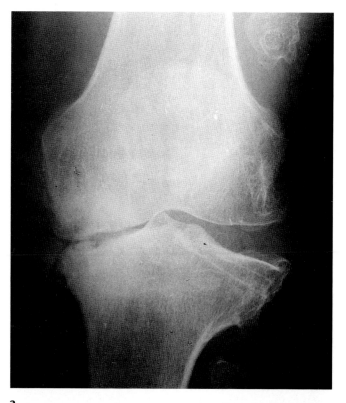

a

b

Figure 2

(a) Anteroposterior radiograph of a 64-year-old woman
showing varus deformity of the knee. She had a high
tibial osteotomy 6 years previously. Note the multiple,
degenerative loose bodies in the knee. (b) Lateral
radiograph of the same patient.

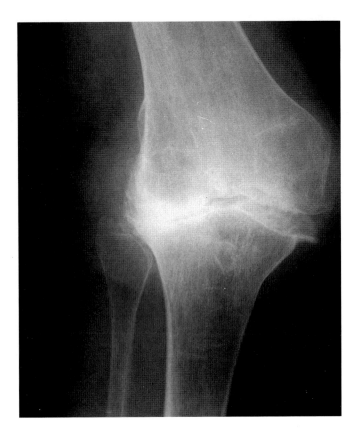

Figure 3

Radiograph showing valgus deformity of the knee in a 68-year-old woman with rheumatoid arthritis.

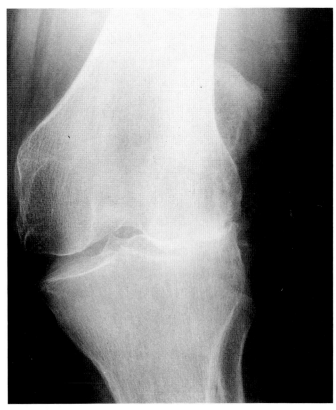

Figure 4

Radiograph of a 65-year-old man with osteoarthritis showing valgus deformity of the knee.

erative day. Manipulation under anaesthesia was undertaken only when the patient had failed to achieve 90° of knee flexion by third postoperative week.

Method of evaluation

The BASK knee function rating system was used. This is a modification of the BOA Knee Function Assessment chart.[11] Of the 100 points for a normal knee, 39 points are given for lack of pain, 25 for range of movement more than 120°, 10 for function, 4 for ability to climb stairs, 4 for walking aids, 2 for subjective stability, and 16 for technical merit of the deformity (4 points each for absence of extension lag and flexion deformity, 4 for valgus alignment between 6° and 10°, and 4 for lateral plane laxity in extension between 0° and 5°).

A score of 91–100 points was rated as excellent; 75–90 as good; 61–74 as fair; and 60 or less as poor.

Weight-bearing anteroposterior radiographs taken on a standard short-film (12 × 16 inches) were

obtained, together with a standard lateral view and a skyline view of the patella at 45°.[12] The prosthesis–bone interfaces at all three components were studied by a zone method.[3] The tilt of the prosthetic components was measured as suggested by Hvid and Nielsen.[13] The various angles measured are shown in Figure 5.

The ideal position for the femoral component was considered to be 6–10° of valgus, with the anterior flange of the femoral prosthesis flush with the anterior cortex. The ideal position for the tibial component was considered to be at 90°±2° to the long axis of the tibia in the frontal plane.

Results

Clinical results

The results were graded as shown in Table 3. The details of clinical results are given in Table 4. The

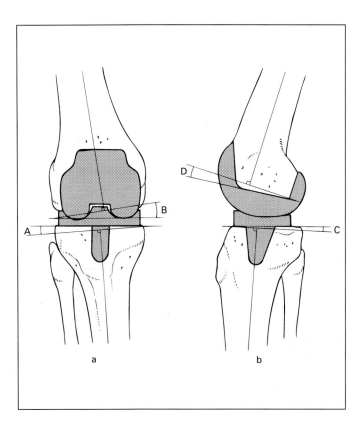

a

b

Figure 5

The angles measured on weight-bearing anteroposterior (a) and lateral (b) radiographs as suggested by Hvid and Nielsen.[13] A, angular deviation of the tibial component from a line at right angles to the tibial axis; B, angular deviation of the femoral component from a line at right angles to the femoral axis. The same method was applied to measure the angular deviations of the tibial (C) and femoral (D) components on the lateral view.

Table 3 Grading of clinical results in 157 knee replacements using BASK scoring system.

Result	BASK score	No. of knees	Percentage of knees
Excellent	91–100	38	24
Good	75–90	97	62
Fair	61–74	16	10
Poor	60 or less	6	4

Table 4 Clinical results in 157 knee replacements given as number and percentage.

	All (No.)	(%)	OA (No.)	(%)	RA (No.)	(%)	Statistical difference (OA vs RA)
Results							
Excellent	38	24	28	27	7	16	
Good	97	62	59	58	34	75	
Fair	16	10	9	9	4	9	
Poor	6	4	6	6	–	–	
Pain							
None	119	76	77	75	37	82	
Mild	35	22	22	22	8	18	NS
Moderate	3	2	3	3	–	–	
Walking							
Unlimited	32	21	22	22	8	18	
500 m–1 km	61	39	40	39	15	33	$P<0.01$
100 m–500 m	43	27	24	23	17	38	
50 m–100 m (outdoors)	19	12	14	14	5	11	
Indoors only	2	1	2	2	–	–	
Stairs							
Normal	35	22	27	27	4	9	
One step at a time	65	42	38	37	21	47	$P<0.05$
With walking aids	54	34	36	35	18	40	
Unable to manage	3	2	1	1	2	4	
Range of movement							
Average flexion	95°		95°		90°		NS
Flexion contracture	3°		2°		5°		$P<0.01$
Postoperative score	79		79		78		NS

NS, not significant.

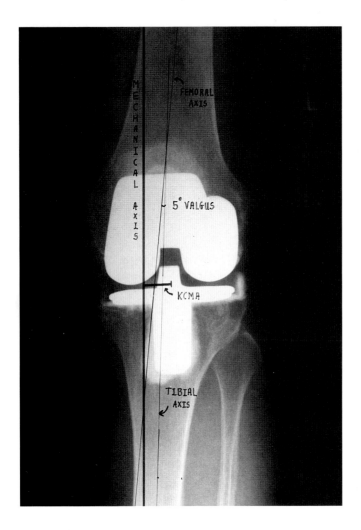

Figure 6

Satisfactory postoperative valgus alignment 3 years after posteriorly stabilized (Insall–Burstein) total condylar knee replacement arthroplasty. KCMA = distance between knee centre to mechanical axis.

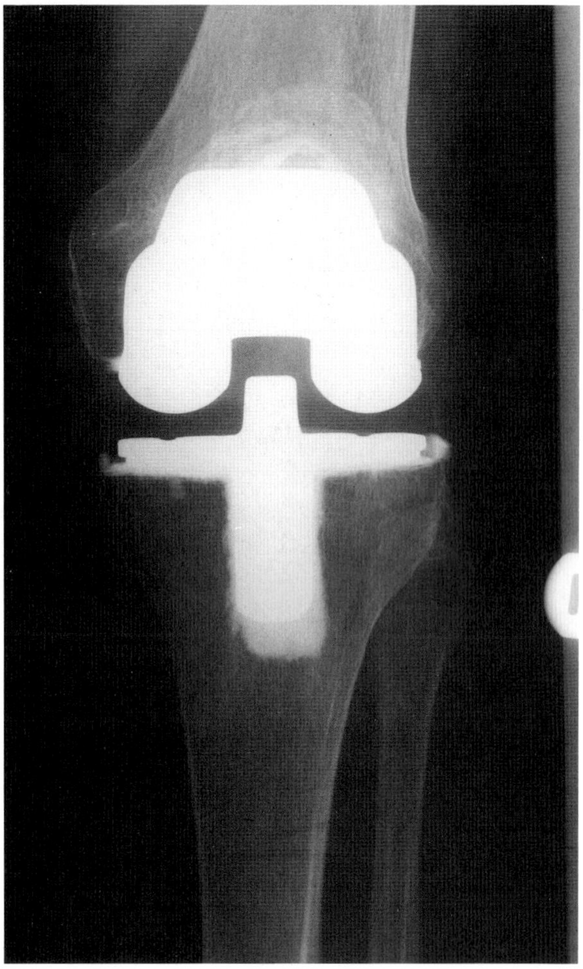

Figure 7

Four-year follow-up of posteriorly stabilized condylar prosthesis.

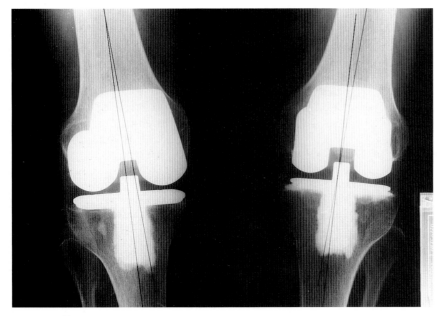

Figure 8

Five-year follow-up of a bilateral condylar knee arthroplasty showing satisfactory valgus alignment. This patient had an excellent clinical result.

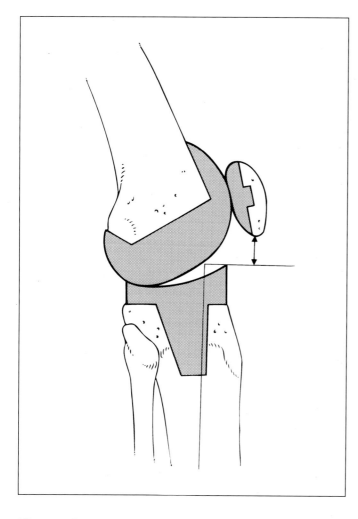

Figure 9

Method of measurement of the relative height of the patella as suggested by Aglietti and Buzzi.[1]

mean postoperative BASK score was 79 points (range 43–98 points). Overall, 86% of the knees had an excellent or good result. Patients with osteoarthritis (OA) had better results as compared to those with rheumatoid arthritis (RA). In all, 76% of the knees were without pain and 22% had only mild and intermittent discomfort.

The walking distance was over 500 m in 70% of the patients with OA and 41% of those with RA. Twenty-five per cent of the patients were able to climb stairs normally; 37% were climbing one step at a time, and 36% required the support of a banister or stick or both. No walking aids were necessary in 76 patients (64%), 30 patients (26%) used walking stick for outdoor activities only, and 12 patients (10%) constantly required support. The average post-operative knee flexion was 95° (range 65–130°). A residual flexion contracture of up to 15° was found in 40 knees (25%), averaging 7°.

Patient satisfaction

Seventy-two per cent of the patients were pleased and 18% were satisfied with the result. Six per cent of the patients expressed reservations and 4% were disappointed.

Radiographic results

A satisfactory postoperative alignment of 6–10° valgus was achieved in 66 knees (42%); 68 knees (43%) were between 0 and 5° of valgus (Figure 6), and 3 knees (2%) had more than 10° of valgus. Twenty knees (13%) were in varus alignment. The average anatomical tibiofemoral angle was 4.6° valgus (range 7° varus to 12° valgus). Figure 7 shows a 4-year follow-up and Figure 8 shows a 5-year follow-up of bilateral posteriorly stabilized (Insall–Burstein) total condylar knee arthroplasties.

An ideal position for the femoral component within 6–10° of valgus was obtained in 116 knees (74%). The femoral prosthesis was within 0–5° valgus in 24 knees (15%) and 11°–15° valgus in 17 knees (11%). The anterior flange of the femoral component was not flush with the distal femoral cortex in 16 knees (10%); the femoral component had been cemented in a slightly flexed position. Ninety-seven per cent of the tibial components were within 2° of varus or valgus, and 96% were within 4° of antero-posterior tilt.

The patellar height (Figure 9) was measured as the distance from its lower pole to the anterior edge of the tibial component.[1] The average height was 9.9 mm (range 1–20 mm), and the knees with impingement symptoms had a significantly lower patella (mean 3.3 mm) than those without similar complaints (mean 10.5 mm, $P<0.05$).

At the patellar interface, an incomplete radiolucent line less than 1 mm wide was seen in 44 knees (28%). Two patients had proximal migration of the patellar component, presumably due to mechanical loosening, and one had stress fracture of the patella.

An accurate radiological assessment of the femoral prosthesis–bone interface was not possible owing to the presence of the metal prosthesis, although there was no evidence of any progression of the observed radiolucent lines around the femoral component.

The incidence of the radiolucent lines beneath the tibial component is shown in Table 5. There were no radiolucent lines below the tibial prostheses in 85 knees (54%); in another 66 knees (42%) they were <1 mm thick, non-progressive and limited to the interface beneath the medial, lateral or both tibial plateaux. In 6 knees (4%), the radiolucent lines were almost complete and reached 2 mm width at some point (Figure 10). Although only two patients had mild pain on clinical examination, we considered that they all probably had mechanical loosening.

Table 5 Incidence of radiolucent lines beneath the tibial component in 157 knees given as number and percentage.

| | Number of knees | Radiolucent lines | | | | | | Statistical significance |
| | | Absent | | 1–2 zones | | Probably loose | | |
		(No.)	(%)	(No.)	(%)	(No.)	(%)	
All	157	85	54	66	42	6	4	
Age								
<60 years	17	12	71	5	29	–	–	P <0.005
60–70 years	68	16	23	48	71	4	6	
>70 years	72	57	79	13	18	2	3	
Sex								
Male	53	13	24	37	70	3	6	
Female	104	72	69	29	28	3	3	
Diagnosis								
OA	102	54	53	46	45	2	2	
RA	45	23	51	18	40	4	9	
Others	10	8	80	2	20	–	–	
Post-op alignment								
Varus 0–5°	17	3	18	12	70	2	12	
Varus 6–10°	3	–	–	1	33	2	67	P <0.001
Valgus 1–5°	68	31	46	36	53	1	1	
Valgus 6–10°	66	50	76	15	23	1	1	
Valgus 11–15°	3	1	33	2	67	–	–	
Tibial component								
>2° varus	6	–	–	4	67	2	33	
2° varus to 2° valgus	140	82	59	56	40	2	1	P <0.01
>2° valgus	11	3	27	6	55	2	18	

The varus alignment of the knee was associated with increased incidence of radiolucent lines, but any valgus alignment was not. Similarly, there was a statistically significant correlation (P<0.01) between varus positioning of the tibial implant and the presence of radiolucent lines around the tibial component.

Complications

The details are given in Table 6. Wound complications were more frequent in knees with RA (24%) than those with OA (9%). Two patients required aspiration of wound haematoma.

Deep infection occurred in a 65-year-old male patient with RA, 4 months after total knee replacement. No causative organism was found on culture. Revision arthroplasty was undertaken using a long-stem constrained Insall prosthesis (Figure 11), 20 months following the primary replacement. At latest review, 30 months following the revision arthroplasty, the knee was quiescent.

One patient (79-year-old male with OA) developed gradual postoperative infection. No causative organism could be detected on cultures from aspiration of the knee joint. After 27 months, arthrotomy and debridement was carried out and the patellar prosthesis was removed 3 months later. At the time of latest follow-up, there was no evidence of active infection and his knee flexion was 85°.

A 79-year-old male patient fell 6 weeks postoperatively, sustaining a supracondylar fracture above the prosthesis. This was treated by open reduction and internal fixation using a condylar plate, and a satisfactory functional result was obtained.

One patient was found to have a stress fracture of the patella which was accidently diagnosed on a routine radiographic examination. However, his knee was clinically asymptomatic and hence no further action was undertaken. A 69-year-old woman with OA complained of repeated patellar subluxation postoperatively. The knee was screened under image intensifier and no patellofemoral maltracking was detected. Now, at 5 years following the knee replacement, the patient is symptom-free.

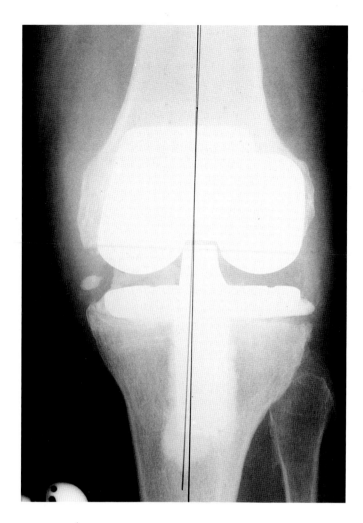

Figure 10

Mechanical loosening of the tibial component, 2.5 years after the operation.

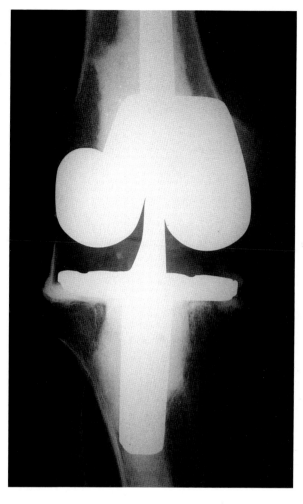

Figure 11

Radiograph showing a 30-month follow-up of a revision arthroplasty using a long-stem constrained prosthesis.

Table 6 Complications.

Complication	Number of knees
Superficial infection	2
Deep infection	1
Delayed wound healing	12
Wound haematoma	7
Wound dehiscence	1
Supracondylar fracture above the prosthesis	1
Superior migration of the patellar component	2
Pulmonary embolism	1
Patellar subluxation	1
Lateral popliteal neurapraxia	1
Patellar impingement	12
Stress fracture of the patella	1
Removal of patellar component	1
Mechanical loosening of the tibial component	2

Patellar impingement symptoms, particularly on extension, were seen in 12 knees (8%). They were mildly painful in 4 patients, moderately painful in 1, and 7 had a painless clicking sensation. Superior migration of the patellar prosthesis was observed in 2 patients (Figure 12). In view of the absence of symptoms, no surgery was advised.

Lateral popliteal nerve palsy occurred in one patient and was associated with correction of a fixed valgus deformity. Complete recovery occurred in 8 weeks.

Discussion

The posteriorly stabilized condylar prosthesis was designed in an effort to increase knee movement and stability. The posterior sloping of the tibial plateau

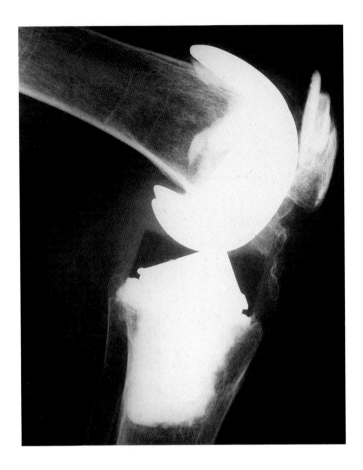

Figure 12

Proximal migration of the patellar component. This was discovered accidently on routine radiological assessment.

and the cam-like action of the central build-up on the tibial component enhances the anteroposterior stability and provides an increased range of knee motion.

Insall et al. reported 88% excellent results using this modified prosthesis at 2–4 years of follow-up.[3] In our series, 86% excellent or good results were obtained at an average follow-up of 42 months (range 24–84 months). Our findings are in comparison with those published previously (Table 7).

Ranawat[14] observed that the posterior stability mechanism may increase the tangential shearing stresses on the tibial component and it has been suggested that it is better to preserve the posterior cruciate ligament, which will transfer stress directly to bone.[15] However, the posterior cruciate-retaining prostheses are more difficult to insert, especially in severely deformed knees. Despite the difference in opinions, various studies have suggested that the clinical results using the various prosthetic designs have been essentially the same.[16–18]

Meticulous surgical technique is essential for a successful functional result. One of the objectives of total knee replacement is the re-establishment of normal tibiofemoral alignment. A valgus alignment of 6–10° is ideal; however, slightly more valgus angulation has no detrimental effects. Varus alignment should be avoided, and this view has been confirmed by clinical experience.[19]

Table 7 Comparative results of posteriorly stabilized total-condylar knee replacement.

	Insall[3]	Scott[5]	Aglietti[1]		Patel et al.	
Knees replaced	133	137	95		180	
Knees evaluated	118	119	85		157	
Osteoarthritis	92%	74%	72%		65%	
Follow-up (years)	2–4	2–8	3–8		2–7	
			OA	*RA*	*OA*	*RA*
Postoperative score	90[a]	90[a]	81[a]	80[a]	79[b]	78[b]
Excellent results	88%	83%	66%	38%	27%	16%
Good results	9%	15%	26%	50%	58%	75%
Unlimited walking	76%	–	49%	12%	22%	18%
Walking 500 m–1 km	–	–	26%	21%	39%	33%
Stairs normal	76%	–	44%	17%	27%	9%
Stairs one step at a time	–	–	42%	46%	37%	47%
Average post-op flexion	115°	107°	98°	98°	95°	90°
Impingement symptoms	2.5%	–	20%		8%	
Patellar stress fracture	11%	5%	0	0	0.6%	
Insignificant tibial radiolucent lines	31%	76%	61%	50%	45%	40%
Probable loosening (radiographic only)	0	10%	5%	4%	2%	9%
Re-operation (loosening)	1%	0.8%	2%	0	–	–

[a]HSS knee score.
[b]BASK score.

In our study, 87% of the knees had valgus alignment and 13% of the knees had varus alignment, postoperatively. Our results are in comparison with Hood et al., who reported on their experience with Insall–Burstein posteriorly stabilized condylar prosthesis and found overall alignment to be within $7°±5°$ of valgus in 89% of the knees.[20]

Radiolucent lines may be present soon after the insertion of the prosthesis.[21] These are not significant and probably not indicative of loosening. Radiolucencies of more than 2 mm width are important only if they span two or more zones and are progressive. In the present series, the radiolucent lines around the tibial implant were absent or insignificant in 96% of the knees, whereas six knees (4%) had complete radiolucent lines beneath the tibial component. Similar incidence of loosening has been reported by various authors using the Total Condylar I prosthesis.[8,22–24]

The alignment of the prosthetic components and overall knee alignment have important effects upon fixation.[7,9,25–30] Sneppen et al. reported that an economical tibial cut at 90° allows optimal fixation of the tibial component.[10] We observed a statistically significant correlation between the incidence of tibial radiolucent lines and varus alignment of the replaced knee ($P<0.001$). A varus position of more than 2° of the tibial component was also associated with increased incidence of radiolucent lines ($P<0.01$) (details in Table 5). Both these findings were more pronounced in the RA group.

Femoral component radiolucencies were difficult to assess. However, the clinical problem of femoral component loosening is negligible and radiolucencies are found to be sparse beneath the femoral components.[21,31] In this study, there was no evidence of progression of the observed radiolucent lines around the femoral prosthesis. The femoral component was positioned between 6° and 10° of valgus in 74% of the knees.

An increased number of patellar complications are reported following the use of Insall–Burstein posteriorly stabilized condylar prosthesis.[1,3] In the present study, a total of 17 patellar complications were noted. The incidence of stress fractures of the patella was low in our series (0.6%) as compared to 11% incidence reported by Insall et al.[3] The higher incidence of patellar stress fractures noted in Insall's series[3] was attributed to a larger patellar component (38 mm), increased knee movement and greater overall functional activity level achieved by their patients.

The impingement symptoms were due to the patella and the peripatellar soft tissues grating against the anterior margin of the femoral component. The patellofemoral impingement symptoms were more common when the patella was lower than usual. The patella is low because the tibial component is thicker than the amount of bone resected.[2]

The need for manipulation under anaesthesia has gradually declined with the advent of continuous passive mobilization. In the present series, the mean postoperative knee flexion was 95°. Eighteen per cent of the knees required manipulation at an average of 2 weeks postoperatively.

Conclusions

One-hundred-and-eighteen patients (157 knees) who underwent Insall–Burstein posteriorly stabilized replacement arthroplasty were reviewed at an average of 42 months postoperatively. Overall, 86% of the knees had excellent or good results. The mean postoperative BASK score was 79 points and the average knee flexion achieved was 95°. Patients with OA did better than those with RA.

We agree with Insall et al.[3] that the posteriorly stabilized prosthetic design does offer some advantages, particularly in terms of movement and function, apparently without compromising fixation. The enhanced anteroposterior stability provided by the prosthesis is useful for correction of severe deformities.

Acknowledgments

The authors thank Miss Dina Stanford for the computer analysis of the data. Our thanks are also extended to the Medical Photography Department of Westminster Hospital for their help with the illustrations.

References

1. **Aglietti P, Buzzi R,** Posteriorly stabilised total-condylar knee replacement: three to eight years' follow-up of 85 knees, *J Bone Joint Surg (Br)* (1988) **70:** 211–216.
2. **Figgie E III, Goldberg VM, Heiple KG et al.,** The influence of tibial-patellofemoral location on function of the knee in patients with the posterior stabilised condylar knee prosthesis, *J Bone Joint Surg (Am)* (1986) **68:** 1035–1040.
3. **Insall JN, Lachiewicz PF, Burstein AH,** The posterior stabilised condylar prosthesis: a modification of the total condylar design: two to four-year clinical experience, *J Bone Joint Surg (Am)* (1982) **64:** 1317–1323.
4. **Kjaersgaard-Andersen P, Hvid I, Wethelund J-O et al.,** Total condylar knee arthroplasty in osteoarthritis: a four to six-year follow-up evaluation of 103 cases, *Clin Orthop* (1989) **238:** 167–173.
5. **Scott WN, Rubinstein M, Scuderi G,** Results after knee replacement with a posterior cruciate-substituting prosthesis, *J Bone Joint Surg (Am)* (1988) **70:** 1163–1173.
6. **Scuderi GR, Insall JN, Windsor RE et al.,** Survivorship of cemented knee replacements, *J Bone Joint Surg (Br)* (1989) **71:** 798–803.

7. **Vince KG, Insall JN, Kelly MA**, The total condylar prosthesis: 10 to 12-year results of a cemented knee replacement, *J Bone Joint Surg (Br)* (1989) **71**: 793–797.

8. **Ranawat CS, Rose HA**, Clinical and radiographic results of total-condylar knee arthroplasty: a 3- to 8-year follow-up, *Total-condylar knee arthroplasty: technique, results and complications*, ed Ranawat CS (New York: Springer-Verlag, 1985) 140–148.

9. **Dorr LD**, Complications: loosening of the cement–bone interface after total knee arthroplasty, *Total-condylar knee arthroplasty: technique, results and complications*, ed Ranawat CS (New York: Springer-Verlag, 1985) 173–185.

10. **Sneppen O, Christensen P, Larsen H et al.**, Mechanical testing of trabecular bone in knee replacement: development of an osteopenetrometer, *Int Orthop* (1981) 5: 251–256.

11. **Aichroth PM, Freeman MAR, Smillie IS et al.**, A knee function assessment chart, *J Bone Joint Surg (Br)* (1978) **60**: 308–309.

12. **Merchant AC, Mercer RL, Jacobsen RH et al.**, Roentgenographic analysis of patellofemoral congruence, *J Bone Joint Surg (Am)* (1974) 56: 1391–1396.

13. **Hvid I, Nielsen S**, Total condylar knee arthroplasty: prosthetic component positioning and radiolucent lines, *Acta Orthop Scand* (1984) 55: 160–165.

14. **Ranawat CS**, Future trends in knee arthroplasty, *Total-condylar knee arthroplasty: technique, results and complications*, ed Ranawat CS (New York: Springer-Verlag, 1985) 168–171.

15. **Sledge CB, Walker PS**, Total knee arthroplasty in rheumatoid arthritis, *Clin Orthop* (1984) **182**: 127–136.

16. **Dorr LD, Scott RD, Ranawat CS**, Importance of retention of the posterior cruciate ligament, *Total-condylar knee arthroplasty: technique, results and complications*, ed Ranawat CS (New York: Springer-Verlag, 1985) 197–202.

17. **Scott RD, Volatile TB**, Twelve years' experience with posterior cruciate-retaining total knee arthroplasty, *Clin Orthop* (1986) **205**: 100–107.

18. **Scott WN, Rubinstein M**, Failure rate of primary total knee replacement, *Total knee revision arthroplasty*, ed Scott WN (New York: Grune and Stratton, 1987) 1–8.

19. **Rand JA, Coventry MB**, Stress fractures after total knee arthroplasty, *J Bone Joint Surg (Am)* (1980) **62**: 226–233.

20. **Hood RW, Vanni M, Insall JN**, The correction of knee alignment in 225 consecutive total condylar knee replacements, *Clin Orthop* (1981) **160**: 94–105.

21. **Ahlberg A, Linden B**, The radiolucent zone in arthroplasty of the knee, *Acta Orthop Scand* (1977) **48**: 687–690.

22. **Aglietti P, Rinonapoli E**, Total condylar knee arthroplasty: a five-year follow-up study of 33 knees, *Clin Orthop* (1984) **186**: 104–111.

23. **Insall JN, Hood RW, Flawn LB et al.**, The total condylar knee prosthesis in gonarthrosis: a five to nine-year follow-up of the first one hundred consecutive replacements, *J Bone Joint Surg (Am)* (1983) **65**: 619–628.

24. **Laskin RS**, Total condylar knee replacement in rheumatoid arthritis: a review of one hundred and seventeen knees, *J Bone Joint Surg (Am)* (1981) **63**: 29–35.

25. **Bargren JH, Blaha JD, Freeman MAR**, Alignment in total knee arthroplasty: correlated biomechanical and clinical observations, *Clin Orthop* (1983) **173**: 178–183.

26. **Cornell CN, Ranawat CS, Burstein AH**, A clinical and radiographic analysis of loosening of total knee arthroplasty components using a bilateral model, *J Arthroplasty* (1986) **1**: 157–163.

27. **Ducheyne P, Kagan A II, Lacey JA**, Failure of total knee arthroplasty due to loosening and deformation of the tibial component, *J Bone Joint Surg (Am)* (1978) **60**: 384–391.

28. **Insall JN**, Total knee replacement, *Surgery of the knee*, ed Insall JN (New York: Churchill Livingstone, 1984) 587–695.

29. **Lotke PA, Ecker ML**, Influence of positioning of prosthesis in total knee replacement, *J Bone Joint Surg (Am)* (1977) **59**: 77–79.

30. **Tew M, Waugh W**, Tibiofemoral alignment and results of knee replacement, *J Bone Joint Surg (Br)* (1985) **67**: 551–556.

31. **Cameron HU, Freeman MAR**, The radiolucent line around bone cement, *Acta Orthop Belg* (1979) **45**: 75–78.

17.5 A radiological study of alignment after total knee replacement: short radiographs or long radiographs?

Dipak V. Patel, Barry D. Ferris and Paul M. Aichroth

The importance of the axial alignment following total knee replacement is well recognized.[1-8] There is controversy concerning the best method of measuring this alignment radiologically. Some authors[9,10] recommend the use of long radiographs, whilst others have suggested that short radiographs are adequate.[11] We compared the short and long radiographs in patients who underwent posteriorly stabilized (Insall–Burstein) condylar knee arthroplasty.

Patients and methods

We measured the anatomical tibiofemoral angle on standard anteroposterior radiographs (12×16 inches) and on long-cassette radiographs (14×38 inches). There were 50 total knee replacement arthroplasties (27 right and 23 left) in 34 patients (24 females and 10 males). Twenty-two patients had osteoarthritis, 11 had rheumatoid arthritis and one had psoriatic arthritis. Their mean age at operation was 69.7 years (range 51–85 years) and the average follow-up was 38.4 months (range 24–74 months). All radiographs were taken with the patient standing and the patellae oriented anteriorly. Patients with flexion deformity at the knee were excluded from this study.

The anatomical tibiofemoral angle was measured by intersecting the femoral anatomical axis with that of the tibia. On the short radiographs, the femoral anatomical axis was found by locating and connecting two points that lie midway between the femoral cortex. One point was chosen as far proximal as the radiograph allowed and the other was chosen 10 cm above the joint-line.

The tibial axis was drawn in the same manner, with two points marked in the centre of the tibial cortex. The upper point was located 10 cm below the joint-line and the lower point was marked as far distal as the radiograph allowed.

On the long radiographs, the femoral axis was drawn by choosing points at the isthmus and at 10 cm proximal to the joint-line in the centre of the femoral cortex. The anatomical axis of the tibia was found by connecting points marked 10 cm distal to the joint-line and at the centre of the dome of the talus (Figure 1).

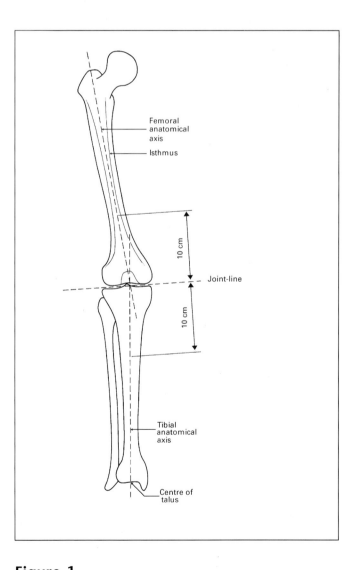

Figure 1

The method of measuring anatomical femoral and tibial axis on both short and long radiographs.

Results

The tibiofemoral angle on short radiographs was 5.3° ± 2.6° (mean ± SD) with a range from 1° varus to 12° valgus. On the long radiographs, the tibiofemoral angle was 6.9°±3° (mean ± SD) with a range from 2° varus to 14° valgus. There was no significant difference between these two groups of measurements. However, when the individual pairs of measurements were compared, they were found to be significantly different from each other ($P<0.0013$, Mann–Whitney U two-tailed test).

Discussion

In the present series, we found a discrepancy of 1.6° in measuring the anatomical tibiofemoral angles on both long and short radiographs. We agree with Petersen and Engh[10] that the short radiographs tend to underestimate the tibiofemoral angle. Dorr et al.[12] and Petersen and Engh[10] reported a similar difference of 1.9° and 1.4°, respectively. The mean difference of 1.6° in this series may seem insignificant. However, with a standard deviation of 2.6°, the short radiograph in any individual case could potentially underestimate tibiofemoral valgus by 6.8° or overestimate by 3.6° (1.6°±2SD = −3.6° to +6.8°).

Restoration of normal alignment following total knee replacement is essential for a successful result. We assumed acceptable alignment to be between 4° and 10° of valgus as suggested by Petersen and Engh[10] and found that on the short radiographs, 13 knees (26%) fell outside this range (10 were below 4° and 3 were above 10°). In comparison, measurements on long radiographs showed that 8 knees (16%) were outside the acceptable range (4 knees were below 4° and 4 were above 10°).

Our study has shown that there is significant difference in the measurement of the tibiofemoral angle on short and long radiographs when the pairs of measurements are compared in an individual case. The short radiographs tend to underestimate the tibiofemoral angle but for practical purposes are probably adequate for routine follow-up of knee replacements in a busy outpatient department.

However, for precise scientific documentation and comparison of studies, the long radiographs are desirable.

Acknowledgments

We are indebted to the Radiology Department of Westminster Hospital for their help with the radiographs. We are grateful to Miss Dina Stanford for her assistance with the computer analysis of the data.

References

1. **Aglietti P, Buzzi R,** Posteriorly stabilised total-condylar knee replacement: three to eight years' follow-up of 85 knees, *J Bone Joint Surg (Br)* (1988) **70:** 211–216.
2. **Bargren JH, Blaha JD, Freeman MAR,** Alignment in total knee arthroplasty: correlated biomechanical and clinical observations. *Clin Orthop* (1983) **173:** 178–183.
3. **Cornell CN, Ranawat CS, Burstein AH,** A clinical and radiographic analysis of loosening of total knee arthroplasty components using a bilateral model. *J Arthroplasty* (1986) **1:** 157–163.
4. **Dorr LD,** Complications: loosening of the cement–bone interface after total knee arthroplasty, *Total-condylar knee arthroplasty: technique, results and complications*, ed Ranawat CS (New York: Springer-Verlag, 1985) 173–185.
5. **Johnson F, Leitl S, Waugh W,** The distribution of load across the knee: a comparison of static and dynamic measurements, *J Bone Joint Surg (Br)* (1980) **62:** 346–349.
6. **Lotke PA, Ecker ML,** Influence of positioning of prosthesis in total knee replacement, *J Bone Joint Surg (Am)* (1977) **59:** 77–79.
7. **Tew M, Waugh W,** Tibiofemoral alignment and results of knee replacement, *J Bone Joint Surg (Br)* (1985) **67:** 551–556.
8. **Vince KG, Insall JN, Kelly MA,** The total condylar prosthesis: 10 to 12-year results of a cemented knee replacement, *J Bone Joint Surg (Br)* (1989) **71:** 793–797.
9. **Moreland JR, Bassett LW, Hanker GJ,** Radiographic analysis of the axial alignment of the lower extremity, *J Bone Joint Surg (Am)* (1987) **69:** 745–749.
10. **Petersen TL, Engh GA,** Radiographic assessment of knee alignment after total knee arthroplasty, *J Arthroplasty* (1988) **3**(1): 67–72.
11. **Kettelkamp DB, Chao EY,** A method for quantitative analysis of medial and lateral compression forces at the knee during standing, *Clin Orthop* (1972) **83:** 202–213.
12. **Dorr LD, Conaty JP, Schreiber R et al.,** Technical factors that influence mechanical loosening of total knee arthroplasty. *The Knee, Papers of the First Scientific Meeting of the Knee Society*, ed Dorr LD (Baltimore: University Park Press, 1985) 121–135.

17.6   The PFC knee

Paul W. Allen and George S.E. Dowd

Principles

The PFC (press-fit condylar) total knee is a surface replacement, with a variety of components, which allows the prosthetic replacement of most primary or revision knees. The system is modular, which offers the choice of posterior cruciate retention or resection. The femoral component is made of cobalt–chrome, which has good wear characteristics, as it is an articulating component, whilst the tibial tray is made of a titanium alloy, for a better modulus of elasticity. The tibial insert and the patellar component are made of high-density polyethylene.

Components

Femoral component

The femoral component is available in primary cruciate retaining or sacrificing versions. The standard cruciate retaining component is available in six sizes from 50 mm A/P × 54 mm M/L to 74 mm A/P × 78 mm M/L. This femoral component may articulate with either of the posterior cruciate retaining tibial insert types. There is a range of tibial tray sizes that fit with each femoral size, allowing good coverage of the femur and tibia even if the latter are of slightly different sizes. The component is provided with two fixation lugs and is available in a porous coated or non-porous coated form. This component is not compatible with the augmentation or stem extension modules.

The primary posterior cruciate sacrificing component is designed to accommodate the condylar augmentation and modular stem extensions and includes a 'box' to house the tibial spine of the posterior cruciate sacrificing tray. This box has a cam feature on its posterior aspect to interact with the tibial spine and prevent roll-back. The stem extensions are fixed to a hole in the roof of the box (Figure 1).

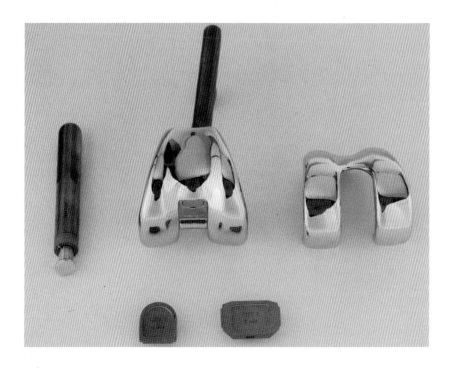

Figure 1

Both femoral components. Cruciate sparing on right, cruciate sacrificing on left with stem extension in place; augmentation wedges in foreground.

Tibial component

The tibial component is available in seven widths. The tray can be used in its standard form for either posterior cruciate preserving or sacrificing knees. There is a cylindrical keel with a slight proximal–distal taper to make removal easier in revision. The keel has a 3° posterior tilt when viewed in the sagittal plane. This allows proper coverage of the upper tibia with central placement of the stem extensions. There are medial, lateral and posterior fins to support the tray and to resist rotation. The trays are available in either normal or porous coated form.

Stem extensions attach to the distal end of the standard stem, which is supplied fitted with a polyethylene plug to seal off the end. The extensions screw into a thread that is exposed when the plug is removed. The extensions are available with large rounded flutes for cemented use, or with sharp flutes to press fit into the tibial canal. The cemented stem extensions are available in two diameters, 13 mm and 15 mm, and in 30- and 60-mm lengths. The larger-diameter variants are to be used with the size 3, 4 and 5 trays. The press-fit stems are available in a larger variety of sizes and do not need to match a particular tray size. They are offered in diameters from 10 to 24 mm and three lengths, 75, 115 and 150 mm (Figure 2).

There is a variety of tibial inserts. All are made of high-molecular-weight polyethylene and snap into the tibial tray. There are two major groups, primary posterior cruciate preserving and primary posterior cruciate resecting. There are two primary posterior cruciate preserving components, the curved and the posterior lipped. The curved component has a higher spine and deeper dishing than the posterior lipped insert, providing additional stability as there is greater congruity between the femoral component and the tibial tray.

There are also two posterior cruciate resection tibial inserts, the stabilized and the constrained. The stabilized component has a lower spine but this is high enough to interact with the cam on the femoral component to resist posterior subluxation. The constrained component is designed for use in knees in which there is a degree of ligamentous instability, and the spine is higher and wider, thus providing some control of varus and valgus stress. The spine is reinforced with a titanium pin in the spine which extends into the keel of the tray when the insert is assembled into the tray. There is a hole for the pin in each tray.

Patellar component

The patellar component is available in different forms for the posterior cruciate retaining and posterior cruciate sacrificing versions. The posterior cruciate retaining patellar component is a modified dome in cross-section and oval when viewed in the coronal plane. It is fixed with cement and has three lugs and a Y-shaped undercut cement groove on its posterior aspect. It is available in three sizes, 35, 38 and 41 mm.

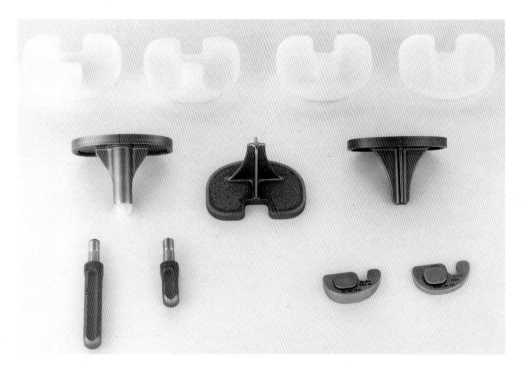

Figure 2

Tibial trays, inserts, stems and wedges. Inserts at top, constrained, stabilized, curved and posterior lipped (from left to right). Trays in centre, stems and wedges in foreground.

The posterior cruciate sacrificing component is hemispherical in shape and sits more deeply in the patellofemoral groove than its posterior cruciate retaining counterpart. The groove on the posterior cruciate sacrificing component is deeper as well. There is a single central peg and an undercut on the posterior surface of the component. This button is available in four sizes: 32, 35, 38 and 41 mm diameters.

The PFC knee may be used with the Mikhail patella, which is similar in cross-section to the posterior cruciate sacrificing component but has a different method of insertion and is available in 25- and 32-mm sizes.

These implants are only available for cemented implantation and are not metal-backed. There have been a number of reports of problems with the separation of the polyethylene from the metal backing and of excessive wear of the polyethylene to expose the metal[1] in joints with a cementless, metal-backed patellar component.

Instrumentation

Femoral

As with most modern total knee systems, the PFC utilizes an intramedullary guide system for the accurate and reproducible implantation of the femoral component (Figure 3). There is provision for the use of a varying degree of valgus, by using 5°, 7° or 9° bushings. The intramedullary alignment may be checked using an extramedullary jig if required. After the distal femoral cut has been made, it is possible to check the size of the femoral component needed in an AP dimension by using a stylus on the jig. Thus, it may be ensured that the planned anterior femoral cut will not notch the anterior cortex; if this were likely to happen, the next size of femoral block would be selected.

The rotation of the anterior–posterior guide is controlled by the size checking jig; after the anterior and posterior cuts are made the chamfer is cut using the appropriate cutting block.

The instruments for the posterior cruciate sacrificing femoral component are initially exactly the same size as the instruments for the cruciate preserving component. The anterior–posterior cutting block is different and is set up on the guide hole used for the intramedullary rod. The block is movable in an AP direction to allow the stylus to ensure that the anterior femoral cortex is not notched.

Once the anterior and posterior cuts are made, the notch cut is made using a simple jig, then the chamfer cut is performed. The two types of femoral component are of the same size and the decision to change from one to the other may be delayed until the femur is almost fully prepared. The notch cutting guide may be used on a femur prepared with the posterior cruciate retaining instruments if it is found necessary to excise the posterior cruciate at a later stage.

Tibial

Both intramedullary and extramedullary tibial instruments are available. They may be used with either posterior cruciate preserving or sacrificing tibial components as the tray is the same but the insert is different. There are tibial blocks to allow the resection of a 5° posterior slope if this is needed for a knee with a residual flexion tightness. The ordinary blocks

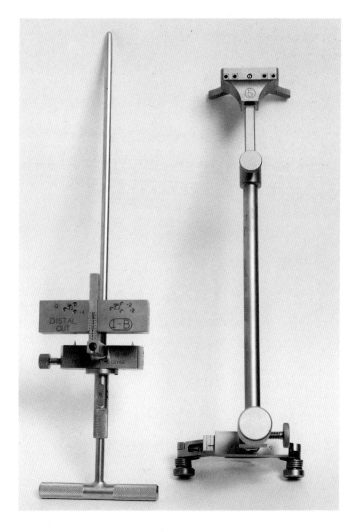

Figure 3

Cutting guides. Intramedullary femoral (left); extramedullary tibial (right).

allow for the resection of 2 mm more or less bone by moving them on the pins transfixing them to the bone.

The tibial stem is inserted into a drill hole in the upper tibia, which is shaped for the tibial fins with a keel punch. The length of the stem is variable.

As with most other surface knee systems, there is a full range of trial implants to allow the selection of the correct size and thickness of components. A trial tibial insert is utilized while the cement is setting and may be easily removed to allow access to the back of the joint for cement removal. This same trial tibial insert is used, after the definitive insertion of the metal femoral and tibial components, to recheck the stability of the knee in flexion and extension. A final check on the correct tibial insert thickness is, thus, possible just prior to implantation.

Patella

The patella is available with three pegs or with a single central peg. The patellar surface is cut and drilled with two simple jigs. It has been suggested that tilting of the patella can predispose to failure.[2]

This problem may be addressed by utilizing the Mikhail patella, which is compatible with the PFC knee. Different instruments are required for this alternative implant. The median ridge is excised and a threaded guide-wire is drilled into the centre of the patella where the bone is thickest, and the patellar hole is then reamed using a reamer over the guide-wire. This allows the easy insertion of the component perpendicular to the mid axis of the patella.

General

The operation is facilitated by the utilization of the Mikhail knee retractors, which help to maintain the tibia subluxed forward and the patella subluxed laterally throughout the procedure. In addition, they provide protection for the posterior cruciate and the collateral ligaments during the division of the posterior femoral condyles.

Modularity

Posterior cruciate retention

The PFC system is modular, as the components are of the same size for the posterior cruciate retaining as well as the posterior cruciate resecting system. The instruments are the same, allowing a decision regarding posterior cruciate retention to be made at the last possible moment. The femur may be prepared with the posterior cruciate retaining instruments, and only the notch cutting guide from the posterior cruciate sacrificing set is required if a late decision is taken to excise the posterior cruciate.

Stems

There are stems of differing lengths available for the tibial components of both systems but the posterior cruciate sacrificing femoral component is the only one available with a stem. These stems simply screw into the components and are tightened with the wrench provided. The additional stem length is reamed during preparation of the appropriate bone.

Wedges

A number of wedges are available to allow augmentation of the standard components to compensate for defects in the bony architecture. There are tibial wedges of two sizes, hemiwedges and quadrant wedges, each available in 10° or 15° sizes. These wedges must be held in place with bone cement prior to implantation; there is an undercut segment of the tibial tray to allow the wedge to be securely fixed. A different tibial cutting block guides an angled cut on one side to allow the wedge to fit. There is biomechanical evidence to support the use of tibial wedges rather than cement, with or without screws, for the management of bone defects.[3]

Femoral condyle augmentation

There are blocks to fill defects in the distal femur or the posterior condyles. These snap into place on prepared sites on the femoral component. It should be noted that, once attached, the femoral component augmentation devices are not removable. Combination blocks are available to fill both distal and posterior defects. These may be particularly useful in revision surgery. Trials are available for these blocks to allow accurate sizing before implantation.

Size compatibility

There is size compatibility across the range of tibial and femoral sizes with the posterior cruciate preserving components, i.e. a size-5 tibial implant may be used with a size-1 femur, although this is an unlikely choice. With the posterior sacrificing components, it is not yet possible to 'mix and match' in this way, although components allowing this feature are under trial.

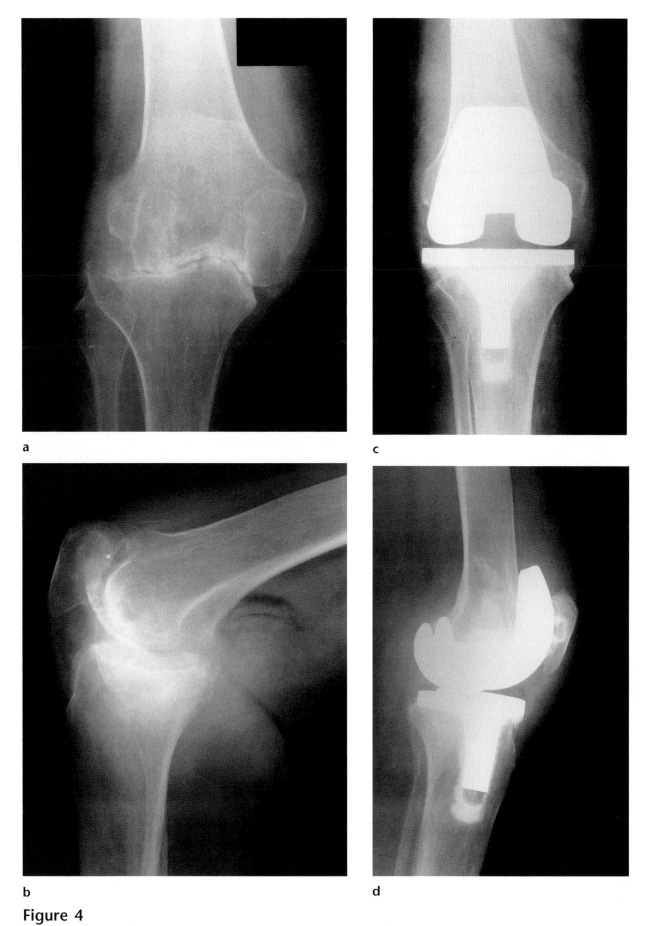

a

b

c

d

Figure 4

(a) Preoperative AP and (b) lateral radiographs. (c) Postoperative AP and (d) lateral radiographs. Posterior cruciate sacrificing components with stabilized 10-mm insert in rheumatoid subluxed knee.

Cement vs no cement

Porous coating

It is inadvisable to use a porous coated component for cemented use. If revision is required, there will be a problem in separating the component from the cement, and consequently bone loss may occur as the component is removed. The PFC system provides femoral components with or without porous coating to allow the choice to be made. It should, however, be noted that there is no recommendation for cementless implantation of any of these components by the FDA.

On the tibial side, there is a similar choice; the porous coated tray is identical to the normal tray, but is coated on the tray surface with sintered Ti-6Al-4V beads, but not coated on the keel or stem. There are two screw holes in the tray located on the medial and lateral sides, and there are recesses in the tray to allow the screws to be encased proximally and distally. The screw holes allow for tilt of the screws of up to 15°. The tray is not coated in the region of the screws, to make the tray stronger at this site. The porous coated tray will accept the full range of tibial extensions and inserts, but is incompatible with the tibial wedges.

The holes in the tray accept 6.0-mm cobalt–chrome alloy cancellous bone screws in lengths of 15–45 mm.

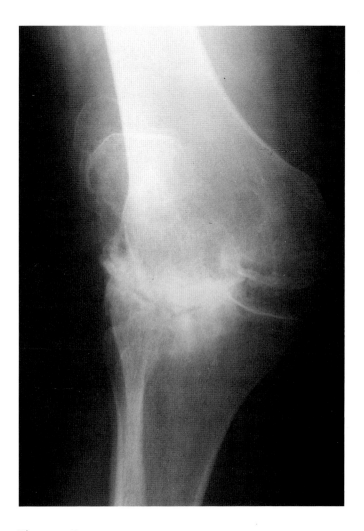

Figure 5

Preoperative radiograph of a 70-year-old woman with osteoarthritis of the knee with gross valgus deformity.

Soft tissues

The satisfactory implantation of a total knee replacement is dependent on an understanding of the soft tissues. Alignment should be corrected by treating any soft-tissue imbalance rather than by bone cuts. This aspect of surface knee replacement is not dependent on the type of prosthesis used. The correct provision of an equal flexion and extension gap is also essential and depends on the cutting jigs. Soft-tissue balancing requires the appropriate releases to be made during surgery. This may be carried out as part of the initial approach to the knee or later during the procedure if imbalance is demonstrated.

Results

This prosthesis is relatively new and, as a consequence, there is relatively little information regarding the results. Recent reports are, by necessity, of short-term follow-up. The first procedure was performed in late 1984. The first 193 cases carried out before the end of 1986 have now been studied at 2 years, with 97% of patients experiencing no pain. There has been one case of tibial component loosening and another

of both components becoming loose; these have been revised.[4] These results are comparable to other series and long-term studies are awaited.

A further study involving the PFC knee has been produced, reviewing the results from 2–4 years after 'hybrid' knee replacement, that is using a cemented tibial and cementless femoral component. The results demonstrate relief of pain in 94% of cases, a range of movement of greater than 100° in 81%, and no evidence of significant loosening.[5]

Problems

There are few problems with the PFC total knee replacement. It provides a reasonably integrated system for primary and revision knee arthroplasty with posterior cruciate retention or sacrifice.

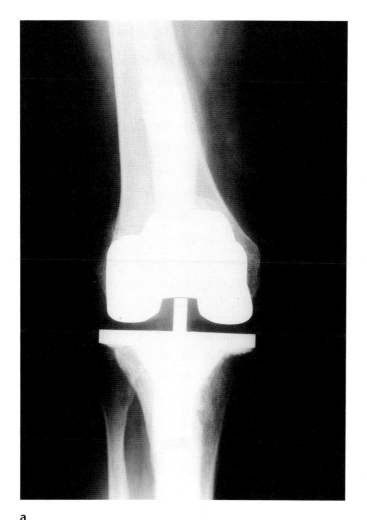
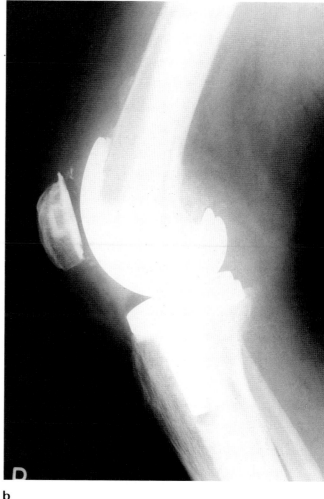

a   b

Figure 6

Postoperative radiographs showing the modular PFC total knee replacement (courtesy of Mr Paul Aichroth and Mr Dipak Patel).

The limitation of size mismatch in the posterior cruciate sacrificing prostheses can be a problem, but this is being addressed. The use of cement to fix the tibial wedges takes rather longer than other forms of fixation.

Summary

The PFC total knee replacement concept offers a versatile, modular system which makes it easy to use even in the complex primary (Figure 4) or revision procedure. There is a wide range of options with variable tibial stems and wedges; stems may be added to the femoral component (Figures 5 and 6). The instrumentation allows reliable, repeatable cuts to be made. The similarity of the components and instrumentation throughout the range allows the decision regarding the retention or sacrifice of the posterior cruciate ligament to be made during the procedure.

References

1. Bayley JC, Scott RD, Ewald FC et al., Failure of the metal-backed patellar component after total knee replacement, *J Bone Joint Surg (Am)* (1988) **70:** 668–674.

2. Stulberg SD, Stulberg BN, Hamati Y et al., Failure mechanisms of metal-backed patellar components, *Clin Orthop* (1988) **236:** 88–105.

3. Brooks PJ, Walker PS, Scott RD, Tibial component fixation in deficient tibial bone stock, *Clin Orthop* (1984) **184:** 302–308.

4. Scott RD and Thornhill TS, Press-fit condylar total knee replacement, *Orthop Clin North Am* (1989) **20:** 89–95.

5. Wright RJ, Lima J, Scott RD et al., 2–4 Year results of posterior cruciate sparing condylar total knee arthroplasty with an uncemented femoral component, *Clin Orthop* (1990) **260:** 80–86.

17.7   Adjustments following the insertion of trial prostheses during total knee arthroplasty surgery

Carroll A. Laurin and David Zukor

In a total knee arthroplasty, the insertion of trial prostheses always precedes the implantation of the definitive implants. It is the best and the last opportunity to verify alignment, range of motion and stability. If all three are acceptable the definitive prostheses are inserted and the wound is closed. Regrettably, this does not always happen and adjustments are then necessary. The rationale of these adjustments is the subject of this contribution.

Adjustments, when necessary, because of malalignment, instability and/or loss of motion, can be made by revising the periarticular soft tissues and/or the bone cuts (or by changing the size and/or design of the implant). Malalignment should always be corrected first. Once the alignments (tibiofemoral and patellofemoral), have been verified (and corrected when necessary), the range of motion and stability should be checked; both will be normal as long as the space, or the gap, between the femur and the tibia corresponds exactly to the dimension, or size, of the implant throughout the range of motion (Figure 1).

Once the femoral and tibial cuts have been completed, the flexion gap (Figure 1) is the space between the posterior coronal cut on the distal femur and the transverse cut on the proximal tibia, while the knee is in flexion. The extension gap (Figure 1) is the space between the transverse cut on the distal femur and the transverse proximal tibial cut while the knee is in complete extension.

The design of most modern implants is such that, if the flexion and extension gaps are correct and equal, with the trial prostheses in place, the range of motion will be complete and the knee will be stable in flexion and in extension. However, following the insertion of the trial prostheses, it may be noted that the gap in flexion and/or in extension may be either too small (with resultant loss of motion), or too large (with resultant instability) (Figures 2 and 3).

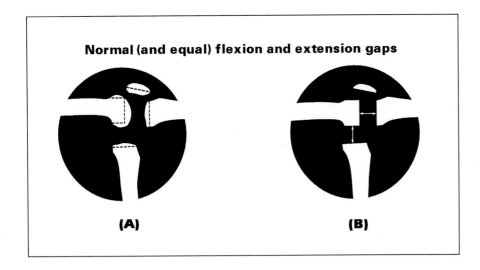

Normal (and equal) flexion and extension gaps

(A)   (B)

Figure 1

The normal knee has a full range of motion and is stable in flexion and extension because the flexion and extension gaps are equal (A). Following soft-tissue adjustments and after the bone cuts (B), the flexion and extension gaps must also be equal so that, following the insertion of the trial prostheses, the range of motion is full and the knee is stable in flexion and in extension. The flexion gap is the space between the posterior coronal cut on the distal femur and the transverse cut on the proximal tibia when the knee is in flexion. The extension gap is the space between the transverse cut on the distal femur and the transverse cut on the proximal tibia when the knee is in complete extension.

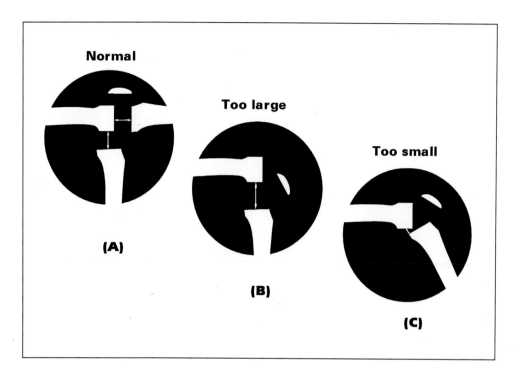

Figure 2

Different flexion gaps. The flexion gap is normal if it is equal to the extension gap (A); following insertion of the trial prostheses, the range of flexion is then normal and the knee is stable in flexion. If the flexion gap is too large (B), the knee is unstable in flexion; on the other hand, if the flexion gap is too small (or too tight) (C), there is loss of flexion.

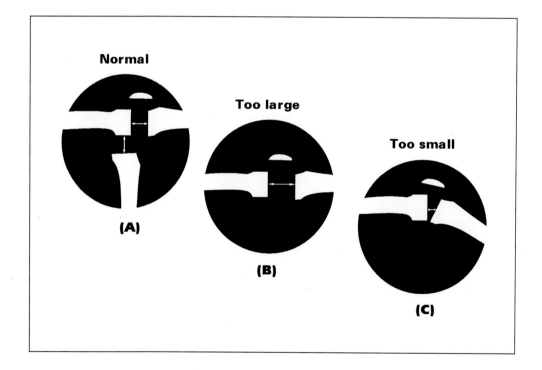

Figure 3

Different extension gaps. The extension gap is normal if it is equal to the flexion gap (A); following insertion of the trial prostheses, the range of extension is then normal and the knee is stable in extension. If the extension gap is too large (B), the knee is unstable in full extension. If the extension gap is too small (or too tight) (C), the knee does not extend completely.

One must also consider the association of different gap problems in flexion and in extension (Figure 4); for example, the extension gap may be too large, with resultant instability in extension, while the flexion gap may be too small, with resultant loss of flexion.

In fact, excluding malalignment problems, there are nine possible permutations (see Figure 5). The flexion gap may be too large (1), in association with an extension gap that is either too large (1–A), too small (or too tight) (1–B) or correct (i.e. just right) (1–C). On the other hand, the flexion gap may be too small (2) in association with an extension gap which is either too large (2–A), too small (2–B), or correct (2–C). Finally, the flexion gap may be correct (3), while the extension gap is either too large (3–A), too small (3–B), or correct (3–C). Only the last situation (i.e. 3–C) is acceptable, while eight of the above nine scenarios are unacceptable.

Since the gap problems may be corrected (Figure 6) by lengthening or shortening soft tissues, by removing bone or adding 'bone' (with a thicker implant or by adding more cement) or by combination of any of the above, there are numerous solutions for different incorrect gap problems. The situation is further complicated by the fact that any adjustments to improve motion in extension can cause instability in flexion and vice versa (Figure 7). For example, an extension gap that is too small with loss of extension, and which has been made larger by incorrectly removing more tibia, will normalize the extension gap but it will also enlarge the flexion gap, with resultant instability in flexion (which did not exist prior to the adjustment; Figure 7(1)).

The following system is an attempt to ensure that the right adjustments are made in the correct sequence. The system may be paraphrased as 'three

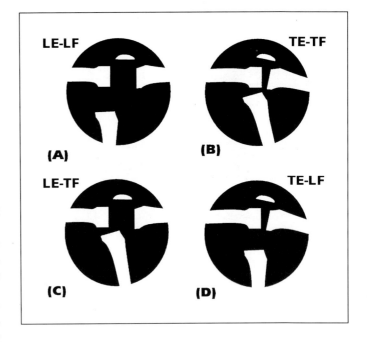

Figure 4

Different gap problems. The gap problems in flexion and in extension are not necessarily identical, i.e. they may be abnormal in extension and/or in flexion and various permutations are possible (see Figure 5). Following insertion of the trial prostheses, the knee may be loose in extension and loose in flexion (A) when both flexion and extension gaps are too large; on the other hand, the knee may be tight in extension and tight in flexion (B), with loss of flexion and extension when both gaps are too small. The knee may also be loose in extension and tight in flexion (C) if the extension gap is too large and the flexion gap is too small; or the knee may be unstable in flexion and too tight in extension (D), with instability in flexion and loss of extension.

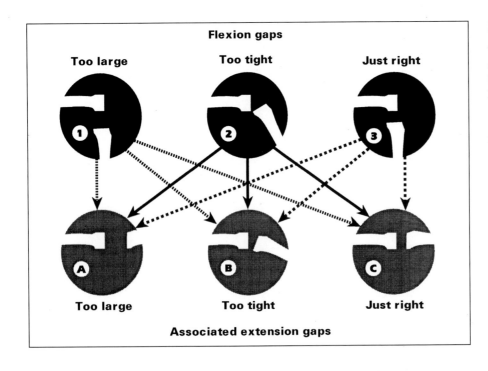

Figure 5

There are nine possible permutations (1A, 1B, 1C, 2A, 2B, 2C, 3A, 3B, 3C) between different flexion gaps (too large (1), too tight (2) or just right (3)), and different extension gaps (too large (A), too tight (B) or just right (C)). Only 3C is acceptable.

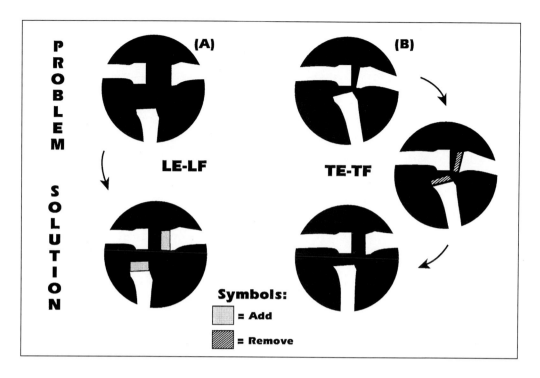

Figure 6

Adjustments following insertion of trial prostheses. Two different symbols will be used to indicate whether the incorrect large gap (A) situation, loose in extension and loose in flexion, is corrected by adding bone (or by inserting a thicker trial prosthesis), or whether a small gap (B), tight in extension and tight in flexion, is corrected by removing more bone or inserting a thinner prosthesis.

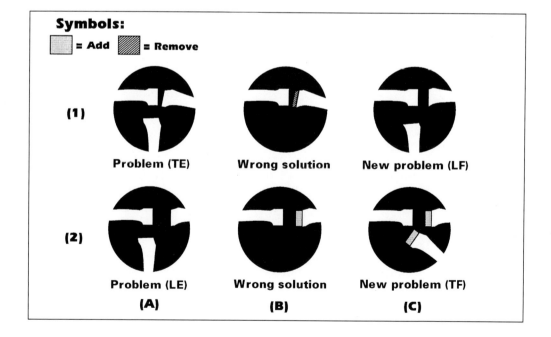

Figure 7

Incorrect solutions. If a gap problem (A) is solved incorrectly (B) (usually by correcting the extension gap first), the result is a new problem (C) that did not exist prior to the adjustment. The top (tight in extension, TE) problem (1A) was a small extension gap (the flexion gap was normal) that was erroneously corrected by removing more tibia (1B), with resultant new instability in flexion (loose in flexion, LF) (1C). The bottom (loose in extension, LE) problem (2A) was a knee that was loose in extension (the flexion gap was normal) (due to a large extension gap) that was incorrectly managed by building up the tibia (2B), which resulted in loss of flexion (tight in flexion, TF) because of a flexion gap which then became too small (2C).

firsts and a *must*': while the 'must' is a reminder that one *must* make a complete diagnosis which refers to both gap situations, the three 'firsts' are the mechanical axis, the soft-tissue adjustments and the flexion gap.

Following insertion of the trial prostheses, the *first* verification is alignment, the single most important factor for long-term survival of the arthroplasty. Since any adjustments to correct malalignment will inevitably affect range of motion and stability, they should be performed first.

The second 'first' refers to soft-tissue adjustments, which must always be made before bone is re-cut; for example, if the extension gap is too small (i.e. the knee does not extend normally), it is vital to release the soft-tissue structures posteriorly (and remove any osteophytes when present) before removing more bone. It will be shown that whether bone is then removed from the femur or the tibia, to improve knee extension, depends on the associated flexion gap problem.

The third 'first' refers to the flexion gap, which should always be normalized first, i.e. before the extension gap. The obvious reason is that the transverse proximal tibial cut affects both gaps while the distal femoral cut affects only the extension gap. It will be shown later (Figure 13) that when both gap problems are incorrect and one inadvertently normalizes the extension gap first, subsequent adjustments to normalize the flexion gap status will create new problems in extension, and the extension gap must again be normalized (i.e. three adjustments). On the other hand, if one normalizes the flexion gap first (e.g. Figure 14), subsequent adjustments of the extension gap, if necessary, will suffice (i.e. two adjustments).

The 'must' refers to the fact that one must make a complete diagnosis and always refer to the status of both gap situations, and not merely refer to one gap problem only. In other words, it is insufficient to diagnose, for example, a small flexion gap problem; one must also refer to the associated extension gap status: if the knee cannot flex normally and is unstable in extension, the correct diagnosis is a small flexion gap and a large extension gap. It would be incorrect (and, as we shall see, misleading) merely to refer to the small flexion gap with loss of knee flexion.

Insertion of the trial prosthesis

If, following the insertion of the trial prostheses, the knee is noted, for example, to be unstable in extension, the possible causes of this instability may be excessive (pathological or iatrogenic) ligament lengthening or excessive removal of bone from the femur, the tibia or both. Which one is it? If one

builds up the tibia when, in fact, the problem is on the femoral side, the surgeon will automatically also decrease the size of the flexion gap and hence the range of knee flexion. One will have then created a new problem that did not exist prior to the adjustment.

The system will be elucidated by dealing with the nine potential scenarios (Figure 5): a flexion gap that is either too large, too small or correct, with an associated extension gap that is too large, too small or correct. One arrives at the same scenarios by considering the extension gap problems that may be associated with the three possible flexion gaps (i.e. refer to Figure 5 and merely reverse the direction of the arrows).

Since one should always normalize the flexion gap first, the scenarios will be considered as variants of three flexion gaps (i.e. too large, too small or correct).

Large flexion gap (instability in flexion)

Let us first consider a knee which is unstable in flexion, i.e. in which the flexion gap is too large (Figure 8). This may be due to a tibial cut which was too distal or, more rarely, to a posterior femoral coronal cut which was too anterior, i.e. removing too much posterior femoral condyle. The associated extension gap may be too large, too small or just right (Figure 8).

If both gaps are too large (Figure 8A) (i.e. the knee is unstable in flexion and in extension), building up the tibia, usually by inserting a thicker trial tibial prosthesis, will suffice since correcting the flexion gap will also correct the extension gap. A similar correction could also be achieved by inserting a larger femoral implant which is thicker distally and posteriorly; however, tibial height adjustments are easier to insert and assess.

On the other hand, if the flexion gap is too large (unstable in flexion) while the extension gap is too small (Figure 8B) (i.e. the knee cannot extend fully), building up the tibia will stabilize the knee in flexion but it will further restrict knee extension. The adjustments are, therefore, then completed by re-cutting the femur more proximally; unlike the previous situation, when only the tibial cut was incorrect, the femoral and tibial cuts were, in this instance, both incorrect and both had to be revised (the flexion gap being normalized first, as always).

The third possibility is a large flexion gap, i.e. a knee that is unstable in flexion but which extends normally and is stable in extension (Figure 8C); i.e. the extension gap is correct. If the instability in flexion is mild, it should be accepted, since the range of motion is normal, the knee is stable in extension, and any revision of the tibial height (to stabilize the flexion gap) will alter the normal extension gap. However, if the instability in flexion is gross, it

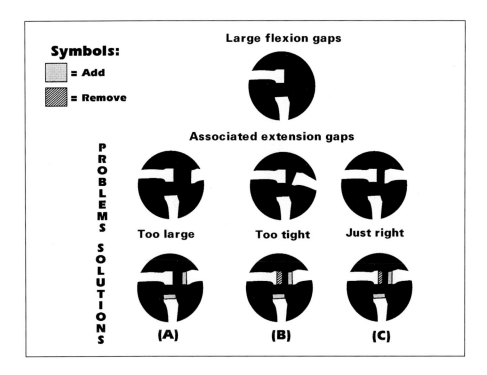

Figure 8

Large flexion gaps (instability in flexion). Correcting the flexion gap first by adjusting the tibial height will automatically also affect the extension gap. Hence, if the extension and flexion gaps are both too large (A), building up the tibia will usually suffice. If the associated extension gap is too small (or too tight) (B), building up the tibia to normalize the flexion gap will further limit knee extension (B), and bone must then be removed from the distal femur to normalize the extension gap. If the large flexion gap is associated with a normal extension gap (C), the latter becomes abnormal after the flexion gap has been normalized (by building up the tibia) and femoral bone must be removed (but less than for the knee (B) that already had a small extension gap). Note that although all three knees (second row) were loose in flexion, the solution to the problems varied and the correct solution to the flexion gap problem could only be identified by referring to the associated extension gap situation.

should be corrected by inserting a thicker tibial implant; the resultant loss of extension is then corrected by re-cutting the distal femur more proximally.

Small flexion gaps (loss of knee flexion)

The causes of incomplete knee flexion are: (1) a tibial cut that is too proximal (Figure 9A,B,C) (the tibial cut may be too proximal and perpendicular to the tibial axis or it may not have a sufficient posterior slope, i.e. the tibial cut is then too proximal posteriorly); (2) a posterior femoral coronal cut which is inadequate, i.e. too posterior (Figure 9D) (thus leaving too much posterior femoral condyle); (3) an anterior femoral coronal cut which is inadequate, i.e. too anterior (Figure 9E); or (4) a patellar cut which is too superficial (Figure 9F), with a resultant increase in total patellar thickness (bone and implant). The latter two, incorrect bone cuts (Figure 9E,F) will only decrease

knee flexion after the patella has been reduced. It is, therefore, important to verify the range of knee flexion, before and after relocating the patella, since the causes of loss of knee flexion are different.

Following insertion of trial prostheses, there are five incorrect bone cuts (the three femoral cuts, the tibial cut and the patellar cut) which may limit knee flexion. Which one is it? The answer will become clear by making a complete diagnosis, i.e. by assessing the associated extension gap status, which may be too small, too large or just right.

If the knee cannot flex and is loose in extension (Figure 9A), both transverse bone cuts, i.e. femoral and tibial, must be revised. It will be shown in a moment that, whenever the gap problems are diametrically opposite (e.g. tight in flexion and loose in extension, or vice versa), the tibial and femoral transverse cuts are both wrong. The knee is first normalized in flexion by recutting the tibia more distally (or inserting a thinner tibial prosthesis); this correction will increase the instability in extension, which is then corrected by building up the femur

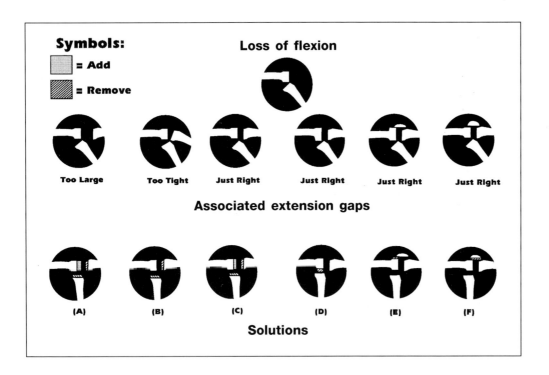

Figure 9

Small flexion gaps (loss of flexion). Loss of flexion is usually due to a small flexion gap and the loss of flexion is then noted prior to relocating the patella (A,B,C,D). Excessive tension on the extensor mechanism because of an excessively anterior femoral coronal cut (E) or a thick patella (F) will only restrict flexion after the patella has been reduced. Whenever the flexion gap is normalized by changing the tibial cut (A,B,C), the extension gap will automatically be modified by that correction; the extension gap will then become abnormal (i.e. too large), requiring build-up of the femur (A,C) (unless both problem gaps were small, e.g. B). Correcting the flexion gap by revising the posterior coronal cut will not modify the extension gap problem (D), nor will achieving normal flexion by revising the anterior femoral coronal cut (E), or the patellar cut (F); hence, no femoral gap adjustments were necessary for the latter three scenarios of loss of flexion (D,E,F).

distally only (i.e. with cement, bone graft, or by using a femoral prosthesis which is thicker distally only).

If the knee cannot flex and cannot extend (Figure 9B), re-cutting the tibia more distally (or inserting a thinner tibial implant) will usually correct both gap problems and should suffice.

The third scenario is a knee which cannot flex and is normal in extension (Figure 9C,D,E,F). This situation may be due to a transverse tibial cut which is too proximal (or with an inadequate posterior slope) (Figure 9C), to a posterior femoral coronal cut which is insufficient, i.e. too posterior (Figure 9D), to an anterior femoral cut which is inadequate, i.e. too anterior (Figure 9E), or to a patella which is too thick (Figure 9F). The latter two scenarios (Figure 9E,F) will only be noted after relocating the patella and revising either cut will not alter the extension gap status (Figure 9E,F). Similarly, if the loss of knee flexion was due to a posterior femoral coronal cut which was too posterior (Figure 9D), revising that cut will normalize knee flexion without affecting the already normal extension gap.

On the other hand, if the loss of flexion was due to a transverse tibial cut which was too proximal (Figure 9C) (the joint-line is then too proximal and the transverse femoral and tibial cuts are both wrong), the extension gap will become too large, with instability in extension, after the tibial cut has been revised to achieve normal knee flexion. If the loss of flexion was due to a tibial cut which had an inadequate posterior slope, re-cutting the tibia more distally to achieve normal flexion will cause instability either in extension or hyperextension due to laxity of the posterior capsular structures. Therefore, once the flexion gap status has been normalized by re-cutting the tibia, the resultant instability in extension is corrected by building up the femur distally, i.e. with cement or by inserting a femoral implant which is thicker distally. The situation is in fact similar to the scenario noted when the knee was loose in extension but could not flex normally (Figure 9A). In both instances (but to different degrees) (Figure 9A,C) the joint-line was too distal, the femoral and tibial cuts were incorrect and both had to be revised.

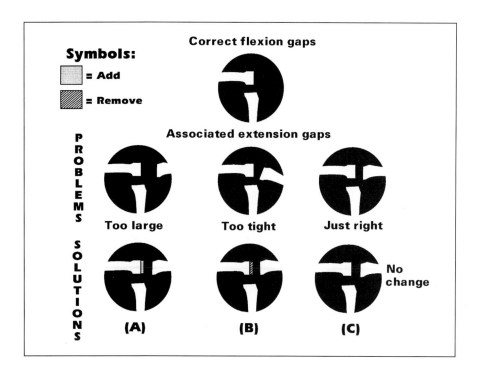

Figure 10

A correct flexion gap, when associated with an abnormal extension gap, corresponds to an isolated extension gap problem, i.e. A and B; if the extension gap is too large (A), building up the distal femur will suffice; if the extension gap is too small (B), with incomplete extension, re-cutting the distal femur more proximally will suffice. If the correct flexion gap is associated with a correct extension gap (C) (i.e. both gaps are correct and equal), the knee is stable in flexion and extension, there is a normal range of motion, no adjustments are necessary and the trial prosthesis may be replaced by the definitive prosthesis.

Correct flexion gap

We have considered flexion gaps which were too large and flexion gaps which were too loose. Let us now envisage the possible scenarios in association with a flexion gap which, following insertion of the trial implants, is correct (Figure 10).

If the associated extension gap is also correct (Figure 10C), there is no problem with range of motion or with stability and the trial implants need only be replaced by the definitive implants. On the other hand, the associated extension gap may be too large (the knee is then unstable in extension) (Figure 10A) or too small (the knee then cannot extend fully with a resultant knee flexion deformity) (Figure 10B). Since the flexion gap is normal, we are then dealing, in both instances, with an isolated extension gap problem (Figure 11). Both will be corrected by simply revising the distal femoral cut, which will have no effect on the already normal flexion gap. Loss of full extension (presuming, of course, that posterior soft tissues

have already been lengthened to their maximum), will be corrected by re-cutting the femur more proximally (Figure 10B). On the other hand, if the knee is normal, except for instability in extension, building up the femur distally (by using cement or inserting a femoral prosthesis that is thicker distally only) will correct the unduly large extension gap (Figure 10A).

Discussion

Following insertion of the trial prostheses, the possible incorrect scenarios are a knee which does not flex and/or does not extend normally, or a knee which is unstable in extension and/or in flexion, i.e. range of motion and/or stability problems. The nine permutations of the above possibilities require different adjustments that can only be identified by first making a complete diagnosis that refers to both gap situations.

Large flexion gaps

A large flexion gap (Figure 8) may be associated with an extension gap which may be too large (unstable in extension), too small (loss of extension), or correct (normal extension and stable in extension). When both gaps are too large, building up a tibia will usually suffice. However, if the large flexion gap is associated with a small extension gap (Figure 8B), or, indeed, with a normal extension gap (Figure 8C), we are then dealing with diametrically opposite situations (i.e. the flexion gap status and the extension gap status are different). When the gap problems are different, both tibial and femoral cuts are wrong. Since we must always normalize the flexion gap first, inserting a thicker tibial implant will stabilize the knee in flexion but will decrease knee extension, which is then corrected by re-cutting the distal femur more proximally.

Small flexion gaps

The second flexion scenario is a small flexion gap (i.e. loss of flexion) (Figure 9); if it is associated with loss of extension, resecting more tibia (or inserting a thinner tibial implant) should normalize both gaps. If gap problems are opposite, i.e. a small flexion gap and a large extension gap, both cuts are incorrect, and the flexion gap should be corrected first. Re-cutting the tibia to increase flexion will increase instability in extension, which, in turn, is corrected by building up the femur.

Whenever the knee cannot flex completely but is normal in extension (i.e. small flexion gap with a normal extension gap), the range of flexion should be verified before and after reducing the patella. If loss of knee flexion is only noted after reducing the patella, normal flexion will be achieved by revising either the anterior femoral coronal cut or the patellar cut. If the loss of flexion is noted in the absence of a relocated patella, the posterior coronal cut is possibly the cause of loss of flexion and its revision will not alter the normal extension gap status. Another cause of loss of flexion (noted with the patella in the dislocated position) is a tibial cut which is too proximal or in recurvatum, i.e. with an inadequate posterior slope. The correction, by re-cutting the tibia to achieve normal flexion, will increase the extension gap with a resultant instability in extension; the latter is then an isolated extension gap problem and building up the femur will suffice.

Correct flexion gap

The final scenario is a flexion gap which is correct (Figure 10) but is associated with an extension gap which may be too large or too small. Since we are

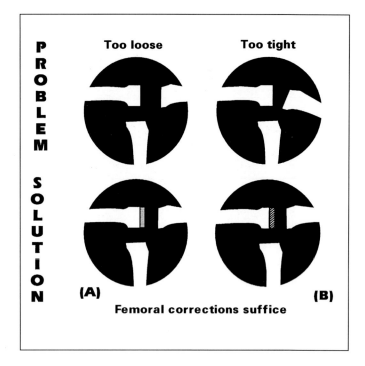

Figure 11

Isolated extension gap problems. Since the flexion gap is already normal, a knee that is only unstable in extension can be corrected by simply building up the distal femur (A). On the other hand, if the only problem is loss of extension, and the posterior structures were already released, resecting more distal femur will suffice (B).

then dealing with an isolated extension gap problem, adjusting the distal femoral cut will suffice (Figure 11).

If the correct flexion gap is associated with a correct extension gap, the range of motion is normal, the knee is stable in flexion and extension; no adjustments are necessary and the definitive implants are inserted.

Similar but not identical gap problems

It has already been stated that when the flexion and extension gaps are identical (i.e. too large or too small, that is too loose or too tight), a tibial correction will usually suffice (Figure 12). However, if the flexion and extension gap problems are similar but are not identical (e.g. too loose in extension but much looser in flexion, or too tight in extension but much tighter in flexion) the effect of tibial adjustments on the extension gap is far more critical, i.e. full extension and stability in extension are vital for

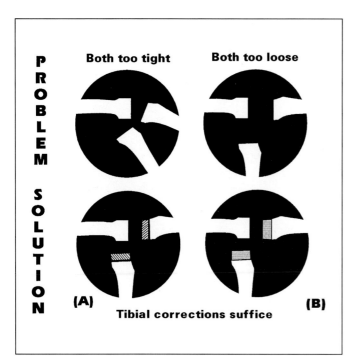

Figure 12

Identical gap problems. If both gaps are too small (A), removing tibia or inserting a thinner tibial implant should normalize both gaps. On the other hand, if both gaps are too large (B) (i.e. the knee is unstable in flexion and in extension), inserting a thicker tibial implant will usually suffice to correct both gap problems.

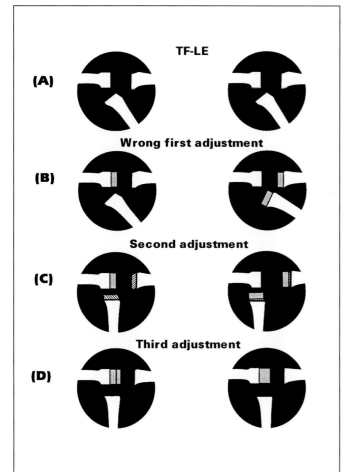

Figure 13

Incorrect sequence of adjustments for different gap problems. Two bad cuts (in this instance, tight in flexion and loose in extension, TF–LE) normalized in the wrong sequence, i.e. by normalizing the extension gap first. In the presence of diametrically opposite gap problems (A), the extension gap problem may be incorrectly normalized first, by revising either the distal femoral cut (left-hand column) or the tibia (right-hand column). Building up the femur distally (left-hand column, B) does not correct the flexion gap problem, which remains abnormal; hence, when the flexion gap is corrected (C) (by removing tibia), instability reappears in extension, requiring a second femoral adjustment (the femur must again be built up, D). If the different gap problems were incorrectly dealt with by first correcting the extension gap by building up the tibia (right-hand column, B), the latter makes the flexion gap tighter and increases the loss of flexion (C); re-cutting the tibia to normalize flexion will make the extension gap abnormal again (C), and the femur must again be built up (D).

weight bearing, while minor loss of knee flexion or mild instability in flexion can be tolerated; priority should always be given to the extension gap adjustments. Although in terms of sequence of adjustments one must always correct the flexion gap first, the extension gap status is functionally more important.

If, in instances of opposite gap problems (Figure 13), one incorrectly normalizes the extension gap problem first, subsequent adjustments to adjust the flexion gap (usually by revising the tibial cut) will inevitably alter the extension gap which must again be normalized (i.e. three adjustments as opposed to two). For that reason, in the presence of different gap problems, one must always correct the flexion gap first (Figure 14).

If the problem is one of loss of knee flexion, and the extension status is normal (Figure 9C,D,E,F), it is important to consider the position of the extensor mechanism when testing for the range of flexion. If the loss of knee flexion only becomes obvious after reducing the patella (Figure 9E,F), the loss of flexion is obviously due to a tight extensor mechanism, i.e. too thick a patella or too anterior a femoral coronal cut.

On the other hand, if there is a loss of flexion while the patella is still dislocated (Figure 9C,D), the cause is either a posterior femoral coronal cut which was too posterior or a tibial cut which was too proximal or in recurvatum; the revision of the posterior femoral coronal cut will not alter the extension gap status but the revision of the tibial cut will, and subsequent revision of the distal femoral cut is then necessary.

Summary

(1) Normalize the alignment first. A correct mechanical axis is the single most important factor affecting long-term results.

(2) Assess both gaps and make a complete diagnosis. It is insufficient to diagnose incomplete knee flexion; the correct diagnosis is one of the following: (a) loss of knee flexion and instability in extension; (b) loss of knee flexion and loss of extension; (c) loss of knee flexion and normal status in extension.

(3) Make soft-tissue corrections first.

(4) When making bony corrections, always normalize the flexion gap first; if knee flexion is incomplete, verify the range of flexion before and after relocating the patella.

(5) Identical flexion and extension gap problems (i.e. both too large or both too small) usually require tibial adjustments only, since the tibial cut affects both gaps.

(6) Diametrically opposite flexion and extension gap problems require tibial and femoral adjustments. Tibial adjustments should always be made first and

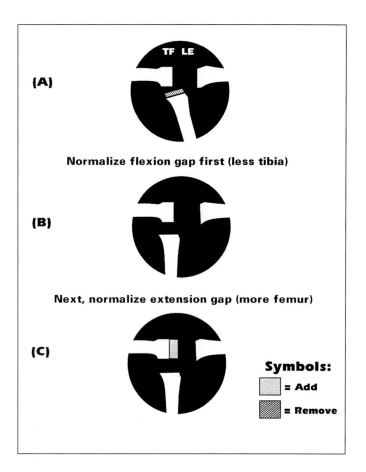

Figure 14

Correct sequence of adjustments for diametrically opposite gap problems. When the gap problems are opposite (in this instance, tight in flexion and loose in extension, TF-LE), both cuts are wrong and both must be revised; the flexion gap is normalized first by re-cutting the tibia (A); the resultant problem in extension (i.e. loose) (Figure 10B), is then corrected by building up the distal femur (Figure 10C), thus normalizing two incorrect bone cuts in the right sequence (i.e. two adjustments as opposed to three adjustments as in Figure 13).

distal femoral adjustments last, since the former affects both gaps while the latter affects the extension gap only. By normalizing the flexion gap first, one is then left with an isolated extension gap problem to deal with.

(7) Isolated extension gap problems require distal femoral adjustments only.

Acknowledgement

The authors gratefully acknowledge the excellent work of the medical illustrator, David Rolling.

17.8   Insall–Burstein Mark II total knee replacement: A prospective, multicentre study of 240 knees

Dipak V. Patel, Manjit Bhamra, Paul M. Aichroth, Peter A. N. Hutton, Brian G. Andrews, James E. Scott and Peter R. E. Baird

The total condylar knee prosthesis was introduced at the Hospital for Special Surgery in 1974.[1-4] In 1978, the total condylar prosthesis was modified into a posteriorly stabilized version by the addition of a tibial polyethylene spine and a transverse femoral cam to provide function of the posterior cruciate ligament. Excision of the posterior cruciate ligament allows easier correction of a fixed flexion deformity. The specific aim in designing the posteriorly stabilized knee prosthesis was to improve stair-climbing, increase the range of movement and prevent posterior subluxation. Satisfactory, short-term as well as long-term results have been reported by various authors using the posteriorly stabilized (Insall–Burstein) Mark I prosthetic design.[5-11]

The posteriorly stabilized (Insall–Burstein) Mark II knee prosthesis is a modular system which provides the surgeon with a number of options during surgery. It incorporates optimal stems for both femur and tibia, metal augmentation blocks for the femur and metal wedges for the tibia. Polyethylene tibial inserts of varying thickness are interchangeable on the metallic tibial tray, and have the capability of either a standard posteriorly stabilized or a constrained condylar design.[12]

With the original prosthetic design, many patients experienced patellar impingement problems. This was attributed to the configuration of the anterior flange of the femoral component, which was subsequently revised in 1983 to incorporate a deeper patellar groove. Further modifications and deepening of this articular surface have been made within the posteriorly stabilized Mark II prosthesis.

The purpose of this study was to assess the preliminary clinical and radiological results of posteriorly stabilized Mark II total knee arthroplasty, with special reference to patellar complications.

Materials and methods

We prospectively studied 212 patients who underwent posteriorly stabilized (Insall–Burstein) Mark II total knee replacement at Westminster Hospital, Queen Mary's University Hospital, the Humana Hospital, Wellington, and the Charing Cross Hospital, London, in the past 4 years. Two patients had died from unrelated causes and two were unable to attend the follow-up owing to associated medical illnesses. Thus, 208 patients were available for detailed clinical and radiological assessment.

There were 52 males and 156 females. The right knee was involved in 126 cases and the left in 114. Thirty-two patients had bilateral knee arthroplasty. The operation was performed by orthopaedic surgeons of varying grade, i.e. consultants, orthopaedic senior registrars and registrars.

The average age of the patients at operation was 67.7 years (range 42–88 years) and the mean follow-up was 31.8 months (range 24–48 months). The details of preoperative diagnosis are shown in Table 1. One hundred and eight patients (52%) had had previous operations on their knees (Table 2). Pre-

Table 1 Preoperative diagnosis in 208 patients (240 knees).

Diagnosis	No. of patients	No. of knees	Percentage of knees
Osteoarthritis	154	166	69
Rheumatoid arthritis	34	54	23
Post-traumatic arthritis	12	12	5
Osteonecrosis	8	8	3

Table 2 Previous operations in 108 patients.

Operation	No. of knees
Open medial meniscectomy	23
Open lateral meniscectomy	7
Arthroscopic debridement and lavage	54
High tibial osteotomy	17
Supracondylar femoral osteotomy	4
Synovectomy	13
Arthrotomy and removal of loose bodies	6

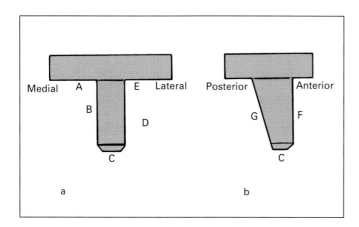

Figure 1

The tibial component was divided into eight zones for assessment of radiolucency: (a) anteroposterior view; (b) lateral view.

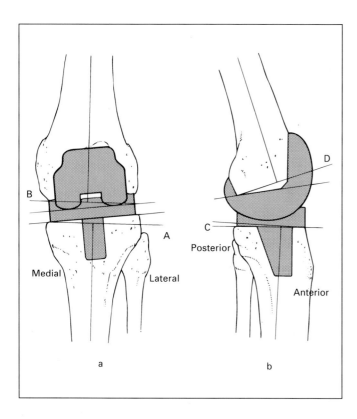

Figure 2

The angles measured on weight-bearing anteroposterior (a) and lateral (b) radiographs as suggested by Hvid and Nielsen (1984).[14] A = angular deviation of the tibial component from a line at right-angles to the tibial axis. B = angular deviation of the femoral component from a line at right-angles to the femoral axis. The same method was applied to measure the angular deviations of the tibial (C) and femoral (D) components on the lateral view.

operatively, 149 knees (62%) had a varus deformity of a mean of 14.8° (range 4–50°), and 91 knees (38%) had a valgus deformity of a mean of 16.3° (range 3–32°). One hundred and fifty-six knees (65%) had a flexion contracture (mean 15.4°, range 5–35°).

The mean preoperative BASK (British Association for Surgery of the Knee) score was 35 points (range 15–60 points), and the average HSS (Hospital for Special Surgery) score was 33 points (range 5–54). The mean preoperative knee flexion was 84.6° (range 30–125°). The majority of the patients had painful, deformed knee that had failed to respond to conservative measures. The walking distance was less than 50 metres (indoors only) in 18% of the knees; between 50 and 100 metres in 53%, between 100 and 500 metres in 21%, and between 500 and 1000 metres in 8% of the knees. Eighty-two per cent of the patients required walking aids preoperatively.

All patients were independently reviewed by one of us (D.V.P.). The clinical and radiological findings were recorded with meticulous detail. The data were analysed using the chi-squared test and Student's t-test. Significance was accepted at $P<0.05$.

Method of evaluation

The results were assessed using two different scoring systems. The BASK score was utilized to enable a valid comparison with our previously reported series using the posteriorly stabilized Mark I prosthesis.[8] The BASK scoring system is a modification of the BOA knee function assessment chart, published by Aichroth et al.[13] Of the 100 points for a normal knee, 39 points are given for lack of pain, 25 for range of movement more than 120°, 10 for function, 4 for ability to climb stairs, 4 for walking aids, 2 for subjective stability, and 16 for technical merit of the deformity (4 points each for absence of extension lag and flexion deformity, 4 for valgus alignment between 6° and 10°, and 4 for lateral plane laxity in extension between zero and 5°). Based on the BASK scoring system, a score of 91–100 points was rated as excellent, 75–90 as good, 61–74 as fair, and 60 or less as poor.[8]

In addition, the HSS knee rating scale[6] was used to allow a future comparison with studies reported from centres in the USA, where the HSS score is popularly used. Patients with a HSS score between 85 and 100 were considered excellent, between 70 and 84 as good, between 60 and 69 as fair, and less than 60 as poor.

Standard weight-bearing anteroposterior, lateral and skyline views were obtained. The prosthesis–bone interfaces at all three components were studied by a zone method[6] (Figure 1). The tilt of the prosthetic components was measured as suggested by Hvid and Nielsen.[14] The various angles measured are shown in Figure 2.

The ideal position for the femoral component was considered to be between 6° and 10° of valgus, with the anterior flange of the femoral prosthesis flush with the anterior cortex. The ideal position for the tibial component was considered to be at 90° ± 2° to the long axis of the tibia in the frontal plane.

Operative technique

The surgical technique is demonstrated in Figures 3 to 17. Some important technical details merit attention.

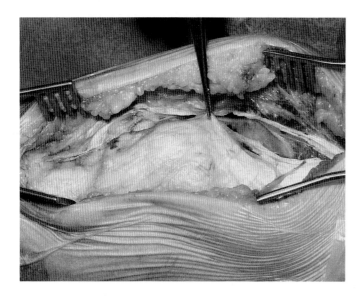

Figure 3

A medial parapatellar arthrotomy incision is made.

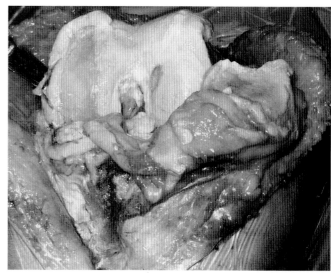

Figure 4

The knee joint showing severe arthritis with eburnated bone.

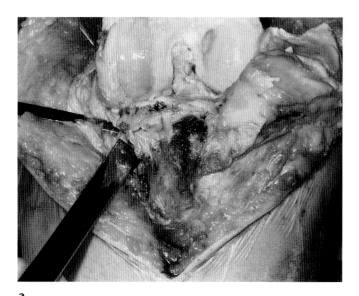

a

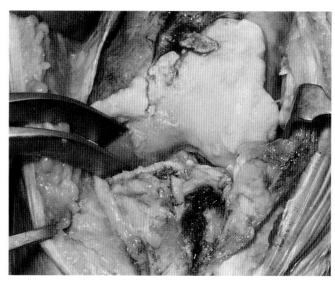

b

Figure 5

(a) Medial soft tissue release is performed to correct the varus malalignment. (b) Satisfactory opening up of the medial joint space is seen following soft-tissue release.

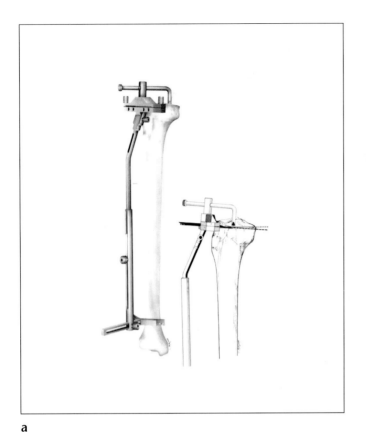

a

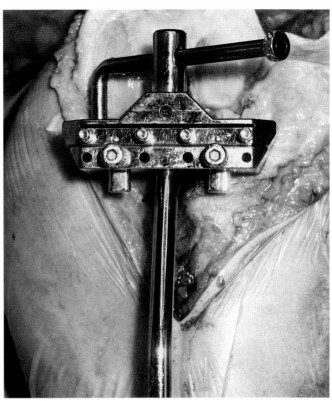

b

Figure 6

Proximal tibial resection is performed using an extramedullary jig. A 5° posterior tilt of the tibial cut is preferred.

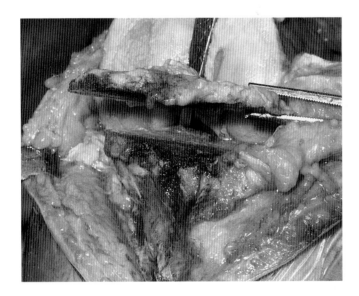

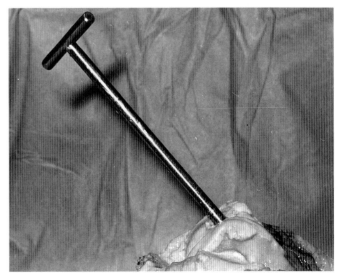

Figure 7

Proximal tibial cut is completed.

Figure 8

An intramedullary rod is inserted into the centre of the distal femur.

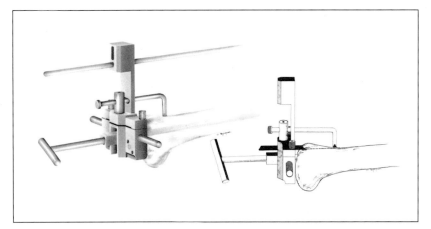

a

Figure 9

Femoral intramedullary alignment guide is inserted and anterior condylar rough cut is made.

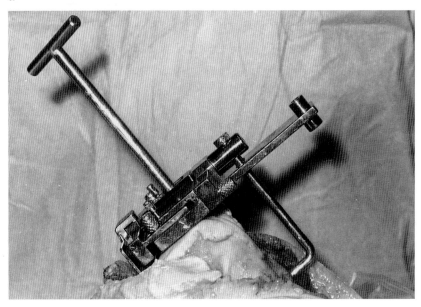

b

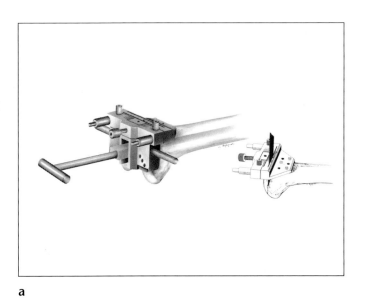

a

b

Figure 10

Distal femoral cut is made.

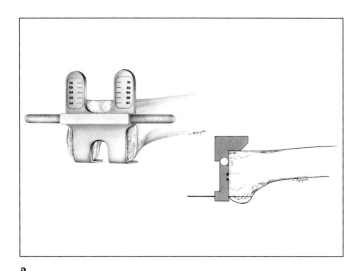
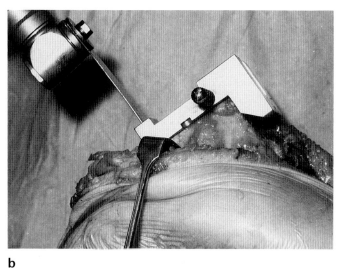

a   b

Figure 11

The size of the femoral component is determined using the measuring guide. Posterior condylar resection is performed.

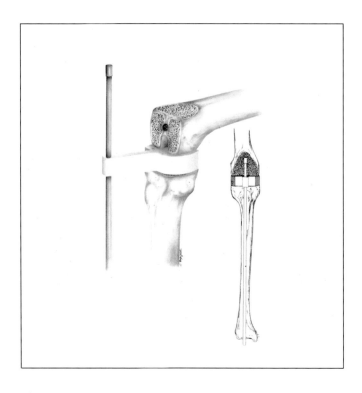

Figure 12

Flexion/extension gap is verified and the correct thickness of the tibial insert is determined, using the spacer block. The alignment and soft-tissue balance are checked using extramedullary rod.

Femoral resection

The anterior femoral cut should be made before removing the intra-medullary grid and pins in order to make an accurate cut. The posterior chamfering cuts should be made first and the surgeon should then work anteriorly in order to avoid displacement of the jig. The hole in the distal femur should be blocked using a bone block to prevent the cement going into the medullary canal.

Patellar resection

The patella was routinely replaced in all the knees in our series. A precise patellar resection should be performed and at least 10–15 mm of the patella should be retained. A patellar jig, which would enable the surgeon to make an accurate patellar resection, is necessary.

Lateral patellar retinacular release was not undertaken routinely; it was usually necessary only for patients with severe valgus deformities.

Postoperative management

A well-padded compression bandage was applied. Continuous passive mobilization was started the next day when the patient was more comfortable. Weight-bearing mobilization with either crutches or a walker was started on the third or fourth postoperative day,

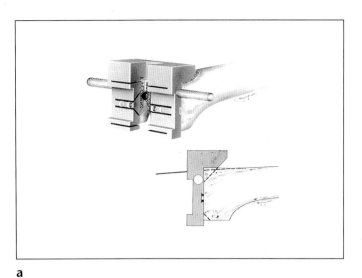

a

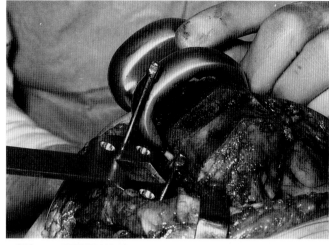

b

Figure 13

The femoral cuts are now completed.

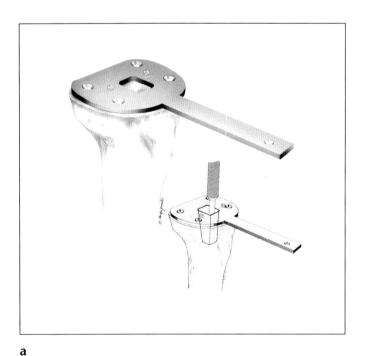

a

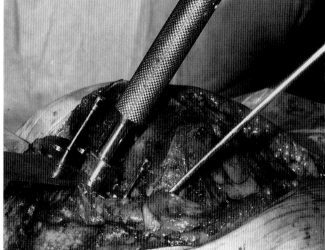

b

Figure 14

The tibial hole is prepared using the correct punch.

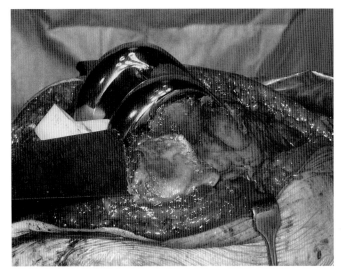

a

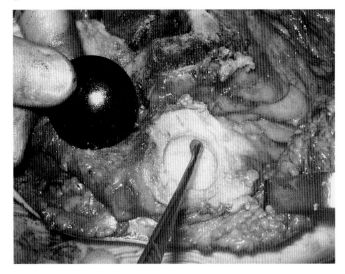

c

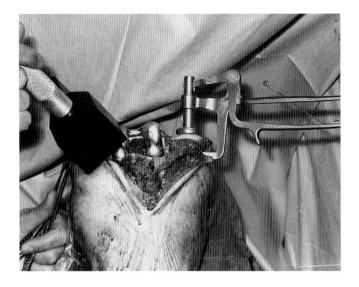

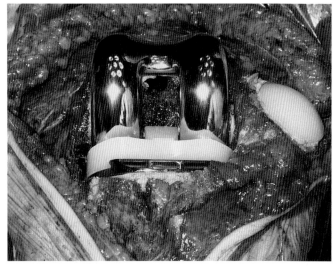

Figure 15

(a) Patellar articular surface is resected. (b) A patellar clamp is used and a hole is made in the centre of the cut surface. (c) A trial patellar component is inserted to determine the correct size of the patellar prosthesis.

Figure 16

The definitive femoral and patellar prostheses are cemented.

Figure 17

The tibial component with high-density polyethylene (HDPE) tibial tray is now cemented in position.

depending upon the patient's comfort. Static quadriceps, active straight leg raising and mobilizing exercises were encouraged from the second post-operative day. Manipulation under anaesthetic was performed only when the patient failed to gain at least 90° of knee flexion by the third postoperative week.

Results

Clinical results

The results were analysed as shown in Tables 3 and 4. The details of the clinical results are given in Table 5. According to the BASK scoring system, 94 knees (39%) had an excellent result, 123 knees (51%) had a good result, 17 knees (7%) had a fair result and 6 knees (3%) had a poor result. The mean postoperative BASK score was 87 points (range 30–99 points).

Based on the HSS scoring system, we found that 116 knees (48%) had an excellent result, 101 knees (42%) had a good result, 17 knees (7%) had a fair result and 6 knees (3%) had a poor outcome. The mean postoperative HSS score was 82 points (26–96 points).

At the time of latest follow-up, 89% of the knees were without pain, 8% had mild, intermittent discomfort, whereas 3% had moderate pain. The walking distance was greater than 1 km in 78% of the knees, between 500 and 1000 metres in 14%, between 100 and 500 metres in 3%, between 50 and 100

Table 3 Grading of clinical results in 240 knee replacements using BASK scoring system.

Result	BASK score	No. of knees	Percentage of knees
Excellent	91–100	94	39
Good	75–90	123	51
Fair	61–74	17	7
Poor	60 or less	6	3

Table 4 Grading of clinical results in 240 knee replacements using HSS scoring system.

Result	BASK score	No. of knees	Percentage of knees
Excellent	85–100	116	48
Good	70–84	101	42
Fair	60–69	17	7
Poor	<60	6	3

Table 5 Clinical results in 240 knee replacements given as number and percentage (percentages in parentheses). The results were graded according to the BASK scoring system.

	All	OA	RA	Statistical difference OA vs RA
Results				
Excellent	94 (39)	65 (39)	20 (37)	
Good	123 (51)	89 (54)	23 (43)	P<0.05
Fair	17 (7)	10 (6)	7 (13)	
Poor	6 (3)	2 (1)	4 (7)	
Pain				
None	214 (89)	159 (96)	39 (72)	
Mild	19 (8)	5 (3)	10 (19)	P<0.01
Moderate	7 (3)	2 (1)	5 (9)	
Walking				
Unlimited	187 (78)	158 (95)	12 (22)	
500 m–1 km	34 (14)	5 (3)	26 (48)	P<0.05
100 m–500 m	7 (3)	–	7 (13)	
50 m–100 m (outdoors)	9 (4)	3 (2)	6 (11)	
Indoors only	3 (1)	–	3 (6)	
Stairs				
Normal	50 (21)	25 (15)	8 (15)	
One step at a time	91 (38)	72 (43)	17 (31)	
With walking aids	96 (40)	68 (41)	27 (50)	P<0.05
Unable to manage	3 (1)	1 (1)	2 (4)	
Range of movement				
Average flexion	97.5°	96.7°	95.4°	NS[a]
Flexion contracture	5.4°	3.2°	6.7°	P<0.01
Postoperative score	87	89.3	82.6	P<0.05

[a]NS = not significant

metres in 4%, and limited to indoors in 1% of the knees.

No walking aids were necessary in 148 patients (71%); 44 patients (21%) used a walking stick only for outdoor activities; and 16 patients (8%) constantly required support. The stair-climbing was normal in 21% of the knees; 38% were climbing one step at a time; 40% required the support of a banister or stick or both; and 3 knees (1%) were unable to ascend stairs.

The average postoperative knee flexion was 97.5° (range 35–135°). Fifty-three knees (22%) had a residual flexion contracture of an average of 5.4° (range 3–25°).

Overall, patients with osteoarthritis (OA) had better results than those with rheumatoid arthritis (RA), as far as the final result was concerned. Patients with RA seemed to fare a little worse when the individual categories in the BASK and the HSS scoring systems were assessed. The walking distance was significantly restricted in patients with RA owing to involvement of multiple joints, thereby reducing the overall knee function score.

Patient satisfaction

Ninety-three per cent of the patients were pleased or satisfied with the result of their knee replacement; 4% expressed reservation about the outcome; and 3% were disappointed.

Radiographic results

A satisfactory postoperative alignment of 6–10° valgus was seen in 113 knees (47%); 109 knees (45%) were between zero and 5° of valgus; and 11 knees (5%) had more than 10° of valgus. Seven knees (3%) were in varus alignment. The average anatomical tibiofemoral angle as measured on the standard radiographs was 5.6° valgus (range 3° varus to 14° valgus).

An ideal position for the femoral component within 6–10° of valgus was obtained in 187 knees (78%). The femoral prosthesis was within zero to 5° valgus in 46 knees (19%) and 11–15° valgus in 7 knees (3%). The anterior flange of the femoral component was not flush with the distal femoral cortex in 32 knees (13%); i.e. the femoral component had been cemented in a slightly flexed position. Ninety-two per cent of the tibial components were within 2° of varus or valgus, 5% were in greater than 2° of valgus and 3% were in greater than 2° of varus. Ninety-three per cent of the tibial prostheses were within 4° of anteroposterior tilt, 5% had greater than 5° of posterior tilt and 2% had greater than 4° of anterior tilt.

An accurate radiological assessment of the femoral prosthesis–bone interface was difficult owing to the presence of the metal prosthesis, although there was no evidence of any progression of the observed radiolucent lines around the femoral component.

There were no radiolucent lines beneath the tibial prostheses in 154 knees (64%); in another 65 knees (27%) they were incomplete, non-progressive and less than 1 mm in thickness limited to the interface beneath the medial or the lateral tibial plateau. Twenty-one knees (9%) showed incomplete, radiolucent lines of 1–2 mm width covering one tibial zone, although none of the patients had clinical symptoms of mechanical loosening. None of the knees had a complete or progressive radiolucency.

Complications

The details of complications are given in Table 6. There were 28 wound complications (12%). Seventeen knees with RA (31%) had wound problems as compared to 11 knees with OA (7%). Twelve knees had a spontaneously resolving wound haematoma. Three patients required secondary suturing for wound dehiscence.

Deep infection occurred in a 66-year-old male patient with OA, 4 weeks after knee replacement; this required arthrotomy, debridement and irrigation of the wound. Septopal beads were inserted for 1 week and secondary closure of the wound was performed. The femoral and tibial prostheses were found to be stable and were therefore left in situ. Broad-spectrum antibiotics were given for 12 weeks. At the time of latest follow-up, the patient was asymptomatic.

Table 6 Complications.

Complication	Number of knees
Superficial infection	3
Deep infection	1
Delayed wound healing	9
Wound haematoma	12
Wound dehiscence	3
Patellar subluxation	7
Patellar dislocation (including one case of patellectomy)	2
Patellar impingement	12
Stress fracture of the patella	0
Mechanical loosening of the patellar component	0
Mechanical loosening of the tibial component	0
Deep vein thrombosis	10
Pulmonary embolism	3
Myocardial infarction	2
Urinary tract infection	18
Lateral popliteal neurapraxia	5

The most notable feature of this series was a 3.8% complication rate of patellofemoral problems. There were no patellar fractures in this series. Seven patients had subluxation of the patella and two had a frank dislocation of the patella. One of the two patients with persistent dislocation of the patella, despite two realignment procedures, underwent patellectomy; the other was left alone as the patient was a poor operative risk owing to associated cardiopulmonary problems. None of the patients had a mechanical loosening of the patellar prosthesis.

None of the patients had clinical evidence of mechanical or aseptic loosening of the tibial component.

The incidence of deep vein thrombosis in this series was 4%. Three patients had non-fatal pulmonary embolisms which were successfully treated.

Lateral popliteal nerve palsy occurred in five patients and was associated with correction of a severe, fixed valgus deformity. Complete recovery occurred in four cases and one patient was noted to have a residual weakness of the dorsiflexors of the ankle, at the time of latest follow-up.

In our series, 41 knees (17%) required manipulation under anaesthesia at an average of 3.3 weeks postoperatively. All patients achieved and maintained a satisfactory range of movement following the manipulation.

Discussion

An increased number of patellar complications is reported following the use of posteriorly stabilized (Insall–Burstein) Mark I condylar prosthesis.[5,6] Although the prosthetic design of the patellofemoral articulation has improved considerably over the past 10 years, a significant number of patients still continue to have patellofemoral problems, which include patellar subluxation and dislocation, patellar fracture, and persistent anterior knee pain due to impingement. Patellar fractures have been attributed to avascular necrosis secondary to the surgical approach (including medial arthrotomy and lateral patellar retinacular release), patellar bone resection, thermal necrosis or anatomical variation.[15]

In our series, seven patients had a patellar subluxation and two had patellar dislocation. All these patients underwent subsequent lateral release of the patella but only four had a satisfactory patellar alignment; three patients still have a patellar subluxation. A 79-year-old female patient with a persistent patellar dislocation, despite two attempts at surgical correction, underwent patellectomy; she had a poor clinical result. One elderly patient with a patellar dislocation was left alone as the patient was a poor operative risk.

We believe that the incidence of patellofemoral problems is related to technical factors. The patellofemoral subluxation was frequently encountered in obese women with severe valgus deformities of the knees. A meticulous soft-tissue release must be accomplished prior to bone resection. In our experience, we have found that the lateral patellar retinacular release is frequently needed for patients with gross valgus deformities of the knee. At operation, prior to the wound closure, the patellofemoral tracking must be verified, and patellar release performed if necessary.

There is no consensus of opinion in the literature on the amount of patellar surface resection. The majority of the authors state that 10–15 mm of the patella should be retained. If too much of the patella is resected, then there is an increased risk of patellar fracture. On the other hand, if minimal patellar resection is performed, and a patellar prosthesis is inserted, the resulting anteroposterior width of the replaced patella could significantly limit knee flexion or produce anterior knee pain due to impingement.

Whether the patella should be routinely resurfaced or not is a question of major international debate, and it is not the primary purpose of this contribution to discuss this controversial subject. In our series, all knees had a routine patellar resurfacing. We believe that the postoperative rehabilitation is much better following patellar replacement. Further, we feel that the issue of patellar replacement is poorly addressed in the literature. Perhaps a patellar jig would be ideal, as it would enable the surgeon to make a precise patellar resection.

Malrotation of the femoral or tibial component can lead to abnormal patellofemoral articulation, with subsequent patellar subluxation or dislocation. Every attempt must be made at operation to ensure that the rotational alignment of both the femoral and the tibial prostheses is ideal.

In patients with persistent patellar subluxation or dislocation, the surgeon must try to identify the underlying causative factor and deal with it accordingly. If femoral or tibial component malrotation is the cause, then a revision procedure may be required to correct the rotational malalignment. This may be a major undertaking, especially in an elderly patient. Proximal realignment or medial transposition of the tibial tuberosity may be required for the correction of patellofemoral subluxation.

Patellar impingement symptoms, particularly on extension of the knee, were seen in 24 knees (10%). They were mildly painful in 4 patients, moderately painful in 3, and 17 had a painless clicking sensation. These symptoms are possibly due to the peripatellar soft-tissue impingement against the anterior margin of the intercondylar box of the femoral component. None of the patients with patellar impingement required surgical intervention.

Insall et al.[6] reported 88% excellent and 9% good results using the posteriorly stabilized Mark I prosthesis at 2–4 years of follow-up. In our series, 90% of the knees had excellent or good results at an average follow-up of 32 months (range 24–48 months).

Summary and conclusions

We report the preliminary results of a prospective, multicentre study of 208 patients (240 knees) who underwent Insall–Burstein Mark II total knee arthroplasty. The mean age of the patients at the time of operation was 67.7 years (range 42–88 years) and the average follow-up was 31.8 months (range 24–48 months).

The results were evaluated using two scoring systems (BASK and HSS). Based on the BASK scoring system, 94 knees (39%) had an excellent result, 123 knees (51%) had a good result, 17 knees (7%) had a fair result and 6 knees (3%) had a poor result. The mean improvement in the BASK score was from 35 points preoperatively (range 15–60) to 87 points postoperatively (range 30–99).

According to the HSS rating scale, 116 knees (48%) had an excellent result, 101 knees (42%) had a good result, 17 knees (7%) had a fair result and 6 knees (3%) had a poor result. The mean improvement in the HSS score was from 33 points preoperatively (range 5–54) to 82 points postoperatively (range 26–96). The average postoperative knee flexion was 97.5° (range 35–135°).

Three patients had a superficial wound infection which settled with a course of antibiotics, and one had deep sepsis requiring arthrotomy and wound drainage. Patellar subluxation was seen in seven cases and patellar dislocation in two. Ninety-three per cent of the patients were pleased or satisfied with the result of their knee arthroplasties.

We conclude that the clinical results of Insall–Burstein Mark II total knee arthroplasty on a short-term basis are encouraging and justify continuation of its use on a long-term basis. Clearly, the patellofemoral problems need to be addressed more critically; the majority of these problems are related to the surgical technique. Using an appropriate patellar jig, these problems should be minimized. A long-term follow-up study is necessary.

Acknowledgments

The authors thank Miss Dina Stanford and Christine Samuel for the computer analysis of the data. Our thanks are also extended to the Medical Photography Department of Westminster Hospital for their help with the illustrations.

References

1. **Insall J, Ranawat CS, Scott WN et al.**, Total condylar knee replacement: preliminary report, *Clin Orthop* (1976) **120**: 149–154.
2. **Insall JN**, Total knee replacement, *Surgery of the knee*, ed Insall JN (New York: Churchill Livingstone, 1984) 587–695.
3. **Ranawat CS, Sculco TP**, History of the development of total knee prosthesis at the Hospital for Special Surgery, *Total-condylar knee arthroplasty: technique, results and complications*, ed Ranawat CS (New York: Springer-Verlag, 1985) 3–6.
4. **Walker PS**, The total-condylar knee and its evolution, *Total-condylar knee arthroplasty: technique, results and complications*, ed Ranawat CS (New York: Springer-Verlag, 1985) 7–16.
5. **Aglietti P, Buzzi R**, Posteriorly stabilised total-condylar knee replacement: three to eight years' follow-up of 85 knees, *J Bone Joint Surg (Br)* (1988) **70**: 211–216.
6. **Insall JN, Lachiewicz PF, Burstein AH**, The posterior stabilised condylar prosthesis: a modification of the total condylar design: two to four-year clinical experience, *J Bone Joint Surg (Am)* (1982) **64**: 1317–1323.
7. **Kjaersgaard-Andersen P, Hvid I, Wethelund J-O et al.**, Total condylar knee arthroplasty in osteoarthritis: a four to six-year follow-up evaluation of 103 cases, *Clin Orthop* (1989) **238**: 167–173.
8. **Patel DV, Aichroth PM, Wand JS**, Posteriorly stabilised (Insall–Burstein) total condylar knee arthroplasty: a follow-up study of 157 knees, *Int Orthop* (1991) **15**: 211–218.
9. **Scott WN, Rubinstein M, Scuderi G**, Results after knee replacement with a posterior cruciate-substituting prosthesis, *J Bone Joint Surg (Am)* (1988) **70**: 1163–1173.
10. **Scuderi GR, Insall JN, Windsor RE et al.**, Survivorship of cemented knee replacements, *J Bone Joint Surg (Br)* (1989) **71**: 798–803.
11. **Vince KG, Insall JN, Kelly MA**, The total condylar prosthesis: 10 to 12-year results of a cemented knee replacement, *J Bone Joint Surg (Br)* (1989) **71**: 793–797.
12. **Scuderi GR, Insall JN**, The Insall–Burstein posterior stabilized knee, *Joint replacement – State of the art*, ed Coombs R, Gristina A, Hungerford D (London: Orthotext, 1990) 221–225.
13. **Aichroth PM, Freeman MAR, Smillie IS et al.**, A knee function assessment chart, *J Bone Joint Surg (Br)* (1978) **60**: 308–309.
14. **Hvid I, Nielsen S**, Total condylar knee arthroplasty: prosthetic component positioning and radiolucent lines, *Acta Orthop Scand* (1984) **55**: 160–165.
15. **Scuderi G, Scharf SC, Meltzer LP et al.**, The relationship of lateral releases to patella viability in total knee arthroplasty, *J Arthroplasty* (1987) **2**: 209–214.

18

Revision arthroplasty of the knee

18.1   Revision total knee arthroplasty

W. Norman Scott, Mark S. McMahon and Susan M. Craig

From 1987 through 1989, 537 000 knee replacements were inserted worldwide. The good news is that there has been about a 95% success rate for virtually all types of surface replacements. Failure rates, which have ranged from 5% to 10%, include patellofemoral problems (2–4%), infection (2–3%), mechanical failure (2–4%), and miscellaneous problems (2%) (Figure 1). With these numbers it is obvious that, worldwide, approximately 19 000 revision arthroplasties will be required annually. From a practical point of view, it means that for every 100 cases that each of us performs we can count on almost 10 revisions being necessary. It is important to note that the numbers quoted reflect the most favorable conditions, i.e., large series at major institutions. Thus, it is imperative for any orthopedic surgeon performing knee replacements to be familiar with all the problems and controversies surrounding revision arthroplasty.[1-5]

The basic problems in revision knee arthroplasty are: (1) exposure, (2) bone loss, (3) prosthetic selection, and (4) rehabilitation. It is important to develop a rational approach and understand the indications

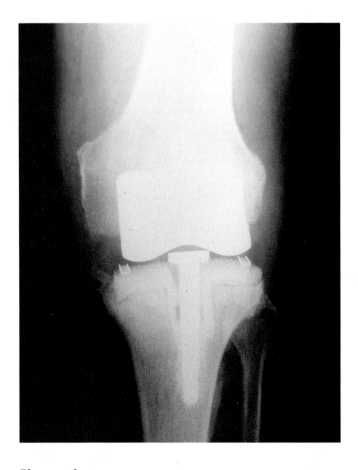

Figure 1

Stabilocondylar prosthesis exhibiting loosening of the tibial component.

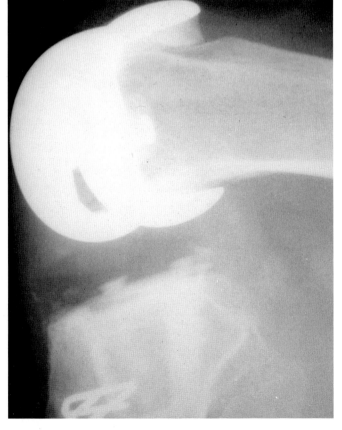

Figure 2

Patellar tendon avulsion with resultant patella alta.

when they are distinct and the theoretical applications as they are evolving.

Exposure in the revision knee includes understanding problems of the skin, capsule, ligaments, and component removal. Unlike total hip arthroplasty, the total knee replacement is almost a subcutaneous implant and thus we must be very careful of multiple skin incisions, the use of skin grafts and muscle flaps. For instance, we should all probably be more aware of how to use fluorescein to ascertain the viability of the skin prior to closure. If there is a question, we should be very aggressive either personally or with the help of a plastic surgeon in performing muscle transfers and split-thickness skin grafts at the time of closure. While a lateral approach has been advocated by some, the standard medial parapatellar capsular approach is the procedure of choice. One of the major problems with revision arthroplasty pertains to the integrity of the insertion of the patellar tendon. It is essential that this should not be avulsed (Figure 2). Since prevention of this potential disaster is the best treatment, it is important to understand the alternative approach if the attachment appears to be under too much tension. These alternatives include a tibial tubercle elevation and transfer,[6] a V–Y quadricepsplasty, or a proximal oblique transection of the quadriceps tendon (Insall modified quadricepsplasty or quadriceps snip).[7]

Deformities include ligamentous and bone involvement. In the varus knee, the medial structures, e.g., pes anserinus tendons and superficial and deep medial collateral ligaments, are often contracted. It is important to diminish abnormal force on the revision replacement and thus it is important to understand how and when to perform the release.

Bone loss is one of the most challenging aspects of a revision knee arthroplasty and has been addressed by the use of screw(s) with cement, bone grafting, and application of wedges to the tibial and femoral components. Probably the best use for screws is for leveling the insertion of components during the cementing stage. They can also be helpful if one has a rotational malalignment of the tibial component and it is difficult to secure the component in the correct rotation. A more permanent reinforcement or correction of bone loss involves bone grafting, harvesting from either autologous or bone-bank sources. Although it is initially successful, a recent review suggests late failure.[8] One of the best advances in recent years has been the availability of systems which will allow for correction of deformities at the time of surgery. These systems, such as the Genesis, PFC, PCA revision, and Insall–Burstein constrained condylar, allow for the use of wedges to correct this bone loss. Controversies pertain to the fixation of these wedges to the undersurfaces to which they are being applied and also to their sizing.

Prosthetic selection in revision arthroplasty is unquestionably a major concern. One has to be familiar with all the systems that are available. As we enter the 1990s, it is safe to say that at this time we have four categories of replacement: the cruciate retaining, sacrificing, and substituting, and the articulated designs. While the posterior cruciate controversy continues to persist, the clinical results support the use of both types of replacements. The question of retention of the posterior cruciate ligament in revision arthroplasty, however, seems to be somewhat moot. Except in certain unicompartment replacements, it is virtually impossible to keep a posterior cruciate ligament and maintain the kinematics of a revision arthroplasty. Cruciate substituting designs have had a rather good track record and are probably the most popular replacements now. From a practical point of view, it is probably the safest type of design to use. One other factor in prosthetic selection is understanding of the kinematics of the joint and how that relates to the flexion and extension spaces, primarily rotation and patellofemoral biomechanics. Do we just augment the proximal tibia, or augment the distal femur, or what combinations should be used?

Rehabilitation of the revision total knee replacement is different from the primary situation because of the compromises that usually have to be made during the procedure. When to begin the continuous passive mobilization depends on the exposure that had to be used and the integrity of the extensor mechanism. Similarly, weight bearing depends on the bone loss that occurred during the procedure and bracing will occasionally be necessary. Strengthening is an important part of the rehabilitation.

For revision of the septic replacement, the basic problems are augmented by specific issues germane to the infection. Diagnosis is not always easy and is something of an eclectic experience. Treatment, ranging from suppression to amputation, is not as successful as revision of the aseptic knee and a rational approach must be developed.

In summary, the knee replacement requiring revision should no longer be the province of a 'special few.' Orthopedists performing primary replacement must be able to handle their own problems.

Exposure and removal of components

The surgeon must be familiar with the particular implant to be removed so that potential problems can be anticipated. Since tissues are scarred, exposure is often difficult. Release of skin bound to the underlying quadriceps mechanism is often helpful. The usual medial parapatellar capsular incision is used, with extensive proximal split of the quadriceps to facilitate exposure. The quadriceps should be freed from the underlying femur, and an extensive proximal medial tibial release should be performed. Patellar eversion can often be difficult, and so lateral subluxation of the patella may have to suffice so as to avoid avulsion of the patellar tendon from the tibial tubercle. As mentioned earlier, a V–Y plasty of the quadriceps mechanism is an excellent alternative, especially in the setting of an extension contracture. Tibial tubercle osteotomy and oblique quadriceps transection are also alternatives.[6,7]

An all-plastic tibial component is removed by first cutting off the stem with an oscillating saw. Osteotomes are then used to pry off the tibial tray without sacrificing bone. The stem is removed with a threaded polyethylene extractor. A polyethylene extractor can also be used to remove plastic from a metal tray. If the tibial tray and stem are metal, the accessible interface between the tray and plateau should be loosened with thin osteotomes or the oscillating saw. A simple impaction tool can then be used to exert a proximal extraction force. The femoral component is removed by first loosening it using thin osteotomes. Any significant prying against bone must be done with care. Once the component is loosened, an extraction force is applied, attempting at all times to minimize bone loss. Cemented femoral or tibial stems may require transection with metal-cutting power tools, followed by use of the hollow drill (trephine) to core out the trapped stem.

Patellar component removal can be accomplished by first transecting the stem with an oscillating saw and then using a high-speed burr to excise the remaining stem. Removal of a metal-backed patellar component is best accomplished with an oscillating saw and osteotomes. Patellar fractures can be treated nonoperatively if the patient is able to straight leg raise. If the fracture results in component loosening, the component is removed without replacement.

After the prosthesis is out, attention is turned to cement removal. Long stem removal osteotomes, cement extraction taps, and cement rongeurs may be necessary. Areas of skin necrosis should be aggressively treated. While simple excision and closure can be successful, occasionally skin grafts or muscle flaps are required.[9]

Bone grafting

Bone grafts can be divided into two categories, minor and major. Minor bone grafts can be done either with autograft generated from previous bone cuts or with small amounts of allograft. Minor bone grafts complete the interface rather than support the prosthesis. While small defects do not require any form of fixation, larger defects may require one or two screws. Peripheral, sloping defects should be converted to a flat bone surface, since the greater the slope, the more the shear at the interface between graft and host. If the prosthesis is to be cemented, the interface between graft and host should be protected by sealing it with a small amount of cement prior to prosthetic seating. The graft should be protected with an even distribution of load—metal baseplates are thus more appropriate.

Many revisions result in loss of tibial cancellous bone stock, with only the cortical shell left intact. Allografts can be shaped and fitted within the empty shell. The prosthesis should rest upon the cortical rim that remains, allowing immediate weight bearing.

Major grafts are those which support the prosthesis. The amount of bone required varies from smaller defects which can be repaired with allograft femoral heads to more massive defects which will require either complete or partial femoral or tibial allografts. When partial, these grafts can be used to replace hemicondyles, etc.—step-cut techniques with screw fixation are often necessary.[10]

When most of the distal femur or tibia is destroyed, the 'femur within a femur' or 'tibia within a tibia' techniques are required. The allograft is shaped to fit within the remaining host bone, with the maximal length of allograft used to increase contact within the host medullary cavity. Intramedullary stems and constrained rotary hinge prostheses are used to prevent postoperative instability.[11]

Custom and modular components

A custom-designed implant is required in the setting of deficient bone stock, usually apparent on preoperative radiographs. Despite careful preoperative planning, however, these devices will on occasion not fit well. Thus modular systems with interchangeable parts evolved (Figure 3). Tibial wedge augments which attach to the undersurface of metal tibial trays are available with a range of angles. Femoral augments to compensate for bone deficiency can be added in the operating room. Intramedullary stems of varying lengths and thicknesses can also be affixed to femoral or tibial components.

The correct intramedullary stem diameter should be chosen to allow uncemented press-fit insertion. The absence of cement around intramedullary stems also facilitates possible subsequent revisions. The sclerotic lines seen about the stems postoperatively are the result of the useful stress transfer from deficient, weak proximal subchondral bone to strong bone distally. The stems carry bending, not axial load. Augmented components provide the theoretical advantage of distributing stress more evenly in areas of deficient bone stock.

Peripheral defects of the proximal tibia are typically medial or posteromedial. Defects less than 13 mm can be managed by cement and/or screws or by shift-

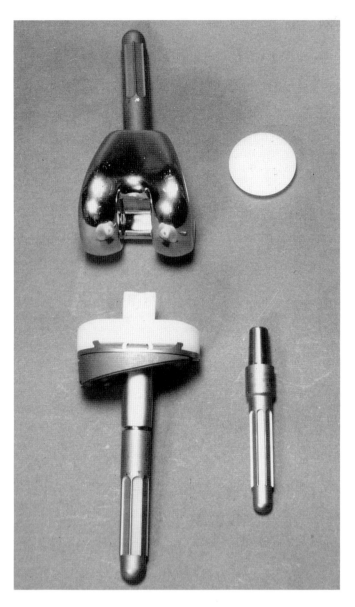

Figure 3

Insall–Burstein modular system.

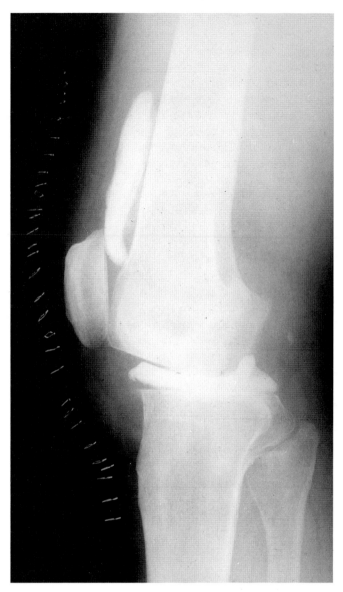

Figure 4

Antibiotic cement spacers in place after removal of components for infected total knee replacement.

ing the component off of the defect. Metallic wedges are useful with defects greater than 13 mm and up to approximately 25 mm.[12] Biomechanical studies[13] have shown that metallic wedges perform well when subjected to axial and varus loading. The size of the wedge required is determined intraoperatively. A wedge cutting block is then used to fashion the defect to optimally conform to the exact wedge size.[12]

Infection

The overall incidence of infected total knee replacement is 2–3%. Predisposing host factors include prior

osteomyelitis, prior septic arthritis, rheumatoid arthritis, previous surgery, concurrent sepsis elsewhere, corticosteroids, diabetes, poor nutrition, old age, and obesity. Errors in surgical technique have also been implicated, including wound contamination, skin necrosis, wound dehiscence, and hematoma. The diagnosis is based on the existence of prolonged pain and effusion, a draining sinus (approximately 1/3 of cases), a positive aspirate (only 50% of infected total knee replacements have a positive aspirate), progressive radiolucencies, and a positive indium scan. ESR and white blood cell count can be highly variable. *Staphylococcus aureus* is the causative organism in approximately half the cases, with *S. epidermidis* (27%) and *Pseudomonas aeruginosa* (16%) frequently responsible.

Although antibiotic suppression will not cure the infection, it remains a treatment option if implant removal is not feasible, the microorganism is relatively avirulent and sensitive to an oral antibiotic, the patient can tolerate the antibiotic, and the prosthesis is not loose. A second alternative, debridement followed by antibiotics, may be performed in the setting of an acute infection, with a low rate of success with a chronic infection.[14] Resection arthroplasty may be indicated in a polyarticular rheumatoid patient with limited ambulatory demands.

Immediate or delayed exchange reimplantation is frequently performed with a susceptible microorganism in the setting of good host tissue factors.[15,16] A typical delayed exchange protocol consists of (1) removal of components and cement, (2) placement of antibiotic cement spacers (Figure 4), (3) intravenous antibiotics for 6 weeks, and (4) reimplantation with antibiotic cement.[17]

Knee arthrodesis is considered when there is unilateral disease, the patient is young or a heavy laborer, or the infecting organism is fungal or otherwise highly resistant. Several techniques, including external fixation or intramedullary rods, have been used. Amputation becomes a last resort in the face of massive bone loss, persistent sepsis, or life-threatening infection.

Results of revision total knee replacement

The success rate of revision total knee arthroplasty is not as good as that of primary replacement.[8,18] This is particularly true in the setting of good bone stock, alignment, and extensor mechanism. Good to excellent results have ranged from 37% to as high as 89%.[19-21] Infection rates average approximately 4–5%. In general, there is a higher incidence of radiolucent lines, less satisfactory alignment, more extensor mechanism complications, and a high revision rate than in primary replacements. Patients with poor bone stock, pseudo-subchondralized bone surfaces, ligamentous instability, or unreconstructible extensor mechanism complications (particularly patellar tendon avulsion) are more likely to have an unsatisfactory result.[22]

References

1. Alexiades M, Sands A, Craig SM et al., Management of selected problems in revision knee arthroplasty, *Orthop Clin N Am* (1989) **20**: 211–219.
2. Jacobs MA, Hungerford DS, Krackow KA et al., Revision total knee arthroplasty for aseptic failure, *Clin Orthop* (1988) **226**: 78–85.
3. Ranawat CS, Revision of total knee replacement, *J Bone Joint Surg (Br)* (1989) **71**: 542.
4. Scott RD, Revision total knee arthroplasty, *Clin Orthop* (1988) **226**: 65–77.
5. Scott WN (ed), *Total knee revision arthroplasty* (Orlando: Grune and Stratton, 1987).
6. Whiteside LA, Ohl MD, Tibial tubercle osteotomy for exposure of the difficult total knee arthroplasty, *Clin Orthop* (1990) **260**: 6–9.
7. Insall JN, Revision of total knee replacement, *Instr Course Lect* (1986) **35**: 290–296.
8. Laskin RS, Presentation at the annual meeting of the Knee Society, September 1990, Laguna Nigel, California.
9. Craig SM, Soft tissue considerations, *Total knee revision arthroplasty*, ed Scott WN (Orlando: Grune and Stratton, 1987) 99–112.
10. Sculco TP, Bone grafting in revision total knee replacement surgery, *Total knee revision arthroplasty*, ed Scott WN (Orlando: Grune and Stratton, 1987) 137–148.
11. Hedley AK, Gruen TA, Ruoff DP, Revision of failed total hip arthroplasties with uncemented porous-coated anatomic components, *Clin Orthop* (1988) **235**: 75–90.
12. Brand MG, Daley RJ, Ewald FC et al., Tibial tray augmentation with modular metal wedges for tibial bone stock deficiency, *Clin Orthop* (1989) **248**: 71–79.
13. Brooks PJ, Walker PS, Scott RD, Tibial component fixation in deficient tibial bone stock, *Clin Orthop* (1984) **184**: 302–308.
14. Schoifet SD, Morrey BF, Treatment of infection after total knee arthroplasty by debridement with retention of the components, *J Bone Joint Surg (Am)* (1990) **72**: 1383–1390.
15. Rand JA, Fitzgerald RH Jr, Diagnosis and management of the infected total knee arthroplasty, *Orthop Clin N Am* (1989) **20**: 201–210.
16. Jacobs MA, Hungerford DS, Krackow KA et al., Revision of septic total knee arthroplasty, *Clin Orthop* (1989) **238**: 159–166.
17. Windsor RE, Insall JN, Urs WK et al., Two-stage reimplantation for the salvage of total knee arthroplasty complicated by infection: further follow-up and refinement of indications, *J Bone Joint Surg (Am)* (1990) **72**: 272–278.
18. Hanssen AD, Rand JA, A comparison of primary and revision total knee arthroplasty using the kinematic stabilizer prosthesis, *J Bone Joint Surg (Am)* (1988) **70**: 491–499.
19. Goldberg VM, Figgie MP, Figgie HE III et al., The results of revision total knee arthroplasty, *Clin Orthop* (1988) **226**: 86–92.
20. Rand JA, Bryan RS, Results of revision total knee arthroplasties using condylar prostheses: a review of 50 knees, *J Bone Joint Surg (Am)* (1988) **70**: 738–745.
21. Friedman RJ, Hirst P, Poss R, et al., Results of revision total knee arthroplasty performed for aseptic loosening, *Clin Orthop* (1990) **255**: 235–241.
22. Moreland JR, Mechanisms of failure in total knee arthroplasty, *Clin Orthop* (1988) **226**: 49–64.

18.2   Revision of total knee arthroplasty

Kevin Hardinge

The long-continued functioning of a knee arthroplasty is dependent upon stable fixation of the components. A range of movement of 90–100° will allow transfer activities such as stair climbing, getting in and out of bed and chair, and comfortable automobile travel.

Standing for long periods is dependent upon being able to fully extend the knee and thus relax the quadriceps muscles, and walking for long periods is dependent upon mobility of the knee in the swing phase, which will only occur if the quadriceps mechanism is sufficiently flexible to allow the patella to glide.

Stiffness in a knee arthroplasty is a more serious constraint to function than stiffness in a hip arthroplasty, this being caused by the long levers (femur and tibia) that actuate the joint. Thus the condition of the quadriceps mechanism has to be taken into account when considering total knee arthroplasty revision.

Lessons in total knee revision have been gained when considering the behavior of early arthroplasties and in this regard a short account of the experiences at Wrightington Hospital is presented—giving first of all a description of the behaviour of John Charnley's load angle inlay and the lessons learnt from that experience and subsequently the failures of total condylar knee arthroplasty in the Wrightington series.

Between 1972 and 1978, a total of 789 load angle inlay arthroplasties were performed. John Charnley envisaged that this was a fairly simple arthroplasty that was suitable for rheumatoid arthritis at the stage when the joint surfaces were just beginning to be damaged so that synovectomy (popular in 1970–4) was unnecessary.

The arthroplasty reversed the normal configuration in that the convex portion was of high-density polyethylene (HDPE). Two curved runners were cemented and recessed into the femoral condyles—articulated with flat metal plates that were cemented into the tibial plateau (Figure 1). A range of flexion between 0° and 50° (which Charnley designated as the 'load angle') could be expected during normal gait, and during this arc the HDPE runners glided over the flat metal plates. It was observed that the

posterior femoral condyles in these cases were not frequently damaged and in the sitting position the relatively normal posterior femoral condyle would articulate with the flat tibial plates. There was no patellar replacement and, as observed, the flat tibial plates had no lateral constraint.

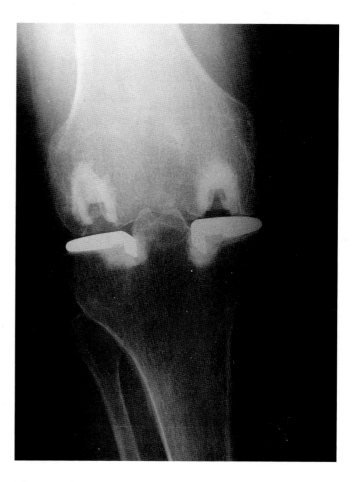

Figure 1

Load angle inlay of John Charnley [Manufacturers: Chas. F Thackray Ltd (Leeds)]. High-density polyethylene curved runners are recessed into the femoral condyles and articulated with flat metal plates on the tibia during the swing phase of the gait, 10–55° of flexion, that Charnley designated the 'load angle'.

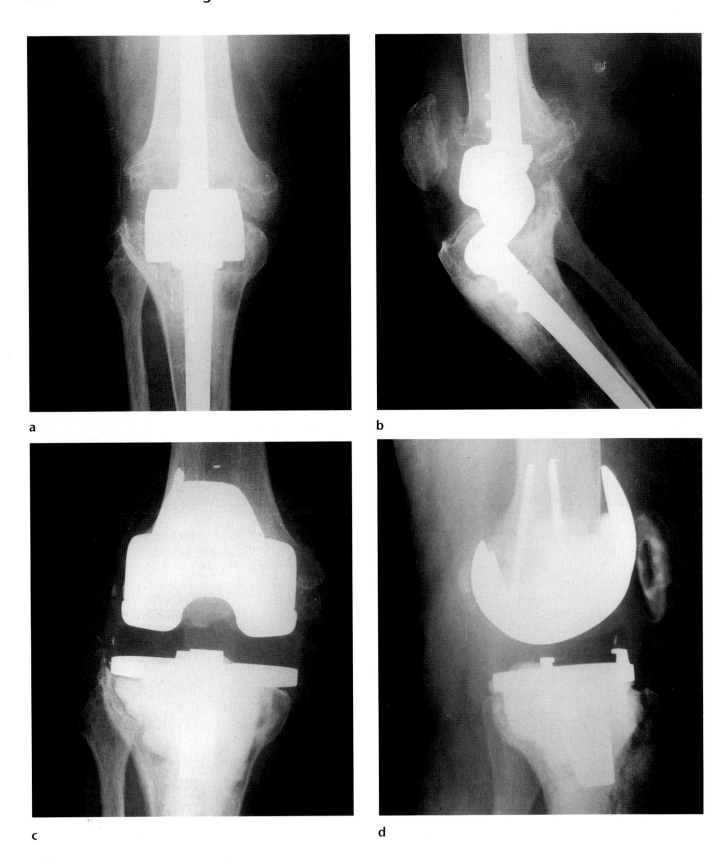

a

b

c

d

Figure 2

(a and b) Shiers and Walldius type of total knee arthroplasty showing massive endosteal cavitation of the tibia and subsidence of the implant due to loosening. (c and d) Revision to a total condylar knee arthroplasty. Supporting screws are inserted into the femur in order to provide a strut support. In this way the implant is held up so that compression can be applied to the cement. The tibial medullary canal is blocked by a cement restrictor (metal marker visible) and cement used to fill the cavity. Despite the bone cement demarcation shown in the lateral view, function has been maintained for nine years.

The success in the early cases led to an extension of the arthroplasties from rheumatoid arthritis to osteoarthrosis. In addition, Charnley did not, at that stage (1972–4), have confidence in the larger arthroplasties available—Shiers and Walldius hinges, which he considered removed too much bone to allow a satisfactory salvage procedure in the event of failure (Figure 2).

In the load angle inlay, the lack of lateral constraint led to instability and the lack of patellar components resulted in stiffness when patellofemoral degeneration developed. It was recognized that the load angle inlay had a narrow application in rheumatoid arthritis in its early stages of joint degeneration and, in 1978, the Attenborough knee arthroplasty was performed for 2 years with a total of 120 cases in all. Patellar problems and the lack of a comprehensive jigging system caused a move gradually to the total condylar knee from 1978 onwards.

The lessons learned from the load angle inlay and the Attenborough arthroplasty brought about an appreciation of the principles of knee arthroplasty which are widely accepted.

1. Medial parapatellar skin and capsular incision offers best exposure and minimal excavation of soft tissue allows best closure with least wound dehiscence.
2. Ligamentous release is important in bringing about soft-tissue balance to allow correct alignment. The soft-tissue release should be sufficient to allow the limb to 'fall' into correct alignment; it should not be held in tension in the 'correct' position by tensors or distracting devices.
3. Arthritis of the knee is progressive and minimal knee arthroplasties replacing only small damaged areas of the bone ends can be overwhelmed by subsequent deterioration of the joint.
4. Tibial components need to have some form of lateral constraint, otherwise subluxation in the coronal plane can occur.
5. Lack of resurfacing of the patella leads to subsequent development of pain and stiffness due to the onset of patellofemoral arthrosis.
6. A poor range of movement in the postoperative phase is usually followed by a stiff knee.
7. Jigging systems of the knee must take account of correct alignment in the sagittal, coronal and rotary planes. The knee flexes, hinges, glides and rotates, so that a jigging system must take account of all these dimensions.

Revision of total condylar knee arthroplasty

Between 1978 and 1989, 2178 total knee arthroplasties of the total condylar type were performed at Wrightington Hospital. There were 314 Mark I polyethylene tibial component total knee arthroplasties from 1978 to 1981, and from 1981 onwards 1864 Mark II total condylars, the tibial components being metal-backed.

A gradual increase in the success of the procedure is reflected in the complication revision rate. There were 44 failures in all—the failure rate in Mark I being 17/314 = 5.4%, but in the Mark II knee cases 31/1864 = 1.66%.

The failures were all due to infection, loosening of the components due to technical error, or loosening due to fracture of the components (tibial plates in the case of kinematic total condylar implants). Of the 12 knees that were infected 8 patients had a rheumatoid arthritis and 4 patients osteoarthrosis. Of the patients with osteoarthrosis, 3 out of 4 had previous surgery—upper tibial osteotomies in all cases.

In the rheumatoid arthritis cases, 6 out of 8 had a late infection, that is an infection that did not manifest itself clinically and radiologically until at least 1 year had elapsed after the operation. Further surgery in this infection group consisted of 2 revisions, 10 pseudarthroses and 2 Kuntscher nail fusions as secondary procedure when 6 months had elapsed after the initial pseudarthrosis (Figure 3).

Complications of the total knee arthroplasty are many and varied but there are special anatomical features that distinguish the superficially placed knee joint from the deeply situated hip joint.

Care of the soft tissues is of paramount importance in knee arthroplasty, as a breakdown of the skin or capsule can lead to infection and disaster. The earlier stemmed hinges (Walldius, Shiers) imparted severe shearing strain to the knee and loosening could occur with consequent endosteal cavitation of the femur and tibia (Figure 2). Loosening of the total condylar type replacement can also occur with loss of bone stock and resort may need to be made to larger implants.

Any resumé of complications will be incomplete, but an approximate scale of complications, rising in severity, is presented with suggested actions:

(1) Dehiscence of skin. Secondary suture after local cleansing with aqueous povidone solution, lavage and soaking with hydrogen peroxide and spraying with topical antimicrobial neomycin or povidone iodine.

(2) Extensor lag and dislocation of patella due to dehiscence of capsular suture line. Secondary suture using interrupted non-absorbable sutures with or without lateral release of the quadriceps mechanism depending upon the tracking of the patella.

(3) Extension loss due to rupture of the ligamentum patellae—a troublesome and potentially intractable problem. Secondary suture using augmenting material such as Gore-Tex ligament that must be passed through drill holes in the anterior tibial tubercle and lower pole of the patella.

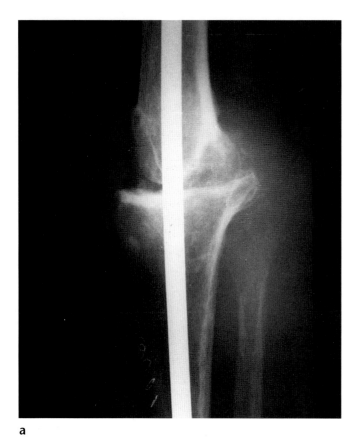

a

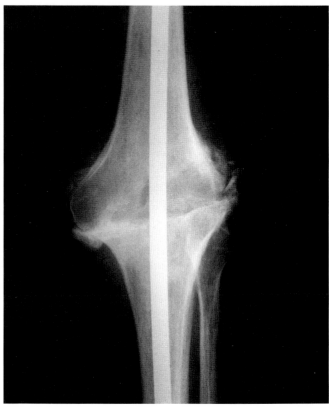

b

Figure 3

(a and b) Kuntscher nail fusion of the knee joint is resorted to where there is severe deficiency of the bone ends and/or marked fibrosis of the quadriceps mechanism. If as a result of sepsis or multiple operations quadriceps fibrosis occurs, a poor range of movement can be forecast in the postoperative phase. A stiff knee arthroplasty (less than 15° of movement) is undesirable as often the knee is flexed and irritable. Kuntscher nail fusion is adopted when the bone ends are ragged and friable and unlikely to hold a compression device.

(4) Subluxation of implant due to rupture of the quadriceps mechanism. This can result in complete dislocation of the implant and is usually accompanied by a traumatic episode, such as a fall downstairs onto the affected limb with consequent rupture of the quadriceps mechanism. It is usually necessary to resort to a constrained implant such as a Gallannaugh, which has a central post that confers anterior–posterior stability (Figure 4).

(5) Loosening of patellar component. This can occur as a result of poor initial fixation or more frequently may be a reflection of high focal loading of the patellar component fixation. This latter condition reflects faulty alignment of the knee components as a whole, and, even though revision of the patellar component may provide a temporary improvement, further problems can be encountered because of component malalignment—the most common of which is internal rotation of the femoral component. Revision of the major component may be necessary if the patella fails to track properly after a revision of its fixation.

(6) Fracture of the tibial component. This has been a problem in some varieties of total condylar components (in our experience the tibial plateau of the kinematic implant). Revision to the Kinemax is possible in many cases but occasionally resort must be made to a stemmed implant such as the Gallannaugh.

(7) Loosening of the tibial or femoral components. If these occur in isolation it is usually due to incorrect initial alignment. This may be corrected at revision. If both components are loose, a suspicion that a low-grade infection is present must be considered and revision must take account of this with complete debridement, sterilization with topical antimicrobials and systemic antibiotics.

(8) Fractures of the femur and tibia around the implant. It is usually necessary to use a stemmed implant to augment the fixation; the Gallannaugh prosthesis is a versatile implant in this respect.

(9) Loss of bone stock of femur and tibia due to absorption histiocytosis and loosening of long-stemmed implants. Bone grafting will need to be

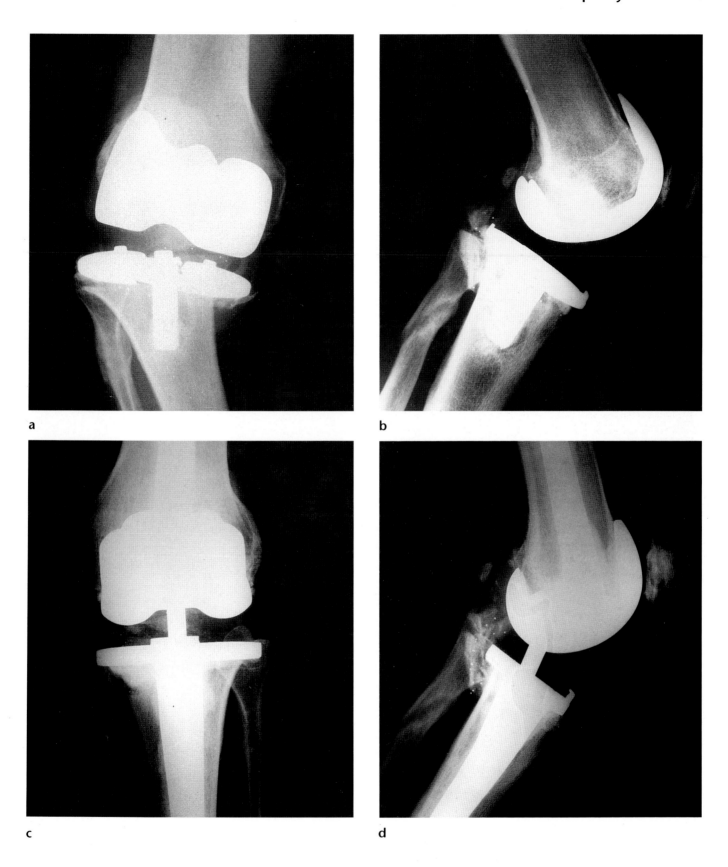

a

b

c

d

Figure 4

Fracture of the tibial plateau of cemented PCA knee arthroplasty. There had previously been an upper tibial osteotomy and a kinematic knee arthroplasty, both of which had been followed by marked coronal instability. (a) The anteroposterior view shows the fracture of the prosthetic medial tibial plateau. (b) The lateral view shows the loosened prosthetic tibial component and fracture of the posterior tibial metaphysis. (c) and (d) show postoperative anteroposterior and lateral views of Gallannaugh knee arthroplasty using stemmed components to produce stability. The central post of the implant confers sagittal and coronal stability in the arthroplasty.

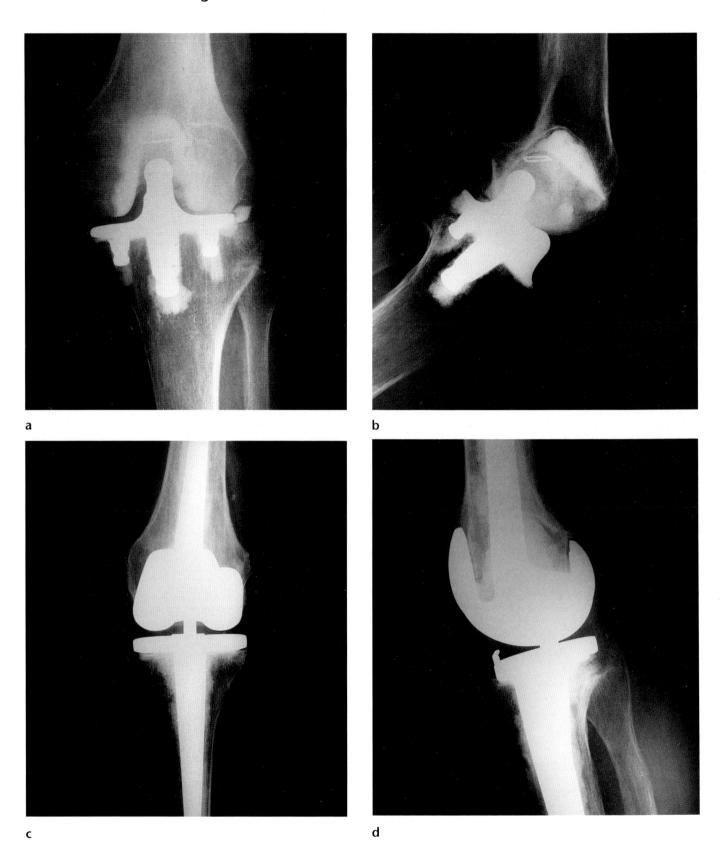

a

b

c

d

Figure 5

Loosening of Deane ball and socket knee arthroplasty. Cystic change in the lateral femoral condyle due to erosion of the high-density polyethylene caused a caseous necrosis in the bone. Revision using the stemmed Gallannaugh implant restores stability in the knee.

considered in addition to stemmed implants as above.

(10) Fibrosis of quadriceps mechanism. Occasionally exploration of an implant that has been installed for some time reveals extreme stiffness of the implant due to fibrosis of the quadriceps mechanism in addition to intra-articular adhesions. If there is severe bony defect requiring grafting and of necessity a slow increase in movement afterwards, it is to be expected that the fibrosis of the quadriceps mechanism will militate against regaining a good range of movement in the arthroplasty. The worst scenario is an arthroplasty with a poor range of movement. In these cases, it is worth considering an arthrodesis which, because of the ragged bone ends, can usefully be performed using a Kuntscher nail (Figure 3).

Technical features of knee arthroplasty revision

(1) Constrained hinges such as the Shiers, Walldius and Guepar cause large torsional forces in the femur and tibia. If they are inadequately fixed, loosening can occur with subsidence of the implant and endosteal cavitation in the femur and tibia (Figure 2a). In revision, the collateral ligaments need to be put under tension by using high tibial components and alignment of the femoral component needs to be maintained by screw struts so that compression can be applied to the femoral component to obtain a high pressure bone cement fixation (Figure 2). Despite the demarcation shown in the tibial fixation, knee function has been maintained over a 9-year period.

(2) The Deane ball and socket knee replacement (Figure 5). Here there is a reversal of the normal configuration in that the femoral component is made out of high-density polyethylene and has a central socket that contains a ball from the metal tibial component. This acts as a pivot to allow flexion along with lateral shoulders. In this case, the high-density polyethylene has deformed and become abraded so that a gross cystic area has occurred in the lower end of the femur (Figure 5a,b). In revision, resort had to be made to a Gallannaugh arthroplasty conferring fixation and stability (Figure 5c,d).

19

Medical management of the rheumatoid knee

19.1 Medical and conservative management of the rheumatoid knee

Edward C. Huskisson

Physicians and surgeons have probably contributed in about equal proportions to the transformation which has occurred in the prognosis of rheumatoid arthritis. It is impossible to fail to notice a huge reduction in the numbers of seriously disabled patients in wheelchairs attending rheumatology clinics and a corresponding increase in the numbers of patients who are active and mobile but who attend regularly for supervision of their therapy. Two things have contributed to the change. First, drugs are now available which control rheumatoid disease; notable among them are penicillamine, azathioprine and methotrexate. Second, joints can be replaced before patients become immobile. In rheumatoid arthritis, serious disability can usually be avoided by replacement surgery, particularly for advanced disease of the hip and knee. Another feature of modern management is the cooperation between physician and surgeon; joint clinics are now considered essential for a properly constituted centre for the treatment of arthritis.

When to choose conservative therapy

With a wide choice of treatment modalities, drugs of different types, surgery and many other possible approaches, it is clearly essential to choose the right treatment for the right patient at the right time in the course of his disease. Patients with rheumatoid disease may be seen first by general practitioners or by rheumatologists or orthopaedic surgeons, sometimes by physiotherapists or less orthodox practitioners. All have the responsibility to ensure that patients get the treatment they need. Early active rheumatoid disease presents an opportunity to achieve good control with drugs—once the disease is established with permanent joint damage and the accompaniments of chronic inflammation (pannus, cartilage deterioration and fibrinous debris in the joint) the possibilities are much less exciting, although drug treatment may still

Table 1 Features which suggest that medical and conservative treatment will be particularly appropriate for a rheumatoid knee.

SYMPTOMS
Prolonged morning stiffness
SIGNS
Warmth; a large effusion
TESTS
High ESR
Minimal change on radiographs

be worthwhile. Similarly, a disabled patient with flexion deformities of both knees who has not walked for years is a less exciting prospect to the orthopaedic surgeon than a patient whose knees are just beginning to threaten his mobility.

Assessment is therefore all-important. Table 1 summarizes those features of rheumatoid disease of the knee which suggest that medical and conservative therapy is particularly appropriate. In essence, these features suggest that symptoms arise predominantly from active inflammation rather than from anatomical damage to the joint.

Pain is a feature of both active inflammation and structural deterioration of joints and its severity is of little help in attributing the pain; in inflammatory situations, the pain tends to be worse in the morning and relieved by activity, while with mechanical damage the pain is relieved by rest and brought on by activity. Morning stiffness is, however, a particularly good guide to the severity of the inflammatory process. Signs similarly reflect the presence or absence of inflammation: warmth and a large effusion are amongst the cardinal signs and the presence or absence of structural deterioration indicated by deformity, instability and crepitus on movement. The ESR is some guide to systemic inflammation and radiographs are of value in assessing the degree of cartilage loss.

The variability of rheumatic disease

The knee is almost always involved in rheumatoid arthritis, and even when it is just part of a generalized inflammatory polyarthritis it is usually an important part. Some aspects of the variability of rheumatoid arthritis are summarized in Table 2.

About 25% of cases of rheumatoid arthritis are monarticular at presentation and the knee is the commonest site of such disease. About half of these cases will go on to develop the more typical bilateral symmetrical polyarthritis. Monarticular diseases often atypical in other respects, may be seronegative and may be relatively benign. It is in these atypical cases that one should consider the differential diagnosis, particularly psoriatic arthropathy (Figure 1) which may be difficult to distinguish, and other inflammatory conditions such as pyrophosphate arthropathy.

While rheumatoid arthritis is usually easy for diagnosis, it is often difficult for prognosis. But it is important to try to predict, in order to decide on appropriate treatment. The cases which do best are those presenting acutely at an older age and with negative tests for rheumatoid factor. The most severe cases are in teenagers, and patients who present after many years of disease tend to have an unpleasant course with a lot of joint destruction and often little in the way of inflammation. Seropositivity is a weak guide to prognosis and other measures like the ESR are of no value at all. Rheumatoid disease can be very benign—some cases never appear in hospital clinics and are discovered only at population surveys. It is more often damaging or disabling and in all its forms is unpleasant and worthy of our best endeavours at treatment.

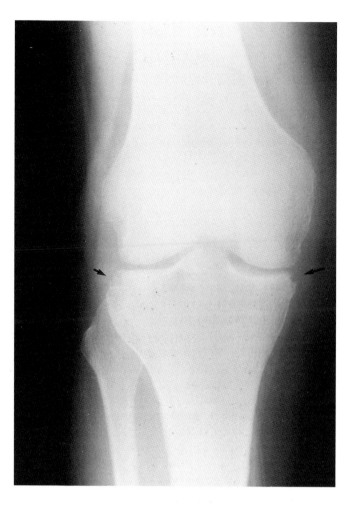

Figure 1

Radiograph of a 75-year-old woman with psoriatic arthropathy of the knee. The black arrows show the peripheral erosions. By kind permission of Mr Paul M. Aichroth and Mr Dipak V. Patel.

Medical treatment of the rheumatoid knee

The physician's instruments are summarized in Table 3. Drugs are of various types; the non-steroidal anti-inflammatory drugs are pre-eminent for the relief of symptoms and the penicillamine-like drugs are of increasing importance in the attempt to control the disease and alter its course. The physician may consider intra-articular therapy, particularly with corticosteroids. Finally, physical measures and psychological aspects must be considered.

Table 2 Some aspects of the variability of rheumatoid disease.

Joint involvement	Outcome	Prognosis
Monarticular 25% at onset; often knees	Unpleasant but with minimal damage in 33%	Better with acute onset, older age and seronegativity
Polyarticular 75% of cases, usually including knees	Unpleasant and deforming in 33% Unpleasant and disabling in 33%	Worse with insidious onset, younger age and seropositivity

Table 3 The physician's instruments.

Drugs
  Penicillamine
  NSAIDs
  Corticosteroids
  Analgesics

Intra-articular therapy

Physical measures
  Rest, splints, exercises, laser therapy

Psychological aspects

Penicillamine-like drugs

This class of drugs is now widely used in rheumatoid arthritis. They have no immediate analgesic or anti-inflammatory activity; they start to work after 4–6 weeks and require 4–6 months to achieve their maximal activity. Their action on joints is accompanied by a reduction in ESR and in the titre of rheumatoid factor. They have the potential to cause serious side-effects and all require careful supervision. Penicillamine is a good choice for the younger patient and it illustrates an important concept which is true of many of these drugs: success requires the skilful management of adverse reactions, for which penicillamine has a considerable potential. Many different problems may arise and it is essential to know the natural history of these drug-related syndromes in order to plan their management. Some are relatively benign, like the loss of taste which recovers despite continued treatment. Surprisingly, this is also true of the immune-complex nephritis which can complicate penicillamine therapy. Provided that proteinuria is not excessive, treatment can therefore be continued. The aim of such treatment is of course the long-term control of the disease—over many years, not just for a year or two. Routine supervision of penicillamine therapy usually requires monthly full blood counts and urine testing for protein. Communication between physician and patient is essential to provide safe supervision.

Methotrexate is probably the most effective treatment currently available for rheumatoid arthritis and has a convenient weekly dosing schedule. It is usually reserved for older patients because of the theoretical hazards of immunosuppressive therapy. Extensive experience of the use of azathioprine in younger patients following renal transplantation suggests that such restriction is no longer necessary for this drug. Such patients had normal pregnancies despite continuing treatment, suggesting that azathioprine can now be used for the younger rheumatoid patient of potential child-bearing age.

It is fortunate that there are many drugs of this type, since side-effects and lack of response limit the usefulness of any single agent. Some are relatively

Table 4 Penicillamine-like drugs for rheumatoid arthritis.

The 'big three'	Penicillamine 250 mg daily Azathioprine 50 mg twice daily Methotrexate 7.5 mg weekly
The rest	Injectable gold Auranofin Hydroxychloroquine Sulphasalazine

safer than the 'big three' and hydroxychloroquine, sulphasalazine and auranofin are notable in this respect. In the difficult case, it is becoming fashionable to combine therapies and the combination of sulphasalazine and penicillamine or an immunosuppressive drug is particularly useful. Drugs of this type are listed in Table 4.

The non-steroidal anti-inflammatory drugs (NSAIDs)

Non-steroidal anti-inflammatory drugs are the cornerstone of symptomatic therapy in rheumatoid arthritis. Early in the course of the disease, it is a good plan to establish an optimal anti-inflammatory regime, recognizing that individual variation in response is the major factor that determines efficacy. A selection of NSAIDs is available, emphasizing the once-a-day drugs which are usually preferred nowadays. The analgesic action of these drugs is sometimes of benefit, particularly in advanced disease and ibuprofen is included as an example of this use. These drugs take no more than a few days to become effective and a week is therefore sufficient to find out whether they will be adequate. It is a good plan to give four of them, each for a week at the onset of the disease, and to choose the best. Modern drugs are well tolerated with only occasional patients having to stop treatment because of indigestion or rarely a rash. There is, however, increasing concern about the frequency of gastric catastrophes, but it is possible to identify patients particularly at risk who should be treated with particular care. Age is the major risk factor and elderly women are particularly at risk. Other risk factors include rheumatoid disease, steroid therapy and smoking. If anti-inflammatory therapy is essential in such patients, and in rheumatoid arthritis it usually is, it should be combined with the prostaglandin analogue misoprostol.

Intra-articular therapy

Although some orthopaedic surgeons dislike and discourage the use of intra-articular steroids, they are widely used by rheumatologists. There is no doubt that overuse is harmful and that such therapy should be used occasionally and in response to clear-cut indications. There are three indications: first to relieve pain, for example in a patient whose arthritis is responding to a penicillamine-like drug but who has a persistently painful and swollen knee. There is the expectation that long-term control will be achieved with drugs, so that the repeated use of intra-articular steroids will not be necessary. Second, as an aid to correcting deformity, for example a flexion deformity of the knee of recent origin in a patient with early disease and no structural deterioration. Third, as an aid to the mobilization of a stiff joint, also resulting from active inflammation rather than structural damage.

A variety of intra-articular medication has been tried in rheumatoid arthritis, including radioactive isotopes and toxic chemicals such as osmium, with the aim of achieving a synovectomy. None of these has been of proven value and none can be recommended.

Physical therapy

The value of physical therapy as an adjunct to other measures in the treatment of rheumatoid arthritis is beyond doubt. Rest is of particular importance early in the course of the disease and splints may be useful to prevent or correct flexion deformity in the knee joint. Quadriceps exercises are an essential part of the restoration of a knee joint once the inflammatory process has been controlled. Ultrasound, laser and other radiations are used to relieve symptoms.

Psychological aspects

Rheumatoid arthritis is a potentially devastating illness which mainly affects young people. Not surprisingly, it has a huge impact on psychological well-being, marriages and social activity, as well as on mobility. The physician or whoever takes on the long-term care of such a patient can make a huge difference to the patient's quality of life, not only by skilful management of the disease but by being a caring and sympathetic guide for a long and sometimes difficult journey.

20

Anterior knee pain

20.1   Anterior knee pain

George S. E. Dowd and George Bentley

Anterior knee pain is a non-specific term encompassing many different clinical disorders. While patients with anterior knee pain may have chondromalacia patellae, the two are not synonymous. This point is emphasized since an accurate diagnosis of the cause of anterior knee pain is essential in order to provide specific and successful treatment.

Whereas some disorders, such as idiopathic symptomatic chondromalacia patellae, may be difficult to treat successfully, others, including thickened synovial plicae, are treatable by surgery.

The techniques of arthroscopy and arthroscopic surgery have greatly improved the diagnostic accuracy and management of anterior knee pain. Arthroscopy has also facilitated postoperative rehabilitation by avoiding the large incisions previously associated with arthrotomy.

Causes of anterior knee pain

Disorders causing anterior knee pain, excluding significant patellar fractures, dislocations and osteoarthritis, include:

Extra-articular
Bursae
   Infrapatellar bursitis
   Prepatellar bursitis
Patellar tendon
   'Jumper's knee'
   Osgood–Schlatter's disease
   Sinding–Larsen–Johansson disease
Patellar disorders
   Subluxation of the patella
   Chondromalacia patellae
   Osteochondritis dissecans patellae
   Bipartite patella
   Excessive lateral pressure syndrome (ELPS)
   Marginal fractures of the patella
   Infrapatellar fat-pad syndrome
Intra-articular disorders
   Synovial plicae
   Anterior horn meniscal tears
   Discoid lateral menisci
   Reflex sympathetic dystrophy

The history

A careful history is an essential basis for further investigation and diagnosis of anterior knee pain.

Often the symptoms are vague and the site of pain is poorly defined. This is especially the case in patients with chondromalacia patellae. Exacerbating factors such as athletic activity and climbing up and down stairs are significant in patellofemoral problems because of the increased loading of the joint in this type of activity. It is rare for the patient to be awakened from sleep by pain. However, prolonged sitting with the knees flexed often exacerbates the pain of chondromalacia patellae, while not affecting such disorders as jumper's knee, plicae or meniscal injuries.

Kneeling may well exacerbate disorders such as bursitis and Osgood–Schlatter's disease.

'Giving-way', due to transient quadriceps inhibition, may occur in many cases of anterior knee pain including chondromalacia and early patellofemoral osteoarthritis. It may also be associated with patellar instability in teenagers and rarely with torn menisci.

While many patients complain of swelling in the knee, it is not usually the classical effusion of the knee with a swollen suprapatellar pouch but a subjective feeling of swelling, often localized to the site of pain. Free fluid in the joint suggests severe cartilage damage or an inflammatory synovitis.

Restriction of movement is not usually a symptom in anterior knee pain but occasionally the patient may describe a feeling of 'stiffness' in the knee. 'Locking' or catching of the knee may also be described by the patient with anterior knee pain during mid-movement, but this is not the true locking of a bucket-handle tear since the symptom does not result in restriction of extension.

Physical signs

Observation of the patient's gait is essential to assess any exaggerated response to pain and to see whether the patient limps.

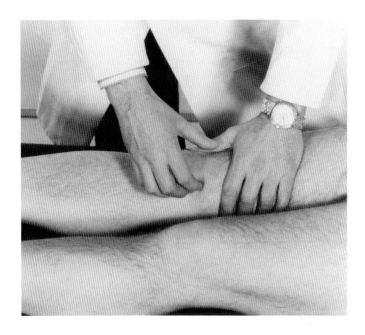

Figure 1

Examination for medial retropatellar tenderness.

The patient should be asked to crouch and return to the erect position to assess loading on the patellofemoral joints. Palpation of the patellae by the examiner may elicit crepitus from the patellofemoral joints during this procedure.

The patient should be requested to sit over the edge of the examining couch, and asked to actively extend and flex the knees; the excursion of the patellae can then be examined for any gross malpositioning or tracking. There is great variability in patellar excursion in normal individuals, so that only gross maltracking is relevant.

Examining for an effusion is essential since its presence, no matter how small, suggests a pathology within the knee. Likewise, the presence of measurable quadriceps wasting greater than 2 cm, at 6 cm above the patella, strongly suggests knee pathology.[1]

Having measured the range of movement in both knees, the knee should be examined for tenderness and an attempt made to correlate the sites of tenderness with the patient's pain.

Gentle medial shift of the patella will allow palpation of the undersurface of the patella over the medial facet, a frequent site of tenderness in chondromalacia patellae (Figure 1).

Tenderness may be elicited along the joint lines in chondromalacia patellae, but must not be confused with that due to a torn meniscus. It is almost certainly due to synovitis at the junction with the margins of the joint. Unfortunately, it has been shown that in chondromalacia patellae tenderness was the vaguest and least reliable sign of the disorder.[2] In jumper's knee the site of tenderness is at the lower pole of the patella and in Osgood–Schlatter's disease, which is confined to teenagers, is over the tibial tubercle. Tenderness may be elicited over the femoral condyle due to a thickened synovial plica, where constant rubbing of the fold over the articular surface of the condyle may have resulted in an area of fibrillation. With a very thick plica, the plica itself may be palpable.

Signs of patellar instability (subluxation and dislocation)

A more detailed examination of the patellofemoral joint must include the passive mobility of the patella with the knee extended and the quadriceps muscle relaxed. Since mobility of the patella varies greatly in individuals, the normal should be compared with the abnormal knee, if possible. The classical finding is a small, high patella which is excessively mobile in a teenage female. This is not diagnostic of instability and many attempts have been made to quantitate instability; few if any are reliable. Kolowich et al.[3] described a patellar glide test with the knee in 30° of flexion to assess either medial or lateral laxity. They considered that a lateral patellar glide of three quadrants was suggestive of an incompetent medial restraint. They measured the Q (quadriceps) angle, the angle between a line drawn proximally from the anterior superior iliac spine passing through the middle of the patella and a line passing down through the centre of the patella to the centre of the tibial tubercle with the knee flexed to 90°. They referred to it as the 90° tubercle–sulcus angle. A Q angle greater than 10° was regarded as abnormal. They also described a patellar tilt test in which the knee is fully extended and the quadriceps relaxed. An excessively tight lateral restraint was demonstrated by a neutral or negative angle between the horizontal and a line drawn across the superior border of the patella when the lateral edge of the patella is lifted from the lateral femoral condyle. The apprehension test, where the knee is gently flexed while applying a lateral force to the patella, should be interpreted with great caution. Classically, sudden resistance to this manoeuvre by the patient indicates patellar instability, since the test reproduces the feeling of giving-way and pain associated with the disorder. However, other causes for a positive test include a forceful examination and the possibility of pain caused by pressure on the medial facet of the patella, which is the site of chondromalacia. It is essential to assess whether the test reproduces the symptoms described by the patient.

These assessments and measurements are notoriously difficult to repeat accurately and we rely, in doubtful cases, on assessment of patellar instability under general anaesthesia, which will demonstrate whether the patella is unstable or dislocatable.[4] The instability described above is due to slackness of the quadriceps mechanism. It is important to realize that abnormal lateral tracking of the patella, which may lead to dislocation in flexion, may occur secondarily to congenital tightness of the lateral quadriceps retinaculum, a condition similar to, if not identical to, the excessive lateral pressure syndrome described by Ficat.[5]

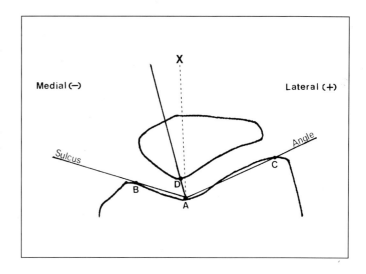

Figure 2

Congruence angle: the angle (XAD) between the line from the lowest point in the sulcus (A) to the lowest point on the patella (D) and the line bisecting the sulcus angle (XA). *Sulcus angle*: the angle (BAC) between the highest point of the medial (B) and lateral (C) condyle and the lowest point in the sulcus. (After ref. 6.)

Radiographic assessment in anterior knee pain

In recent years, many radiographic techniques have been developed in an attempt to aid diagnosis in cases of anterior knee pain. Obviously, in cases of soft-tissue pathology such as jumper's knee or bursitis, no abnormality will be present.

The tangential radiograph

Various methods of visualizing the patellofemoral joint have been described, but the one described by Merchant et al.[6] has probably been used most frequently.

Using this technique, the patient lies flat on his back and the knees are flexed to about 30° with the quadriceps muscle relaxed. Both patellofemoral joints are radiographed in comparable positions on the same plate. Careful positioning by an experienced radiographer is essential in producing useful radiographs for measurement.

Merchant's views can be useful in assessing degrees of lateral subluxation of the patella and may identify old marginal fractures not visualized on routine anteroposterior and lateral radiographs of the knee. However, the authors found that patients with 'idiopathic' chondromalacia patellae demonstrated no such abnormal measurements.[4]

Sulcus angle

The sulcus angle can be measured simply from the tangential radiograph (Figure 2) and, as described by Merchant et al.,[6] is greater in patients with femoral dysplasia. Brattström,[7] using a complicated technique not applicable to routine clinical use, gave a mean sulcus angle of 142°. Merchant et al.[6] described a mean angle of 138° (range 126–150°, SD ±6°) and Aglietti and Cerulli,[8] using the same technique,

presented similar results. In Dowd and Bentley's[4] series of 50 normal knees, the mean was 139° (range 120–150°, SD ±6.3°). In a series of 40 patients with symptomatic subluxation of the patella, the sulcus angle was increased to a mean of 147° (range 137–172°, SD ±7.26°). In 35 patients with symptomatic chondromalacia patellae confirmed by arthroscopy, the measurements were also within normal limits. By contrast, Aglietti and Cerulli,[8] observed a significant difference in the sulcus angle between normals and those with both chondromalacia and subluxation, but they did not distinguish clearly between the groups. The discrepancy may be explained by the fact that in our series, the diagnosis of chondromalacia was based on both clinical and arthroscopic findings, and cases of malalignment associated with chondromalacic changes were separated from those with chondromalacia but no malalignment as proved by examination under general anaesthesia. In Aglietti's series, the diagnosis of chondromalacia was made on clinical grounds only.

Congruence angle

Merchant et al.[6] stated that the congruence angle was useful in identifying minor degrees of patellar subluxation. The angle is measured by bisecting the angle between the highest points on the femoral condyles

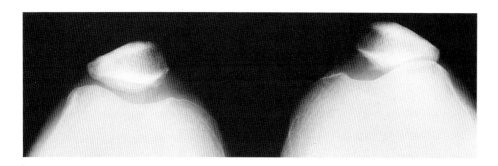

Figure 3

Radiographs of a patient with bilateral dislocating patellae. Both knees demonstrate an abnormal sulcus angle. Only the right knee demonstrates an increased abnormal congruence angle.

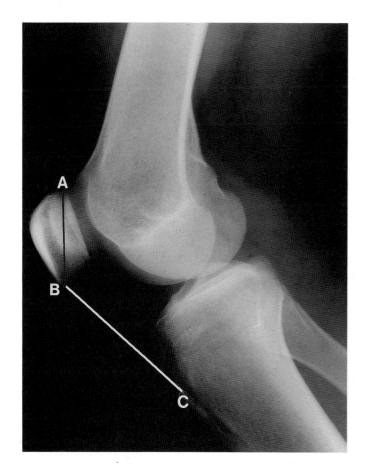

Figure 4

The patellar tendon/patella ratio is the ratio between the length BC to length AB. In this case the ratio is 1.8. (After ref. 9.)

and the lowest point in the sulcus and measuring the angle between the bisector and a line from the lowest point on the patella and the lowest point in the sulcus (Figure 2).

In a study of 200 knees,[6] the mean was −6° and a congruence angle greater than +16° was considered abnormal at the 95th percentile. Aglietti et al.[8] demonstrated a mean congruence angle of −9° in a series of 100 normal knees. They also found a mean value of 0° in 30 patients with chondromalacia and a mean of +17° in patients with recurrent subluxation. In our series of 35 patients with chondromalacia confirmed by arthroscopy, we were unable to confirm these findings.[4] The congruence angle was within the normal range in patients with chondromalacia and in recurrent subluxation, while the mean congruence angle was increased; only 4 out of 33 patients had a congruence angle outside the 95th percentile of the normal group[4] (Figure 3).

Patellar tendon/patella ratio (Figure 4)

Insall and Salvati[9] described a method of measuring the ratio between the greatest diagonal length of the patella and the length of the patellar tendon using a lateral radiograph taken with the knee in about 30–40° of flexion. They found that these two measurements were equal in a normal population and that a variation of greater than ±0.2 represented an abnormal position of the patella.

Lancourt and Cristini,[10] in a series of male and female patients with chondromalacia patellae and recurrent dislocation, claimed that patella alta was a significant factor in both conditions. When further investigations were performed by other authors,[4,11] they showed that if the results in both normals and chondromalacia were matched by sex, there was no difference in the patellar index between the two groups. In our series,[4] patella alta was significant in instability and the presence of a patellar tendon/patellar length ratio of greater than 1.25 indicated patellar instability, especially when associated with a femoral sulcus angle greater than 140°.

Computerized tomography and magnetic resonance imaging

Reikeras and Hoiseth,[12] using computerized tomography (CT), described the relationship of the patellofemoral joint in the adult knee in 43 patients. No significant differences were found between men and women or left and right knees. They showed that instability of the patella was most evident in full extension of the knee and often the abnormal knee was congruent beyond 30° of flexion.

Ihara[13] used double-contrast arthrography with air and contrast together with CT with the knee flexed to 30° in order to study the articular cartilage of the patellofemoral joint. He studied the results in cadaveric specimens in which cartilage defects were made and then used the technique on a series of patients. Computerized tomographic results were compared with arthroscopic or arthrotomy findings. The results showed that the CT diagnosis was accurate in 68 of 70 knees. Similar results were reported by Boven et al.[14] The stated disadvantage of arthroscopy alone was the inability to assess the depth of the patellar articular cartilage and the extent of ulceration in the deep layers. Ihara maintained that combined CT double-contrast arthrography and arthroscopy provided a comprehensive evaluation of the patellofemoral joint cartilage.

Yulish et al.[15] have presented their results of magnetic resonance imaging (MRI) scanning in patients with chondromalacia patellae. MRI showed focal areas of swelling of the patellar cartilage surface, irregularity and thinning. They correlated their results with arthroscopic findings and found MRI to be an accurate method of assessing chondromalacia patellae, but it is not accurate in assessing the extent of the surface of cartilage damage.

Boven et al.[16] described the assessment of synovial plicae by computed tomography following double-contrast arthrography, but such an assessment appears to be inferior to direct visualization by arthroscopy.

Shellock et al.[17] have developed a technique described as kinematic MRI to assess patellar tracking from 0 to 30° of flexion of the knee and this technique may prove valuable for assessing tracking disorders.

The drawback of routine CT and MRI imaging, as of radiography, is the static nature of the investigation. It is possible that with dynamic imaging of the patellofemoral joint more information on the patient with anterior knee pain and no other obvious abnormality may be forthcoming. This is particularly so in minor degrees of patellar instability.

Arthroscopic assessment of patellar alignment

The normal patella, when viewed from the midline below or above, strikes the femoral groove 2–3 mm lateral of 'dead centre'. We employ this method in addition to examination under anaesthesia and radiography to assess patellar tracking. Displacement laterally by more than 5 mm suggests malalignment.

Disorders producing anterior knee pain

Idiopathic chondromalacia patellae

Chondromalacia patellae is a clearly defined syndrome of pain accurately localized to the patella and accompanied by abnormal changes in the articular cartilage on the undersurface of the patella. One group of patients, usually female, complain of aching pain behind the patella, especially after sitting for a period with knees flexed. It is frequently relieved by gentle movement. In more advanced cases, the pain is more persistent and is aggravated by increased activity and often by climbing and descending stairs, when the patellofemoral joint is subjected to increased loading. Frequently, the symptoms are bilateral. Another group are highly athletic individuals who are restricted during activity by anterior knee pain. While the majority of cases of chondromalacia do not have an obvious cause, the disorder may be related to some underlying condition such as subluxation of the patella or excessive lateral pressure syndrome. In this case the chondromalacia affects the lateral patellar facet.[18]

Examination of the knee may reveal tenderness on palpation of the medial undersurface of the patella. While quadriceps wasting may be present, free fluid in the knee joint is unusual. In approximately 50% of patients, palpable crepitus may be felt from the patellofemoral joint on flexion and extension of the knee.[1]

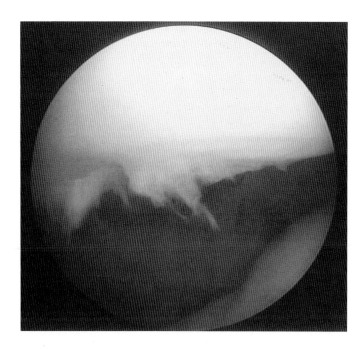

Figure 5

Typical arthroscopic features of fibrillation of articular cartilage over the medial facet of the patella.

It should be stressed that articular cartilage changes of chondromalacia may be present without symptoms, just as osteoarthritic changes may be present on radiographs without symptoms. A clinical diagnosis of chondromalacia must combine the symptom-complex with articular cartilage changes confirmed by arthroscopy. The lack of correlation between symptoms, physical signs and appearance of the articular surface of the patella at arthroscopy was investigated in a prospective study of 78 patients with persistent retropatellar pain by Leslie and Bentley.[1] It was found that only 51% had abnormalities of articular cartilage of the patella at arthroscopy and the remainder had no demonstrable lesion within the knee. When the patients with no demonstrable abnormality were reviewed at 1 year, 58% were symptom-free. In this study, symptoms were unreliable in predicting the presence of chondromalacia and the only useful physical signs were quadriceps wasting of more than 2 cm, the presence of an effusion in the knee joint and obviously palpable crepitus from the patellofemoral joint on knee flexion.

Without the combination of typical symptoms and arthroscopic changes on the patellar surface, a diagnosis of chondromalacia cannot be made and conditions giving rise to anterior knee pain other than chondromalacia patellae must be considered.

The macroscopic appearances of chondromalacia ('softening of cartilage') are well recognized (Figure 5). The articular cartilage may be roughened, softened or fibrillated and is seen most commonly at the junction of the medial and the 'odd' facet on the undersurface of the patella. Outerbridge[19] graded the changes into four grades which indicate the extent of the cartilage changes from small areas of softening and swelling (Grade 1) to fibrillation or fissuring up to 1 cm in size (Grade 2). Grade 3 is fibrillation or fissuring over an area between 1 and 2 cm, and Grade 4 is fibrillation exceeding 2 cm with exposure of bone. Measurements can be made at arthroscopy by comparing the area of damage with a probe of known length. In a recent editorial, Casscells[20] criticized this classification. He argued that it provided too little information on the state of the chondral lesion and that Grade 4, especially, describes any lesion down to bone irrespective of diameter. He advised the use of one of several more comprehensive classifications which take into account depth as well as diameter.[21-23] It would appear impossible to have a consensus on the issue and there is no doubt that the Outerbridge[19] classification is simple and probably the most frequently used.

Aetiology and pathology

The commonest observed lesion of the articular cartilage is fibrillation on the undersurface of the patella at the junction of the medial and 'odd' facets and this may spread to involve wide areas of the medial facet. The histological appearances are those of superficial fibrillation of the cartilage with loss of cells and matrix staining in zones 1 and 2. Small, heavily stained chondrocyte clusters are seen in zone 3 of the cartilage that is believed to be an attempt at repair. At a later stage, there may be thickening of the subchondral bone.

Ficat[5] described involvement of the lateral facet of the patella and defined a critical zone lateral to the medial ridge of the patella. In our series of over 1000 cases, this type of abnormality is rare. It appears to be associated specifically with tightness of the lateral quadriceps expansion, a disorder which Ficat described as the 'excessive lateral pressure syndrome'.[5]

Hirsch[24] demonstrated that articular cartilage over the medial and 'odd' facets of the patella may be as thick as 0.8 cm and can be the thickest in the human skeleton. It is therefore prone to deficient nutrition from synovial fluid and at the same time mechanically vulnerable, especially in conditions of shear. Ficat[5] suggested that the excessive lateral pressure syndrome, which is due to congenital tightness of the lateral quadriceps retinaculum, results in 'hypopression' of the medial facet, resulting in poorer nutrition and subsequently breakdown and fibrillation of the articular cartilage. The breakdown products, including cathepsins, which are proteolytic enzymes, digest and break down the chains of proteoglycan in the matrix. Such an event leads to loss of proteoglycan pressure and water and an increased susceptibility to fissuring and breakdown of the articular cartilage.

The sequence of events in the breakdown of articular cartilage of the patella is disputed.

Goodfellow et al.[25] described a swollen appearance of the articular cartilage and considered that this was due to a degenerative change in zone 2 of the cartilage. This led to secondary superficial change and fibrillation of the surface due to breakdown in the collagen meshwork support in zones 2 and 3 of the cartilage. However, Bentley,[26] in a study employing histological, electron-microscopic and autoradiographic methods, demonstrated that in 20 out of 21 cases the degeneration of the cartilage began on the surface. This study also demonstrated cell division and 'healing' of chondromalacic cartilage, which could explain the resolution of symptoms recorded in many series with conservative treatment.

Progression of chondromalacia patellae to established osteoarthritis appears to be rare. Karlson[27] followed a series of patients for 20 years and found no incidence of osteoarthritis. Clinically, it is uncommon for patients with established osteoarthritis of the knee to give a history of anterior knee pain in their youth.

Meachim et al.[28] found in a necropsy study of the typical distribution of degenerative change in the patellofemoral joint that progressive changes were mainly on the lateral facet of the patella, which is not the common area for chondromalacia. This suggests a different aetiology and pathological process in the medial facet that may be similar to that described in the hip joint by Byers,[29] who observed age-related cartilage changes in the hip which he believed did not have a major potential to progress to bone exposure of the sort seen in surgical specimens from clinical osteoarthritis.

In a further recent study, Bentley (1988) has confirmed that patients with medial facet chondromalacia do not progress to osteoarthritis and also that osteoarthritis occurs principally on the lateral facet of the patella, suggesting that the two conditions are distinct entities.[18]

Treatment (Table 1)

Conservative management is the basis for treatment in the majority of patients with symptomatic chondromalacia patellae. Use of isometric quadriceps exercises with increasing weights is a vital part of conservative treatment. A regime of four periods of 15 minutes per day should be encouraged, preferably under supervision of a physiotherapist, over a period of 6 weeks. Why isometric quadriceps exercises improve symptoms in some patients is not under-

Table 1 Recommended plan of management after 3 months of failed conservative treatment.

1. Exclude patellar subluxation:
   Radiography—sulcus angle, patella/patellar tendon ratio
   Examination under anaesthesia
2. Diagnostic arthroscopy.
3. Teenagers and athletes:
   Grades I–III—matrix support prosthesis or distal quadriceps medial transposition
   Grade IV—distal quadriceps medial transposition or patellectomy
   Adults:
   Grades I–III—matrix support prosthesis
   Grade IV—patellectomy
4. Lateral facet chondromalacia—lateral release/or medial quadriceps transposition

stood. It may improve minor degrees of patellofemoral malalignment by increasing the power and tone of vastus medialis. It may also improve nutrition of the articular cartilage by repetitive compression of the cartilage surface.

If conservative treatment fails, examination of the knee under anaesthesia, together with appropriate radiography, is essential to exclude patellar instability. Arthroscopic examination of the knee is advised to assess the patellofemoral joint and the presence or absence of a specific cartilage abnormality on the undersurface of the patella. Probing of the retropatellar surface is important to check for areas of cartilage softening which may exist without fibrillation.

The value of operative treatment in chondromalacia is constantly debated. There is little doubt that many patients with chondromalacia patellae do respond to conservative treatment or no treatment at all. However, there are others, especially athletes, in which the symptoms can result in a significantly restricted lifestyle. A number of authors have attributed the cause of chondromalacia to minor degrees of malalignment of the patella and, therefore, recommend a procedure to realign the patella more medially in the intercondylar groove, either by lateral release, or by a transposition of the whole patellar apparatus medially.

Osborne and Fulford[30] presented the results of lateral release in 75 patients with chondromalacia patellae in which conservative management had failed. The degree of cartilage irregularity was assessed using Outerbridge's grading system. In the early stages of chondromalacia, release of the lateral retinaculum relieved symptoms for a year or more. Unfortunately, review at 3 years showed a significant number of relapses. The procedure has little value in patellae with widespread chondral damage unless there is definitive evidence of malalignment.

Insall et al.[31] described a realignment procedure in which a lateral release is performed followed by a procedure in which the medial and lateral components of the quadriceps expansion are joined to form a tube to a point where the patella is no longer heavily loaded on the lateral facet. They reported 43 (81%) patients with excellent or good results in 53 patients. Hughston and Walsh[32] advised advancement of the vastus medialis, reporting 71% satisfactory results over a follow-up of up to 15 years. Other surgeons have used a Roux–Goldthwaite type of realignment of the patella or transposition of the tibial tubercle,[33] but in our experience the results of all these procedures are unpredictable.

An alternative approach is to decrease the pressure on the patellofemoral joint by tibial tubercle elevation.[34–36] While good results may be achieved when the procedure is performed carefully,[37] complications such as fracture of the elevated tibial tubercle, resorption of the graft, wound breakdown and a troublesome prominence of the tibial tubercle causing cosmetic problems in females and pain on kneeling, exclude this procedure from current practice.

Recently, there has been a renewed interest in shaving of the patellar lesion by arthroscopic means. Open shaving was described by Wiles et al.[38] with good results, but the experience of Bentley[39] was poor. Milgram[40] reported on a series of five patellae removed from patients who had previously undergone elective shaving procedures for chondromalacia patellae. There was no significant repair response in any of the specimens, which admittedly were derived from failed shaving procedures.

A review comparing four methods of surgical treatment of chondromalacia patellae evaluated over intervals between 2 and 30 years (average 7 years) was carried out by Bentley.[39] A total of 140 operations had been performed in 98 patients. Twenty patients had a medial patellar transfer with lateral release, 20 underwent cartilage excision and drilling of the subchondral bone, 40 patients had open shaving of the patella, and 60 had a patellectomy. Satisfactory results were obtained in only 25% of 40 open shavings of the affected patellar cartilage, 35% after 20 cartilage excisions, 60% after 20 medial transfers of the patellar tendon, and 77% after 60 patellectomies. Thirty-four primary patellectomies gave 82% satisfactory results compared with only 62% in 26 patellectomies after a previously unsuccessful operation or operations. The results were worst in patients below 20 years of age and in those with grade 4 changes in the patellar cartilage. Weakness of the quadriceps muscle after any operation resulted in an unsatisfactory result.

In performing patellectomy it is essential to have good quadriceps preoperatively and to have full cooperation from the patient. Minimal trauma to the quadriceps is achieved by a 'snatch' patellectomy where the patella is carefully enucleated by a small lateral incision. Postoperatively, the leg is enclosed in a cylinder cast for 3 weeks and full weightbearing begins at 48 hours. Mobilization is supervised closely at the hospital or by a physiotherapist until full movement is achieved actively.

Recently, the procedure of cartilage and subchondral bone excision and filling of the defect with a fibre matrix of carbon to support repair by fibrocartilage has been reported to give good results.[41] This method is being evaluated at present by us and early results are encouraging.

It is essential to exclude patellar dislocation before any operative treatment, by assessment of the femoral groove angle on the 30° tangential radiographs and the presence of patella alta on the lateral view.

Overall, the problems associated with the treatment of chondromalacia patellae are related to the difficulty of establishing the diagnosis, identifying any predisposing cause and correlating symptoms with the pathological appearances of the patellar cartilage. While mild degrees of patellar malalignment have been suggested as a cause of chondromalacia and the operations previously described have been used to address this problem, minor degrees of malalignment are difficult to assess and the radiological parameters available are inexact. The relatively new technique of kinematic MRI described by Shellock et al.[17] may provide more accurate information on abnormal patellar tracking (vide infra).

Before any operative treatment other than diagnostic arthroscopy it is essential that the patient fully comprehends that the operation is only part of the overall management and that application by the patient to pre- and postoperative physiotherapy is essential to success.

Inflammation of the infrapatellar fat pad (Hoffa's syndrome)[42]

This condition is associated with pain felt anteriorly over the fat pad immediately below the lower pole of the patella. In some patients, the fat pad is a large structure which may be traumatized by direct injury or by excessive exercise. It may also become inflamed in rheumatoid arthritis. There is characteristic tenderness beneath the patellar tendon and to each side, usually 1–2 cm below the lower pole of the patella. The absence of any other signs of chondromalacia patellae may suggest the diagnosis, and the fat pad can be viewed on arthroscopy from a suprapatellar portal and may show fibrosis or impingement between the femoral condyle and the tibial plateau. It should be emphasized that the syndrome is an uncommon cause of anterior knee pain. Very occasionally when the pad is very bulky, 'debulking' may be indicated.

Patellar instability

Patellar instability can range from a mild degree of abnormal patellar tracking in the femoral trochlear groove to complete recurrent patellar dislocation. Individuals with congenital ligament laxity or Ehlers–Danlos syndrome may have extremely unstable patellae which dislocate during normal walking. There is also a very small group of patients who have congenital lateral dislocation of the patella secondary to tightness of the lateral quadriceps retinaculum.

Clinically, the patient with patellar instability may complain of recurrent giving way of the knee associated with swelling and anterior knee pain in mild cases of subluxation, to complete irreducible patellar dislocation in severe cases. In mild cases of subluxation, there may be obvious patellar laxity on pushing the patella medially or laterally with the knee in full extension. The hypermobility may be associated with apprehension. The patella may be small and relatively high.

Tangential radiographs of both patellae taken at 30° of flexion may demonstrate a flattened intercondylar groove measuring more than 140° and a high-riding patella with a patellar tendon-to-patella ratio of greater than 1.25. However, it should be emphasized that such radiological abnormalities may be present rarely in normal knees without symptoms. It should also be emphasized that the diagnosis of patellar malalignment by physical examination may be difficult and may lead to errors, especially since the history and symptoms may mimic other disorders of the knee. If in doubt the patient should be examined under general anaesthesia, when instability of the patella may be demonstrated.

In patients with definite lateral subluxation of the patella, procedures including lateral release and patellar realignment have been performed.[30,43]

The dynamics of patellar tracking have recently been examined using MRI by Shellock et al.[44] and this technique may provide important objective confirmatory evidence of patellar instability. Kinematic MRI imaging takes tangential pictures of both patellofemoral joints from zero flexion at increasing intervals of 5° to 30° of flexion. The quadriceps muscles are relaxed. The resulting images can be viewed in a static mode or as a continuous cine-loop.

Shellock et al.[17] have subsequently identified patterns of patellar position demonstrating lateral and medial subluxation of the patella and a combined abnormality of lateral-to-medial subluxation. This technique has the potential to greatly improve the diagnosis of patellar subluxation by providing objective information on patellar tracking. In their series of 40 patients (43 knees) treated for patellar subluxation and patellofemoral pain by lateral release who remained symptomatic, kinematic MRI imaging demonstrated that in patients with persistent pain, only 2% of knees had normal patellar alignment. Twenty-three per cent had lateral subluxation of the patella and 63% had medial subluxation of the patella. Nine per cent had lateral-to-medial subluxation and 2% had ELPS. Of 40 patients with unilateral arthroscopic lateral release, 17 had medially subluxating patellae on the unoperated joints. It would appear, therefore, that initial diagnosis of the type of subluxation preoperatively was incorrect and that simple lateral release either made matters worse or failed to correct the subluxation.

We consider that any demonstrable instability of the patella or tightness of the lateral retinaculum should be treated by lateral release in cases of lateral subluxation. Distal quadriceps realignment should be performed in cases of recurrent dislocation, incorporating lateral release, medial reefing and medial repositioning of the patellar tendon.[43]

Jumper's knee

Jumper's knee is a condition associated with localized tenderness at the insertion of the patellar tendon into the patella or the patellar ligament.[45] The symptoms may develop after excessive jumping exercise such as volleyball, basketball or netball. Physical and arthroscopic examinations are negative.

Most patients' symptoms can be resolved by a period of rest and by several injections of local anaesthetic into the tender area. Persistent symptoms may require operative exploration. A small transverse incision is made over the tender area. A longitudinal incision is made over the tendon at the site of tenderness and the site can usually be marked preoperatively. An area of granulation tissue may confirm the site of damage and this area can be curetted or excised. The knee should be rested post-operatively in a plaster cylinder for about 3 weeks, but return to sport should be delayed for approximately 2 months.

Osteochondroses

Osgood–Schlatter's disease is a common cause of anterior knee pain in adolescents[46] who are usually keen on sport. Ogden and Southwick[47] described the cause as an inability of the developing secondary ossification centre to withstand tensile forces, resulting in avulsion of segments of the ossification centre and eventual formation of extra bone between the fragments. Clinically, the patient complains of pain and tenderness over the tibial tubercle, which may feel swollen. Symptoms are exacerbated by activity and when kneeling. Clinically, there is a tender swelling over the tibial tuberosity. The knee joint itself is normal. Patients are encouraged to maintain sporting activity whenever possible. If symptoms are very severe, a short period of rest in a plaster-of-Paris cylinder will usually diminish the pain level. The disorder resolves at the time of skeletal maturity, but the patient will retain the prominent tubercle.

Occasionally a separate ossicle may remain after skeletal maturity. It may cause pain and irritation. Radiographs will confirm the presence of the ossicle and arthroscopy will exclude any intra-articular lesion. The excision of a bony ossicle is perhaps the only indication for operation in Osgood–Schlatter's disease. The ossicle can be dissected out from the patellar tendon, taking care not to damage the tendon.

Sinding–Larsen–Johansson's syndrome is associated with pain at the lower pole of the patella. It may be associated with an accessory ossicle. Considerable morbidity may result from the condition. Rest, occasionally with the knee in plaster, may be necessary. Fortunately, the disorder is usually self-limiting.

Prepatellar bursitis and infrapatellar bursitis

The prepatellar bursa is subcutaneous and lies at the lower pole of the patella. It may become inflamed owing to repetitive trauma or may swell as part of a generalized disease such as gout. The inflamed bursa may be small and tense and creak on flexion and extension of the knee. On the other hand, it may become very large and measure several centimetres in diameter, a condition known formerly as 'housemaid's knee'. In suitable cases where conservative treatment has failed, excision of the bursa may be considered.

A similar disorder may originate from the small infrapatellar bursa ('clergyman's knee'), situated over the patellar ligament, just above the tibial tubercle.

The plica syndrome

There are three main synovial folds in the knee joint. They consist of thin sheets of fibrous tissue covered by synovium. The suprapatellar plica may be large and extend up to two-thirds of the way across the suprapatellar pouch in up to 30% of knees.[48] Occasionally the fold may become thickened and stiff causing pain. It may be palpable as it moves across the femoral condyle on flexion and extension of the knee. Other symptoms include pseudolocking and snapping in flexion and extension of the knee.

The medial synovial shelf, which is the most frequent site of symptoms, varies in its shape and width in normal individuals, but is greater than 1 cm in width in 13% of knees.[48] A third fold, the lateral plica, may be seen in some knees.

It is emphasized that plicae are usually normal anatomical variants and do not cause symptoms. Occasionally, a shelf may become thickened and

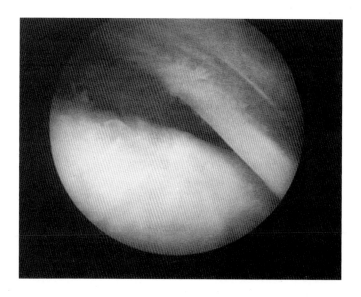

Figure 6

A thickened synovial plica associated with femoral cartilage fibrillation. The patient complained of 'clicking' on flexing the knee associated with pain.

fibrosed (Figure 6). It may rub on the medial femoral condyle in flexion and extension, resulting in fibrillation of the articular cartilage, or impinge between the patella and the femoral condyle. It will produce symptoms of pain and snapping as the fold crosses the condyle. There may be tenderness over the condyle. In these uncommon cases, arthroscopic division should be undertaken[49–51] and if the plica does not retract instantly it should be resected.

Osteochondritis dissecans patellae

Osteochondritis dissecans patellae is a rare disorder, usually presenting after an acute flexion injury. Symptoms may confuse the disorder with chondromalacia patellae. Edwards and Bentley[52] reported a series of 18 cases. The lateral knee radiograph may show a defect in the posterior surface of the patella. A loose body may be seen within the knee joint. Treatment is similar to that of patients with osteochondritis dissecans of the medial femoral condyle. Loose bodies are removed and the defect is multiply-drilled with a fine drill. In large defects with persistent pain despite drilling and debridement, a patellectomy may be necessary.

Bipartite patellae

Bipartite patellae are not uncommon findings on routine radiographs of the knee, seen on the upper lateral aspect of the patella. The majority are asymptomatic. Occasionally, they may become symptomatic, either following a single episode of trauma or after repeated episodes.[53,54] In such cases, the pain over the patella may be associated with localized tenderness over the synchondrosis. Compression of the fragment may reproduce the patient's symptoms. A bone scan may show a hot spot in a painful bipartite patella. It is important to differentiate pain from a congenital bipartite patella and a recent tangential fracture of the patella that may have been missed on initial examination.[55]

Conservative treatment should be advised in the first instance, but occasionally, excision of the fragment may be required. Osborne[30] reported that six patients with anterior knee pain associated with bipartite patella had good results following lateral release.

Summary

Anterior knee pain may be caused by many different pathologies. The aim is to make an accurate diagnosis based on careful clinical assessment and the use of special investigations. Failure of conservative treatment should be followed by arthroscopy to establish the correct diagnosis. Identifiable lesions should be dealt with arthroscopically or in cases of instability by appropriate surgery. Where the diagnosis is uncertain, the patient should be reassured and no operative treatment should be followed. If the patient has symptomatic chondromalacia patellae, then a treatment regimen is recommended that is essentially conservative and the patient can be reassured that osteoarthritis will not occur later in life. Operative treatment can be successful in a high proportion of patients provided they are cooperative in the rehabilitation programme.

References

1. Leslie IJ, Bentley G, Arthroscopy in the diagnosis of chondromalacia patellae, *Ann Rheum Dis* (1978) **37**:540–547.
2. Bentley G, Chondromalacia patellae, *J Bone Joint Surg (Am)* (1970) **52**:221–232.
3. Kolowich PA, Paulos LE, Rosenberg TD et al., Lateral release of the patella: indications and contraindications, *Am J Sports Med* (1990) **18**:359–365.
4. Dowd GSE, Bentley G, Radiographic assessment in patellar instability and chondromalacia patellae, *J Bone Joint Surg (Br)* (1986) **68**:297–300.
5. Ficat PR, Excessive lateral pressure syndrome, *Disorders of the patello-femoral joint*, ed Ficat P, Hungerford DS (Paris: Masson, 1977) 127.
6. Merchant AC, Mercer RL, Jacobsen RH et al., Roentgenographic analysis of patello-femoral congruence, *J Bone Joint Surg (Am)* (1974) **56**:1391–1396.
7. Brattström H, Shape of the intercondylar groove normally and in recurrent dislocation of patella: A clinical and x-ray anatomical investigation, *Acta Orthop Scand* (1964) **68**(suppl):1–148.
8. Aglietti P, Cerulli G, Chondromalacia and recurrent subluxation of the patella, *Ital J Orthop Traumatol* (1979) **5**:187–201.
9. Insall J, Salvati E, Patella position in the normal knee joint, *Radiology* (1971) **101**:101–104.
10. Lancourt JE, Cristini JA, Patella alta and patella infera, *J Bone Joint Surg (Am)* (1975) **57**:1112–1115.
11. Marks KE, Bentley G, Patella alta and chondromalacia, *J Bone Joint Surg (Br)* (1978) **60**:71–73.
12. Reikeras O, Hoiseth A, Patello-femoral relationships in normal subject determined by computed tomography, *Skeletal Radiol* (1990) **19**:591–592.
13. Ihara H, Double-contrast C.T. arthrography of the cartilage of the patello-femoral joint, *Clin Orthop Rel Res* (1985) **198**:50–55.
14. Boven F, Bellemans M-A, Geurts J et al., The value of computed tomography scanning in chondromalacia patellae, *Skeletal Radiol* (1982) **8**:183–185.
15. Yulish BS, Montanez J, Goodfellow DB et al., Chondromalacia patellae: Assessment with M.R. imaging, *Radiology* (1987) **164**:763–766.
16. Boven F, Boeck MD, Potvliege R, Synovial plicae of the knee on computed tomography, *Radiology* (1983) **147**:805–809.
17. Shellock FG, Mink JH, Deutsch A et al., Evaluation of patients with persistent symptoms after lateral retinacular release by kinematic magnetic resonance imaging of the patello-femoral joint, *Arthroscopy* (1990) **6**:226–234.
18. Bentley G, Is chondromalacia patellae a precursor of osteoarthritis of the knee? *J Bone Joint Surg (Br)* (1988) **70**:334.
19. Outerbridge RE, The etiology of chondromalacia patellae, *J Bone Joint Surg (Br)* (1961) **43**:752–757.
20. Casscells SW, Outerbridge's ridges, *Arthroscopy* (1990) **6**:253.
21. Casscells SW, Gross pathological changes in the knee joint of the aged individual: a study of 300 cases, *Clin Orthop Rel Res* (1978) **132**:225–232.
22. Bauer M, Jackson RW, Chondral lesions of the femoral condyles: a system of arthroscopic classification, *Arthroscopy* (1988) **4**:97–102.
23. Noyes FR, Stabler CL, A system for grading articular cartilage lesions at arthroscopy, *Am J Sports Med* (1989) **17**:505–513.
24. Hirsch C, The pathogenesis of chondromalacia of the patella, *Acta Chir Scand Suppl* (1944) **90**:1–106.
25. Goodfellow JW, Hungerford DS, Zindel M, Patello-femoral joint mechanics and pathology. 1. Functional anatomy of the patello-femoral joint, *J Bone Joint Surg (Br)* (1976) **58**:287–290.
26. Bentley G, Articular cartilage changes in chondromalacia patellae, *J Bone Joint Surg (Br)* (1985) **67**:769–774.
27. Karlson S, Chondromalacia patellae, *Acta Chir Scand* (1940) **83**:347–381.
28. Meachim G, Bentley G, Baker R, Effect of age on thickness of adult patellar articular cartilage, *Ann Rheum Dis* (1977) **36**:563–568.
29. Byers P, Contepomi CA, Farkas TA, A post mortem study of the hip joint, *Ann Rheum Dis* (1970) **29**:15–31.
30. Osborne AH, Fulford PC, Lateral release for chondromalacia patellae, *J Bone Joint Surg (Br)* (1982) **64**:202–205.
31. Insall J, Bullough PG, Burstein AH, Proximal 'tube' realignment of the patella for chondromalacia patellae, *Clin Orthop Rel Res* (1979) **144**:63–69.
32. Hughston JC, Walsh WM, Proximal and distal reconstruction of the extensor mechanism for patellar subluxation, *Clin Orthop Rel Res* (1979) **144**:36–42.
33. Devas M, Golski A, Treatment of chondromalacia patellae by transposition of the tibial tubercle, *Br Med J* (1973) **1**:589–591.
34. Maquet P, Advancement of the tibial tuberosity, *Clin Orthop Rel Res* (1976) **115**:225–231.
35. Heatley FW, Allen PR, Patrick JH, Tibial tubercle advancement for anterior knee pain: A temporary or permanent solution? *Clin Orthop Rel Res* (1986) **208**:215–224.
36. Ferguson AB, Brown TD, Fu FH et al., Relief of patello-

femoral contact stress by anterior displacement of the tibial tubercle, *J Bone Joint Surg (Am)* (1979) **61**:159–166.

37. **Leach B**, Tibial tubercle elevation, Paper presented to The International Arthroscopy Association, Toronto, Canada, 27 May 1983.

38. **Wiles P, Andrews PS, Bremner RA**, Chondromalacia of the patella: A study of the later results of excision of the articular cartilage, *J Bone Joint Surg (Br)* (1960) **42**:65–70.

39. **Bentley G**, The surgical treatment of chondromalacia patellae, *J Bone Joint Surg (Br)* (1978) **60**:74–81.

40. **Milgram JW**, Injury to articular cartilage joint surfaces, *Clin Orthop Rel Res* (1985) **192**:168–173.

41. **Pongor P, Betts J, Muckle DS** et al., Surface replacement of the knee with woven carbon, *J Bone Joint Surg (Br)* (1991) **73**(suppl 1): 89.

42. **Hoffa A**, The influence of adipose tissue with regard to the pathology of the knee joint, *J Am Med Assoc* (1904) **43**:795–796.

43. **Goldthwaite JE**, Slipping or recurrent dislocation of the patella with the report of eleven cases, *Boston Med Surg J* (1904) **150**:169–194.

44. **Shellock FG, Mink JH, Fox JM**, Patello-femoral joint: Kinematic M.R. imaging to assess tracking abnormalities, *Radiology* (1988) **168**:551–553.

45. **Blazina ME, Kerlan RK, Jobe FW** et al., Jumper's knee, *Orthop Clin North Am* (1973) **4**:665–678.

46. **Kujala U, Kuist M, Heinonen O**, Osgood–Schlatter's disease in adolescent athletes, *Am J Sports Med* (1985) **13**:236–241.

47. **Ogden JA, Southwick WO**, Osgood–Schlatter's disease and tibial tuberosity development, *Clin Orthop Rel Res* (1976) **116**:180–189.

48. **Dandy DJ**, Anatomy of the medial suprapatellar plica and medial synovial shelf, *Arthroscopy* (1990) **6**:79–85.

49. **Patel D**, Arthroscopy of the plicae—synovial folds and their significance, *Am J Sports Med* (1978) **6**:217–225.

50. **Broom MJ, Fulkerson JP**, The plica syndrome: A new perspective, *Orthop Clin North Am* (1986) **17**:279–281.

51. **Jackson RW, Marshall DJ, Fujisawa Y**, The pathological medial shelf, *Orthop Clin North Am* (1982) **13**:307–312.

52. **Edwards DH, Bentley G**, Osteochondritis dissecans patellae, *J Bone Joint Surg (Br)* (1977) **59**:58–63.

53. **Green WT**, Painful bipartite patellae: A report of three cases, *Clin Orthop Rel Res* (1975) **110**:197–200.

54. **Weaver JK**, Bipartite patellae as the cause of disability in the athlete, *Am J Sports Med* (1977) **5**:137–143.

55. **Dowd GSE**, Marginal fractures of the patella, *Injury* (1982) **14**:287–291.

20.2   Jumper's knee

Zaid Al-Duri

'Jumper's knee' was described first by Blazina et al.[1] as an affliction involving the athlete's knees and the term was used synonymously with patellar (or quadriceps) tendinitis.[1,2] Others have referred to the same condition as patellar apicitis[3] or simply patellar tendinitis.[4,5] Whether it is the quadriceps attachment to the patella, the inferior pole of the patella, the patellar tendon proper, or the patellar tendon attachment to the tibial tubercle, the condition is an expression of overuse involving the patellar ligament unit. It is more appropriate to view jumping as a mechanism rather than a type of sport when considering the term 'jumper's knee'.

Aetiology

The aetiology of this condition is a subject of debate. The most widely accepted concept is that jumper's knee is due to the cumulative effects of repetitive strains during periods of sustained physical activity; in other words, of overuse.[1,4–15] The repetitive actions (stress) concentrate a tremendous load on the extensor mechanism, with the inferior patellar pole being the most commonly involved.[16] Thus, jumping becomes one in the line of many sports that could lead to jumper's knee, such as volleyball, badminton, football, running, skiing, cycling.

Some believe that jumper's knee occurs as a consequence of repeated eccentric loading which exposes the tendon to a stress 200% greater than conventional isometric loading.[45] Others attribute it to muscular imbalance manifesting itself as either a disproportionate strength ratio difference between the agonist and antagonist muscle groups and resulting in dysfunction in the musculotendinous unit of the weaker muscle group[18] or as an imbalance due to preaxial muscles becoming overdeveloped without an equal counterbalancing postaxial force.[6]

Others consider jumper's knee as a secondary part of an impressive picture of chondromalacia and synovitis,[15] whilst Ferretti et al.[9] found no correlation between malalignment of the extensor mechanism or biomechanical derangement and the incidence of jumper's knee. It was concluded, therefore, that the mechanical properties of the tendon (resistance, elasticity, and extensibility) at the tendon–bone junctions were the most significant aetiological factors. Finally, the author of the present contribution agrees with Kujala et al.,[19] that repeated direct striking of the knee on the floor may play a role in the development of jumper's knee.

Predisposing factors

Intriguing controversial opinions exist regarding the predisposing factors. Such factors have been broadly divided into sport-specific ones (such as vertical forces on the ligament insertion, abrupt stops, floor hardness, quality of athletic shoes) and constitutional factors (such as patellofemoral dysplasia, angular deformities, short quadriceps muscles, lateralized patellae, patella alta, and vastus medialis dysplasias).[20] Ferretti et al.[9,21] stressed that the only factors found to correlate positively with the incidence of jumper's knee were hard playing surfaces and the increased frequency of the training sessions. Thirty seven per cent of their athletes participating on a cement surface developed symptoms, whereas only 5% of those participating on softer parquet surface developed symptoms. Similarly, the greater the number of training sessions per week, the higher the percentage of players affected with jumper's knee. Others described patella alta and leg length inequality as particular predisposing factors to jumper's knee.[3,19] They also propose that the repeated jumping activity itself may cause the patella alta to develop.

An interesting profile for the overuse individual in general was described by Lysens et al.[22] The profile is based on physical traits which are a combination of muscle weakness, ligamentous laxity and muscle tightness. Such factors are intensified by a large body weight, a high explosive strength, and malalignment of the lower limbs. There is abundant evidence that joint laxity plays an important role in the pathogenesis of such lesions in sport.[23]

Incidence

The incidence of jumper's knee is variable, depending on the available trials in certain sports. It is 3.0% in Australian ballet dancers,[7] 15.7% in runners,[6] 22% in volleyball players,[9] the incidence being higher (40%) in high-level players.[19]

The patellar tendon–patella junction appears to be the most commonly involved site in the extensor apparatus of the knee. In a study by Martens et al.[4] of 102 cases, the distribution of the cases was quadriceps–patellar junction, 6 knees; patella–patellar tendon junction, 88 knees; tibial tubercle–patellar tendon junction, 14 knees. A similar study of jumper's knee by Ferretti et al.[9] of 109 cases showed quadriceps–patellar junction, 24.8%; patella–patellar tendon junctions, 65.1%; tibial tubercle–patellar tendon junction, 10.1%.

It may be worth mentioning that jumper's knee may affect both knees of the same individual. The reported incidence of bilaterality in jumper's knee varies: Martens et al.,[4] 13.3%; Ferretti et al.,[9] 21.8%; Fritschy et al.,[13] 28%; Myllymäki et al.,[24] 10%.

The natural history

The natural history is controversial owing to factors such as the lack of a uniformly accepted classification of the condition and the variation in the surgical and conservative treatment schemes. It is felt by some authors that jumper's knee is a self-limiting condition.[15] However, others believe that the condition is progressive, occurring in stages, and if inadequately treated can result in irreversible pathological changes and eventual failure of conservative treatment.[16] This leaves highly competitive athletes with a choice of retirement or undergoing surgical treatment.[1,16]

Blazina et al.[1] were rather disappointed with the inadequacy of the conservative treatment methods available at that time and urged for the need of a new look at the conservative methods in the initial phases of the lesion. The conservative treatment regime of the Blazina group was highly recommended by Colosimo et al.[16] Conservative treatment if started early and if given the necessary time could cure the athlete.[2,15,16] Agreement by the patient to reduce the activity level may preclude the necessity for further treatment.[9] An interesting pointer to a good conservative treatment result may be a negative ultrasound in a case that is clinically consistent with patellar tendinitis.[24]

The reported incidence of surgical intervention in patellar tendinitis in various series is 16–17% (Orava et al.[12]); 16.5% (Ferretti et al.[9]); 33.3% (Martens et al.[4]); and 18.7% (Fritschy et al.[13]).

Analysis of the results of the surgical treatment depends on the staging system used by the surgeons (which is equivalent to their surgical indications) and the type of the procedure they prefer. In a review article, Colosimo et al.[16] reported on two consecutive patient series. In the first group, 52 patients were treated surgically by excision of the damaged area of the patellar tendon and the results were that 42 cases had complete relief; 2 cases had no relief and 8 cases required subsequent exploration. In the second group treated using the same procedure in 15 highly competitive athletes the results were that 12 cases obtained complete symptomatic relief and returned to their previous level of activity; 1 case had to give up sport; 1 case modified the type of sport and 1 case had repeated explorations which revealed further areas of necrosis.

Possible complications of jumper's knee

The main complication that can occur with jumper's knee is patellar ligament rupture. Kelly et al.[25] reported that patellar and quadriceps tendon ruptures represent the end-stage of jumper's knee. Such a view has been shared by many, as evidenced by the symptomatic classifications available.[1,4,12,20,26] Jumper's knee is primarily found in healthy individuals.[18,27] Therefore, complete tendon rupture in a healthy individual is rare, but it has been reported.[1,4,20,28] There is a possibility that some ruptures encountered in the cases of jumper's knee are secondary to intrapatellar injection of the tendon with steroids. Four out of five cases of complete ruptures had received steroids injections in the series of Martens et al.[4]

Spontaneous ruptures of the patellar tendon represent a different entity and can occur as the initial presentation in hyperparathyroidism,[27] systemic lupus erythematosus,[29] renal failure,[30] gout,[31] diabetes mellitus,[17] and rheumatoid arthritis.[32–34]

Anatomy

Anatomically, the type of the tissue found in the patellar ligament is collagenic fibres that run more or less in the same plane and direction. Hence the ligament has a great tensile strength and can withstand tremendous pulls in the plane and directions of its fibres without stretching. The cells are nearly all fibrocytes and are located between the parallel bundles of collagenic fibres.[35] According to Ferretti et al.[2] the osteotendinous junction of the patellar tendon and patella is made of four zones: patellar tendon, fibrocartilage, mineralized fibrocartilage, and finally bone. Changes were always observed at the junction of the mineralized fibrocartilage and bone in jumper's knee. It is also said that bone–tendon junctions are poorly supplied with blood because the fibrocartilage creates a barrier.[11] The blood supply of the inferior pole of the patella along the osteotendinous junction is poor.[28]

The force generated by the quadriceps muscle is quite large and increases 6% for every degree of knee flexion.[14] A stress 17.5 times the body weight is needed to rupture the extensor mechanism along one of several points, including the patellar ligament.[27,36]

Pathology

Pathologically the condition can be broadly described as lesions involving the osteotendinous junction of the patella–patellar tendon junction or the patellar tendon proper. The pathology of the condition was described from surgical specimen or ultrasonographic studies. Some stress that jumper's knee is the lesion of the osteotendinous junction and does not include the patellar tendon proper.[2,16] Abnormalities were found at the osteotendinous junction of all the histological specimens of the 18 knees studied and operated on by Colosimo et al. The observed changes included pseudocystic cavities filled with necrotic fragmented tissue or loose areolar tissue with many capillaries. There was increase in the thickness of the insertional fibrocartilage, which often had the appearance of myxomatous tissue or of hyaline cartilage.

Colosimo et al.[16] were the first to correlate pathology with symptomatology. They found that gross pathology noted at the time of surgical exploration varies with the duration of symptoms. Accordingly, they proposed the following scheme for the overall correlation of pathology to symptomatology: (A) In patients with symptoms of less than 6 months' duration there is loss of the finely organized appearance of normal collagen with mucoid degeneration of the collagen. Of note was the lack of inflammatory cells. (B) When symptoms had been present for 6 months to a year, further fibrocartilaginous formation and portions of dense fibrous tissue with degeneration and some calcified cartilage were noted. (C) When symptoms had lasted longer than 1 year, further disorganization and sometimes bone spicules were seen. Also, increased thickness of insertional fibrocartilage was typical.

Fritschy[13] gave an account of the patellar tendinitis pathology based on ultrasonographic analysis and divided the process into three stages: *Stage one*: there is an initial pure inflammatory reaction with oedema leading to thickening of the tendon fibres in segment or as a whole. *Stage two* is called the stage of reversible pathology. Here there may be an inflammatory reaction plus segmental microruptures. There may be some scarring and intratendinous ossification. *Stage three*: the tendon's envelope is irregular, corresponding to nodular zones. The inflammation has disappeared. The surrounding tissue response to these tears fills in the defect. There may be ingrowth of bone, synovium or cartilage within the tear, depending upon which tissue responds.[37]

Diagnosis

The diagnosis of jumper's knee begins by a proper history-taking in an attempt to establish overuse. In 80% of the cases the athlete has only recently taken up the sport or has markedly increased his or her training intensity.[38] A history of a direct blow to the knee may be elicited.[14] In a young athlete, a rapid growth history may be obtained.[1]

Symptoms

The symptoms of jumper's knee may exist alone or be a part of a confusing complex of coexisting entities such as chondromalacia patellae, pes bursitis or even generalized synovitis.[15] The chief complaint, however, is pain of an insidious onset at the extensor tendon attachment to the inferior pole of the patella. Stiffness and pain may be experienced as well after prolonged sitting or following driving, but the symptoms are not disabling at first. There may also be a feeling of deep tenderness by the patient at the site of the lesion. Kujala et al.[19] stressed that pain should be felt where the tenderness is, i.e. at the patellar tendon attachment to the inferior pole of the patella or the quadriceps tendon attachment to the upper pole of the patella.

The pattern of occurrence and progression of the pain has formed the basis for the staging of the lesion and correlation with the progression of pathology. Such classifications have been used extensively in grading and treating patients.[1,4,14,18,39] The author of the present contribution believes that whilst such classifications represent some indication to the progression of the condition, they would only be of true value if correlated with the pathology of the lesion, whether elicited ultrasonographically, histologically or with the use of magnetic resonance imaging. Unfortunately, such work has not been done yet, except the notable article of Colosimo et al.[16]

Clinical examination

A general examination may be needed to assess generalized joint laxity, lower-limb length inequalities and rotational deformities. The diagnosis of the involved knee is made by the location of the point of maximum tenderness at the centre of the bone–tendon junction or along the length of the patellar tendon, and the reproduction of the symptoms during attempts at manually resisted extension. The patellar tendon may be palpated, when a subtle defect may be felt;[15] however, thickening of the tendon itself can sometimes be elicited on comparison with the other knee patellar tendon. Crepitus may be felt in the early stages of the disease. Evidence of a true knee effusion is rare.[16]

Investigation

Plain radiography

Radiographic changes are rare prior to 6 months. Radiolucency of the involved pole of the patella secondary to disuse atrophy or hyperaemia is the most common finding with symptoms that have lasted more than 6 months.[16] Other changes in the adult include irregularity of the involved pole of the patella, fatigue fracture of the involved pole, and calcification of the involved tendon.[1]

In the pre-teens and teenagers there may be a periosteal reaction at the anterior surface of the patella in the involved area.[1] In adolescents, there is visible radiographic lesion which may result in elongation of the lower pole of the patella or even the formation of a separate ossicle (Sinding–Larsen–Johansson syndrome).

Calcification in the patellar tendon can mean transition from acute to chronic or healed lesions, or that it is dystrophic calcification, or that it is a sequel of previous trauma. Calcification increases the fragility of the tendon.[40] Calcification may occur in primary involvement of the tendon with hyperparathyroidism.[27]

Xeroradiography has not been much better than plain radiography.[1]

Scintigraphy

Strobel and Stedtfeld[20] believe that scintigraphy has a definite role in localization of the inflammatory foci as well as pain in the knee, whether of unknown origin or of a chronic nature. Some believe that it has a complementary role to ultrasonography in cases of involvement of the inferior pole of the patella.[13] Kahn et al.[41] reviewed three cases of jumper's knee that were investigated using radioisotope scanning. They were scanned 10 months, 1.5 years and 2 years after the onset of symptoms. In all three cases there was abnormal uptake in the region of the inferior pole of the patella and the intensity of the uptake was approximately equivalent in the three cases.

Ultrasonography

Ultrasound is not only useful in the diagnosis of jumper's knee, but is equally useful for following the progression of jumper's knee and confirming the therapeutic response. It thus provides a sensitive diagnostic technique for evaluating the disorder and monitoring treatment.[13,14,20,24]

Fritschy et al.[13] proposed a staging classification of the patellar tendon pathology based on ultrasonography (see under Pathology).

Computerized tomography

Like ultrasonography, computerized tomography (CT) does not seem to give false positives; however, ultrasound is found to provide a greater distinction of the histological abnormalities and therefore is more informative than CT scanning.[24,42]

Magnetic resonance imaging

Magnetic resonance imaging (MRI) can detect changes in the patellar ligament.[20,43] Bodne et al.[5] evaluated seven patellar tendons in five patients with chronic patellar tendinitis. They concluded that MRI is useful in evaluating chronic patellar tendinitis because it establishes the diagnosis, detects associated chronic tears, and may help determine appropriate rehabilitation. MRI and ultrasonography are useful in preoperative planning for surgical treatment of recalcitrant tendinitis.[14]

Treatment

Conservative treatment

Conservative treatment is most effective in the early phases of jumper's knee.[1,4,15,44] The treatment should be started with the aim of trying to stop the process in its initial phases by preventing the continuation of overuse and stress application to the patellar tendon and allowing the inflammation to abate. In general, a fair trial of conservative treatment should be given to all; surgery, if decided upon, should be the last resort. Chronicity here is a reference to persistence of symptoms and failure of repeated attempts at conservation.

The general outline of conservative treatment includes the following.

Rest in the form of immediate and adequate immobilization. Some would advise a plaster cylinder for mild to moderate cases.[15] Others feel that cast immobilization has been disappointing since it protracts an already long period of inactivity and does not yield a good, lasting result in cases where conservative treatment has failed.[4]

Anti-inflammatory medications include the non-steroidal drugs in tablet form and are recommended by the majority of authors.[1,6,15,44] Sometimes the discomfort may disappear while these medications are being used, only to recur when they are discontinued. At other times there is no response to oral medication.[1]

Physiotherapy is advised after the immobilization or rest period. It includes quadriceps strengthening exercises, i.e. isometrics and straight leg raising at the outset without weight.[15] Others recommend an exercise programme designed to load the muscle tendon unit in an eccentric fashion. They would also advise hamstring stretch as an integral part of attempting to readdress the problem of the muscle imbalance associated with the overuse syndromes.[18,44,45] Ultrasound,[44] moist heat,[1] and ice[15] are also useful modalities. Transcutaneous electrical stimulation is recommended on trial basis in cases of anterior knee pain since it has a very beneficial effect in relieving pain of acute soft-tissue inflammation and perhaps even chondromalacia.[15] Patellar tendon straps and horse-shoe orthoses may be helpful in reducing pain at times.[1,15]

Steroids. Many believe that steroid injections should not be used in the treatment of this condition.[4,10,12,15,44] Others advise occasional use at the site of maximal tenderness.[46] Steroid injections are discouraged because used alone they have never yielded a good, lasting result and they bear the hazard of causing tendon rupture. Such injections may not only weaken the tendon but also permit the athlete to continue to overload and further damage the tendon because of the analgesic effect of the drug.

However, other forms of steroid therapy have been advocated. The topical application of hydrocortisone in addition to oral anti-inflammatory medication is used by Albright.[15] This is accomplished by a phonoporesis process using ultrasound as an energy source to transport 5–10% hydrocortisone lotion transcutaneously to the problem area. This must be accomplished over a 10–14 day period to avoid counterproductive irritation from the energy source. The same opinion is shared by Fulkerson and Hungerford.[47]

Glycosaminoglycanpolysulphate. Recently local injections of this substance have been reported with promising results by Orava et al.,[12] based on the work of Kvist et al.[48] on chronic Achilles paratenonitis.

Surgical treatment of jumper's knee

Surgery is indicated in a small well-defined group of patients with chronic symptoms resistant to non-operative treatment. They include (A) athletes whose goals are to return to action with a reasonably functional level of performance. Colosimo et al.[16] believe that, for highly competitive athletes, only surgical treatment provides long-lasting relief. (B) Those individuals who might prefer a surgical approach because it offers the only chance left for a cure and for whom restrictions required for adaptation to the physical impairment are not tolerable. They refuse to quit sports.[1,15] (C) For establishing the presence of a local lesion on ultrasound.[24]

Surgery is contraindicated in the absence of a specific diagnosis;[8,15] in a patient who maintains unrealistic aims; and in the presence of oedema of the tendon on ultrasound.[44]

Surgically, two broad areas of the patellar ligament are tackled: the patellar tendon–patella junction and the patellar tendon proper. Some authors advocate approaching both.[1]

Four main groups of surgical procedures have been mentioned in the literature as follows.

(A) Placement of multiple drillholes in the affected pole of the patella so as to improve the blood supply to the tendon attachment.[49] Such an operation has had a disappointing outcome according to some.[1] Others have proposed that since the lesion of the patellar tendinitis is situated at a predisposed area in the deep fibres of the tendon near its insertion, operative treatment should be directed towards the affected tendon rather than the patellar bone.[4] Others have considered drilling the inferior pole of the patella plus excision of exostosis as a reasonable procedure.[12]

(B) Excision of the degenerated portion of the tendon and resuturing of the remaining healthy tendon.[15] This approach is favoured by many, alone or in combination with other procedures.[12,15] Blazina et al.[1] believe that excision of the diseased tendon portion has the disadvantage of quite limited visualization of the overall involved area, thus potentially overlooking associated disease on or around the tendon.

(C) Detachment of the entire patellar or quadriceps tendon with resection of the diseased segment, excision of the involved patellar pole and surgical reattachment of the tendon to non-articular patellar surface.[1] Many feel that resection of the lower pole of the patella is not necessary if the bone configuration is normal.[4,12]

(D) Under local anaesthesia, the bone–tendon junction is exposed and the dead tissue is excised and the tendon is resutured on to itself.[16]

Others may combine procedures in treating jumper's knee. Albright's[15] preferred method of treatment is to excise the diseased portion of the tendon, drill the inferior pole of the patella and then resuture the remaining part of the tendon. Some would excise the retinaculum where it is found to be thick and adherent.[12] If malalignment of the patella coexists with patellar tendinitis, then proximal realignment with lateral release and advancement of the vastus medialis has been advised by Ferretti et al.[9]

References

1. Blazina ME, Kerlan RK, Jobe FW et al., Jumper's knee, *Orthop Clin North Am* (1973) 4(3):665–678.

2. Ferretti A, Ippolito E, Mariani P et al., Jumper's knee, *Am J Sports Med* (1983) 11:58–62.

3. Kujala UM, Österman K, Kvist M et al., Factors predisposing to patellar chondropathy and patellar apicitis in athletes, *Int Orthop* (1986) 10(3):195–200.

4. Martens M, Wouters P, Burssens A et al., Patellar tendinitis: pathology and results of treatment, *Acta Orthop Scand* (1982) 53(3):445–450.

5. Bodne D, Quinn SF, Murray WT et al., Magnetic resonance images of chronic patellar tendinitis, *Skeletal Radiol* (1988) 17(1):24–28.

6. Apple DF, Common peri-patellar inflammatory conditions, *South Med J* (1979) 72(11):1377–1379.

7. Quirk R, Ballet injuries: the Australian experience, *Clin Sports Med* (1983) 2(3):507–514.

8. Insall JN, *Surgery of the knee* (New York: Churchill Livingstone, 1984) 228.

9. Ferretti A, Puddu G, Mariani PP et al., The natural history of jumper's knee: patellar or quadriceps tendonitis, *Int Orthop* (1985) 8(4):239–242.

10. Brashear HR, Raney RB, *Handbook of orthopaedic surgery*, 10th edn (St Louis: CV Mosby, 1986) 424.

11. Peterson L, Renström P, *Sports injuries—their prevention and treatment* (London: Martin Dunitz, 1986) 43.

12. Orava S, Osterback L, Hurme M, Surgical treatment of patellar tendon pain in athletes, *Br J Sports Med* (1986) 20(4):167–169.

13. Fritschy D, DeGautard R, Jumper's knee and ultrasonography, *Am J Sports Med* (1988) 16(6):637–640.

14. Teitz CC, Ultrasonography in the knee. Clinical aspects, *Radiol Clin North Am* (1988) 26(1):55–62.

15. Albright JP, Musculotendinous problems about the knee, *Surgery of the musculoskeletal system*, 2nd edn, ed Evarts CM (New York: Churchill Livingstone, 1990) 3520–3525.

16. Colosimo AJ, Bassett FH, Jumper's knee: diagnosis and treatment [Review], *Orthop Rev* (1990) 19(2):139–149.

17. Stern CA, Palmer LH, Simultaneous bilateral rupture of both quadriceps tendons, *Clin Orthop* (1980) 147:188–189.

18. O'Toole ML, Hiller WDB, Smith RA et al., Overuse injuries in ultraendurance triathletes, *Am J Sports Med* (1989) 17(4):514–518.

19. Kujala UM, Aalto T, Österman K et al., The effect of volleyball playing on the knee extensor mechanism, *Am J Sports Med* (1989) 17(6):766–769.

20. Strobel M, Stedtfeld HW, Diagnostic evaluation of the knee (Berlin: Springer-Verlag, 1990) ch. 2.

21. Ferretti A, Epidemiology of jumper's knee, *Sports Med* (1986) 3(4):289–295.

22. Lysens RJ, Ostyn MS, Auweele YV et al., The accident-prone and overuse-prone profiles of the young athlete, *Am J Sports Med* (1989) 17(5):612–619.

23. Beighton P, Soucacos P, Carr W, *Hypermobility of joints*, 2nd edn (London: Springer-Verlag, 1989) 70.

24. Myllymäki T, Bondestam S, Suramo I et al., Ultrasonography of jumper's knee, *Acta Radiol* (1990) 31(2):147–149.

25. Kelly DW, Carter VS, Jobe FW et al., Patellar and quadriceps tendon ruptures—jumper's knee, *Am J Sports Med* (1984) 12(5):375–380.

26. Roels J, Martens M, Mulier J et al., Patellar tendinitis (jumper's knee), *Am J Sports Med* (1978) 6(6):362.

27. Maddox PA, Garth WP, Tendinitis of the patellar ligament and quadriceps (jumper's knee) as an initial presentation of hyperparathyroidism: a case report, *J Bone Joint Surg (Am)* (1986) 68(2):288–292.

28. Podesta L, Sherman MF, Bonamo JR, Bilateral simultaneous rupture of the infrapatellar tendon in a recreational athlete: a case report, *Am J Sports Med* (1991) 19(3):325–327.

29. Martin JR, Wilson CL, Mathews WH, [Bilateral rupture of the ligamentum patellae in a case of disseminated lupus erythematosus.] Ruptura bilateral del ligamentos patellar in un caso de disseminate lupus erythematose, *Arthritis Rheum* (1958) 1:548–552.

30. Cirincione RJ, Baker BE, Tendon ruptures with secondary hyperparathyroidism: a case report, *J Bone Joint Surg (Am)* (1975) 57:852–853.

31. Levy M, Seelenfreund M, Maor P et al., Bilateral spontaneous and simultaneous rupture of the quadriceps tendons in gout, *J Bone Joint Surg (Br)* (1971) 53:510–513.

32. Peiro A, Ferrandis R, Garcia L et al., Simultaneous and spontaneous bilateral rupture of the patellar tendon in rheumatoid arthritis: a case report, *Acta Othop Scand* (1975) 46:700–703.

33. Rao JP, Siwek KW, Bilateral spontaneous rupture of the patellar tendons. A new method of treatment, *Orthop Rev* (1978) 7:49–51.

34. Razzano CD, Wilde AH, Phalen GS, Bilateral rupture of the infrapatellar tendon in rheumatoid arthritis, *Clin Orthop* (1973) 91:158–161.

35. Ham AW, *Histology*, 7th edn (Philadelphia: JB Lippincott, 1976) 368.

36. Zernicke RF, Garhammer J, Jobe FW, Human patellar-tendon rupture: a kinetic analysis, *J Bone Joint Surg (Am)* (1977) 59:179–183.

37. Nance EP, Kaye JJ, Injuries of the quadriceps mechanism, *Radiology* (1982) 142:301–307.

38. Harvey JS, Overuse syndromes in young athletes, *Pediatr Clin North Am* (1982) 64(1):1369–1381.

39. Siwek CW, Rao JP, Ruptures of the extensor mechanism of the knee joint, *J Bone Joint Surg (Am)* (1981) 63:932–937.

40. Fornage BD, Rifkin MD, Touche DH, Segal PM, Sonography of the patellar tendon, *Am J Roentgenol* (1984) 143:179–182.

41. Kahn D, Wilson MA, Bone scintigraphic findings in patellar tendinitis, *J Nucl Med* (1987) 28(11):1768–1770.

42. Mourad K, King J, Guggiana P, Computed tomography and ultrasound imaging of jumper's knee—patellar tendinitis, *Clin Radiol* (1988) 39(2):162–165.

43. Hartzman S, Gold RH, The knee, *MRI Atlas of the Musculoskeletal System*, ed Bassett LW, Gold RH, Seeger LL (London: Martin Dunitz, 1989) 217–218.

44. Fritschy D, Jumper's knee ultrasonography, *Surgery and arthroscopy of the knee: Second European Congress of Knee Surgery and Arthroscopy*, ed Müller W, Hackenback W (Berlin: Springer-Verlag, 1986) 495.

45. Stanish WD, Lamd H, Curwin S, The biomechanical analysis of chronic patellar tendinitis and treatment with eccentric loading, *Müller and Hackenback's surgery and arthroscopy of the knee*, Second European Congress of Knee Surgery and Arthroscopy (Berlin: Springer-Verlag, 1986) 493.

46. Dodson CF, Common peri-patellar inflammatory conditions, *J Arkansas Med Soc* (1979) 75(9):330–332.

47. Fulkerson JP, Hungerford DS, *Disorders of the patellofemoral joint*, 2nd edn (Baltimore: Williams and Wilkins, 1990) 93.

48. Kvist MH, Lehto MUK, Jozsa L et al., Chronic Achilles paratenonitis: an immunohistologic study of fibronectin and fibrinogen, *Am J Sports Med* (1988) 16(6):616–623.

49. Smillie LS, *Diseases of the knee joint* (Edinburgh: Churchill Livingstone, 1974).

20.3 Reflex sympathetic dystrophy of the knee

Zaid Al-Duri and Paul M. Aichroth

Reflex sympathetic dystrophy (RSD) is an aetiologically based term that is meant to describe a complex clinical entity characterized by varying degrees of intractable pain associated with trophic changes and vasomotor disturbance secondary to sympathetic nervous system hyperactivity. The description of RSD was given first by Silas W. Mitchell in a monograph on the results of gunshot injuries of nerves in the US civil war in 1864. Mitchell, however, coined the term causalgia to describe the condition in 1867.[1] Sudeck differentiated osteoporosis of bone from disuse osteoporosis in 1900 and soon after that related the syndrome to a reflex mechanism mediated by the autonomic nervous system.[2] It is essentially an 'immobilization dystrophy'.

Since then, various synonyms have been employed to portray the condition, relating mostly to the possible aetiology to which it was attributed. These terms include causalgic syndrome, minor causalgia, major causalgia, causalgic state, mimcausalgia, algodystrophy, algoneurodystrophy, post-traumatic acute bone atrophy, post-traumatic dystrophy, post-traumatic pain syndrome, post-traumatic osteoporosis, hyperaesthetic neurovascular syndrome, post-traumatic vascular disorders, traumatic vasospastic disease, Sudeck's post-traumatic osteoporosis, Sudeck's atrophy, and shoulder–hand syndrome.[1,3–6] It is evident from these descriptive terms that trauma, the sympathetic nervous system, and major and minor nerve injury were all thought to be intimately connected at one stage or another with this condition. Some terms may refer to the degree of damage to a structure, such as causalgia major (referring to major nerve damage) and causalgia minor (referring to a minor nerve injury). Others chose terms that described a variant of the main clinical presentation, such as reflex sympathetic imbalance used by Ladd et al.[7] stressing an incomplete manifestation of RSD. In this at least one of the four classic signs of RSD—pain, swelling, stiffness and discoloration—is absent.

Currently, however, the accepted term appears to be reflex sympathetic dystrophy.[1,6]

Incidence

It is difficult, indeed, to find the true incidence of the knee joint involvement in RSD in view of the underestimation of the clinical prevalence of the condition by surgeons, the diversity of the conditions and circumstances leading to its development and the multiplicity of the terminology used in describing it. Many of the available series do not specify the joints involved but refer to the limb in general.

Strobel and Stedtfeld[3] believe that the knee joint is the fourth most commonly affected joint, accounting for 10% of all RSD joint involvement. Tietjen[2] remarked that RSD is a seldom-considered diagnosis in knee pain of undetermined aetiology. In a retrospective study of 67 patients with unexplained knee pain, 14 patients met the criteria to establish the diagnosis of RSD, making the incidence of RSD in Tietjen's series 21%. Seale[6] stated that the incidence of RSD in the lower extremity is probably more frequent than is commonly recognized. The clinical signs and symptoms in 441 patients with post-traumatic dystrophy were recorded by Goris et al.[8] They documented involvement twice as often in the arms as in the legs. Katz and Hungerford[9] claim that 65% of the RSD in the knee originates at the patellofemoral joint. They reported 5 cases of RSD after total knee replacement (700 consecutive cases), making it a more common complication than infection.[10]

Females are more commonly involved than males[2,6,8,11] and some believe that RSD of the lower extremity is more frequently seen in the fourth and fifth decades.[6]

It is also believed that the spontaneous forms of RSD are much less common in the knee region than in upper limbs, as most experience in the knee region is that relating the RSD to injury.[10] Bilaterality of lesions has been suggested.[12]

Coughlan et al.[11] reviewed 33 patients with undiagnosed chronic knee pain who had features of autonomic disturbance. The long duration of symptoms, high proportion of young females and the severity of the associated disability were notable. It is suggested that algodystrophy is a more frequent cause of chronic knee pain than previously recognized. Autonomic abnormalities may be less intense in disease at this site, particularly in young females, and may be overlooked. This characteristic of algodystrophy of the knee may contribute to chronicity and subsequent disability.

Aetiology

Pellegrini and McCollister Evarts[4] stated that 'It remains to be demonstrated how a minor injury can cause severe, persistent pain after the injured tissue has healed.' It is not the purpose here to discuss the aetiological theories of the condition in detail. However, it is true to say that several theories exist regarding RSD in general, but there is no single proven one. The main aim of these theories was to explain the intractable pain and the involvement of the sympathetic nervous system. Spurling in 1930 was the first to treat the syndrome successfully by sympathectomy. Before then patients severely affected by RSD were treated as chronic invalids; they became narcotic addicts and many committed suicide.[9] Normally, the body responds to injury with vasoconstriction followed by vasodilatation which facilitates the normal repair. In RSD, an inappropriate hyperactivity of the sympathetic system results in an abnormal feedback mechanism.[6] Some state that sensory and autonomic symptoms resulted from increased sympathetic outflow to the skin and collateral sproutings in the peripheral nerve fibres.[13] Others believe that painful neurogenic syndromes commonly diagnosed as RSD may not be the consequence of sympathetic dysfunction. Recent experimental data on the mechanism of hyperalgesia indicate that the primary pathophysiological mechanism of RSD may be sensitization of either peripheral nociceptors, or central neurons, or both. The sympathetic system might be involved in maintaining this condition, but this is not always the case.[12,14] Serotonin was suggested to play a role in the development of RSD.[15]

Omohundro and Payne[16] grouped the theories along four lines: (1) It is possible that nerve injuries produce abnormal discharges in the sympathetic afferents. (2) There may be sensitization of the peripheral sensory receptor by sympathetic activity. (3) Artificial synapses may form as a consequence of nerve injury. These synapses may allow the shunting of the current from the sympathetic efferent fibres to the somatic afferent fibres at the injury site. (4) At the site of the nerve injury, spontaneous ectopic discharges may develop.

Katz and Hungerford[9] reviewed 36 patients with RSD primarily affecting the knee. Injuries or operations about the patellofemoral joint triggered its onset in 64% of the patients. The events triggering the RSD were surgery in 41% of patients; anterior knee trauma in 47% of patients; twisting injury in 8% of patients; crush injury in 3% of patients. The surgical procedures triggering the onset of RSD were total knee replacement, 5 patients; arthrotomy, lateral release, partial patellar chondrectomy, 4 patients; patellectomy, 1 patient; high tibial osteotomy, 1 patient; medial meniscectomy, 2 patients; tibial tubercle elevation (Maquet), 1 patient; medial arthrotomy, 1 patient.

Ogilvie-Harris and Roscoe[17] reported that 3 out of 19 patients they reviewed develop RSD of the knee joint postoperatively. Meniscectomies were performed on 2 patients, and the Maquet procedure on 1 patient.

Ladd et al.[7] reviewed 11 patients with reflex sympathetic imbalance in 12 knees and one ankle. The associated diagnoses in knee joint lesions included knee sprain, 3 knees; patellofemoral lesions, 5 knees (including patellar malalignment, subluxating patella, two avulsion fractures of the patella, overuse); osteoarthritis of the knee joint, 2 knees (in the same patient); anterior cruciate ligament injury, 1 knee; meniscal injury, 1 knee. Seven patients had undergone previous surgical procedures. In three of these patients surgery clearly triggered reflex sympathetic imbalance.

Surgery may, indeed, be the precipitating factor that initiates the events leading to RSD of the knee joint. However, Fulkerson and Hungerford[10] stress the point that faulty postoperative rehabilitation may provide the trigger. Such rehabilitation may be imposed by the surgeon who undertakes vigorous manipulation, or the physiotherapist who pursues vigorous quadriceps exercises against resistance, causing aggravation of a significant lesion.

RSD can involve a multitude of tissues such as skin, subcutaneous tissue, fascia, ligaments, capsule, muscles, and bones. In patellofemoral involvement, RSD had been most prominent in bone.[10]

Poehling et al.[18] examined the possible relationship between isolated injury to the infrapatellar branch of the saphenous nerve (IPBSN) and the etiology and natural course of RSD. Thirty-five patients with clinically significant sympathetic dystrophy of the knee were examined retrospectively. All patients (100%) had clinical evidence of insult to the IPBSN. Ninety-four per cent were found to have vasomotor instability. All patients in their population of 33 were treated with vasoactive therapies. Eighty per cent of patients treated within 1 year improved with one or more vasoactive therapies, whereas only 44% improved when treatment was started after 1 year.

The personality of the patient has been implicated in the development of RSD. Zucchini et al.[19] emphasized the role of the personality in a review of 13 patients affected by the algodystrophic syndrome of the upper limb. Such patients were found to have higher scores on the Depression, Hysteria and Hypochondria scales. Egle and Hoffmann[20] state that patients suffering from this disease are 'psychically peculiar', i.e. they appear strange or odd. Psychometric examinations show that they suffer from enhanced anxiety, are emotionally rather unstable and display a tendency to depressiveness associated with a marked self-esteem rating problem complex. Studies on children with reflex sympathetic dystrophy likewise confirmed these characteristic features. Others feel that it is the vasomotor nature or make-up of the individual rather than her or his mental state that leads to RSD. Tietjen[2] stated that the reflex sympathetic dystrophy syndrome was related to injury sustained in a compensation or liability accident.

There are various reports that suggest that RSD may occur in association with other conditions or as a consequence of a certain therapy. Arlet et al.[21] reported their observations in three patients with algodystrophy of the foot and stated that biological disorders suggestive of osteomalacia were found in two patients who recovered after receiving vitamin D. Cushing disease was diagnosed in the remaining patient; again algodystrophy disappeared after specific therapy was given. Such conditions should be looked for in all patients with apparently primary algodystrophy of a lower limb.

Munoz-Gomez et al.[22] believe that RSD should be added to the list of complications that may appear in kidney transplant patients who receive cyclosporin-A treatment. In a 36-month period, 240 patients at their institution received kidney transplants from cadaver donors. Cyclosporin-A (CsA) was used as the initial immunosuppressive therapy. Seven patients (5 men and 2 women) developed severe pain, periarticular soft-tissue swelling with no effusion, and vasomotor changes in affected areas. All of their symptoms and radiographic and scintigraphic signs were compatible with definite RSD. Articular symptoms began within 3 months after kidney transplantation in all patients; all but one patient had plasma CsA levels greater than 200 ng/ml at that time. When the dosage of CsA was reduced, there was concomitant improvement in the RSD, which appeared when the plasma CsA levels declined to less than 200 ng/ml. The mean duration of the clinical symptoms of RSD was 8 months.

Histology

Histological work in RSD is based, in general, on bone biopsy from involved regions. Lagier et al.[23] performed a histological study of the biopsy material of a case of algodystrophy of the left knee, and showed the classical image of cortical and cancellous bone atrophy with non-specific remodelling that explained the increased uptake on the scintigraph as well as the repairing of the bone tissue observed on the radiographs.

Arlet et al.[24] reported on 16 cases of reflex sympathetic dystrophy of the knee, in which the authors obtained by drill biopsy 29 bone samples from the epiphyseal and metaphyseal regions of the femur and tibia and 8 cartilaginous samples (including 6 by arthrotomy and 2 after patellectomy). They noted thinning of the cortical bone, lacunae of cortical reabsorption, rarefaction of the trabeculae (of which some were dead), stasis and fibrosis of the bone marrow. The eight cartilage samples were pathological, with fibrosis of the surface cartilage (vascular pannus formation). The association of chondromalacia of the patella with an RSD syndrome of the knee was frequent.

Tietjen[2] reported on the results of synovial biopsies from four patients with knee problems in the process of attempting to establish the diagnosis. They were all retrospectively diagnosed as having RSD of the knee joint. All the biopsies of the synovium of the knee joint were reported as having synovial inflammation.

Staging of RSD

The progression of the RSD has been divided into stages. Whilst a high index of suspicion is the most valuable notion in RSD diagnosis, staging is of value in appreciating the pattern of this disorder and hopefully early planning of a treatment schedule.

Various staging patterns have been proposed.[4,6,7,17] There is a general consensus, however, on dividing RSD into three stages:

Stage I (also described as the acute or early stage) is present for the first 3 months from the onset of symptoms.[6,7] Others define it as present for the first 6 months.[17] In this stage, pain is the presenting symptom.[2] The pain tends to be along a localized nerve or vascular area.[7]

Stage II (also described as the dystrophic stage) lasts from 3 to 6 months.[2,6,7] It is characterized by diffuse radiating pain, stiffness, swelling, and osteoporosis.[4,7] Skin and colour temperature changes would have begun.[2]

Stage III (also described as the atrophic stage): in this stage, the symptoms would have persisted in excess of 6–9 months.[6,7] It is characterized by diminishing pain, irreversible skin and nail changes, and marked demineralization.[7] Some feel that this stage represents relative intractability.[6] In this stage, the changes may involve the knee joint or the entire lower limb, although the knee joint involvement is the most common.[2]

On the same basis, reflex sympathetic *imbalance* was divided into three stages.[7]

1. Acute stage: defined as being present less than 3 months.
2. Subacute stage: corresponds to the dystrophic stage of 3–6 months.
3. Chronic stage: corresponds to the atrophic stage of 6 months or more.

Ogilvie-Harris and Roscoe[17] reviewed a series of 19 patients with RSD of the knee joint. The patients were divided into three groups according to the onset of the RSD. In the 'early' group (less than 6 months from the time of onset of symptoms) there were 7 patients. There was a history of pain after a minor twist or other injury. In the 'late' group (more than 6 months since the onset of symptoms) consisting of 9 patients, the presentation was that of persistent knee pain and dysfunction, often after unsuccessful attempts of rehabilitation. In the 'postoperative' group (in whom symptoms developed postoperatively) consisting of 3 patients, the presentation was that of a stormy postoperative course with persistent pain, stiffness and difficulty in rehabilitation.

Symptoms

In the diagnosis of RSD, a high index of suspicion is essential. Tietjen,[2] in a review of 67 patients with knee complaints, stated that there was a certain number of knee injuries that defied anatomical diagnosis. It was the retrospective review of these knees that established the diagnosis of RSD. This syndrome should be suspected in patients who report excruciating burning pain following an injury or operation. The onset of RSD can be detected either immediately after the insult or late in the course of the treatment. This pain is out of proportion to that expected with such an ailment, whether an injury or a postoperative course.[1-4] This pain is either persistent or intermittent and is aggravated by passive or active movement or weight bearing. Hyperaesthesia to light touch is also characteristic. The intensity of the pain is exaggerated with the passage of time.[1,4] Generally, most surgeons note that pain is the most prominent symptom; however, Tietjen[2] stated that true causalgia was rarely seen in his series, though many patients complained of a burning sensation in and around the extremity.

Katz and Hungerford[9] reviewed 36 patients who were included in their study of reflex sympathetic dystrophy of the knee according to strict diagnostic criteria that included (a) intense, prolonged pain; (b) delayed recovery following injury or surgical procedure to the knee; (c) all patients had undergone lumbar sympathetic blockade as a diagnostic test with at least transient partial relief of symptoms, associated with transient rise of the temperature of the skin of the extremity. They evaluated the level of discomfort and disability both at the time of diagnosis and at follow-up using a 50-point pain and function rating scale as follows:

(A) Frequent rest pain. Severe pain with any activity, thus preventing weight bearing. Analgesics stronger than aspirin required. Cannot perform routine activities because of knee pain (0 points).
(B) Common rest pain. Moderately severe pain with almost any activity. Heavy dependence upon weight-bearing-assistive devices. Unable to do most work because of pain. Unable to do most housework or even simple activities (10 points).
(C) Less frequent rest pain. Routine activities moderately restricted. May require mild or narcotic analgesics (25 points).
(D) Ability to perform most routine activities with slight or tolerable pain. Occasional mild, non-narcotic analgesics or anti-inflammatory analgesics (40 points).
(E) No discomfort with routine activity. Excessive activity provokes discomfort. Rarely taking of analgesics or anti-inflammatory medications (45 points).
(F) No pain with any activity (50 points).

The symptoms of RSD were (a) pain and burning sensation in 67% of patients, aching in 33%; (b) pain location—global in 56% of patients' knees, anterior in 36%, medial in 8%; (c) night pain in 78% of patients.

Fulkerson and Hungerford[10] believe that pain is the sine qua non of RSD, although it is often more severe and persistent than can be attributed to the patellofemoral joint. They support the views of Katz and Hungerford[9] that night pain is characteristic.

Bryan et al.[25] studied prospectively 33 patients with RSD to ascertain the pressure-pain threshold of affected and unaffected limbs. The affected side had a lower threshold, which was found to be statistically significant. In all 18 patients with upper limb involvement, the pain threshold was reduced on the affected side, but this applied to only 11 of 15 with leg involvement. This difference may be because patients with lower limb symptoms had been referred later in the course of the syndrome. They showed by repeated tests that after an average of 49 days there was a slow return to normality. They concluded that the estimation of pressure-pain thresholds may help in the earlier diagnosis of reflex sympathetic dystrophy.

In a review of 14 patients with RSD of the knee joint by Tietjen,[2] the relation of symptoms to the number of patients was: pain, 100% of patients; burning pain, 39%; numbness, 64%; stiffness, 100%; mechanical complaints, 100%; swelling, 71%.

Signs

The signs elicited in the examination of a patient with RSD are discoloration of the skin, vasomotor instability and sensory disturbances.[1,3] It is important to appreciate that progressive trophic and vasomotor changes occur in all tissue layers such as the skin, subcutaneous tissue, muscles, joints, ligaments and bones, leading to atrophy of the skin, muscle and bones and joint stiffness.[6]

Thirty-six patients with RSD were examined by Katz and Hungerford.[9] The percentage of elicitation of various signs were: skin discoloration, 56% of patients; sensitivity to cold, 97% of patients; cutaneous hypersensitivity, 61% of patients.

Ogilvie-Harris and Roscoe[17] reviewed 19 patients and divided them into three groups. Two of these groups were related to the time of onset of the symptoms and attendance and were therefore called 'early' if attendance was within 6 months of the development of symptoms. In the 'late' group, the duration was more than 6 months from the onset of symptoms. The third group was that in which the RSD developed postoperatively.

In the 'early' group (7 patients), there was marked hypersensitivity to touch, loss of quadriceps bulk and flexion contractures that were less than those in the other two groups. Only one patient had dystrophic changes. In the 'late' group (9 patients) the patients had extensive wasting of the quadriceps and considerable loss of flexion. Eight patients had dystrophic changes, often associated with thickening and fibrosis. In the 'post-operative' group (3 patients), two had wasting of the quadriceps and loss of movement particularly terminal flexion and two had dystrophic skin changes.

Schwartzman and Kerrigan[26] presented 43 patients with RSD who manifested abnormalities of movement. The patients had focal dystonia, weakness, spasms, tremor, difficulty in initiating movement, and increased tone and reflexes. These motor signs and symptoms may precede other manifestations of the illness by weeks or months. They most frequently, but not invariably, occur concomitantly with sudomotor or vasomotor changes and pain. They affirmed that in many patients the movement disorder becomes independent of sympathetic innervation.

Stiffness is another characteristic feature of RSD and is a common presentation in knee joint involvement.[2,10] In the beginning of the disorder, stiffness may be due to pain. Later, oedema sets in and aggravates stiffness. Eventually periarticular fibrosis of the soft tissue contributes to the persistence of the stiffness.[1] Stiffness is one of the most important complaints around the knee joint and may simply be a moderate limitation of movement (e.g. up to 90°) or may be total stiffness of the joint, causing pain with any movement.[10] Tietjen[2] emphasized that stiffness seemed to be related to the disease stage. In most of the patients with RSD of the knee joint, examination under anaesthesia before the trophic stage will show a full range of motion. In later stages of the disease, notably the trophic stage, capsular and retinacular thickening contribute to limitation of movement in the knee joint and the patellofemoral joint region.[2,10]

Tenderness is another feature of the tissues involved. Perhaps tenderness is exaggerated by the hyperaesthesia of the skin.

The prevalence of the signs of RSD in the knees of 14 patients who were reviewed by Tietjen[2] was: skin changes, 39% of patients; effusion, 0%; synovitis, 86%, diffuse tenderness, 100%; point tenderness, 39%; atrophy, 100%; dystrophy, 50%; loss of motion, 50%; gait change—limp, 21%, when observed, 64%; none, 14%.

It is interesting to note that the stage of presentation to the physician of RSD of the knee joint in the above series was 'early' in 13 of the patients and 'atrophic' in 1 patient only. Yet the author states that atrophy, as such, was present very early in the course of the syndrome. Point tenderness was common, particularly in the region of the medial capsule and the patellofemoral joint.

Aids to diagnosis

Preliminary investigation may include a full blood count, erythrocyte sedimentation rate and rheumatoid tests.[2] Arthrography and arthroscopy may help in establishing the precipitating pathology and avoid unnecessary arthrotomy. Neither of these modalities yet have an established role in the diagnosis of RSD of the knee joint, but their role in exclusion is helpful.

Plain radiography

Osteoporosis is classically described in RSD. It is due to hyperaemia;[6] the increased bone turnover may be another factor. However, osteoporosis is not an early finding in RSD. Some believe that the radiographic features occur approximately 6–8 weeks after the onset of the symptoms.[4] Strobel and Stedtfeld[3] stress that by the time such a radiographic appearance reveals itself, permanent loss of function may be inevitable. Therefore, the diagnosis should not be delayed in the absence of osteoporosis.[6] Others state that radiographic changes occur within 2–4 weeks from the beginning of the syndrome.[2] The osteoporosis tends to be widespread and extreme. The cortices are extremely thin and scalloped; medullary bone appears to be patchily resorbed, but the joint spaces are preserved.[27] The term Sudeck's atrophy should not be used if the spotty radiographic appearance is not apparent. Such spotty rarefaction, present in the involved bones, is different from the generalized ground-glass appearance seen with disuse atrophy of bone.[4]

It is equally important to note that not all component members of a joint are equally affected by the RSD. Katz and Hungerford[9] reviewed the plain radiographs of 36 patients with RSD of the knee joint. The distribution of osteopenia was: patella, 49%; diffusely through the knee, 39%; distal femur, 9%; patella and distal femur, 3%.

Lagier[28] reported on the involvement of the lateral femoral condyle in this condition. A 62-year-old man presented with intense pain in the right knee, experienced immediately after slipping. The radiograph taken during the following weeks showed the development of a localized radiolucence of the lateral femoral condyle. Bone biopsy excluded an infectious process or tumour and revealed the histological characteristics of Sudeck's bone dystrophy. The clinical, radiological and histological data considered together were consistent with a diagnosis of 'partial algodystrophy', a term these authors preferred to 'transient osteoporosis'. The diagnosis was confirmed on clinical and radiological follow-up.

RSD involving the patella can occur, and is best demonstrated on axial views.[2,10] In the review by Tietjen,[2] all of the 14 patients who were affected by RSD of the knee joint had regional osteoporosis involving the patellofemoral joint. It involved the medial femoral condyle and the medial tibial plateau. It was stressed that the patella was uniformly involved when the knee joint was affected by RSD.

Radioisotope scanning

When radiographic changes are not evident for osteoporosis, many believe that triple-phase radioisotope scanning can be used with success in the early phase. The usual pattern of the scan is one of increased periarticular activity involving multiple joints in the affected extremity.[6,10,27] The cause of the increased uptake of the radioisotope scan in cases of RSD is the non-specific remodelling that occurs in this condition during the healing phase of the trauma.[23] Many believe that radioisotope scanning is sensitive but not specific.[29] Tietjen[2] affirmed that radioisotope bone scan was positive in two-thirds of the patients in his series.

The three-phase technetium bone scan (TPBS), with a combined sensitivity and specificity of greater than 90%, had been recommended for use in the diagnosis of RSD. Davidoff et al.[30] conducted a study to determine the predictive value and usefulness of TPBS in the diagnosis of RSD and to discover how the predictive value might be influenced by demographic and medical factors (e.g. duration of symptoms). A retrospective chart review was conducted of 119 patients who underwent a TPBS as part of a work-up for unexplained limb pain. Twenty-five patients met the Kozin criteria for definite or probable RSD. All patients were injected with technetium-99m methylene diphosphonate and scanned using established criteria. The 3-hour delayed image demonstrated a sensitivity of 44%, a specificity of 92%, a positive predictive value of 61%, and a negative predictive value of 86%. The blood-flow and pool-imaging phases added no further sensitivity or specificity to that achieved by the uptake scan in patients with upper-extremity involvement. Blood-flow and pool-imaging did improve the predictive value of the TPBS in patients with involvement of the lower extremities.

Williame and Sand[31] reported an adult case of reflex sympathetic dystrophy in the lower limb. In contrast to the usual findings in adults, three-phase scintigraphy showed decreased blood-flow and blood-pool with hypofixation on delayed steady-state bone scan of the affected lower limb. In spite of various therapeutic attempts, severe dystrophy developed.

Thermography

It is known that the initial phase of RSD is that of vasodilatation (warmth), which becomes vasoconstriction (cold) as the disease progresses. Thermograms have proved to be helpful but are not diagnostic. Temperature changes of 2°C or greater are highly suggestive of RSD but have to be interpreted in the overall clinical context.[16] Rothschild[32] advised that thermographic examination provided a valuable tool for monitoring the therapeutic response, whilst Tietjen[2] considered that thermography might be helpful in the evaluation of RSD.

Magnetic resonance imaging

Masciocchi et al.[29] compared MRI to radiology, CT scanning and radioisotope scanning in 5 patients with hip and knee pains presumed to be due to RSD. They concluded that MRI proved to be a reliable technique. MRI allows a differential diagnosis between RSD and other bone lesions such as osteonecrosis and tumours. Fulkerson and Hungerford[10] believe that MRI and CT scanning add little in the diagnosis of RSD.

Sympathetic block

Pathophysiologically, a complex disturbance of the sympathetic vasoconstrictor system is involved, which mediates the dominant symptoms of RSD, namely the spontaneous pain and swelling. The early interruption of the neuronal sympathetic activity by means of a sympathetic blockade reduces the pain and at the same time also the vicious circle of RSD.[33] Sympathetic block remains the standard for establishing the diagnosis of RSD.

Cone biopsy, interosseous phlebography, and intramedullary bone pressure readings have been evaluated by Ficat and co-workers;[10] however, such studies are difficult to accomplish clinically and the interpretation of the results is also difficult.[2]

Treatment of RSD

'RSD is not a disorder to be beaten into submission, but rather seduced.'[10]

The treatment of RSD depends on an early diagnosis. The essence of the treatment is to utilize all the modalities available to reduce the pain and initiate a gentle, supervised mobilization programme. A combination of the various methods may be needed to achieve good results. It is very important to establish a good doctor–patient relationship and to provide the patient with as much encouragement as possible.[2] The role of the nurse in early identification of such a syndrome should not be underestimated. The nursing-care plans must be directed towards providing emotional support and encouragement, maintaining and/or restoring mobility and establishing adequate pain control.[34]

Physiotherapy

It is important to instruct the physiotherapist to encourage active and active-assisted exercises below the pain threshold.[2,3] Hydrotherapy is the preferred method. Stimulation of the vascular tree by alternating warmth and cold at 5–10-minute intervals has been recommended.[10]

Transcutaneous electrical stimulation (TENS) has been advocated by many.[4,16] However, electrical stimulation of a neuroma had led to a case of RSD.[10] Robaina et al.[35] presented 35 patients with the diagnosis of reflex sympathetic dystrophy in a late stage that had been treated with transcutaneous electrical nerve stimulation. Six of the 35 were also submitted to spinal cord stimulation (SCS). The follow-up was from 10 to 36 months. The results obtained were: TENS group, 25% excellent, 45% good, 10% fair, 20% poor; SCS group, 16.6% excellent, 66.6% good, 16.6% fair. It was concluded that in the long run these results were better than those obtained with sympathetic blocks and sympathectomy and that TENS and SCS have no effect on osteoporosis or ankylosis.

Trigger-point injections and ultrasound treatments are claimed by some to be useful adjuncts.[4,16] Others believe that the results of these injections were temporary at best and tended to confuse the diagnosis.[2]

It has been stated that failure of the patient to respond to the usual physiotherapy should lead the physiotherapist to suspect RSD.[16]

Manipulation under anaesthesia

Insall[36] advised that knee stiffness due to reflex sympathetic dystrophy may require a manipulation under anaesthesia and affirmed that several manipulations under general anaesthetic may be required, motion being regained in small increments rather than all at once. Others, however, advised against such a procedure, maintaining that a fibrous reaction to the trauma of manipulation makes the situation worse.[10,37]

Drug therapy

A wide variety of pharmacological agents have been described. A few are mentioned here.

A non-steroidal anti-inflammatory drug (e.g. aspirin, naproxen, diflunisal and ibuprofen) can be helpful in providing both pain relief and anti-inflammatory action. A medication combination is used by Hungerford for the treatment of the milder cases of RSD on a trial basis of 6 weeks. It consists of Indocid (or any similar agent) 25 mg t.i.d., Hydergine 1–2 mg t.i.d., and Valium 2–5 mg t.i.d. If the patient shows improvement, the regime can be continued for another 6 weeks.[10]

Oral sympatholytic drugs include alpha- and beta-adrenergic antagonist drugs such as prazocin and phenoxybenzamine. These agents may be useful in the short-term. Their side-effects, particularly orthostatic hypotension, limit their use. Tricyclic antidepressant drugs such as amitriptyline and doxepin are used in the management of chronic pain. Calcium-channel blockers such as nifedepine have been used in the treatment of RSD. Anticonvulsant drugs such as phenytoin and carbamazepine have been used, particularly when paroxysmal pain is a feature.[16]

Lioresal is likely to be most beneficial in patients whose spasticity is a handicap to their activities. Schwartzman and Kerrigan[26] presented 43 patients with RSD who manifested abnormalities of movement. Lioresal was effective in reducing spasms. Early in the course of RSD, the motor manifestation may be alleviated by intense sympathetic blockade or sympathectomy.

Corticosteroids (such as prednisone in doses of 60–80 mg/day) have been used in the treatment of RSD.[4,12,16] Kozin et al.[12] reviewed 11 patients fulfilling criteria for the reflex sympathetic dystrophy syndrome. Corticosteroid therapy predictably resulted in improvement of all treated patients.

Calcitonin has been used in the treatment of RSD on the basis of the evidence of increased bone turnover that is associated with RSD.[4,38-40] Jaeger et al.[39] reported on the results of IV calcitonin treatment in patients suffering from postoperative phantom limb pain (n = 12) or causalgia following peripheral nerve lesions (n = 4). All patients complained of severe pain after a traumatic event or amputation, with disturbed sleep in many cases. After only 1-2 infusions, 10 patients with phantom limb pain (83%) were discharged from hospital pain-free. Pain was effectively reduced by up to five infusions in 2 patients (17%). At a follow-up of 24 months, recurrence of pain occurred in only 4 patients with obvious stump problems or reamputations. Three patients with causalgia also benefitted from a remarkable but transitory pain reduction; in one patient therapy was ineffective. Recurrent pain due to causalgia could not be improved by repeated calcitonin infusion, although this was effective for phantom limb pain. They concluded that the administration of calcitonin was recommended as a valuable treatment for phantom limb pain and causalgias in the early postoperative period. Therapy was effective, with negligible side-effects, and long-term follow-up revealed a long-lasting effect.

Solarova and Kunev[40] reviewed 23 patients with algodystrophy who were treated with calcitonin during the period 1978-88. The age range was 28-82 years. The treatment was carried out with the drug Myacalcic 'Sandoz' in a dose of 100 IU, administered intramuscularly every day in the course of 10 days. The following clinical parameters were followed up: pain, swelling, functional capacity and skin (dystrophic) changes. The patients were classified in two groups in relation to the results: group I = acute stage and group II = chronic stage of the disease. The pain was favourably influenced in both groups by the Myacalcic treatment. In the acute stage, the swelling was favourably influenced in 81% of the patients and the skin changes in 89%; the functional capacity was improved 1.64 times. In the chronic stage, the swelling was reduced in 25% of the patients, there was no effect on the dystrophic changes, and the functional capacity decreased in spite of the treatment.

Bickerstaff and Kanis[38] remarked that calcitonin is widely used in the treatment of algodystrophy but a major disadvantage was the need for its parenteral administration. For this reason, they evaluated the effect of 400 IU of nasal calcitonin in the treatment of post-traumatic algodystrophy in a prospective randomized double-blind study. They found no demonstrable effect on the clinical or skeletal progression of the disorder using sensitive methods of measuring the response to treatment. There was, however, a small but significant hypocalcaemic response in the treatment group despite no change in the other indices of bone turnover.

Sympathetic block

In this procedure, the advice and assistance of colleagues from the anaesthesia department or the neurosurgical department is essential. Apart from its undoubted diagnostic value, the use of prolonged sympathetic blockade as an adjunct increases the margin of safety in surgery for these patients when non-operative measures could not relieve the pain or restore function.[41] Only with the early administration of sympathetic blocks in addition to adjunctive therapies will pain relief and return to normal function be most assured.[42]

Omohundro and Payne[16] described the four methods employed to perform the sympathetic block: (1) intravenous or intra-arterial regional blockade; (2) differential spinal block; (3) paravertebral; (4) epidural.

Regional blocks can be performed using guanethidine (alpha-receptor blocking agent) or reserpine.[16,43,44] The initial block may provide relief lasting only a few hours (paravertebral) to several days (intravenous guanethidine). Cooper et al.[45] retrospectively reviewed the cases of 14 patients who had reflex sympathetic dystrophy of the knee. All 14 were hospitalized, and epidural block anaesthesia was instituted with an indwelling catheter for an average of 4 days, during which continuous passive motion, manipulation (as necessary), stimulation of muscles, and alternating hot and cold soaks were used. The average length of follow-up was 32 months. Eleven patients had complete resolution of the symptoms, two had sufficient intermittent aching with changes in the weather to need medication, and one had no relief. The diagnosis was confirmed if the symptoms were relieved by a lumbar sympathetic block. Pain that was out of proportion to the severity of the injury was the most consistent finding, being present in all 14 patients. However, variation in clinical severity was characteristic of the syndrome. Eleven of the 14 patients had a previous patellar operation. After the onset of the symptoms, 9 patients had two or more arthroscopic examinations, without notable findings. All 14 patients had had extensive physical therapy and medical treatment before the epidural block was performed.

Driessen et al.[43] assessed 20 patients with documented reflex sympathetic dystrophy who were treated with a series of regional intravenous guanethidine blocks. The mean delay between the first clinical symptoms and the start of guanethidine blocks was 3.6 months. The overall result was good in 11 patients, moderate in 2 patients and poor in 7 patients. Poor results were due mainly to incorrect diagnosis and to application either too late in the third phase or too early in the first phase, when only signs of increased blood flow are part of the symptomatology. Side-effects, except pain after the injection, were few and of minor importance. The tolerance of the procedure may be improved by preceding the injection of guanethidine by an injection of a local anaesthetic agent. It was concluded, that with correct diagnosis and indication, guanethidine injections may play an important part in the treatment of reflex sympathetic dystrophy and may replace sympathetic blocks with local anaesthetics because of the longer duration of action and lower incidence of serious side-effects.

Regional intravenous guanethidine blocks and stellate ganglion blocks were compared in a randomized trial by Bonelli et al.[44] Nineteen patients, randomly allocated to two groups of therapy and exhibiting severe reflex sympathetic dystrophy following peripheral nerve lesions, have been treated. The results of this study showed that regional sympathetic block with guanethidine was a good therapeutic tool in the treatment of reflex sympathetic dystrophies, especially on account of its negligible risks and contraindications.

Thermal biofeedback techniques

Barowsky et al.[46] assessed a 12-year-old male unresponsive to therapy for symptoms associated with reflex sympathetic dystrophy. He was treated by thermal biofeedback techniques. Within the first four treatment sessions, transfer of training from digital warming to warming the affected knee area produced skin temperature elevation around the gastrocnemius and patellar areas. Attenuation of localized vasospasm and cold intolerance resulted, followed by total abolition within ten sessions. After alleviation of symptoms, his function returned.

Blanchard[47] reported a patient with chronic pain due to a reflex sympathetic dystrophy in his hand and arm who was successfully treated with temperature biofeedback after several months of conservative standard medical care had brought little relief. Over the 18 treatment sessions the patient learned to emit a reliable hand-warming response of 1–1.5°C. Coincident with his learning, the pain in his hand and arm decreased markedly and remained absent at 1-year follow-up.

Surgical sympathectomy

Permanent interruption of the sympathetic reflex may become necessary.[4] It is suggested that it should be done only when there is an unequivocal but transient benefit from sympathetic blockade.[16] Thompson[48] reviewed a series of 147 patients; 56% required surgical sympathectomy. The rest were treated by sympathetic blocks, physical therapy, and other medical measures. Eighty-two per cent had excellent relief of pain, 11% had good relief, while 7% had no relief. Thirty-one per cent of patients had

residual symptoms resulting from the original injury, or from irreversible occurrences on the basis of pain and trophic changes. Surgical sympathectomy must not be the first line of treatment because there is a small but definite recurrence rate of pain after sympathectomy; in addition, it may be complicated by the development of post-sympathectomy pain.[16]

Psychological therapy

In individuals with chronic pain, psychological assessment and advice may be helpful.

Reflex sympathetic dystrophy and the 'stiff-knee' syndromes

The problem with reflex sympathetic dystrophy is by no means solved. It merits serious consideration and thought. The overall incidence of RSD appears to be underestimated in the aftermath of knee injury. The importance of such a situation lies in the fact that it represents the body's response to injury, be it primary following the injury itself or secondary to surgery and the disability it inflicts on the sufferer. Spontaneous occurrence of RSD in the knee joint has been described as rare.[10] Response to injury in RSD is still vague in terms of the initiation of the disorder.

Stiffness is a term that is both subjective and objective. The two may coincide but can be very deceptive. In RSD of the knee joint, stiffness has been described as being localized to the knee joint or diffusely involving the lower limb.[10] The stiffness referred to in knee injury and/or RSD is basically that related to trauma. This excludes categories such as postinfective stiffness and the stiffness of arthritis. Different dimensions have been added to the diagnosis of post-traumatic knee stiffness by the inclusions of syndromes such as 'infrapatellar contracture syndrome',[49] 'patella infera syndrome',[50] and 'reflex sympathetic imbalance'.[7] All these syndromes endeavour to explain the knee stiffness and reaction to trauma.

Wotjys et al.[51] described the use of immunohistochemical techniques to identify and trace substance-P so as to subsequently identify nociceptive fibres. The study demonstrated that selective tracing of nociceptor pain fibres is possible in and around the knee both in soft tissue and, in some circumstances, in bone. This study demonstrated the possibility of existence of erosion channels not present in a normal patellae in the chondral defects occurring in degenerative disease. Nociceptive fibres found in these defects may explain the origin of symptoms in some patients. The distribution of substance-P in nerve fibres in the soft tissues around the knee suggests that denervation may be the mechanism by which surgical procedures for anterior knee pain produce favourable results. Cheshire and Snyder[52] described a 31-year-old female with intractable RSD who experienced nearly complete, though temporary resolution of pain following 3 weeks of topical capsaicin. They propose that capsaicin may be a useful treatment for RSD either by depleting substance-P from the primary afferent neurons that mediate allodynia, or by modulating sympathetic efferent activity.

RSD has been described affecting the patellofemoral region.[2,10] The knee ligaments are not static stabilizers. They are structures innervated by nerve endings of various descriptions that help adjust the response to the various loads to which the knee is subjected and that beyond certain stress thresholds recruit the quadriceps and hamstrings to accommodate and adjust the load absorption and knee position.[53] It is also evident that medial, and more so lateral, patellar retinacula are not static stabilizers but rather dynamic ones.[10,54] When a balance is maintained between these structures, as is the case in a normal knee, then the patella and the patellar ligament are in line mediolaterally. However, the quadriceps–patellar ligament axis still requires some explanation. The reports describing corrugation of the patellar ligament following high tibial osteotomy highlight the need for further work to understand the extensor mechanism.[55,56] Scuderi et al.[56] thought that the explanation was that the lower position of the patella was probably due to shortening of the patellar tendon after prolonged immobilization in a cast, interstitial scarring of the patellar tendon and new bone formation in the area of insertion of the patellar ligament. Dandy and Gordon[57] proposed the possible presence of an annular knee ligament.

The role of surgery is equally variable. Surgery was frequently the precipitating factor in RSD of the knee joint. Then repeated surgery has to be performed to overcome postoperative stiffness. Such surgery, including manipulation under anaesthesia and arthroscopic arthrolysis, may need to be extensive. Manipulation of the knee under anaesthesia has been rejected by some,[10,37] whilst arthrolysis is technically more exacting but empirical in that retinacular release does not seem to restore the full height of the patella in patella infera. Another valid point is the relation of the fat pad to the patellar tendon. The finding of a fat pad adherent to the patellar ligament post-injury may, indeed, represent an attempt at healing.

Early postoperative mobilization is important in avoiding postoperative stiffness. But the term mobilization is becoming ambiguous as opinions differ on the degree and the type of mobilization. It is important that forceful mobilization is abandoned for a more gradual, persistent programme.[10] Physiotherapy may be combined with non-steroidal anti-inflammatory drugs, and the clue to successful mobilization is a multidiscipline approach by all concerned to make mobilization as pain-free as possible.

References

1. Lankford LL, Reflex sympathetic dystrophy, *Surgery of the musculoskeletal system*, 2nd edn, ed McCollister Evarts C (New York: Churchill Livingstone, 1990) 1265–1296.
2. Tietjen R, Reflex sympathetic dystrophy of the knee, *Clin Orthop* (1986) **209**: 234–243.
3. Strobel M, Stedtfeld HW, *Diagnostic evaluation of the knee* (Berlin: Springer-Verlag, 1990) 57–58.
4. Pellegrini VD, McCollister Evarts C, Complications, *Fractures in adults*, 3rd edn, ed Rockwood CA Jr, Green DP, Bucholz RW (Philadelphia: J.B. Lippincott, Philadelphia, 1991) 383–387.
5. Schott G, Clinical features of algodystrophy: is the sympathetic nervous system involved? *Funct Neurol* (1989) **4**(2): 131–134.
6. Seale K, Reflex sympathetic dystrophy of the lower extremity, *Clin Orthop* (1989) **243**: 80–85.
7. Ladd AL, DeHaven KE, Thanik J et al., Reflex sympathetic imbalance. Response to epidural blockade, *Am J Sports Med* (1989) **17**(5): 660–668.
8. Goris RJ, Reynen JA, Veldman P, [The clinical symptoms in post-traumatic dystrophy] De klinische verschijnselen bij posttraumatische dystrofie, *Ned Tijdschr Geneeskd* (1990) 3: 134 (44): 2138–2141.
9. Katz MM, Hungerford DS, Reflex sympathetic dystrophy affecting the knee, *J Bone Joint Surg (Br)* (1987) **69**(5): 797–803.
10. Fulkerson JP, Hungerford DS, *Disorders of the patellofemoral joint*, 2nd edn (Baltimore: Williams and Wilkins, 1990) 247–264.
11. Coughlan RJ, Hazleman BL, Thomas DP et al., Algodystrophy: a common unrecognized cause of chronic knee pain, *Br J Rheumatol*, (1987) **26**(4): 270–274.
12. Kozin F. McCarty DJ, Sims J et al., The reflex sympathetic dystrophy syndrome. I. Clinical and histologic studies: evidence for bilaterality, response to corticosteroids and articular involvement, *Am J Med* (1976) **60**(3): 321–331.
13. Hakusui S, Iwase S, Mano T et al., [A microneurographic analysis of minor reflex sympathetic dystrophy with increased skin sympathetic activity—report of a case] *Rinsho Shinkeigaku* (1990) **30**(6): 668–671.
14. Marchettini P, Lacerenza M, Ieracitano D et al., Sensitized nociceptors in reflex sympathetic dystrophies, *Funct Neurol* (1989) **4**(2): 135–140.
15. Hanna MH, Peat SJ, Ketanserin in reflex sympathetic dystrophy. A double-blind placebo controlled cross-over trial, *Pain* (1989) **38**(2): 145–150.
16. Omohundro PH, Payne R, Reflex sympathetic dystrophy, *Spine* (1988) **2**(4): 685–698.
17. Ogilvie-Harris DJ, Roscoe M, Reflex sympathetic dystrophy of the knee, *J Bone Joint Surg (Br)* (1987) **69**(5): 804–806.
18. Poehling GG, Pollock FE Jr, Koman LA, Reflex sympathetic dystrophy of the knee after sensory nerve injury, *Arthroscopy* (1988) **4**(1): 31–35.
19. Zucchini M, Alberti G, Moretti MP, Algodystrophy and related psychological features, *Funct Neurol* (1989) **4**(2): 153–156.
20. Egle UT, Hoffmann SO, [Psychosomatic correlations of sympathetic reflex dystrophy (Sudeck's disease). Review of the literature and initial clinical results] Psychosomatische Zusammenhänge bei sympathischer Reflexdystrophie (Morbus Sudeck). Literaturübersicht und erste klinische Ergebnisse, *Psychother Psychosom Med Psychol* (1990) **40**(3–4): 123–135.
21. Arlet P, Arlet J, Riviere R et al., [Pain and inflammation of the foot in metabolic osteopathies: new causes of algodystrophy] Pied douloureux et inflammatoire des osteopathies métaboliques. Nouvelles causes d'algodystrophe, *Sem Hôp Paris* (1982) **58**(22): 1345–1347.
22. Munoz-Gomez J, Collado A, Gratacos J et al., Reflex sympathetic dystrophy syndrome of the lower limbs in renal transplant patients treated with cyclosporin A, *Arthritis Rheum* (1991) **34**(5): 625–630.

23. **Lagier R, Boussina I, Mathies B,** Algodystrophy of the knee. Anatomico-radiological study of a case, *Clin Rheumatol* (1983) 2(1): 71–77.
24. **Arlet J, Ficat P, Durroux R** et al., [Histopathology of bone and cartilage lesions in reflex sympathetic dystrophy of the knee. A propos of 16 cases] Histopathologie des lesions osseuses et cartilagineuses dans l'algodystrophe sympathique reflexe du genou. A propos de 16 observations, *Rev Rheum Mal Osteoartic* (1981) 48(4): 315–321.
25. **Bryan AS, Klenerman L, Bowsher D,** The diagnosis of reflex sympathetic dystrophy using an algometer, *J Bone Joint Surg (Br)* (1991) 73(4): 644–646.
26. **Schwartzman RJ, Kerrigan J,** The movement disorder of reflex sympathetic dystrophy, *Neurology* (1990) 40(1): 57–61.
27. **Renton P,** Orthopaedic radiology. *Pattern recognition and differential diagnosis* (London: Martin Dunitz, 1990) 30–34.
28. **Lagier R,** Partial algodystrophy of the knee. An anatomico-radiological study of one case, *J Rheumatol* (1983) 10(2): 255–260.
29. **Masciocchi, C, Fascetti E, Michelini O** et al., [Reflex sympathetic dystrophy syndrome. Contribution of magnetic resonance] Sindrome distrofica simpatico riflessa (RSDS). Contributo della risonanza magnetica, *Radiol Med (Torino)* (1987) 74(5): 408–412.
30. **Davidoff G, Werner R, Cremer S** et al., Predictive value of the three-phase technetium bone scan in diagnosis of reflex sympathetic dystrophy syndrome, *Arch Phys Med Rehabil* (1989) 70(2): 135–137.
31. **Williame LM, Sand A,** Hypofixation on bone scintigraphy in reflex sympathetic dystrophy syndrome, *Clin Rheumatol* (1991) 10(1): 73–75.
32. **Rothschild B,** Reflex sympathetic dystrophy, *Arthritis Care Res* (1990) 3(3): 144–153.
33. **Blumberg H, Griesser HJ, Hornyak M,** [Neurologic aspects of clinical manifestations, pathophysiology and therapy of reflex sympathetic dystrophy (causalgia, Sudeck's disease)] Neurologische Aspekte der Klinik, Pathophysiologie und Therapie der sympathischen Reflexdystrophie (Kausalgie, Morbus Sudeck), *Nervenartz* (1991) 62(4): 205–211.
34. **Greipp ME, Thomas AF,** Reflex sympathetic dystrophy syndrome: pain that does not stop, *J Neurosci Nurs* (1986) 18(1): 23–25.
35. **Robaina FJ, Rodriguez JL, de Vera JA** et al., Transcutaneous electrical nerve stimulation and spinal cord stimulation for pain relief in reflex sympathetic dystrophy, *Stereotact Funct Neurosurg* (1989) 52(1): 53–62.
36. **Insall JN,** Chronic instability of the knee, *Surgery of the Knee*, ed Insall JN (New York: Churchill Livingstone, 1984) 349.
37. **Feagin JA, Lambert KL, Raymond Cunningham R,** Repair and reconstruction of the anterior cruciate ligament, *Operative orthopaedics* ed Chapman MW (Philadelphia: J.B. Lippincott Company, 1988) 1648–1649.
38. **Bickerstaff DR, Kanis JA,** The use of nasal calcitonin in the treatment of post-traumatic algodystrophy, *Br J Rheumatol* (1991) 30(4): 291–294.
39. **Jaeger H, Maier C, Wawersik J,** [Postoperative treatment of phantom pain and causalgias with calcitonin] Postoperative Behandlung von Phantomschmerzen und Kausalgien mit Calcitonin, *Anaesthesist* (1988) 37(2): 71–76.
40. **Solarova P, Kunev K,** [The calcitonin treatment of patients with algodystrophy] Lechenie s kaltsitonin pri bolni s algodistrofia, *Vutr Boles* (1990) 29(5): 102–105.
41. **Hobelmann CF Jr, Dellon AL,** Use of prolonged sympathetic blockade as an adjunct to surgery in the patient with sympathetic maintained pain, *Microsurgery* (1989) 10(2): 151–153.
42. **Simon D,** Pain syndromes: case studies, *Iowa Med* (1991) 81(3): 109–112.
43. **Driessen JJ, van der Werken C, Nicolai JP** et al., Clinical effects of regional intravenous guanethidine (Ismelin) in reflex sympathetic dystrophy, *Acta Anaesthesiol Scand* (1983) 27(6): 505–509.
44. **Bonelli S, Conoscente F, Movilia PG** et al., Regional intravenous guanethidine vs. stellate ganglion block in reflex sympathetic dystrophies: a randomized trial, *Pain* (1983) 16(3): 297–307.
45. **Cooper DE, DeLee JC, Ramamurthy S,** Reflex sympathetic dystrophy of the knee. Treatment using continuous epidural anesthesia, *J Bone Joint Surg (Am)* (1989) 71(3): 365–369.
46. **Barowsky EI, Zweig JB, Moskowitz J,** Thermal biofeedback in the treatment of symptoms associated with reflex sympathetic dystrophy, *J Child Neurol* (1987) 2(3): 229–232.
47. **Blanchard EB,** The use of temperature biofeedback in the treatment of chronic pain due to causalgia, *Biofeedback Self Regul* (1979) 4(2): 183–188.
48. **Thompson JE,** The diagnosis and management of post-traumatic pain syndromes (causalgia), *Aust N Z J Surg* (1979) 49(3): 299–304.
49. **Paulos LE, Rosenberg TD, Drawbert J** et al., Infrapatellar contracture syndrome. An unrecognized cause of knee stiffness with patella entrapment and patella infera, *Am J Sports Med* (1987) 15(4): 331–341.
50. **Noyes FR, Wotjys EM, Marshall MT,** The early diagnosis and treatment of developmental patella infera syndrome, *Clin Orthop* (1991) 265: 241–252.
51. **Wotjys EM, Beaman DN, Glover RA** et al., Innervation of the human knee joint by substance-P fibers, *Arthroscopy* (1990) 6(4): 254–263.
52. **Cheshire WP, Snyder CR,** Treatment of reflex sympathetic dystrophy with topical capsaicin. Case report, *Pain* (1990) 42(3): 307–311.
53. **Solomonow M, D'Ambrosia R,** Neural reflex arcs and muscle control of knee stability and motion, *Ligament and extensor mechanism injuries of the knee. Diagnosis and treatment*, ed Norman Scott W (St Louis: Mosby–Year Book, Inc., 1991) 389–400.
54. **Hallisey M, Doherty N, Bennett W** et al., Anatomy of the junction of the vastus lateralis tendon and the patella, *J Bone Joint Surg (Am)* (1987) 69: 545.
55. **Berlin RC, Levinsohn EM, Chrisman H,** The wrinkled patellar tendon: an indication of abnormality in the extensor mechanism of the knee, *Skeletal Radiol* (1991) 20(3): 181–185.
56. **Scuderi GR, Windsor RE, Insall JN,** Observations on the patellar height after proximal tibial osteotomy, *J Bone Joint Surg (Am)* (1989) 71(2): 245–248.
57. **Dandy DJ, Gordon RG,** Patellar height following high tibial osteotomy: evidence of an annular ligament at the knee, Paper presented at the British Association for Surgery of the Knee (BASK) Meeting, Cambridge, 26 Sept. 1991.

21

Documentation and evaluation in disorders of the knee

21.1 Documentation and evaluation in disorders of the knee: An overview

Paul M. Aichroth and Dipak V. Patel

Each orthopaedic department will have its own evaluation and documentation system for its prime work. This is important for internal audit but it is difficult to relate one set of parameters with another, for each orthopaedic surgeon will put different emphasis on various assessment features. A consensus is vital among knee surgeons and to this end, the International Knee Documentation Committee and the SICOT-IDES (International Documentation Evaluation System) have been at work.

The International Knee Documentation Committee (IKDC) published its Knee Ligament Injury and Reconstructive Evaluation form in 1991 and the consensus achieved was quite remarkable. Eminent members of the American Orthopaedic Society for Sports Medicine (AOSSM) and ESKA (European Society of Knee Surgery and Arthroscopy) met regularly during the preceding year and this splendid cooperation has produced a form which is brief, workable and certainly comprehensive enough to allow adequate comparison of one set of results with another. Of course, many departments will demand more parameters in their documentation and others will expect a score to be given. These features may be added, but they were not felt to be essential.

An example of an individual knee ligament rating system is that from the Hospital for Special Surgery described by Thomas Wickiewicz in this chapter. It is well established, published and has been scored. However, it is hoped that in the future the consensus which produced the IKDC form will take over in international communication and journal articles. Similarly, Feagin and Blake's[1] ACL Follow-up Form (Tables 4 and 5 in contribution 21.5) was a product of the AOSSM Study Group, and has been used successfully for many years. However, John Feagin and the Study Group have evolved and consented to the shorter and concise IKDC form. Surgical cooperation and consensus are winning through!

There are many surgeons—and certainly many patients—who think that the only important thing about knee problems and their treatment is the *function* of the joint. Lysholm and Gillquist[2] produced a form to assess knee function and produced a score sheet—Table 1 in 21.5. This was simple, quick and could be used in retrospect as well as in prospect. In its modified form the Lysholm-II score (Table 2) became the criterion of knee function assessment and has been used extensively through the 1980s.

A further assessment of knee activity was published by Tegner and Lysholm[3] in 1985, and this is now widely used (Table 3). However, the activities described are those for the Scandinavian scene and each country will need to modify the sports, pastimes and work to suit its own culture. Noyes et al.[4] have an alternative sports/activities rating scale for the American scene.

An attempt to incorporate all features of knee problems and disabilities was published by Noyes, Barber and Mangine[4] in the American *Journal of Bone and Joint Surgery* in 1990. This is comprehensive and scored, and is described in Tables 6 to 9 in 21.5. It represents a method of recording global knee symptoms, signs, function and activity in all diseases and disorders. It is probably better to separate knees with mechanical derangements in athletes from those with arthritic features whose assessment and documentation require many different parameter readings.

Many national societies and knee surgery associations have attempted to produce assessment forms for their patients with arthritic conditions. In an attempt to compare the results of one prosthetic replacement with another, the British *Journal* insisted in the early 1980s that the British Orthopaedic Association Knee Assessment Form[5] be used to record the essential parameters in follow-up examinations. This early form was not scored, but subsequent ones, such as the Hospital for Special Surgery and the BASK (British Association for Surgery of the Knee) forms were. During the 1980s a vast array of assessment forms for arthritic conditions and their prosthetic replacement were used and published, with one country frequently vying with the next for supremacy in quality, brevity or comprehensiveness. This has led to a complete tangle and the IDES was set up by SICOT and the Maurice Müller Foundation to produce an International Consensus in Hip Disorders and Replacements. The philosophy behind this and the Documentation Evaluation Form itself was published in the literature in 1990.[6-8] This has now gained progressive recognition among the hip surgeons of the world. A similar exercise for knee surgery is now under way, with the IDES Knee Documentation Evaluation Subcommittee reporting its draft assessment form in this chapter. The Committee is still sitting and the final form will appear with appropriate publications in 1992. The draft form is the result of international consensus with representatives of the American Academy, the American Knee Society, the International Knee Society, the British Orthopaedic Association, the British Association for Surgery of the Knee, the Guepar Group, the Japanese Orthopaedic Association and the Swiss and German Orthopaedic Groups.

Should the Assessment Form be scored? Graham Apley has written a pertinent editorial in a British journal,[9] pointing out that science is measurement but it is difficult to measure success. It implores us not to substitute bad accounting for good judgment. Mr Apley points out that the most conscientious evaluation will vary with the assessor and we should 'resist the seductive simplicity of numerical scores'. It is more important to define the most important factors in knee function assessment and this will allow the comparison of one series with another. If an individual unit cannot tear itself away from the scoring system, the computerization of the IDES knee form will allow it to occur, but this must be for inter-nal consumption and audit. Scoring in this context is a pseudoscience.

References

1. **Feagin JA Jr, Blake WP,** Postoperative evaluation and result recording in the anterior cruciate ligament reconstructed knee, *Clin Orthop* (1983) **172:** 143–147.
2. **Lysholm J, Gillquist J,** Evaluation of knee ligament surgery results with special emphasis on use of a scoring scale, *Am J Sports Med* (1982) **10:** 150–154.
3. **Tegner Y, Lysholm J,** Rating system in the evaluation of knee ligament injuries, *Clin Orthop* (1985) **198:** 43–49.
4. **Noyes FR, Barber SD, Mangine RE,** Bone–patellar ligament–bone and fascia lata allografts for reconstruction of the anterior cruciate ligament, *J Bone Joint Surg (Am)* (1990) **72:** 1125–1136.
5. **Aichroth P, Freeman MAR, Smillie IS et al.,** A knee function assessment chart, *J Bone Joint Surg (Br)* (1978) **60:** 308–309.
6. **Galante J,** Evaluation of results of total hip replacement, *J Bone Joint Surg (Am)* (1990) **72:** 159–160.
7. **Johnson RC, Fitzgerald RH, Harris WH et al.,** Clinical and radiographic evaluation of total hip replacement, *J Bone Joint Surg (Am)* (1990) **72:** 161–168.
8. **Müller ME, Sledge C, Poss R et al.,** Report of the SICOT Presidential Commission on documentation and evaluation, *Int Orthop* (1990) **14:** 221–229.
9. **Apley AG,** An assessment of assessment, *J Bone Joint Surg (Br)* (1990) **72:** 957–958.

21.2 The philosophical issues of knee documentation

Glenn C. Terry

Webster's dictionary defines philosophy as a critical study of the basic principles and concepts of a particular branch of knowledge, especially with a view to improving or reconstituting them; and it is also defined as a system of principles for guidance in practical affairs. A system is defined as an assemblage or combination of parts forming a complex or unitary whole.

In the case of knee documentation, the whole is an inclusive system of assessment and documentation of the patient's knee disabled from instability, extensor mechanism deficiency, arthritis, or internal derangement. See examinations 1–6.

Historically, the approach to knee documentation has been guided by clinical intuition. Also, different practice interest has stimulated different systems of assessment. In the case of knee instability, clinical experience and anatomy guided early contributors who developed the limits of motion examination tests, which included: (1) abduction–adduction at 0 and 30° knee flexion; (2) anterior and posterior drawer testing with the knee flexed to 90° and the tibia oriented in external, neutral, or internal rotation; (3) the tibial anterior translation test near extension (Lachman's test); (4) posterolateral tibial rotation at 30° of knee flexion; (5) the pivot shift/jerk test; and (6) external rotation recurvatum test.

The 0, +1 (5 mm), +2 (6–10 mm), +3 (>10 mm) method of quantifying displacement recommended by the American Medical Association (AMA) was a step towards objectivity, but when compared to millimeter increments of displacement, the AMA system seems qualitative. Nevertheless, the demonstration of the specific anatomical injuries and their correlation to the abnormal motion limits assessment is a real strength of this earlier system and provides the basis for a classification of knee instability. However, since the limits of motion (examination) tests have been regionally developed, the language utilized as descriptors of tests has tended to be colloquial. This colloquialism, although 'comfortable' to some, has impeded international communication.

An International Knee Documentation Committee (IKDC) was formed in 1987 under the auspices of the European Society of Knee Surgery and Arthroscopy (ESKA) and the American Orthopaedic Society for Sports Medicine (AOSSM) to develop a system of knee documentation that was simple to use and provided the minimum requirements for the objective documentation of knee instability. European committee members include: Pierre Chambat, Albert Van Kampen, Ejnar Eriksson, Jan Gillquist, Fritz Hefti, Roland Jakob, Hans-Ueli Stäubli, Giancarlo Puddu, and Bernard Moyen, under the direction of cochairman Werner Mueller. North American members include: Peter Fowler, William Clancy, Dale Daniel, Kenneth DeHaven, Edward Grood, Frank Noyes, Peter Torzilli, Russell Warren, and Glenn Terry, under the direction of cochairman John Feagin.

In attempting to accomplish its goal, the committee approached the task like a problem in education:

1. Identify the problem.
2. List alternative solutions.
3. List solution strategies.
4. Implement the solution strategies.
5. Evaluate the performance.
6. Revise the strategy as necessary.

In the case of knee instability documentation, the committee decided that the most important issue was to provide a quantitative method of symptom and impairment documentation as well as motion limits documentation.

But before accepting a single method of documentation one must consider many philosophical variables common to any experiment. For example, the internal method of learning utilized by the individual to assimilate information is important. Is the student/experimenter right-brain dominant (more analytical) or left-brain dominant (more artistic and creative). The former individual may favor examination tests and test descriptors based on in-vitro biomechanical studies, while the latter favors tests and test descriptors based on in-vivo clinical experience.

The fact that the examiner is a variable in every experimental process (complementarity) is commonly forgotten. Certainly, the perceptual abilities of the individual will influence his interpretation (outcome) of the experiment. For example, our lack of complete understanding of knee functional anatomy and the appropriate examination method to perfectly test that anatomy may produce an imperfect prospective study design as a consequence of our uncertainty in understanding nature. The results thus obtained, although true to the prospective experimental design, may incompletely explain natural or abnormal knee phenomena, or incomplete information may help create a logic paradox.

A corollary to the uncertainty of our understanding of natural phenomena is special nonsense. Since the test information required to completely evaluate each knee problem is unknown, it is fair to say that all data that are accumulated may be important, even though the relative importance of each part may emerge only from an understanding of the whole.

This concept is of prime importance in understanding the difficulties in designing a knee documentation form in a prospective way when we, as a committee, do not truly know which data are the most important to our future understanding of knee instability treatment. However, since each of us has an opinion, it makes the discussions interesting.

Another variable that influences the acceptability of any data management system involves the descriptors utilized for communication. Such descriptors must be universally accepted by the international community. Thus, the committee has chosen terminology and units of measurement that have an engineering basis or are internationally acceptable rather than using the familiar colloquial terms and English units of measurement which currently are a source of international confusion.

As I considered giving up familiar tests and units of measure, I realized that perception is a process, and that one's mind can mold reality, and that molding can create a logic paradox. Classical logic would offer a single method of knee instability assessment, but quantum logic dictates that every alternative method of assessment exists as a viable possibility. To force an examiner to use a single method of assessment is unacceptable; hence the proposed method is for documentation only and is not offered as a classification system and is not an attempt to restrict any method of assessment currently in use.

The IKDC method of documentation has been formated in a simple way. Since documentation is its purpose, and not assessment, it includes a minimum of examination tests thought to be relevant and relatively objective.

The components of this evaluation system include demographic information; patient knee category, sport, and activity assessment—level, intensity, and exposure. Symptoms and impairments are also assessed. The general examination, limits of motion examination, objective functional testing, knee compartment assessment, and instrumented limits of motion assessment and radiographic assessment complete the included categories.

The limits of motion assessment do not represent a compendium of tests but rather represent a minimum of acceptable tests. These tests were recommended by a consensus of the IKDC committee and are based on biomechanical studies, with each test theoretically representing a test for a single ligament as determined by biomechanical studies.

Functional testing of the patient preoperatively (when possible) and postoperatively was considered important, since the patient's functional assessment thus far has primarily been done by patient history. Obviously, these data may be adversely affected by the acute knee injury. Several additional issues were considered and excluded from the documentation form—radiographic assessment and special testing. Radiographic assessment of the tibiofemoral compartments in a weight-bearing status was thought to be important; however, the objectivity of minor radiographic changes was questioned. Special testing utilizing stress radiographic analysis, KT-1000 or equivalent, three-dimensional magnetic resonance imaging testing and gait analysis were considered but not felt to be a minimum requirement at this early stage.

After a limited trial of utilization of this documentation system by an IKDC subcommittee, several difficulties and omissions were realized. The minor difficulties primarily involved format, lack of familiarity with the descriptors utilized, and examiner time to completion. The elimination of certain variables thought to be important to other conditions affecting the knee were thought to be major deficiencies if a complete system of analysis is the goal. Also, conflicts in perceived reality were noted. Perhaps sharing some thoughts on this experience will explain these problems.

The proposed formats for the documentation data were as varied as the committee members themselves, and there are currently several formats available for data collection. These formats include a categorical assessment, visual analog method, numerical methods, and a computerized version developed by Roland Jakob. The final documentation format decided upon by consensus of the committee in 1991 is presented as contribution 21.3 in this volume.

The omission of certain examination variables thought to be important to a comprehensive knee assessment is in conflict with a holistic or quantum-logic concept, and this omission may have an undesirable effect on outcome comparisons. The largest omission is in the area of the decelerator/extensor mechanism. Also, many 'favorite' but 'qualitative' tests were omitted by the committee in the compromise necessary to develop an objective documentation form.

The issue of a quantitative versus a qualitative method has not been resolved entirely by changing terminology and changing the examination test sequence utilized. At question is whether the IKDC suggested tests can all be validated by an instrumented test method and whether these tests are more important than other examination tests available which offer important although 'qualitative' information. Also, the ability of all examiners to accurately estimate millimeters of displacement has not been consistently demonstrated; is this in fact better than the original 0, +1, +2, +3 method?

The issue of one ligament–one test proposed from biomechanical studies remains unproven in vivo by an examination–anatomic injury correlation, a fact which presents a major obstacle to universal acceptance. Certainly, one of the important objectives of any initial knee evaluation assessment is to arrive at a probability of anatomic injury at the conclusion of the clinical assessment. Whether this may be extrapolated and reproduced from the IKDC documentation tests has yet to be demonstrated in clinical practice. Since many blocking tests, coupled motions tests, and other favorite examination tests utilized to assess the acute knee injury are omitted, the ability of this documentation method of examination to allow each reader to classify the anatomical structures injured remains to be proved.

In spite of its limitations, the acknowledgment that an internationally accepted system of knee documentation is important and timely is a great step forward. However simplified the form may appear, it is a testimony to perseverance in the midst of many potentially conflicting and confounding issues. Since the data that each of us records are representative of our experience, and that experience is used in the daily treatment of patients, there is an advantage to documenting our patient assessments in as objective a way as possible, in order to more closely mimic the reality perceived by the patient. This objective documentation, it is hoped, will allow us to 'let all reasoning be silent when (documented) experience gainsays its conclusion' in our presentations and papers.

21.3   Knee ligament injury and reconstruction evaluation

The International Knee Documentation Committee*

The International Knee Documentation Committee is committed to a system of knee evaluation which will allow comparison of the results of knee ligament surgery. The Committee has met over the past four years and made substantial progress in the rudiments of such a system. What to include, what to leave out, what has been validated, what data are reproducible —these are key questions which have absorbed the energies of a very talented and experienced group of clinicians and scientists. Now is the time to place the preliminary work of this committee in the hands of all knee surgeons so that the data collection system may be further refined through usage. This will serve also to stimulate others to do better in collecting the data. What is presented now has the full confidence of the Committee, and has stood the test of discussion, debate, and usage. Preliminary data are by no means the end of the quest for a universal system, nor are they a completed outcome study; but this methodology, integrated into department's current data-collecting system, will serve it.

The crux of this data collection lies in the assessment of seven variables, each assigned one of four grades. The seven variables are:

Patient subjective assessment
Symptoms
Range of motion
Ligament examination
Compartment findings (crepitus)
Radiographic findings
Functional tests
The four grades are:
A: Normal
B: Nearly normal
C: Abnormal
D: Severely abnormal

For some users, seven variables will prove cumbersome; therefore, we have selected four of these variables as a Quick Knee Profile: patient subjective assessment, symptoms, range of motion, and ligament examination.

For other users, seven variables will prove too limiting. These users should understand that the Committee has considered many more variables but could not at this time establish validity or necessity for others.

These seven variables, each with four grades, serve as discriminators to separate patients and knees into groups that will stand the test of comparison. The Committee believes that this preliminary system will do this for knee surgery as it is today. Progress will require the system to become more sophisticated and more discriminating. It is felt that this rudimentary system is so fundamental that it will stand as a foundation to which more can be added as the need arises.

The Committee has resisted a 'pro-forma'. There are many pro-formas available. Some come close to the seven variables and four grades recommended by the Committee. To endorse one pro-forma would prove restrictive and this is not the Committee's intention. The simplification and computerization of data collection will be the next quest for all concerned, now that the minimal essential data have been identified.

Data evaluation imposes the need for arbitrary committee standards which may require amendment later but which, for now, seem to be a required discipline. The Committee recommends three guidelines:

- The postoperative patient will be graded at the highest activity level he has accomplished – i.e. Level I: jumping, pivoting, hard cutting (football, soccer); II: heavy manual work (skiing, tennis); III: light manual work (jogging, running); IV: sedentary work (ADL). Thus, symptoms and function will be linked to activity level.
- Each of the seven variables will be characterized by the lowest score awarded: normal, nearly normal, abnormal, severely abnormal.
- Short-term results are those followed for a minimum of 2 years; 5 years are required for intermediate-term results; and 10 years minimum for long-term results.

*American Orthopaedic Society for Sports Medicine:
A. Anderson, W. G. Clancy, D. Daniel, K. E. DeHaven, P. J. Fowler, J. Feagin, E. S. Grood, F. R. Noyes, G. C. Terry, P. Torzilli, R. F. Warren
European Society of Knee Surgery and Arthroscopy:
P. Chambat, E. Eriksson, J. Gillquist, F. Hefti, R. Huiskes, R. P. Jakob, B. Moyen, W. Mueller, H. Stäubli, A. Van Kampen

The knee ligament standard evaluation form

The Seven Groups	The Four Grades				Group Grade (see footnotes)

	A: normal	B: nearly normal	C: abnormal	D: sev. abnorm.	A B C D
1 Patient subjective assessment On a scale of 0 to 3 how did you rate your pre-injury activity level?	☐ 0	☐ 1	☐ 2	☐ 3	
On a scale of 0 to 3 how did you rate your current activity level?	☐ 0	☐ 1	☐ 2	☐ 3	
If your normal knee performs 100%, what percentage does your operated knee perform?	_____ %				☐☐☐☐

2 Symptoms	(Grade at highest activity level known by patient)				
	I Strenuous Activities	II Moderate Activities	III ADL/Light Activities	IV ADL Problems	
Pain	☐	☐	☐	☐	
Swelling	☐	☐	☐	☐	
Partial giving way	☐	☐	☐	☐	
Full giving way	☐	☐	☐	☐	☐☐☐☐

3 Range of motion	Flex/Ext: Index side: _/_/_ Opposite side: _/_/_				
Lack of extension (from zero degrees)	☐ <3°	☐ 3–5°	☐ 6–10°	☐ >10°	
△ Lack of flexion	☐ 0–5°	☐ 6–15°	☐ 16–25°	☐ >25°	☐☐☐☐

4 Ligament examination					
△ Lachman (25° flex) (manual, instrumented, x-ray)	☐ 1 to 2 mm	☐ 3 to 5 mm	☐ 6 to 10 mm	☐ >10 mm	
Endpoint: ☐ firm ☐ soft	☐ firm		☐ soft		
△ Total a.p. transl. (70° flex)	☐ 0 to 2 mm	☐ 3 to 5 mm	☐ 6 to 10 mm	☐ >10 mm	
△ Post. sag in 70° flex	☐ 0 to 2 mm	☐ 3 to 5 mm	☐ 6 to 10 mm	☐ >10 mm	
△ Med. joint opening (valgus rotation)	☐ 0 to 2 mm	☐ 3 to 5 mm	☐ 6 to 10 mm	☐ >10 mm	
△ Lat. joint opening (varus rotation)	☐ 0 to 2 mm	☐ 3 to 5 mm	☐ 6 to 10 mm	☐ >10 mm	
Pivot shift	☐ neg.	☐ + (glide)	☐ ++ (clunk)	☐ +++ (gross)	
Reversed pivot shift	☐ equal	☐ glide	☐ marked	☐ gross	☐☐☐☐

5 Compartmental findings					
Crepitus patellofemoral	☐ none		☐ moderate	☐ severe	
Crepitus medial compartment	☐ none		☐ moderate	☐ severe	
Crepitus lateral compartment	☐ none		☐ moderate	☐ severe (palpable & audible)	☐ ☐☐

6 X-ray findings					
Med. joint space narrowing	☐ none		☐ <50%	☐ >50%	
Lat. joint space narrowing	☐ none		☐ <50%	☐ >50%	
Patellofemoral joint space narrowing	☐ none		☐ <50%	☐ >50%	☐ ☐☐

7 Functional test					
△ One leg hop (% of opposite side)	☐ 100–90%	☐ 90–76%	☐ 75–50%	☐ <50%	☐☐☐☐

Final evaluation					☐☐☐☐

Footnotes:
- Group Grade: The lowest grade within a group determines the group grade.
- Final evaluation: The worst group determines the final evaluation.
- In a final evaluation all 7 groups are to be evaluated; for a quick knee profile the evaluation of groups 1–4 are sufficient.

21.4 The Hospital for Special Surgery knee ligament rating form

Thomas L. Wickiewicz

History

It has been the goal of many orthopedic surgeons who are involved in the treatment of knee ligament injuries to establish a standardized evaluation method for their patients. There are many reasons for the need for a standardized evaluation. Such evaluation forms allow the physician to follow specific anatomic lesions and their resultant functional deficits through the course of the prescribed treatment. Since numerous treatment options exist for each of these anatomic deficits, it is essential to have some uniform method for evaluation of the outcome and to allow meaningful comparison of treatments for the same injury. Such forms need to encompass subjective complaints of the individual and objective deficits and instabilities found in the injured knee and in some way to measure success or failure of the treatment modality.

In 1977, the first Hospital for Special Surgery knee ligament evaluation form was published.[1] It was meant to be a comprehensive, standardized evaluation form and was specifically designed for individuals who had suffered ligamentous injuries of the knee. Although it allowed for other problems, such as patellar dysfunction, to be recognized, its intent was not to be a standard measure of such problems but rather an indication for the treatment, both conservative and surgical, of the injured ligament. Its basis was a comprehensive knee discharge summary form. This was designed to mimic a complete medical examination. It was hoped that by using such a form not only would the efficacy of the treatment be revealed but also the natural history of the disease studied. The knee discharge summary was a multi-page form which recorded the specific mechanism of injury, both acute and chronic, including the sport or event in which the injury took place and initial forms of treatment, whether conservative or surgical. The form reviewed both subjective and objective complaints referable to the knee for activities of daily living, work, sports, general medical examination, ability to perform functional tests, overall knee alignment and physical examination of the involved and normal knee. In addition, measures of generalized ligamentous laxity and reviews of procedures, including plain radiographs, arthrography and knee arthroscopy, and examination under anesthesia, were included in this form. It also allowed for recording specific operative procedures performed as well as the postoperative course and a final diagnosis for the individual.

In conjunction with this comprehensive form, a knee score sheet was developed (Figure 1). This follow-up score sheet was an evaluation form that was specifically designed for the postoperative, postinjury evaluation of the patient's progress. It awarded 50 points to a normal knee. Forty percent of those points, or a total of 20, were assigned for objective stability measures of the knee. The remaining 30 points were distributed between subjective complaints, objective physical examination other than ligamentous stability, and functional testing. When it was developed, its specific intention was to review the natural history and response to treatment of the injured anterior cruciate ligament. As a result, one of the primary functional disabilities recorded in the form was a phenomenon known as 'giving way.' This is the specific sensation an individual has who suffers an instability episode due to the absence of the anterior cruciate ligament. The phenomenon is a momentary anterior translation of the tibia from under the femur in association with varying degrees of rotation. An important distinction needed to be made between a true giving-way episode and the sense of an individual experiencing anterior collapse or buckling, which can be caused by numerous other maladies of the knee. At the time of its development, the clinical tests of the Lachman maneuver and the pivot shift maneuver with its variations were not universally accepted or popular. As a result, the objective score for the anterior cruciate examination was left unspecified with regard to how the maneuver was performed. Five points were awarded to a normal knee, 4 points to a slight jog, 3 points to a moderate jog, 2 points when severe in neutral and 0 for severe in neutral and rotation. This latter category included any abnormal tests such as a pivot shift, a Slocum or a jerk test. In addition, a letter-designated category of either A or B for hard end point or soft no end point, respectively, was also included in the evaluation.

Figure 1

The 50-point knee score sheet first used at the Hospital for Special Surgery.

THE HOSPITAL FOR SPECIAL SURGERY KNEE LIGAMENT RATING FORM

NAME _____

DIAGNOSIS ACL   PCL   MM   LM   MCL   LCL   ACUTE   CHRONIC   AGE _____   SEX M   F
HSS # _____   PREVIOUS SURGERY _____

INJURY DATE _____   OPERATIVE DATE _____   TYPE _____

				LEFT						RIGHT			
	Score	pre	6mo	1yr	2yr	3yr	4yr	pre	6mo	1yr	2yr	3yr	4yr

SYMPTOMS (5)

SWELLING:
No 2
Yes 0

LOCKING:
No 3
Yes 0

GIVING WAY (20)
SEVERITY:
None 10
Transient 8
Recovery < 1 day 6
Recovery < 1 week 2
Recovery > 1 week 0
FREQUENCY:
None 10
1 per year 8
2-6 per year 6
1 per month 4
1 per week 2
Daily 0

FUNCTION (20)
ADL AND WORK:
Full return 4
Limited or job change 2
Unable due to knee 0
SPORTS:
Full return 4
Same but modified 3
Different sport 2
No return 0
ABILITY TO:
Decelerate 4
Cut side-to-side 4
Jump 4

EXAMINATION (45)
ROM:
Normal 3
Limited flexion or extension 1
Both 0
EFFUSION:
No 4
Yes 0
THIGH CIRCUMFERENCE:
Equal to 1cm difference 2
> 1cm difference 0
LACHMAN: (note end point)
Negative 4
1+ (0-5mm) 3
2+ (5-10mm) 2
3+ (10-15mm) 0

EXAMINATION (45)

	Score	pre	6mo		LEFT					RIGHT			
				1yr	2yr	3yr	4yr	pre	6mo	1yr	2yr	3yr	4yr

ANTERIOR DRAWER:
Negative 2
1+ (0-5mm) 2
2+ (5-10mm) 0
3+ (10-15mm) 0
POSTERIOR DRAWER:
Negative 5
1+ (0-5mm) 3
2+ (5-10mm) 2
3+ (10-15mm) 0
PIVOT SHIFT:
Negative (or equal to
  unaffected side) 10
Grind, no movement 8
1+, slight movement 4
2+, definite movement 2
3+, movement and locks 0
MCL:
Normal 5
1+ 3
2+ 2
3+ 0
LCL:
Normal 5
1+ 3
2+ 2
3+ 0
REVERSE PIVOT SHIFT:
Negative 5
Positive 0

FUNCTIONAL EXAM (10)
STANDING FORWARD JUMP %
DIFFERENCE BETWEEN LEGS:
90-100% 10
75-90% 7
50-75% 5
50% 0

SCORE: _____

DEDUCTIONS
DEROTATION BRACE:
Security of mind 2
Due to instability 4
PAIN: (if PCL, X3)
None 0
Occasional Aching 2
After stressful sports 5
After daily activities 8
Continuous 10

TOTAL SCORE: _____

SPORTS CATEGORIES (A = Very Stressful, B = Moderately Stressful, C = Mildly Stressful)

A	B	C
Basketball	Professional Dance	X-Country Skiing
Volleyball	Football	Jogging
Gymnastics	Rugby	Tennis (doubles)
Soccer	Racquetball	Swimming
	Squash	Bicycling
	Handball	Fencing
	Tennis (singles)	Boxing
	Downhill Skiing	Golf

Figure 2

The modified 100-point Hospital for Special Surgery knee score sheet.

The form proved to be a reliable tool in the follow-up evaluation of knee ligament surgery. Four categories of subjective success were established: good to excellent (41–50 points), fair(+) (36–40 points), fair(–) (31–35 points), and poor (less than 30 points). Using this form, a population of 233 patients with injuries to their anterior cruciate ligament was studied.[1] The patients were divided into those treated conservatively, those undergoing primary repair of the anterior cruciate and those undergoing late intra-articular reconstruction. The score system was found to be sensitive to differences between these three groups. Of conservatively treated individuals, those with isolated anterior cruciate injuries were seen to have a score of 30 beyond 2 years postinjury and those with combination injuries to have a score of 28 at a similar reference time. In contrast, those undergoing primary repair showed a score of 40, which remained stable beyond 3 years from surgery, and those with late reconstruction were able to change their preoperative score, which averaged 30, to a level of 40 at the 3-year postsurgery mark for isolated anterior cruciate ligament reconstruction and to 36 for those with mixed lesions.

Current Hospital for Special Surgery rating form

In 1982, a revised score sheet was developed for use by the Sports Medicine and Knee services at the Hospital for Special Surgery.[2] This form was a composite of subjective, objective and functional findings. It had a maximum score of 100 points for a normal knee (Figure 2). At the time of its inception, the impression was that the majority of knee ligament injuries included the anterior cruciate, the medial collateral ligament, or a combination thereof. As a result, the evaluation form was developed predominantly to test the anterior cruciate-deficient knee. It was recognized, however, that the form needed to be sensitive enough to detect other knee ligament instabilities and their resultant deficit.

In the revised score system, an excellent scoring or normal knee would have a total score between 90 and 100 points. The good category corresponded to 80–89 points, fair to 70–79 points, and a poor score to less than 70 points.

The form was designed to be kept in the patient's chart and set up in such a way so as to allow easy recording of follow-up scores on the same sheet so that ready comparison could be made to the individual's prior level of function and also to allow ready comparison to the contralateral limb. The top of the form included demographic data; the individual's primary diagnosis; whether the injury, when first evaluated at the Hospital for Special Surgery, was an acute or chronic problem; a listing of any previous surgery to the limb; the date of the index injury to the involved knee; the date of surgery and the type of operative procedure that was performed.

Subjectively, the individual can complain of phenomena of swelling, locking, instability and pain. In the Hospital for Special Surgery system, a total of 5 points is awarded for absence of the symptoms of swelling and locking. In a knee that is suffering from anterior cruciate insufficiency, it is uncommon for swelling to be a predominant feature unless the individual has had a recent episode of instability. Swelling on a more chronic basis usually reflects some other form of intra-articular pathology – meniscal degeneration, articular cartilage wear, or presence of loose bodies. Similarly, locking is a phenomenon that usually indicates either the meniscus or a loose body as its cause. Although any of the combinations of the above are commonly seen in association with an anterior cruciate-deficient knee, it was the intent of the form to record the primary disability due to the absence of the anterior cruciate, and so only 5 points were awarded to these categories. Similarly, the phenomenon of pain is uncommon unless an individual has had an episode of recent instability or there are associated problems. As a result, pain is used in the rating system as a deduction. No positive points are awarded for the absence of pain; rather, when the form has been completed, an individual can have a deduction of up to 10 points for the presence of pain, depending on its frequency and whether it is associated with activities of daily living or occurs only after stressful sports activities.

When this form was revised, however, it was recognized that individuals who suffer from posterior cruciate ligament insufficiency very often have a different clinical course and pattern from those who suffer from anterior cruciate ligament problems. Whereas a person with an anterior cruciate insufficient knee complains of episodic instability, one with a posterior cruciate abnormality rarely reports instability. Rather, these individuals complain primarily of pain, emanating either from the patellofemoral joint or from the medial compartment of the knee. As this pain becomes the hallmark of the disability in a person with posterior cruciate insufficiency, the 100-point rating score was made sensitive to this by trebling the deduction for complaints of pain. Thus an individual who had constant pain in his knee and suffered from posterior cruciate insufficiency would have a total deduction of 30 points from the total score.

Since the hallmark of anterior cruciate insufficiency is an unpredictable instability in the knee, heavy weighting was given to this in the development of the form. A total of 20 points is allocated to the phenomenon of giving way. It was felt that giving way could vary not only in frequency but also in severity. The severity of the event is best reflected by how long it takes the individual to recover from such an event. Thus, if the individual has an episode of instability in which he senses the knee sliding in and out of position, but there is no residual symptom as a result of this (that is, he has no swelling and no subsequent pain and he can return fully to his activities), the full 10 points are awarded under the category of severity and the deduction is based on the frequency with which this phenomenon takes place.

A total of 20 points was allocated to the category of function. This included the ability of the individual to function in activities of daily living, in a job and also participating in sports. Sixteen of 20 points are aimed at evaluating the individual's ability to participate in sports. The majority of the points were awarded to specific maneuvers that are known to stress the knee with anterior cruciate insufficiency. Specifically, these are the ability to decelerate rapidly, an activity that maximizes quadriceps firing and anterior translation of the tibia; the ability to rapidly change direction, as in a side-to-side cut; and the ability to jump and come down on a straight leg. An attempt at a careful assessment of the individual's return to sports function is also made by deciding whether the individual has had to change the preferred sport or is still able to participate in the pre-injury sport but in some way has modified participation – for example a change in position or a change in frequency of playing or a subjective sense of change in intensity of participation.

A total of 45 points is allocated for objective examination of the knee. With regard to range of motion, loss of either flexion or extension causes deductions from the score, but no delineation is made with regard to the amount of range of motion loss; simply, the basis for this decision is whether or not deficits exist compared to the uninvolved knee. The presence or absence of an effusion is noted and deductions are made accordingly. Persistent thigh atrophy causes a deduction. Objective measures of ligament stability are rated on 1–3 basis with 1+ for excursion between 0 and 5 mm greater than that which is seen in the uninvolved knee, 2+ for 5–10 mm and 3+ for 10–15 mm. Thus a negative Lachman would reflect a knee that has the same excursion in millimeters when performed at 30° of flexion as does the uninvolved leg. In addition, on the Lachman maneuver, the absence or presence of an end point is noted but points are not awarded or deducted for either.

In the original 50-point knee score sheet, the anterior drawer sign was the primary measure for the anterior cruciate ligament. At the time of the development of the newer score sheet, less importance was put on the anterior drawer examination. Even under anesthesia, the anterior drawer is often difficult to interpret and the feeling developed that its sensitivity with regard to anterior cruciate function was more suspect. Greater reliance was placed on the Lachman test performed at 30°, which was generally accepted to be the most sensitive position of testing for trans-

lation due to anterior cruciate absence. On both the anterior drawer test and the posterior drawer test, the performance is neutral in rotation.

The pivot shift maneuver is awarded 10 points. A normal knee is one with a negative shift or one that exhibited what was felt to be a physiologic shift. Certain knees, because of their inherent ligamentous laxity, will demonstrate a suggestion of slight slide taking place, which for that individual is normal. This obviously becomes somewhat subjective on the part of the examiner and careful examination with regard to both the normal and involved knees is required. If there is felt to be slight movement, it is rated as 1+; a definitive jump is 2+ and a sense of locking out of position a 3+. In general, insufficiency of the anterior cruciate has been associated with a 2+ and 3+ level of pivot shift maneuver. Those that exhibit a 1+ or slight movement usually examine in a fashion such that there is increased translation on a Lachman maneuver but characteristically have a firm end point. In general, 1+ pivot shifts are usually not correlated with clinical instability.

The category of grind, no movement, often reflects abnormalities of articular cartilage or abnormalities of the lateral meniscus due to compression in the lateral compartment. These are very often present in the knee which has undergone successful reconstruction but had either a very severe pivot shift at the time of the acute injury or repeated episodes of instability when in a chronic setting. Two points are deducted for such a phenomenon.

The presence or absence of a reverse pivot shift is noted. Upon performing a reverse pivot shift maneuver, the examiner must be very attuned to the motion of the tibial plateau relative to the femoral condyle. In a reverse pivot shift, the tibial plateau is subluxed posteriorly relative to the lateral femoral condyle in positions of flexion and, as the knee is brought to an extended position, will jump and reduce under the lateral tibial plateau. This needs to be differentiated from a pivot shift maneuver in which in flexion the tibial plateau is reduced under the lateral femoral condyle and with extension subluxes anteriorly from under the femoral condyle. Individuals may exhibit differences in the degree of pivot shift when the knee is internally or externally rotated. Although this internal and external rotation may, to some degree, accentuate the presence or absence of a pivot shift, the direction of motion of the tibial plateau is still anterior with respect to the femoral condyle and this must be differentiated from the reverse pivot shift in which its direction is posterior.

The final 10 points of the evaluation are on a functional examination. It was felt that a one-legged standing forward broad jump is the best simple measure to test the individual's ability and subjective confidence in the knee with an absent cruciate ligament. The distance jumped with the affected leg becomes the numerator, that with the unaffected leg the denominator, and the percentage dictates the score for that category. The final deduction was for use of a brace. Two points are deducted for the subjective sense of stability afforded by the brace to prevent episodes of instability. Finally, an assessment of the individual's sports categories is recorded with the various sports divided into those that are very stressful for a cruciate-deficient knee, moderately stressful, or only mildly stressful for such an abnormality. There is no point score for this category.

With use of the 100-point knee score sheet, a group of 60 individuals who underwent reconstruction of their anterior cruciate ligament averaged a postoperative score of 88 points.[2] This same group averaged 55 points preoperatively. This score sheet has been shown to be a sensitive measure for functional outcome following treatment for anterior cruciate ligament injuries.

The value of a knee score system depends on recognition of its strengths and weaknesses and the appropriateness of its application. The intention behind the Hospital for Special Surgery's 100-point knee score sheet is evaluation in injury and treatment to one or more of the ligament structures of the knee joint. The score sheet incorporates the commonly accepted tests that reflect the function of a cruciate-deficient knee. Its format has been designed to make it easy to use in the setting of a busy clinical practice. Since its development, greater reliance has been placed on objective measures using instrumented knee testing devices such as KT1000 or Genucom.

The fact that this particular score system does not reflect those measures does not detract from its value. Such objective measures can be used in conjunction with the knee score sheet and objective measures obtained using the KT1000 and Genucom can be used to decide the appropriate category of score for the respective ligament on the knee score sheet.

Potential shortcomings of the form are: (1) inadequate measure of rotational assessments of the knee; (2) the development of arthrofibrosis in a postsurgical knee, with its severe consequences, and yet an artificially high score because few points are deducted for range of motion loss and the fact that the person may function at a high level despite the contracture; (3) the fact that the development of degenerative joint disease in a stoical patient may result in a knee that has an artificially high score. These pitfalls are offset by the proven reliability of this particular score sheet when applied to specific ligamentous problems of the knee and by the ease of use of this particular system.

References

1. **Marshall JL, Fetto JF, Botero PM**, Knee ligament injuries: a standardized evaluation method, *Clin Orthop* (1977) **123:** 115–129.
2. **Windsor RE, Insall JN, Wickiewicz TL et al.**, The Hospital for Special Surgery knee ligament rating form, *Am J Knee Surg* (1988) **1:** 140–145.

21.5 Rating tables

Table 1 Lysholm-I score

Limp (5 points)
None	5
Slight or periodical	3
Severe and constant	0

Support (5 points)
Full support	5
Stick or crutch	3
Weight bearing impossible	0

Stairclimbing (10 points)
No problems	10
Slightly impaired	6
One step at a time	2
Unable	0

Squatting (5 points)
No problems	5
Slightly impaired	4
Not past 90°	2
Unable	0

Walking, running and jumping (70 points)

A. Instability
Never giving way	30
Rarely during athletic or other severe exertion	25
Frequently during athletic or other severe exertion (or unable to participate)	20
Occasionally in daily activities	10
Often in daily activities	5
Every step	0

B. Pain
None	30
Inconstant and slight during severe exertion	25
Marked on giving way	20
Marked during severe exertion	15
Marked on or after walking more than 2 km	10
Marked on or after walking less than 2 km	5
Constant and severe	0

C. Swelling
None	10
With giving way	7
On severe exertion	5
On ordinary exertion	2
Constant	0

Atrophy of thigh (5 points)
None	5
1–2 cm	3
More than 2 cm	0

After ref. 1.

Table 2 Lysholm-II score

Limp
None	5
Slight or periodic	3
Severe and constant	0

Support
None	5
Stick or crutch needed	2
Weight bearing impossible	0

Locking
None	15
Catching sensation, but no locking	10
Locking occasionally	6
Locking frequently	2
Locked joint at examination	0

Instability
Never	25
Rarely during athletic activities	20
Frequently during athletic activities	15
Occasionally during daily activities	10
Often during daily activities	5
Every step	0

Pain
None	25
Inconstant and slight during strenuous activities	20
Marked during or after walking more than 2 km	10
Marked during or after walking less than 2 km	5
Constant	0

Swelling
None	10
After strenuous activities	6
After ordinary activities	3
Constant	0

Stairs
No problem	10
Slight problem	6
One step at a time	3
Impossible	0

Squatting
No problem	5
Slight problem	4
Not beyond 90° of flexion of the knee	2
Impossible	0

Table 3 The Tegner activity scale

10 Competitive sports
        Soccer – national or international level
 9 Competitive sports
        Soccer – lower divisions
        Ice hockey
        Wrestling
        Gymnastics
 8 Competitive sports
        Bandy
        Squash or badminton
        Athletics (jumping, etc.)
        Downhill skiing
 7 Competitive sports
        Tennis
        Athletics (running)
        Motocross or speedway
        Handball or basketball
    Recreational sports
        Soccer
        Bandy or ice hockey
        Squash
        Athletics (jumping)
        Cross-country track finding (orienteering) both
            recreational and competitive
 6 Recreational sports
        Tennis or badminton
        Handball or basketball
        Downhill skiing
        Jogging, at least 5 times weekly
 5 Work
        Heavy labour (e.g. construction, forestry)
    Competitive sports
        Cycling
        Cross-country skiing
    Recreational sports
        Jogging on uneven ground at least twice weekly
 4 Work
        Moderately heavy work (e.g. truck driving, scrubbing
            floors)
    Recreational sports
        Cycling
        Cross-country skiing
        Jogging on even ground at least twice weekly
 3 Work
        Light work (e.g. nursing)
    Competitive and recreational sports
        Swimming
    Walking in rough forest terrain
 2 Work
        Light work
    Walking on uneven ground
 1 Work
        Sedentary work
    Walking on even ground
 0 Sick leave or disability pension because of knee problems

After ref. 2.

Table 4 Anterior cruciate ligament follow-up form – side 1

To be filled out by patient

PLEASE PRINT   Date _____

IDENTIFICATION

Name _____ SS # _____ OFF # _____
     (LAST)   (FIRST)   (INITIAL)

Age _____ Sex ☐ M ☐ F Knee involved ☐ Right ☐ Left

Phone _____ Phone # and name of ⎫ Name: _____
     (AREA CODE)   someone who can reach ⎬ Phone: _____

Sport causing injury _____ you if you have moved ⎭   (AREA CODE)

Date of Surgery _____ Number of months since surgery: 6 12 18 24 36
     (MO)   (DATE)   (YEAR)   (CIRCLE ONE)

POST-OP COURSE

Cast? # weeks in rigid cast _____ # weeks in flexible/hinged cast _____

Brace? ☐ Yes ☐ No **Current Brace Use?** ☐ All the Time ☐ Sports Only ☐ No Longer used

Physical Therapy? # months in supervised program (Cybex Orthotron etc.) _____

           Are you still doing a regular home program ☐ Yes ☐ No

SYMPTOMS

Knee Pain? ④ None ③ Mild ② Moderate (with activity)   Score

         ① Severe (at rest & preventing activity)   _____

Giving Way? ⑧ None ⑥ Only with Cutting (stop & turn) Sports

         ④ Occasional (only with awkward step) ③ With Normal Daily Activities _____

Swelling? ④ None ③ Strenuous Activity ② With Moderate Activity

         ① With Any Activity   _____

Stiffness? ④ None ② Occasional ① Frequent   _____

                                                [_____]

('x' in appropriate box)   Symptom Summary = Total/4

FUNCTION

Activity Level? ① No sports   ③ Active, but different sports [_____]

         ② Sports activities significantly limited ④ Same sports, but lower performance level Function summary
                                                         (Activity level)

Problems with Specific Activities? ③ Equal performance at same sports as

('X' in appropriate box)   before injury

	NONE	MILD	MODERATE	CAN'T DO
Walking	☐	☐	☐	☐
Running	☐	☐	☐	☐
Turn/Cut	☐	☐	☐	☐
Jumping	☐	☐	☐	☐
Stairs	☐	☐	☐	☐

If your prior injury activity level rates at 10, what does your current activity level rate? _____

If your normal knee performs 100%, at what % does your operated knee perform? _____

After ref. 3.

Table 5 Anterior cruciate ligament follow-up form – side 2

To be filled out by physician

SURGICAL H$_x$

Type ACL Injury: ☐Acute (<1 wk) ☐Sub Acute (1–6 wks) ☐Chronic (>6 wks) ☐Acute on Chronic

Associated Injury (acute or chronic): ☐MCL ☐PCL ☐LCL ☐Med Men ☐Lat Men

ACL Surgery: ☐No Repair ☐Primary Repair Aug with _____
☐Primary Repair without Augmentation ☐Reconstruction with _____

Subsequent Injury: ☐None ☐Medial Meniscus ☐Lateral Meniscus
☐ACL ☐MCL ☐LCL ☐PCL

Subsequent Surgery: ☐None ☐Hardware removal ☐MUA ☐Meniscectomy ☐Ligament repair

STABILITY

R   Ant Draw/Lachmans   L

_____ 15° _____

_____ 90° _____

Sublux (Pivot Shift, Jerk, etc.)

_____   _____

record as 0 tr 1⁺ 2⁺ 3⁺

Varus   Valgus   Varus
_____   _____ 0° _____   _____
_____   _____ 30° _____   _____

ROM
−10°
R   0°
140°   45°
90°

−10°
0°   L
45°   140°
90°

ADDITIONAL STUDIES

X-ray:	NONE	MILD	MOD	SEVERE
Med joint DJD	☐	☐	☐	☐
Lat joint DJD	☐	☐	☐	☐
P/F joint DJD	☐	☐	☐	☐
ICN osteophytes	☐	☐	☐	☐

Other (your favorite test):

Cybex/Orthotron
(if available)

Strength _____   Power _____
R rate L   R rate L

Q   Q

H   H

Thigh Circ   R _____   L _____
(10cm ↑ patella)

CAPSULE SUMMARY*

Symptoms _____   Function _____   Stability _____

1) The **Symptom** score is the total score/4 of the entire symptom section
2) The **Function** score is the score of the activity level question only
3) The **Stability** score comes from only the Ant Draw/Lach/Sublux portion of the P.E. as follows: 5 = none of the 3 tests>trace; 4 = none of the 3 tests > 1⁺; 3 = two tests 1⁺ one test 2⁺; 2 = two tests 2⁺ one test 1⁺; 1 = all tests ⩾2⁺.

*The Capsule Summary is intended to give a brief picture of the patient NOT summarize all of the above data.

After ref. 3.

Table 6 Cincinnati Knee Rating System: symptom rating scale[a]

Normal knee; able to do strenuous work/sports with jumping, hard pivoting	10
Able to do moderate work/sports with running, turning, twisting; symptoms with strenuous work/sports	8
Able to do light work/sports with no running, twisting, jumping; symptoms with moderate work/sports	6
Able to do activities of daily living alone; symptoms with light work/sports	4
Moderate symptoms (frequent, limiting) with activities of daily living	2
Severe symptoms (constant, not relieved) with activities of daily living	0

[a]The symptoms that are rated are pain, swelling, partial giving way, and full giving way.
After ref. 4.

Table 7 Cincinnati Knee Rating System: sports activities rating scale

Level I (participates 4–7 days per week)	
Jumping, hard pivoting, cutting (basketball, volleyball, football, gymnastics, soccer)	100
Running, twisting, turning (tennis, racquetball, handball, baseball, ice hockey, field hockey, skiing, wrestling)	95
No running, twisting, jumping (cycling, swimming)	90
Level II (participates 1–3 days per week)	
Jumping, hard pivoting, cutting (basketball, volleyball, football, gymnastics, soccer)	85
Running, twisting, turning (tennis, racquetball, handball, baseball, ice hockey, field hockey, skiing, wrestling)	80
No running, twisting, jumping (cycling, swimming)	75
Level III (participates 1–3 times per month)	
Jumping, hard pivoting, cutting (basketball, volleyball, football, gymnastics, soccer)	65
Running, twisting, turning (tennis, racquetball, handball, baseball, ice hockey, field hockey, skiing, wrestling)	60
No running, twisting, jumping (cycling, swimming)	55
Level IV (no sports)	
Performs activities of daily living without problems	40
Has moderate problems with activities of daily living	20
Has severe problems with activities of daily living – on crutches, full disability	0

After ref. 4.

Table 8 Cincinnati Knee Rating System: assessment of function

Activities of daily living	
Walking	
Normal, unlimited	40
Some limitations	30
Only 3–4 blocks possible	20
Less than 1 block, cane, crutch	0
Stair-climbing	
Normal, unlimited	40
Some limitations	30
Only 11–30 steps possible	20
Only 1–10 steps possible	0
Squatting/kneeling	
Normal, unlimited	40
Some limitations	30
Only 6–10 possible	20
Only 0–5 possible	0
Sports	
Straight running	
Fully competitive	100
Some limitations, guarding	80
Run half-speed, definite limitations	60
Not able to do	40
Jumping/landing on affected leg	
Fully competitive	100
Some limitations, guarding	80
Definite limitations, half-speed	60
Not able to do	40
Hard twisting/cutting/pivoting	
Fully competitive	100
Some limitations, guarding	80
Definite limitations, half-speed	60
Not able to do	40

After ref. 4.

Table 9 Cincinnati Knee Rating System: scheme for final rating[a]

	Excellent	Good	Fair	Poor
Pain	10	8	6–4	2–0
Swelling	10	8	6–4	2–0
Partial giving way	10	8	6–4	2–0
Full giving way	10	8	6–4	2–0
Walking	40	30	20	0
Stairs ⎱ (score lowest) Squatting ⎰	40	30	20	0
Running	100	80	60	40
Jumping	100	80	60	40
Hard twists, cuts, pivots	100	80	60	40
Effusion (ml)	Normal	<25	26–60	>60
Lack of flexion (degrees)	0–5	6–15	16–30	>30
Lack of extension (degrees)	0–3	4–5	6–10	>10
Tibiofemoral crepitus[b]	Normal		Moderate	Severe
Patellofemoral crepitus[b]	Normal		Moderate	Severe
Anterior displacement (KT1000)	<3 mm	3–5 mm	6 mm	>6 mm
Pivot-shift test	Negative	Slip	Definite	Severe
Joint-space narrowing				
Medial tibiofemoral (radiographs)[c]	Normal	Mild	Moderate	Severe
Lateral tibiofemoral (radiographs)[c]	Normal	Mild	Moderate	Severe
Patellofemoral (radiographs)[c]	Normal	Mild	Moderate	Severe
Functional testing (limb symmetry) (%)[d]	100–85	84–75	74–65	<65

[a]Rating for pain, swelling, partial giving way, and full giving way – see Table 6. Rating for walking, stairs, squatting, running, jumping, hard twists, cuts, and pivots – see Table 8.
[b]Moderate indicates definite fibrillation and cartilage abnormality of 25–50°; severe indicates cartilage abnormality of more than 50°.
[c]Moderate indicates narrowing of less than one-half of the joint space; severe indicates of more than one-half of the joint space.
[d]Use average of at least three one-legged hop-type tests.
After ref. 4.

References

1. Lysholm J, Gillquist J, Evaluation of knee ligament surgery results with special emphasis on use of a scoring scale, *Am J Sports Med* (1982) **10:** 150–154.
2. Tegner Y, Lysholm J, Rating system in the evaluation of knee ligament injuries, *Clin Orthop* (1985) **198:** 43–49.
3. Feagin JA Jr, Blake WP, Postoperative evaluation and result recording in the anterior cruciate ligament reconstructed knee, *Clin Orthop* (1983) **172:** 143–147.
4. Noyes FR, Barber SD, Mangine RE, Bone–patellar ligament–bone and fascia lata allografts for reconstruction of the anterior cruciate ligament, *J Bone Joint Surg (Am)* (1990) **72:** 1125–1136.

21.6 IDES/SICOT Knee Documentation/Evaluation Subcommittee draft assessment form

Form A: clinical evaluation

Primary visit	
Follow-up visit	
Right knee	
Left knee	

Name	First name	Language
Country code	Postal/zip code	City
Street	Telephone	Patient number
Occupation	Height (cm)	Weight (kg)	Date of birth (day/month/year)
Admission	Discharge	Date of surgery

Diagnosis

1. OA 2. RA 3. Post-fracture 4. Osteonecrosis 5. Failed Arthroplasty 6. Miscellaneous

Subgroups

1. Primary OA 2. Secondary OA 3. Infection 4. Post-juvenile RA 5. Malalignment 6. Crystal arthropathy 7. Neuropathic 8. Miscellaneous

Previous surgery/injury

1. None 2. Intra-articular steroids 3. Intra-articular fracture 4. Femoral osteotomy 5. Tibial osteotomy 6. Patellectomy 7. Uni-arthroplasty 8. Total knee replacement

	OPEN	ARTHROSCOPIC
9. Meniscus surgery		
10. Ligament surgery		
11. Synovectomy		
12. Debridement		
13. Osteochondral surgery		
14. Patellar realignment		
15. Other		

SEPSIS 1. Yes 2. No

Time after operation 1. 0–12 mths 2. 1–2 years 3. 2–5 years 4. 5+ years

Discharge/drainage 1. Yes 2. No
Sinus 1. Yes 2. No
Fistula 1. Yes 2. No
Organisms 1. Gram +ve 2. Gram −ve 3. Other

General locomotor

Is the patient's disability due to the affected knee?
1. Scarcely 2. Partially 3. Mainly 4. Entirely

State of other joints

	Normal	Slightly affected	Moderately affected	Severely affected	Arthrodesed	Replaced	Other
Other knee							
Ipsilateral hip							
Contralateral hip							
Ipsilateral foot/ankle							
Contralateral foot/ankle							

Other pertinent disabilities

1. Multiple arthritis 2. General mechanical 3. Neurological 4. Vascular 5. Death – related to knee treatment 6. Death – unrelated to knee treatment

Pain

Definition: Minor = not interfering with activities nor sleep. No analgesia.
Moderate = activities reduced or sleep disturbed. Analgesia taken.

	None	Minor	Moderate	Severe
At rest				
On movement				
On weight bearing				
On climbing stairs				

Visual analogue scale: see Appendix 2

Medication for knee

1. None 2. Simple analgesics 3. Prescription analgesics 4. Systemic steroids 4. NSAID

Walking aids

1. None 2. Cane/stick outdoors 3. Cane/stick always 4. Two canes/crutches or walking frame 5. Unable to walk

Walking distance – with or without support

1. Unlimited = >60 min 2. Up to 1 km = up to 30 min 3. Up to 500 m = up to 15 min 4. 50–100 m outdoors = up to 5 min 5. Indoors only

Ability to use stairs

	Normal reciprocal	Use bannister	One step at a time	Unable or bizarre method
Ascend				
Descend				

Arising from chair

1. Normal 2. With difficulty 3. Only with use of arms
4. Unable or with help

Stability – subjective

	Gives way or buckles	Falls
Never		
Occasional		
Frequent		

Activity/employment

1. Bedridden/wheelchair
2. Sedentary – desk job or equivalent
3. Light activity – housekeeping, gardening, yard work
4. Moderate activity – moderate manual work, light sports
5. Heavy activity – heavy manual work, major sports

Visual analogue scale: see Appendix 2

Patient satisfaction

1. Enthusiastic 2. Satisfied 3. Has reservations 4. Disappointed
Visual analogue scale: see Appendix 2

Comparison with last visit

1. Better 2. Same 3. Worse

Examination – physical signs

Gait

1. Normal 2. Limited swing – antalgic limp 3. Stiff knee gait 4. Thrust/instability gait

Standing alignment

Ipsilateral

1. Neutral 2. Varus 3. Valgus 4. Flexion contracture 5. Recurvatum

Contralateral

1. Neutral 2. Varus 3. Valgus 4. Flexion contracture 5. Recurvatum

Skin state

1. Normal 2. Abnormal 3. Sinus 4. Fistula

Effusion

1. Absent 2. Present

Patellar alignment

1. Neutral 2. Subluxed 3. Dislocated 4. Absent

Range of motion – record maximum degrees

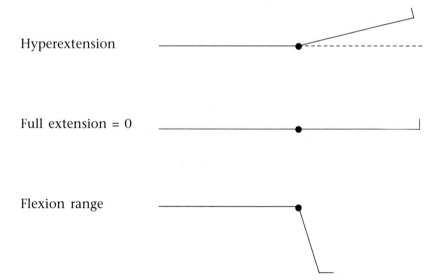

Hyperextension

Full extension = 0

Flexion range

Tick 2 in each line unless ankylosed when 'stiff knee' box to be ticked:

Left knee

Stiff knee ☐

Passive
+16 15–11 10–6 5–1 ☐0☐ 1–5 6–10 11–20 21–30 31–50 51–70 71–85 86–95 96–105 106–115 116–125 126–135 135+

  Hyperextension →   ← Flexion →

Active
+16 15–11 10–6 5–1 ☐0☐ 1–5 6–10 11–20 21–30 31–50 51–70 71–85 86–95 96–105 106–115 116–125 126–135 135+

Right knee

Stiff knee ☐

Passive
+16 15–11 10–6 5–1 ☐0☐ 1–5 6–10 11–20 21–30 31–50 51–70 71–85 86–95 96–105 106–115 116–125 126–135 135+

  Hyperextension →   ← Flexion →

Active
+16 15–11 10–6 5–1 ☐0☐ 1–5 6–10 11–20 21–30 31–50 51–70 71–85 86–95 96–105 106–115 116–125 126–135 135+

Valgus/varus laxity

Left knee

Strained valgus →   ← Strained varus →
41+ 40–21 20–16 15–11 10–6 5–1 0–5 6–10 11–20 21–40 41+

Resting position
41+ 40–21 20–16 15–11 10–6 5–1 0–5 6–10 11–20 21–40 41+

Right knee

Strained valgus →   ← Strained varus →
41+ 40–21 20–16 15–11 10–6 5–1 0–5 6–10 11–20 21–40 41+

Resting position
41+ 40–21 20–16 15–11 10–6 5–1 0–5 6–10 11–20 21–40 41+

AP laxity – gross assessment

Left knee

Total anterior/posterior	Grade	0	1	2	3
translation at 70°:	Excursion (mm)	0–5	6–10	11–15	15+

Right knee

Total anterior/posterior	Grade	0	1	2	3
translation at 70°:	Excursion (mm)	0–5	6–10	11–15	15+

Form B: Operation; in-patient course; complications

Operation

Primary		Date		Right knee	
Revision		Date		Left knee	

Name   First name   Language

Country code   Postal/zip code   City

Street   Telephone   Patient number

Occupation   Height   Weight   Date of birth
                        (cm)   (kg)   (day/month/year)

Admission   Discharge

Technique

1. Arthroscopic debridement 2. Osteotomy 3. Uni-replacement 4. Total replacement 5. Arthrodesis 6. Prosthesis removal for infection 7. Immediate exchange – mechanical 8. Immediate exchange – sepsis 9. Delayed exchange

Osteotomy

1. Tibial 2. Femoral 3. Valgus 4. Varus 5. Flexion 6. Extension

Arthrodesis

1. Primary 2. For salvage – loosening 3. For salvage – infection

Unicompartmental

1. Medial 2. Lateral 3. Patellofemoral

Total replacement

1. Primary 2. Revision for salvage – loosening 3. Revision for salvage – infection

Previous scar

1. Nil 2. Vertical mid-line 3. Parapatellar medial 4. Parapatellar lateral 5. Transverse 6. Other

Skin incision

1. Vertical mid-line 2. Parapatellar medial 3. Parapatellar lateral 4. Transverse 5. Other

Capsulotomy

1. Medial 2. Lateral 3. Trans tubercle osteotomy

Soft-tissue release (– for alignment)

1. Medial 2. Lateral 3. Posterior

State of extensor apparatus

1. Intact 2. Deficient – soft tissue 3. Deficient bone or fractured patella

Bacteriology

1. Negative culture 2. Gram +ve 3. Gram −ve 4. Other

Ligament condition

	Functional	Deficient/incompetent	Contracted
Ant. cruciate			
Post. cruciate			
Med. collat.			
Lat. collat.			

Cruciate spared – anterior—posterior
Cruciate divided – anterior—posterior

Synovium

1. Normal 2. Hypertrophic 3. Fibrotic 4. Metallosis

Synovectomy

1. Near complete 2. Partial 3. Nil

Joint surfaces

		Bone loss	Bone exposed	Widespread fibrillation	Local fibrillation	Soft	Normal
Medial:	Femoral						
	Tibial						
Lateral:	Femoral						
	Tibial						
Patellar							
Trochlear femoral							

If previous prosthetic replacement – state

	Patella	Femoral	Tibial
Migration			
Loosening			
Fracture			
Wear			

New prostheses insertion

	Tibia	Femur	Patella
Cemented			
Porous			
HAC			
Press fit			
Other			

1. Linked   Fully constrained = hinge
                Rotary hinge
2. Unlinked   Semi-constrained
                Meniscal bearing
                Cruciate sparing or reconstruction
                Cruciate sacrificing
                Cruciate substitution - posterior stabilized
                Medial/lateral controlled
                Other

Uni-compartmental

1. Unconstrained 2. Semi-constrained = dished 3. Meniscal bearing 4. Medial 5. Lateral 6. Patellofemoral

Revision

1. Modular (augmented) 2. Custom-made linked 3. Custom-made unlinked

Cement

1. Methylmethacrylate 2. Other 3. Antibiotic loaded 4. No antibiotic

Polyethylene

	Metal-backed	Non-metal-backed
Tibial		
Patellar		

Augmentation materials

1. Metal 2. Auto-graft 3. Allograft 4. Cement 5. Other

Augmentation sites

1   2   3   4   5   6   7   8   9   10   11   12

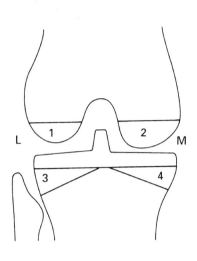
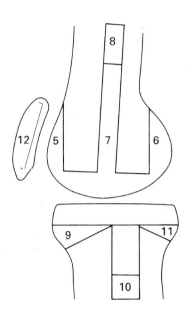

Patella/extensor apparatus

Resurfaced	1. Yes 2. No
Lateral release	1. Yes 2. No
Reefing	1. Yes 2. No
Realignment	1. Proximal 2. Distal
Quadricepsplasty	1. Yes 2. No
Final tracking	1. Central 2. On medial condyle 3. On lateral condyle

If patella is fractured – treatment
1. Wire 2. Screw 3. Button remains 4. Button exchanged 5. Patellectomy

Antibiotic prophylaxis

1. Yes 2. No

Additional antibiotic post-op

1. Yes 2. No

CPM

1. Yes 2. No
Day start
1, 2, 3+

MUA

1. No 2. Yes
Date post-op – week 2, 3, 4–6, 7–10, 10+

DVT prophylaxis

1. Systemic 2. Mechanical 3. Nil

Drains

0 1 2 3

Tourniquet

1. Yes 2. No 3. Reinflated

Final operative state

Flexion contracture 0 1–5 6–10 10+
Medial structures 1. Stable 2. Lax 3. Unstable
Lateral structures 1. Stable 2. Lax 3. Unstable.
Angle of deviation from mechanical axis
(i.e. angle γ – see Radiology for explanation)

Complications – intra-operative

Fracture

1. Tibial 2. Femoral 3. Patellar 4. Tibial tubercle

Perforation

1. Tibial diaphysis 2. Femoral diaphysis

Patellar tendon avulsion

1. Yes 2. No

If yes – reinsertion with

1. Screw 2. Wire 3. Staple 4. Augmentation/reconstruction

Complications – post-operative

General

1. DVT 2. Pulmonary embolus 3. Respiratory 4. Cardio-vascular 5. GI tract 6. Urological 7. CNS 8. Pressure sore

Local

Significant haematoma

1. Yes 2. No 3. Operative evacuation 4. Rehab. modification

Discharge/drainage

1. Yes 2. No 3. Sterile 4. Infected

Wound healing

1. Perfect 2. Delayed 3. Skin necrosis 4. Major dehiscence

Infection

Primary surgical 1. Yes 2. No
Organisms 1. Gram +ve 2. Gram −ve 3. Other

Nerve palsy

1. Damaged intra-operatively 2. Discovered post-op
Repaired? 1. Yes 2. No 3. Primarily 4. Secondarily
Recovered spontaneously? 1. Yes 2. No 3. Complete 4. Incomplete

Reflex sympathetic dystrophy

1. Yes 2. No 3. Recovered completely 4. Recovered incompletely

Form C: Radiology pre-op/post-op

Name   First name   Language

Country code   Postal/zip code   City

Street   Telephone   Patient number

Occupation   Height   Weight   Date of birth
                              (cm)   (kg)   (day/month/year)

Admission   Discharge

Pre-op	
Post-op	

Weight bearing X-ray

Indicate most severe involvement
Narrowing 0. Nil 1. Minor 2. Moderate 3. Severe = contact
Bone loss = Bone attrition with loss of mechanical integrity and may
include necrosis, cyst or erosion;
0. Nil 1. Minor 2. Moderate 3. Severe

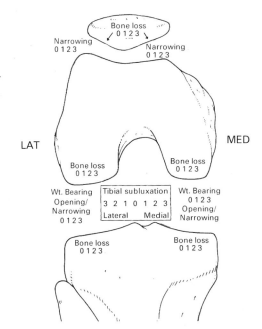

Long-standing film

XZ = mechanical axis
WYZ = tibio-femoral angle

Angle WYZ
<160 161–170 171–175 176–179 ⟨180⟩ 181–185 186–190 191–200 >200

Angle γ
>20 20–16 15–11 10–6 5–1 ⟨0⟩ 1–5 6–10 11–15 16–20 20+
       ← Valgus   ← Varus →

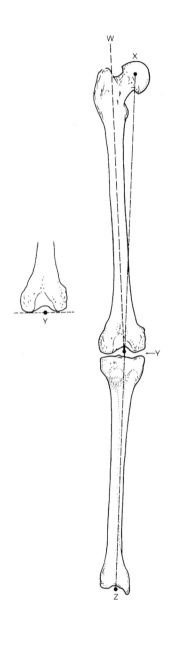

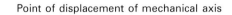
Point of displacement of mechanical axis

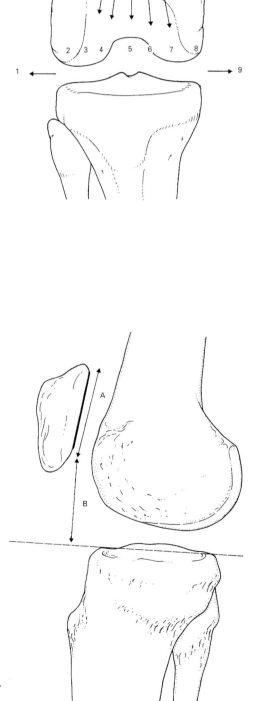

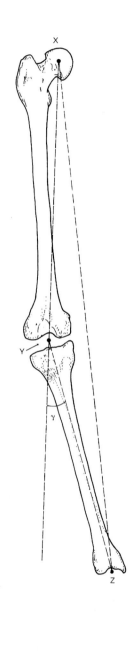

Patella

Normal A = B
Alta B > A
Infera B < A

Patella skyline view

1. Normal 2. Minor tilt 3. Significant displacement 4. Dislocated

Prosthesis positions – radiology

NB. These diagrams show malposition.

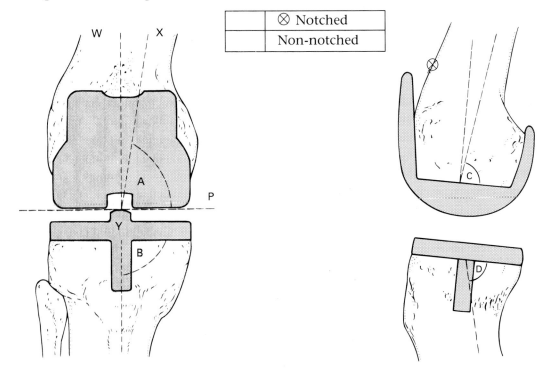

	⊗ Notched
	Non-notched

Angles

A: use Short-film WYP [   ]

     Long-film XYP [   ]

     81–83 84–86 87–89 |90| 91–93 94–96 97–99 100–102 103–105

B	85–90	91–95	96–100	101+	
C	90–85	84–80	79–75	74–	
D	75–80	81–85	86–90	91–95	96+

Percentage cover – tibia

AP	100%	99–90	89–80	<80
LAT	100%	99–90	89–80	<80

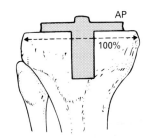

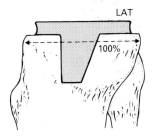

The patellar prosthesis

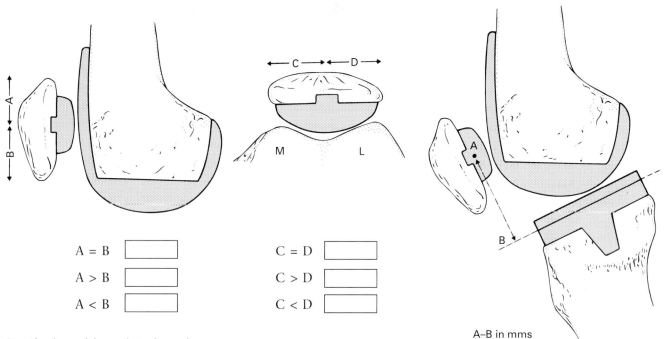

A = B		C = D			
A > B		C > D			
A < B		C < D			

A–B in mms

Prosthesis and bone interface changes

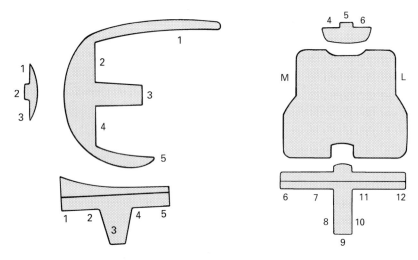

Patella: Points 2 and 5 are at any or all of the pegs.
Tibia: Points 3 and 9 are the tips of any or all pegs.

Loosening	No	Doubtful	Definite	Fracture
Femoral				
Tibial				
Patellar				

Interface change	Patella						Femur					Tibia											
	1	2	3	4	5	6	1	2	3	4	5	1	2	3	4	5	6	7	8	9	10	11	12
None visible																							
Linear translucency 1 mm																							
Linear translucency 2 mm																							
Wide translucency >2 mm																							
Major bone disruption																							

Sinkage

Best undertaken by RSA

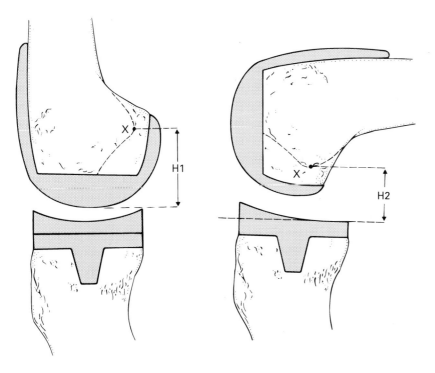

Point X: Where Blumensaat's line crosses the posterior intercondylar line.
Femoral: Measure H1 and H2 in mm.
Tibial: Assess by RSA or radiograph superimposition.

Appendix 1

Passive rotation at 70° flexion – tibia on femur

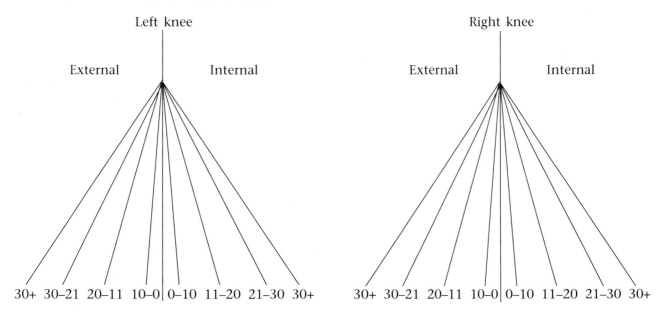

Appendix 2

Visual analogue scale for pain

None   Minor   Moderate   Severe

(Patient to indicate pain intensity:
At rest
On movement
On weight bearing
On climbing stairs)

Visual analogue scale for activity

Bedridden   Light activity   Heavy manual work
Wheelchair   Housekeeping   Major sports
                     Gardening

(Patient to indicate level of activity)

Visual analogue scale for patient satisfaction

Disappointed   Reservations   Satisfied   Enthusiastic

(Patient to indicate the amount of satisfaction)

Index

References to illustrations are in *italic* type